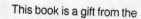

COLORECTAL CANCER

CURRENT CLINICAL ONCOLOGY

Maurie Markman, MD, SERIES EDITOR

COLORECTAL CANCER

Multimodality Management

Edited by

LEONARD B. SALTZ, MD

Memorial Sloan-Kettering Cancer Center,
New York, NY

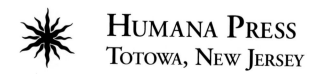

HUMANA PRESS
TOTOWA, NEW JERSEY

Cover illustration: Fig. 2 from Chapter 7, Fig. 2 from Chapter 9, Fig. 3 from Chapter 11, and Fig. 5 from Chapter 1.

Production Editor: Jessica Jannicelli.
Cover design by Patricia F. Cleary.

For additional copies, pricing for bulk purchases, and/or information about other Humana titles, contact Humana at the above address or at any of the following numbers: Tel: 973-256-1699; Fax: 973-256-8341; E-mail: humana@humanapr.com or visit our website at www.humanapress.com

Due diligence has been taken by the publishers, editors, and authors of this book to ensure the accuracy of the information published and to describe generally accepted practices. The contributors herein have carefully checked to ensure that the drug selections and dosages set forth in this text are accurate in accord with the standards accepted at the time of publication. Notwithstanding, as new research, changes in government regulations, and knowledge from clinical experience relating to drug therapy and drug reactions constantly occurs, the reader is advised to check the product information provided by the manufacturer of each drug for any change in dosages or for additional warnings and contraindications. This is of utmost importance when the recommended drug herein is a new or infrequently used drug. It is the responsibility of the health care provider to ascertain the Food and Drug Administration status of each drug or device used in their clinical practice. The publisher, editors, and authors are not responsible for errors or omissions or for any consequences from the application of the information presented in this book and make no warranty, express or implied, with respect to the contents in this publication.

This publication is printed on acid-free paper. ∞
ANSI Z39.48-1984 (American National Standards Institute)
Permanence of Paper for Printed Library Materials.

Printed in the United States of America. 10 9 8 7 6 5 4 3 2 1

Library of Congress Cataloging-in-Publication Data

Colorectal cancer : multimodality management / edited by Leonard B. Saltz.
    p. ; cm. -- (Current clinical oncology)
  Includes bibliographical references and index.
  ISBN 0-89603-935-8 (alk. paper)
    1. Colon (Anatomy)--Cancer. 2. Rectum--Cancer. I. Saltz, Leonard B. II. Current
clinical oncology (Totowa, N.J.)
    [DNLM: 1. Colorectal Neoplasms--therapy. 2. Colorectal Neoplasms--diagnosis. 3.
Colorectal Neoplasms--prevention & control. WI 529 C71912 2002]
  RC280.C6 C6685 2002
   616.99'4347--dc21
                                                        2002190225

PREFACE

The rapid growth in the number of options available for the management of colorectal cancer presents the clinician with new opportunities and new complexities. An explosion of understanding in the basic science that underlies both the disease and its potential therapies has translated into remarkable technological advances that can now be applied. So many specialties and subspecialties have now been brought to bear that it is appropriate to attempt to bring the expertise from these areas together in one volume, so that practitioners in one aspect of colorectal cancer management can maintain knowledge and expertise regarding the capabilities of other colleagues working in this disease.

Colorectal Cancer: Multimodality Management provides a concise, focused, and current review of the methodological and technological advances that have recently occurred in the management of colorectal cancer. The book has been divided into six basic parts. The first part, dealing with epidemiology and prevention, focuses on the molecular genetic events that occur in the development of colorectal cancer, as well as on our understanding of dietary and environmental factors, and possible strategies for prevention. Part II focuses on both diagnostic and therapeutic radiology in the management of colorectal cancer, dealing with innumerable advances in imaging, and with the progress in the science and art of radiation therapy. The third section deals with the surgical aspects of management of colorectal cancer, starting with surgical pathology. Specifics of surgery for the colon and rectum, the role of minimal access surgery, management of early stage disease, and issues of resection of metastatic disease are discussed. Also, ablative techniques such as cryosurgery and radiofrequency ablation are reviewed. The fourth main area is medical oncology. This part starts with a review of fluorouracil and biomodulation, and moves forward into a thorough discussion of the currently available drugs for first and second line management of metastatic colorectal cancer. Issues of chemotherapy for adjuvant management are discussed, and local regional therapies, such as intrahepatic and intraperitoneal chemotherapy, are reviewed. Part V, entitled Supportive Management, deals with aspects of pain syndromes and pain control, issues of sexuality and fertility, and complementary and alternative medicine approaches. Finally in a forward-looking conclusion, Part VI discusses some of the new agents in development in colorectal cancer, including targeted therapies, vaccine strategies, and gene therapy.

The aim of *Colorectal Cancer: Multimodality Management* is to provide a well-balanced, authoritative, evidence-based review of the current approaches to the prevention, diagnosis, and treatment of colorectal cancer. We have seen decreases in both incidence and mortality from this disease over the past several decades. It is hoped that this book will further facilitate the dissemination of information to practitioners, and will thereby help contribute to further progress in the prevention and treatment of colorectal cancer.

Leonard B. Saltz, MD

Contents

PART IV. MEDICAL ONCOLOGY

PART V. SUPPORTIVE MANAGEMENT

PART VI. NEW AGENTS IN COLORECTAL CANCER

CONTRIBUTORS

STEVEN R. ALBERTS, MD, MPH, *Department of Medical Oncology, Mayo Clinic, Rochester, MN*

MATTHEW BALLO, MD, *M.D. Anderson Cancer Center, Houston, TX*

MONICA M. BERTAGNOLLI, MD, *Division of Surgical Oncology, Brigham and Women's Hospital, Boston, MA*

RANDALL W. BURT, MD, *Division of Gastroenterology, University of Utah, Salt Lake City, UT*

BARRIE R. CASSILETH, PHD, *Chief, Integrative Medicine Service, Memorial Sloan-Kettering Cancer Center, New York, NY*

NATHAN I. CHERNY, MBBS, FRACP, *Cancer Pain and Palliative Medicine Service, Department of Medical Oncology, Shaare Zedek Medical Center, Jerusalem, Israel*

CAROLYN C. COMPTON, MD, PHD, *Department of Pathology, McGill University, Montreal, Quebec, Canada*

CHRISTOPHER CRANE, MD, *M.D. Anderson Cancer Center, Houston, TX*

ALFRED T. CULLIFORD IV, MD, *Department of Surgery, Memorial Sloan-Kettering Cancer Center, New York, NY*

DAVID CUNNINGHAM, MD, FRCP, *Department of Medicine and Gastrointestinal Unit, Royal Marsden Hospital, Surrey, UK*

ABRAHAM H. DACHMAN, MD, *Department of Radiology, University of Chicago, Chicago, IL*

PETER V. DANENBERG, *Department of Biochemistry and Molecular Biology, USC School of Medicine, Los Angeles, CA*

MARC DELCLOS, MD, *M.D. Anderson Cancer Center, Houston, TX*

ROBERT B. DIASIO, MD, *Department of Pharmacology and Toxicology, University of Alabama at Birmingham, Birmingham, AL*

ROBERT J. DOWNEY, MD, *Division of Thoracic Surgery, Memorial Sloan-Kettering Cancer Center, New York, NY*

MEGAN P. FLEMING, PHD, *Department of Pain Medicine and Palliative Care, Beth Israel Medical Center, New York, NY*

YUMAN FONG, MD, *Department of Surgery, Memorial Sloan-Kettering Cancer Center, New York, NY*

KENNETH A. FOON, MD, *Abgenix Inc., Fremont, CA; and Stanford University Medical Center, Stanford, CA*

HUGO E. R. FORD, MB, BCHIR, MRCP, *Department of Medicine and Gastrointestinal Unit, Royal Marsden Hospital, Surrey, UK*

DOUGLAS L. FRAKER, MD, *Department of Surgery, University of Pennsylvania Medical Center, Philadelphia, PA*

CHARLES S. FUCHS, MD, MPH, *Department of Adult Oncology, Dana-Farber Cancer Institute, Boston, MA*

JULIO GARCIA-AGUILAR, MD, PHD, *Division of Colon and Rectal Surgery, Department of Surgery, University of Minnesota, Minneapolis, MN*

RICHARD M. GOLDBERG, MD, *Department of Medical Oncology, Mayo Clinic, Rochester, MN*

STANLEY J. GOLDSMITH, MD, *Division of Nuclear Medicine, Department of Radiology, New York Presbyterian Hospital-Weill Cornell Medical Center, New York, NY*

JEAN L. GREM, MD, *NCI-Navy Medical Oncology, Cancer Therapeutics Branch, Center for Cancer Research, National Cancer Institute, National Naval Medical Center, Bethesda, MD*

SPIROS HIOTIS, MD, PHD, *Department of Surgery, Memorial Sloan-Kettering Cancer Center, New York, NY*

KYLE HOLEN, MD, *Gastrointestinal Oncology Division, Memorial Sloan-Kettering Cancer Center, New York, NY*

STACY D. JACOBSON, MD, *Department of Medical Oncology, Mayo Clinic, Rochester, MN*

NORA A. JANJAN, MD, *M.D. Anderson Cancer Center, Houston, TX*

WILLIAM R. JARNAGIN, MD, *Department of Surgery, Memorial Sloan-Kettering Cancer Center, New York, NY*

M. MARGARET KEMENY, MD, *Queen's Cancer Center, Queen's Hospital Center, Mt. Sinai School of Medicine, Queens, NY*

NANCY E. KEMENY, MD, *Memorial Sloan-Kettering Cancer Center, New York, NY*

GREGORY D. KENNEDY, MD, *Department of Surgery, University of Wisconsin, Madison, WI*

LALE KOSTAKOGLU, MD, *Division of Nuclear Medicine, Department of Radiology, New York Presbyterian Hospital-Weill Cornell Medical Center, New York, NY*

PETER J. K. KUPPEN, PHD, *Department of Surgery, Leiden University Medical Center, Leiden, The Netherlands*

SCOTT K. KUWADA, MD, *Division of Gastroenterology, University of Utah, Salt Lake City, UT*

FRED T. LEE, JR., MD, *Chief Section of Body Imaging, University of Wisconsin School of Medicine, Madison, WI*

WILLIAM W. LI, MD, *The Angiogenesis Foundation, Cambridge, MA; and Harvard Medical School, Boston, MA*

DAVID MAHVI, MD, *Chief, Division of Surgical Oncology, University of Wisconsin School of Medicine, Madison, WI*

ARNOLD J. MARKOWITZ, MD, *Gastroenterology Service, Memorial Sloan-Kettering Cancer Center, New York, NY*

JOHN L. MARSHALL, MD, *Lombardi Cancer Center, Washington, DC*

ANAND G. MENON, MD, *Department of Surgery, Leiden University Medical Center, Leiden, The Netherlands*

BRUCE D. MINSKY, MD, *Department of Radiation Oncology, Memorial Sloan-Kettering Cancer Center, New York, NY*

DEBORAH W. NEKLASON, PHD, *Oncological Sciences, University of Utah, Salt Lake City, UT*

HEIDI NELSON, MD, *Division of Colon and Rectal Surgery, Mayo Clinic and Mayo Foundation, Rochester, MN*

ALFRED I. NEUGUT, MD, PHD, *Division of Oncology, New York Presbyterian Hospital, New York, NY*

JOHN E. NIEDERHUBER, MD, *Departments of Surgery and Oncology, University of Wisconsin School of Medicine, Madison, WI*

PHILIP B. PATY, MD, *Department of Surgery, Memorial Sloan-Kettering Cancer Center, New York, NY*

NICHOLAS J. PETRELLI, MD, *State University of New York at Buffalo, Roswell Park Cancer Institute, Buffalo, NY*

MITCHELL C. POSNER, MD, *Department of Surgery, University of Chicago, Chicago, IL*

JOHN M. ROBERTSON, MD, *Department of Radiation Oncology, William Beaumont Hospital, Royal Oak, MI*

MIGUEL A. RODRIGUEZ-BIGAS, MD, *Department of Surgical Oncology, Roswell Park Cancer Institute, Buffalo, NY*

LEE S. ROSEN, MD, *Department of Medicine, UCLA Jonsson Cancer Center, Los Angeles, CA*

DAVID A. ROTHENBERGER, MD, *Division of Colon and Rectal Surgery, Department of Surgery, University of Minnesota Cancer Center, Minneapolis, MN*

ERIC K. ROWINSKY, MD, *Institute for Drug Development, Cancer Therapy and Research Center, San Antonio, TX*

DAVID T. RUBIN, MD, *Section of Gastroenterology, Department of Medicine, University of Chicago, Chicago, IL*

LEONARD B. SALTZ, MD, *Gastrointestinal Oncology Division, Department of Medicine, Memorial Sloan-Kettering Cancer Center, New York, NY*

AARON R. SASSON, MD, *Section of Surgical Oncology, Department of Surgery at University of Nebraska Medical Center, Omaha, NE*

WERNER SCHEITHAUER, MD, *Department of Internal Medicine, Division of Clinical Oncology, Vienna University Medical School, Vienna, Austria*

ELIN R. SIGURDSON, MD, PHD, *Department of Surgical Oncology, Fox Chase Cancer Center, Philadelphia, PA*

GLENN D. STEELE, JR., MD, PHD, *Geisinger Health System, Danville, PA*

PAUL H. SUGARBAKER, MD, *Washington Cancer Institute, Washington, DC*

SUSAN M. TALBOT, MBBS, FRACP, *Herbert Irving Comprehensive Cancer Center, College of Physicians and Surgeons, Columbia University, New York, NY*

BERNARDO TISMINEZKY, MD, *Division of Colon and Rectal Surgery, Mayo Clinic and Mayo Foundation, Rochester, MN*

MARJOLIJN M. VAN DER EB, MD, *Department of Surgery, Leiden University Medical Center, Leiden, The Netherlands*

CORNELIS J. H. VAN DE VELDE, MD, PHD, FRCS, *Department of Surgery, Leiden University Medical Center, Leiden, The Netherlands*

ANDREW J. VICKERS, MD, DPHIL, *Integrative Medicine Service, Memorial Sloan-Kettering Cancer Center, New York, NY*

DAVID J. VINING, MD, *Department of Radiology, Wake Forest University School of Medicine, Winston-Salem, NC*

SHARON WEBER, MD, *Department of Surgery, Memorial Sloan-Kettering Cancer Center, New York, NY*

W. DOUGLAS WONG, MD, *Department of Surgery, Memorial Sloan-Kettering Cancer Center, New York, NY*

I EPIDEMIOLOGY/PREVENTION

1

Biology and Molecular Genetics of Colorectal Cancer

Scott K. Kuwada, Deborah W. Neklason, and Randall W. Burt

CONTENTS

1. INTRODUCTION

A little over a decade ago, a molecular genetic model of colonic tumorigenesis was proposed by Vogelstein et al. *(1)*. This paradigm ushered in an explosion of investigations into the molecular genetics and biology of colon cancer. We now understand much of the pathogenesis of colon cancer* at the cellular level, and this has led to and will continue to result in improved rationales for diagnosis, treatment, and even prevention.

Colon cancer involves three broad classes of genes (tumor suppressor genes, oncogenes, and DNA mismatch repair genes), the function of which is perturbed primarily through genetic mutations. Epigenetic mechanisms capable of altering the expression of certain genes in the absence of mutations are operative in some colon cancers as well and will be discussed.

Cyclooxygenase (COX)-2 is a protein that is frequently overexpressed in colorectal cancers and plays an important role in their genesis. Because COX-2 overexpression is not a consequence of COX-2 gene mutations, it is discussed separately from the other classes of colon cancer genes.

---

*The term "colon cancer" is loosely defined in this chapter and several of the references cited. There are actually several types of colon cancers that are defined by the tissues (e.g., muscle, epithelium, neural) from which they originated. In this chapter, the term "colon cancer" refers specifically to colorectal "adenocarcinoma," which originates from colon epithelial cells and comprises the vast majority of all colon cancers.

From: *Colorectal Cancer: Multimodality Management*
Edited by: L. Saltz © Humana Press Inc., Totowa, NJ

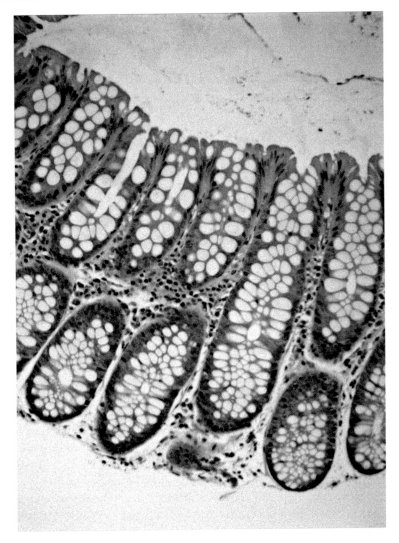

Fig. 1. Normal colonic mucosa oriented with the intestinal lumen at the top of the figure. Note the crypt structures lined by columnar colonic epithelial cells and opening into the intestinal lumen.

2. BIOLOGY

An understanding of the molecular genetics and biology of colon cancer must begin with an introduction to the normal biology of the colonic epithelial cells, because they are the cells that give rise to colon adenocarcinomas.

2.1. Colonic Crypts

2.1.1. NORMAL BIOLOGY

The colon is lined by a single layer of columnar epithelial cells that are organized into invaginations called crypts (Fig. 1). Each crypt can be broadly subdivided into two functional zones: a proliferative compartment that is comprised of cells in the bottom portion of the crypts and a differentiated compartment comprising cells in the upper portion of the crypts. There are several stem cells in the bottom of the colonic crypts that are capable of dividing and giving rise to the four different cell types comprising the crypts: absorptive, Paneth cells, goblet cells, and enteroendocrine cells *(2)*. Stem cells, residing near the bottom of the crypts, divide and give rise to undifferentiated cells that undergo several rounds of division and then migrate up the crypts, with the exception of Paneth cells, which migrate to the bottom of the crypts. As newly divided cells migrate up the crypt, they cease to divide and differentiate into mature enterocytes (absorptive cells), enteroendocrine cells, and goblet cells. Unlike the small intestine, there are no villi in the colon. Instead, cells form a hexagonal "cuff" at the opening at the top of colonic crypts. Intestinal crypts are clonal in adults, meaning that all cells within a particular crypt arise from the same progenitor stem cell. After the cells differentiate, they undergo senescence and, finally, programmed cell death or apoptosis near and at the top of the crypts *(3,4)*. There is limited evidence as to whether the cells at the mouth of the crypts are "pushed" off or simply slough off into the lumen. There is some evidence that senescent cells can be engulfed at the mouth of crypts as well *(5)*. The entire life-span of colonic epithelial cells is approx 4–5 d, except for Paneth cells, which live for about 4 wk. This rapid turnover of intestinal epithelial cells is believed to be, in part, a protective mechanism against the mutagenic effects of intestinal carcinogens. The end result of the regulation of these dynamic cellular events is that the total number of colonic epithelial cells at any given point in time is fairly constant.

2.2. Polyps

A polyp is defined as any growth arising from the intestine and protruding into the lumen. Polyps have classically been defined as lesions visible to the naked eye. Polyps can arise from subepithelial tissues, but in this section, the focus is on polyps arising from the intestinal epithelium, because they can be the precursors to colorectal adenocarcinomas and account for the vast majority of all colorectal polyps.

Polyps can be either benign or malignant and are classified according to their histology. Epithelial polyps can arise from any of the various types of cell comprising the colonic epithelium. Although most epithelial polyps do not transform into malignant neoplasms, a few can and are the subject of the following discussion.

2.2.1. NON-NEOPLASTIC

The non-neoplastic epithelial polyps that are most commonly encountered in the colon are hyperplastic polyps. Although these polyps do not carry a high risk for malignant transformation, patients with hyperplastic polyposis do have an increased risk of forming colorectal cancers *(6)*. In addition, hyperplastic polyps containing adenomatous changes and even colorectal cancers have been reported rarely.

2.2.2. NEOPLASTIC

Adenomatous polyps are neoplastic by definition and are known precursors to colon cancers. These polyps are subclassified as low-, medium-, and high-grade dysplasia depending on several architectural features, the most important being pseudostratification of nuclei, which are basal in location in normal colonic epithelial cells. High-grade dysplasia and adenocarcinoma are found more frequently in polyps larger than 1 cm in diameter and that have a villous histology *(7)*. Multiple colonic adenomas increase the risk for colon cancer as well *(8)*. In the era preceding endoscopy, barium enemas performed on patients who had polyps or cancers removed by rigid sigmoidoscopy were used to follow synchronous polyps in the more proximal colon *(9)*. Studies such as this showed that it took approx 11 yr for some small polyps to develop into a cancer.

Adenomatous polyps may start as microscopic lesions known as aberrant crypt foci. A recent study demonstrated a strong correlation between the presence of dysplastic aberrant crypt foci (ACF) in the colorectum and increasing age, as well as the risk for synchronous macroadenomas and colorectal adenocarcinomas (10). In addition, these dysplastic ACF regressed in patients treated orally with sulindac, which is well known for its chemopreventive qualities in the colon (11).

At the molecular level, the issue of whether adenomas are monoclonal or polyclonal is at the heart of how normal colonic epithelial cells transform into neoplasms. Studies using restriction fragment-length polymorphisms (RFLPs) on colorectal adenomas and adenocarcinomas demonstrated monoclonality (12). This suggested that adenomas and adenocarcinomas arose from a single progenitor stem cell. However, polyclonal adenomatous colon polyps have been demonstrated in a man with familial adenomatous polyposis (FAP) and who was also an XY/XO mosaic (13). Although the intestinal crypts were monoclonal, the majority of adenomas in this man's colon were polyclonal; that is, individual adenomas contained cells that had XY or XO genotypes. Although the adenomas may have had the appearance of being polyclonal due to the loss of Y chromosomes from certain cells comprising the polyps, another potential explanation is a cooperativity between crypts in the formation of adenomatous polyps. This debate over whether adenomas are polyclonal or monoclonal will continue to be waged and keeps us wondering about the molecular genesis of adenomas.

2.3. Adenoma–Carcinoma Sequence

The majority of colorectal adenocarcinomas arise from adenomatous polyps. The evidence for this comes from epidemiological and histological data, which are presented in this subsection.

2.3.1. EVIDENCE

2.3.1.1. Epidemiological. Several studies demonstrated a strong correlation between the incidence and location of colon polyps and cancers (14–18). In developed nations, where colon polyps and cancers are much more common, both occur mostly in the left side of the colon. A recent study showed that close relatives of index cases with adenomatous polyps are at increased risk for colon cancers compared with close relatives of index cases without colonic adenomas (19). Finally, a prospective study demonstrated that the removal of adenomatous colon polyps could prevent the vast majority of colon cancers in those individuals as compared with historical controls (20).

2.3.1.2. Histological. Colon cancers with adjacent adenomatous polyp tissue have been commonly found (21). Furthermore, patients with familial polyposis develop hundreds to thousands of adenomatous colon polyps and almost all develop colorectal adenocarcinomas if the colon is not removed (22,23). These findings suggest that adenomas are the predecessors to colon adenocarcinomas.

3. GENETICS OF COLORECTAL CANCER

Colon cancers arise from mutations in multiple cancer-causing genes in colonic epithelial cells. The actual molecular steps involved in the adenoma–carcinoma sequence are described in Section 3.3.

Certain mutations in cancer-causing genes can be inherited, which is best exemplified by the rare familial colorectal cancer syndromes. The identification of the mutated genes inherited in these rare syndromes provided the foundation needed to achieve our current understanding of the molecular mechanisms underlying colorectal tumorigenesis. However, heredity plays a role in colorectal cancers not belonging to the rare familial syndromes.

3.1. Heredity

It is well established that heredity plays a strong role in colon cancer. The rare colon cancer syndromes, familial polyposis and hereditary nonpolyposis colorectal cancer, are excellent examples of the role of heredity in this disease and are fully discussed in other chapters in this book.

Several studies have demonstrated the role of heredity in sporadic colorectal cancers *(24–29)*. One such study utilized 34 kindreds (670 persons) to demonstrate that colorectal adenoma and cancer occurrence best fit a dominant inheritance pattern with a gene frequency of 19% *(29)*. A recent large study comparing over 44,000 pairs of fraternal and identical twins showed that approximately 35% of colorectal cancers can be attributed to underlying hereditary factors *(30)*. The risk for colorectal cancer is even increased in close relatives of individuals with adenomatous polyps *(19)*. Thus, it is very clear that heredity plays a large role in colorectal cancer risk.

3.1.1. GERMLINE VS SOMATIC MUTATIONS

Mutations in the colon cancer-causing genes can be broadly categorized into two groups. Germline mutations are present within germ cells, which are then passed on to offspring. Germline mutations are present in every cell of the individual inheriting a particular germline mutation.

Somatic mutations are acquired in individual cells. Once a somatic mutation is acquired in a particular cell, it is then passed on through cell divisions to its progeny.

As previously mentioned, the molecular genesis of colorectal cancers is the result of mutations in multiple colon cancer-causing genes. Thus, individuals with a germline mutation in one of these genes are already one step farther along the multistep genetic pathway to colorectal cancer than individuals who must acquire all the necessary mutations. Such germline mutations are responsible for the rare but dramatic familial colorectal cancer syndromes that are discussed later in this chapter and in more detail elsewhere in this book.

Based on hereditary features, colon cancers can be subdivided into a number of categories. Figure 2 is a graphic representation of colorectal cancers divided into separate categories according to hereditary presentations. We have arguably learned the most about colon cancer, one of the most common cancers in humans, from studies of rare familial colon cancer syndromes. The involvement of large numbers of family members facilitated the identification of the genes involved in these rare syndromes. As will be shown, these genes are also central to the much more common sporadic colorectal tumors as well.

3.1.2. FAMILIAL COLORECTAL CANCER SYNDROMES

The best known hereditary colon cancer syndromes are FAP and hereditary nonpolyposis colorectal cancer (HNPCC). Both conditions are inherited in an autosomal dominant fashion and begin with germline mutations. FAP accounts for less than 1% of all colorectal cancer cases and HNPCC for slightly more *(22)*. Thus, they are both rare syndromes, but the penetrance for colorectal cancers in mutation carriers is nearly 100% for FAP *(22)* and between 70% and 80% for HNPCC *(31,32)*.

3.1.2.1. Familial Polyposis. Familial adenomatous polyposis results from germline mutations in the adenomatous polyposis coli *(APC)* gene *(33,34)*. Affected individuals

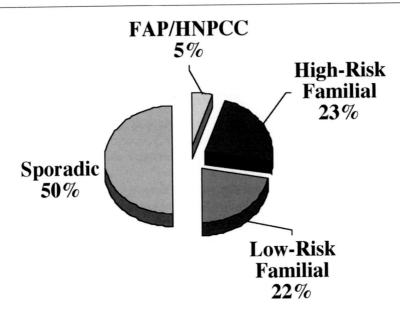

Fig. 2. Types of colorectal cancers divided according to patterns of heredity. Previous population-based estimates determined a familial pattern of inheritance in approximately half of all colorectal cancers.

develop hundreds to thousands of colonic adenomatous polyps beginning in their early teens. The average age of colon cancer is 39 yr, with some occurring much earlier *(22)*. There is also a 10% lifetime risk of developing duodenal cancers. Other extraintestinal manifestations of this syndrome are epidermoid cysts, sebaceous cysts, osteomas, CHRPE (congenital hypertrophy of the retinal pigmented epithelium) lesions, supernumerary teeth, thyroid cancer, hepatoblastoma, and desmoid tumors.

    3.1.2.2. Hereditary Nonpolyposis Colorectal Cancer. Hereditary nonpolyposis colorectal cancer arises from germline mutations in the DNA mismatch repair genes *(35)*. Although the most common cancer in HNPCC families is colon cancer, uterine, gastric, ovarian, small bowel, pancreatic, renal cell, uroepithelial, and biliary tract adenocarcinomas occur at a much higher frequency than in the general population *(36)*.

    3.1.2.3. Turcot's and Crail's Syndromes. Recently, analysis of families with Turcot's syndrome, previously believed to be part of FAP, revealed that this syndrome (colorectal cancers and primary central nervous system tumors) was, in fact, the result of germline mutations either in the *APC* or DNA mismatch repair genes (discussed later) *(37)*. The germline mutations found in Turcot's syndrome families were found to segregate the two most common types of brain tumors in these families. Families with germline *APC* gene mutations were primarily found to have medulloblastomas, whereas those with germline mutations in either the *MLH1* or *MSH2* DNA mismatch repair genes predominantly expressed glioblastomas. Thus, the family Turcot originally described actually had HNPCC. The families with *APC* germline mutations were originally described by Crail *(38)* and it has been proposed that these families be called Crail's syndrome.

    3.1.2.4. High-Risk Familial Colorectal Cancer. Heredity plays a significant role in colorectal adenocarcinomas not arising within FAP or HNPCC families as well *(24)*. Multiple studies showed that having a close relative with colon cancer significantly increases one's risk of colon cancer. Thus, we have used the term "high-risk familial colon cancer" to describe families with at least two affected first-degree relatives or early onset of colorectal cancer (at age 50 yr or less).

Our research, utilizing a large colon cancer database with thorough ascertainment of family histories, suggests that high-risk familial colorectal cancers account for approx 23% of all colorectal cancers (Fig. 2) *(39)*. The genes responsible for susceptibility in these families are unknown, but they are most likely common and less penetrant than those involved in FAP and HNPCC.

3.1.2.5. Sporadic Colorectal Cancer. The majority of colon cancers occur in the absence of a known family history of colon cancer. The sequence of genetic events leading to sporadic colon cancers has been well studied *(1)* and the mutations in key colon cancer-causing genes are acquired rather than inherited.

3.2. Colorectal Cancer Genes

Vogelstein and others first characterized commonly occurring genetic mutations in colonic tumorigenesis *(1)*. This landmark study formed the foundation for the characterization of the major molecular pathways most commonly operative in colon cancers. The development of colon cancer requires the acquisition of multiple mutations in cancer-causing genes. The genes most commonly mutated in colon cancers control key cellular activities and behaviors, such as proliferation, migration, and survival. The involvement of multiple cellular pathways has led to a new understanding of why cancers in general are difficult to treat.

The molecular genetic alterations leading from normal colorectal epithelium to colorectal adenocarcinoma can be broadly categorized as two major pathways: the CIN (chromosomal instability) and MSI (microsatellite instability) pathways (Fig. 3).

In the CIN pathway, mutations in tumor suppressor genes, such as *APC, p53,* and *DCC,* as well as protooncogenes, such as *Ras* occur. The mutations in this pathway are typically manifested by deletions of large regions of chromosomes that contain the tumor suppressor genes involved. The vast majority of all colon cancers, including those in FAP, arise via the CIN pathway and demonstrate early mutation of *APC,* which has thus been coined the "gatekeeper" of this pathway.

Tumors arising from the MSI pathway demonstrate replication errors in DNA nucleotide repeats (microsatellites) that are scattered throughout the genome. MSI is the result of errors in DNA replication and a failure to correct such errors resulting from mutations in DNA mismatch (MMR) repair genes. Subsequent mutations in a different set of colon-cancer-causing genes than the CIN pathway, such as *TGFβIIr* (TGF-β receptor II), *IGFR2* (insulin-like growth factor receptor-2), and *BAX,* and even the DNA mismatch repair genes, *hMSH3* and *hMSH6,* occur in the MSI pathway. The HNPCC colorectal cancers and approx 15% of sporadic colorectal cancers arise via the MSI pathway.

Each of the major colon cancer-causing genes in these pathways will be discussed in the following subsections.

3.2.1. TUMOR SUPPRESSOR GENES

Knudson first hypothesized that mutational inactivation of both alleles of a tumor suppressor gene ("two-hit" hypothesis) was sufficient for the genesis of familial cancers. We now know that in colon cancer, multiple tumor suppressor genes are mutated in this fashion. The most commonly mutated tumor suppressor gene in colon cancer is the *APC* gene, which is mutated in 80% or more of adenomatous polyps as well as adenocarcinomas of the colon *(40,41)*.

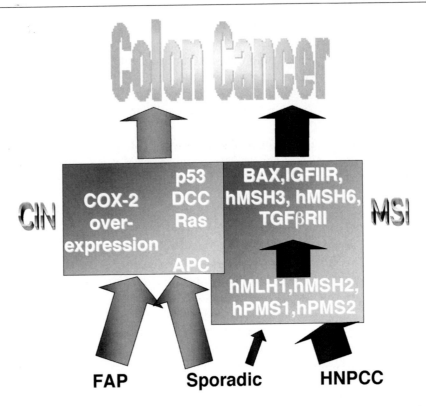

Fig. 3. Summary of the major molecular genetic pathways involved in colonic tumorigenesis. The two major pathways are the chromosomal instability (CIN) and microsatellite instability (MSI) pathways. Note that there is some overlap between these two pathways, as depicted in the figure, since some colorectal cancers possess mutations in genes involved in both pathways. Cyclooxygenase-2 (COX-2) overexpression occurs in a majority of colorectal cancers, but its aberrant expression is not directly due to mutations in the COX-2 gene. COX-2 overexpression is found commonly in CIN pathway but not MSI colorectal cancers. The majority of the approx 15% of sporadic colorectal cancers that display MSI arise through hypermethylation-induced silencing of *hMLH1* rather than mutations in this gene.

3.2.1.1. Adenomatous Polyposis Coli Gene. Two separate groups simultaneously linked the germline mutation responsible for FAP to the long arm of chromosome 5 *(33,34)*. This led to the identification of the *APC* gene at this locus *(42–45)*. *APC* is mutated in approx 80% of colorectal adenomas and cancers *(41)*. Further studies of the function of the APC protein revealed that its major function was to cause the degradation of a cytoplasmic protein called β-catenin *(46,47)*. β-catenin is an abundant protein found primarily along the intercellular junctions of intestinal epithelial cells. β-catenin exists in the cytoplasm for only short periods of time because of its rapid proteasomal degradation (*see* Fig. 4) *(46,48,49)*.

Under normal conditions, cytoplasmic β-catenin binds to the APC protein, GSK-3β, and axin *(50)*. The formation of this complex leads to the phosphorylation of β-catenin by GSK-3β. This specific phosphorylation of β-catenin results in its recognition by proteins that conjugate it to ubiquitin. This, in turn, signals β-catenin for degradation by the proteasome.

There is an important and physiological role for β-catenin-mediated signaling in epithelial cells. In *Drosophila* and mice, Wingless and Wnt, respectively, are homologous growth factors that bind to and stimulate a homologous cell membrane receptor called Frizzled

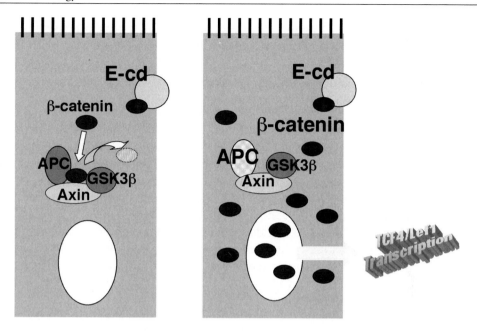

Fig. 4. The normal intestinal epithelial cell on the left shows degradation of cytoplasmic β-catenin by the APC/Axin/GSK-3β complex. Phosphorylation of β-catenin by GSK-3β leads to its degradation by the proteasome (not shown). The intestinal epithelial cell on the right shows a mutated form of APC, which leads to a failure of the APC/Axin/ GSK-3α complex to bind to, phosphorylate, and initiate the degradation the β-catenin. This leads to increasing cytoplasmic concentrations of β-catenin, which translocates to the nucleus and activates specific genes in concert with the TCF4/Lef1 protein.

in *Drosophila*. Activation by Wnt or Wingless of their respective receptors causes the phosphorylation and inhibition of GSK-3β that prevents GSK-3β from phosphorylating β-catenin *(51)*. This then inhibits the degradation of β-catenin in the cytoplasm, leading to its translocation into the nucleus, where it binds to a transcription factor called TCF (T-cell factor) or Lef (lymphoid enhancer factor) *(52–54)*. Binding of β-catenin to the TCF/Lef protein activates the transcription of genes with TFC/Lef recognition sites within their promoter regions. Genes whose transcription is driven by the β-catenin/TCF complex include *c-Myc, cyclin D1, PPARδ, matrilysin, Fra-1, uPAR* (urokinase-type plasminogen activator receptor), *c-jun,* and *gastrin (55–59),* all of which have been implicated in the development of cancer.

The vast majority of mutations found in the *APC* gene in colorectal cancer result in the truncation of the resulting APC protein *(60)*. This leads to a loss of function of the APC protein, which, in turn, results in an accumulation of cytoplasmic β-catenin and an increase in translocation of β-catenin into the nucleus, where it constitutively activates the transcription of specific genes in concert with the TCF4/Lef1 protein. The end result of constitutive β-catenin-induced gene transcription is an inhibition of apoptosis and stimulation of cell proliferation *(61)*—cellular attributes contributing to a selective growth advantage. Recent articles demonstrated that another role for the APC protein is the export of β-catenin from the nucleus *(62,63)*.

The cellular control of β-catenin is not the only function of the APC protein. A recent study showed that APC interacts with Asef, a guanine nucleotide exchange factor, and that APC-mediated stimulation of Asef is important for cell morphology and migration *(64)*.

The *APC* gene is large, containing 15 exons, and encodes a protein consisting of 2843 amino acids. Amino acid repeat domains in the APC protein that interact with β-catenin are found between amino acids 1020–1169 and 1324–2075. Somatic mutations in the *APC* gene cluster in the region of codons 1250–1450, which overlaps with the β-catenin-binding domains *(40,65,66)*.

The locations of mutations in the *APC* gene produce strong genotype–phenotype correlations. Germline mutations in exons 3 and 4 *(67,68)*, exon 9 *(69)*, and downstream of codon 1595 *(70)* of the *APC* gene result in a subset of FAP families called attenuated adenomatous polyposis coli (AAPC) *(67,68,71)*. Individuals from AAPC families are predisposed to fewer adenomatous polyps of the colon (the range is zero to hundreds), a predominance of colonic adenomas in the proximal colon, absence of CHRPE lesions, and a later onset of colon cancers than seen in classical FAP. Although patients with AAPC are also predisposed to a much higher than expected incidence of duodenal cancers and express fundic gland polyps, as do classical FAP patients *(22)*. Germline mutations between codons 463–1444 or stop mutations in codons 215–217 result in the appearance of CHRPE lesions. There does not appear to be a strong link between the site of *APC* gene mutations and the presence of extracolonic tumors seen in FAP families.

A major question is why is there a large variation in the numbers of colonic polyps among FAP and AAPC patients from the same kindreds. Interestingly, in a mouse model of FAP, a modifying allele called *MOM1*, which codes for phospholipase A2, acts to inhibit the number of polyps when present *(72)*. No mutations have been found in the phospholipase A2 gene in AAPC patients *(73–75)*, but the search for other modifying genes is still active.

A fascinating relationship between an *APC* gene polymorphism found in Ashkenazi Jews and an increased colorectal cancer risk was recently discovered. The I1307K polymorphism, which is a T to A transversion at nucleotide 3920, results in an approximately twofold increased risk of colon cancer *(76,77)*. Interestingly, the development of tumors in patients with this polymorphism arise from inactivating mutations of *APC* on the same allele carrying the polymorphism. Furthermore, these inactivating mutations occur in close proximity to the polypmorphism itself. Thus, this polymorphism appears to cause instability, through an unknown mechanism, in the adjacent DNA, which promotes the nearby inactivating *APC* mutations *(76,77)*.

In colon cancers with normal *APC* alleles, about 50% have mutations in the β-catenin gene (*CTNNB1*) *(78)*. These β-catenin mutants are capable of transforming cells through constitutively activating genes driven by TCF promoter elements. *CTNNB1* mutants are found in approx 4–15% of all sporadic colorectal adenomas and carcinomas *(78)*. This means that the vast majority of all colon cancers possess abnormal regulation of β-catenin through mutations in either *CTNNB1* or *APC*. Mutations in *GSK-3*β or *axin* have not been found in colorectal tumors without mutations in *APC* or β-catenin.

3.2.1.2. *p53*. p53 is a protein with a molecular weight of 53 kDa that is encoded by the *p53* gene on chromosome 17 and is the most commonly mutated tumor suppressor gene in all types of human cancers. *p53* gene mutations found in cancers result in inactivation of the p53 protein. As with other tumor suppressor genes, deletions of the wild-type allele typically occur in colorectal tumorigenesis. However, because p53 proteins function as oligomers, a mutation in one *p53* allele can result in p53 oligomer dysfunction through a so-called "dominant-negative" effect.

The main function of p53 is to recognize DNA damage and inhibit cell-cycle progression to allow time for DNA repair *(79,80)*. If the DNA damage is too great for cell survival, p53 can trigger apoptosis of the cell. Recently, p53 has been shown to participate in the DNA repair process as well *(81)*. The half-life of the p53 protein is short, but when the *p53* gene is mutated, the half-life is greatly increased. *p53* gene mutations occur late in the adenoma–carcinoma sequence *(1)*.

3.2.1.3. Deleted in Colon Cancer Gene. 18q deletions were described in colorectal cancers by Vogelstein and others *(1)*. Shortly thereafter, the *DCC* (deleted in colorectal cancer) gene was identified as a candidate tumor suppressor on 18q *(82)*. Multiple investigators studying a vertebrate protein called netrin-1, which guides axons during development, discovered that the *DCC* gene encodes the netrin-1 receptor *(83–85)*.

Transgenic mice hemizygous for *DCC* failed to develop intestinal tumors, which appeared to be evidence against the role of *DCC* as a tumor suppressor gene *(86)*. Recent work showed that expression of DCC in cell lines, including one colon cancer cell line, caused caspase-mediated apoptosis *(87)*. Interestingly, cleavage of the artificially expressed DCC was necessary for DCC-induced apoptosis. Furthermore, this DCC-induced apoptosis could be prevented by the presence of netrin-1. Thus, it appears that DCC can conditionally act as a tumor suppressor by being a dependence receptor that induces apoptosis in the absence of a ligand. This model is consistent with reports that both the expression of DCC suppresses tumorigenicity in vitro *(88)*, and loss of DCC expression in colon cancers is associated with a poorer prognosis *(89)*. SMAD2 and SMAD4, two colon-cancer-associated genes that will be discussed later, also share the 18q21 location of *DCC*. Thus, it remains to be seen which of these genes, or if all of them, is responsible for the poor prognosis in colon cancers with loss of this chromosomal region.

3.2.2. ONCOGENES

In work that would eventually win a Nobel prize, Varmus and others first described how an obscure chicken virus could infect and transform chicken cells into tumors. The transforming agent was found to be a viral gene termed the *src* "oncogene." What was shocking was the finding of similar DNA sequences in human DNA. This then led to the discovery of yet other oncogene-like sequences in human DNA. Curiously, many of these oncogene-like DNA sequences in humans encoded genes whose function was to regulate cell growth. When these genes were mutated in a fashion similar to their viral oncogene counterparts, they too became transforming. Hence, these "protooncogenes" were literally hijacked from the DNA of higher life-forms by infectious viruses, which then utilized them to their advantage. Unlike tumor suppressor genes, "proto"-oncogenes can be activated by mutations. Because protooncogenes typically encode for growth regulatory proteins, activating mutations usually result in constitutive growth signals.

3.2.2.1. Ras. *Ras* is a protooncogene that is mutated in approximately half of both colorectal adenomas and cancers *(1)*. The Ras protein is a GTPase that can be activated by a number of receptors. The mutations in the *Ras* gene found in human colon cancers cluster in regions called "hot spots" and result in constitutive Ras activity. Because Ras activates signal transduction pathways that can drive cell proliferation, activating mutations in *Ras* lead to constitutive growth signals.

3.2.3. DNA MISMATCH REPAIR GENES

The syndrome of HNPCC is caused by germline mutations in at least five DNA mismatch repair genes (*hMLH1, hMSH2, hMSH6, hPMS1,* and *hPMS2*) *(90–92)*. Approximately 90% of HNPCC families harbor germline mutations in the *hMLH1* or *hMSH2* gene. The DNA mismatch repair (MMR) genes encode proteins that recognize base pair mismatches resulting from errors during DNA replication, genetic recombination, and chemical modification of DNA and DNA precursors (93–95). DNA mismatches frequently occur as a result of "slippage" of DNA strands in regions with nucleotide repeats or "microsatellites." DNA microsatellites are regions of nucleotide repeats scattered throughout the human genome.

The DNA MMR proteins both recognize and correct these abnormalities, thus preventing mutations resulting from replication errors. The mechanisms by which these proteins function has been largely gleaned by research in bacteria and yeast. MSH2/MSH6 and MSH2/MSH3 protein complexes recognize base pair mismatches, insertions, and deletions (94,95). The MLH1 and PMS2 proteins then excise the mismatched nucleotides within the newly synthesized DNA strand.

When both alleles of one of the DNA MMR genes are inactivated, errors in DNA replication occur. A manifestation of germline mutations in the DNA MMR genes is MSI in the tumor tissue. When DNA from noncancerous tissue is compared with DNA from cancer tissue of the same individual, MSI can be detected as a change in the length of specific DNA microsatellite repeat sequences. For example, CACACACACA (10 nucleotides) will become CACACACA (8 nucleotides). MSI is readily detectable by performing polymerase chain reaction (PCR) on microsatellites. A consensus panel of five microsatellite markers is currently used for the establishment of the presence of the MSI phenotype in tumors (93). If more than one of these microsatellites exhibit MSI, the tumor is classified as MSI-H (high). If only one microsatellite exhibits MSI, then the tumor is classified as MSI-L (low). If none of the microsatellites exhibits MSI, then the tumor is classified as MSS (stable).

Microsatellite instability occurs in approx 15% of sporadic colorectal tumors; however, DNA MMR gene mutations have been found only in a minority of these cancers (96–99). The majority of these sporadic cancers are due to inactivation of hMLH1 through an epigenetic mechanism. Many gene promoters contain regions containing –CG– repeats termed CpG islands. DNA methyltransferases add methyl groups to the cytosines in CpG islands, which greatly inhibits transcription (called "silencing") of that gene.

Hypermethylation of CpG islands in the hMLH1 promoter region have been found in approx 80% of MSI-positive sporadic colorectal tumors (100). The evidence that such hypermethylation of the hMLH1 promoter may be of significance to colon cancer came from work in colon cancer cell lines demonstrating MSI and hypermethylation of the promoters of both hMLH1 alleles, but lacking mutations in DNA MMR genes (100,101). When the cells were treated with 5-azacytidine, a demethylating agent, the expression of the hMLH1 genes and DNA MMR activity were restored. Furthermore, offspring from a cross between familial polyposis mice (Apc^min) with mice lacking the major eukaryotic DNA methyltransferase gene Dnmt1 showed a major decrease in the expected number of intestinal polyps (102). Key questions now remaining to be answered are what regulates DNA methylation and how is its regulation altered in tumorigenesis?

Interestingly, MSI colorectal cancers demonstrate a predilection for the proximal colon and a much better prognosis than sporadic colon cancers (stage-matched) that are MSS (103). In Turcot's syndrome families with underlying DNA MMR gene germline mutations, the survival of family members with glioblastomas is much longer than is seen in patients with sporadic glioblastomas (37). Thus, the biology of MSI tumors may be intrinsically different from those that are MSS.

Although many DNA microsatellite repeats exist in noncoding regions of chromosomes, some occur within important genes, such as the TGFβIIr (104,105). Mutations in a specific short polyadenine or GT repeat sequence within the *TGFβIIr* gene result in the lack of TGFβII receptor protein expression. In normal epithelial cells, the receptor for the TGFβ peptide is formed by the TGFβI and TGFβII receptor subunits *(106)*. When TGFβ binds to its receptor in epithelial cells, it normally causes inhibition of cell proliferation *(107)*. However, colon cancer cells derived from patients with DNA mismatch repair defects, MSI, and HNPCC demonstrate mutations in the *TGFβIIr* gene that renders them unresponsive to TGFβ *(104,105)*. A more recent study found that 15% of MSS colon cancers have inactivating *TGFβIIr* gene mutations as well *(108)*.

Of 19 MSS colon cancer cell lines tested in one study, 14 (74%) were unresponsive to TGFβ, but expressed the TGFβII receptor. These TGFβ-unresponsive cell lines have mutations in the *SMAD* genes, which are the downstream targets of TGFβ receptor signaling *(108)*. *SMAD* gene mutations have been found in some sporadic colon cancers as well. Indeed, 55% of MSS colon cancer cell lines tested showed defects in the TGFβ receptor signaling pathway downstream of the receptor. Because the *TGFβIIr* gene mutations occur late in the adenoma–carcinoma sequence, it is unlikely that escape from the antiproliferative effects of TGFβ is the major advantage afforded to colon cancers by these mutations.

Other genes targeted for mutation in MSI colon cancers are *IGFR2 109*, *hMSH3 (109)*, *hMSH6 (109)*, BAX *(110)*, and RIZ *111*.

3.2.4. MISCELLANEOUS COLON CANCER GENES

3.2.4.1. Cyclooxygenases. Multiple epidemiological studies and a few prospective trials demonstrated a significant reduction in colon cancer mortality by aspirin. The aspirin-related nonsteroidal anti-inflammatory drug (NSAID) sulindac caused large reductions in polyps in FAP patients as well *(11)*. Later research showed that aspirin and NSAIDs caused colon cancer cells to undergo apoptosis *(112)*.

At the same time, investigators noted that one of the targets of inhibition by NSAIDs, the enzyme cyclooxygenase-2 (COX-2), was overexpressed in approx 85% of colon cancers and 40% or more of adenomas *(113,114)*. The evidence for COX-2 as a major target for NSAIDs in colon tumors came from a number of studies. Inhibition of COX-2 by selective COX-2 inhibitors reduced the number of colonic neoplasms in carcinogen-treated mice and rats *(115–119)*. A dramatic reduction in colonic adenomas occurred when mice with FAP were crossed with mice lacking COX-2 expression *(120)*. In humans, high doses of the COX-2-selective inhibitor celecoxib caused a significant reduction in colonic polyps in FAP patients *(121)*.

What regulates COX-2 expression in colon cancers is currently under study. Interestingly, two recent studies demonstrated the specific lack of COX-2 overexpression in colon cancer cells with MSI *(122,123)*.

COX-2 may not be the only target of NSAIDs and aspirin in colonic tumorigenesis. The doses of NSAIDs needed to achieve inhibition of colonic tumors is much higher than the dose needed to inhibit COX-2 enzymatic activity. The sulindac sulfone metabolite causes apoptosis of colon cancer cells through a mechanism independent of COX-1 or COX-2 *(124)*. Studies have demonstrated COX-2 overexpression not in the colonic epithelial cells but in the submucosal cells of the colon *(125,126)*. Embryonic cells from transgenic mice without COX-2 expression can still be inhibited in vitro by NSAIDs. Finally, PPARδ, whose expression is regulated by the APC–β-catenin pathway, appears to be a major target for NSAIDs in colon cancer cells *(55)*. Thus, NSAIDs and aspirin appear to have multiple targets in colon cancer cells with regard to their antitumor effects.

It will be important to study whether the expression of the targets of NSAIDs in colon tumors, such as COX-2, are related to mutations in tumor suppressors, DNA MMR genes, or oncogenes. Recently, the US FDA has approved a drug (celecoxib), for the first time, for chemoprevention in FAP patients with subtotal colectomies *(127)*.

4. CONCLUSIONS

The major molecular genetic pathways involved in colorectal tumorigenesis can be summarized to a large degree (*see* Fig. 3). The vast majority (over 80%) of sporadic adenocarcinomas arise through the FAP or chromosomal instability (CIN) pathway in which acquired mutations in the *APC* gene occur early and are commonplace. This is followed by mutations in other genes such as *Ras*, *p53*, and *DCC*. In about half of colorectal adenocarcinomas without APC gene mutations, mutations in β-catenin are found. These mutations in β-catenin may functionally substitute for *APC*-gene-inactivating mutations. In the absence of COX-2 gene mutations, COX-2 protein overexpression occurs in a major proportion of MSS colorectal adenomas and adenocarcinomas. COX-2 overexpression appears to play a role early on in the adenoma–carcinoma sequence, but it is currently not known what regulates its expression in tumors. Somatic mutations in the *TGFβIIr* and SMAD genes are common in MSS colon cancer cell lines as well.

Both HNPCC and microsatellite unstable colorectal cancers arise through DNA mismatch repair dysfunction. In this MSI pathway, CIN is infrequent and genes, such as *TGFβIIr*, *IGFIIR*, *hMSH3*, *hMSH6*, and *BAX*, are targeted for mutation. However, approx 10–15% of sporadic adenocarcinomas show MSI, and 80% of these tumors show inactivation of hMLH1 through hypermethylation rather than mutation.

In addition to genotypic distinctions between the CIN and MSI colon cancers pathways, phenotypic distinctions are apparent as well. Cancers arising from the CIN pathway tend to be in the left colon and associated with a poorer prognosis, whereas those arising from the MSI pathway tend to be right sided, associated with a better prognosis, and display tumor infiltrating lymphocytes.

The CIN and MSI pathways are not mutually exclusive, as there is some overlap. Finally, despite the different genes involved in the two major pathways, the end results of both pathways are the the dysregulation of cellular functions such as proliferation, differentiation, and apoptosis.

Tremendous progress has been made with regard to our understanding of the molecular biology of colorectal cancers. This has already led to clinical trials of chemopreventive agents, genetic tests for FAP and HNPCC, improvements in staging, and more targeted chemotherapies. However, the complexity of the multiple cellular pathways deranged in colon tumors has also revealed the difficulty in developing and applying broad clinical strategies for colorectal adenocarcinomas. The immediate challenge will be to formulate preventive care for the earliest stages of colonic tumorigenesis when only one or two cellular pathways are dysfunctional and can thus be easily and effectively targeted.

Other chapters in this book will discuss the environmental forces that may predispose us to the genetic mutations leading to colon cancer. Now that we have good knowledge of the various genes involved in colon cancer, the scientific challenges will be to understand how intestinal genes are mutated in the first place and what hereditary factors predispose certain individuals to these mutations.

REFERENCES

1. Vogelstein B, Fearon ER, Hamilton SR, et al. Genetic alterations during colorectal-tumor development. *N. Engl. J. Med.*, **319** (1988) 525–532.
2. Potten CS and Loeffler M. Stem cells: attributes, cycles, spirals, pitfalls and uncertainties. Lessons for and from the crypt. *Development*, **110** (1990) 1001–1020.
3. Gavrieli Y, Sherman Y, and Ben-Sasson SA. Identification of programmed cell death in situ via specific labeling of nuclear DNA fragmentation. *J. Cell Biol.*, **119** (1992) 493–501.
4. Strater J, Koretz K, Gunthert AR, and Moller P. In situ detection of enterocytic apoptosis in normal colonic mucosa and in familial adenomatous polyposis. *Gut*, **37** (1995) 819–825.
5. Hall PA, Coates PJ, Ansari B, and Hopwood D. Regulation of cell number in the mammalian gastrointestinal tract: the importance of apoptosis. *J. Cell Sci.*, **107** (1994) 3569–3577.
6. Rashid A, Houlihan PS, Booker S, Petersen GM, Giardiello FM, and Hamilton SR. Phenotypic and molecular characteristics of hyperplastic polyposis. *Gastroenterology*, **119** (2000) 323–332.
7. Appel MF, Spjut HJ, and Estrada RG. The significance of villous component in colonic polyps. *Am. J. Surg.*, **134** (1977) 770–771.
8. Atkin WS, Morson BC, and Cuzick J. Long-term risk of colorectal cancer after excision of rectosigmoid adenomas [see comments]. *N. Engl. J. Med.*, **326** (1992) 658–662.
9. Stryker SJ, Wolff BG, Culp CE, Libbe SD, Ilstrup DM, and MacCarty RL. Natural history of untreated colonic polyps. *Gastroenterology*, **93** (1987) 1009–1013.
10. Takayama T, Katsuki S, Takahashi Y, et al. Aberrant crypt foci of the colon as precursors of adenoma and cancer. *N. Engl. J. Med.*, **339** (1998) 1277–1284.
11. Giardiello FM, Hamilton SR, Krush AJ, et al. Treatment of colonic and rectal adenomas with sulindac in familial adenomatous polyposis. *N. Engl. J. Med.*, **328** (1993) 1313–1316.
12. Fearon ER, Hamilton SR, and Vogelstein B. Clonal analysis of human colorectal tumors. *Science*, **238** (1987) 193–196.
13. Novelli MR, Williamson JA, Tomlinson IP, et al. Polyclonal origin of colonic adenomas in an XO/XY patient with FAP. *Science*, **272** (1996) 1187–1190.
14. Vatn MH and Stalsberg H. The prevalence of polyps of the large intestine in Oslo: an autopsy study. *Cancer*, **49** (1982) 819–825.
15. Williams AR, Balasooriya BA, and Day DW. Polyps and cancer of the large bowel: a necropsy study in Liverpool. *Gut*, **23** (1982) 835–842.
16. Coode PE, Chan KW, and Chan YT. Polyps and diverticula of the large intestine: a necropsy survey in Hong Kong. *Gut*, **26** (1985) 1045–1048.
17. Johannsen LG, Momsen O, and Jacobsen NO. Polyps of the large intestine in Aarhus, Denmark. An autopsy study. *Scand. J. Gastroenterol.*, **24** (1989) 799–806.
18. Eide TJ and Stalsberg H. Polyps of the large intestine in Northern Norway. *Cancer*, **42** (1978) 2839–2848.
19. Winawer SJ, Zauber AG, Gerdes H, et al. Risk of colorectal cancer in the families of patients with adenomatous polyps. National Polyp Study Workgroup [see comments]. *N. Engl. J. Med.*, **334** (1996) 82–87.
20. Winawer SJ, Zauber AG, Ho MN, et al. Prevention of colorectal cancer by colonoscopic polypectomy. The National Polyp Study Workgroup [see comments]. *N. Engl. J. Med.*, **329** (1993) 1977–1981.
21. Lev R and Grover R. Precursors of human colon carcinoma: a serial section study of colectomy specimens. *Cancer*, **47** (1981) 20070x2015.
22. Kuwada SK and Burt RW. The clinical features of the hereditary and nonhereditary polyposis syndromes. *Surg. Oncol. Clin. North Am.*, **5** (1996) 553–567.
23. Burt RW. Polyposis syndromes. In *Textbook of Gastroenterology.* Yamada T (ed.), JB Lippincott, Philadelphia, 1995, pp. 1944–1966.
24. Burt RW, Bishop DT, Cannon LA, Dowdle MA, Lee RG, and Skolnick MH. Dominant inheritance of adenomatous colonic polyps and colorectal cancer. *N. Engl. J. Med.*, **312** (1985) 1540–1544.
25. Fuchs CS, Giovannucci EL, Colditz GA, Hunter DJ, Speizer FE, and Willett WC. A prospective study of family history and the risk of colorectal cancer [see comments]. *N. Engl. J. Med.*, **331** (1994) 1669–1674.
26. Planck M, Anderson H, Bladstrom A, Moller T, Wenngren E, and Olsson H. Increased cancer risk in offspring of women with colorectal carcinoma: a Swedish register-based cohort study. *Cancer*, **89** (2000) 741–749.
27. Slattery ML and Kerber RA. Family history of cancer and colon cancer risk: the Utah Population Database [published erratum appears in *J. Natl. Cancer Inst.*, **86(23)** (1994) 1802]. *J. Natl. Cancer Inst.*, **86** (1994) 1618–1626.

28. St. John DJ, McDermott FT, Hopper JL, Debney EA, Johnson WR, and Hughes ES. Cancer risk in relatives of patients with common colorectal cancer. *Ann. Intern. Med.*, **118** (1993) 785–790.

29. Burt RW, Bishop DT, Lee RG, Albright LC, and Skolnick MH. Inheritance of colonic adenomatous polyps and colorectal cancer. *Prog. Clin. Biol. Res.*, **279** (1988) 189–194.

30. Lichtenstein P, Holm NV, Verkasalo PK, et al. Environmental and heritable factors in the causation of cancer—analyses of cohorts of twins from Sweden, Denmark, and Finland [see comments]. *N. Engl. J. Med.*, **343** (2000) 78–85.

31. Aarnio M, Sankila R, Pukkala E, et al. Cancer risk in mutation carriers of DNA-mismatch-repair genes. *Int. J. Cancer*, **81** (1999) 214–218.

32. Vasen HF, Wijnen JT, Menko FH, et al. Cancer risk in families with hereditary nonpolyposis colorectal cancer diagnosed by mutation analysis [published erratum appears in *Gastroenterology*, **111(5)** (1996) 1402]. *Gastroenterology*, **110** (1996) 1020–1027.

33. Bodmer WF, Bailey CJ, Bodmer J, et al. Localization of the gene for familial adenomatous polyposis on chromosome 5. *Nature*, **328** (1987) 614–616.

34. Leppert M, Dobbs M, Scambler P, et al. The gene for familial polyposis coli maps to the long arm of chromosome 5. *Science*, **238** (1987) 1411–1413.

35. Lynch HT, Smyrk T, and Lynch JF. Overview of natural history, pathology, molecular genetics and management of HNPCC (Lynch syndrome). *Int. J. Cancer*, **69** (1996) 38–43.

36. Lynch HT and Lynch JF. 25 years of HNPCC. *Anticancer Res.*, **14** (1994) 1617–1624.

37. Hamilton SR, Liu B, Parsons RE, et al. The molecular basis of Turcot's syndrome [see comments]. *N. Engl. J. Med.*, **332** (1995) 839–847.

38. Crail H. Multiple primary malignancies arising in rectum, brain, and thyroid: report of a case. *US Naval Med. Bull.*, **49** (1949) 123–128.

39. Khandekar S, Kuwada SK, Khullar S, Mineau G, Kerber R, and Burt RW. The frequency of high-risk familial colorectal cancer. *Gastroenterology*, **114** (1988) 621A.

40. Miyoshi Y, Nagase H, Ando H, et al. Somatic mutations of the APC gene in colorectal tumors: mutation cluster region in the APC gene. *Hum. Mol. Genet.*, **1** (1992) 229–233.

41. Smith KJ, Johnson KA, Bryan TM, et al. The APC gene product in normal and tumor cells. *Proc. Natl. Acad. Sci. USA*, **90** (1993) 2846–2850.

42. Groden J, Thliveris A, Samowitz W, et al. Identification and characterization of the familial adenomatous polyposis coli gene. *Cell*, **66** (1991) 589–600.

43. Joslyn G, Carlson M, Thliveris A, et al. Identification of deletion mutations and three new genes at the familial polyposis locus. *Cell*, **66** (1991) 601–613.

44. Kinzler KW, Nilbert MC, Su LK, et al. Identification of FAP locus genes from chromosome 5q21. *Science*, **253** (1991) 661–665.

45. Nishisho I, Nakamura Y, Miyoshi Y, et al. Mutations of chromosome 5q21 genes in FAP and colorectal cancer patients. *Science*, **253** (1991) 665–669.

46. Munemitsu S, Albert I, Souza B, Rubinfeld B, and and Polakis P. Regulation of intracellular beta-catenin levels by the adenomatous polyposis coli (APC) tumor-suppressor protein. *Proc. Natl. Acad. Sci. USA*, **92** (1995) 3046–3050.

47. Rubinfeld B, Souza B, Albert I, Munemitsu S, and Polakis P. The APC protein and E-cadherin form similar but independent complexes with alpha-catenin, beta-catenin, and plakoglobin. *J. Biol. Chem.*, **270** (1995) 5549–5555.

48. Aberle H, Bauer A, Stappert J, Kispert A, and Kemler R. Beta-catenin is a target for the ubiquitin-proteasome pathway. *EMBO J.*, **16** (1997) 3797–3804.

49. Orford K, Crockett C, Jensen JP, Weissman AM, and Byers SW. Serine phosphorylation-regulated ubiquitination and degradation of beta-catenin. *J. Biol. Chem.*, **272** (1997) 24,735–24,738.

50. Peifer M and Polakis P. Wnt signaling in oncogenesis and embryogenesis–a look outside the nucleus. *Science*, **287** (2000) 1606–1609.

51. Cook D, Fry MJ, Hughes K, Sumathipala R, Woodgett JR, and Dale TC. Wingless inactivates glycogen synthase kinase-3 via an intracellular signalling pathway which involves a protein kinase C. *EMBO J.*, **15** (1996) 4526–4536.

52. Korinek V, Barker N, Morin PJ, et al. Constitutive transcriptional activation by a beta-catenin-Tcf complex in APC–/– colon carcinoma [see comments]. *Science*, **275** (1997) 1784–1787.

53. Morin PJ, Sparks AB, Korinek V, et al. Activation of beta-catenin–Tcf signaling in colon cancer by mutations in beta-catenin or APC [see comments]. *Science*, **275** (1997) 1787–1790.

54. Rubinfeld B, Robbins P, El-Gamil M, Albert I, Porfiri E, and Polakis P. Stabilization of beta-catenin by genetic defects in melanoma cell lines [see comments]. *Science*, **275** (1997) 1790–1792.

55. He TC, Chan TA, Vogelstein B, and Kinzler KW. PPARdelta is an APC-regulated target of nonsteroidal anti-inflammatory drugs. *Cell*, **99** (1999) 335–345.

56. He TC, Sparks AB, Rago C, et al. Identification of c-MYC as a target of the APC pathway [see comments]. *Science*, **281** (1998) 1509–1512.

57. Koh TJ, Bulitta CJ, Fleming JV, Dockray GJ, Varro A, and Wang TC. Gastrin is a target of the beta-catenin/TCF-4 growth-signaling pathway in a model of intestinal polyposis [in process citation]. *J. Clin. Invest.*, **106** (2000) 533–539.

58. Mann B, Gelos M, Siedow A, et al. Target genes of beta-catenin–T cell-factor/lymphoid-enhancer-factor signaling in human colorectal carcinomas. *Proc. Natl. Acad. Sci. USA*, **96** (1999) 1603–1608.

59. Tetsu O and McCormick F. Beta-catenin regulates expression of cyclin D1 in colon carcinoma cells. *Nature*, **398** (1999) 422–426.

60. Powell SM, Petersen GM, Krush AJ, et al. Molecular diagnosis of familial adenomatous polyposis [see comments]. *N. Engl. J. Med.*, **329** (1993) 1982–1987.

61. Peifer M. Beta-catenin as oncogene: the smoking gun [comment]. *Science*, **275** (1997) 1752–1753.

62. Henderson BR. Nuclear-cytoplasmic shuttling of APC regulates beta-catenin subcellular localization and turnover. *Nat. Cell. Biol.*, **2** (2000) 653–660.

63. Rosin-Arbesfeld R, Townsley F, and Bienz M. The APC tumour suppressor has a nuclear export function [in process citation]. *Nature*, **406** (2000) 1009–1012.

64. Kawasaki Y, Senda T, Ishidate T, et al. Asef, a link between the tumor suppressor APC and G-protein signaling. *Science*, **289** (2000) 1194–1197.

65. Miyaki M, Tanaka K, Kikuchi-Yanoshita R, Muraoka M, and Konishi M. Familial polyposis: recent advances. *Crit. Rev. Oncol. Hematol.*, **19** (1995) 1–31.

66. Polakis P. The adenomatous polyposis coli (APC) tumor suppressor. *Biochim. Biophys. Acta*, **1332** (1997) F127–F147.

67. Spirio L, Olschwang S, Groden J, et al. Alleles of the APC gene: an attenuated form of familial polyposis. *Cell*, **75** (1993) 951–957.

68. Spirio L, Otterud B, Stauffer D, et al. Linkage of a variant or attenuated form of adenomatous polyposis coli to the adenomatous polyposis coli (APC) locus. *Am. J. Hum. Genet.*, **51** (1992) 92–100.

69. van der Luijt RB, Vasen HF, Tops CM, Breukel C, Fodde R, and Meera Khan P. APC mutation in the alternatively spliced region of exon 9 associated with late onset familial adenomatous polyposis. *Hum. Genet.*, **96** (1995) 705–710.

70. van der Luijt RB, Meera Khan P, Vasen HF, et al. Germline mutations in the 3' part of APC exon 15 do not result in truncated proteins and are associated with attenuated adenomatous polyposis coli. *Hum. Genet.*, **98** (1996) 727–734.

71. Leppert M, Burt R, Hughes JP, et al. Genetic analysis of an inherited predisposition to colon cancer in a family with a variable number of adenomatous polyps. *N. Engl. J. Med.*, **322** (1990) 904–908.

72. Dietrich WF, Lander ES, Smith JS, et al. Genetic identification of Mom-1, a major modifier locus affecting Min-induced intestinal neoplasia in the mouse. *Cell*, **75** (1993) 631–639.

73. Dobbie Z, Muller H, and Scott RJ. Secretory phospholipase A2 does not appear to be associated with phenotypic variation in familial adenomatous polyposis. *Hum. Genet.*, **98** (1996) 386–390.

74. Spirio LN, Kutchera W, Winstead MV, et al. Three secretory phospholipase A(2) genes that map to human chromosome 1P35–36 are not mutated in individuals with attenuated adenomatous polyposis coli. *Cancer Res.*, **56** (1996) 955–958.

75. Tomlinson IP, Beck NE, Neale K, and Bodmer WF. Variants at the secretory phospholipase A2 (PLA2G2A) locus: analysis of associations with familial adenomatous polyposis and sporadic colorectal tumours. *Ann. Hum. Genet.*, **60** (1996) 369–376.

76. Laken SJ, Petersen GM, Gruber SB, et al. Familial colorectal cancer in Ashkenazim due to a hypermutable tract in APC. *Nat. Genet.*, **17** (1997) 79–83.

77. Woodage T, King SM, Wacholder S, et al. The APCI1307K allele and cancer risk in a community-based study of Ashkenazi Jews [see comments]. *Nat. Genet.*, **20** (1998) 62–65.

78. Sparks AB, Morin PJ, Vogelstein B, and Kinzler KW. Mutational analysis of the APC/beta-catenin/Tcf pathway in colorectal cancer. *Cancer Res.*, **58** (1998) 1130–1134.

79. Lane DP. Cancer. p53, guardian of the genome [news; comment] [see comments]. *Nature*, **358** (1992) 15–16.

80. Yew PR and Berk AJ. Inhibition of p53 transactivation required for transformation by adenovirus early 1B protein. *Nature*, **357** (1992) 82–85.

81. Tanaka H, Arakawa H, Yamaguchi T, et al. A ribonucleotide reductase gene involved in a p53-dependent cell-cycle checkpoint for DNA damage [see comments]. *Nature*, **404** (2000) 42–49.

82. Fearon ER, Cho KR, Nigro JM, et al. Identification of a chromosome 18q gene that is altered in colorectal cancers. *Science*, **247** (1990) 49–56.

83. Keino-Masu K, Masu M, Hinck L, et al. Deleted in Colorectal Cancer (DCC) encodes a netrin receptor. *Cell*, **87** (1996) 175–185.

84. Kennedy TE, Serafini T, de la Torre JR, and Tessier-Lavigne M. Netrins are diffusible chemotropic factors for commissural axons in the embryonic spinal cord. *Cell*, **78** (1994) 425–435.

85. Serafini T, Colamarino SA, Leonardo ED, et al. Netrin-1 is required for commissural axon guidance in the developing vertebrate nervous system. *Cell*, **87** (1996) 1001–1014.

86. Fazeli A, Dickinson SL, Hermiston ML, et al. Phenotype of mice lacking functional Deleted in colorectal cancer (Dcc) gene. *Nature*, **386** (1997) 796–804.

87. Mehlen P, Rabizadeh S, Snipas SJ, Assa-Munt N, Salvesen GS, and Bredesen DE. The DCC gene product induces apoptosis by a mechanism requiring receptor proteolysis. *Nature*, **395** (1998) 801–814.

88. Klingelhutz AJ, Hedrick L, Cho KR, and McDougall JK. The DCC gene suppresses the malignant phenotype of transformed human epithelial cells. *Oncogene*, **10** (1995) 1581–1586.

89. Shibata D, Reale MA, Lavin P, et al. The DCC protein and prognosis in colorectal cancer [see comments]. *N. Engl. J. Med.*, **335** (1996) 1727–1732.

90. Jass JR. Pathology of hereditary nonpolyposis colorectal cancer. *Ann. NY Acad. Sci.*, **910** (2000) 62–73; discussion 73–74.

91. Jiricny J and Nystrom-Lahti M. Mismatch repair defects in cancer. *Curr. Opin. Genet. Dev.*, **10** (2000) 157–161.

92. Lynch HT and Lynch JF. Hereditary nonpolyposis colorectal cancer. *Semin. Surg. Oncol.*, **18** (2000) 305–313.

93. Boland CR, Thibodeau SN, Hamilton SR, et al. A National Cancer Institute Workshop on Microsatellite Instability for cancer detection and familial predisposition: development of international criteria for the determination of microsatellite instability in colorectal cancer. *Cancer Res.*, **58** (1998) 5248–5257.

94. Kolodner R. Biochemistry and genetics of eukaryotic mismatch repair. *Genes Dev.*, **10** (1996) 1433–1442.

95. Modrich P and Lahue R. Mismatch repair in replication fidelity, genetic recombination, and cancer biology. *Annu. Rev. Biochem.*, **65** (1996) 101–133.

96. Borresen AL, Lothe RA, Meling GI, et al. Somatic mutations in the hMSH2 gene in microsatellite unstable colorectal carcinomas. *Hum. Mol. Genet.*, **4** (1995) 2065–2072.

97. Bubb VJ, Curtis LJ, Cunningham C, et al. Microsatellite instability and the role of hMSH2 in sporadic colorectalcancer. *Oncogene*, **12** (1996) 2641–2649.

98. Liu B, Nicolaides NC, Markowitz S, et al. Mismatch repair gene defects in sporadic colorectal cancers with microsatellite instability. *Nat. Genet.*, **9** (1995) 48–55.

99. Gryfe R, Kim H, Hsieh ET, et al. Tumor microsatellite instability and clinical outcome in young patients with colorectal cancer [see comments]. *N. Engl. J. Med.*, **342** (2000) 69–77.

100. Herman JG, Umar A, Polyak K, et al. Incidence and functional consequences of hMLH1 promoter hypermethylation in colorectal carcinoma. *Proc. Natl. Acad. Sci. USA*, **95** (1998) 6870–6875.

101. Veigl ML, Kasturi L, Olechnowicz J, et al. Biallelic inactivation of hMLH1 by epigenetic gene silencing, a novel mechanism causing human MSI cancers. *Proc. Natl. Acad. Sci. USA*, **95** (1998) 8698–8702.

102. Laird PW, Jackson-Grusby L, Fazeli A, et al. Suppression of intestinal neoplasia by DNA hypomethylation. *Cell*, **81** (1995) 197–205.

103. Thibodeau SN, Bren G, and Schaid D. Microsatellite instability in cancer of the proximal colon [see comments]. *Science*, **260** (1993) 816–819.

104. Markowitz S, Wang J, Myeroff L, et al. Inactivation of the type II TGF-beta receptor in colon cancer cells with microsatellite instability [see comments]. *Science*, **268** (1995) 1336–1338.

105. Wang J, Sun L, Myeroff L, et al. Demonstration that mutation of the type II transforming growth factor beta receptor inactivates its tumor suppressor activity in replication error-positive colon carcinoma cells. *J. Biol. Chem.*, **270** (1995) 2,2044–2,2049.

106. Massague J. Receptors for the TGF-beta family. *Cell*, **69** (1992) 1067–1070.

107. Massague J and Weinberg RA. Negative regulators of growth. *Curr. Opin. Genet. Dev.*, **2** (1992) 28–32.

108. Grady WM, Myeroff LL, Swinler SE, et al. Mutational inactivation of transforming growth factor beta receptor type II in microsatellite stable colon cancers. *Cancer Res.*, **59** (1999) 320–324.

109. Souza RF, Appel R, Yin J, et al. Microsatellite instability in the insulin-like growth factor II receptor gene in gastrointestinal tumours [letter] [published erratum appears in *Nat. Genet.*, **14(4)** (1996) 488]. *Nat. Genet.*, **14** (1996) 255–257.

110. Rampino N, Yamamoto H, Ionov Y, et al. Somatic frameshift mutations in the BAX gene in colon cancers of the microsatellite mutator phenotype. *Science*, **275** (1997) 967–969.

111. Chadwick RB, Jiang GL, Bennington GA, et al. Candidate tumor suppressor RIZ is frequently involved in colorectal carcinogenesis. *Proc. Natl. Acad. Sci. USA*, **97** (2000) 2662–2667.

112. Shiff SJ, Qiao L, Tsai LL, and Rigas B. Sulindac sulfide, an aspirin-like compound, inhibits proliferation, causes cell cycle quiescence, and induces apoptosis in HT-29 colon adenocarcinoma cells. *J. Clin. Invest.*, **96** (1995) 491–503.

113. Eberhart CE, Coffey RJ, Radhika A, Giardiello FM, Ferrenbach S, and DuBois RN. Up-regulation of cyclooxygenase 2 gene expression in human colorectal adenomas and adenocarcinomas. *Gastroenterology*, **107** (1994) 1183–1188.

114. Kutchera W, Jones DA, Matsunami N, et al. Prostaglandin H synthase 2 is expressed abnormally in human colon cancer: evidence for a transcriptional effect. *Proc. Natl. Acad. Sci. USA*, **93** (1996) 4816–4820.

115. Fukutake M, Nakatsugi S, Isoi T, et al. Suppressive effects of nimesulide, a selective inhibitor of cyclooxygenase-2, on azoxymethane-induced colon carcinogenesis in mice. *Carcinogenesis*, **19** (1998) 1939–1942.

116. Rao CV, Kawamori T, Hamid R, and Reddy BS. Chemoprevention of colonic aberrant crypt foci by an inducible nitric oxide synthase-selective inhibitor. *Carcinogenesis*, **20** (1999) 641–644.

117. Reddy BS, Rao CV, and Seibert K. Evaluation of cyclooxygenase-2 inhibitor for potential chemopreventive properties in colon carcinogenesis. *Cancer Res.*, **56** (1996) 4566–4569.

118. Yoshimi N, Kawabata K, Hara A, Matsunaga K, Yamada Y, and Mori H. Inhibitory effect of NS-398, a selective cyclooxygenase-2 inhibitor, on azoxymethane-induced aberrant crypt foci in colon carcinogenesis of F344 rats. *Jpn. J. Cancer Res.*, **88** (1997) 1044–1051.

119. Yoshimi N, Shimizu M, Matsunaga K, et al. Chemopreventive effect of *N*-(2-cyclohexyloxy-4-nitrophenyl)methane sulfonamide (NS-398), a selective cyclooxygenase-2 inhibitor, in rat colon carcinogenesis induced by azoxymethane. *Jpn. J. Cancer Res.*, **90** (1999) 406–412.

120. Oshima M, Dinchuk JE, Kargman SL, et al. Suppression of intestinal polyposis in Apc delta716 knockout mice by inhibition of cyclooxygenase 2 (COX-2). *Cell*, **87** (1996) 803–809.

121. Steinbach G, Lynch PM, Phillips RK, et al. The effect of celecoxib, a cyclooxygenase-2 inhibitor, in familial adenomatous polyposis. *N. Engl. J. Med.*, **342** (2000) 1946–1952.

122. Karnes WE Jr, Shattuck-Brandt R, Burgart LJ, et al. Reduced COX-2 protein in colorectal cancer with defective mismatch repair. *Cancer Res.*, **58** (1998) 5473–5477.

123. Sinicrope FA, Lemoine M, Xi L, et al. Reduced expression of cyclooxygenase 2 proteins in hereditary nonpolyposis colorectal cancers relative to sporadic cancers. *Gastroenterology*, **117** (1999) 350–358.

124. Thompson WJ, Piazza GA, Li H, et al. Exisulind induction of apoptosis involves guanosine 3′,5′-cyclic monophosphate phosphodiesterase inhibition, protein kinase G activation, and attenuated beta-catenin. *Cancer Res.*, **60** (2000) 3338–3342.

125. Hull MA, Booth JK, Tisbury A, et al. Cyclooxygenase 2 is up-regulated and localized to macrophages in the intestine of Min mice. *Br. J. Cancer*, **79** (1999) 1399–1405.

126. Shattuck-Brandt RL, Varilek GW, Radhika A, Yang F, Washington MK, and DuBois RN. Cyclooxygenase 2 expression is increased in the stroma of colon carcinomas from IL-10(–/–) mice. *Gastroenterology*, **118** (2000) 337–345.

127. Smigel K. Arthritis drug approved for polyp prevention blazes trail for other prevention trials [news]. *J. Natl. Cancer Inst.*, **92** (2000) 297–299.

2 Epidemiological Trends in Colorectal Cancer

Susan M. Talbot and Alfred I. Neugut

CONTENTS

1. INTRODUCTION

Colorectal cancer is the fourth most common cancer worldwide, accounting for approximately 10% of the world total with 782,800 new cases in 1990 (Table 1) *(1)*. In 1990, it accounted for 437,000 deaths *(2)*. It is particularly common in North America, Australia, New Zealand, and parts of Europe, is rare in Asia, and is uncommon in Africa. In developed countries, the lifetime probability of developing colorectal cancer is 4.6% in men and 3.2% in females *(2)*. It affects men and women almost equally, with a similar incidence and number of deaths in the two sexes *(3,4)*. As we enter the new millennium, the incidence and mortality rates for colorectal cancer overall are now declining *(5)*. Rectal cancer incidence, however, as a separate entity, has remained relatively stable over this same time period.

Ethnic and racial differences in colon cancer, as well as studies on migrants, suggest that environmental factors play a major role in the etiology of the disease. In the last decade, multiple genetic mutations have been discovered that play a critical role in colorectal tumorigenesis, in what has become termed the adenoma–carcinoma sequence.

The association between the risk of colorectal cancer and specific conditions such as inflammatory bowel disease, environmental factors such as diet, occupation, smoking, alcohol intake, body mass, and physical activity, and reproductive factors will also be addressed in this chapter.

From: *Colorectal Cancer: Multimodality Management*
Edited by: L. Saltz © Humana Press Inc., Totowa, NJ

Table 1
Estimate of New Cancer Cases Occurring in 1990 Worldwide

Tumor site	Number of cases	Percentage of total
Lung	1,036,900	12.8
Stomach	798,300	9.9
Breast	795,600	9.8
Colon/rectum	782,800	9.7
Liver	437,400	5.4
Prostate	396,100	4.9
Cervix uteri	371,200	4.6
Esophagus	315,800	3.9
Bladder	260,700	3.2
Leukemia	231,200	2.9
Total	8,083,300	100

Adapted from ref. *1*.

2. DESCRIPTIVE EPIDEMIOLOGY

2.1. Incidence and Mortality in the United States

There were an estimated 93,800 new colon cancer cases in the United States in 2000: 43,400 in men and 50,400 in women *(6)*. It was the fourth most common cancer overall, and the third leading form of cancer specifically among both men and women. Estimated new rectal cancer cases for the same time period were 36,400, with 20,200 occurring in males and 16,200 in females. Rectal cancer was the eighth most common cancer overall, seventh most common among men, and eighth most common among women.

There were an estimated 47,700 colon cancer deaths in the United States in 2000, with 23,100 in men and 24,600 in women. It was the second most common cause of death resulting from cancer (after lung cancer), ranking third among both men and women. Rectal cancer accounted for an additional 8600 deaths, with 4700 men and 3900 women. It was ranked 15th among the leading causes of cancer deaths, 12th among men, and 13th among women.

Between 1986 and 1997, there was a decline in the overall cancer incidence and mortality rates within the United States *(5)*, as depicted in Fig. 1 *(7)*.

There is variability in colorectal cancer incidence rates in different states within the United States. This state-to-state variation ranged from 32.4 new cases per 100,000 in Utah to 51.9 cases per 100,000 in Rhode Island *(5)*. During the same time period, the same state-to-state variation in death rates from colorectal cancer ranged from 12.3 per 100,000 in Utah to 20.0 per 100,000 in New Jersey *(5)*. These state-to state variations may reflect different subject demographics, such as race and ethnicity, differences in cancer registration, as well as differences in environmental factors, such as diet and occupation.

2.2. International Variations

International variations in the incidence and mortality rates from colon and rectal cancer differ. Colon cancer varies approx 20-fold internationally *(8)*. Although there is evidence for genetic predisposition to colon cancer, most of this variation is attributed to differences in dietary habits and other environmental factors.

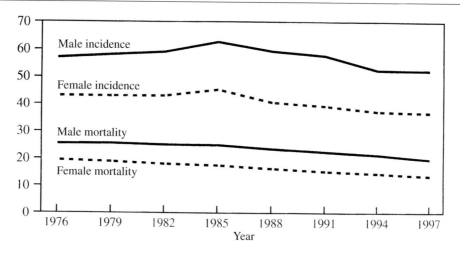

Fig. 1. Age-adjusted mortality rates (per 100,000) for colon and rectal cancer. *SEER Cancer Statistics Review, 1973–1997 (7).*

The estimated age-standardized incidence rates of colon and rectal cancer (per 100,000) by region, and gender are shown in Table 2 *(9)*. The highest rates are seen in Western countries, such as Australia/New Zealand (45.8 male, 34.8 female), North America (44.3 male, 32.8 female), and western Europe (39.8 male, 29.0 female), with lower rates in all parts of Africa (except South Africa) and South Central Asia (5.0 male, 3.8 female).

Incidence rates have risen in most regions since 1985, except for North America, where they have decreased. The estimated number of cases has increased by 15.5% between 1985 and 1990 (21% in men, 10% in females) *(9)*.

Age-adjusted mortality rates per 100,000 population for 45 countries for 1994 to 1997 indicate the highest rates in Western countries, such as New Zealand (26.4 male, 19.1 female), Australia (20.2 male, 13.3 female), United Kingdom (18.0 male, 11.6 female), United States (15.2 male, 10.4 female), and eastern European countries such as the Czech Republic (34.3 male, 17.3 female) and Hungary (34.3 male, 18.7 female), with low rates in Asian countries, such as China (7.9 male, 6.4 female) and South America (Table 3) *(6)*.

Cancers of the colon and rectum are similar with respect to their geographical distribution. In high-risk populations, the ratio of colon cancer to rectal cancer is greater than or equal to 2:1, whereas in low-risk countries, the rates are similar *(2)*.

Within countries, there is also a variation in incidence between urban and rural centers, with an increased incidence in urban regions *(10)*.

2.3. Age

The probability of developing invasive colorectal cancer in the United States in 2000 increased with increasing age, irrespective of gender *(6)*. Colorectal cancer is uncommon among those less than 40 yr of age, with a rapid increase in incidence after age 50 yr *(11)*. This has implications for screening, which is most cost-effective for those at higher risk.

During the period 1994–1996, the risk of developing colorectal cancer for men was 1 in 1579 from birth to age 39, 1 in 124 for ages 40–59, and 1 in 29 for ages 60–79. For women, the risk was 1 in 1947 from birth to age 39, 1 in 149 for ages 40–59, and 1 in 33 for ages 60–79 *(6)*.

Table 2
Estimated Age Standardized Rates of Colon/Rectum Cancer Incidence
by Sex and Area, 1990 (per 100,000)

Site	Male	Female
Eastern Africa	8.1	4.2
Middle Africa	2.3	3.4
Northern Africa	6.0	4.2
Southern Africa	11.2	8.4
Western Africa	4.7	3.9
Caribbean	16.0	15.5
Central America	8.8	7.9
South America (temperate)	27.2	24.4
South America (tropical)	15.0	13.6
North America	44.3	32.8
Eastern Asia: China	13.3	10.2
Eastern Asia: Japan	39.5	24.6
Eastern Asia: Other	21.3	14.1
South Eastern Asia	11.9	8.9
South Central Asia	5.0	3.8
Western Asia	8.8	7.6
Eastern Europe	25.3	18.5
Northern Europe	34.4	26.1
Southern Europe	28.8	20.2
Western Europe	39.8	29.0
Ausatrlia/New Zealand	45.8	34.8
Melanesia	11.1	5.3
Micronesia/Polynesia	17.6	11.3
Developed Countries	35.9	25.4
Developing Countries	10.2	8.1
All areas	19.4	15.3

Adapted from ref. 9.

For patients ≥ 50 yr, colorectal cancer incidence rates were higher for men than women *(5)*. For patients < 50 yr of age, the incidence rates were similar for men and women.

2.4. Gender

In the Annual Report to the Nation on the Status of Cancer 1973–1997, colorectal cancer rates were higher in men than women, regardless of race *(5)*. The colorectal cancer incidence rate was greater than 40% higher in men than women.

The overall sex ratio for colon cancer worldwide is nearly equal. This is in contrast to rectal cancer, for which there is a male predominance, especially with increasing age *(2)*.

In terms of incidence, colorectal cancer is the third most frequent cancer among males and ranks second for women *(2)*. It is the fourth leading cause of cancer mortality for both sexes, with a more favorable outcome than some cancers at other sites *(2)*. In males, age-standardized rates range from 25.3 per 100,000 (Eastern Europe) to 45.8 (Australia/New Zealand). For females, the rates range from 18.5 (Eastern Europe) to 34.8 (Australia/New Zealand) (Table 2) *(9)*.

Table 3
Cancer Around the World: Age-Adjusted Death Rates per 100,000 Population
for Colon and Rectal Cancer for Different Countries, 1994–1997*

Country	Male	Female
United States[a]	15.2 (27)	10.4 (23)
Australia[b]	20.2 (10)	13.3 (10)
Austria[a]	21.7 (8)	12.2 (14)
Bulgaria[c]	17.2 (20)	11.4 (19)
Canada[b]	16.1 (26)	10.3 (25)
Chile[c]	7.0 (38)	6.7 (36)
China[c]	7.9 (36)	6.4 (37)
Colombia[c]	4.8 (44)	5.1 (40)
Croatia[d]	22.5 (6)	11.5 (18)
Cuba[b]	9.4 (34)	11.3 (20)
Czech Republic[e]	34.3 (1)	17.3 (3)
Denmark[e]	22.7 (5)	15.6 (4)
France[b]	16.6 (22)	9.6 (29)
Germany[a]	20.8 (9)	14.0 (7)
Greece[e]	8.0 (35)	6.2 (38)
Hungary[f]	34.3 (2)	18.7 (2)
Ireland[b]	22.5 (7)	13.3 (9)
Israel[e]	17.9 (18)	13.8 (8)
Japan[g]	17.1 (21)	9.9 (28)
Mexico[b]	3.6 (45)	3.3 (45)
New Zealand[c]	26.4 (3)	19.1 (1)
Russian Fed[b]	18.2 (14)	12.6 (12)
United Kingdom[a]	18.0 (17)	11.6 (17)

Adapted from ref. 6.
*Rates are age-adjusted to the World Health Organization world standard population:
[a]1994–1997; [b]1994–1995; [c]1994 only; [d]1995–1996; [e]1994–1996; [f]1996–1997; [g]1995–1997.

2.5. Time Trends

Colorectal cancer mortality rates have been decreasing among women since 1950 *(5)*. The death rates for men did not begin to decrease until the 1980s. Time trends with respect to subsite distribution generally show an increase in right-sided and sigmoid tumors, with stability in the incidence rate of rectal tumors *(12)*.

Time trends in the United States from 1973 to 1997 demonstrate that after a 13-yr increase in the incidence of colorectal cancer, incidence rates began to fall in 1986 for the first time and have continued their downward trend since that time *(5)*, as depicted in Fig. 1 *(7)*. Colorectal cancer incidence rates have decreased an average of 1.6% per year *(5)*. This decline was predominantly in the distal colon and rectum and was almost equal in males and females. From 1973 to 1994, the age-adjusted incidence rate of cancer had decreased in the distal colon and rectum by 24% in white males and by 26% in white females. A decrease in incidence rates was also seen in the proximal colon, with 12% in white males and 14% in white females. Rates among African-Americans were variable, showing no clear pattern of decline, and an increase in the incidence of cancers in the proximal colon in both sexes has occurred since 1986.

In contrast, the incidence rate of colorectal cancer in England and Wales has been gradually rising and is most marked for colon cancer in males, irrespective of age *(13)*. Similar trends were found in the rest of Europe, in particular eastern Europe, where an average increase of greater than 14% in age-specific incidence rates per 5-yr period was seen between 1973 and 1987.

A rise in the age-specific incidence of colorectal cancer per 5-yr period of more than 35% in males and 27% in females was also seen in Japan between 1973 and 1987.

From 1990 to 1996, colon and rectal cancer death rates in the United States decreased significantly, an average of 1.7% per year. Colon and rectum cancer deaths among men were at their highest level in 1990, at 28,635, and had declined to 28,075 in 1997. Although the recorded number of cancer deaths for women have continued to increase, colorectal cancer deaths as a subset have declined, falling from a peak of 29,237 in 1995 to 28,621 in 1997.

Early detection through appropriate screening may be partly responsible for these changes in incidence and mortality. Improvements in mortality may also reflect improvements in definitive therapy, such as surgical techniques and adjuvant therapy *(14)*. Other possible factors contributing to the decline in incidence rates may be changes in diet *(14)* and physical activity *(15)*. Although not in widespread use, chemoprevention with aspirin *(16)* and other nonsteroidal anti-inflammatory drugs (NSAIDs) *(17,18)* is also continuing to show promise

2.6. Race/Ethnicity

Among US women, colorectal cancer was more common for Hispanic, American Indians/Alaska Natives, and Asian/Pacific Islanders, ranking second only to breast cancer, whereas it ranked third after both breast and lung cancer for white and black women *(5)*. Black women are more likely than white women to develop cancers of the colon and rectum *(5,19)*.

Between 1990 and 1996, the age-adjusted incidence rate for cancers of both the colon and rectum was 44.9 per 100,000 for black women compared with 36.8 per 100,000 for white women *(6)*. The incidence rates were lower for Asian/Pacific Islanders, American Indians, and Hispanic Americans (Table 4) *(6)*.

The incidence rate for colorectal cancer increased until 1984 for white women, but has subsequently decreased *(5)*. The colorectal cancer incidence rate for black women also increased until 1980, but has been approximately level since then.

Black women are more likely to die of colon and rectal cancers than women of other ethnic and racial groups. During the same time period, the mortality rates were 20.0 per 100,000 for black women and 14.5 per 100,000 for white women *(6)*. Mortality rates were also lower for Asian/Pacific Islanders, American Indians, and Hispanic Americans *(5)* (Table 5) *(6)*.

There was a decline in death rates for colorectal cancer for white women between 1973 and 1997. The decline was more rapid after 1984 *(5)*. The mortality rates for black women first began to decline in 1985. This decline was less marked for black women than for white women.

Black men have the highest rates for cancers of the colon and rectum, as well as for lung and prostate cancers. Between 1990 and 1996, the male incidence rates for cancers of both the colon and rectum was 58.1 per 100,000 for black men compared with 53.2 per 100,000 for white men *(6)*. Similar to the incidence rates in women, rates among men were lower among Asian/Pacific Islanders, American Indians, and Hispanic Americans *(5)* (Table 4) *(6)*.

Table 4
Incidence Rates of Colon and Rectum Cancer by Race and Ethnicity, US, 1990–1996*

	White	Black	Asian/Pacific Islander	American Indian	Hispanic[a]
Total	43.9	50.4	38.6	16.4	29.0
Male	53.2	58.1	47.5	21.5	35.7
Female	36.8	44.9	31.4	12.4	24.0

Adapted from ref. *6*.
*Rates are per 100,000 population and are age-adjusted to the 1970 US standard population.
[a]Hispanic is not mutually exclusive of white, black, Asian/Pacific Islander, or American Indian.

Table 5
Mortality Rates for Colon and Rectum Cancer by Race and Ethnicity, US, 1990–1996*

	White	Black	Asian/Pacific Islander	American Indian	Hispanic[a]
Total	17.4	23.1	10.9	9.9	10.4
Male	21.5	27.8	13.4	11.0	13.2
Female	14.5	20.0	9.0	8.9	8.4

Adapted from ref. *6*.
*Rates are per 100,000 population and are age-adjusted to the 1970 US standard population.
[a]Hispanic are not mutually exclusive of white, black, Asian/Pacific Islander, or American Indian.

Colorectal cancer incidence rates among white men began decreasing after 1985, with the most rapid decline between 1991 and 1995. Rates in black men increased by an average of 4.4% per year between 1973 and 1980, but have remained level since that time *(5)*. Between 1973 and 1990, estimated incidence rates for colorectal cancer were lower for black men than white men. Since 1990, colorectal cancer incidence rates have been lower for white men than black men.

Colorectal cancer incidence rates among white men began decreasing after 1985, with the most rapid decline occurring between 1991 and 1995. Rates in black men increased by an average of 4.4% per year between 1973 and 1980 but have remained level since that time *(5)*.

Black men also have the highest mortality rates from these cancers. Between 1973 and 1990, the mortality rates were 27.8 per 100,000 for black men and 21.5 per 100,000 for white men *(6)*. The mortality rates among men were lower for Asian Pacific Islanders, American Indians, and Hispanic Americans (Table 5) *(6)*.

Colorectal mortality rates began to decline by 0.6% per year between 1978 and 1986 for white men. Since 1986, the decrease per year has been even more rapid. Colorectal cancer incidence rates among white men were level between 1973 and 1978 and began to decline between 1978 and 1986 by 0.6% per year *(5)*. Death rates among black men rose until 1989 and have leveled off since that time. Prior to 1980, mortality rates for colorectal cancer were lower for black men than white men.

2.7. Migrants

Migrant data suggest a 20-fold international difference in the incidence ratio of colorectal cancer *(8)*. Studies looking at the incidence of colorectal cancer among migrants, Japanese living in the United States and Europeans living in either the United States or Australia, indicate that migrants from low-risk areas to high-risk areas, exposed to the environment of the host population, develop the same cancer risk as that population *(12,20)*.

Among Japanese in Japan, colorectal cancer has a very low incidence rate, although it is rising *(21)*. In Japan, the fat intake is low in comparison to Western countries. Dietary fiber intake was high and is now decreasing *(22)*. Japanese migrating to Hawaii and California experience increases in colorectal cancer incidence, with first-generation immigrants having about double the frequency of cancers of the sigmoid colon and rectum as their white neighbors *(21,23)*. In another study, US-born Japanese men had incidence rates of colorectal cancer twice that of foreign-born Japanese men and about 60% higher than those of US-born white men *(24)*. United States-born Japanese women had a colorectal cancer incidence rate that was about 40% higher than among Japanese women born in Japan or US-born white women.

Similarly, colorectal cancer rates among were four to seven times higher than rates in China; this was most striking among men and with increasing age *(25)*.

3. PATHOLOGIC ISSUES

3.1. Adenoma–Carcinoma Sequence

The adenoma–carcinoma sequence was originally proposed by Hill and colleagues in 1978 *(26)*. It is generally believed that almost all colorectal adenocarcinomas arise from adenomas.

Vogelstein and colleagues have provided evidence for a series of specific chromosomal and somatic genetic changes that occur during the transition from normal colonic mucosa to invasive carcinoma *(27–29)*. The most common changes are point mutations of the K-ras protooncogene, and mutations in three growth suppressor genes, *p53* on chromosome 17p *(30)*, the adenomatous polyposis coli (APC) gene on chromosome 5q *(31)*, and DCC (deleted in colon cancer) gene on chromosome 18q *(29)*. Both alleles of the three tumor suppressor genes must be lost or defective for phenotypic expression to occur, whereas in the case of the protooncogene, K-ras, mutation need only occur in one allele for phenotypic expression to occur *(32)*. No gene has been implicated as occurring in all cases of colorectal cancer. Figure 2 depicts a proposed sequence of allelic losses during colorectal cancer development, although the exact number and sequence of genetic mutations necessary for carcinoma formation remain to be determined.

The APC gene has been mapped to the tumor supressor locus (5q21–q22) *(33)*, and it is thought to be involved in the initiation of adenoma formation *(34)*. Inactivation of the APC gene by two mutations is involved in the development of adenomas, and loss of heterozygosity of the APC gene is associated with further progression to carcinoma *(35)*. It is mutated in between 30% and 75% of sporadic adenomas and adenocarcinomas *(32,33,35)*. The mutation is apparent even in early adenomas, and it remains constant throughout the malignant transformation *(33)*. Mutation of the APC gene is the most frequent genetic mutation seen in colorectal cancer *(29)*. Germline mutations of the APC gene are also responsible for the formation of multiple adenomas in familial adenomatous polyposis (FAP) *(31,35)*.

The APC protein may be involved in a series of interactions between proteins involved in cell signaling *(36)*, apoptosis *(37)*, and cell adhesion *(38)*.

K-ras is thought to promote tumorigenesis by causing hyperproliferation of colorectal cells, both at the early adenoma stage and later at the time of malignant transformation. Expression of the protooncogene is less in small adenomas, becoming more pronounced at

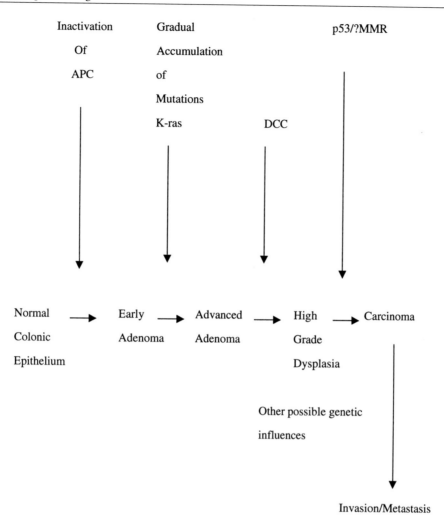

Fig. 2. A model of genetic events in colorectal carcinogenesis.

around 50% in larger adenomas (>1 cm in size) and adenocarcinomas *(27,39)*. The role of the K-ras mutation in tumorigenesis is not entirely clear, as mutations have also been found in normal colonic epithelium *(40)* and aberrant crypt foci *(41)*.

The DCC gene is located on chromosome 18q *(27,42)*, and is a neural cell adhesion molecule. It may play a role in tumor progression, invasion, and metastasis. Allelic loss of this chromosome is seen in 50% of advanced adenomas and more than 70% of carcinomas.

The *p53* gene is located on chromosome 17p. It appears to be involved late in malignant transformation, during the conversion from adenoma to focal carcinoma *(30,43)*. Loss of the *p53* gene is uncommon in adenomas but occurs in greater than 75% of carcinomas *(27,30)*. Mutation of *p53* may also have multiple effects, including a decreased ability to detect DNA damage, karyotypic instability, impaired G1 cell-cycle arrest, and decreased apoptosis *(44–46)*.

Germline mismatch repair (MMR) mutations occur in hereditary nonpolyposis colon cancer (HNPCC). The MMR mutations are thought to increase the overall mutation rate, but they may also play a role in the initiation of tumorigenesis *(46)*. MMR mutations are also found to occur in about 15% of sporadic colorectal cancers *(47,48)*. MMR mutations seem to occur at the stage of late adenoma or transformation to carcinoma *(49)*.

Microsatellite genetic instability has been demonstrated at the benign adenoma stage of HNPCC tumors. Carcinoma is more likely to occur in adenomas with a greater rate of genetic instability *(50)*. This finding supports the hypothesis of adenoma–carcinoma progression in HNPCC.

Other possible tumor suppressor genes have also been identified. These genes may be involved in later stages of tumorigenesis. An example is mutation at the p16 (MTS1) locus, resulting in failure of cell-cycle arrest *(51)*.

There may also be genetic changes specific for invasion and metastasis *(46)*.

3.2. Subsite Distribution

Surveillance, Epidemiology, and End Results Program (SEER) data show that left-sided tumors outnumber right-sided tumors throughout the United States *(52)*. There is evidence to support a progressive left-to-right shift in cancer distribution within the colon during the latter part of the last century *(52,53)*. SEER data show that the ratio of right-sided cancer to total colorectal cancer has increased from 1970 to 1990 among all age-, sex-, and race-matched cohorts *(52)*.

In the Annual Report to the Nation on the Status of Cancer between 1973 and 1997, all anatomic subsites demonstrated a decline in incidence rates except the right side of the colon, incorporating the cecum, appendix, ascending colon, and hepatic flexure *(5)*.

For whites, increased age has been associated with a progressive decline in the proportion of distal colorectal cancer for both genders, as evidenced by SEER incidence data from 1977, 1986, and 1994 *(54)*. The greatest and most consistent decline was seen in 1994. Distal colorectal cancer became less prevalent at about age 72 for women and age 82 for men. Among the younger age cohorts, distal colorectal cancer was more prevalent than proximal disease for both genders. There was no similar trend in subsite distribution among African-Americans, regardless of gender or age, although proximal disease is generally more prevalent than among whites.

There appears to be a relative increase in the incidence of right-sided tumors after age 70 *(55)*. This trend is more striking in females in higher-risk areas *(53)*. The relative risk for right-sided tumors also increases among males after the age of 70 in high-risk nations, but the ratio is usually less than 1.0 *(52,53)*.

A retrospective review of 1694 consecutive cases of colorectal cancer diagnosed at the University of Chicago Medical Center during a 25-yr period (1960–1984) demonstrated a 10.2% increase in cancers originating in the cecum or ascending colon and a 15.8% decline in rectal and rectosigmoid carcinomas during this period *(56)*.

A review of the National Cancer Registry registration data for colorectal cancer in New Zealand from 1972 to 1975 (4678 cases) showed an excess of right-sided colonic tumors in females compared with males, with males having a higher incidence of rectal cancers *(57)*. Environmental factors that may contribute to colon carcinogenesis may produce specific segmental effects within the large bowel.

In a study from western New York, total energy intake and dietary fat disproportionately increased the risk for left-sided tumors *(58)*. In contrast, other studies have demonstrated an increase in right-sided tumors in the setting of high-fat diets both for men *(59)* and women *(60)*.

An association between cholecystectomy and an increased risk of colon cancer has been suggested. Two meta-analyses found a slightly increased risk for right-sided colon cancers

(61,62). Possible explanations for this observation include changes in bile acid composition and flow and concomitant risk factors for both diseases, such as obesity *(63)*.

This increase in proximal colon cancers and change in subsite distribution within the large bowel add to the evidence for the need for full colonoscopic visualization as the optimal technique for detection of colorectal neoplasms.

4. RISK FACTORS

4.1. Diet

The large international variation in the incidence of colorectal cancer may be the result in part of genetic predisposition to colon cancer, but it may largely be related to differences in dietary habit. However, it remains difficult to interpret the impact of any one dietary constituent in isolation on the risk of colon cancer.

A thorough depiction of diet as a risk factor for colorectal cancer is beyond the scope of this chapter. An in-depth analysis of the literature with respect to the global impact of food and nutrition was recently published *(64)*.

There is convincing evidence that diets high in vegetables decrease the risk of colorectal cancer. Consumption of diets high in red meat probably increases the risk of colorectal cancer *(64)*. It is not clear that there is an association between the intake of dietary fiber and the risk of colorectal cancer *(65)*.

Dietary influences on colon cancer development are covered in detail in Chapter 3.

4.2. Family History and Genetics

Family history is an important risk factor for colorectal cancer. Epidemiological case-control studies of family history suggest that there is about a twofold to threefold risk of the development of colorectal cancer for an individual with a single first-degree relative suffering with the disease *(66–68)*. The risk becomes greater if more relatives are affected *(68)*. Rozen and colleagues studied 471 asymptomatic adults with first-degree relatives who had adenomatous polyps and/or cancer *(68)*. Those screened had a significant linear trend of increasing risk of colorectal neoplasia with increasing number of affected relatives. When considering cancer cases only, the risk was threefold if only one relative was affected, whereas the risk increased to ninefold with more than one affected relative. An increased risk was also seen in a reconstructed cohort study specifically addressing the risk of colorectal cancer among patients of colorectal adenomas, the relative risk being 1.74 (95% confidence interval [CI], 1.24–2.45) among first-degree relatives of patients with newly diagnosed adenomas compared with the risk among first-degree relatives of controls *(69)*.

A prospective cohort study of subjects from both the Nurses' Health Study and the Health Professionals Follow-up Study was analyzed specifically for whether a family history of colorectal cancer (in first-degree relatives) was an independent risk factor for colorectal cancer *(66)*. The age-adjusted relative risk of colorectal cancer for men and women with affected first-degree relatives, compared to those without a family history of the disease, was 1.72 (95% CI: 1.34–2.19). The relative risk for subjects with two or more affected first-degree relatives was 2.75 (95% CI: 1.34–5.63). The risk was greatest for patients under 45 yr with one or more affected first-degree relatives, with a relative risk of 5.37 (95% CI: 1.98–14.6).

Hereditary colon cancer syndromes will be mentioned only briefly. A more detailed discussion is provided in a later chapter.

Familial adenomatous polyposis is an autosomally dominant inherited disease, which predisposes to the development of colorectal cancer *(70)*. The colon is involved with innumerable adenomatous polyps that occur early in life. Virtually all individuals affected will develop colorectal cancer unless they undergo a prophylactic colectomy, with 75% of subjects developing colorectal cancer by the age of 35 yr. APC is the germline mutation in FAP, involving a large deletion on chromosome 5q *(31,35)*. Carcinoma associated with FAP accounts for about 1% of all colorectal cancer cases *(71)*. Colorectal cancer cases in subjects with FAP have a left-sided predominance *(72)*.

Hereditary nonpolyposis colorectal cancer (Lynch syndrome) is an autosomally dominant inherited syndrome with an increased incidence of colorectal cancer. The associated germline mutations in mismatch repair genes have been identified as *MSH2, MLH1, PMS1*, and *PMS2*. Recently, the newly identified *hMLH3* gene has also been considered as another possible mismatch repair gene *(73)*. HNPCC probably accounts for at least 5% of all colorectal cancers. It is characterized by an earlier age of cancer onset, proximal predominance of disease, the development of multiple synchronous and metachronous cancers, and an excess of certain extra-colonic tumors *(74)*.

4.3. Inflammatory Bowel Disease

Long-standing ulcerative colitis is associated with an increased risk of colorectal cancer; reported relative risks compared to the general population vary between 1 and 20 *(75–77)*. Carcinomas begin to appear 5–8 yr after the onset of ulcerative colitis, with an absolute risk of colorectal cancer of 30% after 35 yr *(78)*. Incidence rates for the development of colorectal cancer in the setting of ulcerative colitis are not the same universally, with reports of lower rates in Scandinavia and Europe *(79,80)*.

The cumulative risk of colorectal cancer appears to vary according to the extent of colitis, with a significantly higher risk seen with pancolitis rather than just left-sided disease *(22,77)*. There is a higher proportion of right-sided and transverse colon carcinomas in patients with ulcerative colitis compared to patients without colitis *(81)*. Younger age at diagnosis of ulcerative colitis may be an independent risk factor for the development of colorectal cancer *(77)*. Additional risk factors may include the presence of primary sclerosing cholangitis *(82,83)*, the severity of the colitis and frequency of attacks *(84)*, the effect of medications for the disease *(85)*, and folate deficiency and folate supplementation *(86)*. The incidence of colorectal cancer is equal for both sexes. Often, the lesions are aggressive and poorly differentiated at the time of diagnosis. APC gene mutations have also been reported to occur at a lower frequency in colorectal cancers associated with ulcerative colitis than in sporadic cancers *(87)* and may not be the initiating event for malignant transformation *(88)*.

Patients with pancolitis of more than 8 yr duration should consider periodic colonoscopic surveillance or prophylactic colectomy *(89)*. Surveillance programs to detect dysplastic lesions prior to the development of colorectal cancer may be a method of preventing prophylactic colectomy. However, colorectal cancers that develop in ulcerative colitis patients often are infiltrative and schirrous, and their flat nature may make them more difficult to be detected at the time of endoscopy *(81)*.

The evidence for an increased incidence of colorectal cancer among people afflicted with Crohn's disease is less clear *(90)*. Actuarial data suggest that the risk of developing colorectal cancer as a complication of long-standing Crohn's disease may be 4.3–20 times that in the general population *(91,92)*.

4.4. Medications

Aspirin and other NSAIDs have recently been implicated as potential protective agents against the development of colorectal cancer and adenomatous polyps. This evidence is not yet conclusive. There is evidence supporting the beneficial effect of these drugs in chemically induced colon cancer in rodent models *(93–97)* and in patients with FAP *(17,18)*. There are several possible mechanisms by which these drugs may inhibit tumor development. NSAIDs appear to induce apoptosis *(98,99)* as well as inhibit cyclooxygenase-2 *(18)*.

Two randomized clinical trials showed a decrease in the number and size of colorectal polyps in patients with FAP treated with sulindac *(17,100)*. Polyps did not fully resolve, and they recurred on cessation of therapy.

Recently celecoxib, a selective cyclooxygenase-2 inhibitor, was shown to significantly reduce the number of colorectal polyps in patients with FAP in a double-blind, placebo-controlled study *(18)*. Treatment with celecoxib consisted of 100 mg or 400 mg twice daily for 6 mo. After 6 mo, the patients receiving 400 mg twice daily celecoxib had a 28% reduction in the mean number of colorectal polyps and a 30.7% reduction in the polyp burden (the sum of polyp diameters). The reductions in the group receiving 100 mg celecoxib twice a day were not statistically significant.

The first evidence to suggest that aspirin might reduce the risk of colorectal cancer was from a retrospective exploratory analysis published in 1988 by a group from Melbourne, Australia *(101)*. A 40% lower risk of incident colon cancer was found among people who regularly used aspirin, although the frequency of use was not specified. Decreased risk was also seen for subjects using NSAIDs other than aspirin.

The Boston Collaborative Drug Study conducted an epidemiologic study specifically to test the aspirin–colon cancer hypothesis *(102)*. They identified an approximately 50% lower risk of incident colorectal cancer among people who regularly used aspirin. Regular use was defined as at least 4 d a week for at least 3 mo.

The relation of aspirin use to fatal colon cancer was assessed in Cancer Prevention Study II (CPS II), a prospective cohort study that enrolled 1,185,239 Americans between 1982 and 1988 *(16)*. Death rates from colon cancer decreased in both men and women with more frequent use of aspirin. The trend of decreasing relative risk was similar after controlling for other potential risk factors for colon cancer *(103)*. For rectal cancer, aspirin use was associated with a greater reduction in risk in men than in women. Several other epidemiologic studies and clinical trials provide additional data on the aspirin–colon cancer hypothesis *(104–108)*.

These findings are in contrast to those of the U.S. Physicians Health Study, a randomized clinical trial of aspirin (325 mg every other day) in preventing cardiovascular disease. It was also the first randomized, placebo-controlled study of whether aspirin can reduce colon cancer incidence *(109)*. Male physicians given aspirin for 5 yr had a slightly higher risk of invasive colorectal cancer (relative risk [RR] = 1.15; range; 0.80–1.65) and lower risk of *in situ* cancer or polyps (RR = 0.86; range; 0.68–1.10), although they had no systematic screening for colorectal cancer or polyps. It is not clear why this result conflicts with findings from other studies. The every-other-day dosage is somewhat unusual, and it is possible that the duration of therapy may have been insufficient to demonstrate a protective effect.

Another prospective exploratory study assessing the risk of incident colon cancer among approx 14,000 elderly American daily aspirin users reported a small increased risk *(110)*. Overall the relative risk of colon cancer was 1.5 (95% CI = 1.1–2.2).

4.5. Occupation

Among asbestos workers, colorectal cancer is the third most common malignancy after lung cancer and mesothelioma *(111)*. There is a reported increased relative risk for colon cancer in the range of 1.4–3.0 *(111–115)*. There was no evidence for synergy between asbestos exposure and smoking for colon cancer, in contrast to the definite relationship seen with lung cancer *(113)*. The increased risk of colon cancer among asbestos workers is probably secondary to exposure of the colonic mucosa to swallowed asbestos-contaminated sputum *(113)*. There is a temporal relationship, with exposure predating the development of malignancy by at least 20 yr, and evidence to support a dose-response relationship *(111)*. Identification of asbestos bodies among colon cancer cells in an asbestos worker add supportive experimental evidence to the concept that occupational asbestos exposure is a colorectal cancer risk factor *(116)*. A case-control study conducted in New York City found an elevated risk for both adenomatous polyps and colorectal cancer among subjects with a significant exposure to asbestos *(117)*.

Acrylonitrile is a gaseous monomer widely used for the synthesis of plastic and synthetic rubber and fiber polymers. Two historical cohort studies of acrylonitrile workers showed increases in both the proportional mortality ratio (PMR) *(118)* and the standardized mortality rate (SMR) *(119)*. All of the cases of colorectal cancer occurred in workers who had more than 6 mo of exposure and with a long latency period of up to 10–30 yr.

Ethylacrylate and methyl methacrylate are monomers capable of conversion into versatile transparent polymers that were widely used during World War II in the manufacture of airplanes. An historical cohort study of mortality among workers employed at a manufacturing plant between 1933 and 1946 found an increased colorectal cancer SMR, with at least a 10–yr latency period *(111)*.

Dibromochloropropane (DMCP) and related halogenated organic compounds have a causal association with rectal cancer, with an increase in PMR documented by the National Institute for Occupational Safety and Health (NIOSH) *(111)* and two other historical cohort studies *(120,121)*.

An increased SMR for colon cancer has been reported among printing workers *(122)* and an excess of rectal cancers in a study of commercial pressmen over 65 yr of age *(123)*. Statistically significant SMRs were also found for colorectal cancer among automotive workers making wooden models and patterns *(124,125)*.

Two historical cohort studies of synthetic rubber workers demonstrated an increase in mortality from colorectal cancer as well as other cancers *(126,127)*. A British study failed to confirm this association, despite demonstrating increases in lung cancer and gastric cancer *(128)*.

An historical cohort study also demonstrated statistically significant SMRs for colon and rectal cancer among paint and varnish workers employed for at least 1 yr *(129)*. Colon and rectal cancer had the highest risks of any neoplasm studied.

4.6. Smoking and Alcohol

Smoking has not been conclusively shown to be a risk factor for colorectal cancer, but it has been consistently associated with adenomatous polyps. Cigarettes have been associated with an approximately twofold increase in risk of colon adenomas or polyps *(130–137)*.

In a large case-control study based on colonoscopy results in New York, there was a statistically increased risk between heavy cigarette smoking (smokers with $\geq$ 40 pack-years of smoking) and risk of adenoma, but no increased colorectal cancer risk *(138)*. An hypothesis to explain the paradox of this finding was that the association between cigarette smoking and risk for colorectal cancer might have been masked by inclusion in the control group of subjects with adenomas. The authors also concluded that the major effect of smoking on the adenoma–carcinoma sequence occurred in the earlier stages of adenoma formation. It is likely in the causal relationship between smoking and colorectal adenomas, in contrast to cancers, that the effect of smoking on progression from an adenoma to invasive carcinoma is less evident as a result of other factors impacting on the malignant transformation *(139)*. Similar results were found in a case-control study from France *(140)*. Smoking was associated with a risk of adenomas in men, but there was no association between tobacco and cancer risk, adding support to the concept of an independent effect of tobacco in men at early steps of the adenoma–carcinoma sequence. In women, no association was observed between smoking and the risk for adenoma or cancer.

In a cohort study of 248,046 American male veterans followed prospectively over a 26-yr period, the risk of death was significantly increased for both colon and rectal cancer among current and former cigarette smokers in comparison with veterans who had never used tobacco *(141)*. The patterns of risk were less marked among pipe and cigar smokers. Risk of rectal cancer was also significantly increased among tobacco chewers or users of snuff. Risk increased significantly for both sites with number of pack-years, earlier onset of tobacco use, and total number of cigarettes smoked per day. A limitation of the study was that data were not available for other potential risk factors for colorectal cancer, in particular diet and total physical activity. In addition, mortality rather than incidence of colorectal cancer was the measure of effect, with death certificates being used to determine the type of cancer.

Five prior case-control studies using population controls had reported increased risks of colon cancer with cigarette smoking *(142–146)*, in contrast to earlier case-control and cohort studies that have not consistently shown an association between tobacco use and the incidence of colorectal cancer *(147–152)*.

The results of a large cohort study (the Physicians' Health Study I) recently reported on the association between lifetime cigarette smoking and colorectal cancer incidence *(14)*. A cohort of 22,000 healthy men aged between 40 and 84 yr were followed for more than 12 yr. Cigarette smoking was found to be an independent risk factor for the development of colorectal cancer. The strongest risk was found among current smokers of greater than or equal to 20 cigarettes a day. Cumulative lifetime exposure was also found to increase the risk of colorectal cancer.

Among smokers compared with nonsmokers, colorectal cancers appear to be diagnosed at a later stage *(153–155)* and also at an earlier age *(155)*.

Alcohol is inconsistently associated with an increased risk of colon cancer *(4)*. Similar to the findings for colon cancer, results are varied with respect to an association between alcohol consumption and risk of rectal cancer.

Cohort studies investigating the association between alcohol and colon cancer among alcoholics *(156,157)* and brewery workers *(158)* failed to show any significant increased risk. For rectal cancer, only one of seven cohort studies addressing a possible association among alcoholics or brewery workers showed a significant association—in brewery workers in Dublin, Ireland *(158)*. In contrast, cohort studies of the general population, investigating the effect of alcohol consumption on colon cancer risk showed a significant association *(159–163)*. A dose-response relationship between alcohol and rectal cancer was observed in three of these studies *(161–163)*.

Case-control studies investigating the association between alcohol and colon cancer have had mixed results, both positive *(147,164–166)* and negative *(142,149,150,167–169)*. Similar results were seen for studies specifically looking at rectal cancer, with both positive associations *(169,170)* and no association seen *(149,168)*. Beer appeared to have a stronger relationship to cancer of the rectum in men than in women *(171)*.

4.7. Obesity and Physical Activity

Diet and lifestyle factors are thought to have important roles in the carcinogenic process. Obesity as well as lack of physical activity has been associated with an increased risk of colon cancer *(172,173)*.

The correlation between obesity and colon cancer incidence may reflect the association between obesity and increased intake of energy or fat. Increased body mass has been associated with an increased mortality rate from cancer, including colon cancer *(174,175)*.

There have been conflicting results with respect to the association between obesity and colon adenomas. One case-control study found that an increased body mass index (BMI) in women was a risk factor for colonic adenomas, but the same did not apply for men *(176)*. In contrast, a German study showed no relationship between being overweight and the incidence of colorectal adenomas for either sex, but there was an increased risk of high-risk adenomas among obese men *(177)*.

In an American Cancer Society study, a cohort of 419,080 men and 336,442 women was followed to ascertain the relationship between body weight and a variety of illnesses *(178)*. Increased body weight was associated with an increased PMR from colon cancer among men. No association was found for women in this study.

In the Framingham study of 5200 men and women who were followed for 18 yr, there was no association between being overweight by 20% and an increased incidence of colorectal cancer *(179)*.

Body weight in adolescence has also been evaluated as a predictor of colon cancer development in later life. Data from the Harvard Growth Study, which recorded heights and weights of 3000 children aged between 13 and 18 yr, examined the effects of being overweight during adolescence on health 55 yr later *(180)*. There was a significant association between a high BMI during adolescence and an increased risk of colorectal cancer among men (although this was based on only six deaths), but not among women.

A similar study of Harvard University alumni relied on questionnaires completed in 1962 and 1966 that gathered information on height, weight, sociodemographic characteristics, and medical history *(181)*. Of the 17,595 subjects who were followed for more than 20 yr, the 20% who were heaviest on entering college and during the period of the questionnaires had nearly 2.5 times the risk for colon cancer when compared to the leanest 20% among the group. After adjustment for degree of physical activity, the increased risk of colon cancer in the overweight group was evident only in the setting of less physical activity.

A third study followed a cohort of 52,539 men born between 1913 and 1927 in Hawaii and linked them to the Hawaii Tumor Registry, investigating the role of obesity in early adulthood *(182)*. Between 1972 and 1986, 737 cases of colon cancer were identified, and each case was matched with an average of 3.8 control subjects. Increased body weight during early and middle age was associated with an increased risk of developing cancer of the sigmoid colon, but no increased risk of cancer for other segments of the colon.

There is evidence to support an association between physical activity and risk of colon cancer *(4,64)*. Physical activity is inversely associated with risk of colon cancer. The majority of studies evaluating this association have concentrated on occupational activity

(25,164,183,184), although there have been some studies examining leisure time and total activity *(25,173,185,186)*. These studies have demonstrated a reduced risk of colon cancer with increased physical activity.

Lee and colleagues showed that individuals who reported high levels of physical activity throughout their lives were at a lower risk of developing colorectal cancer than individuals who had only a short duration of physical activity *(173)*.

4.8. Reproductive Factors

Studies on the potential protective effect of postmenopausal estrogen replacement therapy on the incidence of colon cancer have been contradictory. A meta-analysis of observational studies published between 1974 and 1993 reported that the overall risk of colorectal cancer, in the setting of estrogen hormone replacement therapy, was 0.92 (95% CI: 0.74–1.5) *(187)*.

A multicenter population-based case-control study in the United States found that the use of hormone replacement therapy had a significant inverse relationship to the risk of colorectal carcinoma, with the effect limited to women who were recent users of therapy *(188)*.

A cohort study of over 40,000 postmenopausal women originally participating in the Breast Cancer Detection Demonstration Project (BCDDP) in the United States had a small reduction in risk of colorectal cancer for recent hormone therapy, especially if therapy had been for 5 or more years in duration *(189)*.

A clinical review assessed 35 studies, including 3 meta-analyses *(190)*. Twenty-three suggested some degree of protective effect of hormone replacement therapy, 11 reported null results, and 1 suggested a negative impact. Confounding factors were as follows: There was only one prospective randomized controlled trial with small numbers; studies did not uniformly specify hormone type, dose, duration of therapy, or provide a subset analysis of impact on right- versus left-sided tumors; estrogen and progesterone effects were usually not considered separately; and many studies did not adequately control for confounding variables, such as family history or indication for colonoscopy.

In a case-control study from New York, reproductive variables such as parity, history of spontaneous or induced abortion, infertility, type of menopause, age at menopause, use of oral contraceptives, and use of menopausal hormone replacement therapy had no statistically significant association with risk of colorectal adenomas *(191)*. A lower risk of colorectal adenomas was found for women who had menarche before age 13 yr.

Prospective studies are still needed to determine whether a protective effect from hormone replacement therapy exists, the extent of this effect, and the mechanism of the effect.

5. CONCLUSION

Colorectal cancer remains the fourth most common cancer worldwide. Colon cancer occurs almost equally for both men and women. The probability of developing invasive colorectal cancer increases with increasing age, irrespective of gender.

The highest incidence rates are found in Australasia, Western Europe, and the United States, with the lowest rates in south-central Asia and all areas of Africa except South Africa.

Time trends indicate a fall in both incidence and mortality rates for colorectal cancer in the United States at the very end of the last century. This decline was most evident among white men and women.

Migrant data suggest a 20-fold international difference in the incidence rates of colorectal cancer. Migrants from low-risk areas to high-risk areas develop the same cancer risk as that population. This observation may reflect genetic differences, but is also probably largely a result of environmental and dietary differences.

The concept of an adenoma–carcinoma sequence is widely accepted and appears to occur for both familial and sporadic forms of colorectal cancer. The idea of screening for colorectal cancer becomes important in this context. The subsite distribution of colorectal cancers tends to suggest a trend toward increased right-sided colon lesions, suggesting that full visualization of the colon with colonoscopy, rather than flexible sigmoidoscopy, is desirable *(192,193)*. Inflammatory bowel disease has also been shown to result in an increased rate of colorectal cancer, necessitating surveillance and therapeutic interventions.

Much has been written about the relationship between diet and colorectal cancer incidence rates. There appears to be an increased risk of colorectal cancer with increasing consumption of fat, protein, and meat. The inverse result can also be seen with increased consumption of fruit and vegetables. The impact of fiber intake on the incidence rate of colorectal cancer is less certain. The most recently published large cohort study suggested no positive impact on colorectal cancer incidence *(65)*. Two recent randomized trials with adenoma recurrence as the outcome have also shed doubt on the role of fiber *(194,195)*. Mixed results have been reported regarding the role of other dietary factors such as calcium and caffeine on the incidence rate of colorectal cancer. The association between smoking and alcohol consumption, and the relative risk of colorectal cancer have shown mixed results.

There is increasing evidence to suggest that chemopreventive strategies with either aspirin or NSAIDs may have a major role to play in the prevention of colorectal cancer, both in sporadic and familial cases.

The recently published reports of a decline in both the incidence and mortality rates for colorectal cancer, in conjunction with an ever-increasing genetic understanding of the disease and ongoing advances in the area of chemoprevention of the disease, render colorectal cancer an area of great ongoing epidemiological interest.

REFERENCES

1. Parkin D. Epidemiology of cancer: global patterns and trends. *Toxicol. Lett.*, **102–103** (1998) 227–234.
2. Parkin D, Pisani P, and Ferlay J. Global cancer statistics. *CA: Cancer J. Clin.*, **49** (1999) 33–64.
3. Pisani P, Parkin D, Bray F, et al. Estimates of worldwide mortality from 25 cancers in 1990. *Int. J. Cancer*, **83** (1999) 18–29.
4. Potter J, Slattery M, Bostick R, et al. Colon cancer: a review of the epidemiology. *Epidemiol. Rev.*, **15** (1993) 499–535.
5. Ries L, Wingo P, Miller D, et al. The annual report to the nation on the status of cancer, 1973–1997, with a special section on colorectal cancer. *Cancer*, **88** (2000) 2398–2424.
6. Greenlee R, Murray T, Bolden S, et al. Cancer statistics, 2000. *CA Cancer J. Clin.*, **50** (2000) 7–33.
7. Ries L, Eisner M, Kosary C, et al. *SEER Cancer Statistics Review, 1973–1997*. National Cancer Institute, Bethesda, MD, 2000.
8. Parkin D. *Cancer Incidence in Five Continents*. IARC Scientific Publications, Lyon, 1997.
9. Parkin D, Pisani P, and Ferlay J. Estimates of the worldwide incidence of 25 major cancers in 1990. *Int. J. Cancer*, **80** (1999) 827–841.
10. Correa P and Haenszel W. The epidemiology of large bowel cancer. *Adv. Cancer Res.*, **26** (1978) 1–141.
11. Sandler R. Epidemiology and risk factors for colorectal cancer. *Gastroenterol. Clin. North Am.*, **25** (1996) 717–735.
12. Crespi M and Caperle M. Trends in epidemiology of colorectal cancer. *J. Surg. Oncol.*, **2(Suppl.)** (1991) 1–3.
13. Wilmink A. Overview of the epidemiology of colorectal cancer. *Dis. Colon Rectum*, **40** (1997) 483–493.
14. Sturmer T, Glynn R, Lee I-M, et al. Lifetime cigarette smoking and colorectal cancer incidence in the Physicians' Health Study I. *J. Natl. Cancer Inst.*, **92** (2000) 1178–1181.
15. Colditz G, Cannuscio C, and Frazier A. Physical activity and reduced risk of colon cancer: implications for prevention. *Cancer Causes Control*, **8** (1997) 649–667.

16. Thun M, Namboodiri M, and Heath C. Aspirin use and reduced risk of fatal colon cancer. *N. Engl. J. Med.*, **325** (1991) 1593–1596.

17. Giardello F, Hamilton S, Krush A, et al. Treatment of colonic and rectal adenomas with sulindac in familial adenomatous polyposis. *N. Engl. J. Med.*, **328** (1993) 1313–1316.

18. Steinbach G, Lynch P, Phillips K, et al. The effect of celecoxib, a cyclooxygenase-2 inhibitor, in familial adenomatous polyposis. *N. Engl. J. Med.*, **342** (2000) 1946–1952.

19. SEER. *SEER Cancer Statistics Review, 1972–1996.* National Cancer Institute, Bethesda, MD, 1997.

20. Kune S, Kune G, and Watson L. The Melbourne Colorectal Cancer Study: incidence findings by age, sex, site, migrants and religion. *Int. J. Epidemiol.*, **15** (1986) 483–493.

21. Walker A and Segal I. Puzzles in the epidemiology of colon cancer. *J. Clin. Gastroenterol.*, **11** (1989) 10–11.

22. Levin K and Dozois R. Epidemiology of large bowel cancer. *World J. Surg.*, **15** (1991) 562–567.

23. Shimizu M, Mack T, Ross R, et al. Cancer of the gastrointestinal tract among Japanese and white immigrants in Los Angeles County. *J. Natl. Cancer Inst.*, **78** (1987) 223–228.

24. Flood D, Weiss N, Cook L, et al. Colorectal cancer incidence in Asian migrants in the United States and their descendants. *Cancer Causes Control*, **11** (2000) 403–411.

25. Whittemore A, Wu-Williams A, Lee M, et al. Diet, physical activity, and colorectal cancer among Chinese in North America and China. *J. Natl. Cancer Inst.*, **82** (1990) 915–926.

26. Hill M, Morson B, and Bussey H. Aetiology of adenoma–carcinoma sequence in large bowel. *Lancet*, **1** (1978) 245–247.

27. Vogelstein B, Fearon E, Hamilton S, et al. Genetic alterations during colorectal-tumor development. *N. Engl. J. Med.*, **319** (1988) 525–532.

28. Fearon E, Cho K, Nigro J, et al. Identification of a chromosome 18q gene that is altered in colorectal cancers. *Science*, **247** (1990) 49–56.

29. Fearon E and Vogelstein B. A genetic model for colorectal tumorigenesis. *Cell*, **61** (1990) 759–767.

30. Ohue M, Tomita N, Monden T, et al. A frequent alteration of p53 gene in carcinoma in adenoma of colon. *Cancer Res.*, **54** (1994) 4798–4804.

31. Bodmer W, Bailey C, Bodmer J, et al. Localization of the gene for familial adenomatous polyposis on chromosome 5. *Nature*, **328** (1987) 614–616.

32. Kim E and Lance P. Colorectal polyps and their relationship to cancer. *Gastroenterol. Clin. North Am.*, **26** (1997) 1–17.

33. Powell S, Zilz N, Beazer-Barclay Y, et al. APC mutations occur early during colorectal tumorigenesis. *Nature*, **359** (1992) 235–237.

34. Boland C, Sato J, Appelman H, et al. Microallelotyping defines the sequence and tempo of allelic losses at tumour suppressor gene loci during colorectal cancer progression. *Nature Med.*, **1** (1995) 902–909.

35. Miyaki M, Konishi M, Kikuchi-Yanoshita R, et al. Characteristics of somatic mutation of the adenomatous polyposis coli gene in colorectal tumors. *Cancer Res.*, **54** (1994) 3011–3020.

36. Baeg G, Matsumine A, Kuroda T, et al. The tumor suppressor gene product APC blocks cell cycle progression from G0/G1 to S phase. *EMBO J.*, **14** (1995) 5618–5625.

37. Browne S, Williams A, Hague A, et al. Loss of APC protein expressed by human colonic epithelial cells and the appearance of a specific low-molecular-weight form is associated with apoptosis in vitro. *Int. J. Cancer*, **59** (1994) 56–64.

38. Burchill S. The tumour suppressor APC product is associated with cell adhesion. *Bioassays*, **16** (1994) 225–227.

39. Smith A, Stern H, Penner M, et al. Somatic APC and K-ras codon 12 mutations in aberrant crypt foci from human colons. *Cancer Res.*, **54** (1994) 5527–5530.

40. Minamoto T, Yamashita N, Ochiai A, et al. Mutant K-ras in apparently normal mucosa of colorectal cancer patients. Its potential as a biomarker of colorectal tumorigenesis. *Cancer*, **75** (1995) 1520–1526.

41. Pretlow T. Aberrant crypt foci and K-ras mutations: earliest recognised players or innocent bystanders in colon carcinogenesis? *Gastroenterology*, **108** (1995) 600–603.

42. Jen J, Kim H, Piantadosi S, et al. Allelic loss of chromosome 18q and prognosis in colorectal cancer. *N. Engl. J. Med.*, **331** (1994) 213–221.

43. Cunningham J, Lust J, Schaid D, et al. Expression of p53 and allelic loss in colorectal carcinoma. *Cancer Res.*, **52** (1992) 1974–1980.

44. Lane D. Cancer, p53, guardian of the genome. *Nature*, **358** (1992) 15–16.

45. Donehower L and Bradley A. The tumor suppressor p53. *Biochem. Biophys. Acta*, **1155** (1993) 181–205.

46. Tomlinson I, Ilyas M, and Novelli M. Molecular genetics of colon cancer. *Cancer Metastasis Rev.*, **16** (1997) 62–79.

47. Liu B, Nicolaides N, Markowitz S, et al. Mismatch repair gene defects in sporadic colorectal cancers with microsatellite instability. *Nat. Genet.*, **9** (1995) 48–55.

48. Liu B, Parsons R, Papadopoulos N, et al. Analysis of mismatch repair genes in hereditary non-polyposis colorectal cancer patients. *Nature Med.*, **2** (1996) 148–156.

49. Young J, Leggett B, Gustafson C, et al. Genomic instability occurs in colorectal carcinomas but not in adenomas. *Hum. Mutat.*, **2** (1993) 351–354.

50. Jacoby R, Marshall D, Kailas S, et al. Genetic instability associated with adenoma to carcinoma progression in hereditary nonpolyposis colon cancer. *Gastroenterology*, **109** (1995) 73–82.

51. Herman J, Merlo A, Mao L, et al. Inactivation of the CDKN2/p16/MTS1 gene is frequently associated with aberrant DNA methylation in all common human cancers. *Cancer Res.*, **55** (1995) 4525–4530.

52. Devesa S and Chow W-H. Variation in colorectal cancer incidence in the United States by subsite of origin. *Cancer*, **71** (1993) 3819–3826.

53. Adami H. Aspects of descriptive epidemiology and survival in colorectal cancer. *Scand. J. Gastroenterol.*, **23** (1988) 6–20.

54. Nelson R, Persky V, and Turyk M. Time trends in distal colorectal cancer subsite location related to age and how it affects choice of screening modality. *J. Surg. Oncol.*, **69** (1998) 235–238.

55. Cooper G, Yuan Z, Landefeld C, et al. A national population-based study of incidence of colorectal cancer and age. Implications of screening in older Americans. *Cancer*, **75** (1995) 775–781.

56. Ghahremani G and Dowlatshahi K. Colorectal carcinomas: diagnostic implications of their changing frequency and anatomic distribution. *World J. Surg.*, **13** (1989) 321–325.

57. Stewart R, Stewart A, Turnbull P, et al. Sex differences in subsite incidence of large-bowel cancer. *Dis. Colon Rectum*, **26** (1983) 658–660.

58. Graham S, Marshall J, Haughey B, et al. Dietary epidemiology of cancer of the colon in western New York. *Am. J. Epidemiol.*, **128** (1988) 409–503.

59. West D, Slattery M, Robison L, et al. Dietary intake and colon cancer. Sex and anatomic site-specific associations. *Am. J. Epidemiol.*, **130** (1989) 883–894.

60. McMichael A and Potter J. Diet and colon cancer. Integration of the descriptive, analytic and metabolic epidemiology. *J. Natl. Cancer Inst.*, **69** (1985) 223–228.

61. Giovannucci E, Colditz G, and Stampfer M. Cholecystectomy and the risk for colorectal cancer: a meta-analysis. *Gastroenterology*, **105** (1993) 130–141.

62. Talley N. Cholecystectomy and the risk of colorectal cancer. *Ann. Intern. Med.*, **120** (1994) 24–25.

63. Neugut AI, Murray T, Garbowski GC, et al. Cholecystectomy as a risk factor for colorectal adenomatous polyps and cancer. *Cancer*, **68** (1991) 1644–1647.

64. Cancers, nutrition and food. Colon, rectum. In *Food, Nutrition and the Prevention of Cancer: A Global Perspective*. Potter J (ed.), American Institute for Cancer Research, Washington, DC, 1997, pp. 216–251.

65. Fuchs C, Giovannucci E, Colditz G, et al. Dietary fiber and the risk of colorectal cancer and adenoma in women. *N. Engl. J. Med.*, **340** (1999) 169–176.

66. Fuchs C, Giovannucci E, Colditz G, et al. A prospective study of family history and the risk of colorectal cancer. *N. Engl. J. Med.*, **331** (1994) 1669–1674.

67. Petersen G. Genetic epidemiology of colorectal cancer. *Eur. J. Cancer*, **31A** (1995) 1047–1050.

68. Rozen P, Fireman Z, Figer A, et al. Family history of colorectal cancer as a marker of potential malignancy within a screening program. *Cancer*, **60** (1987) 248–254.

69. Ahsan H, Neugut AI, Garbowski GC, et al. Family history of colorectal adenomatous polyps and increased risk for colorectal cancer. *Ann. Intern. Med.*, **128** (1998) 900–905.

70. Lal G and Gallinger S. Familial adenomatous polyposis. *Semin. Surg. Oncol.*, **18** (2000) 314–323.

71. Mecklin J. Frequency of hereditary colorectal carcinoma. *Gastroenterology*, **93** (1987) 1021–1025.

72. Bulfill J. Evidence for distinct genetic categories based on proximal distal tumor location. *Ann. Intern. Med.*, **113** (1990) 779–788.

73. Jiricny J and Nystrom-Lahti M. Mismatch repair defects in cancer. *Curr. Opin. Genet. Dev.*, **10** (2000) 157–161.

74. Lynch H, Smyrk T, and Lynch J. An update of HNPCC (Lynch syndrome). *Cancer Genet. Cytogenet.*, **93** (1997) 84–99.

75. Langholz E, Munkholm P, and Binder V. Colorectal cancer risk and mortality in patients with ulcerative colitis. *Gastroenterology*, **103** (1992) 1444–1451.

76. Gilat T, Fireman Z, Grossman A, et al. Colorectal cancer in patients with ulcerative colitis. A population study in central Israel. *Gastroenterology*, **94** (1988) 870–877.

77. Ekbom A, Helmick C, Zack M, et al. Ulcerative colitis and colorectal cancer: a population-based study. *N. Engl. J. Med.*, **323** (1990) 1228–1233.

78. Bernstein C, Shanahan F, and Weinstein W. Are we telling the truth about surveillance colonoscopy in ulcerative colitis? *Lancet*, **343** (1994) 71–74.
79. Hordijk M and Shivonanda S. Risk of cancer in inflammatory bowel disease: why are the results in the reviewed literature so varied? *Scand. J. Gastroenterol.*, **170** (1989) 70–74, 81–82.
80. Isbell G and Levin B. Ulcerative colitis and colon cancer. *Gastroenterol. Clin. North Am.*, **17** (1988) 733–791.
81. Ohman U. Colorectal carcinoma in patients with ulcerative colitis. *Am. J. Surg.*, **144** (1982) 344–349.
82. Choi P, Nugent F, and Rossi R. Relationship between colorectal neoplasia and primary sclerosing cholangitis in ulcerative colitis. *Gastroenterology*, **103** (1992) 1707–1709.
83. D'Haens G, Lashner B, and Hanauer S. Pericholangitis and sclerosing cholangitis are risk factors for dysplasia and cancer in ulcerative colitis. *Am. J. Gastroenterol.*, **88** (1993) 1174–1178.
84. Katzka I, Brody R, Morris E, et al. Assessment of colorectal risk in patients with ulcerative colitis: experience from a private practice. *Gastroenterology*, **85** (1983) 22–29.
85. Connell W, Kamm M, Dickson M, et al. Long-term neoplasia risk after azathioprine treatment in inflammatory bowel disease. *Lancet*, **343** (1994) 1249–1252.
86. Lashner B, Provencher K, Seidner D, et al. The effect of folic acid supplementation on the risk of cancer or dysplasia in ulcerative colitis. *Gastroenterology*, **107** (1997) 117–120.
87. Tarmin L, Yin J, Harpaz N, et al. Adenomatous polyposis gene mutations in ulcerative colitis-associated dysplasia and cancers versus sporadic colon neoplasms. *Cancer Res.*, **55** (1995) 2035–2038.
88. Brentnall T, Crispin D, Rabinovitch P, et al. Mutations in the p53 gene: an early marker of neoplastic progression in ulcerative colitis. *Gastroenterology*, **107** (1994) 369–378.
89. Snapper S, Syngal S, and Friedman L. Ulcerative colitis and colon cancer: more controversy than clarity. *Dig. Dis.*, **16** (1998) 81–87.
90. Persson P, Karlen P, Bernell O, et al. Crohn's disease and cancer: a population-based cohort study. *Gastroenterology*, **107** (1994) 1675–1679.
91. Hamilton S. Colorectal carcinoma in patients with Crohn's disease. *Gastroenterology*, **89** (1985) 398–407.
92. Ekbom A, Helmick C, Zack M, et al. Increased risk of large bowel cancer in Crohn's disease with colonic involvement. *Lancet*, **336** (1990) 357–359.
93. Pollard M and Luckert P. Treatment of chemically-induced intestinal cancers with indomethacin. *Proc. Soc. Exp. Biol. Med.*, **167** (1981) 161–164.
94. Reddy B, Maruyama H, and Kelloff G. Dose-related inhibition of colon carcinogenesis by dietary piroxicam, a nonsteroidal anti-inflammatory drug, during different stages of rat colon tumor development. *Cancer Res.*, **47** (1987) 5340–5346.
95. Rubio C, Wallin B, Ware J, et al. Effect of indomethacin in autotransplanted colonic tumors. *Dis. Colon Rectum*, **32** (1989) 488–489.
96. Skinner S, Penney A, and O'Brian P. Sulindac inhibits the rate of growth and appearance of colon tumors in the rat. *Arch. Surg.*, **126** (1991) 1094–1096.
97. Craven P and Derubertis F. Effects of aspirin on 1,-dimethylhydrazine-induced colonic carcinogenesis. *Carcinogenesis*, **13** (1992) 541–546.
98. Barnes C, Cameron I, Hardman W, et al. Non-steroidal anti-inflammatory drug effect on crypt cell proliferation and apoptosis during initiation of rat colon carcinogenesis. *Br. J. Cancer*, **77** (1998) 573–580.
99. Gupta R and DuBois R. Aspirin, NSAIDs, and colon cancer prevention: mechanisms [editorial]. *Gastroenterology*, **114** (1998) 1095–1098.
100. Labayle D, Fischer D, Vielh P, et al. Sulindac causes regression of rectal polyps in familial adenomatous polyposis. *Gastroenterology*, **101** (1991) 635–639.
101. Kune G, Kune S, and Watson L. Colorectal cancer risk, chronic illnesses, operations, and medications: case control results from the Melbourne Colorectal Cancer Study. *Cancer Res.*, **48** (1988) 4399–4404.
102. Rosenberg L, Palmer J, Zauber A, et al. A hypothesis: nonsteroidal anti-inflammatory drugs reduce the incidence of large-bowel cancer. *J. Natl. Cancer Inst.*, **83** (1991) 355–358.
103. Thun M, Namboodiri M, Calle E, et al. Aspirin use and risk of fatal cancer. *Cancer Res.*, **53** (1993) 1322–1327.
104. Logan R, Little J, Hawkin P, et al. Effect of aspirin and non-steroidal anti-inflammatory drugs on colorectal adenomas: case-control study of subjects participating in the Nottingham faecal occult blood screening programme. *Br. Med. J.*, **307** (1993) 285–289.
105. Peleg I, Maibach H, Brown S, et al. Aspirin and nonsteroidal anti-inflammatory drug use and the risk of subsequent colorectal cancer. *Arch. Intern. Med.*, **154** (1994) 394–399.
106. Suh O, Mettlin C, and Petrelli N. Aspirin use, cancer, and polyps of the large bowel. *Cancer*, **72** (1993) 1171–1177.

107. Greenberg E, Baron J, Freeman D, et al. Reduced risk of large-bowel adenomas among aspirin users. *J. Natl. Cancer Inst.*, **85** (1993) 912–916.

108. Schreinemachers D and Everson R. Aspirin use and lung, colon, and breast cancer incidence in a prospective study. *Epidemiology*, **5** (1994) 138–146.

109. Gann P, Manson J, Glynn J, et al. Low-dose aspirin and incidence of colorectal cancers in a randomized trial. *J. Natl. Cancer Inst.*, **85** (1993) 1220–1224.

110. Paganini-Hill A, Chao A, Ross R, et al. Aspirin use and chronic disease: a cohort study of the elderly. *Br. Med. J.*, **229** (1989) 1247–1250.

111. Lashner B and Epstein S. Industrial risk factors for colorectal cancer. *Int. J. Health Serv.*, **20** (1990) 459–483.

112. Neugut AI and Wylie P. Occupational cancers of the gastrointestinal tract, Part I: colon, stomach, and esophagus. *Occup. Med. State-of-the-Art-Rev.*, **2** (1987) 109–135.

113. Levine D. Does asbestos exposure cause gastrointestinal cancer? *Dig. Dis. Sci.*, **30** (1985) 1189–1198.

114. Morgan R, Foliart D, and Wong O. Asbestos and gastrointestinal cancer. *West. J. Med.*, **143** (1985) 60–65.

115. Miller A. Asbestos fiber dust and gastrointestinal malignancies. Review of literature with regard to a cause/effect relationship. *J. Chronic Dis.*, **31** (1978) 23–33.

116. Ehrlich A, Rohl A, and Holstein E. Asbestos bodies and carcinoma of colon in an insulation worker with asbestos. *JAMA*, **254** (1985) 2932–2933.

117. Neugut AI, Murray TI, Garbowski GC, et al. Association of asbestos exposure with colorectal adenomatous polyps and cancer. *J. Natl. Cancer Inst.*, **83** (1991) 1827–1828.

118. O'Berg M. Epidemiological study of workers exposed to acrylonitrile. *J. Occup. Med.*, **22** (1980) 245–252.

119. Werner J and Carter J. Mortality of United Kingdom acrylonitrile polymerization workers. *Br. J. Ind. Med.*, **38** (1981) 247–253.

120. Wong O, Brocker W, Davis H, et al. Mortality of workers potentially exposed to organic and inorganic brominated chemicals, DBCP, TRIS, PBB, and DDT. *Br. J. Ind. Med.*, **41** (1984) 15–24.

121. Ditraglia D, Brown D, Namekata T, et al. Mortality study of workers employed at organochlorine pesticide manufacturing plants. *Scand. J. Work Environ. Health,* **7** (1981) 140–146.

122. Greene M, Hoover R, Eck R, et al. Cancer mortality among printing plant workers. *Environ. Res.*, **20** (1979) 66–73.

123. Lloyd J, Decouffle P, and Salvin L. Unusual mortality experience of printing pressmen. *J. Occup. Med.*, **19** (1977) 543–550.

124. Swanson G and Belle S. Cancer morbidity among woodworkers in the U.S. automotive industry. *J. Occup. Med.*, **24** (1982) 315–319.

125. Swanson G, Belle S, and Burrows R. Colon cancer incidence among model makers and patternmakers in the automotive manufacturing industry. *J. Occup. Med.*, **27** (1985) 567–569.

126. Delzell E and Monson R. Mortality among rubber workers: processing workers. *J. Occup. Med.*, **24** (1982) 539–545.

127. McMichael A, Spirtas M, and Kupper L. An epidemiologic study of mortality within a cohort of rubber workers: 1964–1972. *J. Occup. Med.*, **16** (1974) 458–464.

128. Parkes H, Veys C, Waterhouse J, et al. Cancer mortality in the British rubber industry. *Br. J. Ind. Med.*, **39** (1982) 209–220.

129. Morgan R, Kaplan S, and Gaffey W. A general mortality study of workers in the painting and coating manufacturing industry. *J. Occup. Med.*, **23** (1981) 13–21.

130. Lee WC, Neugut AI, Garbowski GC, et al. Cigarettes, alcohol, coffee, and caffeine as risk factors for colorectal adenomatous polyps. *Ann. Epidemiol.*, **3** (1993) 239–244.

131. Hoff G, Vatn M, and Larsen S. Relationship between tobacco smoking and colorectal polyps. *Scand. J. Gastroenterol.*, **22** (1987) 13–16.

132. Kikendall J, Bowen P, Burgess M, et al. Cigarettes and alcohol as independent risk factors for colonic adenomas. *Gastroenterology*, **97** (1989) 660–664.

133. Zahm S, Cocco P, and Blair A. Tobacco smoking as a risk factor for colon polyps. *Am. J. Public Health*, **81** (1991) 846–849.

134. Monnet E, Allemand H, Farina H, et al. Cigarette smoking and the risk of colorectal adenoma in men. *Scand. J. Gastroenterol.*, **26** (1991) 758–762.

135. Kune G, Kune S, Watson L, et al. Smoking and colorectal adenomatous polyps [letter]. *Gastroenterology*, **103** (1992) 1370–1371.

136. Honjo S, Kono S, Shinchi K, et al. Cigarette smoking, alcohol use and adenomatous polyps of the sigmoid colon. *Jpn. J. Cancer Res.*, **83** (1992) 806–811.

137. Giovannucci E and Martinez M. Tobacco, colorectal cancer, and adenomas: a review of the evidence. *J. Natl. Cancer Inst.*, **88** (1996) 1717–1730.

138. Terry MB and Neugut AI. Cigarette smoking and the colorectal-adenoma sequence: a hypothesis to explain the paradox. *Am. J. Epidemiol.*, **147** (1998) 903–910.

139. Terry MB, Neugut AI, Schwartz S, et al. Risk factors for a causal intermediate and an endpoint: reconciling differences. *Am. J. Epidemiol.*, **151** (2000) 339–345.

140. Boutron M, Faivre J, Dop M, et al. Tobacco, alcohol, and colorectal tumors: a multistep process. *Am. J. Epidemiol.*, **141** (1995) 1038–1046.

141. Heineman E, Zahm S, McLaughlin J, et al. Increased risk of colorectal cancer among smokers: results of a 26-year follow-up of US veterans and a review. *Int. J. Cancer*, **59** (1995) 728–738.

142. Slattery M, West D, Robison L, et al. Tobacco, alcohol, coffee, and caffeine as risk factors for colon cancer in a low-risk population. *Epidemiology*, **1** (1990) 141–145.

143. Martinez I, Torres R, Frias Z, et al. Factors associated with adenocarcinomas of the large bowel in Puerto Rico. In *Advances in Medical Oncology, Research, and Education*. Pergamon, Oxford, 1978, pp. 45–52.

144. Vobecky J, Caro J, and Devroede G. A case-control study of risk factors for large-bowel carcinoma. *Cancer*, **51** (1983) 1958–1963.

145. Jarebinski M, Adanja B, and Vlajinac H. Case-control study of relationship of some biosocial correlates to rectal cancer patients in Belgrade, Yugoslavia. *Neoplasma*, **36** (1989) 369–374.

146. Kune G, Kune S, Vitetta L, et al. Smoking and colorectal cancer risk: data from the Melbourne Colorectal Cancer Study and brief review of the literature. *Int. J. Cancer*, **50** (1992) 369–372.

147. Williams R and Horm J. Association of cancer sites with tobacco and alcohol consumption and socioeconomic status of patients: interview study from the Third National Cancer Survey. *J. Natl. Cancer Inst.*, **58** (1977) 525–547.

148. Haenszel W, Locke F, and Segi M. A case-control study of large-bowel cancer in Japan. *J. Natl. Cancer Inst.*, **64** (1980) 17–22.

149. Ferraroni M, Negri E, La Vecchia C, et al. Socioeconomic indicators, tobacco, and alcohol in the aetiology of digestive tract neoplasms. *Int. J. Epidemiol.*, **18** (1989) 556–562.

150. Choi S and Kahyo H. Effect of cigarette smoking and alcohol consumption in the etiology of cancer of the digestive tract. *Int. J. Cancer*, **49** (1991) 382–386.

151. Chute C, Willett W, Colditz G, et al. A prospective study of body mass, height, and smoking on the risk of colorectal cancer in women. *Cancer Causes Control*, **2** (1991) 117–124.

152. Tverdal A, Thelle D, Stensvold I, et al. Mortality in relation to smoking history: 13 years' follow-up of 68,000 Norwegian men and women 35–49 years. *J. Clin. Epidemiol.*, **46** (1993) 475–487.

153. Daniell H. More advanced colonic cancer among smokers. *Cancer*, **58** (1986) 784–787.

154. Longnecker M, Clapp R, and Sheahan K. Associations between smoking status and stage of colorectal cancer at diagnosis in Massachusetts between 1982 and 1987. *Cancer*, **64** (1989) 1372–1374.

155. Anton-Culver H. Smoking and other risk factors associated with the stage and age of diagnosis of colon and rectum cancers. *Cancer Detect. Prev.*, **15** (1991) 345–350.

156. Robinette C, Hrubec Z, and Fraumeni JF Jr. Chronic alcoholism and subsequent mortality in World War II veterans. *Am. J. Epidemiol.*, **109** (1979) 687–700.

157. Schmidt W and Popham R. The role of drinking and smoking in mortality from cancer and other causes in male alcoholics. *Cancer*, **47** (1981) 1031–1041.

158. Dean G, MacLennan R, McLoughlin H, et al. Causes of death of blue-collar workers at a Dublin brewery. *Br. J. Cancer*, **40** (1979) 581–590.

159. Giovannucci E, Rimm E, Ascherio A, et al. Alcohol, low-methionine–low-folate diets and the risk of colon cancer in men. *J. Natl. Cancer Inst.*, **87** (1995) 265–273.

160. Gordon T and Kannel W. Drinking and mortality: the Framingham study. *Am. J. Epidemiol.*, **120** (1984) 97–107.

161. Klatsky A, Armstrong M, Friedman G, et al. The relations of alcoholic beverage use to colon and rectal cancer. *Am. J. Epidemiol.*, **128** (1988) 1007–1015.

162. Hirayama T. Association between alcohol consumption and cancer of the sigmoid colon: observations from a Japanese cohort study. *Lancet*, **334** (1989) 725–727.

163. Stemmermann G, Nomura A, Chyou P, et al. Prospective study of alcohol intake and large bowel cancer. *Dig. Dis. Sci.*, **35** (1990) 1414–1420.

164. Peters R, Pike M, Garabrant D, et al. Diet and colon cancer in Los Angeles County, California. *Cancer Causes Control*, **3** (1992) 457–473.

165. Potter J and McMichael A. Diet and cancer of the colon and rectum: a case-control study. *J. Natl. Cancer Inst.*, **76** (1986) 557–569.

166. Tuyns A, Kaaks R, and Haelterman M. Colorectal cancer and the consumption of foods: a case-control study in Belgium. *Nutr. Cancer*, **11** (1988) 189–204.

167. Miller A, Howe G, Jain M, et al. Food items and food groups as risk factors in a case-control study of diet and colorectal cancer. *Int. J. Cancer*, **32** (1983) 155–161.

168. Tuyns A, Pequignot G, Gignoux M, et al. Cancers of the digestive tract, alcohol and tobacco. *Int. J. Cancer*, **30** (1982) 9–11.

169. Kune S, Kune G, and Watson L. Case-control study of alcoholic beverages as etiologic factors: the Melbourne Colorectal Cancer Study Group. *Nutr. Cancer*, **9** (1987) 43–56.

170. Freudenheim J, Graham S, Marshall J, et al. A case-control study of diet and rectal cancer in western New York. *Am. J. Epidemiol.*, **131** (1990) 612–624.

171. Potter J. Nutrition and colorectal cancer. *Cancer Causes Control*, **7** (1995) 127–146.

172. Kohl H, LaPorte R, and Blaire S. Physical activity and cancer. An epidemiological perspective. *Sports Med.*, **6** (1988) 222–237.

173. Lee I-M, Paffenbarger RJ, and Hsieh C. Physical activity and risk of developing colorectal cancer among college alumni. *J. Natl. Cancer Inst.*, **83** (1991) 1324–1329.

174. Mann G. The influence of obesity on health. *N. Engl. J. Med.*, **291** (1974) 178–232.

175. Simonopoulos A and Van Itallie T. Body weight, health and longevity. *Ann. Intern. Med.*, **100** (1984) 285–295.

176. Neugut AI, Lee WC, Garbowski GC, et al. Obesity and colorectal adenomatous polyps. *J. Natl. Cancer Inst.*, **83** (1991) 359–361.

177. Bayerdorffer E, Mannes G, Ochsenkuhn T, et al. Increased risk of "high-risk" colorectal adenomas in overweight men. *Gastroenterology*, **104** (1993) 137–144.

178. Lee E and Garfinkel L. Variations in mortality by weight among 750,000 men and women. *J. Chronic Dis.*, **32** (1979) 563–576.

179. Williams S, Sorlie P, Feinlieb M, et al. Cancer incidence by levels of cholesterol. *JAMA*, **245** (1981) 247–252.

180. Must A, Jacques P, Dallard G, et al. Long-term morbidity and mortality of overweight adolescents. A follow-up of the Harvard Growth Study of 1922 to 1935. *N. Engl. J. Med.*, **327** (1992) 1350–1355.

181. Lee I-M and Paffenbarger RJ. Quetelet's index and risk of colon cancer in college alumni. *J. Natl. Cancer Inst.*, **84** (1992) 1326–1331.

182. Le Marchand L, Wilkens L, and Ming-Pi M. Obesity in youth and middle age and risk of colorectal cancer in men. *Cancer Causes Control*, **3** (1992) 349–354.

183. Slattery M, Abd-Elghany N, Kerber R, et al. Physical activity and colon cancer: a comparison of various indicators of physical activity to evaluate the association. *Epidemiology*, **1** (1990) 481–485.

184. Gerhardsson de Verdier M, Broderus B, and Norell S. Physical activity and colon cancer risk. *Int. J. Epidemiol.*, **17** (1988) 743–746.

185. Slattery M, Schumacher M, Smith K, et al. Physical activity, diet and risk of colon cancer in Utah. *Am. J. Epidemiol.*, **128** (1988) 989–999.

186. Gerhardsson de Verdier M, Hagman U, Steineck G, et al. Diet, body mass and colorectal cancer: a case-referent study. *Int. J. Cancer*, **46** (1990) 832–838.

187. MacLennan S, MacLennan A, and Ryan P. Colorectal cancer and oestrogen replacement therapy: a meta-analysis of epidemiological studies. *Med. J. Aust.*, **162** (1995) 491–493.

188. Kampman E, Potter J, Slattery M, et al. Hormone replacement therapy, reproductive history, and colon cancer: a multi-center case-control study in the United States. *Cancer Causes Control*, **8** (1997) 146–158.

189. Troisi R, Schairer C, Chow W-H, et al. A prospective study of menopausal hormones and risk of colorectal cancer in the United States. *Cancer Causes Control*, **8** (1997) 130–138.

190. Crandall C. Estrogen replacement and colon cancer: a clinical review. *J. Women's Health Gender-Based Med.*, **8** (1999) 1155–1166.

191. Jacobson JS, Neugut AI, Garbowski GC, et al. Reproductive risk factors for colorectal adenomatous polyps (New York City, NY, United States). *Cancer Causes Control*, **6** (1995) 513–518.

192. Neugut AI and Forde KA. Screening colonoscopy: has the time come? *Am. J. Gastroenterol.*, **83** (1988) 295–297.

193. Lieberman D, Weiss D, Bond J, et al. Use of colonoscopy to screen asymptomatic adults for colorectal cancer. Veteran's Affairs Cooperative Study Group 380. *N. Engl. J. Med.*, **343** (2000) 162–168.

194. Schatzkin A, Lanza E, Corle D, et al. Lack of effect of a low-fat, high-fiber diet on the recurrence of colorectal adenomas. Polyp Prevention Trial Study Group. *N. Engl. J. Med.*, **342** (2000) 1149–1155.

195. Alberts D, Martinez M, Roe D, et al. Lack of effect of a high-fiber cereal supplement on the recurrence of colorectal adenomas. Phoenix Colon Cancer Prevention Physicians' Network. *N. Engl. J. Med.*, **342** (2000) 1156–1162.

3

Dietary and Lifestyle Influences on Colorectal Carcinogenesis

Charles S. Fuchs

The field of nutritional epidemiology has offered considerable insight into our understanding of human disease. In previous centuries, deficiency states of essential nutrients, such as scurvy and rickets, were the primary interest of nutritional research. In contrast, contemporary nutritional epidemiology has principally focused on the major diseases of Western civilization, particularly heart disease and cancer. Unlike nutritional deficiencies, these diseases almost always have multiple causes, including not only diet but also genetic, occupational, and environmental influences. Nonetheless, advances in methodology have allowed for the study of chronic diseases, such as colorectal cancer, which have relatively long latency periods as well as multiple causes.

Doll and Peto suggested that up to 90% of US deaths from cancer of the large bowel might be avoidable through alterations in diet (1). In the past four decades, remarkable progress has been made in identifying factors that either enhance or reduce the risk of colorectal cancer. In this chapter, we summarize the available descriptive and analytic data supporting a role for diet and other lifestyle factors in the etiology of colorectal cancer and its precursor lesion, adenomatous polyps.

From: *Colorectal Cancer: Multimodality Management*
Edited by: L. Saltz © Humana Press Inc., Totowa, NJ

1. EPIDEMIOLOGICAL APPROACHES
TO DIET AND COLORECTAL CANCER

Our understanding of the relation between diet and colorectal cancer is derived from many sources (Table 1). Experiments in laboratory animals have assessed the extent to which various dietary factors and nutrients modulate chemically induced colorectal tumors. Although such studies may generate new hypotheses, animal experiments cannot necessarily be extrapolated directly to human carcinogenesis.

In humans, ecological or correlation studies have compared colon cancer rates in various populations with the population per capita consumption of specific dietary factors. Many of the correlations based on such information are remarkably strong. For example, the correlation between meat intake and the incidence of colon cancer is 0.85 for men and 0.89 for women (2). Unfortunately, many potential determinants of disease other than the dietary factor under consideration may vary between areas with high and low incidences of colorectal cancer. For example, similar relations between colon cancer incidence and population ownership of motor vehicles (3) as well as the Gross National Product (2) suggest that affluence may be as good as the dietary variables in predicting international variation.

Migration and time-trend studies have been particularly useful in addressing the possibility that correlations observed in the ecological studies are due to environmental rather than genetic factors. Numerous studies indicate that populations migrating from low to high incidence areas achieve the incidence rate of the host country within one or two generations, even within the migrating generation (4–6). In addition, with the introduction of Western diet and lifestyle into Japanese populations, the mortality from colorectal cancer has increased 44% in men and 40% in women (7). Such secular trends clearly demonstrate that environmental factors, possibly including diet, are important causes of colorectal cancer even though genetic factors may influence who becomes affected, given an adverse environment.

The largest body of epidemiological data relating dietary factors to risk of colon cancer is based primarily on case-control studies, in which the recalled past diet of individuals diagnosed with colon cancer is compared with the recalled diet of a control group without a diagnosis of colon cancer. Such studies may be limited by the potential for differential recall of past diet between cases and controls. Moreover, the selection of an appropriate control group for a study of diet and disease is often problematic.

In prospective cohort studies, dietary data are obtained from a large group of individuals before the diagnosis of colorectal cancer. Because dietary information is collected prospectively, illness cannot affect the recall of diet and, moreover, the issue of an appropriate control group is eliminated. The majority of such studies use some form of food frequency questionnaire, although only a few such questionnaires have been examined for their reproducibility and comparability with other methods such as diet records.

Finally, interventional studies (clinical trials) investigate the effect of a specific nutrient supplement or more broad-based dietary change on colorectal neoplasia. Because of the long latency period of colorectal carcinogenesis, such studies usually focus on the risk of adenoma recurrence among individuals who have undergone a colonoscopic polypectomy. Randomized clinical trials are particularly practical for evaluating hypotheses for specific nutrients such as trace elements or vitamins that can be formulated into pills or capsules. Interventional studies minimize the possibility of confounding by extraneous factors. Nonetheless, the time between change in the level of a dietary factor and any expected change in the incidence of colorectal neoplasia is typically uncertain. Therefore, null intervention studies can be criticized for an insufficient duration of supplementation. Furthermore, studies

Table 1
Epidemiological Approaches to Diet and Colorectal Cancer

Ecological (correlation) studies
Migration studies
Time-trend (secular trend) studies
Retrospective case-control studies
Prospective cohort studies
Randomized clinical trials

of adenoma recurrence will potentially miss factors that influence the progression from adenoma to cancer rather than from normal epithelium to polyp.

2. FIBER

The rarity of colorectal cancer in Africa suggested to Burkitt that the high-fiber diet of Africans is protective against colorectal cancer (8). Since then, dietary fiber has been postulated to prevent colorectal cancer by diluting or adsorbing fecal carcinogens, reducing colonic transit time, altering bile acid metabolism, reducing colonic pH, or increasing production of short-chain fatty acids (9).

Despite the intuitive appeal of Burkitt's hypothesis, epidemiologic studies of a possible link between dietary fiber and colorectal cancer have been inconclusive (10). A meta-analysis of case-control studies demonstrated a combined odds ratio of 0.58 between the highest and lowest quintiles of fiber intake (11). However, when this analysis was restricted to studies that used validated diet questionnaires and incorporated qualitative data into nutrient estimation, the risk estimates for dietary fiber and colorectal cancer were closer to the null (12). The retrospective design of the previous case-control studies may have introduced recall and selection biases. Furthermore, many of these studies had limited data on other dietary factors, thereby preventing clear distinctions between the effects of fiber and other constituents of plant foods.

In six large prospective studies (13–18), inverse associations between intake of fiber and risk of colon cancer have been weak or nonexistent. Using a limited dietary questionnaire, Thun et al. did observe a significant inverse relation between intake of "citrus fruit, vegetable, and high-fiber grains" and colon cancer, although dietary fiber intake was not specifically analyzed (19). In the largest cohort study of dietary fiber, Fuchs and colleagues analyzed 88,757 women over a 16-yr follow-up period and found no association between dietary fiber intake and risk of colorectal cancer; the relative risk for the highest as compared to the lowest quintile of fiber intake was 0.95 (95% confidence interval [CI] 0.73–1.25) (18). Moreover, no significant association between fiber intake and risk of colorectal adenoma was seen. Another prospective study of 16,448 US men also failed to demonstrate a significant association between total dietary, cereal, or vegetable fiber intake and colorectal adenomas, although a modest reduced risk was observed with increasing fruit fiber intake (20).

Three large, randomized, controlled trials have examined the rates of adenoma recurrence among individuals who had undergone a colonoscopic removal of an adenomatous polyp (Table 2). In all three studies, participants randomized to a high-fiber diet or supplement did not experience any significant reduction in adenoma recurrence (21–23). In fact, Bonithon-Kopp and colleagues observed a significant increase in the rate of adenoma recurrence among participants randomized to the fiber supplement (21).

Table 2
Randomized Controlled Trials of Fiber in the Prevention of Recurrent Adenomatous Polyps

Author	Intervention	No. of patients	Rate of adenoma recurrence (%)		Risk ratio for intervention (95% CI)
			Intervention	Control	
Schatzkin et al. *(22)*	Low-fat, high-fiber diet	1905	39.7	39.5	1.00 (0.90–1.12)
Alberts et al. *(23)*	High-fiber supplement	1303	47.0	51.2	0.88 (0.70–1.11)
Bonithon-Kopp et al. *(21)*	High-fiber supplement	552	29.3	20.2	1.67 (1.01–2.76)

Although ongoing research continues to assess the influence of fiber intake on the risk of colorectal neoplasia, the preponderance of the evidence would indicate that dietary fiber exerts a minimal, if any, influence on colorectal carcinogenesis. There are cogent reasons for increasing fiber intake, particularly the inverse association observed with coronary heart disease in many studies *(24,25)*. However, dietary measures to reduce colorectal cancer risk must include other strategies beyond increasing dietary fiber intake.

3. VEGETABLES AND FRUITS

Consumption of fruit and vegetables could reduce colorectal cancer risk through anticarcinogenic components, such as antioxidants (in particular, carotenoids and vitamin C), folic acid, flavonoids, organosulfides, and isothiocyanates, the induction of detoxification enzymes by cruciferous vegetables, and protease inhibitors that might influence DNA damage and thus reduce mutations *(26,27)*. The association of fruit and vegetable intake with colon and/or rectal cancer incidence has been considered in numerous previous epidemiologic studies, and many of these studies have concluded that strong evidence exists for a benefit *(28)*. At least 22 retrospective case-control studies have evaluated the association of vegetable and fruit consumption with colon cancer risk *(28,29)*. Of these studies, 18 found some degree of risk reduction with higher-level consumption of at least one category of vegetable or fruit. A decreased risk with higher-level consumption of cruciferous vegetables was seen in 8 of 13 studies in which such an association was reported, and a protective association with intake of green vegetables was reported in 5 of 6 studies. Less data are available on the association between fruit consumption alone and colon cancer risk; most case-control studies have found no substantial association. In case-control studies, however, diet is assessed retrospectively; hence, such studies are prone to recall or reporting bias because case patients and control subjects are likely to differ in their reporting of their dietary habits.

Prospective studies of fruit and vegetable intake generally have produced more modest *(30–32)* or nonsupportive *(33,34)* results. A recent analysis of two large cohorts observed no protective benefit of fruit or vegetable intake on the risk of colorectal cancer *(34)*. Similarly for adenomas, some *(35–41)*, but not all, studies *(42–44)* have supported the role of fruits and vegetables.

Despite the lack of support for a strong protective effect for vegetables in recent studies, vegetable consumption has been among the most consistent protective factors for colorectal carcinogenesis across all epidemiologic studies *(45)*. The WRCF report *(28)* concluded that "evidence that diets rich in vegetables protect against cancers of the colon and rectum is convincing," whereas "the data on fruit are more limited and inconsistent; no judgement is possible." Nonetheless, vegetables are a heterogeneous mix of various compounds that may influence colorectal carcinogenesis (including carotenoids, ascorbate, and folate). Further studies on these micronutrient constituents of plant foods may better elucidate the influence of vegetable consumption.

4. FOLATE

Folate is essential for regenerating methionine, the methyl donor for DNA methylation, and for producing the purines and pyrimidines required for DNA synthesis. Inadequate availability of folate may contribute to aberrations in DNA methylation and lead to abnormalities in DNA synthesis or repair, either of which may influence colon carcinogenesis. Consistent with animal studies *(46)*, epidemiologic evidence supports a potential role for folate in reducing risk of colorectal cancer. Five case-control studies found a higher risk of colon cancer among individuals with low folate intakes *(47–51)*. Three of three prospective studies demonstrated an inverse association between higher folate intake and lower colon cancer risk *(52–54)*; another prospective study showed an inverse association between plasma folate and risk of colon cancer *(55)*. In a prospective cohort study of 88,756 women, participants who consumed more than 400 µg of folic acid per day experienced a relative risk for colon cancer of 0.69 (95% CI = 0.52–0.93) when compared to women who consumed 200 µg or less per day *(54)*. Moreover, women who used folate-containing multivitamin supplements for at least 15 yr were 75% less likely to develop colon cancer than women who never took multivitamins. A population-based case-control study also demonstrated a 50% reduction in risk of colon cancer among men and women who reported daily multivitamin use *(51)*. The potentially greater protection of folic acid from multivitamins may be the result of the higher dose and bioavailability of folic acid found in multivitamins *(54)*.

Low dietary folate or erythrocyte folate levels have been associated with an increased risk of colorectal adenomas *(38,56,57)*. Among small studies of individuals with chronic ulcerative colitis, a similar inverse relationship between folate and large bowel dysplasia or cancer has been reported *(58–60)*.

Several plausible mechanisms by which folate may influence colorectal carcinogenesis are available. Folate is an important factor in DNA methylation, and DNA methylation is an important determinant of gene expression, maintenance of DNA integrity and stability, and development of mutations *(61–63)*. Genomic and protooncogene-specific DNA hypomethylation seems to be an early and consistent event in carcinogenesis, particularly in colon cancer *(64–68)*. Folate is also required to convert deoxyuridylate (dUMP) into thymidylate (dTMP). When levels of folate are low, misincorporation of uracil for thymidine may occur during DNA synthesis *(69)*, potentially increasing spontaneous mutation rates *(70)*, sensitivity to DNA-damaging agents *(71)*, frequency of chromosomal aberrations *(72,73)*, errors in DNA replication *(73–75)*, and abnormalities in DNA excision *(76)* and mismatch repair *(77)*. Blount et al. demonstrated that folate deficiency was related to massive misincorporation of uracil into human DNA and increased chromosomal breaks, and these changes were reversible with folate supplementation *(78)*.

Additional evidence for the importance of folic acid in colorectal carcinogenesis comes from studies of individuals with an inherited polymorphism in methylene tetrahydrofolate reductase (MTHFR), a critical enzyme in folate metabolism *(79,80)*. Prospective studies show that homozygotes for a polymorphism of the MTHFR gene, which correlates with reduced activity, have a significantly lower risk for colon cancer, possibly because low activity of this enzyme maintains higher cellular levels of 5,10-methylene tetrahydrofolate, thereby reducing misincorporation of uracil into human DNA *(55,81)*. This relation between a functional polymorphism for this folate-metabolizing gene and risk for colon cancer provides independent evidence for a role of folate that cannot be attributed to confounding by another dietary variable.

Overall, the consistent findings from case-control studies, cohort studies, and the findings associated with polymorphisms of the MTHFR gene suggest an important role for folic acid in colon carcinogenesis, possibly through its effect on DNA synthesis and methylation.

5. CALCIUM AND VITAMIN D

Animal studies have suggested that calcium may be involved in the etiology of colon cancer *(82–85)*. Calcium can bind secondary bile acids and ionized fatty acids, which can promote epithelial cell proliferation in the colon *(86–88)*, and calcium may also directly decrease epithelial cell proliferation *(89)*.

Although epidemiological studies on this association are inconsistent, the majority of studies have found weak but statistically nonsignificant inverse associations between high calcium intake and colorectal or colon cancer risk *(90–96)*. In two male prospective cohorts, higher calcium intake was significantly associated with lower risk of colorectal cancer *(97,98)*. A meta-analysis of 24 studies assessing the relation between calcium intake and colorectal adenoma or cancer found a modest inverse association between calcium intake and risk of colorectal cancer (pooled relative risk = 0.86; 95% CI = 0.74–0.98), but not colorectal adenoma (pooled relative risk = 1.13; 95% CI = 0.91–1.39) *(99)*.

Randomized, placebo-controlled trials of adenoma recurrence have also suggested a small benefit for supplemental calcium use. In a trial of 930 individuals with a history of colorectal adenoma in the United States, calcium supplementation resulted in a statistically significant, albeit moderate, decreased risk of recurrent adenomas (relative risk = 0.81; 95% CI = 0.67–0.99) *(100)*. Another trial from Europe also observed a modest, though nonsignificant, decreased risk of colorectal adenoma recurrence with calcium supplementation (relative risk = 0.66; 95% CI = 0.38–1.17) *(21)*.

In vitro studies have demonstrated that $1,25(OH)_2$-vitamin D, the active metabolite of vitamin D, inhibits proliferation and induces differentiation of human colorectal cells *(101,102)*, and animal studies suggested that $1,25(OH)_2$-vitamin D reduces tumor growth *(103)*. Ecologic studies in humans showed that areas with higher sunlight exposure are associated with lower rates of colorectal cancer incidence and death, leading investigators to suggest a possible role for vitamin D by virtue of higher rates of ultraviolet light photoconversion of skin precursors to vitamin D in areas of greater sunlight *(104,105)*. In prospective cohort studies, the relation between vitamin D and colorectal cancer has been less striking *(106)*. Although four *(107–110)* of the five prospective studies have reported modest inverse associations for dietary vitamin D and colon or colorectal cancer, the association was significant in only one study *(107)*. In the Nurses' Health Study *(110)*, a significant inverse association was seen when total (dietary plus supplemental) vitamin D intake was analyzed. However, many of the women in the highest category of vitamin D were taking multivitamin supplements, so that other constituents of multivitamins could potentially explain these findings.

In summary, the available evidence suggests that calcium and vitamin D may reduce the risk of colon cancer, although the effect appears to be modest.

6. RED MEAT AND FAT

Within human ecological studies, rates of colon cancer are strongly correlated with national per capita disappearance of animal fat and meat (2,111). Moreover, rates of colon cancer have risen sharply in Japan since 1945, paralleling a 2.5-fold increase in meat and fat intake in that country (7). Sixteen of 26 case-control studies have reported a positive association between red meat and the risk of colon cancer (28). Among prospective studies, three of seven cohort studies have reported a positive association between red meat and colon cancer (28). The Nurses' Health Study reported that women who consumed red meat frequently had a statistically significant 2.5-fold increase in the risk of colon cancer when compared with women who consumed red meat rarely (112). Although, the authors also noted a higher risk of colon cancer in association with animal fat intake, a multivariate model, which included both red meat and animal fat intakes, indicated a statistically significant risk of colon cancer for red meat, whereas the association with animal fat was eliminated. Data from the Health Professionals Follow-up Study, a cohort study of men, demonstrated a direct association between red meat consumption and risk of colon cancer and adenoma, but no association was observed with other sources of fat (113). Two other cohort studies observed a significant direct association between intake of processed meats and risk of colon cancer (114,115).

Assessing the specific role of dietary fat, Howe et al. conducted a pooled analysis of 13 case-control studies and found no evidence of any increased risk of colon cancer with dietary fat intake after adjustment for total energy intake (116). Furthermore, there were no statistically significant associations for any type of fat in subgroup analyses by age, sex, or anatomic location of the cancer.

This evidence suggests that consumption of red meat is associated with an increased risk of colon cancer, independent of animal fat. Several possible explanations exist for these findings. First, a specific fatty acid present in red meat may be particularly harmful, independent of total fat. Second, high consumption of red meat may increase concentrations of fecal iron, which could influence the risk of colon cancer by generation of hydroxyl radicals (10). Third, initiators or promoters of carcinogenesis may be formed when red meat is cooked, particularly at high temperatures. Several studies suggested a higher risk of colon cancer (117,118) or adenoma (119) when meat was either fried to a heavily browned surface or cooked "well done." Mutagenic heterocyclic amines are formed when meat is fried, grilled, or broiled at high temperatures for substantial periods (120–122). These compounds and their genetically variable metabolism are being evaluated in ongoing laboratory and epidemiologic investigations.

7. ALCOHOL

Although not entirely consistent, most epidemiologic studies support a positive association between alcohol intake and the risk of colorectal cancer, particularly for cancers originating in the distal colon or rectum (123). Eighteen case-control studies have examined alcohol consumption and colon cancer; alcohol consumption was associated with an increased risk in nine of these studies (124). In addition, 9 of 17 studies of rectal cancer reported an elevated risk in association with alcohol consumption (124). Five prospective cohort studies have reported on the influence of alcohol consumption; four have shown statistically significant positive associations with alcohol *(124)*. Three of these studies explored the association with rectal cancer and each found a positive association.

Although there are studies showing both increased risk as well as no association with alcohol, there are essentially no studies showing reduced risk with higher intake. The inconsistencies among studies may reflect small sample sizes, study methods, differences in patterns of alcohol consumption, or differences in metabolism of alcohol among divergent study populations. The WCRF report concluded that, "high alcohol consumption probably increases the risk of cancers of the colon and rectum"*(28)*.

8. SMOKING

In previous studies, tobacco has been consistently associated with an increased risk for colorectal adenoma. However, among earlier studies, the findings for colorectal cancer had been contradictory *(125)*. In the Iowa Women's Health Study, the relative risks for colon cancer for current and former smokers were 1.09 and 0.92, respectively, and there was no relation between colorectal cancer and pack-years smoked *(115)*. In the New York University Women's Health Study, the relative risks for colorectal cancer were 0.97 for current and 0.99 for past smokers relative to nonsmokers *(126)*. Subsequently, results from both the Nurses' Health Study and the Health Professionals Follow-up Study suggested that the earlier studies of colorectal cancer and smoking were inconsistent because they failed to allow for an adequate induction period. Among both studies, the risk of small adenomas (less than 1 cm) was significantly associated with recent smoking, whereas an elevated risk for larger adenomas required 20 yr following smoking initiation, and colorectal cancers required at least 35 yr from initial exposure *(127,128)*. In the Nurses' Health Study, an increased risk of colorectal cancer was only observed among women who had begun smoking more than 35 yr in the past, with the relative risk increasing from 1.47 for 35–39 yr in the past to 2.00 for more than 45 yr in the past.

Since then, the majority of published studies have reported positive associations between cigarette smoking and colorectal cancer *(129–139)*, although a few studies did not support an association *(140–143)*. The long latency period between initiation of smoking and elevation in colorectal cancer risk and the consistent relationship seen for recent smoking and adenoma risk suggest that smoking may act as an early initiator of colorectal carcinogenesis, causing mutations in genes that occur early in the adenoma–carcinoma sequence (e.g., K-*ras*) (*see* Chapter 1). In one study of colorectal adenomas, Fernandez-Martos et al. observed a significant increase in the prevalence of K-*ras* mutations among past or current smokers *(144)*. In another study, Slattery and colleagues observed a significant increase in the prevalence of microsatellite instability (MSI) in colorectal cancers among smokers *(145)*. The association between MSI-positive cancers and cigarette smoking was strongest among patients who started smoking at a young age or smoked for 35 or more years.

9. OBESITY AND PHYSICAL ACTIVITY

Studies in laboratory animals suggest that energy restriction can reduce the incidence of intestinal tumors. In humans, evidence for a deleterious effect of obesity, assessed by body mass index (BMI), on the risk of colon cancer is derived from prospective *(107,115,129,146–155)* and retrospective *(156–160)* studies. In the Nurses' Health Study, BMI was positively associated with the risk for colon cancer *(161)* and large (≥1 cm) adenomas *(162)*, whereas BMI was not related to small (<1 cm) adenoma risk. Similarly, in the Health Professionals Follow-up Study *(147)*, the risk for colon cancer was significantly associated with both waist-to-hip ratio (relative risk = 3.41) and waist circumference (relative risk = 2.56). Similar associations were observed for adenomas of 1 cm or greater, but no association was observed for smaller adenomas. Of interest, two studies among women reported suggestive but not statistically significant positive associations between waist-to-hip ratio and risk of colon cancer *(115,163)*. Among many studies, measures of central adiposity (e.g., waist-to-hip ratio) are stronger predictors of colon cancer risk for men than for women, which may be indicative of the higher prevalence of central obesity in men compared to women *(147,162)*.

The association between adiposity and risk of colon cancer and large adenoma but not small adenoma suggests that obesity may act relatively late in the pathway of colon carcinogenesis, enhancing the progression to large adenomas and cancer.

The relationship between physical activity and a reduced risk of colon cancer is among the most consistent findings in the epidemiologic literature, reported in studies of occupational activity, leisure activity, and total activity *(124)*. Results of prospective *(129,146,155, 164–171)* and retrospective *(36,156,157,172–181)* studies support an inverse association between physical inactivity and risk of colon, but not rectal cancer *(146,156,167,168,170, 181–183)*. In the Nurses Health Study, women who were in the upper quintile of leisure-time physical activity were less likely to develop colon cancer (relative risk [RR] = 0.54; 95% CI = 0.33–0.90) *(163)* and large adenomas (RR = 0.57, 95% CI = 0.30–1.08) *(162)* compared to nonactive women. In the Health Professionals Follow-up Study, physical activity was inversely associated with colon cancer risk (RR=0.53; 95% CI = 0.32–0.88) *(184)*. When physical activity and BMI are assessed jointly, the highest risk of colon cancer occurs among those both physically inactive and with high BMI levels *(147,185)*. Based on a review of the literature, Colditz et al. reported an approx 50% reduction in incidence of colon cancer among the most active individuals *(186)*.

Maintaining high levels of physical activity throughout life appears to impart the greatest protection *(146,157)*. In the Harvard Alumni Study, men who were at least moderately active at two assessments were 48% less likely to develop colon cancer when compared to men who were inactive at both assessments *(146)*. Nonetheless, among men who were sedentary at the initial assessment, those who increased their activity during follow-up were 13% less likely to develop colon cancer than those who remained sedentary.

Several biologic mechanisms have been proposed for the inverse association between physical activity and colon cancer *(187)*. Martínez et al. showed that a higher level of leisure-time activity was significantly inversely related to the concentration of prostaglandin E_2 (PGE$_2$) in the rectal mucosa, suggesting a potential mechanism through PGE$_2$ synthesis *(188)*. In addition, hyperinsulinemia is related to physical inactivity, high body mass index, and central deposition of adipose, and insulin is mitogenic for normal and neoplastic colonic epithelial cells *(189)*. Insulin has been shown to be a colon tumor promoter in animal models *(190)* and high insulin levels are positively related to risk of colon cancer in humans *(191)*. Adult-onset diabetes mellitus, typically associated with a prolonged history of insulin resistance and hyperinsulinemia, also appears to be a significant risk factor for colon cancer *(192)*. Moreover, insulin-like growth factors (IGFs) have been linked to colon cancer risk. IGF-1 stimulates cellular proliferation and inhibits apoptosis *(193)*. Conversely, IGF-binding proteins (IGFBPs) can oppose the actions of IGF-1, in part by binding and sequestering IGF-1 *(194)* and by inhibitory effects mediated by specific IGFBP-3 membrane-associated receptors *(195)*. In a prospective study of US male physicians, men in the top quintile of IGF-1 had a relative risk for colon cancer of 2.51 (95% CI = 1.15–5.46). For IGFBP-3, the

Table 3
Summary of Selected Dietary and Lifestyle Risk Factors for Colon and Rectal Cancer

Probability of association	Decreases risk	Increases risk
Likely	Physical activity Folate Vegetables	Obesity Smoking Red meat
Possible	Fruit Calcium Vitamin D Methionine	Alcohol Processed meat Heavily cooked meat Iron
Uncertain	Fiber	

relative risk for the top vs bottom quintile was 0.28 (95% CI = 0.12–0.66). High IGF-1 and low IGFBP-3 levels were similarly associated with an increased risk of colorectal cancers and large adenomas (≥1 cm in diameter) among women in the Nurses' Health Study *(196)*.

Overall, these results strongly suggest that both physical inactivity and obesity increase the risk of colon cancer, perhaps by increasing circulating insulin and IGFs and thereby promoting tumorigenesis in the large bowel.

10. CONCLUSION

Epidemiologic studies over the past 20 yr have dramatically improved our understanding of the dietary and lifestyle risk factors for colorectal neoplasia. Although further work is needed to clarify the dietary predictors of colorectal cancer, practical recommendations for the primary prevention of colorectal cancer and adenoma can be offered (Table 3). The available evidence would suggest that a diet high in fruits and vegetables and low in red meat, in conjunction with regular physical activity and avoiding obesity, smoking, and heavy alcohol use will significantly reduce the risk of colorectal cancer. In addition, regular use of multivitamins that contain folate may also substantially reduce colorectal cancer risk. Of note, these guidelines are prudent not only in the prevention of colorectal cancer but also in the prevention of other chronic diseases in Western populations, specifically coronary heart disease *(25)*.

Coupled with our increasing understanding of the genetic events associated with colorectal neoplasia, future models of carcinogenesis will need to account for environmental factors, genetic predisposition, and the molecular events involved in tumorigenesis. It is apparent that although colorectal cancers appear relatively homogenous histologically, the genetic and epigenetic background may differ substantially among tumors. In addition, although relevant data are relatively sparse at present, in vitro, animal, and limited correlative human data indicate that specific exogenous factors may cause (or prevent) specific molecular alterations. The most obvious examples are chemical carcinogens that in some settings cause quite specific mutations. Ongoing studies are examining suspected etiologic factors in relation to mutations in certain genes (e.g., *p53* tumor suppressor gene, the K-*ras* protooncogene), including specific types of mutations (e.g., transition mutations at a specific codon). A better understanding of the causes of colorectal carcinogenesis requires the ability to correlate exogenous factors with markers of colorectal cancer progression. Examples of such studies are just beginning to emerge in the literature *(139,145,197)*. By linking certain exposures to specific genetic alterations, we may enhance our ability to reach firmer conclusions from epidemiologic investigations and better define the mechanistic influence of environmental exposures on the pathogenesis of colorectal neoplasia.

REFERENCES

1. Doll R and Peto R. The causes of cancer: quantitative estimates of avoidable risks of cancer in the United States today. *J. Natl. Cancer. Inst.*, **66** (1981) 1191–1308.
2. Armstrong B and Doll R. Environmental factors and cancer incidence and mortality in different countries, with special reference to dietary practices. *Int. J. Cancer*, **15** (1975) 617–631.
3. Draser B and Irving D. Environmental factors and cancer of the colon and breast. *Br. J. Cancer,* **27** (1973) 167–172.
4. Haenszel W. Cancer mortality among the foreign born in the United States. *J. Natl. Cancer Inst.*, **26** (1961) 37–132.
5. Wynder EL and Shigematsu T. Environmental factors of cancer of the colon and rectum. *Cancer*, **20** (1967) 1520–1561.
6. McMichael AJ and Giles GG. Cancer in migrants to Australia: extending the descriptive epidemiological data. *Cancer Res.*, **48** (1988) 751–756.
7. Aoki K, Hayakawa N, Kurihara M, and Suzuki S. *Death Rates for Malignant Neoplasms for Selected Sites by Sex and Five-year Age Group in 33 Countries, 1953–57 to 1983–87. International Union Against Cancer.* University of Nagoya Coop, Nagoya, 1992.
8. Burkitt D. Epidemiology of cancer of the colon and rectum. *Cancer*, **28** (1971) 3–13.
9. Kritchevsky D. Epidemiology of fibre, resistant starch and colorectal cancer. *Eur. J. Cancer Prev.*, **4** (1995) 345–352.
10. Giovannucci E and Willett WC. Dietary factors and risk of colon cancer. *Ann. Med.*, **26** (1994) 443–452.
11. Howe G, Benito E, Castelleto R, et al. Dietary intake of fiber and decreased risk of cancers of the colon and rectum: evidence from the combined analysis of 13 case-control studies. *J. Natl. Cancer Inst.*, **84** (1992) 1887–1896.
12. Friedenreich C, Brant R, and Riboli E. Influence of methodologic factors in a pooled analysis of 13 case-control studies of colorectal cancer and dietary fiber. *Epidemiology*, **5** (1994) 66–79.
13. Giovannucci E, Rimm E, Stampfer M, Colditz G, Ascherio A, and Willett W. Intake of fat, meat, and fiber in relation to risk of colon cancer in men. *Cancer Res.*, **54** (1994) 2390–2397.
14. Goldbohm RA, Van den Brandt PA, Van 't Veer P, Dorant E, Sturmans F, and Hermus RJ. Prospective study on alcohol consumption and the risk of cancer of the colon and rectum in the Netherlands. *Cancer Causes Control*, **5** (1994) 95–104.
15. Heilbrun L, Nomura A, Hankin J, and Stemmermann G. Diet and colorectal cancer with special reference to fiber intake. *Int. J. Cancer*, **44** (1989) 1–6.
16. Kato I, Akhmedkhanov A, Koenig K, Toniolo P, Shore R, and Riboli E. Prospective study of diet and female colorectal cancer: the New York University Women's Health Study. *Nutr. Cancer*, **28** (1997) 276–281.
17. Steinmetz KA, Kushi LH, Bostick RM, Folsom AR, and Potter JD. Vegetables, fruit, and colon cancer in the Iowa Women's Health Study [see comments]. *Am. J. Epidemiol.*, **139** (1994) 1–15.
18. Fuchs CS, Giovannucci EL, Colditz GA, et al. Dietary fiber and the risk of colorectal cancer and adenoma in women [see comments]. *N. Engl. J. Med.*, **340** (1999) 169–176.
19. Thun M, Calle E, Namboodiri M, et al. Risk factors for fatal colon cancer in a large prospective study. *J. Natl. Cancer Inst.*, **84** (1992) 1491–1500.
20. Platz E, Giovannucci E, Rimm E, et al. Dietary fiber and distal colorectal adenoma in men. *Cancer Epidemiol. Biomakers Prev.*, **6** (1997) 661–670.
21. Bonithon-Kopp C, Kronborg O, Giacosa A, Rath U, and Faivre J. Calcium and fibre supplementation in prevention of colorectal adenoma recurrence: a randomised intervention trial. European Cancer Prevention Organisation Study Group. *Lancet*, **356** (2000) 1300–1306.
22. Schatzkin A, Lanza E, Corle D, et al. Lack of effect of a low-fat, high-fiber diet on the recurrence of colorectal adenomas. Polyp Prevention Trial Study Group. *N. Engl. J. Med.*, **342** (2000) 1149–1155.
23. Alberts DS, Martinez ME, Roe DJ, et al. Lack of effect of a high-fiber cereal supplement on the recurrence of colorectal adenomas. Phoenix Colon Cancer Prevention Physicians' Network. *N. Engl. J. Med.*, **342** (2000) 1156–1162.

24. Rimm E, Ascherio A, Giovannucci E, Spiegelman D, Stampfer M, and Willett W. Vegetable, fruit, and cereal fiber intake and risk of coronary heart disease among men. *JAMA*, **275** (1996) 447–451.

25. Willett W. *Nutritional Epidemiology*. Oxford University Press, New York, 1998.

26. Steinmetz KA and Potter JD. Vegetables, fruit and cancer. I. Epidemiology. *Cancer Causes Control*, **2** (1991) 325–357.

27. Frei B. Reactive oxygen species and antioxidant vitamins: mechanisms of action. *Am. J. Med.*, **97** (1994) 5S–13S; discussion 22S–28S.

28. World Cancer Research Fund (WCRF) Panel. *Food, Nutrition and the Prevention of Cancer: A Global Perspective*. American Institute for Cancer Research, Washington, DC, 1997.

29. Franceschi S, Parpinel M, La Vecchia C, Favero A, Talamini R, and Negri E. Role of different types of vegetables and fruit in the prevention of cancer of the colon, rectum, and breast. *Epidemiology*, **9** (1998) 338–341.

30. Thun MJ, Calle EE, Namboodiri MM, et al. Risk factors for fatal colon cancer in a large prospective study. *J. Natl. Cancer Inst.*, **84** (1992) 1491–1500.

31. Shibata A, Paganini-Hill A, Ross RK, and Henderson BE. Intake of vegetables, fruits, beta-carotene, vitamin C and vitamin supplements and cancer incidence among the elderly: a prospective study. *Br. J. Cancer*, **66** (1992) 673–679.

32. Voorrips LE, Goldbohm RA, van Poppel G, Sturmans F, Hermus RJ, and van den Brandt PA. Vegetable and fruit consumption and risks of colon and rectal cancer in a prospective cohort study: The Netherlands Cohort Study on Diet and Cancer. *Am. J. Epidemiol.*, **152** (2000) 1081–1092.

33. Phillips RL and Snowdon DA. Dietary relationships with fatal colorectal cancer among Seventh-Day Adventists. *J. Natl. Cancer Inst.*, **74** (1985) 307–317.

34. Michels KB, Edward G, Joshipura KJ, et al. Prospective study of fruit and vegetable consumption and incidence of colon and rectal cancers. *J. Natl. Cancer Inst.*, **92** (2000) 1740–1752.

35. Macquart-Moulin G, Riboli E, Cornee J, Kaaks R, and Berthezene P. Colorectal polyps and diet: a case-control study in Marseilles. *Int. J. Cancer*, **40** (1987) 179–188.

36. Kato I, Tominaga S, Matsuura A, Yoshii Y, Shirai M, and Kobayashi S. A comparative case-control study of colorectal cancer and adenoma. *Jpn. J. Cancer Res.*, **81** (1990) 1101–1108.

37. Kune GA, Kune S, Read A, et al. Colorectal polyps, diet, alcohol, and family history of colorectal cancer: a case-control study. *Nutr. Cancer*, **16** (1991) 25–30.

38. Benito E, Cabeza E, Moreno V, Obrador A, and Bosch FX. Diet and colorectal adenomas: a case-control study in Majorca. *Int. J. Cancer*, **55** (1993) 213–219.

39. Sandler RS, Lyles CM, Peipins LA, McAuliffe CA, Woosley JT, and Kupper LL. Diet and risk of colorectal adenomas: macronutrients, cholesterol and fiber. *J. Natl. Cancer Inst.*, **85** (1993) 884–891.

40. Witte JS, Longnecker MP, Bird CL, Lee ER, Frankl HD, and Haile RW. Relation of vegetable, fruit, and grain consumption to colorectal adenomatous polyps. *Am. J. Epidemiol.*, **144** (1996) 1015–1025.

41. Platz EA, Giovannucci E, Rimm EB, et al. Dietary fiber and distal colorectal adenoma in men. *Cancer Epidemiol. Biomarkers Prev.*, **6** (1997) 661–670.

42. Kono S, Imanishi K, Shinchi K, and Yanai F. Relationship of diet to small and large adenomas of the sigmoid colon. *Jpn. J. Cancer Res.*, **84** (1993) 13–19.

43. Neugut AI, Garbowski GC, Lee WC, et al. Dietary risk factors for the incidence and recurrence of colorectal adenomatous polyps: a case-control study. *Ann. Int. Med.*, **118** (1993) 91–95.

44. Little J, Logan RFA, Hawtin PG, Hardcastle JD, and Turner ID. Colorectal adenomas and diet: a case-control study of subjects participating in the Nottingham faecal occult blood screening programme. *Br. J. Cancer*, **67** (1993) 177–184.

45. Potter JD. Nutrition and colorectal cancer. *Cancer Causes Control*, **7** (1996) 127–146.

46. Cravo ML, Mason JB, Dayal Y, et al. Folate deficiency enhances the development of colonic neoplasia in dimethylhydrazine-treated rats. *Cancer Res.*, **52** (1992) 5002–5006.

47. Benito E, Stiggelbout A, Bosch FX, et al. Nutritional factors in colorectal cancer risk: a case-control study in Majorca. *Int. J. Cancer*, **49** (1991) 161–167.

48. Meyer F and White E. Alcohol and nutrients in relation to colon cancer in middle-aged adults. *Am. J. Epidemiol.*, **138** (1993) 225–236.

49. Ferraroni M, La Vecchia C, D'Avanzo B, Negri E, Franceschi S, and Decarli A. Selected micronutrient intake and the risk of colorectal cancer. *Br. J. Cancer*, **70** (1994) 1150–1155.

50. Freudenheim JL, Graham S, Marshall JR, Haughey BP, Cholewinski S, and Wilkinson G. Folate intake and carcinogenesis of the colon and rectum. *Int. J. Epidemiol.*, **20** (1991) 368–374.

51. White E, Shannon JS, and Patterson RE. Relationship between vitamin and calcium supplement use and colon cancer. *Cancer Epidemiol. Biomarkers Prev.*, **6** (1997) 769–774.

52. Glynn SA, Albanes D, Pietinen P, et al. Colorectal cancer and folate status: a nested case-control study among male smokers. *Cancer Epidemiol. Biomarkers Prev.*, **5** (1996) 487–494.

53. Giovannucci E, Rimm EB, Ascherio A, Stampfer MJ, Colditz GA, and Willett WC. Alcohol, low-methionine-low-folate diets, and risk of colon cancer in men. *J. Natl. Cancer Inst.*, **87** (1995) 265–273.

54. Giovannucci E, Stampfer MJ, Colditz GA, et al. Multivitamin use, folate, and colon cancer in women in the Nurses' Health Study. *Ann. Intern. Med.*, **129** (1998) 517–524.

55. Ma J, Stampfer MJ, Giovannucci E, et al. Methylenetetrahydrofolate reductase polymorphism, dietary interactions, and risk of colorectal cancer. *Cancer Res.*, **57** (1997) 1098–1102.

56. Bird CL, Swendseid ME, Witte JS, et al. Red cell and plasma folate, folate consumption, and the risk of colorectal adenomatous polyps. *Cancer Epidemiol. Biomarkers Prev.*, **4** (1995) 709–714.

57. Giovannucci E, Stampfer MJ, Colditz GA, et al. Folate, methionine, and alcohol intake and risk of colorectal adenoma. *J. Natl. Cancer Inst.*, **85** (1993) 875–884.

58. Lashner BA, Heidenreich PA, Su GL, Kane SV, and Hanauer SB. Effect of folate supplementation on the incidence of dysplasia and cancer in chronic ulcerative colitis: a case-control study. *Gastroenterology*, **97** (1989) 255–259.

59. Lashner BA. Red blood cell folate is associated with the development of dysplasia and cancer in ulcerative colitis. *J. Cancer Res. Clin. Oncol.*, **119** (1993) 549–554.

60. Lashner BA, Provencher KS, Seidner DL, Knesebeck A, and Brzezinski A. The effect of folic acid supplementation on the risk for cancer or dysplasia in ulcerative colitis. *Gastroenterology*, **112** (1997) 29–32.

61. Kim YI. Folate and carcinogenesis: evidence, mechanisms and implications. *J. Nutr. Biochemistry*, **10** (1999) 66–88.

62. Choi SW and Mason JB. Folate and carcinogenesis: an integrated scheme. *J. Nutr.*, **130** (2000) 129–132.

63. Choi SW and Mason JB. Folate and colorectal carcinogenesis: is DNA repair the missing link? [editorial; comment]. *Am. J. Gastroenterol.*, **93** (1998) 2013–2016.

64. Feinberg AP and Vogelstein B. Hypomethylation distinguishes genes of some human cancers from their normal counterparts. *Nature*, **301** (1983) 89–92.

65. Cravo M, Fidalgo P, Pereira AD, et al. DNA methylation as an intermediate biomarker in colorectal cancer: modulation by folic acid supplementation. *Eur. J. Cancer Prev.*, **3** (1994) 473–479.

66. Goelz SE, Vogelstein B, Hamilton SR, and Feinberg AP. Hypomethylation of DNA from benign and malignant human colon neoplasms. *Science*, **228** (1985) 187–190.

67. Feinberg AP, Gehrke CW, Kuo KC, and Ehrlich M. Reduced genomic 5-methylcytosine content in human colonic neoplasia. *Cancer Res.*, **48** (1988) 1159–1161.

68. Makos M, Nelkin BD, Lerman MI, Latif F, Zbar B, and Baylin SB. Distinct hypermethylation patterns occur at altered chromosome loci in human lung and colon cancer. *Proc. Natl. Acad. Sci. USA*, **89** (1992) 1929–1933.

69. Wickramasinghe SN and Fida S. Bone marrow cells from vitamin B12- and folate-deficient patients misincorporate uracil into DNA. *Blood*, **83** (1984) 1656–1661.

70. Weinberg G, Ullman B, and Martin DW Jr. Mutator phenotypes in mammalian cell mutants with distinct biochemical defects and abnormal deoxyribonucleoside triphosphate pools. *Proc. Natl. Acad. Sci. USA*, **78** (1981) 2447–2451.

71. Meuth M. Role of deoxynucleoside triphosphate pools in the cytotoxic and mutagenic effects of DNA alkylating agents. *Somatic Cell Genet.*, **7** (1981) 89–102.

72. Sutherland GR. The role of nucleotides in human fragile site expression. *Mutat. Res.*, **200** (1988) 207–213.

73. Fenech M and Rinaldi J. The relationship between micronuclei in human lymphocytes and plasma levels of vitamin C, vitamin E, vitamin B12 and folic acid. *Carcinogenesis*, **15** (1994) 1405–1411.

74. Hunting DJ and Dresler SL. Dependence of u.v.-induced DNA excision repair on deoxyribonucleoside triphosphate concentrations in permeable human fibroblasts: a model for the inhibition of repair by hydroxyurea. *Carcinogenesis*, **6** (1985) 1525–1528.

75. James SJ, Basnakian AG, and Miller BJ. In vitro folate deficiency induces deoxynucleotide pool imbalance, apoptosis, and mutagenesis in Chinese hamster ovary cells. *Cancer Res.*, **54** (1994) 5075–5080.

76. Choi SW, Kim YI, Weitzel JN, and Mason JB. Folate depletion impairs DNA excision repair in the colon of the rat. *Gut*, **43** (1998) 93–99.

77. Cravo ML, Albuquerque CM, Salazar de Sousa L, et al. Microsatellite instability in non-neoplastic mucosa of patients with ulcerative colitis: effect of folate supplementation [see comments]. *Am. J. Gastroenterol.*, **93** (1998) 2060–2064.

78. Blount BC, Mack MM, Wehr CM, et al. Folate deficiency causes uracil misincorporation into human DNA and chromosome breakage: implications for cancer and neuronal damage. *Proc. Natl. Acad. Sci. USA*, **94** (1997) 3290–3295.

79. Frosst P, Blom HJ, Milos R, et al. A candidate genetic risk factor for vascular disease: a common mutation in methylenetetrahydrofolate reductase (letter). *Nature Genet.*, **10** (1995) 111–113.

80. Goyette P, Sumner JS, Milos R, et al. Human methylenetetrahydrofolate reductase: isolation of cDNA, mapping and mutation identification. *Nature Genet.*, **7** (1994) 195–200.

81. Chen J, Giovannucci E, Kelsey K, et al. A methylenetetrahydrofolate reductase polymorphism and the risk of colorectal cancer. *Cancer Res.*, **56** (1996) 4862–4864.

82. Vinas-Salas J, Biendicho-Palau P, Pinol-Felis C, Miguelsanz-Garcia S, and Perez-Holanda S. Calcium inhibits colon carcinogenesis in an experimental model in the rat. *Eur. J. Cancer*, **34** (1998) 1941–1945.

83. Pence BC and Buddingh F. Inhibition of dietary fat-promoted colon carcinogenesis in rats by supplemental calcium or vitamin D3. *Carcinogenesis*, **9** (1988) 187–190.

84. Pence BC. Role of calcium in colon cancer prevention: experimental and clinical studies. *Mutat. Res.*, **290** (1993) 87–95.

85. Pence BC, Dunn DM, Zhao C, Patel V, Hunter S, Landers M. Protective effects of calcium from nonfat dried milk against colon carcinogenesis in rats. *Nutr. Cancer*, **25** (1996) 35–45.

86. Wargovich MJ, Eng VW, and Newmark HL. Calcium inhibits the damaging and compensatory proliferative effects of fatty acids on mouse colon epithelium. *Cancer Lett.*, **23** (1984) 253–258.

87. Van der Meer R, Kleibeuker JH, and Lapre JA. Calcium phosphate, bile acids and colorectal cancer. *Eur. J. Cancer Prev.*, **1 (Suppl 2)** (1991) 55–62.

88. Newmark HL, Wargovich MJ, and Bruce WR. Colon cancer and dietary fat, phosphate, and calcium: a hypothesis. *J. Natl. Cancer Inst.*, **72** (1984) 1323–1325.

89. Buset M, Lipkin M, Winawer S, Swaroop S, and Friedman E. Inhibition of human colonic epithelial cell proliferation in vivo and in vitro by calcium. *Cancer Res.*, **46** (1986) 5426–5430.

90. Kearney J, Giovannucci E, Rimm EB, et al. Calcium, vitamin D, and dairy foods and the occurrence of colon cancer in men. *Am. J. Epidemiol.*, **143** (1996) 907–917.

91. Macquart-Moulin G, Riboli E, Cornee J, Charnay B, Berthezene P, and Day N. Case-control study on colorectal cancer and diet in Marseilles. *Int. J. Cancer*, **38** (1986) 183–191.

92. Martinez ME, Giovannucci EL, Colditz GA, et al. Calcium, vitamin D, and the occurrence of colorectal cancer among women. *J. Natl. Cancer Inst.*, **88** (1996) 1375–1382.

93. Zaridze D, Filipchenko V, Kustov V, Serdyuk V, and Duffy S. Diet and colorectal cancer: results of two case-control studies in Russia. *Eur. J. Cancer*, **29A** (1992) 112–115.

94. Bostick RM, Potter JD, Fosdick L, et al. Calcium and colorectal epithelial cell proliferation: a preliminary randomized, double-blinded, placebo-controlled clinical trial. *J. Natl. Cancer Inst.*, **85** (1993) 132–141.

95. Lee HP, Gourley L, Duffy SW, Esteve J, Lee J, and Day NE. Colorectal cancer and diet in an Asian population—a case-control study among Singapore Chinese. *Int. J. Cancer*, **43** (1989) 1007–1016.

96. Kato I, Akhmedkhanov A, Koenig K, Toniolo PG, Shore RE, and Riboli E. Prospective study of diet and female colorectal cancer: the New York University Women's Health Study. *Nutr. Cancer*, **28** (1997) 276–281.

97. Garland C, Shekelle RB, Barrett-Connor E, Criqui MH, Rossof AH, and Paul O. Dietary vitamin D and calcium and risk of colorectal cancer: a 19-year prospective study in men. *Lancet*, **1** (1985) 307–309.

98. Pietinen P, Malila N, Virtanen M, et al. Diet and risk of colorectal cancer in a cohort of Finnish men. *Cancer Causes Control*, **10** (1999) 387–396.

99. Bergsma-Kadijk JA, van 't Veer P, Kampman E, and Burema J. Calcium does not protect against colorectal neoplasia. *Epidemiology*, **7** (1996) 590–597.

100. Baron J, Beach M, Mandel JS, et al. Calcium supplements for the prevention of colorectal adenomas. Calcium Polyp Prevention Study Group. *N. Eng. J. Med.*, **340** (1999) 101–107.

101. Lointier P, Wagowich MJ, Saez S, Levin B, Widrick DM, and Boman BM. The role of vitamin D3 in the proliferation of human colon cancer cell lines in vitro. *Anticancer Res.*, **7** (1987) 817–822.

102. Shabahang M, Buras RR, Davoodi F, et al. Growth inhibition of HT-29 human colon cancer cells by analogues of 1,25-dihydroxyvitamin D3. *Cancer Res.*, **54** (1994) 407–464.

103. Eisman JA, Barkla DH, Tutton PJM. Supression of in vivo growth of human cancer solid tumor xenographs by 1,25-dihydoxyvitamin D3. *Cancer Res.*, **47** (1987) 21–25.

104. Garland CF and Garland FC. Do sunlight and vitamin D reduce the likelihood of colon cancer? *Int. J. Epidemiol.*, **9** (1980) 227–231.

105. Emerson JC and Weiss NS. Colorectal cancer and solar radiation. *Cancer Causes Control*, **3** (1992) 95–99.

106. Martinez ME and Willett WC. Calcium, vitamin D, and colorectal cancer: a review of the epidemiologic evidence. *Cancer Epidemiol. Biomarkers Prev.*, **7** (1998) 163–168.

107. Garland C, Shekelle RB, Barrett-Conner E, Criqui MH, Rossof AH, and Paul O. Dietary vitamin D and calcium and risk of colorectal cancer: A 19-year prospective study in men. *Lancet*, **1** (1985) 307–309.

108. Bostick RM, Potter JD, Sellers TA, McKenszie DR, Kushi H, and Folsom AR. Relation of calcium, vitamin D, and dairy food intake to incidence of colon cancer in older women. *Am. J. Epidemiol.*, **137** (1993) 1302–1317.

109. Kearney J, Giovannucci E, Rimm EB, et al. Calcium, vitamin D and dairy foods and the occurrence of colon cancer in men. *Am. J. Epidemiol.*, **143** (1996) 907–917.

110. Martínez ME, Giovannucci EL, Colditz GA, et al. Calcium, vitamin D, and the occurrence of colorectal cancer among women. *J. Natl. Cancer Inst.*, **88** (1996) 1375–1382.

111. Rose DP, Boyar AP, and Wynder EL. International comparisons of mortality rates for cancer of the breast, ovary, prostate, and colon, and per capita food consumption. *Cancer*, **58** (1986) 2263–2271.

112. Willett WC, Stampfer MJ, Colditz GA, Rosner BA, and Speizer FE. Relation of meat, fat, and fiber intake to the risk of colon cancer in a prospective study among women. *N. Engl. J. Med.*, **323** (1990) 1664–1672.

113. Giovannucci E, Rimm EB, Stampfer MJ, Colditz GA, Ascherio A, and Willett WC. Intake of fat, meat, and fiber in relation to risk of colon cancer in men. *Cancer Res.*, **54** (1994) 2390–2397.

114. Goldbohm RA, van den Brandt PA, van't Veer P, et al. A prospective cohort study on the relation between meat consumption and the risk of colon cancer. *Cancer Res.*, **54** (1994) 718–723.

115. Bostick RM, Potter JD, Kushi LH, et al. Sugar, meat, and fat intake, and non-dietary risk factors for colon cancer incidence in Iowa women (United States). *Cancer Causes Control*, **5** (1994) 38–52.

116. Howe GR, Aronson KJ, Benito E, et al. The relationship between dietary fat intake and risk of colorectal cancer—evidence from the combined analysis of 13 case-control studies. *Cancer Causes Control*, **8** (1997) 215–228.

117. Gerhardsson de Verdier M, Hagman U, Peters RK, Steineck G, and Overik E. Meat, cooking methods and colorectal cancer: A case-referent study in Stockholm. *Int. J. Cancer*, **49** (1991) 520–525.

118. Lee HP, Gourley L, Duffy SW, Esteve J, Lee J, and Day NE. Colorectal cancer and diet in an Asian population—a case-control study among Singapore Chinese. *Int. J. Cancer*, **43** (1989) 1007–1016.

119. Sinha R, Chow WH, Kulldorff M, et al. Well-done, grilled red meat increases the risk of colorectal adenomas. *Cancer Res.*, **59** (1999) 4320–4324.

120. Sugimura T, Sato S. Mutagens-carcinogens in foods. *Cancer Res.*, **43** (1983) 2415S–2421S.

121. Sugimura T. Carcinogenicity of mutagenic heterocyclic amines formed during the cooking process. *Mutat. Res.*, **150** (1985) 33–41.

122. Wakabayashi K, Nagao M, Esumi H, and Sugimura T. Food-derived mutagens and carcinogens. *Cancer Res.*, **52** (1992) 2092s–2098s.

123. Kune GA and Vitetta L. Alcohol consumption and the etiology of colorectal cancer: a review of the scientific evidence from 1957 to 1991. *Nutr. Cancer*, **18** (1992) 97–111.

124. Potter JD. Colorectal cancer: molecules and populations. *J. Natl. Cancer Inst.*, **91** (1999) 916–932.

125. Giovannucci E and Martinez ME. Tobacco, colorectal cancer, and adenomas: a review of the evidence. *J. Natl. Cancer Inst.*, **88** (1996) 1717–1730.

126. Kato I, Akhmedkhanov A, Koenig K, Toniolo PG, Shore RE, and Riboli I. Prospective study of diet and female colorectal cancer: The New York University Women's Health Study. *Nutr. Cancer*, **28** (1997) 276–281.

127. Giovannucci E, Colditz GA, Stampfer MJ, et al. A prospective study of cigarette smoking and risk of colorectal adenoma and colorectal cancer in US women [see comments]. *J. Natl. Cancer Inst.*, **86** (1994) 192–199.

128. Giovannucci E, Rimm EB, Stampfer MJ, et al. A prospective study of cigarette smoking and risk of colorectal adenoma and colorectal cancer in U.S. men [see comments]. *J. Natl. Cancer Inst.*, **86** (1994) 183–191.

129. Wu AH, Paganini-Hill A, Ross RK, and Henderson BE. Alcohol, physical activity and other risk factors for colorectal cancer: a prospective study. *Br. J. Cancer*, **55** (1987) 687–694.

130. Slattery ML, West DW, Robison LM, et al. Tobacco, alcohol, coffee, and caffeine as risk factors for colon cancer in a low-risk population. *Epidemiology*, **1** (1990) 141–145.

131. Heineman EF, Zahm SH, McLaughlin JK, and Vaught JB. Increased risk of colorectal cancer among smokers: results of a 26-year follow-up of US veterans and a review. *Int. J. Cancer*, **59** (1994) 728–738.

132. Newcomb PA, Storer BE, and Marcus PM. Cigarette smoking in relation to risk of large bowel cancer in women. *Cancer Res.*, **55** (1995) 4906–4909.

133. Slattery ML, Potter JD, Friedman GD, Ma K-N, and Edwards S. Tobacco use and colon cancer. *Int. J. Cancer*, **70** (1997) 259–264.

134. Hsing AW, McLaughlin JK, Chow W-H, et al. Risk factors for colorectal cancer in a prospective study among U.S. white men. *Int. J. Cancer*, **77** (1998) 549–553.
135. Knekt P, Hakama M, Järvinen R, Pukkala E, and Heliövaara M. Smoking and risk of colorectal cancer. *Br. J. Cancer*, **78** (1998) 136–139.
136. Le Marchand L, Wilkens LR, Kolonel LN, Hankin JH, and Lyu L-C. Associations of sedentary lifestyle, obesity, smoking, alcohol use, and diabetes with the risk of colorectal cancer. *Cancer Res.*, **57** (1997) 4787–4794.
137. Yamada K, Araki S, Tamura M, et al. Case-control study of colorectal carcinoma *in situ* and cancer in relation to cigarette smoking and alcohol use (Japan). *Cancer Causes Control*, **8** (1997) 780–785.
138. Chyou P-H, Nomura AMY, and Stemmermann GN. A prospective study of colon and rectal cancer among Hawaii Japanese men. *Ann. Epidemiol.*, **6** (1996) 276–282.
139. Freedman AN, Michalek AM, Marshall JR, et al. The relationship between smoking exposure and p53 overexpression in colorectal cancer. *Genet. Epidemiol.*, **12** (1995) 333.
140. Baron JA, Gerhardsson de Verdier M, and Ekbom A. Coffee, tea, tobacco, and cancer of the large bowel. *Cancer Epidemiol. Biomarkers Prev.*, **3** (1994) 565–570.
141. Nordlund LA, Carstensen JM, and Pershagen G. Cancer incidence in female smokers: a 26-year follow-up. *Int. J. Cancer*, **73** (1997) 625–628.
142. Nyrén O, Bergström R, Nyström L, et al. Smoking and colorectal cancer: a 20-year follow-up study of Swedish construction workers. *J. Natl. Cancer Inst.*, **88** (1996) 1302–1307.
143. Tavani A, Pregnolato A, La Vecchia C, Negri E, Talamini R, and Franceschi S. Coffee and tea intake and risk of cancers of the colon and rectum: a study of 3,530 cases and 7,057 controls. *Int. J. Cancer*, **73** (1997) 193–197.
144. Fernandez-Martos C, Llombart-Cussaic A, Dasi F, et al. Cigarette smoking, colorectal neoplasia, APC and K-*ras* mutations in men. *Proc. Am. Soc. Clin. Oncol.*, **19** (2000) 249a.
145. Slattery ML, Curtin K, Anderson K, et al. Associations between cigarette smoking, lifestyle factors, and microsatellite instability in colon tumors. *J. Natl. Cancer Inst.*, **92** (2000) 1831–1836.
146. Lee IM, Paffenbarger RS Jr., Hsieh CC. Physical activity and risk of developing colorectal cancer among college alumni. *J. Natl. Cancer Inst.*, **83** (1991) 1324–1329.
147. Giovannucci E, Ascherio A, Rimm EB, Colditz GA, Stampfer MJ, and Willett WC. Physical activity, obesity, and risk for colon cancer and adenoma in men. *Ann. Intern. Med.*, **122** (1995) 327–334.
148. Lew EA and Garfinkel L. Variations in mortality by weight among 750,000 men and women. *J. Chronic Dis.*, **32** (1979) 563–576.
149. Waaler HT. Height, weight and mortality. The Norwegian experience. *Acta Med. Scand.*, **679(Suppl.)** (1984) 1–56.
150. Phillips RL and Snowdon DA. Dietary relationships with fatal colorectal cancer among Seventh-Day Adventists. *J. Natl. Cancer Inst.*, **74** (1985) 307–317.
151. Klatsky AL, Armstrong MA, Friedman GD, and Hiatt RA. The relations of alcoholic beverage use to colon and rectal cancer. *Am. J. Epidemiol.*, **128** (1988) 1007–1015.
152. Must A, Jacques PF, Dallal GE, Bajema CJ, and Dietz WH. Long-term morbidity and mortality of overweight adolescents. A follow-up of the Harvard Growth Study of 1922 to 1935. *N. Engl. J. Med.*, **327** (1992) 1350–1355.
153. Le Marchand L, Wilkins LR, and Mi MP. Obesity in youth and middle age and risk of colorectal cancer in men. *Cancer Causes Control*, **3** (1992) 349–354.
154. Chute CG, Willett WC, Colditz GA, Stampfer MJ, Rosner B, and Speizer FE. A prospective study of reproductive history and exogenous estrogens on the risk of colorectal cancer in women. *Epidemiology*, **2** (1991) 201–207.
155. Martinez ME, Giovannucci E, Spiegelman D, et al. Physical activity, body size, and colorectal cancer in women. *Am. J. Epidemiol.*, **143** (1996) S73.
156. Whittemore AS, Wu-Williams AH, Lee M, et al. Diet, physical activity and colorectal cancer among Chinese in North America and China. *J. Natl. Cancer Inst.*, **82** (1990) 915–926.
157. Kune G, Kune S, and Wason L. Body weight and physical activity as predictors of colorectal cancer risk. *Nutr. Cancer*, **13** (1990) 9–17.
158. Graham S, Marshall J, Haughey B, et al. Dietary epidemiology of cancer of the colon in western New York. *Am. J. Epidemiol.*, **128** (1988) 490–503.
159. West DW, Slattery ML, Robison LM, et al. Dietary intake and colon cancer: sex- and anatomic site-specific associations. *Am. J. Epidemiol.*, **130** (1989) 883–894.
160. Dietz AT, Newcomb PA, Marcus PM, and Strer BE. The association of body size and large bowel cancer risk in Wisconsin (United States) women. *Cancer Causes Control*, **6** (1995) 30–36.

161. Martinez ME, Giovannucci E, Spiegelman D, Hunter DJ, Willett WC, and Colditz GA. Leisure-time physical activity, body size, and colon cancer in women. Nurses' Health Study Research Group. *J. Natl. Cancer Inst.*, **89** (1997) 948–955.

162. Giovannucci E, Colditz GA, Stampfer MJ, and Willett WC. Physical activity, obesity, and risk of colorectal adenoma in women (United States). *Cancer Causes Control*, **7** (1996) 253–263.

163. Martinez ME, Giovannucci E, Spiegelman D, Hunter DJ, Willett WC, and Colditz GA. Leisure-time physical activity, body size, and colon cancer in women. Nurses' Health Study Research Group. *J. Natl. Cancer Inst.*, **89** (1997) 948–955.

164. Thun MJ, Calle EE, Namboodiri MM, et al. Risk factors for fatal colon cancer in a large prospective study. *J. Natl. Cancer Inst.*, **84** (1992) 1491–1500.

165. Ballard-Barbash R, Schatzkin A, Albanes D, et al. Physical activity and risk of large bowel cancer in the Framingham Study. *Cancer Res.*, **50** (1990) 3610–3613.

166. Albanes D, Blair A, and Taylor PR. Physical activity and risk of cancer in the NHANES I population. *Am. J. Public Health*, **79** (1989) 744–750.

167. Severson RK, Nomura AMY, Grove JS, and Stemmermann GN. A prospective analysis of physical activity and cancer. *Am. J. Epidemiol.*, **130** (1989) 522–529.

168. Lynge E and Thygesen L. Use of surveillance systems for occupational cancer: data from the Danish national system. *Int. J. Epidemiol.*, **17** (1988) 493–500.

169. Gerhardsson M, Floderus B, and Norell SE. Physical activity and colon cancer risk. *Int. J. Epidemiol.*, **17** (1988) 743–746.

170. Paffenbarger RSJ, Hyde RT, and Wing AL. Physical activity and incidence of cancer in diverse populations: a preliminary report. *Am. J. Clin. Nutr.*, **45(Suppl)** (1987) 312–317.

171. Gerhardsson M, Norell SE, Kiviranta H, Pedersen NL, and Ahlbom A. Sedentary jobs and colon cancer. *Am. J. Epidemiol.*, **123** (1986) 775–780.

172. Markowitz S, Morabia A, Garibaldi K, and Wynder E. Effect of occupational and recreational activity on the risk of colorectal cancer among males: a case-control study. *Int. J. Epidemiol.*, **21** (1992) 1057–1062.

173. Slattery ML, Schumacher MC, Smith KR, West DW, and Abd-Elghany N. Physical activity, diet, and risk of colon cancer in Utah. *Am. J. Epidemiol.*, **128** (1988) 989–999.

174. Peters RK, Garabrant DH, Yu MC, and Mack TM. A case-control study of occupational and dietary factors in colorectal cancer in young men by subsite. *Cancer Res.*, **49** (1989) 5459–5468.

175. Brownson RC, Zahm SH, Chang JC, and Blair A. Occupational risk of colon cancer. An analysis of anatomic subsite. *Am. J. Epidemiol.*, **130** (1989) 675–687.

176. Benito E, Obrador A, Stiggelbout A, et al. A population-based case-control study of colorectal cancer in Majorca. I. Dietary factors. *Int. J. Cancer*, **45** (1990) 69–76.

177. Kato I, Tominaga S, and Ikari A. A case-control study of male colorectal cancer in Aichi Prefecture, Japan: with special reference to occupational activity level, drinking habits and family history. *Jpn. J. Cancer Res.*, **81** (1990) 115–121.

178. Gerhardsson de Verdier M, Hagman U, Steineck G, Rieger A, and Norell SE. Diet, body mass and colorectal cancer: a case-referent study in Stockholm. *Int. J. Cancer*, **46** (1990) 832–838.

179. Fredriksson M, Bengtsson NO, Hardell L, and Axelson O. Colon cancer, physical activity, and occupational exposures. A case-control study. *Cancer*, **63** (1989) 1838–1842.

180. Fraser G and Pearce N. Occupational physical activity and risk of cancer of the colon and rectum in New Zealand males. *Cancer Causes Control*, **4** (1993) 45–50.

181. Longnecker MP, Gerhardsson de Verdier M, Frumkin H, and Carpenter C. A case-control study of physical activity in relation to risk of cancer of the right colon and rectum in men. *Int. J. Epidemiol.*, **24** (1995) 42–50.

182. Vena JE, Graham S, Zielezny M, Swanson MK, Barnes RE, and Nolan J. Lifetime occupational exercise and colon cancer. *Am. J. Epidemiol.*, **122** (1985) 357–365.

183. Garabrant DH, Peters JM, Mack TM, and Berstein L. Job activity and colon cancer risk. *Am. J. Epidemiol.*, **119** (1984) 1005–1014.

184. Giovannucci E, Ascherio A, Rimm EB, Colditz GA, Stampfer MJ, and Willett WC. Physical activity, obesity, and risk for colon cancer and adenoma in men. *Ann. Intern. Med.*, **122** (1995) 327–334.

185. Slattery ML, Potter J, Caan B, et al. Energy balance and colon cancer—beyond physical activity. *Cancer Res.*, **57** (1997) 75–80.

186. Colditz G, Cannuscio C, and Frazier A. Physical activity and reduced risk of colon cancer: implications for prevention. *Cancer Causes Control*, **8** (1997) 649–667.

187. Bartram HP and Wynder EL. Physical activity and colon cancer risk? Physiological considerations. *Am. J. Gastroenterol.*, **84** (1989) 109–112.

188. Martinez ME, Heddens D, Earnest DL, et al. Physical activity, body mass index, and prostaglandin E2 levels in rectal mucosa. *J. Natl. Cancer Inst.*, **91** (1999) 950–953.

189. Giovannucci E. Insulin and colon cancer. *Cancer Causes Control*, **6** (1995) 164–179.

190. Tran TT, Medline A, and Bruce R. Insulin promotion of colon tumors in rats. *Cancer Epidemiol. Biomarkers Prev.*, **5** (1996) 1013–1015.

191. Schoen RE, Tangen CM, Kuller LH, et al. Increased blood glucose and insulin, body size, and incident colorectal cancer. *J. Natl. Cancer Inst.*, **91** (1999) 1147–1154.

192. Hu FB, Manson JE, Liu S, et al. Prospective study of adult onset diabetes mellitus (Type 2) and risk of colorectal cancer in women. *J. Natl. Cancer Inst.*, **91** (1999) 542–547.

193. Aaronson S. Growth factors and cancer. *Science*, **254** (1991) 1146–1153.

194. Rechler M. Growth inhibition by insulin-like growth factor (IGF) binding protein-3—what's IGF got to do with it? *Endocrinology*, **138** (1997) 2645–2647.

195. Rajah R, Valentinis B, and Cohen P. Insulin-like growth factor (IGF)-binding protein-3 induces apoptosis and mediates the effects of transforming growth factor-β1 on programmed cell death through a p53 and IGF-independent mechanism. *J. Biol. Chem.*, **272** (1997) 12,181–12,188.

196. Giovannucci E, Pollak MN, Platz EA, et al. Plasma insulin-like growth factor-1 and binding protein-3 and risk of colorectal cancer and adenoma in women. American Association for Cancer Research 90th Annual Meeting Proceedings, Philadelphia, 1999, Vol. 40 (abstract).

197. Martinez ME, Maltzman T, Marshall JR, et al. Risk factors for Ki-ras protooncogene mutation in sporadic colorectal adenomas. *Cancer Res.*, **59** (1999) 5181–5185.

4

Screening and Surveillance

Arnold J. Markowitz

1. INTRODUCTION

The cumulative lifetime risk of developing colorectal cancer for men and women in the United States is about 6% *(1)*. In 2001, colorectal cancer is expected to be the fourth most common cause of cancer, accounting for over 135,000 new cases, and the second most common cause of cancer death, resulting in approx 57,000 deaths, among Americans *(1)*. The detection of early-stage disease at diagnosis is associated with significantly improved survival, with a 5-yr survival rate of greater than 90% for those with localized disease *(2)*.

Routine screening of asymptomatic individuals in the general population will lead to a reduction in the incidence and mortality of colorectal cancer. The colonoscopic removal of adenomatous colorectal polyps, its premalignant precursor lesion, has been demonstrated to reduce the incidence of developing colorectal cancer *(3)* (Fig. 1).

Early detection and endoscopic polypectomy can prevent the development of colorectal cancer. Recommendations for screening and surveillance for colorectal cancer are based on the individual's risk for the development of this disease. This chapter will review currently recommended screening and surveillance guidelines based on individual risk stratification for those at average risk and increased risk, including those at particularly high risk as a result of underlying hereditary predisposition syndromes.

2. AVERAGE RISK

Average-risk individuals are asymptomatic men and women over age 50 with no personal history of colorectal cancer or adenomatous polyps, no history of inflammatory bowel disease (ulcerative or Crohn's colitis), or a family history of colorectal cancer or adenomatous polyps.

From: *Colorectal Cancer: Multimodality Management*
Edited by: L. Saltz © Humana Press Inc., Totowa, NJ

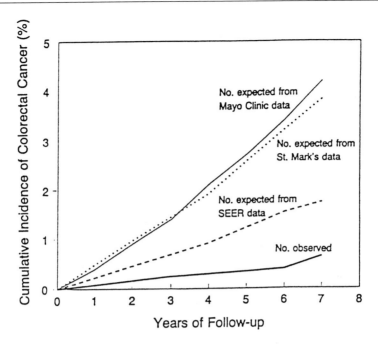

Fig. 1. Cumulative incidence of colorectal cancer in the National Polyp Study Cohort. The observed incidence is compared with the expected incidence based on data from the three reference groups: the Mayo Clinic cohort (US), the St. Mark's cohort (UK), and the SEER Program (US) *(4–6)*. (From ref. *3*, with permission.)

2.1. Evidence for Screening Tests

2.1.1. FECAL OCCULT BLOOD TEST

There are three prospective, randomized, controlled trials, from Minnesota *(7)*, the United Kingdom *(8)*, and Denmark *(9)*, that have demonstrated the effectiveness of fecal occult blood testing in reducing colorectal cancer mortality (Table 1). The British and Danish studies were population-based trials. A prospective, nonrandomized, controlled study from New York also demonstrated a benefit from stool blood testing *(10)*. There are also two retrospective, case-control studies from northern California and Germany that have provided additional evidence to support the effectiveness of fecal occult blood testing *(11,12)*. Furthermore, the Minnesota group recently demonstrated that fecal occult blood testing also reduces the incidence of colorectal cancer *(13)*.

2.1.2. SIGMOIDOSCOPY

The current evidence for sigmoidoscopy is provided by two retrospective, case-control studies that demonstrated a significant reduction in rectosigmoid cancer mortality. A study from northern California *(14)* found that only 8.8% of 261 case patients had had a screening rigid sigmoidoscopy during the 10-yr period prior to their diagnosis of rectosigmoid cancer, as compared to 24.2% of the 868 matched controls (odds ratio = 0.41; 95% confidence interval [CI] = 0.25–0.69). This study demonstrated a 59% reduction in rectosigmoid cancer mortality and that this risk-reduction benefit continued for 10 yr after a single screening examination. A second, smaller, retrospective, case-control study from Wisconsin *(15)* provided additional support for screening sigmoidoscopy, demonstrating an 80% reduction

Table 1
Prospective Controlled Trials of Fecal Occult Blood Testing

Study	Year	N	Duration of follow-up	Mortality reduction
Minnesota (Mandel et al.) *(7)*	1993	46,551	13 yr	33%
United Kingdom (Hardcastle et al.) *(8)*	1996	152,850	7.8 yr	15%
Denmark (Kronborg et al.) *(9)*	1996	140,000	10 yr	18%

in rectosigmoid cancer (odds ratio = 0.21; 95% CI = 0.08–0.52) in patients who had had a single preceding screening sigmoidoscopy examination.

Currently, two prospective screening sigmoidoscopy trials of are actively in progress. In the United States, flexible sigmoidoscopy is being evaluated in the colorectal component of the National Cancer Institute-sponsored Prostate, Lung, Colorectal, and Ovarian (PLCO) screening trial *(16)*. In the United Kingdom, there is an active screening trial specifically designed to assess the efficacy of a once-only sigmoidoscopy examination *(17)*.

2.1.3. COLONOSCOPY

Although there is no prospective randomized, controlled data to demonstrate that screening colonoscopy can reduce colorectal cancer mortality or incidence in average-risk individuals, there is substantial indirect evidence to suggest that this test is an effective screening modality; thus, it is currently endorsed by the American Cancer Society and several major US gastroenterology and colorectal surgery societies as a screening option in this patient population *(18–20)*.

Colonoscopy offers several significant advantages over other available screening tests. Colonoscopy is very sensitive for the detection of small and large adenomas, in contrast to fecal occult blood testing, which has a low sensitivity for the detection of small adenomas. Colonoscopy provides a complete examination of the colon and rectum, whereas sigmoidoscopy, at best, generally examines only the distal third of the large bowel. Colonoscopy also provides the opportunity for the removal of adenomas and biopsy of suspicious mass lesions.

Indirect evidence for the effectiveness of screening colonoscopy in average-risk individuals can be extrapolated from the randomized and nonrandomized controlled screening trials of fecal occult blood testing, in which colonoscopy was used to evaluate those patients who tested positive for occult blood, that demonstrated a reduction in colorectal cancer mortality in this population. In addition, colonoscopy is similar in both performance and effectiveness to sigmoidoscopy, a screening test that has been demonstrated to reduce rectosigmoid cancer mortality. Furthermore, colonoscopy offers the potential for colonoscopic polypectomy and, as demonstrated by the US National Polyp Study (NPS), the removal of adenomas detected at colonoscopy decreases the incidence of colorectal cancer *(3)* (Fig. 1).

There are now multiple published reports in the literature regarding the utility of screening colonoscopy in asymptomatic individuals. A recent large multicenter US Veterans Administration cooperative trial described the findings of a screening colonoscopy in 3196 asymptomatic individuals (97% men) between the ages of 50 and 75 (mean age = 62.9) *(21)*.

Of note, however, fecal occult blood testing was not reported and the study included some increased-risk individuals with a positive family history of colorectal cancer. One or more colorectal neoplasms were detected in 37.5% of patients in this cohort. An adenoma that was large, 1 cm or more, and/or demonstrated villous histology was detected in 7.9% of patients, an adenoma with severe dysplasia in 1.6%, and an invasive cancer in 1.0%. In addition, in 48 of the 1765 patients (2.7%) who had no polyps in the distal colon (beyond the splenic flexure), an advanced neoplasm (large adenoma, 1 cm or more, villous histology, severe dysplasia, or invasive cancer) was detected in the proximal colon. Furthermore, 52% of the 128 patients that had a proximal advanced neoplasm had no distal adenomas, thus demonstrating significant proximal colon neoplasia that would likely have gone undetected following a negative flexible sigmoidoscopy examination. Similar findings from another large study of 1994 asymptomatic men and women, age 50 or older, who underwent a screening colonoscopy, as part of an employer-sponsored screening program offered by their company, demonstrated that colonoscopy detected a considerable number of advanced proximal colon neoplasms that would not have been detected by flexible sigmoidoscopy *(22)*.

In addition, the CONCERN Trial is presently evaluating the efficacy of screening colonoscopy in average-risk, asymptomatic women at US Regional Navy/Army Medical Centers. Furthermore, a prospective, randomized, national screening colonoscopy trial designed to investigate whether the performance of a single screening colonoscopy would be effective in decreasing the incidence and mortality of colorectal cancer in the average-risk general population, between the ages of 50 and 64, is actively being organized and its pilot feasibility trial is currently underway.

2.1.4. DOUBLE-CONTRAST BARIUM ENEMA

There are no studies that directly evaluate the effectiveness of double-contrast barium enema (DCBE) to screen for colorectal cancer in the average-risk population. As compared to colonoscopy, DCBE has several significant drawbacks as a screening modality. DCBE is not as sensitive for detecting small or flat lesions. It may misinterpret retained stool as a false-positive result. Also, DCBE does not allow for the possible removal of polyps or diagnostic biopsies. Furthermore, because the rectal balloon used in the barium enema exam limits visualization of the distal rectum, a flexible sigmoidoscopy should also be performed to avoid missing a potential distal rectal neoplasm.

Several DCBE studies report sensitivity rates in the range of 50–80% for detecting small polyps, <1 cm, 70–90% for large polyps, >1 cm, and 55–85% for early stage (Dukes A and B) cancers *(23–26)*. Reported false-positive rates, as a result of retained stool and/or non-neoplastic mucosal irregularities, range from about 50% for small polyps *(26)*, 5–10% for large polyps, and less than 1% for cancers *(26–28)*.

Nonetheless, because DCBE evaluates the entire colon and will likely detect most clinically significant neoplastic lesions, it may be considered as an alternative screening option in asymptomatic average-risk individuals who are unable or unwilling to undergo colonoscopy.

3. INCREASED RISK

3.1. Risk Factors

Risk factors associated with an increased risk for colorectal cancer include age greater than 50, a personal or family history of colorectal cancer or adenoma, and a personal history of long-standing inflammatory bowel disease (ulcerative colitis and Crohn's colitis). Very

Table 2
Factors Associated with Increased Risk of Colorectal Cancer

Increased risk
    Age greater than 50 yr
    Prior colorectal cancer or adenomatous polyp
    Family history of colorectal cancer or adenomatous polyp
    Long-standing inflammatory bowel disease (ulcerative or Crohn's colitis)
High risk
    Hereditary nonpolyposis colorectal cancer syndrome (HNPCC)
    Familial adenomatous polyposis syndrome (FAP)
    Gardner's syndrome (GS)
    Turcot's syndrome (TS)
    Peutz–Jeghers syndrome (PJS)
    Familial juvenile polyposis (FJP)

high-risk individuals include those with an underlying genetic predisposition as a result of an hereditary polyposis or nonpolyposis syndrome (Table 2).

3.1.1. HISTORY OF COLORECTAL ADENOMA

Adenomas are the most common type of polyp detected at colonoscopy. In the National Polyp Study (NPS), 68% of the polyps removed at the initial colonoscopy examination were adenomas, whereas the remainder included hyperplastic (11%) and other non-neoplastic polyps (29). Several colonoscopy studies have demonstrated that greater than 60% of adenomas are located distal to the splenic flexure (29,30). It is not unusual for patients to have synchronous adenomas. In one colonoscopy study, 60% of patients in whom an adenoma was detected had a single adenoma, whereas 40% had multiple polyps (31). Increased age is associated with an increased risk of multiple synchronous adenomas (32).

The precise time-course of the adenoma to carcinoma pathway is not certain. However, through indirect evidence, it appears to be a relatively slow process that, in most cases, occurs over many years. Data from both the NPS (33) and the St. Mark's Hospital study (34), which described the long-term observation of unresected colorectal adenomas, support an average time-course of about 10–15 yr for the progression from a small adenoma to a cancer.

In hereditary nonpolyposis colorectal cancer (HNPCC) syndrome, however, there is some suggestion that adenomas may progress to cancer over a shorter time interval than that seen in common sporadic colorectal cancers (35,36). The study from the Netherlands (35) reported an unexpectedly high incidence of advanced colorectal cancers detected within 3.5 yr after a negative screening examination (colonoscopy or barium enema) in a large number of HNPCC patients who participated in a national screening program. These findings suggest that HNPCC tumors may demonstrate an accelerated adenoma to carcinoma sequence.

3.1.2. FAMILY HISTORY OF COLORECTAL CANCER OR ADENOMA

Familial factors are associated with a significant proportion of colorectal cancer cases (Fig. 2). In the general population, approx 10% of individuals have a first-degree relative (FDR) who has been affected with colorectal cancer, which increases their relative risk of developing a colorectal cancer by twofold to threefold (37). Furthermore, such an individual's risk is even greater if the patient has more than one affected FDR or if the affected relative

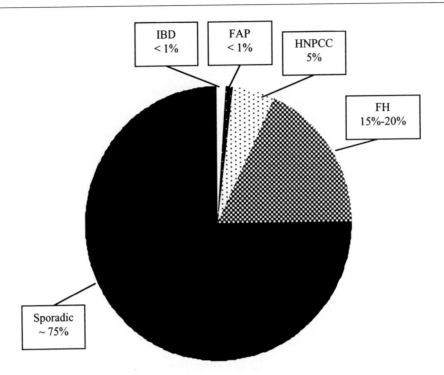

Fig. 2. Factors associated with new cases of colorectal cancer. Sporadic = average-risk individuals age 50 or greater; IBD = inflammatory bowel disease; FAP = familial adenomatous polyposis; HNPCC = hereditary nonpolyposis colorectal cancer; FH = family history of colorectal cancer.

was diagnosed at a young age. In fact, if one encounters a patient with two or more affected FDRs or one with an affected relative diagnosed less than 40 yr of age, one should consider the possibility of an underlying hereditary syndrome in that patient's family. Recently, the NPS demonstrated that an individual's risk of colorectal cancer is also increased if the patient has a FDR (sibling or child) who has had an adenoma, especially if the adenoma was diagnosed prior to age 60 *(38)*.

3.1.3. HISTORY OF INFLAMMATORY BOWEL DISEASE

A long-standing history of ulcerative colitis is associated with an increased risk for colorectal cancer, and its cumulative incidence is increased relative to the duration and anatomic extent of the disease. The risk of cancer appears to begin after about 8–10 yr of disease, and thereafter the cancer risk increases at a rate of about 0.5–1.0% per year. The risk of cancer is greatest in those with pan-colitis, which is typically defined as disease involvement extending proximal to the splenic flexure *(39–50)*.

A review of surveillance colonoscopy trials in patients with chronic ulcerative colitis reported that 15% of patients had dysplasia and 20% of these were subsequently found to have colon cancer *(51)*. One percent of patients had a diagnosis of cancer made by direct mucosal biopsy; however, of concern, 10% of those with cancer did not have dysplasia in any of their biopsies. One study has reported a reduction in colon cancer mortality as a result of colonoscopic screening and biopsy for dysplasia *(52)*.

The risk of colorectal cancer is also increased in long-standing Crohn's colitis, and, until recently, it has remained underappreciated. In fact, the increased risk of cancer is equivalent for both Crohn's and ulcerative colitis of similar duration and anatomic extent *(53–55)*.

3.1.4. History of Colorectal Cancer

Individuals with a history of colorectal cancer are at increased risk for both synchronous and metachronous neoplastic lesions. In patients with a colorectal malignancy, the rate for a synchronous colorectal cancer is 2–6%, and for an adenoma, it is 25–40% (56,57). After curative resection, reported rates of subsequent metachronous cancer are 3–8% and adenoma 25–40% (58,59). However, published rates of metachronous colorectal cancer in these patients are from precolonoscopy era data, whereas now, with colonoscopic clearance of adenomas, it is uncommon to find a metachronous primary colorectal cancer.

The primary goal of postsurgical surveillance is to clear the colon of potentially missed synchronous and subsequent new metachronous adenomas. There is no evidence that there is a more rapid progression along the adenoma to carcinoma sequence in patients with a history of colorectal cancer; thus, once the colon has been cleared of synchronous neoplastic lesions, the surveillance interval can be every 3 yr. However, no prospective, controlled, randomized trials have yet been performed to address the issue of appropriate surveillance intervals after curative resection of colorectal cancer.

3.2. Hereditary Colorectal Cancer Syndromes

Of the cases of colorectal cancer newly diagnosed each year in the United States, only a small percentage are accounted for by rare inherited colorectal cancer syndromes (Fig. 2). These syndromes are commonly classified into hereditary polyposis and nonpolyposis syndromes (Table 2). Families associated with these syndromes carry a particularly high risk for the development of colorectal cancer.

3.2.1. Familial Adenomatous Polyposis and Gardner's Syndrome

Familial adenomatous polyposis (FAP) is an autosomal dominant disorder characterized by the progressive development of hundreds to thousands of colorectal adenomas. FAP accounts for about 1% of all cases of colorectal cancer. Affected patients have a germline mutation in the adenomatous polyposis coli (APC) gene on chromosome 5 (60–63). Adenomas typically begin to present early in the second decade of life. If the colon is left intact, colorectal cancer will inevitably occur by the fourth to fifth decade of life. The average age of cancer occurrence is 39 yr. This syndrome is present in approx 1 in every 8000 births.

Gardner's syndrome (GS), a variant of FAP, is characterized by colorectal adenomas and extraintestinal manifestations, including osteomas, particularly of the mandible and skull, soft tissue tumors such as lipomas, fibromas, and epidermoid and sebaceous cysts, supernumerary teeth, desmoid tumors, mesenteric fibromatosis, and congenital hypertrophy of the retinal pigmentation epithelium (CHRPE). Thyroid cancers and adrenal adenomas and cancers have also been associated with this syndrome. Turcot's syndrome, another variant of FAP, is characterized by colorectal adenomas and brain tumors.

An "attenuated" form of FAP has been described in which affected family members express only a few colonic adenomas, even at an age where complete expression of the colonic phenotype would have been expected. Attenuated FAP has been related to specific mutations in the APC gene. Thus, it appears that occasional variability of expression occurs even with FAP.

3.2.2. Peutz–Jeghers Syndrome

The Peutz–Jeghers syndrome (PJS) is an autosomal dominant inherited disorder characterized by multiple gastrointestinal hamartomatous polyps and mucocutaneous melanin pigmentation (64). The gene responsible for PJS was recently identified on chromosome 19p (65,66).

A review of the Johns Hopkins Polyposis Registry showed that the relative risk of a PJS patient developing a cancer was 18 times greater than expected in the general population *(67)*. A review of the St. Mark's Polyposis Registry found that 22% developed cancer and that the relative risk of death from gastrointestinal cancer was 13, and from all cancers, it was 9 *(68)*.

3.2.3. FAMILIAL JUVENILE POLYPOSIS SYNDROME

Familial juvenile polyposis (FJP) syndrome is an autosomal dominant condition that is characterized by multiple juvenile polyps, ranging in number from 25 to 40 or more, located throughout the gastrointestinal tract *(69–71)*. Extraintestinal congenital abnormalities may also occur. Patients commonly present during childhood with anemia caused by chronic gastrointestinal blood loss, crampy abdominal pain, recurrent intussusceptions, or rectal bleeding.

Although the juvenile polyps found in FJP are typically benign, affected patients are now recognized to have an increased risk of colorectal cancer of at least 9% *(72)* and perhaps even much higher *(73)*. The mean age of cancer onset is 40 yr. Unaffected family members are also thought to have an increased risk for colorectal cancer *(72)*.

3.2.4. HEREDITARY NONPOLYPOSIS COLORECTAL CANCER SYNDROME

Hereditary nonpolyposis colorectal cancer (HNPCC) is an autosomal dominantly inherited disorder in which affected patients develop small numbers of colorectal adenomas and are at increased risk for colorectal cancer. HNPCC accounts for about 5% of all cases of colorectal cancer.

The diagnosis of HNPCC has been primarily based on family history. The Amsterdam criteria define an HNPCC family as one in which three or more close relatives, one being a first-degree relative of the other two, from two or more generations, are affected with colorectal cancer, with at least one cancer diagnosed before age 50, in the absence of gastrointestinal polyposis *(74)*.

The HNPCC patients are at increased risk for early-onset colorectal cancer, at an average age of diagnosis of 40–45 yr. The colon cancers are predominantly right sided, with 60–70% proximal to the splenic flexure. Patients often present with multiple primary colon cancers and are at increased risk for metachronous cancers. HNPCC is also associated with extracolonic cancers of the endometrium, ovary, stomach, small intestine, renal pelvis and ureter (transitional cell cancer), and the pancreaticobiliary system *(75)*. In fact, a newly updated set of Amsterdam criteria were recently published that include associated extracolonic malignancies in the clinical definition of this syndrome *(76)*.

Germline mutations have been identified in five DNA mismatch repair genes in HNPCC patients, including *hMSH2* on chromosome 2p16, *hMLH1* on chromosome 3p21, *hPMS1* on chromosome 2q31–33, *hPMS2* on chromosome 7p22, and *hMSH6* (GTBP) on chromosome 2p16 *(77–81)*. Mutations in these genes result in genomic instability in these patients. Gene testing for HNPCC is currently available.

A long-term Finnish study evaluated the effectiveness of screening in HNPCC patients and their families *(82)*. This trial compared a group of 251 at-risk individuals from 22 HNPCC families who had screening examinations (colonoscopy or flexible sigmoidoscopy and barium enema) every 3 yr to a control group who had no screening, and it demonstrated a significant reduction in incidence ($p = 0.03$) and a reduction in mortality ($p = 0.08$) of colorectal cancer in the screened group. The reduction in colon cancer risk was likely the result of the colonoscopic removal of adenomas. Preliminary data from Memorial

Sloan–Kettering on long-term follow-up of a smaller group of patients at high risk for HNPCC showed that screening colonoscopy reduced the incidence of colorectal cancer to a rate close to that of the unscreened general population *(83)*.

4. COLORECTAL CANCER SCREENING AND SURVEILLANCE GUIDELINES

The initial approach to colorectal cancer screening relies on a thorough risk assessment of the patient. Asymptomatic average-risk individuals are candidates for routine screening, whereas those at increased risk as a result of a personal or family history of colorectal cancer or adenoma, inflammatory bowel disease, or a hereditary colon cancer syndrome are at high risk and require individualized risk-specific recommendations for screening and surveillance.

4.1. Average-Risk Guidelines

Average-risk men and women should begin routine colorectal cancer screening at age 50. Several average-risk screening options are currently recommended *(18–20)*.

The standard option includes a stool occult blood test annually and a flexible sigmoidoscopy every 5 yr. With this screening approach, if a positive stool blood test is detected, the patient should undergo a complete colon evaluation by colonoscopy. Colonoscopy provides the opportunity for direct visualization of the colon and allows for polypectomy or biopsy of suspicious lesions that may be detected.

Furthermore, if a small benign-appearing polyp is detected during a routine screening sigmoidoscopy, a biopsy is taken and further management depends on the histological assessment of the polyp. If the polyp is an adenoma, then a colonoscopy should be scheduled to perform polypectomy and assess the more proximal colon for potential synchronous neoplastic lesions. In contrast, if the polyp is a benign hyperplastic polyp, no additional tests are necessary. If, however, on screening sigmoidoscopy, either a large polyp or multiple polyps are detected, then a biopsy is not necessary and the patient should be scheduled directly for colonoscopy and polypectomy.

A second approach to screening the average-risk individual is the choice of a complete colorectal evaluation by colonoscopy, which can be repeated at 10-yr intervals if negative for neoplasia. Although there are currently no prospective randomized trials to support the effectiveness of this option, it is currently believed that the indirect evidence of its benefits and effectiveness support it as an appropriate screening option for this population *(18–20)*.

A third, although less desirable and also unsupported, screening option in this population would be a DCBE, plus flexible sigmoidoscopy, every 5–10 yr. Any positive test should be followed up by a colonoscopy.

4.2. Increased-Risk Guidelines

4.2.1. HISTORY OF COLORECTAL ADENOMA

Colonoscopy is the preferred surveillance examination in patients who have had a colorectal adenoma removed in the past *(18,20,84)*. The recurrence rate of adenomas in patients after initial polypectomy is high enough to justify periodic follow-up. Ideally, all synchronous adenomas are removed at the time of the initial polypectomy. However, the frequency of missed synchronous lesions, primarily small and tubular, has been suggested to be in the range of 10–15% *(24)*. A surveillance program should, therefore, offer the opportunity to find these potentially missed neoplastic lesions and new metachronous adenomas, yet it must be designed to protect the patient from the risk and cost of unnecessary or too frequent examinations.

The patient's colon must be cleared of all adenomas prior to embarking on routine long-term surveillance follow-up. Based on findings of the NPS, after removal of a colorectal adenoma, a repeat examination can be performed in 3 yr for most patients *(85)*. A shorter follow-up interval may be necessary after removal of multiple adenomas, excision of an adenoma with invasive cancer, incomplete or piecemeal removal of a large sessile adenoma, or a suboptimal examination because of a poor colonic preparation. Longer intervals may be appropriate for patients with a single, small, tubular adenoma.

New data suggest that longer intervals between follow-up surveillance examinations may be appropriate for the management of patients after polypectomy *(86)*. In fact, after colonoscopic polypectomy of an adenoma, if the 3-yr follow-up examination is negative, the surveillance interval can be increased to every 5 yr. Individual considerations such as significant medical comorbidities or pathological predictive factors will also affect the decision regarding continued follow-up.

Following complete colonoscopic removal of an adenoma with invasive cancer ("malignant polyp"), judged by combined gross endoscopic and histological grounds, most endoscopists perform a repeat examination in 3–6 mo, and then again at 1 yr, before reverting back to 3-yr follow-up intervals. Surgical resection is indicated if the polyp has cancer invading close to the cautery margin, demonstrates lymphatic or blood vessel invasion, or is poorly differentiated.

4.2.2. Family History of Colorectal Cancer or Adenoma

Individuals who have one or two FDRs who have been affected with colorectal cancer or adenomas are at increased risk. These patients should undergo screening of their entire large bowel beginning at 40 yr of age, or, if earlier, 10 yr younger than the earliest diagnosed cancer in their affected family member(s). Screening options include the same as those for average-risk individuals, but just beginning at an earlier age. However, the high lifetime probability of colorectal cancer in such families has led to the more aggressive option of colonoscopy, particularly in those families in which the affected FDR was diagnosed with cancer before the age of 55 or an adenoma before age 60.

For patients who have more than two FDRs affected with colon cancer and no history of a polyposis syndrome, one should consider a diagnosis of HNPCC and recommend screening guidelines as outlined for HNPCC, along with formal genetic counseling and possible gene testing. In addition, if a patient has a FDR affected with colon cancer at an age less than 40 yr, an inherited syndrome, such as one of the polyposes or HNPCC, should be suspected and shorter surveillance intervals and formal genetic counseling should be considered.

4.2.3. History of Inflammatory Bowel Disease

Patients with long-standing inflammatory bowel disease are at increased risk for colorectal cancer and should undergo routine surveillance examinations *(18,20)*. Because the cancer risk in chronic Crohn's colitis appears to be the same as that in ulcerative colitis, these patients should be approached similarly. In patients with pan-colitis, typically defined as disease extending proximal to the splenic flexure, surveillance colonoscopy should begin after 8 yr of symptoms. Whereas in patients with left-sided colitis, typically defined as disease involvement distal to the splenic flexure, colonoscopy may start after 12–15 yr of symptoms. The frequency of surveillance colonoscopy examinations should be every 1–2 yr.

At colonoscopy, mucosal biopsies should be routinely taken from grossly normal-appearing mucosa at 10- to 12-cm intervals throughout the colon. In addition, biopsies should also be taken from any areas of mucosal irregularity or plaquelike lesions. Expert pathological consultation should be obtained. If the biopsies are classified as negative or indefinite for dysplasia, surveillance should be continued at 1- to 2-yr intervals.

Colectomy is indicated for findings of confirmed unequivocal low-grade or high-grade dysplasia. In addition, colectomy should also be considered in patients with colitis that is difficult to control medically and in those patients who will not comply with surveillance.

4.2.4. Personal History of Colorectal Cancer

In patients who have recently undergone a curative resection for colorectal cancer, the entire colon should be cleared of any potential synchronous cancers or adenomas by colonoscopy. If this was not performed preoperatively or if this examination was suboptimal, then the first surveillance colonoscopy should be performed within 1 yr after resection. If this postoperative examination is normal, then subsequent follow-up surveillance colonoscopies can be performed at 3-yr intervals.

Routine surveillance follow-up in asymptomatic patients who have undergone curative resection for colorectal cancer should also include periodic outpatient visits with physical examinations every 3 mo within the first 2 yr postresection and then annually, serial digital rectal examinations and proctoscopies in those patients postresection of rectal cancer, annual chest X-rays, and serial serum CEA levels every 3 mo during the first 2 yr postresection and then annually *(87)*. The need for additional surveillance tests such as routine blood tests (complete blood count and liver chemistries) and computed tomography scans should decided on an individual basis for selected patients.

4.2.5. Hereditary Colorectal Cancer Syndromes

4.2.5.1. Familial Adenomatous Polyposis and Gardner's Syndrome. In FAP and GS families, routine colon screening for adenomatous polyposis should be performed by annual flexible sigmoidoscopy in all at-risk individuals beginning at about age 12 and may be decreased in frequency to every 3 yr after age 40. Genetic counseling and gene testing should also be offered to members of these families. Surveillance for gastric, duodenal, and periampullary adenomas should begin at the time of diagnosis of colonic polyposis and continue every 1–3 yr thereafter. At the time of routine upper gastrointestinal endoscopy, a side-viewing endoscope should also be used to assess the periampullary region of the duodenum and to provide optimal visualization of the major papilla (ampulla of Vater).

4.2.5.2. Peutz–Jeghers Syndrome and Familial Juvenile Polyposis Syndrome. In symptomatic patients with PJS or FJP, rectal bleeding or gastrointestinal symptoms require thorough evaluation. Presymptomatic screening in at-risk individuals should begin in the second decade of life and includes stool occult blood testing annually and flexible sigmoidoscopy every 3 yr. Once the diagnosis is made, surveillance endoscopic evaluation of the upper and lower gastrointestinal tract is indicted every 3–5 yr to remove any detected large, grossly abnormal, or bleeding polyps. A small bowel X-ray should be done at similar intervals.

4.2.5.3. Hereditary Nonpolyposis Colorectal Cancer. Colorectal screening in HNPCC patients should be performed by colonoscopy because of the increased incidence of proximal cancers and adenomas. At-risk individuals should have colonoscopy every 1–2 yr beginning at age 20. Additionally, special screening for extracolonic malignancies is recommended. HNPCC families should also be referred for genetic counseling and possible gene testing.

5. COST-EFFECTIVENESS AND INSURANCE COVERAGE

Despite the abundant evidence for the efficacy of screening and surveillance in reducing colorectal cancer incidence and mortality, relatively few individuals in the United States take advantage of these benefits. One significant part of the problem is that most health insurance plans do not recognize the potential benefits of tests for cancer prevention and therefore do not reimburse for the costs of these examinations. As of January 1998, however, a newly enacted US law now provides American citizens, at both average risk and high risk, with the benefit of Medicare coverage for routine colorectal cancer screening (included in provisions of the US Balanced Budget Act of 1997). In addition, legislation has recently been introduced in the US Congress that would require private insurers to cover the cost of colorectal cancer screening—its outcome is currently pending.

A report on the cost-effectiveness of colorectal cancer screening in average-risk individuals was prepared by the Office of Technology Assessment (OTA) of the US Congress *(88)*. The OTA devised a model to calculate the potential costs and effects of 16 different screening strategies, including stool blood testing, flexible sigmoidoscopy, double-contrast barium enema, and colonoscopy, either individually or in combination, at various frequency intervals that would occur in the remaining lifetimes of large cohort of 100,000 average-risk individuals starting at age of 50 and stopping at age 85. This report concluded that colorectal cancer screening in the average-risk population is well within the commonly accepted range of cost-effectiveness accepted for preventive screening modalities for other diseases, with a calculated cost of less than $20,000 per year of life saved, for each of the different screening strategies.

Although there is very limited published data regarding the cost-effectiveness of colorectal cancer screening in high-risk individuals, there was one study in which a mathematical model was utilized to estimate this information for individuals at increased risk because of having an FDR affected with colorectal cancer *(89)*. This study calculated that in these high-risk individuals, annual screening examinations after age 40 may result in the following approximate reductions in colorectal cancer mortality: 30% with annual stool blood testing, 40% with 60-cm flexible sigmoidoscopy, and 85% with either annual colonoscopy or double-contrast barium enema. In addition, they found that screening intervals of 3–5 yr maintained 70–90% of the effectiveness of annual screening. Furthermore, the effectiveness of screening in this high-risk population appeared to be decreased by 5–10% if screening was not initiated until age 50.

6. CONCLUSIONS

Colorectal cancer is the second most common cause of cancer death among American men and woman. Currently available screening and surveillance techniques are effective in detecting early-stage colorectal cancer and its premalignant precursor lesion, the adenoma. Evidence demonstrates that screening examinations reduce colorectal cancer mortality. Removal of adenomas by colonoscopic polypectomy has been demonstrated to significantly reduce the incidence of colorectal cancer.

Appropriate screening and surveillance recommendations should be based on the individual's colorectal-cancer-risk stratification. Average-risk individuals should begin colorectal cancer screening at age 50. Increased-risk individuals should be identified and offered more aggressive screening recommendations, beginning at an earlier age. High-risk groups, such as hereditary nonpolyposis colorectal cancer (HNPCC) and familial adenomatous polyposis (FAP), should be offered genetic counseling and specialized screening recommendations for colorectal and associated extracolonic malignancies.

At the present time, patients need to be encouraged to engage in and benefit from currently proven and available screening and surveillance strategies in order to reduce their risk of developing and dying from colorectal cancer.

ACKNOWLEDGMENTS

This work was supported in part by the Tavel-Reznik Fund for Colon Cancer Research.

REFERENCES

1. Greenlee RT, Hill-Harmon MB, Murray T, et al. Cancer Statistics, 2001. *CA: Cancer J. Clin.*, **51** (2001) 15–36.
2. Ries LAG, Kosary CL, Hankey BF, Miller BA, and Edwards BK (eds.). *SEER Cancer Statistics, 1973–1995.* National Cancer Institute, Bethesda, MD, 1998.
3. Winawer SJ, Zauber AG, Ho MN, et al. Prevention of colorectal cancer by colonoscopic polypectomy. *N. Engl. J. Med.*, **329** (1993) 1977–1981.
4. Stryker SJ, Wolff BG, Culp CE, et al. Natural history of untreated colonic polyps. *Gastroenterology*, **93** (1987) 1009–1013.
5. Atkin WS, Morson BC, and Cuzick J. Long-term risk of colorectal cancer after excision of rectosigmoid adenomas. *N. Engl. J. Med.*, **326** (1992) 658–662.
6. Gloeckler-Ries LA, Hankey BF, and Edwards BK (eds.). *Cancer Statistics Review, 1973–1987.* Department of Health and Human Services, Bethesda, MD, DHHS publication no. (NIH) 90-2789, 1990.
7. Mandel JS, Bond JH, Church TR, et al. Reducing mortality from colorectal cancer by screening for fecal occult blood. *N. Engl. J. Med.*, **328** (1993) 1365–1371.
8. Hardcastle JD, Chamberlain JO, Robinson MHE, et al. Randomised controlled trial of faecal-occult-blood screening for colorectal cancer. *Lancet*, **348**, 1472–1477.
9. Kronborg O, Fenger C, Olsen J, et al. Randomised study of screening for colorectal cancer with faecal-occult-blood test. *Lancet*, **348** (1996) 1467–1471.
10. Winawer SJ, Flehinger BJ, Schottenfeld D, et al. Screening for colorectal cancer with fecal occult blood testing and sigmoidoscopy. *J. Natl. Cancer Inst.*, **85** (1993) 1311–1318.
11. Selby JV, Friedman GD, Quesenberry CP, et al. Effect of fecal occult blood testing on mortality from colorectal cancer: a case-control study. *Ann. Intern. Med.*, **118** (1993) 1–6.
12. Wahrendorf J, Robra B-P, Wiebelt H, et al. Effectiveness of colorectal cancer screening: results from a population-based case-control evaluation in Saarland, Germany. *Eur. J. Cancer Prev.*, **2** (1993) 221–227.
13. Mandel JS, Church TR, Bond JH, et al. The effect of fecal occult-blood screening on the incidence of colorectal cancer. *N. Engl. J. Med.*, **343** (2000) 1603–1607.
14. Selby JV, Friedman GD, Quesenberry CP, et al. A case-control study of screening sigmoidoscopy and mortality from colorectal cancer. *N. Engl. J. Med.*, **326** (1992) 653–657.
15. Newcomb PA, Norfleet RG, Storer BE, et al. Screening sigmoidoscopy and colorectal cancer mortality. *J. Natl. Cancer Inst.*, **84** (1992) 1572–1575.
16. Gohagen JK, Prorok PC, Kramer BS, et al. The prostate, lung, colorectal, and ovarian cancer screening trial of the National Cancer Institute. *Cancer*, **75** (1995) 1869–1873.
17. Atkin WS, Hart A, Edwards R, et al. Uptake, yield of neoplasia, and adverse effects of flexible sigmoidoscopy screening. *Gut*, **42** (1998) 560–565.
18. Winawer SJ, Fletcher RH, Miller L, et al. Colorectal cancer screening: clinical guidelines and rationale. *Gastroenterology*, **112** (1997) 594–642.
19. Rex DK, Johnson DA, Lieberman DA, et al. Colorectal cancer prevention 2000: screening recommendations of the American College of Gastroenterology. *Am. J. Gastroenterol.*, **95** (2000) 868–877.
20. Smith RA, von Eschenbach AC, Wender R, et al. American Cancer Society guidelines for the early detection of cancer: update of early detection guidelines for prostate, colorectal, and endometrial cancers and update 2001: testing for early lung cancer detection. *CA: Cancer J. Clin.*, **51** (2001) 38–75.

21. Lieberman DA, Weiss DG, Bond J, et al. Use of colonoscopy to screen asymptomatic adults for colorectal cancer. *N. Engl. J. Med.*, **343** (2000) 162–168.
22. Imperiale TF, Wagner DR, Lin CY, et al. Risk of advanced proximal neoplasms in asymptomatic adults according to the distal colorectal findings. *N. Engl. J. Med.*, **343** (2000) 169–174.
23. Fork FT. Double contrast enema and colonoscopy in polyp detection. *Gut*, **22** (1981) 971–977.
24. Hixson LJ, Fennerty MB, Sampliner RE, et al. Prospective study of the frequency and size distribution of polyps missed by colonoscopy. *J. Natl. Cancer Inst.*, **82** (1990) 1769–1772.
25. Hixson LJ, Fennerty MB, Sampliner RE, et al. Prospective blinded trial of the colonoscopic miss-rate of large colorectal polyps. *Gastrointest. Endoscopy*, **37** (1991) 125–127.
26. Steine S, Stordahl A, Lunde OC, et al. Double-contrast barium enema versus colonoscopy in the diagnosis of neoplastic disorders: aspects of decision-making in general practice. *Fam. Pract.*, **10** (1993) 288–291.
27. Jaramillo E and Slezak P. Comparison between double-contrast barium enema and colonoscopy to investigate lower gastrointestinal bleeding. *Gastrointest. Radiol.*, **17** (1992) 81–83.
28. Jensen J, Kewenter J, Asztely M, et al. Double contrast barium enema and flexible rectosigmoidoscopy: a reliable diagnostic combination for detection of colorectal neoplasm. *Br. J. Surg.*, **77** (1990) 270–272.
29. O'Brien MJ, Winawer SJ, Zauber AG, et al. The National Polyp Study: patient and polyp characteristics associated with high-grade dysplasia in colorectal adenomas. *Gastroenterology*, **98** (1990) 371–379.
30. Shinya H and Wolff WI. Morphology, anatomic distribution and cancer potential of colonic polyps: an analysis of 7,000 polyps endoscopically removed. *Ann. Surg.*, **190** (1979) 679–683.
31. Winawer SJ, Zauber AG, O'Brien MJ, et al. The National Polyp Study: design, methods, and characteristics of patients with newly diagnosed polyps. *Cancer*, **70** (1992) 1236–1245.
32. Rickert RR, Auerbach O, Garfinkel L, et al. Adenomatous lesions of the large bowel: an autopsy study. *Cancer*, **43** (1979) 1847–1857.
33. The National Polyp Study Workgroup, Winawer SJ, Zauber A, Diaz B. The National Polyp Study: temporal sequence of evolving colorectal cancer from the normal colon. *Gastrointest. Endoscopy*, **33** (1987) 167.
34. Muto T, Bussey HJR, and Morson BC. The evolution of cancer of the colon and rectum. *Cancer*, **36** (1975) 2251–2270.
35. Vasen HFA, Nagengast FM, and Meera Khan P. Interval cancers in hereditary non-polyposis colorectal cancer (Lynch syndrome). *Lancet*, **345** (1995) 1183–1184.
36. Markowitz AJ, Winawer SJ, Zauber AG, et al. Rapid appearance of colorectal cancer following negative colonoscopy in HNPCC. *Gastroenterology*, **116** (1999) A458 (abstract).
37. Burt RW and Petersen GM. Familial colorectal cancer: diagnosis and management. In *Prevention and Early Detection of Colorectal Cancer*. Young GP, Rozen P, Levin B (eds.), WB Saunders, London, 1996, pp. 171–194.
38. Winawer SJ, Zauber AG, Gerdes H, et al. Risk of colorectal cancer in the families of patients with adenomatous polyps. *N. Engl. J. Med.*, **334** (1996) 82–87.
39. Sachar DB. Cancer in inflammatory bowel disease. In *Inflammatory Bowel Disease—Basic Research and Clinical Implications*. Goebell H, Peskan BM, and Malchow H, (eds.), MTP Press, Boston, 1988, pp. 289–294.
40. Butt JH and Lennard-Jones JE. A practical approach to the cancer risk in inflammatory bowel disease. *Med. Clin. North Am.*, **64** (1980) 1203–1220.
41. Johnson W, McDermott F, Hughes E, et al. Carcinoma of the colon and rectum in inflammatory disease of the intestine. *Surg. Gynecol. Obstet.*, **156** (1983) 193–197.
42. Gyde SN, Prior P, Allan PN, et al. Colorectal cancer in ulcerative colitis: a cohort study of primary referrals from three centers. *Gut*, **29** (1988) 206–217.
43. Katzka I, Brody R, Morris E, et al. Assessment of colorectal cancer risk in patients with ulcerative colitis: experience from a private practice. *Gastroenterology*, **85** (1983) 22–29.
44. Lennard-Jones JE, Melville DM, Morson BC, et al. Precancer and cancer in extensive ulcerative colitis: findings among 401 patients over 22 years. *Gut*, **31** (1990) 800–806.
45. Brostrom O, Lofberg R, Nordenvall B, et al. The risk of colorectal cancer in ulcerative colitis: an epidemiologic study. *Scand. J. Gastroenterol.*, **221** (1987) 1193–1199.
46. Gilat T, Fireman Z, Grossman A, et al. Colorectal cancer in patients with ulcerative colitis: a population study in central Israel. *Gastroenterology*, **94** (1988) 870–877.
47. Ransohoff DF. Colon cancer in ulcerative colitis. *Gastroenterology*, **94** (1988) 1089–1091.
48. Lennard-Jones JE. Cancer risk in ulcerative colitis: surveillance of surgery. *Br. J. Surg.*, **72** (1985) 584–586.
49. MacDougall IPM. Cancer risk in ulcerative colitis. *Lancet*, **2** (1964) 655–658.
50. Greenstein A, Sachar D, Smith H, et al. Cancer in universal and left-sided ulcerative colitis: factors determining risk. *Gastroenterology*, **77** (1979) 290–294.

51. Waye JD. Screening for cancer in ulcerative colitis. *Front. Gastrointest. Res.*, **10** (1986) 243–256.
52. Choi PM, Nugent FW, Schoetz DJ, et al. Colonoscopic surveillance reduces mortality from colorectal cancer in ulcerative colitis. *Gastroenterology*, **105** (1993) 418–424.
53. Greenstein AJ, Sachar DB, Smith H, et al. A comparison of cancer risk in Crohn's disease and ulcerative colitis. *Cancer*, **48** (1981) 2742–2745.
54. Ekbom A, Helmick C, Zack M, et al. Increased risk of large bowel cancer in Crohn's disease with colonic involvement. *Lancet*, **336** (1990) 357–359.
55. Sachar DB. Cancer in Crohn's disease: dispelling the myths. *Gut*, **35** (1994) 1507–1508.
56. Moertel CG, Bargen JA, and Dockerty MB. Multiple carcinomas of the large intestine: a review of the literature and a study of 261 cases. *Gastroenterology*, **34** (1958) 85–98.
57. Nava HR and Pagana TJ. Postoperative surveillance of colorectal carcinoma. *Cancer*, **49** (1982) 1043–1047.
58. Howard ML and Greene FL. The effect of preoperative endoscopy on recurrence and survival following surgery for colorectal carcinoma. *Am. Surg.*, **56** (1990) 124–127.
59. Brahme F, Ekelund G, Norden JG, et al. Metachronous colorectal polyps: comparison of development of colorectal polyps and carcinomas with and without history of polyps. *Dis. Colon Rectum*, **17** (1974) 166–171.
60. Bodmer WF, Bailey CJ, Bodmer J, et al. Localization of the gene for familial adenomatous polyposis on chromosome 5. *Nature*, **328** (1987) 614–616.
61. Leppert M, Dobbs M, and Scambler P. The gene for familial polyposis coli maps to the long arm of chromosome 5. *Science*, **238** (1987) 1411–1413.
62. Kinzler KW, Nilbert MC, Su Li-Kuo, et al. Identification of FAP locus genes from chromosome 5q21. *Science*, **253** (1991) 661–665.
63. Groden J, Thliveris A, Samowitz W, et al. Identification and characterization of the familial adenomatous polyposis coli gene. *Cell*, **66** (1991) 589–600.
64. Jeghers H, McKusick VA, and Katz KH. Generalized intestinal polyposis and melanin spots of the oral mucosa, lips and digits: a syndrome of diagnostic significance. *N. Engl. J. Med.*, **241** (1949) 993–1005.
65. Jenne DE, Reimann H, Nezu J, et al. Peutz–Jeghers syndrome is caused by mutations in a novel serine threonine kinase. *Nature Genet.*, **18** (1998) 38–43.
66. Hemminki A, Markie D, Tomlinson I, et al. A serine/threonine kinase gene defective in Peutz–Jeghers syndrome. *Nature*, **391** (1998) 184–187.
67. Giardiello FM, Welsh SB, Hamilton SR, et al. Increased risk of cancer in the Peutz–Jeghers syndrome. *N. Engl. J. Med.*, **316** (1987) 1511–1514.
68. Spigelman AD, Murday V, and Phillips RKS. Cancer and the Peutz–Jeghers syndrome. *Gut*, **30** (1989) 1588–1590.
69. Watanabe A, Nagashima H, Motoi M, and Ogawa K. Familial juvenile polyposis of the stomach. *Gastroenterology*, **77** (1979) 148–151.
70. Grotsky HW, Rickert RR, Smith WD, and Newsome JF. Familial juvenile polyposis coli: a clinical and pathologic study of a large kindred. *Gastroenterology*, **82** (1982) 494–501.
71. Sachatello CR, Pickren JW, and Grace JT Jr. Generalized juvenile gastrointestinal polyposis: a hereditary syndrome. *Gastroenterology*, **58** (1970) 699–708.
72. Haggitt RC and Reid BJ. Hereditary gastrointestinal polyposis syndromes. *Am. J. Surg. Pathol.*, **10** (1986) 871–887.
73. Jarvinen H and Franssila KO. Familial juvenile polyposis coli: increased risk of colorectal cancer. *Gut*, **25** (1984) 792–800.
74. Vasen HF, Mecklin JP, Khan PM, et al. The International Collaborative Group on Hereditary Non-Polyposis Colorectal Cancer (ICG-HNPCC). *Dis. Colon Rectum*, **34** (1991) 424–425.
75. Watson P and Lynch HT. Extracolonic cancer in Hereditary Nonpolyposis Colorectal Cancer. *Cancer*, **71** (1993) 677–685.
76. Vasen HFA, Watson P, Mecklin JP, et al. New clinical criteria for hereditary non-polyposis colorectal cancer (HNPCC, Lynch syndrome) proposed by the International Collaborative Group on HNPCC. *Gastroenterology*, **116** (1999) 1453–1456.
77. Peltomaki P, Aaltonen LA, Sistonen P, et al. Genetic mapping of a locus predisposing to human colorectal cancer. *Science*, **260** (1992) 810–812.
78. Fishel R, Lescoe MK, Rao MRS, et al. The human mutator gene homolog, MSH2 and its association with hereditary nonpolyposis colon cancer. *Cell*, **75** (1993) 1027–1038.
79. Leach FS, Nicolaides NC, Papadopoulos N, et al. Mutations of a muts homolog in hereditary nonpolyposis colorectal cancer. *Cell*, **75** (1993) 1215–1235.

80. Bronner CE, Baker SM, Morrison PT, et al. Mutation in the DNA mismatch repair gene homologue hMLH1 is associated with hereditary nonpolyposis colon cancer. *Nature*, **368** (1994) 258–261.

81. Akiyama Y, Sato H, Yamada T, et al. Germ-line mutation of the hMSH6/GTBP gene in an atypical hereditary nonpolyposis colorectal cancer kindred. *Cancer Res.*, **57** (1997) 3920–3923.

82. Jarvinen HJ, Mecklin JP, and Sistonen P. Screening reduces colorectal cancer rate in families with hereditary nonpolyposis colorectal cancer. *Gastroenterology*, **108** (1995) 1405–1411.

83. Breite I, Markowitz A, Zauber A, et al. Colonoscopy screening of patients at high familial risk for colorectal cancer. *Gastroenterology*, **110** (1996) 495 (abstract).

84. Bond JH. Polyp guideline: diagnosis, treatment, and surveillance for patients with colorectal polyps. Practice Parameters Committee of the American College of Gastroenterology. *Am. J. Gastroenterol.*, **95** (2000) 3053–3063.

85. Winawer SJ, Zauber AG, O'Brien MJ, et al. Randomized comparison of surveillance intervals after colonoscopic removal of newly diagnosed adenomatous polyps. *N. Engl. J. Med.*, **328** (1993) 901–906.

86. Zauber AG, Winawer SJ, Bond JH, et al. Can surveillance intervals be lengthened following colonoscopic polypectomy? *Gastroenterology*, **112** (1997) A50 (abstract).

87. Zauber AG, Bond JH, and Winawer SJ. Surveillance of patients with colorectal adenomas or cancer. In *Prevention and Early Detection of Colorectal Cancer*. Young GP, Rozen P, and Levin B (eds.), WB Saunders, London, 1996, pp. 195–215.

88. Wagner JL, Tunis S, Brown M, et al. The cost effectiveness of colorectal cancer screening in average-risk adults. In *Prevention and Early Detection of Colorectal Cancer*. Young G and Levin B (eds.), WB Saunders, New York, 1996.

89. Eddy DM, Nugent FW, Eddy JF, et al. Screening for colorectal cancer in a high-risk population: results of a mathematical model. *Gastroenterology*, **92** (1987) 682–692.

5 Chemoprevention of Colorectal Cancer

Monica M. Bertagnolli

CONTENTS

1. INTRODUCTION

Recent advances in our understanding of the environmental and dietary influences upon carcinogenesis have made prevention one of the most exciting areas of cancer research. As little as 15 yr ago, few would have thought that drugs as common as aspirin or treatments as simple as dietary supplementation with calcium and vitamin D could produce a meaningful reduction in colorectal cancer (CRC). Chemoprevention studies began in the 1950s with observations from human cancer epidemiology and advanced steadily in parallel with the field of cancer chemotherapy as a variety of natural and synthetic compounds were found to alter the growth of tumor cells. A wealth of data now suggests that cancer-preventing agents halt the progression of the adenoma–carcinoma sequence and may ultimately provide the key to the next major advance in cancer management.

Colorectal cancer is preventable, yet this disease still claims more than 55,000 lives per year in the United States because the optimal method for achieving prevention is not known. Precursor lesions in the form of adenomatous polyps can be identified and removed by endoscopic polypectomy, a practice that results in a significant reduction in CRC incidence and mortality *(1)*. Unfortunately, wide application of this life-saving procedure is limited because it is invasive, costly, and uncomfortable. The appearance of a visible adenoma is probably a late event in the carcinogenesis process, because their formation likely requires the acquisition of multiple cancer-causing genetic events *(2)*. This suggests that earlier intervention by dietary or pharmacological means to prevent advancement of cancer-associated mutations would substantially reduce the development of precursor lesions and thereby prevent their progression to CRC.

Epidemiological studies show a strong negative association between routine nonsteroidal anti-inflammatory drug (NSAID) use and CRC incidence and mortality (reviewed in

From: *Colorectal Cancer: Multimodality Management*
Edited by: L. Saltz © Humana Press Inc., Totowa, NJ

ref. *3*). This observation holds across a wide range of case-control and cohort studies, making NSAIDs the most promising class of candidate agents for CRC chemoprevention. In addition, a diverse body of research shows that a variety of other dietary and pharmacologic agents may prevent carcinogenesis of the lower gastrointestinal tract *(4,5)*. Through the study of human cancer predisposition syndromes and animal models for CRC, a mechanistic understanding of colorectal carcinogenesis and its prevention is emerging.

Chemoprevention is defined as the prevention, reversal, or inhibition of carcinogenesis before the development of invasive cancer by the use of chemical agents. This field broadly includes interruption of carcinogenesis by either dietary or pharmacological means. This chapter will outline our present understanding of the nature of intestinal tumor formation and progression and the ways that chemoprevention strategies can interrupt this process.

2. BIOLOGY OF EARLY COLORECTAL CARCINOGENESIS

Colorectal carcinogenesis is a multistage process characterized by the successive accumulation of cancer-associated gene mutations, with eventual progression of an initiated enterocyte to an invasive phenotype (*see* Chapter 1) *(6)*. This process likely begins 10–20 yr before the development of invasive behavior. Changes in oncogenes and tumor suppressor genes, such as mutations in *APC*, K-*ras*, or mismatch repair genes, or abnormalities in DNA methylation, likely occur during the initiating stage of tumor formation in the colon or rectum (reviewed in ref. *7*). These changes may occur before the development of architectural irregularities in the intestinal mucosa *(8,9)*. At these early stages of tumorigenesis, detection of cancer-associated events is not possible in the clinical setting and, therefore, the incidence of such changes in the population and the frequency of their progression to invasive cancer is unknown.

The earliest visible evidence of neoplasia in the colorectum are alterations of crypt morphology known as aberrant crypt foci (ACF). ACF occur more commonly in individuals with adenomatous polyps or CRC *(10)*, suggesting that they are either precursor lesions for these tumors or indicators of susceptibility to tumor formation. Adenomatous polyps, which are lesions that precede the development of most or all CRCs, are present in approx 40% of the US population by age 60 *(11,12)*. The rate at which adenomatous polyps progress to cancer is estimated at about 2.5 polyps per 1000 per year *(13)*. The risk of transformation of adenomas to invasive CRC varies according to the histologic subtype and also increases with increasing size and multiplicity *(14)*. It is clear that not all initiated cells, ACF, or adenomas progress to CRC; however, the risk of cancer progression increases with each successive stage of tumor formation. Studies of tumor progression show that there is also a rough correlation between tumor-associated mutations and phenotype. For example, mutations in APC are a very early event, perhaps occurring before microscopically visible adenomas, whereas a p53 mutation is a later event, marking the transition from adenoma to dysplasia *(6,8)*.

3. EVIDENCE FROM CANCER EPIDEMIOLOGY

The biology of CRC presents a strong case for the existence of gene–environment interactions that influence tumor formation (*see* Chapter 2). Evidence that environment plays a major role in colon carcinogenesis began with the observation that colon cancer incidence rates varied significantly between different parts of the world. In general, industrialized nations had up to eight times higher rates of CRC than those of developing nations *(15)*. Although this may be ascribed to either environmental or genetic factors, an environmental role is strongly supported by evidence showing that immigrants moving from countries of low incidence to regions of high incidence developed a risk of CRC similar to the inhabitants of the new country of residence *(16)*. In addition to the human migration data, both human and animal studies show that altering the environment of an individual at high genetic risk for cancer can decrease the incidence of neoplasia. The best example of this is the observed regression of adenomatous polyps in patients with familial adenomatous polyposis (FAP), a CRC predisposition syndrome caused by germline mutation of the *APC* tumor suppressor gene. Adenomas in the rectum of patients with FAP occasionally undergo spontaneous regression, but regression can also be induced by changes in diet *(17)*, by postsurgical changes in fecal composition *(18)*, and by pharmacologic agents such as NSAIDs *(19,20)*.

Most of the data related to environmental influences on CRC concerns dietary constituents, such as fat or red meat intake, and lifestyle factors, such as activity level or alcohol and medication use (*see* Chapter 3) *(21)*. Epidemiological studies show that diet is a major etiologic factor in CRC development *(5)*. Determining the relationship between diet and cancer is difficult, however, because of the long interval required for carcinogenesis and the multiple confounding interactions between dietary constituents. As a result, findings in studies of the relationship between single dietary constituents and CRC are sometimes inconsistent. In spite of this, strong cumulative data from both human epidemiology and animal studies link consumption levels of several dietary components to increased CRC risk. These include high consumption of saturated fats and red meat and low consumption of fruits and vegetables *(22,23)*. Insufficient dietary intake of several micronutrients, such as selenium, calcium, folate, and vitamin D, may also be a factor in CRC development *(24–31)*. Human cancer epidemiology also identifies some nondietary means of decreasing CRC risk. Most striking is the association between NSAID use and CRC incidence, as mentioned previously. Other nondietary influences that increase CRC include low physical activity, high alcohol consumption, and tobacco use *(4)*.

4. CLINICAL TRIALS OF COLORECTAL CANCER PREVENTION

4.1. Study Populations

Translating the results of human cancer epidemiology into an effective chemopreventive therapy is a difficult challenge. Optimally, the efficacy of a chemopreventive agent should be documented by a prospective, randomized, placebo-controlled trial with cancer as the endpoint. For CRC prevention, this level of evidence is virtually impossible to achieve. One reason for this is the long latency period from cancer initiation to the development of invasive disease, a process that may take 10–20 yr *(2)*. In addition, even though CRC is relatively common, the correlation between disease development and known risk factors is low. The most important impediment to cancer as a trial end point, however, is the success of endoscopic polypectomy as a prevention method for CRC. The National Polyp Study found that 5 out of 1400 patients treated with polypectomy developed cancer in 5.9 yr of follow-up. Given the success rate of this standard treatment, a two-arm, prospective, randomized, controlled trial comparing endoscopic polypectomy alone to endoscopic polypectomy plus a second cancer-preventing intervention would require 300,000 subjects per arm. This assumes a 2-yr accrual period, 5-yr total study duration, 30% participant dropout rate, $\alpha = 0.05$, and 80% power. A similar study of 150,000 participants would require a 1-yr accrual interval and 10 yr of total duration.

Because of the above-listed constraints, the generally accepted method of evaluating a potential CRC prevention strategy, either pharmacologic agent or procedure based, is a trial

Table 1
Colorectal Cancer Risk Factors and Clinical Trial Cohorts

Risk factor	CRC incidence or RR[a] associated with this risk factor	Proportion of CRC cases with this risk factor	Proportion of general population with this risk factor
Residence in an industrialized nation	20 : 100,000		
Age over 50	Age: 50–60: 1 : 1000 60–70: 2.5 : 1000 70–80: 4 : 1000	95%	
History of CRC	RR 2–4	1–2%	5%
History of adenomatous polyps	RR 1.5–4		Age 50–60: 30% 60–70: 40% 70–80: 55%
Significant family history, not FAP or HNPCC	RR 2–3	20%	10%
Familial adenomatous polyposis (FAP)	100%	<1%	1 : 10,000
Hereditary nonpolyposis CRC	Varies greatly	5%	1 : 200
Chronic ulcerative colitis	RR 1.45	<1%	1 : 1500

Data from refs. *35–38.*
[a]RR = relative risk.

comparing colonoscopy with polypectomy to the new intervention, with the occurrence of an adenomatous polyp at follow-up colonoscopy as the primary endpoint. This endpoint can be further graded by severity depending on the number, size, and histologic type of the recurrent adenoma(s). Study participants can be selected to include those at highest risk for CRC by designing inclusion criteria according to the data presented in Table 1. Trials should carefully control for familial risk. For example, although the molecular biology of CRC suggests that FAP represents an accelerated form of sporadic CRC, the 5–15% of patients with hereditary nonpolyposis colorectal cancer (HNPCC) or mismatch repair deficient tumors may respond differently to tumor-preventing agents. Depending on the demographics of the study population, these studies may also need to control for dietary and lifestyle factors that may affect outcome, particularly the use of concomitant medications such as aspirin and NSAIDs. If multiple clinical sites of broad geographic or cultural distribution are used to conduct large trials of this type, the study should be stratified by site to minimize the effects of regional differences. Finally, the available data concerning the natural history of adenoma development suggest that adenoma recurrence endpoints should be assessed a minimum of 1 yr following index colonoscopy and polypectomy, with more solid support from available studies for an endpoint at 3 yr following polypectomy *(32–34).*

The optimal trial design varies according to the patient population chosen for study. Studies of high-risk populations, such as patients with FAP and HNPCC, yield important information about the biology of malignant transformation and its potential for modulation by various interventions. Information from these high-risk populations can then be used to design larger trials of sporadic disease. Because trials to study sporadic cancers require large numbers of subjects and are expensive and time-consuming, it is important to continue to develop and validate endpoints of shorter duration or more effective cancer-risk prediction. Nested cohort studies within larger clinical trials can examine the reliability of measuring

Table 2
Endpoints for Colorectal Cancer Prevention Studies

SEB description	Status
Adenomatous polyp	These lesions carry a spectrum of CRC risk depending on their degree of dysplasia, histologic subtype, size, multiplicity, and the genetic background of the individual in which they arise. Adenomatous polyps are presently used as validated end points in CRC prevention trials.
Aberrant crypt foci	Investigation of these lesions as indicators of CRC risk are ongoing. A relationship between number and persistence of these lesions and increased adenoma and CRC risk is suggested, but ACF have not yet been tested as an indicator of CRC or adenoma treatment outcome.
Cell growth and differentiation markers	Although studies of enterocyte proliferation, apoptosis, and differentiation antigen expression suggest a correlation between these markers and cancer or adenoma risk, these markers have not been validated as indicators of CRC or adenoma treatment outcome.
Cancer-associated mutations and other forms of DNA modification	Tumors frequently contain particular mutations, such as those in *APC*, K-*ras*, and *p53*, or DNA modifications, such as specific promoter region methylation changes. Unfortunately, there are little or no data concerning the prevalence of these modifications in non-neoplastic mucosa or for the modifications in isolation. Studies addressing these issues are central to development of prevention strategies.

ACF or other surrogate endpoint biomarkers for CRC development (SEBs) and then correlate the results of these studies with the primary outcome of the main trial. SEBs for CRC currently under study include measurement of intestinal cell hyperplasia, hyperproliferation, apoptosis resistance, or increased production of tumor-promoting metabolic products or expression of differentiation-associated antigens *(9)*. Although the ideal SEB for CRC has yet to be identified, these studies of early neoplasia provide valuable insight into the nature of early colorectal carcinogenesis (Table 2).

A final issue that must be addressed in CRC prevention trials is the durability of response to a chemopreventive intervention. Important unanswered questions include the following: (1) Which patients will have significant recurrent neoplasia following endoscopic polypectomy, requiring short follow-up intervals? (2) Can patients with no evidence of neoplasia by a given age safely discontinue CRC screening? (3) Will adenoma-preventing interventions such as calcium, vitamin D, and/or NSAIDs require lifetime use? The answers to these questions are not likely to come from nested cohort studies and will require either randomized trials or long-term follow-up of treated cohorts.

5. AGENTS

Because chemopreventive therapy may require administration to otherwise healthy individuals over long periods of time, potential agents are subject to several constraints. The agents must be extremely safe for administration to a patient population with a broad range of overall health, and they must be cost-effective for prolonged administration. Possible interactions with common concomitant medications such as antihypertensives and cardioprotective aspirin must be considered. Finally, to foster long-term compliance, chemopreventive agents must provide minimal impact upon lifestyle.

Dietary intervention is a relatively straightforward approach to CRC prevention and one likely to have other significant health benefits such as reduction in diabetes and cardiovascular

Table 3
Selected Prospective, Randomized Trials of Colorectal Adenoma Reduction

Agent	Evidence	Ref.
Dietary counseling	No improvement in adenoma recurrence rate following endoscopic polypectomy in sporadic adenoma patients	39
Sulindac	Regression of adenomas in patients with FAP	19,40
Celecoxib	Regression of adenomas in patients with FAP	20
ASA	No direct studies: as a secondary endpoint, ASA 325 mg qod provided no ↓ in adenoma formation or CRC	41
Calcium	A 20% reduction in sporadic adenoma recurrence following polypectomy	30
Antioxidants	No difference in sporadic adenoma recurrence following polypectomy	42
Selenium	Reduced incidence of CRC and adenomas following selenium supplementation in an area of low soil selenium concentration	43
Fiber	No difference in adenoma recurrence rate following endoscopic polypectomy for two supplemental doses of wheat-bran fiber	44

risk. In almost all respects, dietary intervention is the ideal chemoprevention strategy, as it is safe, cost-effective, and readily available. A recent study of dietary intervention examined the effect of a low-fat, high-fiber diet on the recurrence of colorectal adenomas in 2079 men and women following endoscopic polypectomy. The intervention group underwent intensive counseling to achieve an optimal cancer-preventing diet, and the control group was asked to follow their usual diet. Repeat colonoscopy documented the recurrence of adenomas at 1 and 4 yr following initiation of the intervention. This study found no difference in the risk of recurrence of colorectal adenomas between the intervention and the study group. The reasons for this negative result are unclear, but at least a partial explanation is the complex nature of diet, a component of human behavior that is refractory to long-term change.

The field of chemoprevention has so far focused primarily on the development of pharmacological therapies. These treatments arose from studies of epithelial carcinogenesis and target specific steps in the process of tumor formation (Fig. 1). The following subsections describe a few of the best-studied chemopreventive agents for CRC.

5.1. NSAIDs

At the present time, NSAIDs are the most promising class of agents for CRC prevention. Consistent results showing NSAID-associated reduction in CRC incidence, precursor adenoma formation, and even CRC mortality are evident in a wide variety of case-control and cohort studies (reviewed in ref. 45). Assessment of the available studies indicates that NSAID use is associated with an approx 50% decrease in the incidence of colorectal adenomas or polyps and a 40% decrease in the incidence of CRC (Table 4). Most striking is the finding of decreased CRC mortality among NSAID users, a result reported in at least three separate studies (46–48). The first direct evidence of NSAID-associated modulation of colorectal tumors came from studies of patients with FAP. As a result of germline APC mutation, these patients develop hundreds to thousands of colorectal adenomas. FAP patients were first given the NSAID, sulindac, for treatment of desmoid tumors, an APC-related neoplasm characterized by an extensive fibrosis suggesting inflammation (49). Although sulindac did little to alter the natural history of desmoids, FAP patients taking sulindac at anti-inflammatory doses showed regression of coexisting rectal polyps, a result that was later confirmed by randomized trials (19,40,50). Similar adenoma regression was recently

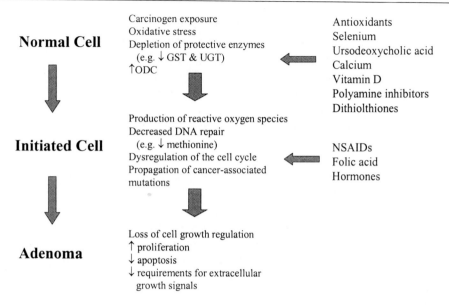

Fig. 1. Chemopreventive agent activity.

Table 4
CRC Epidemiology: Association with NSAID Use

Study endpoint	Adenoma/polyp incidence	Colorectal cancer incidence	Colorectal cancer mortality
Avg. relative risk	0.50	0.59	0.59
No. of studies included	7	23	3

reported following treatment of FAP patients with celecoxib, a selective cyclooxygenase-2 (COX-2) inhibitor *(20)*. These studies are important for two reasons. First, they show that therapeutic modulation of the adenoma–carcinoma sequence can occur relatively late, as these patients showed significant regression, rather than simply prevention, of premalignant lesions. Second, because *APC* loss also occurs in the majority of sporadic CRCs, results in FAP patients may be relevant to prevention of sporadic disease. Clinical trials are underway to determine whether NSAIDs such as aspirin or selective COX-2 inhibitors prevent the development of sporadic colorectal adenomas.

The exact mechanism of NSAID-associated cancer prevention is unknown. NSAIDs exert many effects on the pathways governing cell growth, differentiation, and mobility that may be related to tumor development. For example, NSAIDs alter arachidonic acid metabolism, one result of which is suppression of prostaglandin (PG) synthesis. Certain prostaglandins, such as PGE_2 and $PGF_{2\alpha}$, are associated with epithelial tumorigenesis *(51,52)*, possibly by inducing cell proliferation and inhibiting apoptosis *(52)*. PGE_2, the arachidonic acid metabolite most prevalent in intestinal tissue, also has immunosuppressive effects that may reduce tumor immune surveillance *(53)*. A substantial body of data suggests that the tumor-preventing activity of NSAIDs results from inhibition of COX-2, one of the key enzymes of arachidonic acid metabolism. COX-2 is the product of an intermediate–early response gene that is induced in response to inflammation or mitogenic stimuli *(8,54,55)*. COX-2 expression is increased during the course of tumor development in a variety of epithelial tissues (reviewed in ref. *56*). Many colorectal tumors overexpress COX-2 as well as PGE_2 *(52,57)*. A critical link between COX-2 activity and intestinal tumor prevention is provided by a study of COX-2 expression in *Apc*-deficient mice *(58)*. Animals homozygous for a germline mutation in murine *Apc* develop multiple intestinal tumors, each exhibiting loss of wild-type *Apc*. When these animals are crossed with a mouse altered by genetic knockout of COX-2, intestinal tumor incidence is dramatically decreased. This tumor reduction is also observed for *Apc*-deficient mice treated with selective inhibitors of COX-2 *(58,59)*.

Other NSAID effects may be independent of prostaglandin suppressive activity. Several NSAIDs, including aspirin, indomethacin, and selective COX-2 inhibitors, block the carcinogen-induced activation of AP-1, a transcription factor regulating growth-associated genes *(60,61)*. Aspirin and sodium salicylate alter cell growth by inhibiting the activity of the NFκB-activating enzyme, IκB kinase β, in a prostaglandin-independent fashion *(62)*. Sulindac sulfone, a metabolite of sulindac that does not alter prostaglandin synthesis, protects against carcinogen-induced tumors in rodents *(63)*. These studies suggest that continued study to characterize the mechanism of NSAID-induced tumor regression is important for improving the efficacy and safety of these chemopreventive agents.

5.2. Calcium and Vitamin D

Data from human epidemiology and animal intestinal tumor models suggest that diets deficient in calcium and vitamin D increase spontaneous intestinal tumor formation *(13,14)*. The role of calcium in chemoprevention may be through its ability to counteract the genotoxic effects of intestinal bile acids. Secondary bile acids increase enterocyte proliferation in human CRC cell lines and in carcinogen-induced and spontaneous rodent intestinal tumor models *(64)*. The microflora of the intestine convert luminal secondary bile acids to diacylglycerol (DAG). DAG is an activator of protein kinase C (PCK), a key inducer of the MAP kinase signal transduction cascade and an important promoter of cell growth and tumor formation *(41)*. Bile acids are mucosal irritants and induce epithelial cell proliferation, possibly through activation of PKC *(65,66)*. Bile acids may also contribute to tumor initiation by inhibiting the activity of xenobiotic metabolizing enzymes such as glutathione-*S*-transferase (GST) and UDP-glucuronyltransferase (UGT) *(67)*. The production of secondary bile acids is increased by high dietary fat intake and is therefore a possible mechanism of carcinogenesis associated with the diet of Western nations. Calcium binds to bile acids and reduces their reactivity with intestinal epithelial cells. In rodents with intestinal tumors caused by carcinogens *(68)* or high-fat diets *(69)*, calcium reduces epithelial cell proliferation and decreases tumor formation. In humans with sporadic colorectal adenomas, calcium significantly decreases fecal bile acids *(70)*, and ingestion of approx 1 g of elemental calcium daily decreases colonic epithelial cell proliferation and normalizes the distribution of proliferating cells to the lower colonic crypt *(71)*. These potentially protective effects were confirmed in a recent randomized trial, where patients with a history of colorectal adenomas who received 1200 mg of elemental calcium daily achieved a small but significant decrease in recurrent adenoma formation *(30)*.

Vitamin D is an important regulator of intestinal cell differentiation that supports efficient calcium uptake and may also directly modulate tumorigenesis by regulating PKC activity *(72,73)*. With calcium, vitamin D suppresses Ornithine decroboxylase activity and inhibits the epithelial proliferation produced by bile acids and fatty diets in rodent tumor models *(64)*. Administered alone, vitamin D protects against tumors in azoxymethane-induced rodent tumor models *(73,74)*. At present, clinical trials are underway to test the contribution of calcium and vitamin D for prevention of colorectal carcinogenesis.

5.3. Ursodeoxycholic Acid

As mentioned earlier, evidence from animal tumor models and cancer cell-line studies suggests that bile acids influence intestinal tumor formation. The precise mechanism for this activity is unknown. Ursodeoxycholic acid is a 7β-epimer of chemodeoxycholic acid that is commonly used to treat gallstones or biliary stasis resulting from primary biliary sclerosis. Unlike other bile acids, ursodeoxycholic acid may inhibit intestinal tumorigenesis. Ursodeoxycholic acid decreased carcinogen-induced intestinal tumors in rodents *(75)*, an activity associated with suppression of the specific isoforms of PKC that are activated during epithelial tumorigenesis *(76)*. Other possible mechanisms of chemoprevention by ursodeoxycholic acid are related to its anti-inflammatory activities, including inhibition of epithelial cell PGE_2 and inducible nitric oxide synthase (iNOS) *(77,78)*. Clinical trials are underway to determine whether ursodeoxycholic acid supplementation will prevent colorectal adenoma recurrence following endoscopic polypectomy.

5.4. Folic Acid

Folate or folic acid is a micronutrient present in fruits and vegetables and is particularly abundant in leafy green vegetables such as spinach. An adequate supply of folic acid is important for proper methylation of DNA. Diets deficient in folate potentially produce defects such as hypomethylation of CCGG sites *(79)*, as well as changes in deoxynucleotide availability that are characterized by methionine deficiency. These changes may alter DNA function or repair capability or may inhibit efficient DNA transcription enough to foster the acquisition of tumor-associated mutations *(80)*. Evidence from human epidemiology strongly supports a role for dietary folate in CRC prevention. In the Nurses' Health Study, individuals taking folate supplements demonstrated a significant reduction of CRC risk (relative risk [RR] = 0.25) after 15 yr of supplement use *(31)*.

The chemopreventive benefits of folate supplementation may be most important for patients carrying increased genetic risk for CRC because of inefficient DNA repair or related polymorphisms. The importance of folic acid metabolism to CRC risk is illustrated by the presence of a particular polymorphism of methylene tetrahydrofolate reductase (MTHFR). In certain individuals, MTHFR facilitates the conversion of 5,10-methylene tetrahydrofolate to 5-methyltetrahydrofolate, which then serves as a methyl donor for methionine synthase, allowing the conversion of homocysteine to methionine. Patients who are homozygous for particular polymorphisms of MTHFR or of the enzyme methionine synthase have an approx 50% decreased risk of CRC *(81–83)*. The association of these polymorphisms to altered folate synthesis is further supported by the observation that this genotype-specific benefit is lost for individuals with inadequate dietary folate intake *(84)*.

5.5. Hormones

Although males and females develop CRCs with approximately the same frequency, women in developed countries who are normally at high risk for CRC have recently experienced a substantial decline in mortality from this disease *(21,85)*. This decline has been attributed to the use of menopausal hormone replacement therapy (HRT), a practice which began in the 1970s *(86)*. Numerous studies of CRC incidence show a protective effect of menopausal HRT. A recent meta-analysis of studies published up to December 1996 suggests that HRT reduces colon cancer risk by as much as 25%, with a summary relative risk of 0.85 (95% confidence interval [C.I.] = 0.73–0.99). Studies identifying the duration of HRT use also suggest a dose-response, with a RR among current or recent HRT users of 0.69 (95% CI = 0.52–0.91) compared to 0.88 (95% CI = 0.64–1.21) for short-term users

(87,88). In the C57BL/6J-Min/+ mouse, an animal model for FAP, intestinal tumor formation was increased by 77% following ovariectomy *(89)*. When the ovariectomized animals in this study were treated with replacement doses of estradiol, however, the tumor number decreased to baseline levels. These data suggested that endogenous hormones may protect against CRC and that HRT can counteract spontaneous intestinal tumor formation in the setting of gonadal hormone loss.

The mechanism responsible for HRT-associated reduction in CRC incidence is unknown. One possibility is that estrogens influence intestinal carcinogenesis by an indirect mechanism. Estrogens are metabolized to a variety of compounds that have different half-lives and receptor affinities, and they produce varying effects upon cell growth. Studies of cancer cell lines and animal tumor models suggest that some of these metabolites may have tumor-promoting activity, whereas others may be chemopreventive *(90–92)*. Estrogen receptor ligands other than endogenous hormones may alter intestinal tumor formation. A diet high in fruits and vegetables contains a variety of phytoestrogens that are capable of modulating estrogen receptor activity and may also produce effects on cell growth that are estrogen receptor independent *(93,94)*. The best known nonsteroidal phytoestrogens include the isoflavones, genistein and diadzein, which are present in soybean seeds and flour, and the coumestan, coumestrol, which is found in alfalfa. Several phytoestrogens produce antitumor activity in animal models of epithelial carcinogenesis *(95,96)*.

5.6. Antioxidants

Normal cell function requires a careful balance of intracellular and extracellular oxidantion and reduction. Dysregulation of cellular metabolism produces reactive oxygen species that can damage DNA directly or can lead to tumor-promoting alterations in cell-cycle control (reviewed in ref. *97*). A healthy cell contains enzymes, such as GST, to protect the cell against significant oxidative damage. Certain states of "oxidative stress," however, can overcome the cell's ability to eliminate genotoxic metabolites. In addition, polymorphisms of genes encoding proteins governing oxidative balance, such as those encoding GST, can alter the ability to process carcinogenic substances without sustaining harm *(98)*. Antioxidant compounds enhance the resistance of cultured cells to oxidative stress. These compounds include antioxidant vitamins, such as vitamins A, C, and E, as well as a variety of plant-derived compounds, including those present in curry (phenolics such as curcumin), onion and garlic (sulfides such as allyl sulfide), and tea (catechins). Most of these substances are also anti-inflammatory, as they exhibit varying degrees of cyclooxygenase and lipoxy-genase inhibition *(99)*. Data from human cancer cell lines, animal cancer models, and human epidemiology all suggest that nutrients with antioxidant properties prevent tumors *(100–102)*.

Prospective trials determining the effect of antioxidants upon human cancer development have, unfortunately, yielded disappointing results. A prospective, randomized trial to evaluate the effects of β-carotene, vitamins C and E, or the combination of all three failed to show a decrease in colorectal adenoma recurrence following 1 and 4 yr of antioxidant use *(42)*. The Physicians Health Study revealed no decrease in CRC incidence with the use of vitamin E (α-tocopherol) and β-carotene *(103–105)* and there was no benefit to vitamin E supplementation in the Polyp Prevention Study *(42)*. Although a trial of vitamin C plus fiber showed a modest decrease in tumors in FAP patients *(17)* and in a study of sporadic adenoma patients *(106)*, no benefits were seen with vitamin C supplementation in the Polyp Prevention Study *(42)*.

5.7. Selenium

Selenium, in the form of selenocysteine, is a trace metal required for the activity of the antioxidant enzyme, glutathione peroxidase. This enzyme detoxifies hydrogen peroxide and lipoperoxides that are generated by free radicals and other reactive oxygen species, thus limiting the possible DNA damage produced by inflammatory states *(107)*. Several epidemiological studies suggest that adequate amounts of dietary selenium are important for epithelial cancer prevention *(108,109)*. The Nutritional Prevention of Cancer Trial (NPC) was a randomized, placebo-controlled trial of 1312 men and women that tested whether selenium supplementation of 200 µg/d reduced cancer incidence. The primary end point was a reduction in nonmelanoma skin cancer, and subjects were selected from regions of the United States with high rates of these tumors and low levels of soil selenium. Secondary end points included lung, colon, and prostate cancer incidence *(43,110)*. This study found a significant reduction in CRC incidence among subjects in the selenium-supplemented group compared to placebo *(110)*. Despite these favorable results, caution must be exercised in interpreting the results of selenium studies and before recommending selenium supplementation as a chemopreventive therapy. Background dietary selenium levels vary considerably, based on local soil concentrations in areas of food production. The NPC trial, for instance, was conducted in a region of low selenium concentration, possibly contributing to the positive effect. Another important factor governing the use of selenium as a chemopreventive agent is its narrow therapeutic range. A typical selenium intake in healthy populations is 100 µg/d, but toxicity as evidenced by hair and nail brittleness develops at doses of approx 400 µg/d *(111)*. In spite of these concerns, the available studies suggest that selenium supplementation is important for areas where the diet lacks sufficient levels of this micronutrient.

5.8. Polyamine Inhibitors

Ornithine decroboxylase (ODC) is an enzyme induced in response to mitogenic stimuli and is also increased by oncogenic viruses, chemical carcinogens, and malignant transformation *(112)*. ODC is essential for in the synthesis of polyamines, which, in turn, are required for the growth and function of epithelial cells. Blockade of polyamine synthesis by drugs causes an inhibition of cell growth that can be restored by the addition of exogenous polyamines. Inhibition of polyamine synthesis alters epidermal growth factor signaling activity and disrupts the epithelial cell cytoskeleton *(113)*.

Difluoromethylornithine (DFMO) is an irreversible inhibitor of ODC *(114)* that has potent tumor-preventing activity against cancer cell lines and in animal cancer models *(115,116)*. DFMO inhibits intestinal tumor formation in rats treated with the chemical carcinogens, azoxymethane (AOM) and dimethylhydrazine *(117)*. Consistent with the observed effects of polyamine depletion, DFMO decreases cell motility by altering the epithelial cell cytoskeleton *(113)* and suppressing matrilysin expression *(118)*. In a phase II trial of patients with adenomas, DFMO administration decreased polyamine levels in the lower intestinal mucosa *(119)*. Unfortunately, 12.5% of subjects receiving low-dose DFMO (0.5 g/m^2/d) developed reversible hearing loss. Although its mechanism of activity makes DFMO a promising chemopreventive agent, further human trials of DFMO will require the development of safer dosing schedules.

5.9. Dithiolthiones (Olitpraz)

Phase II detoxification enzymes, such as GST, catalyze the conjugation of certain carcinogens with glutathione, thereby neutralizing their genotoxic effects. The importance of phase II enzymes to CRC prevention is illustrated by several case-control studies showing that polymorphisms in the genes encoding GST enzymes, particularly GSTM-1, were associated with increased CRC risk (reviewed in ref. *98*). Dithiolthiones induce phase II detoxification enzymes such as GST. Several dithiothiones are naturally occurring in diets high in fruits and vegetables, and these compounds are abundant in cruciferous vegetables such as cauliflower, broccoli, brussels sprouts, and cabbage. Epidemiological studies suggest that for GSTM-1 null individuals, an inverse association exists between colon cancer and high dietary intake of cruciferous vegetables *(120)*.

Studies of a synthetic dithiothione, olitpraz, suggest that members of this class of agents prevent intestinal tumor formation. Oltipraz inhibits a variety of epithelial tumors in animal models, including AOM-induced rodent colon tumors *(121)* and may be particularly active against tobacco-related carcinogens. This agent is currently under study in preclinical and phase I studies for the prevention of a variety of epithelial cancers *(122)*. Because of its unique mechanism of activity, oltiprax may be useful in combination with other chemopreventive agents for subsets of the population with phase II enzyme deficiency.

5.10. Fiber

One of the striking differences between the diets of countries with a low incidence and that of the Western world is the amount of dietary fiber. This observation led to the hypothesis that high fiber intake protects against CRC, presumably by binding or diluting carcinogenic luminal contents. Although several case-control studies found that the high intake of dietary fiber is associated with decreased CRC incidence, this result failed confirmation in several prospective trials. In the largest study, the Polyp Prevention Trial, 2079 patients with a history of colorectal adenomas were randomized following endoscopic polypectomy to counseling to achieve a low-fat, high-fiber diet or to receive no intervention other than an informational brochure. Colonoscopy after 1 and 4 yr showed no difference between the two groups *(39)*. A randomized study by the Phoenix Colon Cancer Prevention Physicians Network directly addressed fiber intake by randomizing adenoma patients postpolypectomy to receive either 2.0 g or 13.5 g of supplemental fiber daily *(44)*. Follow-up colonoscopy performed after 3 yr of treatment showed no difference in recurrent adenoma formation between the low- and high-fiber groups.

6. CURRENT RECOMMENDATIONS

Overall health is promoted by a lifestyle that includes a diet rich in fruits and vegetables, low in fat, and that contains adequate amounts of important micronutrients, including selenium, vitamin D, and calcium. Regular exercise, maintenance of ideal body weight, and abstinence from smoking are also contributors to health that play a role in CRC prevention. For postmenopausal women, calcium supplementation is already recommended for the prevention of osteoporosis, and its modest effect in preventing colorectal neoplasia adds to its overall benefit. Although not directly confirmed by randomized trials, the epidemiological evidence that 400 µg of folate daily prevents CRC is strong enough to advise a daily multivitamin containing this agent, particularly for older individuals or patients whose diet may be inadequate. The routine supplementation of other dietary agents, however, must be approached with caution and cannot be universally recommended at this time.

The most potent nondietary preventive agents for CRC appear to be NSAIDs, as a substantial body of data indicates that the long-term regular use of NSAIDs protects against colorectal neoplasia. What is not clear, however, is which NSAID and what dose most effectively balances the risks of NSAID use with chemopreventive efficacy. For instance, epidemiological data suggest that a minimum of 10 yr of regular aspirin use is required to achieve a significant decrease in CRC, admittedly a late point in the process of carcinogenesis. Multiple case-control and cohort studies also suggest a dose-response for aspirin, with minimal efficacy at a dose of approx 325 mg at a frequency of three times per week, and greater efficacy at 5–7 doses per week *(47,123)*. When aspirin use is increased from 325 qod to 325 qd, however, the risk of complications, particularly significant gastrointestinal (GI) bleeding, increases fourfold *(124)*. The potential advantage of the selective COX-2 inhibitors over the nonselective NSAIDs is an improved safety profile. Because the protective effects of prostaglandins on GI mucosa are mediated via COX-1, whereas the states of inflammation and neoplasia are potentiated by COX-2, these agents may be safer for the long-term administration required for chemoprevention *(125)*. Pending the results of randomized trials of selective COX-2 inhibitors for prevention of colorectal adenomas, the safest, most effective NSAID for CRC prevention is aspirin, administered at a standard cardioprotective dose of 81 mg qd or 325 mg qod in enteric-coated form.

Finally, even though this review focuses on chemoprevention, the important contribution of colorectal screening to CRC prevention must be emphasized (*see* Chapter 4). A recent analysis reported by the American Gastroenterological Association suggested that colonoscopy with polypectomy at 10-yr intervals for individuals at average risk for CRC would reduce the incidence of CRC in this population by 72% *(126)*. CRC prevention is also best achieved by the identification and understanding of additional risk factors that may lead a patient to begin screening or aspirin use earlier. These include risks suggested by a family history of CRC or adenomas, or a personal history of adenomatous polyps, particularly multiple or presenting at an early age. At this time, risk identification, chemoprevention, and screening must be used together if our society is to achieve a significant reduction in this disease in the near future.

REFERENCES

1. Winawer SJ, Zauber AG, O'Brien MJ, Ho MN, Gottlieb LS, Sternberg SS, et al. Prevention of colorectal cancer by colonoscopic polypectomy. The National Polyp Study Workgroup. *N. Engl. J. Med.*, **329** (1993) 1977–1981.
2. Kelloff GJ. Perspectives on cancer chemoprevention research and drug development. *Adv. Cancer Res.*, **78** (2000) 199–334.
3. Janne PA and Mayer RJ. Primary care: chemoprevention of colorectal cancer. *N. Engl. J. Med.*, **342** (2000) 1960–1968.
4. Slattery ML, Edwards SL. Boucher KM, Anderson K, and Caan BJ. Lifestyle and colon cancer: an assessment of factors associated with risk. *Am. J. Epidemiol.*, **150** (1999) 869–877.
5. Giovannucci E and Willett WC. Dietary factors and risk of colon cancer. *Ann. Med.*, **26** (1994) 443–452.
6. Kinzler KW and Vogelstein B. Lessons from hereditary colorectal cancer. *Cell*, **87** (1996) 159–170.
7. Ilyas M, Straub J, Tomlinson IPM, and Bodmer WF. Genetic pathways in colorectal and other cancers. *Eur. J. Cancer*, **35** (2000) 1986–2002.
8. Fearon ER and Vogelstein B. A genetic model for colorectal tumorigenesis. *Cell*, **61** (1990) 759–767.
9. Kelloff GJ, Sigman CC, Johnson KM, Boone CW, Greenwald P, Crowell JA, et al. Perspectives on surrogate end points in the development of drugs that reduce the risk of cancer. *Cancer Epidemiol. Biomarkers Prev.*, **9** (2000) 127–137.
10. Takayama T, Katsuki S, Takahashi Y, Ohi M, Nojiri S, Sakamaki S, et al. Aberrant crypt foci of the colon as precursors of adenoma and cancer. *N. Engl. J. Med.*, **339** (1998) 1277–1284.
11. Blatt LJ. Polyps of the colon and rectum: incidence and distribution. *Dis. Colon Rectum* **4** (1961) 277–282.
12. Bernstein MA, Feczko PJ, Halpert RD, Simms SM, and Ackerman LV. Distribution of colonic polyps: increased incidence of proximal lesions in older patients. *Radiology*, **155** (1985) 35–38.
13. Eide TJ. Risk of colorectal cancer in adenoma-bearing individuals within a defined population. *Int. J. Cancer*, **38** (1985) 173–176.
14. Konishi F and Morson BC. Pathology of colorectal adenomas. A colonoscopic survey. *J. Clin. Pathol.* **35** (1982) 830–841.

15. Armstrong B and Doll R. Environmental factors and cancer incidence and mortality in different countries with special reference to dietary practices. *Int. J. Cancer*, **15** (1975) 617–631.

16. Sherlock P, Lipkin M, and Winawer SJ. Predisposing factors in carcinoma of the colon. *Adv. Intern. Med.* **20** (1975) 121–150.

17. DeCosse JJ, Miller HH, and Lesser ML. Effect of wheat fiber and vitamins C and E on rectal polyps in patients with familial adenomatous polyposis. *J. Natl. Cancer Inst.*, **81** (1989) 1290–1297.

18. Feinberg SM, Jagelman DG, Sarre RG, McGannon E, Fazio VW, Lavery IC, et al. Spontaneous resolution of rectal polyps in patients with familial polyposis following abdominal colectomy and ileorectal anastomosis. *Dis. Colon Rectum*, **31** (1988) 169–175.

19. Giardiello FM, Hamilton, SR, Krush, AJ, Piantadosi, S, Hylind, LM, Celano, P, et al. Treatment of colonic and rectal adenomas with sulindac in familial adenomatous polyposis. *N. Engl. J. Med.*, **328** (1993) 1313–1316.

20. Steinbach G, Lynch PM, Phillips RK, Wallace MH, Hawk E, Gordon GB, et al. The effect of celecoxib, a cyclooxygenase-2 inhibitor, in familial adenomatous polyposis. *N. Engl. J. Med.*, **342** (2000) 1946–1952.

21. Potter JD, Slattery ML, Bostick RM, and Gapstur SM. Colon cancer: a review of the epidemiology. *Epidemiol. Rev.*, **15** (1993) 499–545.

22. Newmark HL, Wargovich MJ, and Bruce WE. Colon cancer and dietary fat, phosphate, and calcium: a hypothesis. *J. Natl. Cancer Inst.*, **72** (1984) 1323–1325.

23. Morotomi M, Guillem J, LoGerfo P, and Weinstein IB. Production of diacylglycerol, an activator of protein kinase C, by human intestinal microflora. *Cancer Res.*, **50** (1990) 3595–3599.

24. Haenszel W, Berg JW, Segi M, Kurihara M, and Locke FB. Large bowel cancer in Hawaiian Japanese. *J. Natl. Cancer Inst.*, **51** (1973) 1765–1799.

25. Van Tassell RL, Kingston DGI, and Wilkins TD. Metabolism of dietary genotoxins by the human colonic microflora: The fecapentaenes and heterocyclic amines. *Mutat. Res.*, **238** (1990) 209–221.

26. Richter F, Newmark HL, Richter A, Leung D, and Lipkin M. Inhibition of Western-diet induced proliferation and hyperplasia in mouse colon by two sources of calcium. *Carcinogenesis*, **16** (1995) 2685–2689.

27. Buset M, Lipkin M, Winawer S, Swaroop S, and Friedman E. Inhibition of human colonic epithelial cell proliferation in vivo and in vitro by calcium. *Cancer Res.*, **46** (1986) 5426–5430.

28. Appleton GVN, Owen RW, Wheeler EE, Challacombe DN, and Williamcon RCN. Effect of dietary calcium on the colonic luminal environment. *Gut*, **32** (1991) 1374–1377.

29. Shabahang M, Buras RR, Davoodi F, Schumaker LM, Nauta RJ, and Evans SR. 1,25-Dihydroxyvitamin D_3 receptor as a marker of human colon carcinoma cell line differentiation and growth inhibition. *Cancer Res.*, **53** (1993) 3712–3718.

30. Baron JA, Beach M, Mandel JS, van Stolk RU, Haile RW, Sandler RS, et al. Calcium supplements for the prevention of colorectal adenomas. Calcium polyp prevention study group. *N. Engl. J. Med.*, **340** (1999) 101–107.

31. Giovannucci E, Stampfer ME, Colditz GA, Hunter DJ, Fuchs C, Rosner BA, et al. Multivitamin use, folate, and colon cancer in women in the Nurses' Health Study. *Ann. Intern. Med.*, **129** (1998) 517–524.

32. Winawer SJ, Zauber AG, O'Brien MJ, Ho MN, Gottlieb L, Sternber SS, et al. Randomized comparison of surveillance intervals after colonoscopic removal of newly diagnosed adenomatous polyps. *N. Engl. J. Med.*, **328** (1993) 901–906.

33. Muller AD and Sonnenberg A. Prevention of colorectal cancer by flexible endoscopy and polypectomy. A case-control study of 32,702 veterans. *Ann. Intern. Med.*, **123** (1995) 904–910.

34. Thiis-Evensen E, Hoff GS, Sauar J, Langmark F, Majak BM, and Vatn MH. Population-based surveillance by colonoscopy: effect on the incidence of colorectal cancer. Telemark Polyp Study I. *Scand. J. Gastroenterol.*, **34** (1999) 414–420.

35. Cali RL, Pitsch RM, Thorson AG, Watson P, Tapie P, Blatchford GJ, et al. Cumulative incidence of metachronous colorectal cancer. *Dis. Colon Rectum*, **36** (1993) 388–393.

36. Williams AR, Palasooriya BAW, and Day DW. Polyps and cancer of the large bowel: a necropsy study in Liverpool. *Gut*, **123** (1982) 835–842.

37. National Cancer Institute Surveillance, Epidemiology and End Results (SEER) Program, SEER Cancer Statistics Review, 1973–1995.

38. Fuchs CS, Giovannucci EL, Colditz GA, Hunter DJ, Speizer FE, and Willet WC. A prospective study of family history and risk of colorectal cancer. *N. Engl. J. Med.*, **331** (1994) 1669–1674.

39. Schatzkin A, Lanza E, Corle D, Lance P, Iber F, Caan B, et al. Lack of effect of a low-fat, high -fiber diet on the recurrence of colorectal adenomas. *N. Engl. J. Med.*, **342** (2000) 1149–1155.

40. Labayle D, Fischer D, Vielh P, Drouhin F, Pariente A, Bories C, et al. Sulindac causes regression of rectal polyps in familial adenomatous polyposis. *Gastroenterology*, **101** (1991) 635–639.

41. Physicians' Health Study Group. Final report on the aspirin component of the ongoing Physicians' Health Study. *N. Engl. J. Med.*, **321** (1995) 129–135.

42. Greenberg ER, Baron JA, Tosteson TD, Freeman DH Jr, Beck GJ, Bond JH, et al. A clinical trial of antioxidant vitamins to prevent colorectal adenomas. *N. Engl. J. Med.*, **331** (1994) 141–147.

43. Clark LC, Combs GF, Turnbull BW, Slate EH, Chalker DK, Chow J, et al. Effects of selenium supplementation for cancer prevention in patients with carcinoma of the skin. *JAMA*, **276** (1996) 1957–1963.

44. Alberts DS, Martinez ME, Roe DJ, Guillen-Rodriguez JM, Marchall JR, van Leeuwen JB, et al. Lack of effect of a high-fiber cereal supplement on the recurrence of colorectal adenomas. Phoenix Colon Cancer Prevention Physicians' Network. *N. Engl. J. Med.*, **342** (2000) 1156–1162.

45. Baron JA and Sandler RS. Nonsteroidal anti-inflammatory drugs and cancer prevention. *Annu. Rev. Med.* **51** (2000) 511–523.

46. Thun MJ, Namboodiri MM, and Heath CWJ. Aspirin use and reduced risk of fatal colon cancer. *N. Engl. J. Med.*, **325** (1991) 1593–1596.

47. Giovannucci E, Rimm EB, Stampfer MJ, Colditz GA, Ascherio A, and Willett WC. Aspirin use and the risk for colorectal cancer and adenomas in male health professionals. *Ann. Intern. Med.*, **121** (1994) 241–246.

48. Bansal P and Sonnenberg A. Risk factors of colorectal cancer in inflammatory bowel disease. *Am. J. Gastroenterol.*, **91** (1996) 44–48.

49. Waddell WR and Loughry RW. Sulindac for polyposis of the colon. *J. Surg. Oncol.*, **24** (1983) 83–87.

50. Pasricha PJ, Bedi A, O'Connor K, Rashid A, Akhtar AJ, Zahurak ML, et al. The effects of sulindac on colorectal proliferation and apoptosis in familial adenomatous polyposis. *Gastroenterology*, **109** (1995) 994–998.

51. Furstenberger G, Gross M, and Marks F. Eicosanoids and multistage carcinogenesis in NMRI mouse skin: role of prostaglandins E and F in conversion (first stage of tumor promotion) and promotion (second stage of tumor promotion). *Carcinogenesis*, **10** (1989) 91–96.

52. Sheng H, Shao J, Morrow JD, Beauchamp RD, and DuBois RN. Modulation of apoptosis and Bcl-2 expression by prostaglandin E2 in human colon cancer cells. *Cancer Res.*, **58** (1998) 362–366.

53. Botti C, Seregni E, Ferreri L, Martinetti A, and Bombardieri E. Immunosuppressive factors: role in cancer development and progression. *Int. J. Biol. Markers*, **13** (1998) 51–69.

54. Kujubu DA, Fletcher BS, Varnum BC, Lim RW, and Herschman HR. TIS 10, a phorbol ester tumor promoter-inducible mRNA from Swiss 3T3 cells, encodes a novel prostaglandin synthase/cyclooxygenase homologue. *J. Biol. Chem.*, **266** (1991) 12,866–12,872.

55. Jobin C, Morteau O, Han DS, and Sartor RB. Specific NF-κB blockade selectively inhibits tumor necrosis factor-α-induced COX-2 but not constitutive COX-1 gene expression in HT-29 cells. *Immunology*, **95** (1998) 537–543.

56. Marks F and Furstenberger G. Cancer chemoprevention through interruption of multistage carcinogenesis: the lessons learnt by comparing mouse skin carcinogenesis and human large bowel cancer. *Eur. J. Cancer*, **36** (2000) 314–329.

57. Smalley WE and DuBois RN. Colorectal cancer and nonsteroidal anti-inflammatory drugs. *Adv. Pharmacol.*, **39** (1997) 1–20.

58. Oshima M, Dinchuk JE, Kargman SL, Oshima H, Hancock B, Kwong E, et al. Suppression of intestinal polyposis in APC$^{\Delta716}$ knockout mice by inhibition of cyclooxygenase-2 (COX-2). *Cell*, **83** (1995) 493–501.

59. Jacoby RF, Seibert K, Cole CE, Kelloff G, and Lubet RA. The cyclooxygenase-2 inhibitor celecoxib is a potent preventive and therapeutic agent in the min mouse model of adenomatous polyposis. *Cancer Res.*, **60** (2000) 5040–5044.

60. Huang C, Ma WY, Hahnenberger D, Cleary MP, Bowden GT, and Dong Z. Inhibition of untraviolet B-induced activator protein-1 (AP-1) activity by aspirin in AP-1-luciferase transgenic mice. *J. Biol. Chem.*, **272** (1997) 26,325–26,331.

61. Xie W and Herschman HR. Transcriptional regulation of prostaglandin-2 gene expression by platelet-derived growth factor and serum. *J. Biol. Chem.*, **271** (1996) 31,742–31,748.

62. Kipp E and Gosh S. Inhibition of NF-kappa B by sodium salicylate and aspirin. *Science*, **265** (1994) 956–959.

63. Piazza GA, Alberts DS, Hixson LJ, Paranka NS, Li H, Finn T, et al. Sulindac sulfone inhibits azoxymethane-induced colon carcinogenesis in rats without reducing prostaglandin levels. *Cancer Res.*, **57** (1997) 2909–2915.

64. Pence BC, Dunn DM, Zhao C, Landers M, and Wargovich MJ. Chemopreventive effects of calcium but not aspirin supplementation in cholic acid-promoted colon carcinogenesis: correlation with intermediate endpoints. *Carcinogenesis*, **16** (1995) 757–765.

65. Ochsenkuhn T, Bayerdorffer E, Maining A, Schinket M, Thiede C, Nussler V, et al. Colonic mucosal proliferation is related to serum deoxycholic acid levels. *Cancer*, **85** (1999) 1664–1669.

66. Martinez JD, Stratagoules ED, LaRue JM, Powell AA, Gause PR, Craven MT, et al. Different bile acids exhibit distince biological effects: the tumor promoter deoxycholic acid induces apoptosis and the chemopreventive agent ursodeoxycholic acid inhibits cell proliferation. *Nutr. Cancer*, **31** (1998) 111–118.

67. Baijal PK, Fitzpatrick DW, and Bird RP. Modulation of colonic xenobiotic metabolizing enzymes by feeding bile acids: comparative effects of cholic, deoxycholic, lithocholic, and ursodeoxycholic acids. *Food Chem. Toxicol.*, **36** (1998) 601–607.

68. Pence BC. Role of calcium in colon cancer prevention: experimental and clinical studies. *Mutat. Res.*, **290** (1993) 87–95.

69. Lipkin M, Yang K, Edelmann W, Xue L, Fan K, Risio M, et al. Preclinical mouse models for cancer chemoprevention studies. *Ann. NY Acad. Sci.*, **889** (1999) 14–19.

70. Alberts DS, Ritenbaugh C, Story JA, et al. Randomized, double-blinded, placebo-controlled study of effect of wheat bran fiber and calcium on fecal bile acids in patients with resected adenomatous colon polyps. *J. Natl. Cancer Inst.*, **88** (1996) 81–92.

71. Bostick R, Potter J, Fosdick L, Grambsch P, Lampe JW, Wood JR, et al. Calcium and colorectal epithelial cell proliferation: a preliminary randomized, double-blinded, placebo-controlled clinical trial. *J. Natl. Cancer Inst.*, **85** (1993) 132–141.

72. Slater SJ, Kelly MB, Taddeo FJ, Larkin JD, Yeager MD, McLane JA, et al. Direct activation of protein kinase C by 1,25-dihydroxy Vitamin D3. *J. Biol. Chem.*, **270** (1995) 6639–6643.

73. Sitrin MD, Halline AG, Abrahams C, and Brasitus TA. Dietary calcium and vitamin D modulate 1,2 dimethylhydrazine-induced colonic carcinogenesis in the rat. *Cancer Res.*, **51** (1991) 5608–5613.

74. Belleli A, Shany S, Levy J, Guberman R, and Lamprecht SA. A protective role of 1,25 dihydroxy vitamin D3 in chemically induced rat colon carcinogenesis. *Carcinogenesis*, **13** (1992) 2293–2298.

75. Earnest DL, Holubec H, Wali RK, Jolley CS, Bissonnette M, Bhattacharyya AK, et al. Chemoprevention of azoxymethane-induced colonic carcinogenesis by supplemental dietary ursodeoxycholic acid. *Cancer Res.*, **54** (1994) 5071–5074.

76. Wali RK, Frawley BP Jr, Hartmann S, Roy HK, Khare S, Scaglione-Sewell BA, et al. Mechanism of action of chemoprotective ursodeoxycholate in the azoxymethane model of rat colonic carcinogenesis: Potential roles of protein kinase c-alpha -beta II, and -zeta. *Cancer Res.*, **55** (1995) 5257–5264.

77. Ikegami T, Matsuzaki Y, Shoda J, Kano M, Hirabayashi N, and Tanaka N. The chemopreventive role of ursodeoxycholic acid in azoxymethane-treated rats: suppressive effects on enhanced group II phospholipase A2 expression in colonic tissue. *Cancer Lett.*, **134** (1998) 129–139.

78. Invernizzi P, Salzman AL, Szabo C, Ueta I, O'Connor M, and Stechell KD. Ursodeoxycholate inhibits induction of NOS in human intestinal epithelial cells and in vivo. *Am. J. Physiol.*, **273** (1997) G131–G138.

79. Christman JK, Sheikhnejad G, Diznik M, Abileah S, and Wainfan E. Reversibility of changes in nucleic acid methylation and gene expression induced in rat liver by severe dietary methyl deficiency. *Carcinogenesis*, **14** (1993) 551–557.

80. Song J, Sohn KJ, Medline A, Ash C, Gallinger S, and Kim YI. Chemopreventive effects of dietary folate on intestinal polyps in Apc+/–Msh2–/– mice. *Cancer Res.*, **60** (2000) 3191–3199.

81. Ma J, Stampfer MJ, Giovannucci E, Artigas C, Hunter DJ, Fuchs C, et al. Methylenetetrahydrofolate reductase polymorphism, dietary interactions, and risk of colorectal cancer. *Cancer Res.*, **57** (1997) 1098–1102.

82. Ma J, Stampfer MJ, Christensen B, Giovannucci E, Hunter DJ, Chen J, et al. A polymorphism of the methionine synthase gene: association with plasma folate, vitamin B12, homocyst(e)ine, and colorectal cancer risk. *Cancer Epidemiol. Biomarkers Prev.*, **8** (1999) 825–829.

83. Slattery ML, Potter JD, Samowitz W, Schaffer D, and Leppert M. Methylenetetrahydrofolate reductase, diet, and risk of colon cancer. *Cancer Epidemiol. Biomarkers Prev.*, **8** (1999) 513–518.

84. Chen J, Giovannucci E, Hankinson SE, Ma J, Willett WC, Spiegelman D, et al. A prospective study of methylenetetrahydrofolate reductase and methionine synthase gene polymorphisms, and risk of colorectal adenoma. *Carcinogenesis*, **19** (1998) 2129–2132.

85. Potter JD. Hormones and colon cancer. *J. Natl. Cancer Inst.*, **87** (1995) 1039–1040.

86. McMichael AJ and Potter JD. Reproduction, endogenous and exogenous sex hormones, and colon cancer: a review and hypothesis. *J. Natl. Cancer Inst.*, **65** (1980) 1201–1207.

87. Hebert-Croteau, N. A meta-analysis of hormone replacement therapy and colon cancer in women. *Cancer Epidemiol. Biomarkers Prev.*, **7** (1998) 653–659.

88. Grodstein F, Newcomb PA, and Stampfer MJ. Postmenopausal hormone therapy and the risk of colorectal cancer: a review and meta-analysis. *Am. J. Med.*, **106** (1999) 574–582.

89. Weyant MJ, Carothers AM, Mahmoud NN, Bradlow HL, Remotti H, Bilinski RT, et al. Estrogen-mediated modulation of *Apc*-associated intestinal tumorigenesis. *Cancer Res.*, **61** (2001) 2547–2551.

90. Zhu BT and Conney AH. Is 2-methoxyestradiol an endogenous estrogen metabolite that inhibits mammary carcinogenesis? *Cancer Res.*, **58** (1998) 2269–2277.
91. Telang NT, Suto A, Wong GY, Osborne MP, and Bradlow HL. Induction by estrogen metabolite 16α-hydroxyestrone of genotoxic damage and aberrant proliferation in mouse mammary epithelial cells. *J. Natl. Cancer Inst.*, **84** (1992) 634–638.
92. Klauber N, Paragni S, Flynn E, Hamel E, and D'Amato RJ. Inhibition of angiogenesis and breast cancer in mice by the microtubule inhibitors 2-methoxyestradiol and taxol. *Cancer Res.*, **57** (1997) 81–86.
93. Kuiper GGJM, Lemmen JG, Carlsson B, Corton JC, Safe SH, van der Saag PT, et al. Interaction of estrogenic chemicals and phytoestrogens with estrogen receptor β. *Endocrinology*, **139** (1998) 4252–4263.
94. Patisaul HB, Whitten PL, and Young LJ. Regulation of estrogen receptor beta mRNA in the brain: opposite effects of 17β estradiol and the phytoestrogen, coumestrol. *Molec. Brain Res.*, **67** (1999) 165–171.
95. Davies MJ, Bowey EA, Aldercreutz H, Rowland IR, and Rumsby PC. Effects of soy or rye supplementation of high-fat diets on colon tumor development in azoxymethane-treated rats. *Carcinogenesis*, **20** (1999) 927–931.
96. Kato K, Takahashi S, Cui L, Toda T, Suzuki S, Futakuchi M, et al. Suppressive effects of dietary genistein and diadzein on rat prostate carcinogenesis. *Jpn. J. Cancer Res.*, **91** (2000) 786–791.
97. Aw TY. Molecular and cellular responses to oxidative stress and changes in oxidation–reduction imbalance in the intestine. *Am. J. Clin. Nutr.*, **70** (1999) 557–565.
98. Hengstler JG, Arand M, Herrero ME, and Oesch F. Polymorphisms of *N*-acteyltransferases, glutathione *S*-transferases, microsomal epoxide hydrolase and sulfotransferases: influence on cancer susceptibility. *Recent Results Cancer Res.*, **154** (1998) 47–85.
99. Bravo L. Polyphenols: chemistry, dietary sources, metabolism, and nutritional significance. *Nutr. Rev.*, **56** (1998) 317–333.
100. Tanaka T. Effect of diet on human carcinogenesis. *Crit. Rev. Oncol. Hematol.*, **25** (1997) 73–95.
101. Enger SM, Longnecker MP, Chen MJ, Harper JM, Lee ER, Frankl HD, et al. Dietary intake of specific carotenoids and vitamins A, C, and E, and the prevalence of colorectal adenomas. *Cancer Epidemiol. Biomarkers Prev.*, **5** (1996) 147–153.
102. Lupulescu A. The role of hormones, growth factors, and vitamins in carcinogenesis. *Crit. Rev. Oncol. Hematol.*, **23** (1996) 95–130.
103. Hainonen O and Albanes D. The effect of vitamin E and beta-carotene on the incidence of lung cancer and other cancers in male smokers. *N. Engl. J. Med.*, **330** (1994) 1029–1035.
104. Hennekens CH, Buring JE, Manson JE, Stampfer M, Rosner B, Cook NR, et al. Lack of effect of long-term supplementation with beta-carotene on the incidnece of malignant neoplasms and cardiovascular disease. *N. Engl. J. Med.*, **334** (1996) 1145–1149.
105. Omenn GS, Goodman GE, Thornquist MD, Balmes J, Cullen MR, Glass A, et al. Effects of a combination of beta carotene and vitamin A on lung cancer and cardiovascular disease. *N. Engl. J. Med.*, **334** (1996) 1150–1155.
106. McKeown-Eyssen G. A randomized trial of vitamins C and E in the prevention of recurrence of colorectal polyps. *Cancer Res.*, **48** (1988) 4701–4705.
107. Combs GF Jr. Chemopreventive agents: selenium. *Pharmacol Ther.*, **79** (1998) 179–192.
108. Nomura A, Heilbrun LK, Morris S, and Stemmerman GN. Serum selenium and the risk of cancer, by specific sites: case-control analysis of prospective data. *J. Natl. Cancer Inst.*, **79** (1987) 103–108.
109. Ghadirian P, Masionneuve P, Perret C, Kennedy G. Boyle P, Krewski D, et al. A case-control study of toenail selenium and cancer of the breast, colon, and prostate. *Cancer Detect. Prev.*, **24** (2000) 305–313.
110. Clark LC, Dalkin B, Krongrad A, Combs GF, Turnbull BW, Slate EH, et al. Decreased incidence of prostate cancer with selenium supplementation: results of a double-blind cancer prevention trial. *Br. J. Urol.*, **81** (1998) 730–734.
111. Mayne ST and Lippman SM. Cancer prevention: chemopreventive agents. Retinoids, carotenoids, and micronutrients. In *Principles and Practice on Oncology*, 6th ed. DeVita VT Jr, Hellman S, and Rosenberg SA (eds.), Lippincott Williams & Wilkins, Philadelphia, 2000.
112. Killinken S, Castilla M, and Thorgiersson S. Effect of inhibitors of ornithine decarboxylase on retrovirus induced transformation of murine erythroid precursors in vitro. *Cancer Res.*, **46** (1986) 6246–6249.
113. McCormack SA, Blanner PM, Zimmerman BJ, Ray R, Poppelton HM, Patel TB, et al. Polyamine deficiency alters EGF receptor distribution and signalling effectiveness in IEC-6 cells. *Am. J. Physiol.*, **274** (1998) C192–C205.
114. Kelloff GJ, Boone CW, Steele VE, Fay JR, Lubet RA, Crowell JA, et al. Mechanistic considerations in chemopreventive drug development. *J. Cell. Biochem.*, **20(Suppl.)** (1994) 1–24.
115. Thompson H and Ronan A. Effect of D,L-2-difluoromethylornithine and endocrine manipulation on the induction of mammary carcinogenesis by 1-methyl-1-nitrosourea. *Carcinogenesis*, **7** (1986) 2003–2006.

116. Reddy B, Nayini J, Tokumo K, Rigotty J, Zhang E, and Kelloff G. Chemoprevention of colon carcinogenesis by concurrent administration of piroxicam, a nonsteroidal antiinflammatory drug with D,L-*a*-difluoromethylornithine, an ornithine decarboxylase inhibitor, in diet. *Cancer Res.*, **50** (1990) 2562–2568.

117. Tsunoda A, Shibusawa M, Tsunoda Y, Yasuda N, and Koide T. Reduced growth rate of dimethylhydrazine-induced colon tumors in rats. *Cancer Res.*, **52** (1992) 696–700.

118. Wallon UM, Shassetz LR, Cress AE, Bowden GT, and Gerner EW. Polyamine-dependent expression of the matrix metalloproteinase matrilysin in a human colon cancer-derived cell line. *Mol. Carcinog.*, **11** (1994) 138–144.

119. Love RR, Jacoby R, Newton MA, Tutsch KD, Simon K, Pomplun M, et al. A randomized, placebo-controlled tiral of low-dose alpha-difluoromethylornithine in individuals at risk for colorectal cancer. *Cancer Epidemiol. Biomarkers Prev.*, **7** (1998) 989–992.

120. Slattery ML, Kampman E, Samowitz W, Caan BJ, and Potter JD. Interplay between dietary inducers of GST and the GSTM-1 genotype in colon cancer. *Int. J. Cancer*, **87** (2000) 728–733.

121. Rao CV, Tokomo K, Katicoalla M, Kelloff GJ, and Reddy BS. Chemopreventive effect of oltipraz during different stages of experimental colon carcinogenesis induced by azyoymethane in male F344 rats. *Cancer Res.*, **53** (1993) 3499–3504.

122. Benson AB III, Olopade OI, Fatain MJ, Rademaker A, Mobarhan S, Stucky-Marshall L, et al. Chronic daily low dose of 4-methyl-5-(2-pyrazinyl)-1,2-dithiole-3-thione (oltipraz) in patients with previously resected colon polyps and first-degree female relatives of breast cancer patients. *Clin. Cancer Res.*, **6** (2000) 3870–3877.

123. Giovannucci E, Egan KM, Hunter DJ, Stampfer MJ, Colditz GA, Willett WC, et al. Aspirin and the risk of colorectal cancer in women. *N. Engl. J. Med.*, **333** (1995) 609–614.

124. Langman M and Boyle P. Chemoprevention of colorectal cancer. *Gut*, **43** (1998) 578–585.

125. Fournier DB and Gordon GB. Cox-2 and colon cancer: Potential targets for chemoprevention. *J. Cell Biochem.*, **34(Suppl.)** (2000) 97–102.

126. Winawer SJ, Fletcher RH, Miller L, Godlee F, Stolar MH, Mulrow CD, et al. Colorectal cancer screening: clinical guidelines and rationale. *Gastroenterology*, **112** (1997) 594–642.

6

Management of Hereditary Colon Cancer Syndromes

Miguel A. Rodriguez-Bigas
and Nicholas J. Petrelli

Hereditary cancers account for approximately 10% of the overall cancer burden. As such, colorectal cancer is no different. The most common hereditary colorectal cancers are hereditary nonpolyposis colorectal cancer (HNPCC) or the Lynch syndrome and familial adenomatous polyposis (FAP). There are, however, other less well-known inherited syndromes for which the colon and rectum are at risk, such as familial juvenile polyposis, Peutz–Jeghers syndrome, and Cowden syndrome.

As discussed in Chapter 2, germline mutations in different genes have been described that are responsible for these syndromes. If an affected individual in a kindred is identified as a carrier of a germline mutation, genetic testing can then be used to screen at-risk individuals in that kindred. However, if a mutation has not been identified in an affected individual, genetic testing will not be beneficial for screening at-risk individuals in that kindred; thus, every at-risk individual must be considered as a potential carrier of the mutation and, as such, surveilled accordingly.

The surgical options in patients with hereditary colorectal cancer syndromes include both therapeutic and prophylactic procedures. Each syndrome presents distinct issues which need to be considered prior to a final surgical recommendation. In this chapter, we will address those surgical issues.

1. FAMILIAL ADENOMATOUS POLYPOSIS

Familial adenomatous polyposis (FAP) is a syndrome characterized by hundreds to thousands of colorectal polyps that left untreated will invariably turn into malignancy. In the milder phenotypic variant, attenuated adenomatous polyposis coli (AAPC), colorectal polyps are less numerous, and colorectal carcinoma will occur at a later age. As previously

From: *Colorectal Cancer: Multimodality Management*
Edited by: L. Saltz © Humana Press Inc., Totowa, NJ

discussed, the syndrome also includes extracolonic manifestations. In this syndrome, the penetrance is close to 100%; therefore, in those individuals carrying a germline mutation, polyposis will invariably develop.

The surgical management of FAP relies on prophylactic colorectal surgery. Prophylactic abdominal colectomy and surveillance has been shown to increase survival by approx 30 yr compared to untreated FAP patients (1). There is no ideal surgical procedure in the management of FAP. Segmental resections, total proctocolectomy and ileostomy, abdominal colectomy with ileorectal anastomosis (IRA), total abdominal colectomy, mucosal proctectomy and ileoanal pouch anastomosis (IPAA) are procedures which have been described in the management of FAP patients (2). The most common procedures are IRA and IPAA. There is debate over which of these procedures is best. Both procedures have advantages and disadvantages. Several factors must be considered prior to a final surgical recommendation, including symptomatology, extent of the polyposis, extracolonic manifestations, age of the patient, presence of carcinoma, social and psychological factors such as the ability to handle a potential temporary or even permanent stoma, compliance of the patient, morbidity of the procedure, experience of the surgeon, and results. The genotype of the patient, if available, prior to surgical prophylaxis should also be considered in the decision-making process (3–5).

1.1. Segmental Resections

Rarely should segmental resection be used in the management of FAP. Occasionally, they may be of use in patients with advanced carcinoma who are bleeding or obstructed or in the patient with a high surgical risk for any other procedure. If a segmental resection performed, if possible, a segment of bowel with minimal or no involvement with polyps should be chosen for anastomosis to minimize the risks anastomotic leaks.

1.1.1. TOTAL PROCTOCOLECTOMY AND ILEOSTOMY

Total proctocolectomy and ileostomy (TPC) is a procedure that should be offered only to selected patients with FAP and invasive distal rectal adenocarcinoma. The technique as described by Brooke in 1952 includes removal of the colon and rectum and immediate maturation of the ileal mucosa to the skin (6). In 1969, Kock described the use reversed ileal segments to construct a reservoir that evolved into the construction of a valve mechanism with an intussuscepted portion of the small bowel (7). Table 1 illustrates the advantages and disadvantages of this procedure compared to other procedures available in the management of FAP.

1.1.2. ABDOMINAL COLECTOMY AND ILEORECTAL ANASTOMOSIS

This procedure was originally described by Mayo and Wakefield in 1936 (8). It consists of removing the entire colon and performing an anastomosis in the true rectum (9). Ideal candidates for this procedure are young patients who present with sparse polyposis or with polyps in the rectum easily controlled endoscopically. These patients must be compliant patients who will adhere to rigorous surveillance programs. The main disadvantage of this procedure is the subsequent cancer risk in rectal stump. As illustrated in Table 2, the cumulative incidence of rectal cancer at 20 yr after IRA has been reported to be between 13% and 37% (5,10–14). However, this risk has been reported to be as high as 55% at 30 yr postcolectomy (15). In the latter study, the high cancer rate could have been the result of potential ileosigmoid anastomosis as well as to the fact that not all patients underwent surveillance. Age has been implicated as a factor in rectal cancer risk after IRA. In Scandinavia and at the St. Mark's Registry, the cumulative rectal cancer risk increased

Table 1
Advantages and Disadvantages of Surgical Procedures in the Management of Familial Adenomatous Polyposis

Procedure	Advantages	Disadvantages
Total proctocolectomy and ileostomy (Brooke)	No specific training needed; colorectal cancer risk eliminated	Permanent stoma; peristomal skin problems; Bladder and sexual dysfunction; potential psychological effects on patient and family members
Total proctocolectomy and ileostomy (Kock pouch)	Colorectal cancer risk eliminated; continent reservoir	More complex procedure; similar to Brooke ileostomy; potential for pouchitis
Abdominal colectomy and ileorectal anastomosis (IRA)	No specific training needed; avoids stoma; relatively normal bowel function; sexual and bladder function usually preserved; ease of exam of residual rectum	Rectal cancer risk
Abdominal colectomy, mucosal proctectomy, ileoanal pouch anastomosis (IPAA)	Virtual elimination of colorectal mucosa; avoidance of permanent stoma; relatively good bowel function; acceptable continence; sexual and bladder function usually preserved	Complex surgery; minimal rectal cancer risk, but still present

Table 2
Cumulative Risk of Rectal Cancer After Abdominal Colectomy and Ileorectal Anastomosis

Investigators	Cancer/ patients	Follow-up (yr)	Mucosa at-risk length (cm)	Rectal cancer risk (%)				Rectal excision cumulative rate
				10 yr	20 yr	25 yr	30 yr	
Mayo Clinic (10)	46/143	19.1[a]	19.5	13	26	34	55	NS
Cleveland Clinic (11)	10/133	5.4[b]	NS	4	12			NS
Scandinavian Study (12)	14/294	NS	NS	4.5	9.4	13		44% (25 yr)
St. Mark's (13)	22/224	13.6[b]	10.3[c]			15		NS
Japanese Registry (14)	105/320	NS	15[a]	13	37			NS
Finnish Registry (15)	9/100	10[b]	15[a]	5.8	25			74% (29 yr)
Toronto Registry (23)	5/60	7.7[b]	15					37%
Italian Registry (5)	27/371	6.8[a]	NS	7.7	23			NS

[a]Median.
[b]Mean.
[c]230 of 320 patients; NS = not stated.

sharply from 5% and 10% at age 50, to 14% and 29% by age 60 respectively *(11,12)*. This was not noted in the Finnish Registry in which seven of nine patients developed rectal cancer before age 50 *(14)*. Other factors implicated in an increase rectal cancer risk after IRA include the number of rectal adenomas at the time of colectomy, the presence of colon cancer, the length of the rectal stump, and the length of follow-up after IRA *(5,11,12,15,17–19)*. The genotype of the patient has also been implicated with increased rectal cancer risk. Mutations implicated with increased rectal cancer risk and eventual excision of the rectum after IRA include mutations downstream exon 15 codon 1250, exon 15 codon 1309 and 1328, and exon 15 mutations between codons 1250 and 1464 *(3–5)*. Patients with such mutations will benefit from an IPPA rather than an IRA as their prophylactic surgery. The spontaneous regression of rectal polyps after ileorectal anastomosis has been reported to be as high as 33% *(10)*. The adenoma regression correlates with the number of rectal adenomas at the time of IRA *(20)*. However, the adenomas may reappear *(20)*. Although it is not known why this regression occurs, some authors have suggested decreased secondary bile acid excretion as a possible mechanism *(21)*.

Even though IRA is considered a less complex procedure than IPAA, it is not a procedure to be taken lightly. Complications can occur following this procedure. Thompson reported 10% morbidity and 1% mortality in 215 patients undergoing abdominal colectomy and ileorectal anastomosis at St. Mark's Hospital *(22)*. Thirty-six patients (16.7%) developed 55 episodes of bowel obstruction during follow-up, of whom 24 required surgery *(22)*. Table 3 illustrates the largest published series comparing functional outcome between IRA and IPAA *(23)*. From these data, it appears that the functional outcome is better after IRA than IPAA. The groups at St. Mark's Hospital and the Toronto Registry have published similar functional results, whereas the Mayo Clinic group reported no difference in function between the two procedures *(16,24,25)*. The experience van Duijvendijk et al. as well as others suggests that there is no difference in function between those patients undergoing IPAA as the initial procedure for FAP versus those undergoing IPAA after rectal excision after and IRA *(23,26)*.

1.1.3. TOTAL ABDOMINAL COLECTOMY, MUCOSAL PROCTECTOMY, AND ILEOANAL POUCH ANASTOMOSIS

Total abdominal colectomy, mucosal proctectomy, and ileoanal pouch anastomosis virtually removes the whole colorectal mucosa at risk. The current practice is to leave a 1- to 2-cm rectal muscular cuff just above the levators *(27)*. However, there have been case reports of carcinoma developing in the pouch *(28–30)*. In addition, two separate group of investigators have reported an 18% and 42% incidence of pouch adenomas after IPAA, respectively *(31,32)*. Therefore, lifetime surveillance of the pouch is mandatory after this procedure. Ideal candidates for this procedure include patients with numerous rectal adenomas, patients with a family history of desmoid tumors, and patients with mutations that have been implicated with increased rectal cancer risk, as described earlier. Advantages and disadvantages of this procedure are illustrated in Table 1.

Ileal reservoirs creating a double (J), triple (S), or quadruple reservoir (W) pouch have been described *(33–35)*. The difference between these is the amount of distal ileum utilized for construction of the pouch, the capacity of the pouch, and the type of pouch–anal anastomosis. The most commonly used pouches are the J and S pouches. The former requires 30 cm of distal ileum to be folded in two 15-cm segments whereas the latter requires 47 cm of distal ileum to be folded into three 15-cm limbs with a 2-cm exit conduit. The main advantage of the S pouch over the J pouch is that the S pouch will reach farther (approx

Table 3
Functional Results After Surgery for Familial Adenomatous Polyposis

	IRA[a] n = 145	IPAA[b] n = 106
Responders	88%	84%
Mean age	41 ± 14	37 ± 12
Mean age at surgery	29 ± 13	30 ± 11
Mean follow-up (yr)	12 ± 7.5	6.8 ± 4.9
Male/female (%)	48/52	57/43
Daytime stool frequency	4.7 ± 2	6.0 ± 2.2
Nighttime stool frequency	1.4 ± 1.9	2.0 ± 2
Soiling	37.3%	64.6%
Passive incontinence	9.4%	25.7%
Antidiarrheal medication	14.9%	27.5%
Flatus continence	79.8%	63.0%
Ability to distinguish flatus/feces	44.4%	32.1%
Perianal skin irritation	72.9%	86.4%

Note: All were statistically significant ($p < 0.05$ IRA vs IPAA) except responders, age at surgery, and gender.
[a]Abdominal colectomy ileorectal anastomosis.
[b]Abdominal colectomy mucosal proctectomy and ileoanal pouch anastomosis.
Source: ref. *23.*

2–4 cm) than the J pouch, thus decreasing the chances of anastomotic tension *(36).* The anastomosis in the J pouch is side to end (pouch to anus), whereas it is end to end in the S pouch. The anastomosis can either be hand-sewn or stapled. The disadvantage of the stapled anastomosis is the retention of rectal mucosa proximal to the dentate line. Table 4 illustrates functional results after IPAA for FAP.

Ileoanal pouch anastomois is more complex than IRA. It, therefore, has a higher morbidity. The morbidity after IPAA has been reported to be 10% to as high as 60%, including morbidity from temporary ileostomy closure *(2,38,39).* However, there are some centers at which IPAA is performed without a protecting ileostomy. The morbidity after IPAA in 94 FAP patients who underwent the procedure at the Mayo Clinic series was reported to be 28% compared to 17% morbidity after IRA *(25).* The incidence of small bowel obstruction requiring reoperation was 5% after IPAA and 6% after IRA. These differences, overall morbidity, and small bowel obstruction requiring laparotomy were not statistically significant *(25).* In an updated report from the Mayo Clinic in 187 patient undergoing IPAA, the overall complication rate was 24% with 25 (13%) patients developing small bowel obstruction *(37).* Twenty-five percent of these patients underwent reoperation *(37).* Kartheuser et al. reported on 171 patients with FAP who underwent IPAA as their initial operations *(38).* The postoperative morbidity was 10% *(38).* The overall incidence of small bowel obstruction was 15%, with 13 patients undergoing 14 operations *(38).* In that study, 11 of the 15 episodes of obstruction that occurred after ileostomy closure required surgery *(38).* Van Duijvendijk et al. reported 15/161 (9%) patients experiencing small bowel obstruction after IRA versus 17/118 (14%) after IPAA for FAP *(23).* Three patients developed an anastomotic leak and 20 patients (12%) required reoperation after IRA, whereas 12 patients had an anastomotic and 29 patients (25%) required reoperation after IPAA *(23).* These differences were statistically

Table 4
Functional Outcome After IPAA

	van Duijvendijk (23) (n = 118)	Nyam (37) (n = 187)	Kartheuser (38) (n = 101)
Follow-up (yr)	6.8 ± 4.9	5[a] (range 0.4–14)	>1
Stool frequency per 24 h	6.0 ± 2.2	4[a] (range 1–12)	4.2 ± 0.2
Nightime stools	2.0 ± 2.0	1[a] (range 0–4)	26%
Soiling	64.6%		
Daytime continence			
Complete		84%	98%
Spotting		12%	1%
Incontinence		4%[b]	1%
Nighttime continence			
Complete		74%	96%
Spotting		22%	3%
Incontinence		4%[c]	1%
Protective pads			
Sometimes/always			1%
Never			99%
Perianal skin irritation	84.6%		5%
Antidiarrheal medication	27.5%		18%
Sometimes			9%
Always			9%
Sexual dysfunction		4.3%[d]	0%[e]

[a]Median.
[b]"Severe" in one patient.
[c]Nocturnal soiling.
[d]Five men (impotency n = 3, retrograde ejaculation n = 2); three women dyspareunia.
[e]One patient transient impotence.

significant *(23)*. The authors do not mention how many reoperations were due to small bowel obstruction *(23)*.

The use of a sodium hyalouronate-based bioresorbable membrane to prevent postoperative adhesions after IPAA was evaluated in a prospective, randomized, double-blind multicenter study utilizing standardized direct peritoneal visualization *(40)*. Patients who received the bioresorbable membrane had a significantly reduced incidence of postoperative abdominal adhesions at 8–12 wk post-IPAA compared to those patients who did not received the membrane *(40)*.

Sexual dysfunction (impotence, retrograde ejaculation, and dyspareunia) was reported to be 4% in the Mayo Clinic experience *(37)*. In that series, urinary dysfunction was reported to be less than 1% (38%). These problems can be avoided by dissection close to the rectal wall *(41)*. However, this may not be possible in patients with rectal cancer. A study of 48 teenagers undergoing IPAA revealed that the procedure was safe and had few effects on social, sexual, sport, housework, recreation, family, travel, and work activities *(42)*.

Pouchitis is another source of morbidity after IPAA in FAP patients and occurs rarely. In fact, some authors even question its existence in FAP patients *(43)*. In the Mayo Clinic experience, it was reported to be 3% *(39)*. Pouch excision after IPAA in FAP has also been reported *(18,39)*.

Both IRA and IPAA have distinct advantages and disadvantages. In some centers, the morbidity and functional results after IPAA for FAP did not differ from those for IRA, leading the investigators to propose IPAA as the initial procedure in the management of FAP *(14,16,37,38)*. None of these procedures is an ideal procedure that eliminates the risk of cancer with minimal interference with physiologic functions and minimal morbidity and mortality. Chemoprevention ads discussed in Chapter 5 may play a role in delaying surgical procedures. Therefore, the choice of which procedure to perform as well as the timing of the procedure needs to be individualized and must be made by the patients in conjunction with a team of individuals (surgeons, gastroenterologists, genetic counselors, psychologists, and social workers) who have in-depth knowledge of the natural history syndrome.

2. HEREDITARY NONPOLYPOSIS COLORECTAL CANCER

Hereditary nonpolyposis colorectal cancer is characterized as by early-onset colorectal cancer, right-sided predominance, excess synchronous or metachronous neoplasms, and extracolonic neoplasms such as endometrial, transitional cell carcinoma of the renal pelvis and ureter, and small bowel adenocarcinoma and others. The management of HNPCC can be divided as follows: management of an affected individual with untreated colorectal cancer, management of an affected individual with colorectal cancer treated with less than an abdominal colectomy, management of the yet unaffected individual with a germline mismatch repair mutation, and the management of individuals who have developed adenomas, but not carcinoma (Table 5).

The treatment of choice for a newly diagnosed untreated HNPCC individual with colon cancer is an abdominal colectomy and ileorectal anastomosis. The risk of metachronous colorectal cancers has been estimated to be as high as 40% at 10 yr after less than an abdominal colectomy and up to 72% at 40 yr after the diagnosis of colorectal cancer *(44,45)*. At our institution, at a median of 12 yr after the diagnosis of colorectal cancer, 22% of HNPCC patients treated with less than an abdominal colectomy at their initial presentation developed metachronous colorectal cancers *(46)*. However, as discussed in the surgical management of FAP, an abdominal colectomy and ileorectal anastomosis is not an innocuous procedure and individualization may be required in special circumstances. Because of the potential morbidity, this procedure may not be ideal in patients whose procedure is palliative or in those with resectable metastatic disease. Such patients may be best served with segmental resection and surveillance. Occasionally, there will be a patient who will flatly refuse the procedure in lieu of a segmental resection. It must be recognized that a TAC-IRA will not eliminate rectal cancer risk in HNPCC patients. The incidence of rectal cancer risk after abdominal colectomy and ileorectal anastomosis has been reported to be from 6% to 20% *(47–49)*. This incidence is similar to that reported for FAP.

The management of a female presenting with colon cancer presents the issue of whether or not a prophylactic total abdominal hysterectomy and bilateral salpingoophorectomy (TAH-BSO) should be performed at the time of colectomy. Endometrial cancer is the most common extracolonic tumor in HNPCC, being the index cancer in up to 30% of affected females *(44,50)*. The cumulative incidence of endometrial cancer in putative gene carriers has been reported to be 30% by 70 yr *(51)*. An even higher risk was reported by Dunlop et al. *(52)*. These authors reported a 42% risk of developing endometrial cancer vs a 30% risk of developing colorectal cancer in HNPCC-affected female patients *(52)*. Thus, the decision for prophylactic TAH-BSO should be individualized. In female patients with colorectal and a family history of endometrial cancer who are postmenopausal or who have completed their

Table 5
Treatment Options in Hereditary Nonpolyposis Colorectal Cancer

Options	Treatment of choice	Other
Affected patient with colon cancer[a] Segmental resection	Abdominal colectomy ileorectal anastomosis	
Affected patient with rectal cancer[a] Anterior resection, abdominoperineal resection, total proctocolectomy	Abdominal colectomy, mucosal proctectomy, ileoanal pouch anastomosis	Low
Affected patient treated with less than completion colectomy abdominal colectomy	Surveillance, enrollment in chemoprevention study	
Mismatch repair gene carrier that has prophylactic colectomy? not yet developed colorectal cancer	Surveillance, enrollment in chemoprevention study	
Mismatch repair gene carrier or at risk Abdominal colectomy individual with adenomas endoscopically resectable	Surveillance, enrollment in chemoprevention trial	
Mismatch repair gene carrier or at-risk individual with adenomas not amenable to endoscopic resection	Abdominal colectomy	
At-risk individual with no colonic manifestation	Surveillance	

[a]Female patients consider total abdominal hysterectomy and bilateral salpingoophorectomy if history of endometrial cancer in the family and family completed or postmenopausal.

families, consideration should be given for prophylactic TAH-BSO. However, there is no data to support this recommendation.

Rectal carcinoma can be the index colorectal cancer in 20–31% of HNPCC patients (49,53). Efforts should be made for sphincter preservation in these patients. The preferred surgical options for patients with HNPCC presenting with rectal cancer are total colectomy mucosal proctectomy and ileoanal pouch anastomosis and total proctocolectomy and ileostomy. Möslein et al. reported that 54% of HNPCC patients presenting with rectal cancer as their index colorectal cancer developed a metachronous colonic cancer at a mean of 7.4 yr after the diagnosis (49). At our institution 17% of HNPCC patients with index rectal cancer developed metachronous colon cancer at a median of 17.5 yr after their diagnosis of rectal cancer (53). Less preferred options include segmental resections such as low anterior resection, coloanal anastomosis, and abdominoperineal resection. However, the latter options should be individualized depending on the circumstances such as comorbidities, reliability of the patient for subsequent surveillance, and curative or palliative nature of the procedure.

The HNPCC patients treated with less than an abdominal colectomy at the time of their index cancer should be on a surveillance program of colonoscopy every 1–2 yr. Prophylactic completion colectomy could be an option in these individuals; however, there are no data to support it. Extracolonic cancer surveillance recommendations have been proposed, but their efficacy remains to be proven (54).

Prophylactic abdominal colectomy should be strongly considered in mismatch repair gene mutation carriers or at-risk individuals who have phenotypically expressed adenomas, especially if these are not controllable by colonoscopy, if they are numerous, or if they are frequently recurring. Adenomas in HNPCC have been reported to be larger, more advanced histologically (tubulovillous or villous), and more dysplastic than adenomas in the general population, suggesting that the adenoma carcinoma sequence is hastened in HNPCC (55,56). Further refinement in an at-risk individual prior to surgery may be possible because most adenomas in HNPCC-affected patients will have microsatellite instability and loss of expression of hMLH1 or hMSH2 protein (57).

The role of prophylactic colectomy in an HNPCC-affected individual with a completely normal colon is controversial (58,59). As opposed to FAP, where the penetrance is close to 100%, the penetrance in HNPCC is 80–85%, which means that between 15% and 20% of mutation gene carriers in HNPCC will not develop colorectal cancer during their lifetime (44,60,61). Prophylactic abdominal colectomy eliminates the majority of the colon at risk for cancer, may provide a psychological benefit to the patient in terms of knowing that most of the main target organ for cancer has been removed, as well as eliminates colonoscopic examinations with the potential complications. However, the cancer risk will not be completely eliminated in these patients. Patients undergoing prophylactic abdominal colectomy will still have rectal mucosa at risk as well as cancer risk in other extracolonic organs, which, in turn, may even be potential target for subsequent surgical prophylaxis. As discussed in the FAP section, there is morbidity associated with this procedure. In addition, there is the potential for psychological trauma in terms of body image and sexuality after an invasive procedure in a young individual, as well as the effect on at-risk family members.

There have been mathematical models utilized to calculate the survival benefits of prophylactic surgery in gene carriers (61,62). None of these models demonstrated a survival advantage of more than 24-mo with surgical prophylaxis, as opposed to endoscopic surveillance assuming 100% compliance (61,62). In these patients, colonoscopic surveillance has proven to be effective. Järvinen et al. reported a 62% decrease in colorectal cancer incidence and a 65% reduction in overall death rate in HNPCC at-risk individuals who underwent surveillance with flexible sigmoidoscopy and barium enema or colonoscopy every 3 yr over a 15-yr period compared to those HNPCC at-risk individuals who refused surveillance (63). Therefore, colonoscopy every 2–3 yr is an effective option in the management of at-risk individuals and in those individuals with a germline mismatch repair gene mutation who have not yet developed colorectal cancer. Surgical prophylaxis should not be an option in individuals who are at risk and have not developed any colorectal manifestations (adenomas or carcinoma). In these authors' opinion, prophylactic colectomy should be offered only in highly selected situations such as in a mutation carrier with a normal colon where colonoscopic surveillance is technically not possible or in a patient who completely refuses colonoscopic surveillance. In both situations, the patient must realize that endoscopic rectal surveillance should be performed after prophylactic colectomy. There is no evidence against or in favor of prophylactic colectomy in a germline mutation gene carrier in HNPCC.

Chemoprevention as discussed in Chapter 5 should be considered in at-risk individuals, mutation carriers, and patients who have undergone abdominal colectomy. However, chemoprevention will not and should not be used as a substitute for surveillance in HNPCC.

3. HAMARTOMATOUS POLYPOSIS SYNDROMES

The hamartomatous polyposis syndromes are characterized by overgrowth of cells native to the area in which they normally arise. These syndromes comprise less than 1% of hereditary colorectal cancer syndromes. These syndromes are autosomal dominant with variable penetrance and, therefore, surveillance of the proband and at-risk relatives are warranted. The most common of these syndromes are juvenile polyposis and Peutz–Jeghers. Other hamartomatous syndromes include Cowden's disease and the less common Rubalcava–Myhre–Smith syndrome. The management of these syndromes depends on the presentation of the patients and will be discussed next.

3.1. Juvenile Polyposis Syndromes

Juvenile polyposis syndrome is defined as any patient with greater than three or more colorectal juvenile polyps, and/or any number of juvenile polyps throughout the gastrointestinal tract, and/or any number of polyps with a family history of juvenile polyposis *(64,65)*. As opposed to the solitary juvenile polyps of infancy, which have no malignant potential, patients with juvenile polyposis syndrome are at increased risk of developing colorectal, gastric, and small bowel carcinoma *(66–68)*. In patients under 35 yr of age, the incidence of colorectal cancer has been reported to be 35%, whereas the cumulative risk of colorectal cancer by age 60 was 68% *(64,69,70)*. Diarrhea, gastrointestinal bleeding, intussusception, rectal prolapse, and/or protein losing enteropathy characterize juvenile polyposis of the infancy *(71)*. Gastrointestinal blood loss is the characteristic presentation in older patients.

The management and surveillance of juvenile polyposis patients will depend on the symptomatology and extent of the polyposis as well as to their increased risk of gastrointestinal malignancies. In patients who present with severe clinical manifestations of the syndrome, supportive measures such as fluid and electrolyte replacement, blood transfusion, and nutritional support will need to be addressed prior to definitive therapy. The symptomatology, extent of the polyposis, and reliability of the patient should guide definitive surgical therapy. Prior to elective surgical therapy, upper and lower endoscopy should be performed with biopsies when indicated to document the extent of the polyposis. Consideration should be given to enteroscopy where available or to a small bowel contrast study.

There will be patients with sparse polyps and no symptomatology for whom the colonic juvenile polyps will be able to be controlled endoscopically. In these patients, endoscopic polypectomy and surveillance will suffice. The interval of endoscopic surveillance should be no longer than 2–3 yr in these patients. Not all authors agree with this approach. Järvinen and Franssila *(72)* have recommended prophylactic colectomy in affected patients over age 20, whereas others suggest that as long as the polyps can be controlled endoscopically and the patient is compliant, colonoscopic surveillance is a reasonable option *(65,73)*.

In patients with colonic polyps that can not be controlled endoscopically, surgical therapy should be instituted. The surgical procedures available to these patients are similar to those for patients with familial adenomatous polyposis. For patients in which the rectum is not involved, an abdominal colectomy and ileorectal anastomosis should be recommended. If the rectum is involved with polyps and there is no evidence of invasive adenocarcinoma precluding a sphincter-sparing procedure, then consideration should be given to a colectomy with an ileoanal pouch anastomosis. At the time of surgery, a careful exploration of the abdomen should be performed with special attention on palpation of the small bowel for additional juvenile polyps. We have used intraoperative enteroscopy as well as enterotomies to remove larger polyps *(66)*. In patients with frank carcinoma, the extent of the surgical procedure should be dictated by the clinical findings.

It is important not to forget the management of at-risk family members. There are little data in the literature regarding surveillance on familial juvenile polyposis. Based on the fact that colorectal cancer has been reported in the second decade in patients with familial juvenile polyposis *(64)*, it is not unreasonable to begin colonoscopic surveillance in the teenage years and tailor subsequent exams according to the findings. In our practice, we perform colonoscopies every 2–3 yr and upper endoscopies every 3 yr. As previously discussed, surveillance can be tailored if there are positive results from genetic testing.

3.2. Peutz–Jeghers Syndrome

Peutz–Jeghers syndrome is characterized by hamartomatous polyps of the gastrointestinal tract, mainly the jejunum, and pigmentation in the perioral region, buccal mucosa, genitalia, or hands and feet *(74)*. The most common presentation is intussusception or gastrointestinal bleeding *(74)*. There is an increased malignancy rate both for intestinal and extraintestinal malignancies *(75–78)*; the former mainly in the small bowel, but also the colon and rectum. The latter include breast, ovarian, pancreatic, and testicular carcinoma as well as adenoma malignum (well-differentiated multicystic adenocarcinoma) of the cervix.

Because of the rarity of this syndrome, management of intestinal polyps in the Peutz–Jeghers syndrome has been controversial. Some authors advocate multiple laparotomies with enterotomies and polypectomies, whereas others have advocated the use of enteroscopy and polypectomy, both at the time of laparotomy and as surveillance in an attempt to reduce number of potential relaparotomies *(79–81)*. Pennazio and Rossini reported their experience with surveillance of seven patients with Peutz–Jeghers syndrome *(81)*. Over a 13-yr period, patients were under surveillance with upper and lower endoscopy every 2–3 yr, with surgery reserved for bowel obstruction. Five of seven patients underwent emergency small bowel resection. Two patients underwent re-exploration. Subsequently, over the last 6 yr, these patients have undergone enteroclysis with push enteroscopy and/or intraoperative enteroscopy based on the radiological findings *(81)*. Intraoperative enteroscopy was reserved for patients who had multiple large polyps throughout the small bowel. Push enteroscopy was performed approximately every 2 yr. Three of four patients with diffuse polyposis underwent intraoperative enteroscopy and polypectomy, whereas the other underwent push enteroscopy and polypectomy. These four patients are reported to be asymptomatic at a mean of 50 mo. The other three patients had polyps in the proximal small bowel. They underwent periodic push enteroscopy and polypectomy and remained asymptomatic at a mean of 47 mo *(81)*. These authors concluded that clearance for small bowel polyps by enteroscopy will reduce the need for emergency procedures and potential small bowel resection in these patients *(81)*.

The appropriate surveillance in Peutz–Jeghers syndrome affected individuals, and their at-risk family members has not been extensively studied or validated. At the St. Mark's Hospital, surveillance recommendations include annual history and physical exam, complete blood counts, upper and lower endoscopies every 2 yr and enteroclysis every 2 yr, with laparotomy and intraoperative enteroscopy for small bowel polyps greater than 1.5 cm in diameter *(82)*. Extensive small bowel resections should be avoided. In addition, extraintestinal sites should be evaluated with breast exams, mammography, pelvic exams, PAP smears, pelvic ultrasonography, and testicular exams and ultrasonography.

3.3. Cowden Syndrome

Cowden syndrome is a rare autosomal dominant hereditary disorder where hamartomatous gastrointestinal polyps may be present. Gastrointestinal polyps are present in approx 35% of Cowden syndrome patients *(83)*. These polyps are not only hamartomas, but can be lipomas, ganglioneuromas, or inflammatory polyps *(83)*. Other manifestations of the disease include trichilemmomas, neurologic manifestations, and breast and thyroid pathology *(84)*.

Because of the rarity of this syndrome, there are no clear-cut recommendations in terms of surveillance. The malignant potential for gastrointestinal polyps is low however, periodic endoscopic surveillance, both upper and lower, should be undertaken. Surveillance should also be performed for thyroid and breast malignancies.

REFERENCES

1. Nugent KP, Spigelman AD, and Phillips RKS. Life expectancy after colectomy and ileorectal anastomosis for Familial Adenomatous Polyposis. *Dis. Colon Rectum*, **36** (1993) 1059–1062.
2. Rodriguez-Bigas MA, Bertario L, and Herrera L. Management of follow-up of patients with familial adenomatous polyposis. In *Cancer of the Colon, Rectum, and Anus*. Cohen AM, Winawer SJ, Friedman MA, and Gunderson LL (eds.), McGraw-Hill, New York, 1995, pp. 391–397.
3. Vasen HFA, van der Luijt RB, Slors JF, et al. Molecular genetic tests as a guide to surgical management of familial adenomatous polyposis. *Lancet*, **348** (1996) 433–435.
4. Wu JS, Paul P, McGannon EA, and Church JM. APC genotype, polyp number, and surgical options in familial adenomatous polyposis. *Ann. Surg.*, **227** (1998) 57–62.
5. Bertario L, Russo A, Radice P, et al. Genotype and phenotype factors as determinants for rectal stump cancer in patients with familial adenomatous polyposis. *Ann. Surg.*, **231** (2000) 538–543.
6. Brooke BN. Management of ileostomy including its complications. *Lancet*, **2** (1952) 102–104.
7. Kock NG. Intra-abdominal "reservoir" in patients with permanent ileostomy: Preliminary observations on a procedure resulting in fecal "continence" in five ileostomy patients. *Arch. Surg.*, **99** (1969) 223–231.
8. Mayo CW and Wakefield EG. Disseminated polyposis of the colon: new surgical treatment in selected cases. *J. Am. Med. Assoc.*, **107** (1936) 324–348.
9. Jagelman DG. Familial polyposis coli. *Surg. Clin. North Am.*, **63** (1983) 117–128.
10. Sarre RG, Jagelman DG, Beck GJ, et al. Colectomy with ileorectal anastomosis for familial adenomatous polyposis: the risk of rectal cancer. *Surgery*, **101** (1983) 20–26.
11. De Cosse JJ, Bulow S, Neale K, et al. Leeds Castle Polyposis Group. Rectal cancer risk in patients treated for familial adenomatous polyposis. *Br. J. Surg.*, **79** (1992) 1372–1375.
12. Nugent KP and Phillips RKS. Rectal cancer risk in older patients with familial adenomatous polyposis and ileorectal anastomosis: a cause for concern. *Br. J. Surg.*, **79** (1992) 1204–1206.
13. Iwama T, Mishima Y, and Utsunomiya J. The impact of familial adenomatous polyposis on the tumorigenesis and mortality at several organs: its rational treatment. *Ann. Surg.*, **217** (1993) 101.
14. Heiskanen I and Järvinen HJ. Fate of the rectal stump after colectomy and ileorectal anastomosis for familial adenomatous polyposis. *Int. J. Colorect. Dis.*, **12** (1997) 9–13.
15. Bess MA, Adson MA, Elveback LR, and Moertel CG. Rectal cancer following colectomy for polyposis. *Arch. Surg.*, **115** (1980) 460–467.
16. Soravia C, Klein L, Berk T, O'Connor BI, Cohen Z, and Mcleod RS. Comparison of ileal pouch anastomosis and ileorectal anastomosis in patients with familial adenomatous polyposis. *Dis. Colon Rectum*, **42** (1999) 1028–1034.
17. Iwama T and Mishima Y. Factors affecting the risk of rectal cancer following rectum-preserving surgery in patients with polyposis coli. *Dis. Colon Rectum*, **37** (1994) 1024–1026.
18. Setti-Carraro P and Nicholls RJ. Choice of prophylactic surgery for the large bowel component of familial adenomatous polyposis. *Br. J. Surg.*, **83** (1996) 885–892.
19. Iwama T and Nishima Y. Factors affecting the risk of rectal cancer following rectum-preserving surgery in patients with familial adenomatous polyposis. *Dis. Colon Rectum*, **37** (1994) 1024–1026.
20. Feinberg SM, Jagelman DG, Sarre RG, et al. Spontaneous resolution of rectal polyps in patients with familial adenomatous polyposis following abdominal colectomy and ileorectal anastomosis. *Dis. Colon Rectum*, **31** (1988) 169–175.
21. Cats A, Kleibeuker JH, Kuipers F, et al. Changes in rectal epithelial cell proliferation and intestinal bile acids after subtotal colectomy in familial adenomatous polyposis. *Cancer Res.*, **52** (1992) 3552–3557.
22. Thompson JPS Familial adenomatous polyposis: the large bowel. *Ann. R. Coll. Surgeons England*, **72** (1990) 177–190.
23. van Duijvendjik P, Slors JF, Taat CW, Oosterveld P, and Vasen HFA. Functional outcome after colectomy and ileorectal anastomosis compared with proctocolectomy and ileal pouch–anal anastomosis in familial adenomatous polyposis. *Ann. Surg.*, **230** (1999) 648–654.
24. Madden MV, Neale KF, Nicholls RJ, et al. Comparison of morbidity and function after colectomy with ileorectal anastomosis or restorative proctocolectomy for familial adenomatous polyposis. *Br. J. Surg.*, **78** (1991) 789–792.

25. Ambroze WL Jr, Dozois RR, Pemberton JH, Beart RW Jr, and Ilstrup DM. Familial adenomatous polyposis: results following ileal pouch-anal anastomosis and ileorectostomy. *Dis. Colon Rectum*, **35** (1992) 12–15.

26. Penna C, Kartheuser A, Parc R, et al. Secondary proctectomy and ileal pouch-anal anastomosis after ileorectal anastomosis for familial adenomatous polyposis. *Br. J. Surg.*, **80** (1993) 1621–1623.

27. Fazio VW, Tiandra JJ, and Lavery IC. Techniques of pouch construction. In *Restorative Proctocolectomy*. Nicholls J, Bartolo D, and Mortensen N (eds.), Blackwell Scientific, Oxford, 1993, pp. 13–33.

28. Palkar VM, deSouza LJ, Jagannath P, and Naresh KN. Adenocarcinoma arising in "J" pouch after total proctocolectomy for familial polyposis coli. *Indian J. Cancer*, **34** (1997) 16–19.

29. Hoehner JC and Metcalf AM. Development of invasive adenocarcinoma following colectomy with ileoanal anastomosis for familial polyposis coli. Report of a case. *Dis. Colon Rectum*, **37** (1994) 824–828.

30. von Herbay A, Stern J, and Herfarth C. Pouch–anal cancer after restorative proctocolectomy for familial adenomatous polyposis. *Am. J. Surg. Pathol.*, **20** (1996) 995–999.

31. Wu JS, McGannon EA, and Church JM. Incidence of neoplastic polyps in the ileal pouch of patients with familial adenomatous polyposis after restorative proctocolectomy. *Dis. Colon Rectum*, **41** (1998) 552–556.

32. van Duijvendijk P, Vasen HF, Bertario L, et al. Cumulative risk of developing polyps or malignancy at the ileal pouch-anal anastomosis in patients with familial adenomatous polyposis. *J. Gastrointest. Surg.*, **3** (1999) 325–330.

33. Parks AG and Nicholls RJ. Proctocolectomy without ileostomy for ulcerative colitis. *Br. Med. J.*, **2** (1978) 85–88.

34. Utsunomiya J, Iwama T, Imajo M, et al. Total colectomy, mucosal proctectomy and ileoanal anastomosis. *Dis. Colon Rectum*, **23** (1980) 459–466.

35. Harms BA, Hamilton JW, Yamamoto DT, and Starling JR. Quadruple-loop (W) ileal pouch reconstruction after proctocolectomy: analysis and functional results. *Surgery*, **102** (1987) 561–567.

36. Smith LE, Friend W, and Medwell S. The superior mesenteric artery: the critical factor in pouch-pull through procedure. *Dis. Colon Rectum*, **27** (1984) 741–744.

37. Nyam DC, Brillant PT, Dozois RR, Kelly KA, Pemberton JH, and Wolff BG. Ileal pouch-anal anastomosis for familial adenomatous polyposis: early and late results. *Ann. Surg.*, **226** (1997) 514–539.

38. Kartheuser AH, Parc R, Penna CP, et al. Ileal–pouch–anal anastomosis as the first choice operation in familial adenomatous polyposis: a ten-year experience. *Surgery*, **119** (1996) 615–623.

39. Pemberton JH. Complications, management, failure and revisions. In *Restorative Proctocolectomy*. Nicholls J, Bartolo D, and Mortensen N (eds.), Blackwell Scientific, Oxford, 1993, pp. 34–52.

40. Becker JM, Dayton MT, Fazio VW, et al. Prevention of postoperative abdominal adhesions by a sodium hyalouronate-bioresorbable membrane: a prospective, randomized, double-blind multicenter study. *J. Am. Coll. Surg.*, **183** (1996) 297–306.

41. Dozois RR, Berk T, Bulow S, et al. Surgical aspects of familial adenomatous polyposis. *Int. J. Colorect. Dis.*, **3** (1988) 1–16.

42. Parc Y, Moslein G, Dozois RR, Pemberton JH, Wolff BG, and King JE. Familial adenomatous polyposis. Results after ileal pouch-anal anastomosis in teenagers. *Dis. Colon Rectum*, **43** (2000) 893–902.

43. Shepherd NA, Jass JR, Duval I, Moskowitz RL, Nicholls RJ, and Morson BC. Restorative proctocolectomy with ileal reservoir: pathological and histochemical study of mucosal biopsy specimens. *J. Clin. Pathol.*, **40** (1987) 601–607.

44. Aarnio M, Mecklin JP, Aaltonen L, Nystrom Lahti M, and Järvinen HJ. Life-time risk of different cancers in hereditary nonpolyposis colorectal cancer (HNPCC) syndrome. *Int. J. Cancer*, **64** (1995) 430–433.

45. Fitzgibbons R, Lynch HT, Stanislav G, et al. Recognition and treatment of patients with hereditary nonpolyposis colon cancer (Lynch syndromes I and II). *Ann. Surg.*, **206** (1987) 289–295.

46. Box JC, Rodriguez-Bigas MA, Weber TK, and Petrelli NJ. Clinical implications of multiple colorectal carcinoma in hereditary nonpolyposis colorectal carcinoma. *Dis. Colon Rectum*, **42** (1999) 717–721.

47. Rodriguez-Bigas MA, Vasen HFA, Mecklin JP, et al. Rectal cancer risk in hereditary nonpolyposis colorectal cancer after abdominal colectomy. *Ann. Surg.*, **225** (1997) 202–207.

48. Baba S. Hereditary nonpolyposis colorectal cancer, an update. *Dis. Colon Rectum*, **40(Suppl.)** (1997) S86–S95.

49. Moslein G, Nelson H, Thibodeau S, and Dozois RR. Rectal Carcinoma in HNPCC. *Lagenbecks Arch. Chirurgie*, **115** (1998) 1467–1469 (in German).

50. Watson P and Lynch HT. Extracolonic cancer in hereditary nonpolyposis colorectal cancer. *Cancer*, **71** (1993) 677–685.

51. Watson P, Vasen HFA, Mecklin JP, Järvinen H, and Lynch HT. The risk of endometrial cancer in hereditary nonpolyposis colorectal cancer. *Am. J. Med.*, **96** (1994) 561–620.

52. Dunlop MG, Farrington SM, Carothers AD, et al. Cancer risk associated with germline DNA mismatch repair gene mutations. *Hum. Mol. Genet.*, **6** (1997) 105–110.

53. Lee JS, Petrelli NJ, and Rodriguez-Bigas MA. Rectal cancer in hereditary nonpolyposis colorectal cancer. *Am. J. Surg.*, **181** (2001) 207–210.

54. Burke W, Petersen GM, Lynch P, et al. Recommendations for follow-up care of individuals with an inherited predisposition to cancer: hereditary nonpolyposis colorectal cancer. *JAMA*, **277** (1997) 915–919.

55. Jass JR, Stewart SM, Stewart J, and Lane MR. Hereditary nonpolyposis colorectal cancer: morphologies, genes, and mutations. *Mutat. Res.*, **290** (1994) 125–133.

56. Jass JR, Smyrk TC, Stewart SM, Lane MR, Lanspa SJ, and Lynch HT. Pathology of hereditary nonpolyposis colorectal cancer. *Anticancer Res.*, **14** (1994) 1631–1635.

57. Iino H, Simms L, Young J, et al. DNA microsatellite instability and mismatch repair protein loss in adenomas presenting in hereditary nonpolyposis colorectal cancer. *Gut*, **47** (2000) 37–42.

58. Lynch HT. Is there a role for prophylactic subtotal colectomy among hereditary nonpolyposis colorectal cancer germline mutation carriers? *Dis. Colon Rectum*, **39** (1996) 109–10.

59. Rodriguez-Bigas MA. Prophylactic colectomy in gene carriers in hereditary nonpolyposis colorectal cancer; has the time come? *Cancer*, **78** (1996) 199–201.

60. Lynch HT, Albano WA, Ruma TA, Schimtz GD, Costello KA, and Lynch JF. Surveillance/management of an obligate gene carrier: the cancer family syndrome. *Gastroenterology*, **84** (1983) 404–408.

61. Vasen HFA, Wijnen JT, Menko FH, et al. Cancer risk in families with hereditary nonpolyposis colorectal cancer diagnosed by mutation analysis. *Gastroenterology*, **110** (1996) 1020–1027.

62. Syngal S, Weeks JC, Schrag D, Garber JE, and Kuntz KM. Benefits of colonoscopic surveillance and prophylactic colectomy in patients with hereditary nonpolyposis colorectal cancer mutations. *Ann. Intern. Med.*, **15** (1998) 787–796.

63. Järvinen HJ, Aarnio M, Mustonen H, et al. Controlled 15-year trial on screening for colorectal cancer in families with hereditary nonpolyposis colorectal cancer. *Gastroenterology*, **118** (2000) 829–834.

64. Jass JR, Williams CB, Bussey HJR, and Morson BC. Juvenile Polyposis-a precancerous condition. *Histopathology*, **13** (1988) 619–630.

65. Giardiello FM, Hamilton SR, Kern SE, et al. Colorectal neoplasia in juvenile polyposis or juvenile polyps. *Arch. Child. Dis.*, **66** (1991) 971–975.

66. Hofting I, Pott G, and Stolte M. Das syndrom der juvenillen polyposis. *Leber. Magen. Darm.*, **23** (1993) 107–112.

67. Rodriguez-Bigas MA, Penetrante RB, Herrera L. and Petrelli NJ. Intraoperative small bowel enteroscopy in familial adenomatous and familial juvenile polyposis. *Gastrointest. Endosc.*, **42** (1995) 560–564.

68. Coburn MC, Pricolo VE, DeLuca FG, and Bland KI. Malignant potential in juvenile polyposis syndromes. *Ann. Surg. Oncol.*, **2** (1995) 386–391.

69. Murday V and Slack J. Inherited disorders associated with colorectal cancer. *Cancer Surv.*, **8** (1989) 139–157.

70. Desai DC, Neale KF, Talbot IC, Hodgson SV, and Phillips RKS. Juvenile polyposis. *Br. J. Surg.*, **8** (1995) 14–17.

71. Sachatello CR, Hahn IS, and Carrington CB. Juvenile gastrointestinal polyposis in a female infant: report of a case and review of the literature of a recently recognized syndrome. *Surgery*, **75** (1974) 107–114.

72. Järvinen H and Franssila KO. Familial juvenile polyposis coli; increased risk of colorectal cancer. *Gut*, **25** (1984) 792–800.

73. Sturniolo GC, Montino MC, Dall'Igna F, et al. Familial juvenile polyposis coli: results of endoscopic treatment and surveillance in two sister. *Gastrointest, Endoscopy*, **39** (1993) 561–565.

74. Jeghers H, Mckusick VA, and Katz KH. Generalized intestinal polyposis and melanin spots of the oral mucosa, lips, and digits: a syndrome of diagnostic significance. *N. Engl. J. Med.*, **241** (1949) 992–1005.

75. Giardiello FM, Welsh MD, Hamilton SR, et al. Increased risk of cancer in the Peutz–Jeghers syndrome. *N. Engl. J. Med.*, **316** (1987) 1511–1514.

76. Spigelman AD, Murday V, and Phillips RKS. Cancer and the Peutz–Jeghers syndrome. *Gut*, **30** (1989) 1588–1590.

77. Hizawa K, Iida M, Matsumoto T, et al. Cancer in Peutz–Jeghers syndrome. *Cancer*, **72** (1993) 2777–2781.

78. Boardman LA, Thibodeau SN, Schaid DJ, et al. Increased risk for cancer in the Peutz–Jeghers syndrome. *Ann. Intern. Med.*, **128** (1998) 896–869.

79. Foley TR, McGarrity TJ, and Abt AB. Peutz–Jeghers syndrome: a clinicopathologic survey of the "Harrisburg family" with a 49-year follow-up. *Gastroenterology*, **95** (1988) 1535–1540.

80. Spigelman AD, Thompson JPS, and Phillips RKS. Towards decreasing the relaparotomy rate in the Peutz–Jeghers syndrome: the role of preoperative small bowel endoscopy. *Br. J. Surg.*, **77** (1990) 301–302.

81. Pennazio M and Rossini FP. Small bowel polyps in Peutz–Jeghers syndrome: management by combined push enteroscopy and intraoperative enteroscopy. *Gastrointest. Endoscopy*, **51** (2000) 304–308.
82. Spigelman AD, Arese P, and Phillips RKS. Polyposis: the Peutz–Jeghers syndrome. *Br. J. Surg.*, **82** (1995) 1311–1314.
83. Guillem JG, Smith AJ, Puig-La Calle J, and Ruo L. Gastrointestinal polyposis syndromes. *Curr. Probl. Surg.*, **36** (1999) 228–323.
84. Eng C. Cowden syndrome. *J. Genet. Counsel.*, **6** (1997) 181–191.

II DIAGNOSTIC AND THERAPEUTIC RADIOLOGY

7

Overview of CT, MRI, and Ultrasound in the Imaging and Staging of Colorectal Cancer

David J. Vining

Contents

1. INTRODUCTION

Recent technological advances in computed tomography (CT), ultrasound (US), and magnetic resonance imaging (MRI) have made these modalities standards of care in every aspect of colorectal cancer (CRC) management, including screening, staging, and surveillance.

Computed tomography remains a mainstay for the primary workup and staging of colorectal cancer, as well as assessment of treatment response. The basic CT principle is that a rotating X-ray beam is directed through a patient, and thousands of X-ray attenuation values are collected on a circular detector array. A cross-sectional image, or slice of anatomy, is generated from these "raw data." Since its origins in the 1960s, CT technology has undergone significant evolution. Early-generation scanners relied on the incremental movement of a patient in a gantry in order to obtain a collection of "single slices," a process that required substantial time and was prone to missing small lesions because of respiratory misregistration and motion artifact. In the late 1980s, helical CT scanning allowed a patient to be moved through a scanner at a constant speed while the X-ray beam revolved continuously around the patient. An uninterrupted helix of X-ray data was obtained from which a "volume of slices" could be constructed. The late 1990s saw yet another advance with the introduction of multislice helical CT. Rather than obtaining a single helix of X-ray data, multiple slices could be acquired simultaneously, thereby decreasing scan time (on the order of less than 1 min to cover the chest, abdomen, and pelvis), improving spatial resolution, and lowering radiation exposure *(1)*. In addition, multislice helical CT scanning has spawned

From: *Colorectal Cancer: Multimodality Management*
Edited by: L. Saltz © Humana Press Inc., Totowa, NJ

many new and exciting applications, including virtual colonoscopy for CRC screening and CT angiography for surgical planning.

Ultrasound imaging is often reserved for specific purposes, such as local tumor staging with endoscopic ultrasound, or biopsy guidance for suspected liver metastases. The last two decades have also seen important technological advances with this modality, including the development of specialized transducers, color and power Doppler imaging, harmonic and compound imaging, panoramic and three-dimensional (3D) viewing, and even inexpensive, hand-held equipment. Ultrasound contrast agents, which are essentially small microbubbles injected intravenously, are under development that could better distinguish subtle lesions within the liver, thereby allowing ultrasound to be used earlier in the management of CRC patients *(2,3)*.

Magnetic resonance imaging avoids the stigma of ionizing radiation and provides superior tissue contrast resolution, compared to CT or ultrasound, in the evaluation and characterization of suspected liver metastases. Unfortunately, costs, limited availability, and lower patient compliance have limited MRI's widespread use. Specialized techniques, such as endorectal MRI for staging rectal tumors and MRI virtual colonoscopy, are proving beneficial *(4)*. The development of novel MRI contrast agents and MRI spectroscopy for colorectal cancer imaging remain goals for future exploration.

2. SCREENING

Endorsement of endoscopic CRC screening has decreased the impact of radiologic methods in the last few years, particularly with respect to the barium enema. However, virtual colonoscopy (VC), first described in 1994, is emerging as a strong contender to endoscopic screening *(see* Chapter 8) *(5)*. Virtual colonoscopy combines volume scanning (helical CT or MRI) with computer visualization techniques to enable minimally invasive screening. As a total colon examination, VC offers several advantages over conventional colonoscopy, including better patient compliance, less risks, avoidance of unnecessary endoscopy, potentially lower cost, and earlier diagnosis and management of disease both inside and outside the colon.

Virtual colonoscopy consists of three basic steps: (1) bowel preparation, (2) helical CT or MRI scanning, and (3) image analysis *(6)*. Effective bowel preparation remains the most critical step in a VC examination. Residual feces can simulate polyps and masses, and retained fluid or collapsed bowel segments can obscure subtle lesions. Many VC investigators use conventional bowel preparation methods, such as a polyethylene glycol colonic lavage and hand-bulb air insufflation of the colon. However, refinements to bowel preparation have been advocated, including the use of oral sodium phosphate, an oral iodinated contrast agent administered prior to CT scanning, and the use of a CO_2 insufflator for controlled bowel distention *(7)*. When MRI is employed for VC, the use of a dimeglumine gadopentetate enema following bowel cleansing has been suggested *(8)*. Virtual colonoscopy research has focused on the exclusive use of oral contrast agents to opacify the fecal stream and eliminate conventional bowel cleansing altogether *(9–11)*.

Volume scanning of a patient's abdomen and pelvis is achieved with either helical CT or MRI. Regardless of the imaging modality, a caveat is that image datasets are obtained using the thinnest slices possible during a single breath-hold acquisition. Scanning patients in both supine and prone positions facilitates visualization of the entire colon. Although helical CT and MRI are capable of detecting small polyps, both modalities remain limited in their ability to fully characterize the histology of lesions or accurately stage local disease.

A radiologist's primary goal is to identify sites of colorectal polyps and masses within the helical CT or MRI image data (Fig. 1). Image analysis requires that a radiologist interpret hundreds of CT or MRI images using a dedicated computer workstation and 3D imaging tools for problem-solving (e.g., determining whether a suspicious finding represents a polyp or complex haustra). With proper training and an adequate computer system, most investigators can interpret an examination in 10–15 min. The value of identifying diseases outside the colon on the source helical CT or MRI images is an added benefit that is not possible with conventional endoscopic screening.

The ability to interact with simulated anatomy and navigate through the colon is the essence of VC. More advanced computer techniques are being developed to aid in-flight-path planning, splitting or unfolding colon models, and computer-assisted polyp detection (CAPD). One form of CAPD uses measurements of the colon's wall thickness at regularly spaced intervals and mathematical analysis of the colon's shape in order to detect potential polyp sites *(12)*. In this manner, CAPD assists a radiologist in identifying subtle lesions. Rapid image analysis affords a patient an option of undergoing a therapeutic colonoscopy procedure on the same day if deemed necessary.

Preliminary results from clinical trials comparing VC to direct colonoscopy (DC) indicate that the sensitivity and specificity of VC ranges from 75% to 100% and 87% to 90%, respectively, for the identification of polyps 1 cm or greater (i.e., those deemed significant lesions) *(13–18)*. As outcomes studies emerge, it is important for the medical community to realize that the accuracy of VC relative to DC may hinge on the selected bowel preparation and that false-positive VC findings might actually represent false-negative DC results. In the future, a national consensus will be needed to determine what polyp size detected by VC necessitates therapeutic colonoscopy.

3. STAGING

After initial CRC diagnosis, accurate staging is the next important step in cancer management. For rectal tumors, endorectal ultrasound and endorectal MRI have been beneficial in discriminating T1 and T2 lesions from T3 lesions, and prompting presurgical radiation and/or chemotherapy to downstage more advanced lesions in order to permit sphincter-sparing curative surgery *(see* Chapter 9) *(19,20)*.

Despite advances in CT and MRI, both remain limited with regard to determining regional lymph node status: Normal-sized lymph nodes may contain tumor, whereas enlarged nodes may only be reactive (Fig. 2). In the future, position-emission tomography (PET) and novel nuclear medicine techniques may play a greater role in determining nodal metastases *(see* Chapter 10) *(21)*.

For the evaluation of distant metastases, helical CT is the current standard of care because of its speed, availability, and superiority over conventional CT scanning. In the early 1990s, CT arterioportography (i.e., bolus injection of iodinated contrast via an arterial catheter placed in the celiac artery followed by helical CT scanning) was promoted for the detection of subtle liver lesions, but this has been replaced by multislice helical CT imaging and MRI in recent years *(22,23)*.

Often, helical CT scanning detects small, indeterminate liver lesions that require ultrasound or MRI for better characterization. When available, MRI is superior for distinguishing small cysts and hemangiomas from metastases (Fig. 3). Furthermore, the development of MRI contrast agents shows promise for imaging occult liver disease *(24,25)*. Unfortunately, MRI

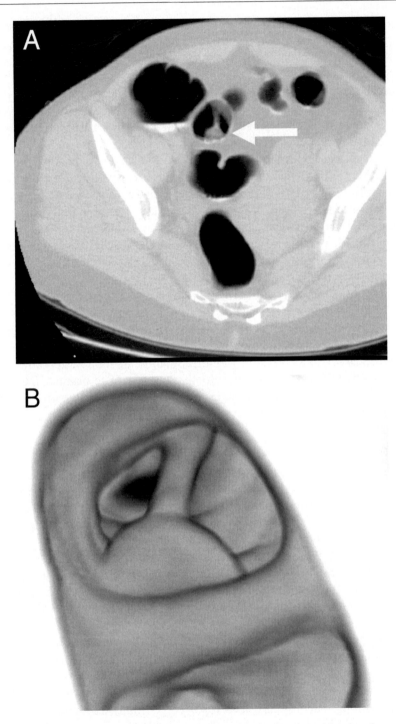

Fig. 1. (**A**) Virtual colonoscopy reveals a pedunculated polyp in the sigmoid colon (arrow). (**B**) Three-dimensional rendering of the CT data better illustrates the polyp.

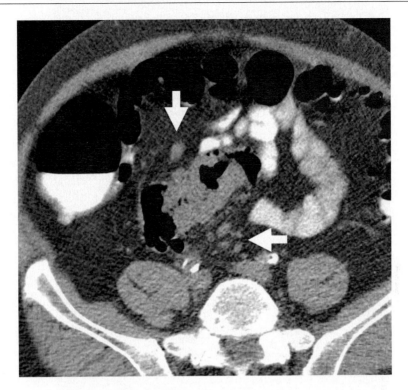

Fig. 2. Multislice helical CT image of a sigmoid colon neoplasm. Note the small regional lymph nodes that are suspicious for metastatic disease (arrows).

remains time-consuming, less available, subject to patient apprehension and claustrophobia, and limited in its ability to image potential carcinomatosis as a result of bowel peristalsis. Despite what imaging methods are employed during staging, an important caveat is that patients must be imaged in proximity to a planned surgical date in order to record accurate results.

When suspicious but indeterminate liver lesions are identified, ultrasound-guided biopsy of such lesions may be required for definitive diagnosis (Fig. 4). Ultrasound is generally better for guiding these procedures because it images the liver in "real time," which is especially advantageous when trying to biopsy small lesions in a moving liver. Ultrasound is hindered by its ability to image small or subtle lesions, but technical developments like harmonic imaging and ultrasound-specific contrast agents are overcoming this barrier *(26–28)*.

Finally, when anatomical guidance is required for performing intraoperative cyrotherapy or radio-frequency ablation of liver lesions, portable ultrasound units are proving to be valuable. In addition, preoperative CT angiography utilizing multislice helical CT and intravenous iodinated contrast boluses can assist in road-mapping hepatic vasculature prior to placement of intra-arterial chemotherapy catheters (Fig. 5).

4. SURVEILLANCE

After treatment, patients must undergo serial monitoring of treatment response with tumor markers and imaging. No steadfast rules apply as to how frequently a patient should undergo

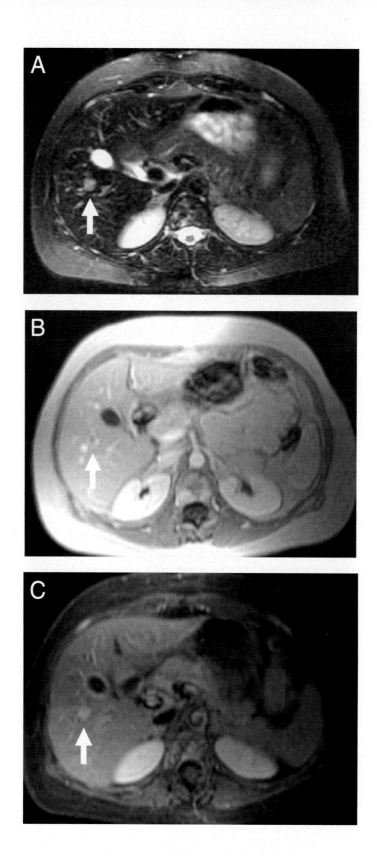

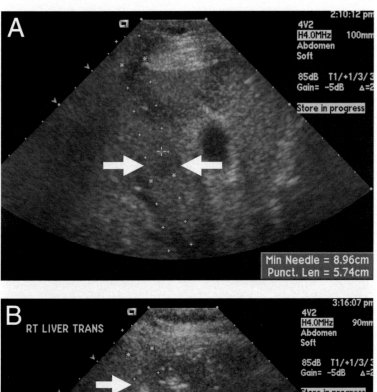

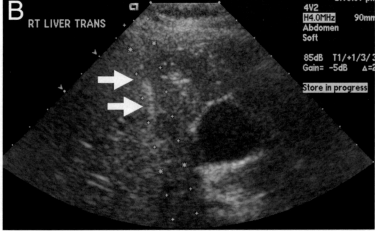

Fig. 4. Ultrasound-guided biopsy of the lesion shown in Fig. 3. (**A**) The 1-cm liver lesion appears as a subtle sonolucency (arrows). (**B**) Ultrasound guidance directs an echogenic needle (arrows) toward the lesion that subsequently proved to be a colon cancer metastasis.

followup imaging. If elevations in tumor markers such as carcinoembryonic antigen (CEA) indicate recurrent disease, then imagining can be applied as deemed appropriate.

5. FUTURE INITIATIVES

The future of CRC imaging is focused on functional and molecular imaging with the aim of identifying tissue characteristics on a cellular or molecular level, thus overcoming the

---

Fig. 3. *(opposite page)* MRI is useful for characterization of small liver lesions. (**A**) T2-weighted image indicates a hyperintense (bright) lesion in the right hepatic lobe (arrow). (**B**) Contrast-enhanced gradient image shows the lesion with ring enhancement. (**C**) Delayed postcontrast T1-weighted image with fat suppression reveals that the lesion enhances abnormally, thus indicating a metastasis.

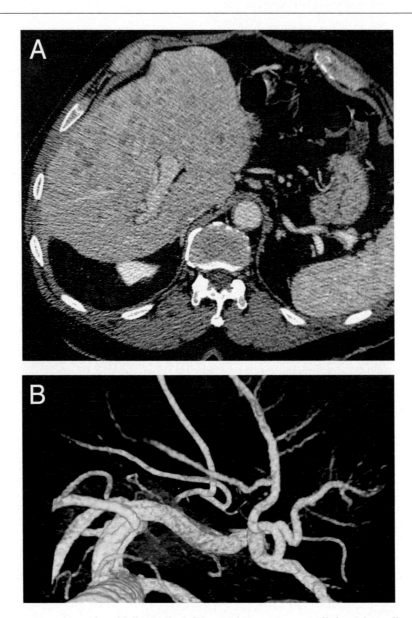

Fig. 5. (A) Contrast-enhanced multislice helical CT reveals numerous small, hypodense liver metastases. **(B)** CT angiography was performed to outline the hepatic artery anatomy in preparation for placement of an intra-arterial chemotherapy catheter.

limited whole-organ view offered by today's modalities *(29)*. Nuclear medicine techniques, such as single-photon-emission computed tomography (SPECT), combined with specific monoclonal antibody tagging agents, have stimulated interest in this area *(30,31)*. In addition, recent reports of positron emission tomography (PET) ability to detect earlier metastases and to monitor tumor response to chemotherapeutic agents has made this one of the most exciting technologies in the radiologic armamentarium *(32,33)*.

Basic scientists have generated important information about tissue processes (e.g., angiogenesis, growth kinetics, drug delivery), cellular dynamics (e.g., tumor markers, drug targeting), and genetics (e.g., gene mutations, gene therapy) that imaging scientists need to harvest. Future research will be directed at developing imaging markers, targeting and delivery systems, signal amplification strategies, and dedicated imaging systems to take advantage of these discoveries. The formation of imaging strategies aimed at evaluating disease initiation, progression, and selection of the best treatment regimen remains an essential goal.

REFERENCES

1. Hu H. Multi-slice helical CT: scan and reconstruction. *Med. Phys.*, **26** (1999) 5–18.
2. Harvey CJ and Albrecht T. Ultrasound of focal liver lesions. *Eur. Radiol.*, **11** (2001) 1578–1593.
3. Leen E. Ultrasound contrast harmonic imaging of abdominal organs. Semin. Ultrasound CT MR, 22 (2001) 11–24.
4. Thoeni RF. Colorectal cancer. Radiologic staging. *Radiol. Clin. North Am.*, **35** (1997) 457–485.
5. Vining DJ and Gelfand DW. Noninvasive colonoscopy using helical CT scanning, 3D reconstruction, and virtual reality. Society of Gastrointestinal Radiologists Annual Meeting, Maui, HI, February 13–18, 1994.
6. Vining DJ. Nuts and bolts of virtual endoscopy. In *Syllabus for Categorical Course in Diagnostic Radiology: Gastrointestinal*. Balfe DM and Levine MS (eds.), RSNA, Oak Brook, IL 1997, pp. 123–127.
7. Vining DJ and Pineau BC. Improved bowel preparation for virtual colonoscopy examinations. *Gastroenterology*, **116** (1999) A524 (abstract).
8. Luboldt W, Steiner P, Bauerfeind P, et al. Detection of mass lesions with MR colonography: preliminary report. *Radiology*, **207** (1998) 59–65.
9. Teigen EL, Vining DJ, McCorquodale D, et al. Improving virtual colonoscopy with a fecal contrast agent. Society of Gastrointestinal Radiologists Annual Meeting, Cancun, Mexico, March 9–14, 1997.
10. Patak MA, Weishaupt D, Froehlich J, et al. Fecal tagging with Gd-DOTA: a path to eliminate the need for colonic cleansing prior to MR colonography. *Radiology*, **213** (1999) 340 (abstract).
11. Wax MR, Bitter I, May S, et al. Optimizing bowel preparation for virtual colonoscopy electronic cleansing. *Radiology*, **221** (2001) 578 (abstract).
12. Vining DJ, Ge Y, Ahn D, Stelts D, et al. Enhanced virtual colonoscopy system employing automatic detection of colon polyps. *Gastroenterology*, **114** (1998) 698 (abstract).
13. Fenlon HM, Nunes DP, Schroy PC, et al. A comparison of virtual and conventional colonoscopy for the detection of colorectal polyps. *N. Engl. J. Med.*, **341** (1999) 1496–1503.
14. Hara AK, Johnson CD, Reed JE, et al. Detection of colorectal polyps with CT colography: initial assessment of sensitivity and specificity. *Radiology*, **205** (1997) 59–65.
15. Akerkar GA, Hung RK, and Yee, J. Sensitivity and specificity of virtual colonoscopy for detection of colorectal neoplasia. *Gastroenterology*, **116** (1999) A44 (abstract).
16. Pineau BC, Mikulaninec C, and Vining DJ. Ability of virtual colonoscopy to detect patients with colorectal polyps. *Gastroenterology*, **116** (1999) A485.
17. Lees WR and Gillams AR. Is CT colography a reliable method for detecting colorectal cancer in symptomatic patients? *Radiology*, **221** (2001) 307 (abstract).
18. Laghi A, Iannaccone R, Carbone I, et al. Multi-slice spiral CT colonography for the detection of colorectal polyps and neoplasms. *Radiology*, **221** (2001) 307 (abstract).
19. Schnall MD, Furth EE, Rosato EF, Kressel HY. Rectal tumor stage: correlation of endorectal MR imaging and pathologic findings. *Radiology*, **190** (1994) 709–714.
20. Kim NK, Kim MJ, Yun SH, et al. Comparative study of transrectal ultrasonography, pelvic computerized tomography, and magnetic resonance imaging in preoperative staging of rectal cancer. *Dis. Colon Rectum*, **42** (1999) 770–775.
21. Blend MJ and Abdel-Nabi H. New methods for the staging of colorectal cancer using noninvasive techniques. *Semin. Surg. Oncol.*, **12** (1996) 253–263.
22. Choi D, Kim SH, Lim JH, Cho JM, Lee WJ, Lee SJ, Lim HK. Detection of hepatocellular carcinoma: combined T2-weighted and dynamic gadolinium-enhanced MRI versus combined CT during arterial portography and CT hepatic arteriography. *J. Comput. Assist. Tomogr.*, **25** (2001) 777–785.
23. Seneterre E, Taourel P, Bouvier Y, et al. Detection of hepatic metastases: ferumoxides-enhanced MR imaging versus unenhanced MR imaging and CT during arterial portography. *Radiology*, **200** (1996) 785–792.
24. Alger JR, Harreld JH, Chen S, et al. Time-to-echo optimization for spin echo magnetic resonance imaging of liver metastasis using superparamagnetic iron oxide particles. *J. Magn. Reson. Imaging*, **14** (2001) 586–594.
25. Said B, McCart JA, Libutti SK, Choyke PL. Ferumoxide-enhanced MRI in patients with colorectal cancer and rising CEA: surgical correlation in early recurrence. *Magn. Reson. Imaging*, **18** (2000) 305–309.

26. Lassau N, Paturel-Asselin C, Guinebretiere JM, et al. New hemodynamic approach to angiogenesis: color and pulsed Doppler ultrasonography. *Invest. Radiol.*, **34** (1999) 194–198.
27. Leen E. The role of contrast-enhanced ultrasound in the characterisation of focal liver leasions. *Eur. Radiol.*, **11** (2001) E27–E34.
28. Bartolozzi C and Lencioni R. Contrast-specific ultrasound imaging of focal liver lesions. Prologue to a promising future. *Eur. Radiol.*,**11** (2001) E13–E14.
29. Weissleder R and Mahmood U. Molecular imaging. *Radiology*, **219** (2001) 316–333.
30. Ward RL, Packham D, Smythe AM, et al. Phase I clinical trial of the chimeric monoclonal antibody (c30.6) in patients with metastatic colorectal cancer. *Clin. Cancer Res.*, **6** (2000) 4674–4683.
31. Willkomm P, Bender H, Bangard M, et al. FDG PET and immunoscintigraphy with 99mTc-labeled antibody fragments for detection of the recurrence of colorectal carcinoma. *J. Nucl. Med.*, **41** (2000) 1657–1663.
32. Bar-Shalom R, Valdivia AY, Blaufox MD. PET imaging in oncology. *Semin. Nucl. Med.*, **30** (2000) 150–185.
33. Tempero M, Brand R, Holdeman K, Matamoros A. New imaging techniques in colorectal cancer. *Semin Oncol.*, **22** (1995) 448–471.

8

Virtual Colonoscopy for Colorectal Cancer Screening and Surveillance

David T. Rubin and Abraham H. Dachman

CONTENTS

1. INTRODUCTION

Although colorectal cancer remains a significant cause of morbidity and mortality in industrialized nations, compliance with screening recommendations is poor. This is because existing tests are feared by patients and misunderstood by practitioners. Computed tomography (CT) colonography (CTC) or virtual colonoscopy (VC) offers the hope of rapid, minimally invasive imaging of the entire colon and possibly offers improved patient acceptance. In addition, this evolving technology may be useful in a variety of other situations, including incomplete colonoscopy and surveillance in patients at increased risk of neoplasia. This chapter describes the current state of CTC, with particular emphasis on its use for colorectal cancer screening.

2. RATIONALE AND APPROACH TO CURRENT SCREENING TESTS FOR COLORECTAL CANCER

Despite the fact that colorectal cancer (CRC) remains the second leading cause of cancer mortality in industrialized nations, accounting for more than 10% of all cancer deaths *(1)*, compliance with proven prevention strategies is poor. Current screening and prevention recommendations are based on our understanding of the adenoma–carcinoma sequence of CRC development. Therefore, secondary prevention of colorectal cancer involves the detection and removal of polyps before they transform into adenocarcinoma *(2)*. Current methods of screening for colorectal cancer include fecal occult blood testing (FOBT), flexible sigmoidoscopy, double-contrast barium enema, and colonoscopy, but all suffer from some limitations. FOBT and flexible sigmoidoscopy are limited by incomplete views of

From: *Colorectal Cancer: Multimodality Management*
Edited by: L. Saltz © Humana Press Inc., Totowa, NJ

the colon and low sensitivities and specificities. Both barium enema and colonoscopy offer complete views of the colon, but are limited by the need for a cathartic bowel cleansing, a small but important risk of perforation, and fear of embarrassment and discomfort by patients. Colonoscopy is considered the gold standard for CRC screening and it offers the advantages of biopsy and polypectomy, but it requires sedation and is also the most expensive screening test.

The approach to CRC screening has been moving in the direction of total colonic examination and away from the limited views and insensitive tests of flexible sigmoidoscopy and FOBT. Recently published studies have supported the use of colonoscopy over flexible sigmoidoscopy for colorectal screening (3,4). National screening recommendations support this approach as well. The 1997 American Gastroenterology Association guidelines offer colonoscopy or barium enema as options for total colonic evaluation in average-risk individuals (asymptomatic, ≥50 yr old) (5). In 2000, the American College of Gastroenterology proposed colonoscopy every 10 yr as the preferred examination for screening average-risk patients (6). These recommendations have culminated in the United States government approving Medicare coverage of colonoscopy for CRC screening of patients at average-risk. It is anticipated that other third-party payers will follow this lead.

Despite the evidence and these recommendations, many physicians do not offer colorectal cancer screening and less than 40% of eligible patients ever have obtained fecal occult blood tests (7,8). There are a number of reasons for this persistently poor rate of screening. Polyps and early colorectal cancer are asymptomatic and therefore may be forgotten by busy physicians or patients seeking treatment for other problems. Patients dislike the bowel cleansing necessary for the imaging tests, and there is a great deal of embarrassment and fear of discomfort from the exams.

Recognition of the benefit of colonoscopy for colorectal cancer screening combined with the currently poor rate of screening compliance has led researchers to seek a total colonic examination that is minimally invasive, fast, and offers increased patient acceptance. CTC is a novel imaging modality that may address many of these needs.

3. CT COLONOGRAPHY

Computed tomography colonography (also called virtual colonoscopy) is a technique that uses helical CT data to create standard axial and reformatted two-dimensional (2D) or three-dimensional (3D) images of the colon. In 1994, Vining and colleagues at Wake Forest University excited the gastrointestinal community with the first report of this technique, in which they used volumetric CT data to create three-dimensional endoluminal images of the colon (9).

3.1. Technique

Although the technique by which virtual colonoscopy is performed continues to evolve, the basic approach is now fairly uniform at major centers (Table 1). The technical performance of this imaging modality relies on a combination of complete bowel preparation, dedicated hardware for data collection, and specialized software for data processing. Finally, CTC requires observer interpretation, image manipulation and problem-solving, and standardized result reporting. These functions have been performed by radiologists who are experienced in reading abdominal CT scans. Since the technique is still evolving, a learning curve and recommended number of procedures to determine competence has not been determined.

Because stool or liquid may complicate the interpretation of virtual colonoscopy, investigators have attempted to minimize these sources of error with a cathartic bowel

Table 1
Virtual Colonoscopy: The University of Chicago Technique

Identification of patient (average risk = asymptomatic, >50 yr)
Bowel preparation [poly(ethylene glycol) preparation]
Glucagon, 1 mg intravenous (optional)
Digital rectal exam
Placement of rectal tube, insufflation until minimal patient discomfort
Scout film to assess bowel distension
Breath hold and supine scanning of patient with multislice spiral CT (approx 30 s) helical technique;
    2.5 mm collimation; table speed 15 cm/s, HS (high speed) mode; reconstruction index, 1.5 mm,
    60–100 mA)
Reposition patient, additional insufflation
Breath hold and prone scanning of patient with multislice spiral CT (approx 30 s)
Data processing at computer workstation
Radiologist reading
    Simultaneous reading of supine/prone axial and coronal images
    Multiplanar reconstructions and 3D problem-solving for unclear lesions
    Soft-tissue windows for wall thickening and extracolonic findings
Recording and reporting data

preparation similar to that used for conventional colonoscopy (e.g., a standard polyethylene glycol electrolyte solution). Next, insufflation of the colon is necessary in order to distinguish collapsed loops of bowel from polyps or masses. We perform a careful digital rectal exam to examine the distalmost area of the rectum, which may be obscured by the insufflation tube. Next, a flexible tip catheter is inserted into the rectum and room air or carbon dioxide is infused either to a set volume (1.5–2 L) or to patient tolerance. Our approach is to use room air and insufflate the colon to minimal discomfort of the patient. Other centers use manometers (such as laparoscopic carbon dioxide pumps) and insufflate to a set pressure. Scout views are obtained to confirm the adequacy of bowel distension before scanning is performed. Despite these rather imprecise methods of bowel distension, image quality is quite good because of the high contrast between the air-filled colon and the soft tissue of the colonic wall. The only complication of this method in our institution was a single patient with mild postprocedure bloating and discomfort.

Bowel spasm causes pain and can complicate interpretation in the sigmoid colon, so glucagon is used as a bowel-relaxing agent. We have found that glucagon minimizes patient discomfort and provides better images, although it also may result in ileocecal valve relaxation and unwanted refluxing of air into the small bowel *(10)*. Some investigators do not use glucagon however, and one study has shown no significant difference in colonic distension when comparing CTC exams done with and without glucagon *(10)*.

Most centers now use the newer multislice CT. This technology permits the rapid collection of volumetric data of the abdomen and pelvis in less than 30 s. Currently up to four slices can be acquired in one gantry rotation and eight-slice scanners are expected to be on the market shortly. Patients are now able to hold their breath during the entire scan and therefore minimize motion artifact. In addition, scans are obtained with the patient in supine and prone positions to allow shifting of gravity-dependent material and minimize errors in interpretation *(11)*.

A number of investigators have described their results with differing CT scanning parameters. The goal of these parameters is to obtain maximum sensitivity with the least amount of data collection (faster and less computer resources) and a safe amount of radiation exposure. Adequate image quality requires a collimation of 2.5–5 mm or less, pitch between 1 and 2, and reconstruction intervals of 1–3 mm. At 70 mA with these settings, the radiation dose administered is substantially less than that required for standard-body CT settings and approx 20% less than the standard films obtained during a double-contrast barium enema *(12)*. Some researchers now advocate 1 mm collimation at a reduced mA in order to achieve isotopic voxels for high resolution multiplanar reconstruction at an acceptable radiation dose.

3.2. Three-Dimensional vs Two-Dimensional Images

Early virtual colonoscopy techniques attempted to simulate the perspective of conventional colonoscopy with endoluminal views and navigated "fly-throughs." These 3D perspectives were obtained by two different techniques, *volume rendering* and *surface rendering*. Volume rendering allows a multiplanar display of extraluminal soft tissues and attenuation data but is computationally more demanding, expensive, and time-consuming than surface rendering. Surface rendering eliminates the extraluminal data and uses the endoluminal surface data only, thereby offering somewhat limited information but using less computer resources. Advances in computational speed have made volume rendering more available, but optimal processing parameters remain undefined *(13,14)*.

In order to "navigate" through the 3D endoluminal images and "fly through" the colon, a centerline can be calculated. This allows the viewer to traverse the colon while inspecting pathology without focusing on navigation. Newer computers permit rapid navigation without a centerline by using simultaneous multiplanar images to map colon position. However, poor data quality can substantially distort 3D endoluminal images and result in artificial floating "debris." The difficulties with this approach for primary reading of CTC have supported the primary use of 2D images and selective use of 3D computations for problem-solving. Improved software and semiautomated segmentation of the colon supplemented by automated centerline navigation may make 3D endoluminal views an important component of CTC primary interpretation.

Two-dimensional images are the standard CT images with which radiologists are most familiar. Numerous investigators have demonstrated that 2D images (usually magnified axial images) are equally effective at polyp detection as 3D endoluminal constructions *(15,16)* (Figs. 1 and 2). In addition, navigation through 2D images is more rapid than 3D reconstruction and navigation *(17)*. Optimal 2D images require lung window settings, but soft-tissue windows may be necessary to assess areas of bowel collapse, bowel wall thickening, and incidental extracolonic findings. Lipomas also are distinguished more clearly with soft-tissue windows. Intermediate window/level settings may permit both polyp detection and detection of wall thickening at the same time. A separate soft-tissue window/level setting review is necessary to detect extracolonic findings and confirm wall thickening.

A potentially significant advantage of CTC is that data interpretation occurs after the patient's exam is completed. Most centers now employ user-friendly workstations that allow easy scrolling between cine-loop 2D images and 3D images-on-demand. Several independent companies as well as academic centers are developing more specialized software for CTC interpretation. Rapid interpretation would be important if CTC were to be applied in the screening setting, not only for optimal utilization of radiologists but also in order for the already-prepped patient to be sent to conventional colonoscopy if there are findings on the CTC.

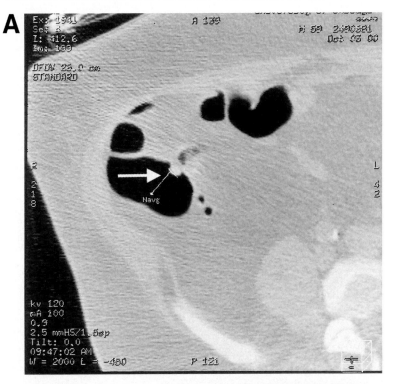

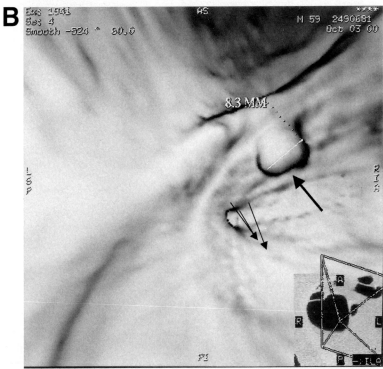

Fig. 1. (A) Axial image from a supine scan shows a nondependent 8-mm soft-tissue polyp (arrow) in the ascending colon. (B) Endoluminal perspective image shows a sessile polyp (arrows) behind a normal colonic fold.

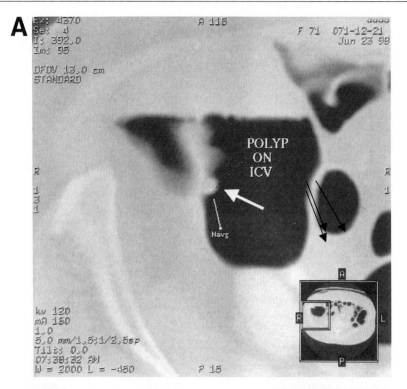

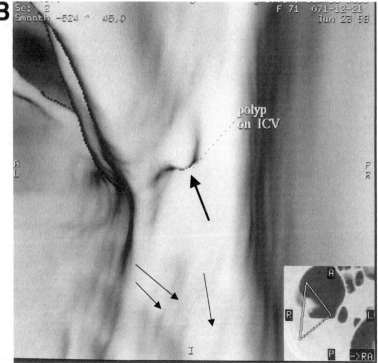

Fig. 2. (A) Axial image from a prone scan displayed on a lung window (W = 2000, L = −450) shows a small polyp (arrow) projecting off a medially-oriented ileocecal valve. **(B)** Endoluminal perspective view shows the polyp on the valve.

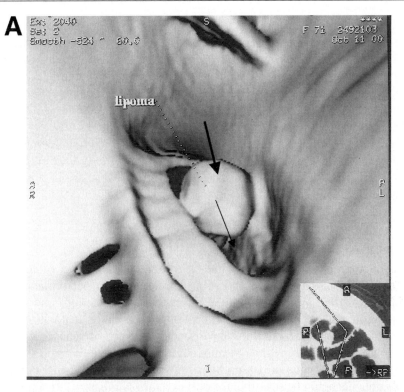

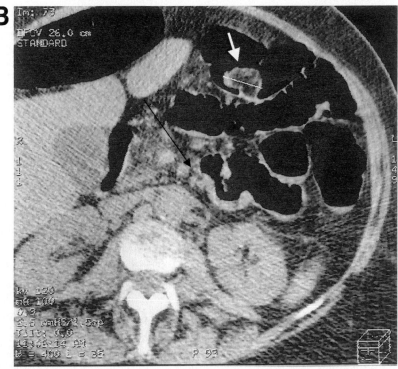

Fig. 3. Patient with a large lesion found at colonoscopy. **(A)** Endoluminal perspective view shows a polypoid mass. **(B)** Axial image from the cleansed, air-distended colon, displayed using soft-tissue window ($W = 400$, $L = 40$) shows a large lobular fatty mass (arrow) in the transverse colon, diagnostic of a submucosal lipoma. No additional intervention was needed based on this diagnosis.

At The University of Chicago, we use a commercially available workstation to view magnified prone and supine images simultaneously in a 4-on-1 format showing both the axial and coronal images *(18)*. Endoluminal views are used on-demand primarily to problem-solve and occasionally to rapidly view straight segments of the colon to search for additional lesions. This method adds little to reading time and increases confidence of interpretation *(18)*. One can rapidly change the endoluminal viewing angle and navigate the colon using simultaneous multiplanar images, or we use software that keeps the "camera's eye" on a centerline or fixed on an area targeted for problem-solving. Other centers describe a similar approach and studies have shown better sensitivity and specificity for polyp detection using this method than 2D or 3D images alone *(16)*. Various investigators now report reading times of approx 5–15 min per exam.

3.3. Performance

3.3.1. TOTAL COLONIC EXAMINATION

Computed tomography colonography has been studied at a number of centers to evaluate sensitivity and specificity for polyp detection. Comparison of performance in these trials is difficult due to differences in technique, threshold for detection, and interpretation of results. In addition, newer helical scanners have improved image acquisition and resolution, and changes in computer workstations have made the work of reading CT colonography different in many institutions. Although most investigators have targeted polyps of 1 cm or larger, there are some investigators who believe that in order for virtual colonoscopy to be widely applicable, it should be sensitive for polyps 5 mm or greater *(19)*. Table 2 summarizes the diagnostic performance of virtual colonoscopy for polyps >10 mm in size.

It is generally accepted that analyzing performance in a "by-patient" manner is acceptable, and eliminates errors in real-world management that may occur in a purely by-polyp analysis. In other words, identifying when a patient requires a conventional colonoscopy based on the results of the virtual colonoscopy is the goal, rather than identifying every polyp. However, the concern with this analysis is the question of the patient with a single small index polyp that is below the threshold of detection. This question requires additional study, and will affect recommendations for screening intervals.

The by-patient sensitivity for patients with polyps ≥10 mm ranges from 75–100% in most series, and was 100% in the two largest series published to date *(20,21)*. A by-polyp sensitivity for polyps ≥10 mm ranges from 50–100%, and was 89–90% in the two largest series. If the threshold of detection is decreased to 5–9 mm, sensitivity and specificity fall significantly, and the number of false positive lesions is greatly increased.

The American College of Radiology Imaging Network (ACRIN) is conducting a multi-center retrospective study in a large, well-defined cohort. We estimate that about 10,000 examinations have been performed by investigators as of early 2000. In addition, a national multicenter study comparing virtual colonoscopy to conventional colonoscopy and to barium enema has started (NIH, Don Rockey, principal investigator). The study includes patients with any approved indication for colonoscopy, and includes detailed surveys of patient preference. This study will recruit approx 4000 patients and be completed in 2004.

Although the results of these early studies are encouraging, no large study has yet been published on an average risk screening population. Studies to determine the effectiveness of this technology on average risk individuals need to be performed. A multicenter trial to assess asymptomatic patients is now under way (Department of Defense, Peter Cotton, principal investigator).

Table 2
Virtual Colonoscopy Exam Performance Data for ≥10 mm Polyps[a]

Author, ref. no., year published	Total no. of patients	No. of patients w/lesions ≥1 cm	Sensitivity % (by patient)	Specificity % (by patient)	No. of lesions ≥1 cm	Sensitivity % (by polyp)	Reading method	Inclusion criteria
Yee (21) 2001	300	≥49	100		82	90	2D and 3D	96 screening, 204 symptomatic
Spinzi (49) 2001	96	10[f]	80[f]	100[f]	13	61.5	2D and 3D	High risk
Hara (20) 2001	237	5	100	90[a]	9	89[d]	2D and 3D	High risk
Mendelson (50) 2000	53[b]				11	73	2D and 3D	High risk
Macari (17) 2000	42	4 (≥7 mm)	100	100	1	100	2D, 3D problem solving	High risk
Hopper (51) 2001	100		Obs B: 37		9	100	2D and 3D	High risk. Supine and select prone/decub
Pescatore (52) 2000	50		Obs A: 62	74	11	62[c]	2D and 3D	High risk
Fletcher (53) 2000	180	96	85.4	93	121	75.2	2D, 3D problem solving	Very high risk, 20 surveillance patients
Morrin (54) 2000	33[e]	6	86	100	12	91	2D and 3D	High risk
Fenlon (27) 1999	100		96	96	22	91	2D and 3D	High probability
Kay (55) 2000	38		90	82.1	11		3D only	High risk. Supine ONLY
Rex (56) 1999	46	10	80	89	14	50	3D (best)	Screening
Pineau (57) 1999	88	10	100	87			2D, 3D problem solving	High risk
Dachman (18) 1998	44	6	83	100	6	83	2D, 3D problem solving	High risk. Supine and prone
Royster (15) 1997	20	20	100		22	100	2D and 3D	All 20 patients had known masses
Hara (58) 1997	70	12	Obs. A: 75 / Obs. B: 75	Obs. A: 91 / Obs. B: 90	15	Obs. A: 73 / Obs. B: 67	2D, 3D problem solving	35 known polyps, 35 high probability Supine only

Adapted from Diagnostic Performance of Virtual Colonoscopy (59), with permission. *Note:* Blank cells indicate data not available or not applicable, *see* text. Obs., Observer; ref., reference number in reference section.

[a]Large masses (≥3 cm) and occlusive carcinomas excluded unless indicated. Patient data for Macari et al., is for ≥7 mm.

[b]Only those with both prone and supine shown.

[c]Includes 2 stoning carcinomas.

[d]High probability is indicated by (1) family or personal history of colorectal cancer, (2) personal history of adenomatous polyps, (3) positive fecal occult blood test, (4) rectal bleeding, (5) iron deficiency anemia, (6) weight loss, (7) recent sigmoidoscopy demonstrating one or more polyps, or (8) altered bowel habit.

[d]Single detector CT (multidetector had 80% sensitivity for polyps >1 cm and a patient specificity of 93%).

[e]Only patients without IV contrast and only polyps 1–2 cm shown.

[f]Additional data by personal communication.

3.3.2. CT Colonography vs Barium Enema

Early reports of the efficacy of virtual colonoscopy have compared this imaging modality to the sensitivity of barium enema. The reported performance of CTC for polyp detection is better than that previously described for barium enema, although only one specific study has yet reported a direct comparison of these tests (22). However, several studies have demonstrated that CTC is superior to barium enema for viewing colonic segments proximal to obstructing lesions (23–26).

3.3.3. CT Colonography for Incomplete Colonoscopy

Virtual colonoscopy offers the unique application in cases of incomplete colonoscopy resulting from technical difficulties, patient discomfort, or obstructing lesions. Morrin and colleagues reported their experience with 40 patients in whom the cecum could not be reached during routine colonoscopy (24). CTC revealed 96% of all colonic segments, and identified the probable reason for the incomplete colonoscopy in 74% of the cases. The same group of investigators recently reported a prospective study of 200 patients with similar results (25). Additionally 19% (33) of those 200 patients also underwent barium enema that adequately demonstrated 91% of segments. A similar study by Fenlon and colleagues evaluated the utility of CTC in 29 patients with occlusive colon carcinoma. They found that CTC identified the obstructing lesion in all of the patients and synchronous lesions in 18/20 patients compared to either colonoscopy or barium enema and visualized the proximal colon in 26/29 patients, whereas barium enema failed in all 29 patients (27). These results suggest that CTC may be the study of choice in patients with an incomplete colonoscopy due to an obstructing mass.

3.3.4. CTC for Colorectal Cancer Staging

It has been proposed that the unique nature of CTC images may not only provide information about the intraluminal lesions but also simultaneously provide information about the stage of a colorectal cancer. Morrin's group studied 34 patients with colorectal cancers and obstructing colorectal lesions and found that CTC correctly staged 13/16 cancers and identified 16/17 synchronous polyps. Ninety-seven percent of the colonic segments were visualized, compared to only 60% with barium enema. In addition, CTC correctly identified the surgical anastomosis of nine patients, but local tumor recurrence could not be distinguished from surgical changes in one patient (26). When colonoscopy is incomplete because of a constricting mass, a same-day CT scan can combine CTC for evaluation of the remainder of the colon and an intravenous contrast-enhanced CT for staging. Some investigators now perform a rapid wet reading of the CTC study while the patient is still on the CT table, and if a polyp or mass is seen, an infused study is done (Morrin, personal communication). Further study is required in this area.

3.3.5. Extraintestinal Findings

Because data collection for virtual colonoscopy involves CT scanning of the abdomen and pelvis, a proposed benefit (and risk) of this exam is the ability to identify extraintestinal abnormalities of clinical significance. Hara and colleagues reported the extraintestinal findings in 264 patients who had a CTC (28). Half of these patients had an abnormality identified and 11% had highly significant findings (abdominal aortic aneurysm, renal adenocarcinoma, and inguinal hernia with bowel). In a retrospective review of 228 consecutive cases, Rosen et al. reported that CTC detected extracolonic abnormalities in 26% of cases and 36% of these had a major impact on patient care (29). Investigators remain excited by the possibility of total-body scans and identifying these extraintestinal lesions, but outcomes and cost-analysis studies of the impact of these "incidentalomas" need to be performed. In addition, the potential for finding such unintended abnormalities should be included in the patient consent process. Finally, if radiologists who read and interpret CTC are required to review the additional abdominal organs, reading time will be significantly increased and population-level screening may be adversely affected.

3.4. Problems and Pitfalls

Despite the major advances that have occurred in the field of CTC, there remain a number of problems and pitfalls requiring future improvement. Although the learning curve for CTC has not been defined, it is understood that interpretation errors can be minimized with experience and the application of the common principles of barium radiography. In fact, the levels of experience of the investigators may be one explanation for the difference in sensitivity and specificity among the published CTC studies. The challenge remains in decreasing the reading time while maintaining appropriate sensitivity and specificity for neoplasms in order to effect cost and mortality benefits.

False-negative results ("pitfalls") decrease sensitivity of this exam and may occur as a result of retained fluid or fecal material as well as from collapsed portions of bowel. These problems are addressed, but not eliminated, by the addition of prone scanning and shifting of gravity-dependent material *(11,30)*. The balloon cuff on the tip of the insufflation catheter theoretically might obscure a distal rectal lesion, so we recommend a careful digital rectal exam prior to placement of the rectal catheter. Other investigators have proposed using intravenous contrast to better distinguish polyps or masses from stool *(31–33)*. One center describes removal of the rectal insufflation tube and additional scanning in order to evaluate the distal rectum *(21)*. The ileocecal valve can be mistaken for a polyp. In addition, some villous adenomas may appear as stool because of their surface architecture. Flat adenomas and infiltrating cancers need to be distinguished from collapsed bowel folds and this may be accomplished by comparison to adjacent folds. In addition, the heterogeneous texture of ulcerated mass lesions may be misinterpreted as stool. False-negative results are potentially costly because they result in missed lesions and possibly cancer. Factoring in additional cancers and associated therapies must be considered in any cost-effectiveness analysis.

False-positive readings ("pseudolesions") reduce specificity and occur from misinterpretations of folds or retained stool. The larger the size threshold of interpretation, the fewer false-positive readings will result. This error may be minimized by recognizing that retained stool appears heterogeneous on CT imaging because of a mixture of air and fecal material. Stool does not have an obvious attachment to the bowel wall when prone images are obtained *(30)*. The problem of false-positive readings is less dangerous (although not less expensive) than that of false-negative readings, because patients with false-positive errors will undergo colonoscopy and presumably, subsequent correction of this mistake. The impact of false positives would be a large number of unnecessary conventional colonoscopies with the accompanying financial and psychological costs, in addition to potential complications.

Patient-related factors affecting reading include retained fluid or fecal material, breathing artifacts, patient motion, and streak artifact from metallic prostheses or surgical clips. Although right hemicolectomy might affect colonic distension during CTC, we have not found this to be a problem in our experience. It may be necessary to include these factors and assign confidence levels to the exam, similar to gastroenterologists' description of the quality of preparation to determine recommendations for future exams.

3.5. Unsettled Issues and Future Applications

There are a number of areas that require clarification before CTC can reach its potential. Performance in screening populations needs to be evaluated. Researchers are developing methods of automated polyp detection in order to minimize reading time and potentially increase accuracy *(34,35)*. Alternate methods of display and advances in dedicated CTC software are likely to further reduce interpretation time. The role of intravenous contrast in screening or surveillance CTC is unclear.

Detailed cost and resource analysis needs to be performed, including cost and outcome analysis for workup of incidental findings. Sonnenberg and colleagues published a model that assumed a hypothetical population of 100,000 people who had screening virtual colonoscopy every 10 yr and underwent conventional colonoscopy for abnormalities, with surveillance exams subsequently. Their model suggests that in order for virtual colonoscopy to have cost-effectiveness similar to colonoscopy, it needs to be 54% less expensive or have compliance rates 15–20% higher than conventional colonoscopy (even if it is 100% sensitive) *(36)*. However, the numerous assumptions required to model cost effectiveness are a subject of controversy.

Computed tomography colonography remains unproven in patients in high-risk groups, such as inherited forms of colorectal cancer *(37)*. Patients with inflammatory bowel disease (IBD) have an increased risk of developing colorectal cancer, but it is via dysplasia of (flat) inflamed mucosa, and CTC is unlikely to offer an alternative to conventional colonoscopy surveillance and biopsies. More recent work has examined the utility of CTC for mapping of involved intestine in a small number of patients with IBD *(38)*, and other investigators in Europe have explored the possibility of magnetic resonance colonography for IBD *(39,40)*.

Early work has demonstrated that patients may prefer the minimally invasive CTC to barium enema or to conventional colonoscopy *(41,42)*. Current CTC methods do not eliminate the need for a bowel prep, which is described by some patients as the most uncomfortable part of colorectal cancer screening tests. In fact, if the CTC has positive findings, an additional bowel cleansing will then be required for the subsequent conventional colonoscopy. Institutions will need to offer immediate image interpretation and subsequent colonoscopy for positive findings to eliminate the unpleasantness of requiring a repeat bowel preparation. Development of computer-assisted automated polyp detection and standardized reporting methods to inform a gastroenterologist of the location and size of a suspected lesion are necessary. Pilot work using a proprietary detection algorithm has been encouraging *(43)*.

Physicians and patients alike eagerly await development of a "virtual preparation." A pilot study using barium as a contrast agent instead of a cathartic preparation had fair results *(44)*. A combination of a low-fiber diet and stool tagging with barium and a minimal preparation with magnesium citrate alone is under study and is now being marketed by industry *(45)*. Stool tagging offers the possibility of computer thresholding and electronic subtraction of stool which might permit CTC without any preparation *(46)*. Other studies have suggested that different contrast agents or magnetic resonance (MR) colonography might hold promise in this area *(47)*, but it does not yet offer comparable sensitivity to the cleansed colon. MR colonography in the prepared colon has shown accuracy similar to CTC *(48)*.

4. CONCLUSIONS

Computed tomography colonography offers a minimally invasive view of the entire colon that may address some of the inadequacies of current screening and prevention strategies and improve population compliance with CRC screening. Current approaches to this exciting technology appear to be safe, well tolerated, and sensitive for detection of polyps or masses larger than 1 cm. In addition, the current techniques may offer the ability to perform preoperative cancer staging and same-day identification of synchronous lesions after incomplete or obstructed colonoscopic examinations. Routine use of CTC for screening purposes is limited by the absence of population studies, unclear cost and resource allocation, an undefined learning curve for radiologists, and possibly uncertain sensitivity for polyps 6–9 mm. Advances in technology and ongoing research hold promise for the widespread use of this test in the future.

REFERENCES

1. Landis SH, et al. Cancer statistics, 1999 [see comments], *CA Cancer J. Clin.*, **49(1)** (1999) 8–31.
2. Winawer SJ, et al. Prevention of colorectal cancer by colonoscopic polypectomy. The National Polyp Study Workgroup [see comments]. *N. Engl. J. Med.*, **329(27)** (1993) 1977–1981.
3. Lieberman DA, et al. Use of colonoscopy to screen asymptomatic adults for colorectal cancer. Veterans Affairs Cooperative Study Group 380 [see comments]. *N. Engl. J. Med.*, **343(3)** (2000) 162–168.
4. Imperiale TF, et al. Risk of advanced proximal neoplasms in asymptomatic adults according to the distal colorectal findings. *N. Engl. J. Med.*, **343(3)** (2000) 169–174.
5. Winawer SJ, et al. Colorectal cancer screening: clinical guidelines and rationale [see comments] [published errata appear in *Gastroenterology*, **112(3)** (1997) 1060 and **114(3)** (1998) 625]. *Gastroenterology*, **112(2)** (1997) 594–642.
6. Rex DK, et al. Colorectal cancer prevention 2000: screening recommendations of the American College of Gastroenterology. American College of Gastroenterology. *Am. J. Gastroenterol.*, **95(4)** (2000) 868–877.
7. From the Centers for Disease Control and Prevention. Screening for colorectal cancer—United States, 1997. *JAMA*, **281(17)** (1999) 1581–1582.
8. Vernon SW. Participation in colorectal cancer screening: a review [see comments]. *J. Natl. Cancer Inst.*, **89(19)** (1997) 1406–1422.
9. Vining D and Gelfand D. Noninvasive colonoscopy using helical CT scanning, 3D reconstruction, and virtual reality. *The Society of Gastrointestinal Radiologists.* Maui, Hawaii, 1994.
10. Yee J, et al. Colonic distention and colorectal polyp detection with and without glucagon on virtual colonoscopy. *The Society of Gastrointestinal Radiologists.* Palm Beach, FL, 1999.
11. Chen SC, et al. CT colonography: value of scanning in both the supine and prone positions. *AJR Am. J. Roentgenol.*, **172(3)** (1999) 595–599.
12. Hara AK, et al. Reducing data size and radiation dose for CT colonography. *AJR Am. J. Roentgenol.*, **168(5)** (1997) 1181–1184.
13. McFarland EG, et al. Visualization of colorectal polyps with spiral CT colography: evaluation of processing parameters with perspective volume rendering. *Radiology*, **205(3)** (1997) 701–707.
14. Reed J. Display/navigation: Mayo Clinic experience. *First International Symposium on Virtual Colonoscopy*, 1998.
15. Royster AP, et al. CT colonoscopy of colorectal neoplasms: two-dimensional and three-dimensional virtual-reality techniques with colonoscopic correlation. *AJR Am. J. Roentgenol.*, **169(5)** (1997) 1237–1242.
16. Hara AK, et al. Colorectal polyp detection with CT colography: two- versus three-dimensional techniques. Work in progress [see comments]. *Radiology*, **200(1)** (1996) 49–54.
17. Macari M, et al. Comparison of time-efficient CT colonography with two- and three-dimensional colonic evaluation for detecting colorectal polyps. *AJR Am. J. Roentgenol.*, **174(6)** (2000) 1543–1549.
18. Dachman AH, et al. CT colonography with three-dimensional problem solving for detection of colonic polyps. *AJR Am. J. Roentgenol.*, **171(4)** (1998) 989–995.
19. Rex D. Virtual Colonoscopy. *Digestive Disease Week.* San Diego, CA, 2000.
20. Hara AK, et al. CT colonography: single- versus multidetector row imaging. *Radiology*, **219(2)** (2001) 461–465.
21. Yee J, et al. Colorectal neoplasia: performance characteristics of ct colonography for detection in 300 patients. *Radiology*, **219(3)** (2001) 684–692.
22. Hara AK, et al. Computed tomographic colography (virtual colonoscopy) for polyp detection: early comparison against barium enema. *Gastroenterology*, **112(Suppl.)** (1997) A575.
23. Fenlon HM, et al. Occlusive colon carcinoma: virtual colonoscopy in the preoperative evaluation of the proximal colon. *Radiology*, **210(2)** (1999) 423–428.

24. Morrin MM, et al. Endoluminal CT colonography after an incomplete endoscopic colonoscopy. *AJR Am. J. Roentgenol.*, **172(4)** (1999) 913–918.

25. Morrin MM, et al. Experience with 200 CT colonography examinations after incomplete endoscopic colonoscopy. *Radiology*, **217(Suppl.)** (2000) 582.

26. Morrin MM, et al. Role of virtual computed tomographic colonography in patients with colorectal cancers and obstructing colorectal lesions. *Dis. Colon Rectum*, **43(3)** (2000) 303–311.

27. Fenlon HM, et al. A comparison of virtual and conventional colonoscopy for the detection of colorectal polyps [see comments] [published erratum appears in N. Engl. J. Med. 2000 Feb. 17;342(7):524]. *N. Engl. J. Med.*, **341(20)** (1999) 1496–1503.

28. Hara AK, et al. Incidental extracolonic findings at CT colonography. *Radiology*, **215(2)** (2000) 353–357.

29. Rosen MP, Morrin MM, and Raptopoulos V. Prevalence of findings unrelated to the colon detected during CT colonography (abstract). *Radiology*, **217(Suppl.)** (2000) 583.

30. Fletcher JG, et al. CT colonography: potential pitfalls and problem-solving techniques [see comments]. *AJR Am. J. Roentgenol.*, **172(5)** (1999) 1271–1278.

31. Luz O, et al. Enhancement of colonic polyps in high-resolution CT colonography following bolus injection of IV contrast (abstract). *Radiology*, **217(Suppl.)** (2000) 583.

32. Neri E, et al. Contrast-enhanced CT colonography after incomplete fyberoptic (sic.) colonoscopy in the preoperative management of colorectal cancer (abstract). *Radiology*, **217(Suppl.)** (2000) 582.

33. Vining D. *Discussion at MUSC multi-center VC trial investigators' meeting*. Rubin DT (ed.) Charleston, SC,1999.

34. Summers RM, et al. Automated polyp detector for CT colonography: feasibility study. *Radiology*, **216(1)** (2000) 284–290.

35. Yoshida H, et al., Detection of colonic polyps in CT colonography based on geometric features (abstract). *Radiology*, **217(Suppl.)** (2000) 582.

36. Sonnenberg A, Delco F, and Bauerfeind P. Is virtual colonoscopy a cost-effective option to screen for colorectal cancer? *Am. J. Gastroenterol.*, **94(8)** (1999) 2268–2274.

37. Macari M, et al. Diagnosis of familial adenomatous polyposis using two-dimensional and three-dimensional CT colonography. *AJR Am. J. Roentgenol.*, **173(1) (1999) 249–250.**

38. Tarjan Z, et al. Spiral CT colonography in inflammatory bowel disease [In Process Citation]. *Eur. J. Radiol.*, **35(3)** (2000) 193–198.

39. Luboldt W, et al. Contrast optimization for assessment of the colonic wall and lumen in MR colonography. *J. Magn. Reson. Imaging*, **9(5)** (1999) 745–750.

40. Luboldt W, et al. [New perspectives in 3D MR colonography]. *Schweiz. Rundsch. Med. Prax.*, **88(3)** (1999) 73–79.

41. Hara AK, Johnson CD, and Reed JE. Colorectal polyp detection with CT colography (virtual colonoscopy): a blinded prospective study (abstract). *Radiology*, **201** (1996) A252.

42. Farrell RJ, et al. Virtual colonoscopy in patients undergoing elective colonoscopy: diagnostic accuracy and patient tolerance (abstract). *Gastroenterology*, **118(4part2)** (2000) A258.

43. Yoshida H, et al. Computerized Detection of Colonic Polyps in CT Colonography Based on Volumetric Features: A Pilot Study (in print). *Radiology*, (2001).

44. Callstrom MR, et al. CT colonography of the unprepped colon: an early feasibility study of "virtual preparation" (abstract). *Gastroenterology*, **118(4)(Suppl.)** (2000) A257.

45. Gryspeerdt SS, et al. Dietary fecal tagging enables reduced colon cleansing and improves diagnosis in virtual CT colonoscopy (abstract). *Radiology*, **217** (2000) 170.

46. Zalis ME, et al. Improving patient tolerance of colon cancer screening: digital bowel subtraction in CT colonography. *Radiology*, **217** (2000) 370.

47. Weishaupt D, et al. Faecal tagging to avoid colonic cleansing before MRI colonography [letter]. *Lancet*, **354(9181)** (1999) 835–836.

48. Saar B, et al. Virtual MR-colonosocopy: prospective evaluation vs. endoscopic colonoscopy (abstract). *Radiology*, **217** (2000) 583.

49. Spinzi G, et al. Computed tomographic colonography and conventional colonoscopy for colon diseases: a prospective, blinded study. *Am. J. Gastroenterol.*, **96(2)** (2001) 394–400.

50. Mendelson RM, et al. Virtual colonoscopy compared with conventional colonoscopy: a developing technology. *Med. J. Aust.*, **173(9)** (2000) 472–475.

51. Hopper KD, Khandelwal M., and TC. CT colonoscopy: experience of 100 cases using volumetric rendering. *Proceedings of SPIE*, **12** (2001) 489–494.

52. Pescatore P, et al. Diagnostic accuracy and interobserver agreement of CT colonography (virtual colonoscopy). *Gut*, **47(1)** (2000) 704–711.

53. Fletcher JG, et al. Optimization of CT colonography technique: prospective trial in 180 patients. *Radiology*, **216(3)** (2000) 704–711.
54. Morrin MM, et al. Utility of intravenously administered contrast material at CT colonography. *Radiology*, **217(3)** (2000) 765–771.
55. Kay CL, et al. Virtual endoscopy—comparison with colonoscopy in the detection of space-occupying lesions of the colon. *Endoscopy*, **32(3)** (2000) 226–232.
56. Rex DK, Vining D, and Kopecky KK. An initial experience with screening for colon polyps using spiral CT with and without CT colography (virtual colonoscopy) [see comments]. *Gastrointest. Endosc.*, **50(3)** (1999) 309–313.
57. Pineau BC and Vining D. Ability of virtual colonoscopy to detect patients with colorectal polyps (abstract). *Gastroenterology*, **116(4part2)** (1999) A485.
58. Hara AK, et al. Detection of colorectal polyps with CT colography: initial assessment of sensitivity and specificity. *Radiology*, **205(1)** (1997) 59–65.
59. Dachman AH. Diagnostic Performance of Virtual Colonoscopy, in press.

9 Preoperative Staging of Rectal Cancer

Endorectal Ultrasound and Endorectal MRI

Spiros Hiotis, Sharon Weber, and W. Douglas Wong

Contents

1. RATIONALE

The treatment algorithm for rectal cancer has changed markedly over the last decade. Radical surgery, either low anterior resection or abdominal perineal resection, is no longer the initial or only therapy for the majority of patients with rectal carcinoma. The reason for this is twofold: First, in both nonrandomized and randomized studies, preoperative multimodality treatment has been found to decrease the local recurrence rate and result in significant downstaging in patients with rectal tumors; second, local excision of rectal tumors has become the preferred treatment in highly selected, early-stage patients. Because of this, preoperative staging has become increasingly important in order to direct patients into the appropriate treatment arm. In addition, in patients who are downstaged after undergoing preoperative chemoradiation, postoperative decisions regarding further chemotherapy are often dependent on the preoperative stage alone. Therefore, it is imperative to have easily available, accurate preoperative imaging studies in order to assess not only the depth of penetration but also the presence of involved lymph nodes. In addition, before embarking on expensive and often physically demanding preoperative therapies, it is important to assure the absence of metastatic disease.

Staging patients with rectal carcinoma by digital rectal examination is unreliable, with overall accuracy rates of 40–80% *(1,2)*. In addition, digital exam is unable to reliably assess for the presence of involved lymph nodes. The identification of pathologic nodes is particularly important in the evaluation of early (T1/T2) tumors because these patients should be excluded for consideration of local therapy.

From: *Colorectal Cancer: Multimodality Management*
Edited by: L. Saltz © Humana Press Inc., Totowa, NJ

Although computed tomographic (CT) scans are 80–90% accurate in assessing transmural penetration *(3,4)* and are also accurate in determining adjacent organ invasion, the rectal wall layers cannot be resolved on CT. Therefore, this is not effective in distinguishing early-stage tumors. Conventional magnetic resonance imaging (MRI) results in accuracy rates of 58–82% for assessing the depth of penetration *(1,5,6)*. In a prospective comparison of CT and MRI in staging patients with rectal lesions, CT was found to be more accurate than MRI in assessing penetration of the muscularis propria (74% vs 58%, respectively). In a separate study, there was no difference in assessing transmural penetration using these techniques *(7)*. There appears to be no difference between the two modalities in assessing nodal status, with sensitivities of 40% and specificities of 70–90% *(5,7)*.

Because neither of these modalities provides the accuracy needed to select patients for either neoadjuvant therapy or local excision, both endorectal ultrasound and endorectal coil MRI have been increasingly used.

2. ENDORECTAL ULTRASOUND

2.1. Introduction

Introduced in 1983, endorectal ultrasound (ERUS) has become the standard preoperative imaging modality for rectal carcinoma *(8,9)*. ERUS is performed in the office setting and is well tolerated without sedation. As with many varieties of ultrasonography, ERUS requires a fair amount of expertise on the part of the ultrasonographer. Still images are easily printed and saved for later review, but a great deal of information can be obtained during the real-time acquisition of images. The precise relationships of tumors to anatomical landmarks are best determined by actually performing the ultrasound and studying the images in real-time.

For the right-handed ultrasonographer, the procedure is best performed with the patient in the left lateral decubitus position. Gentle insertion of the lubricated transducer is easily accomplished with minimal discomfort to the patient. Most commonly, the transducer is inserted through a rigid proctoscope, thus facilitating both proctoscopic and ultrasound evaluation of the rectum at a single setting *(10)*. The ultrasonographer should be seated in a comfortable position to manipulate the transducer with two hands. The right hand should be used to control the degree of insertion into the rectum and the left hand should be used to center the transducer. Maintaining the transducer in the center of the rectal lumen is important because it affords clear imaging of the entire 360° circumference of the bowel and prevents loss of contact between the transducer and the rectal surface.

There are many manufacturers who produce high-quality ultrasound devices, but probes that acquire 360° images are preferable for endorectal imaging. Such probes acquire several images per second of the complete endorectal luminal circumference. Ultrasonic signals travel best in water, thus (in the most common imaging setting) a balloon covering the transducer is filled with water following the insertion of the transducer into the rectum. A sufficient quantity of water is instilled to prevent any separation of the balloon from the rectal wall; this prevents the interposition of nonconductive air between the probe and the rectum. The balloon is not used in certain situations. For example, the entire rectum can be filled with water (usually 180 cm^3 instilled via a Foley catheter) for imaging selected lesions when it is anticipated that the balloon may cause distortion of the lesion preventing adequate imaging. In this case, the transducer is covered with a sonolucent plastic cap filled with water that does not cause compression of the rectal wall as with the balloon. Additionally, when precise imaging of the anal canal is desired, this water-filled plastic cap is simply placed over the transducer. The transducer covered by a small plastic cap is moved through the anal canal with greater ease than one covered by the larger balloon.

Interpreting ERUS images requires some experience, but most physicians who are familiar with the anatomy of the lower pelvis learn to read these images quickly. Structures such as the seminal vesicles and prostate in males and the vagina in females serve as useful landmarks. These structures may help in properly orienting the ultrasonographer to anterior/posterior direction and also in determining the level of insertion of the probe. Generally, high-quality images cannot be acquired above 12–15 cm from the anal verge. Lower anorectal landmarks such as the puborectalis muscle as well as the internal and external anal sphincters are clearly demonstrated on ERUS and serve as useful distal landmarks. High-quality images can be acquired as low as the distal anal canal.

2.2. Interpreting the Images

Five layers of the rectal wall are clearly demonstrated by ERUS; familiarity with each of these leads to proper interpretation of the images *(11,12)*. These layers are recognized by the alternating hyperechoic (bright) and hypoechoic (dark) appearance of each. The first layer visualized (from the center of the image to the periphery) is hyperechoic and represents the interface of the balloon with the rectal mucosal surface. The second layer is hypoechoic and represents the mucosa and muscularis mucosa. The third layer is hyperechoic and represents the submucosa. The fourth layer is hypoechoic and represents the muscularis propria. In more distal images, the muscularis propria increases in thickness as it transitions into the internal anal sphincter. The fifth layer is hyperechoic and represents the interface of the rectum with the perirectal fat.

2.3. Staging Rectal Cancers

Rectal tumors are identified by their hypoechoic (dark) appearance on ERUS. Distinguishing between superficial (T1/T2) tumors (Figs. 1–3) and deep (T3/T4) tumors (Fig. 4) is relatively easy *(13)*. Superficial tumors will not cause distortion in the outer, dark layer of the muscularis propria, and this layer will be clearly visible around 100% of the rectal circumference. Difficulty arises when attempting to distinguish a deep T2 tumor from an early T3 *(14)*. Deep T2 lesions abut the outer portion of the muscularis propria and minimal tumor penetration beyond this layer may be difficult to visualize because of distortion of the muscularis at areas of maximal tumor involvement. The distinction between T2 and T3 lesions is important because, under current recommendations and in the absence of nodal disease, T2 tumors are treated differently than T3 tumors. Most patients diagnosed with T3N0 lesions will be advised to undergo multimodality therapy, in accordance with the National Cancer Institute's (NCI) consensus statement about these lesions. Patients with T3N0 disease will receive preoperative chemoradiation in many centers, followed by resection, whereas patients with T2N0 disease will be treated with resection alone *(15)*.

Endorectal ultrasound can reliably distinguish T1 from deep T2 lesions. However, the distinction between T1 and superficial T2 lesions is often difficult to make by ERUS. Neither of these superficial tumors cause distortion of the muscularis propria. In the absence of nodal involvement, T1 lesions may be satisfactorily treated with transanal, full thickness excision, as transanal resection of these lesions yields similar results when compared to more radical resection. However, current evidence reveals that transanal excision of T2 lesions leads to a high local recurrence rate, as high as 42%, and therefore should not be routinely employed as definitive therapy for T2 lesions in good-risk patients *(16)*. Hence, patients identified by ERUS to have deep T2 lesions should undergo major resection. However,

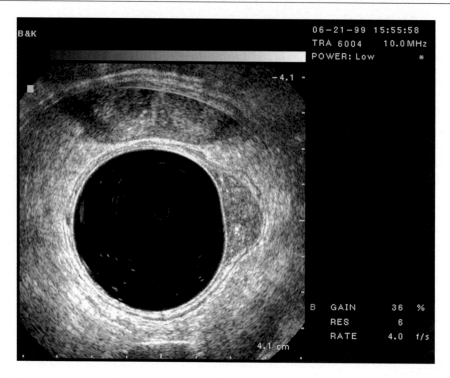

Fig. 1. Endorectal ultrasound image of a patient with a T1 lesion. The lesion is located in the left lateral position and invades into but not beyond the hyperechoic submucosal layer. This is characterized by irregularity but not disruption of the hyperechoic middle line.

for patients who are staged by ERUS to have a T1 or superficial T2 lesion where reliable distinction is difficult, then transanal excision is an appropriate initial step in treatment *(17)*. If the final pathology confirms a T1 lesion, then no further therapy is necessary, and careful ERUS follow-up alone is recommended. However, if the final pathology reveals a significant T2 lesion, then radical resection, such as low anterior resection or abdomino-perineal resection, should be considered in the acceptable-risk patient. Another consideration is to treat locally excised T2 lesions with postoperative chemoradiation, but resultant local recurrence rates approach 20% *(18,19)*.

2.4. Determining Nodal Involvement

Lymph nodes may be visible in the mesorectum during ERUS imaging *(20–22)*. Nodes are usually visualized as round, hypoechoic (dark) structures within the mesorectum. Lymph nodes are categorized as pathologic or benign according to their size and ultrasound characteristics. If no lymph nodes are visualized within the mesorectum, then the patient is staged as N0. Hypoechoic nodes that are 5 mm or greater in diameter are generally felt to harbor metastatic disease (Fig. 4) *(23)*. This is especially true of lymph nodes located adjacent or proximal to the level of the cancer. Hyperechoic mesorectal nodes usually contain benign inflammatory changes. A hyperechoic focus within the center of an otherwise hypoechoic node or mixed echogenicity within a mesorectal node suggests a benign node *(24)*.

One must exercise caution when diagnosing nodal disease, as blood vessels within the mesorectum will often appear similar to enlarged nodes in a still image. Imaging these structures in real-time allows one to easily distinguish blood vessels from lymph nodes.

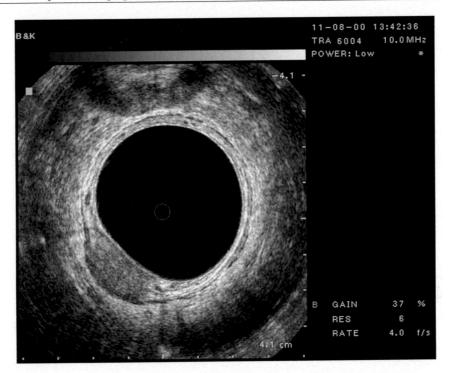

Fig. 2. Endorectal ultrasound image of a patient with a posteriorly located T2 lesion. The tumor extends into but not beyond the muscularis propria and is characterized by disruption of the hyperechoic middle line.

Any hypoechoic structure in the mesorectum that can be imaged while moving the probe in a proximal to distal fashion for a distance greater than the diameter of that structure is probably a blood vessel that is being seen in cross-section. Lymph nodes are generally round in shape and will disappear from the image when the probe is moved for a distance greater than its diameter. Unfortunately, ERUS is limited in its ability to detect the presence of micrometstatic disease in mesorectal lymph nodes.

2.5. Determining Proximity of Tumor to the Sphincter Muscles and Adjacent Structures

Additional information that may be obtained on ERUS is a tumor's precise relationship to the sphincter muscles. This information is relevant when attempting to make proper decisions regarding sphincter-preserving resection. As stated earlier, the puborectalis muscle can be identified with ease. This structure has a striated, hyperechoic appearance is distinguished by its slinglike shape travels downward from the anterior lower pelvis, and envelopes the rectum posteriorly. Similarly, the external anal sphincter is also distinguished by its striated, hyperechoic character. The internal sphincter is hypoechoic and does not have striations. It is developed from the muscularis propria in the distal rectum. ERUS is an exquisitely accurate method of visualizing involvement or close proximity of a low-lying rectal tumor to the sphincter muscles.

Involvement of surrounding pelvic structures with tumor can also be easily assessed with ERUS. The vagina is clearly identifiable in its relationship to the anterior rectum in women, as are the prostate and seminal vesicles in men. T4 tumors that infiltrate these structures can be

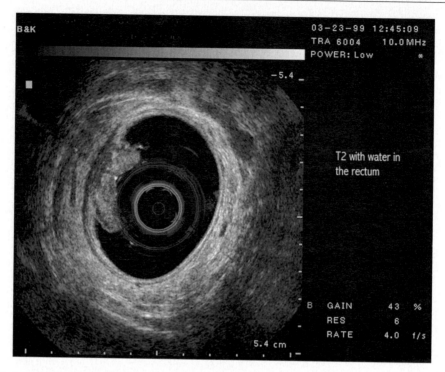

Fig. 3. Endorectal ultrasound image of a patient with a T2 lesion. This image was acquired without the use of a water-filled balloon around the probe. Instead, the rectum was filled with water and a sonolucent hard cap covered the transducer.

identified with precision. Thus, decisions regarding the need for preoperative chemoradiation or radical resection with possible pelvic exenteration can be appropriately made.

2.6. Utility of ERUS Following Chemoradiation

Among those patients who receive preoperative chemoradiation, restaging prior to resection may be desirable. However, regardless of the response to chemoradiation, surgical resection should be offered to all acceptable-risk patients. Only one study has supported nonoperative observation for complete responders (25). However, data from Memorial Sloan-Kettering suggests that assessing complete response after chemoradiation is highly inaccurate, and patients who appear to have had a complete response usually harbor occult foci of tumor (25a). Restaging by ERUS is not reliable following treatment with chemoradiation. Scar develops in the rectal wall, and discriminating scar from tumor is often not possible (26). In one prospective study, the positive predictive value for ERUS determination of residual rectal wall penetration and lymph node involvement following preoperative chemoradiation was only 72% and 56%, respectively, although the negative predictive value of ERUS in this setting was significantly better (100% for wall penetration and 82% for lymph node involvement) (27). However, given the currently available technology and current recommendations for treatment, restaging patients with ERUS following chemoradiation is not recommended (28). Imaging in this setting is inaccurate and the treatment plan should not be altered, even if the patient is believed to have experienced a complete response to chemoradiation.

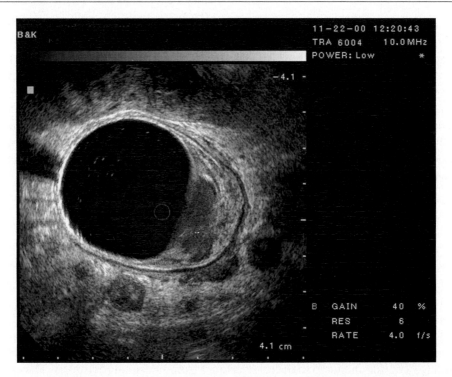

Fig. 4. Endorectal ultrasound image of a patient with a T3N1 lesion. The tumor clearly extends beyond the muscularis propria. Several pathologic nodes are seen in this image. The enlarged pathologic lymph node located at the 6 o'clock position demonstrates hyperechoic foci within an otherwise hypoechoic node.

2.7. Surveillance

Endorectal ultrasound may be used in a variety of settings for surveillance purposes. Most commonly, ERUS may prove useful following endoscopic or transanal resection of superficial cancers or benign lesions with suspicious histologic features. When used in combination with digital rectal examination and endoscopic surveillance, ERUS may significantly improve the sensitivity of detection of recurrent lesions *(29,30)*. Although little reported experience with ERUS exists in this setting, its potential value in imaging small, early lesions that cannot be felt or seen is implicit. The correct interval in between imaging studies is not clearly understood, although imaging every 4 mo may be appropriate. Additionally, the proper duration of surveillance following endoscopic or transanal resection is not clear, although continuing regular surveillance for a minimum of 3 yr may be appropriate, with less frequent ERUS surveillance until 5 yr.

2.8. ERUS Accuracy Rates

Endorectal ultrasound is most accurate in assessing transmural penetration, with a sensitivity of up to 95% *(3,4,31,32)*. Overall accuracy rates are lower, however, because ultrasound tends to incorrectly overstage some T2 tumors *(31)*. ERUS is 83–88% specific in separating patients with T1–T2 rectal cancers from patients with T3–T4 cancer *(33)*. Two recent series found very similar accuracy rates for T1 and T2 lesions. T1 tumors were correctly staged in 54–58% of patients, and for T2 tumors, accuracy was 70–75% *(31)*. In

Adams' series, T1 lesions were equally understaged and overstaged, whereas T2 lesions were primarily overstaged *(31)*.

The accuracy of ERUS for transmural penetration has been equal to or better than computed tomography (CT) when they have been directly compared *(3,4)*. However, both modalities are less reliable in assessing nodal positivity, with an accuracy of 70% *(3)* and 80% *(24,32)*, respectively. It is important to remember that even small errors in specificity may commit an incorrectly overstaged patient to several additional months of treatment with minimal benefit. Because of its accuracy, particularly in identifying T3 or deeper tumors, ERUS should be considered an invaluable diagnostic modality in staging patients with resectable rectal tumors.

3. ENDORECTAL MRI

3.1. Introduction

The accuracy of MRI improves markedly when an endorectal coil is used instead of conventional imaging with a body coil. The endorectal coil is a rigid instrument with a receive-only loop coil covered with a balloon. The device is 15 cm in length. The coil is inserted into the rectum with the patient in the lateral position. Air is inflated into the balloon to allow adequate distension of the rectum. Sagittal localizing images assure correct placement of the coil, then multiple images are obtained in the sagittal and axial planes. Glucagon may be administered to decrease artifact from intestinal peristalsis. The endorectal coil improves the signal-to-noise (S/N) ratio and allows imaging with a small field of view, which improves resolution. This is essential for accurate visualization of the rectal wall layers and accurate interpretation of tumor T stage.

Additional use of a pelvic coil improves S/N at distances greater than 3 cm from the endorectal coil *(34)*. This also results in an increased size of the field of view, which improves detection of pelvic nodes. The combined use of two coils allows greater resolution local extension of tumors greater than 3 cm in depth. It is, therefore, important to distinguish the technique used when interpreting the results of preoperative staging with endorectal MRI.

It has been argued that the use of these techniques may overcome one criticism of ERUS—that it is extremely operator dependent. However, some series evaluating endorectal coil MRI have found it to have poor correlation between radiologists when images are reviewed by blinded examiners *(35,36)*. One problem with the endorectal coil is that images of the rectal wall layers are often only seen clearly from part, but not all, of the circumference of the rectum *(37)*. This may be the result of the compression of the layers of the rectal wall by the coil itself and may result in errors in interpretation of the depth of invasion. Poor contact between larger tumors and the coil may also limit image interpretation *(38)*. In addition, although ERUS can usually be performed with minimal discomfort in 10–15 min, endorectal coil MRI is often uncomfortable and imaging may take up to 60 min *(35)*.

3.2. Interpreting the Images

The T2-weighted MRI images performed with the endorectal coil distinguish three layers of the rectal wall. The initial layer of high signal density is the result of mucus and fluid between the coil and the rectal wall. The first rectal wall layer, the mucosa and muscularis mucosa, is of low signal intensity. The second, the submucosal, layer is of high signal intensity, followed by the third layer containing the muscularis propria, which is of low signal intensity. The outermost layer of perirectal adipose tissue is of high signal intensity.

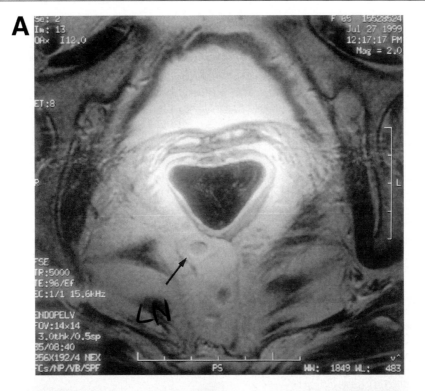

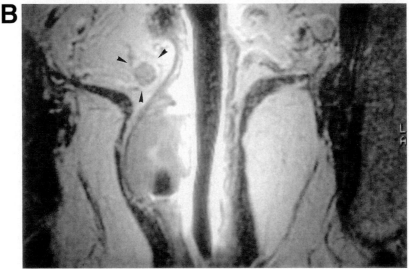

Fig. 5. Endorectal MRI of a patient with node positive disease (arrows) on axial (**A**) and sagital (**B**) views. (MRI images courtesy of Dr. Ron Bleday, Boston MA.)

On T2-weighted images, rectal tumors have a low-to-medium signal intensity higher than that of the muscularis propria.

Nodal tissue in the perirectal fat appears as rounded, nontubular structures (Fig. 5A, B). It is not possible to distinguish inflammatory from metastatic nodes, and there are no well-defined characteristics that classify a metastatic node. Therefore, when interpreting results from studies examining nodal status, it is important to determine the criteria for nodal positivity.

Table 1
Overall Results of Accuracy of Endorectal MRI in Preoperative Staging of Primary Rectal Cancer
in Patients Who Did Not Receive Neoadjuvant Therapy (Comparison to ERUS When Available)

Author	Date	n	Criteria for nodal positivity	Technique[a]	MRI T (%)	MRI N (%)	ERUS T (%)	ERUS N (%)
Schnall et al. (37)	1994	36	Structure[b]	ECMRI	81	78		
Murano et al. (38a)	1995	22	Structure	ECMRI	73	82		
Drew et al. (35)	1999	29	Structure, size[c]***	MMRI, Gd	31	66		
Kim et al. (39)	1999	73	Structure, size**	ECMRI	81	63	81	64
Maldjian et al. (40)	2000	14	Structure, size*	MMRI	71	77	71	54
Gualdi et al. (38)	2000	26	All visible[d]	ECMRI	85	73	77	76

[a]ECMRI = endorectal coil MRI, MMRI = multicoil MRI (endorectal coil with pelvic multicoil array),
Gd = gadolinium-contrast enhanced.
[b]Structure = all nodes with abnormal appearance (loss of fat at the hilum, heterogeneous, or irregular)
considered positive.
[c]Size = all nodes greater a particular size were considered positive (* >1 cm, ** >3 mm, *** >5 mm).
[d]All visible = all nodes detected were considered positive.

3.3. Endorectal MRI Accuracy Rates

Overall accuracy rates for endorectal coil MRI preoperative staging, as compared to pathologic stage in patients who did not receive neoadjuvant therapy, are seen in Table 1. In most series, the accuracy for T stage varies from 70% to 85% and for N stage from 60% to 80%. When endorectal coil MRI is examined according to its ability to accurately assess T3 disease, between 70% (35) and 100% of patients are correctly staged as T3, with most series between 85% and 100% accurate (34,36,37,39,41).

Several studies are limited by the small number of patients and the use of neoadjuvant therapy in subsets of the entire patient group examined, and are therefore not included in Table 1 (34,41–43). Imaging with the endorectal coil, like other imaging modalities, is difficult after preoperative chemoradiation and does not reliably predict response to treatment (44).

Endorectal coil MRI is limited in its ability to distinguish T1 (Fig. 6) and T2 tumors; one study that utilized gadolinium-enhanced images overstaged 10/14 T2 tumors as T3 and 4/4 T1 tumors as either T2 or T3 (35). In most series, the degree of overstaging is not as severe, but it is still far more likely than understaging tumor (37–39). This is likely the result of peritumoral inflammation, which also limits distinction of early T-stage tumors with ERUS. Although overstaging will assure that patients are not undertreated, it also commits patients with potentially early stage tumors to more radical therapy, either a course of neoadjuvant therapy or a more extensive operation (e.g., low anterior resection instead of local excision).

Correctly determining nodal positivity is dependent on the criteria used to evaluate a node as pathologically involved with tumor. Large (>1 cm) nodes can be inflammatory and small

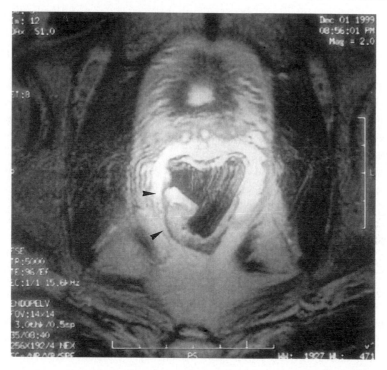

Fig. 6. Endorectal MRI revealing T1 rectal lesion (arrows). (Image courtesy of Dr. Ron Bleday, Boston MA.)

Table 2
Accuracy Rates Between Endorectal MRI and ERUS for Individual T Stages

Author	Technique	T1 (%)	T2 (%)	T3 (%)	T4 (%)
Kim et al. *(39)*	ERUS	100[a]	50	87	100
	ECMRI		57	89	100
Gualdi et al. *(38)*	ERUS	100	40	82	
	ECMRI	100	60	96	

[a]All patients underwent local excision only.

nodes (<2 mm) metastatic *(37)*. Thus, using size alone as the criteria for nodal positivity often results in erroneous readings. Structural characteristics, such as loss of fat at the hilum of the node, are also inaccurate. Because no preoperative staging system can accurately detect micrometastases, it is not surprising that accuracy for detecting metastatic nodes decreases compared to the assessment of T stage. Most series have shown almost equal numbers of patients that are overstaged and understaged with regard to nodal status *(35,37,39,40)*. This is problematic because a high sensitivity (accurately determining all patients with positive nodes) is more important than specificity, both in order to appropriately treat patients with stage III disease with chemoradiation and to exclude patients with early T-stage but node-positive disease from local excision.

Direct comparison to ERUS was performed prospectively in the last three studies listed in Table 1 and therefore are particularly important in comparing these two modalities. All of the studies found nearly equivalent rates of detection of depth of invasion, with little difference between accuracy rates in detection of individual T stages (Table 2). Only one study suggested a small improvement in the ability of endorectal MRI to correctly determine nodal status, with MRI accurate in 10/13 cases compared to 7/13 cases with ERUS (40). Overall, both techniques resulting in overstaging of patients with early T-stage tumors and low accuracy rates for detecting nodal disease.

The use of endorectal coil MRI in evaluating patients with recurrent disease may result in improved detection of small lesions and enhanced ability to differentiate posttherapeutic fibrotic change from tumor, because of the increased spatial resolution of the endorectal coil over both conventional, body coil MRI, and CT (36,45–47). The ability to detect recurrent diseases improved from 60% using conventional MRI techniques to nearly 80% with the endorectal coil (48). When the criteria for distinguishing recurrent tumor from fibrosis were evaluated, the combination of high signal intensity on T2-weighted images, round margins, and >40% contrast enhancement were most predictive of recurrence. When these three criteria were combined, the accuracy was 92%, with a sensitivity and specificity of 100% and 85%, respectively. Interestingly, the specificity was dependent on time from surgery, with patients who were more than 1 yr postoperative having an improved specificity to 100% (49). Endorectal coil MRI is only slightly less sensitive in detecting recurrence than PET scanning (50), but it adds the ability to assess extent of pelvic disease for preoperative planning.

An ideal preoperative imaging modality would not only be easily and readily available but also inexpensive. It is clear that the use of endorectal MRI will be limited by both of these factors. In Gualdi's study, although the accuracy of endorectal MRI and ERUS were comparable, MRI cost 2.5 times as much (38). In addition, many centers do not routinely offer this technique. Also, MRI is often not possible in patients with metal implants. Because of all of these factors, this technology is unlikely to become either widely available or cost-effective compared to transrectal ultrasound.

4. CONCLUSION

In preoperative staging of patients with rectal carcinoma, it is extremely important to assess both depth of penetration and nodal spread because these factors will dictate entrance into neoadjuvant and adjuvant protocols. Also, accurately determining early T1/N0 tumors is essential in considering patients for local excision. Both ERUS and endorectal coil MRI offer similar accuracy rates when performed at centers with extensive experience in using these techniques. ERUS is less costly, less uncomfortable, and not limited in patients with metal implants. Because of these factors, patients with rectal carcinoma should be staged with ERUS as the procedure of choice. However, in experienced hands and when ERUS is not available, endorectal MRI is an equivalent alternative.

REFERENCES

1. Starck M, Bohe M, Fork FT, Lindstrom C, and Sjoberg S. Endoluminal ultrasound and low-field magnetic resonance imaging are superior to clinical examination in the preoperative staging of rectal cancer. *Eur. J. Surg.*, **161(11)** (1995) 841–845.
2. Nicholls RJ, Mason AY, Morson BC, Dixon AK, and Fry IK. The clinical staging of rectal cancer. *Br. J. Surg.*, **69(7)** (1982) 404–409.
3. Beynon J, Mortensen NJ, Foy DM, Channer JL, Virjee J, and Goddard P. Pre-operative assessment of local invasion in rectal cancer: digital examination, endoluminal sonography or computed tomography? *Br. J. Surg.*, **73(12)** (1986) 1015–1017.
4. Holdsworth PJ, Johnston D, Chalmers AG, Chennells P, Dixon MF, Finan PJ, et al. Endoluminal ultrasound and computed tomography in the staging of rectal cancer. *Br. J. Surg.*, **75(10)** (1988) 1019–1022.

5. Zerhouni EA, Rutter C, Hamilton SR, Balfe DM, Megibow AJ, Francis IR, et al. CT and MR imaging in the staging of colorectal carcinoma: report of the Radiology Diagnostic Oncology Group II. *Radiology*, **200(2)** (1996) 443–451.

6. Thaler W, Watzka S, Martin F, La Guardia G, Psenner K, Bonatti G, et al. Preoperative staging of rectal cancer by endoluminal ultrasound vs. magnetic resonance imaging. Preliminary results of a prospective, comparative study. *Dis. Colon Rectum*, **37(12)** (1994) 1189–1193.

7. Guinet C, Buy JN, Ghossain MA, Sezeur A, Mallet A, Bigot JM, et al. Comparison of magnetic resonance imaging and computed tomography in the preoperative staging of rectal cancer. *Arch. Surg.*, **125(3)** (1990) 385–388.

8. Hildebrandt U, Feifel G, Schwarz HP, and Scherr O. Endorectal ultrasound: instrumentation and clinical aspects. *Intl. J. Colorect. Dis.*, **1(4)** (1986) 203–207.

9. Beynon J, Foy DM, Roe AM, Temple LN, and Mortensen NJ. Endoluminal ultrasound in the assessment of local invasion in rectal cancer. *Br. J. Surg.*, **73(6)** (1986) 474–477.

10. Orrom WJ, Wong WD, Rothenberger DA, Jensen LL, and Goldberg SM. Endorectal ultrasound in the preoperative staging of rectal tumors. A learning experience. *Dis. Colon Rectum*, **33(8)** (1990) 654–659.

11. Beynon J, Mortensen NJ, Foy DM, Channer JL, Virjee J, and Goddard P. Endorectal sonography: laboratory and clinical experience in Bristol. *Intl. J. Colorect. Dis.*, **1(4)** (1986) 212–215.

12. Boscaini M, Moscini PL, and Montori A. Transrectal ultrasonography: interpretation of normal intestinal wall structure for the preoperative staging of rectal cancer [published erratum appears in *Scand. J. Gastroenterol.* **(9) preceding 1025**]. *Scand. J. Gastroenterol.*, **123(Suppl.)** (1986) 87–98.

13. Hildebrandt U and Feifel G. Preoperative staging of rectal cancer by intrarectal ultrasound. *Dis. Colon Rectum*, **28(1)** (1985) 42–46.

14. Wang KY, Kimmey MB, Nyberg DA, Mack LA, Haggitt RC, Shuman WP, et al. Colorectal neoplasms: accuracy of US in demonstrating the depth of invasion. *Radiology*, **165(3)** (1987) 827–829.

15. Schaldenbrand JD, Siders DB, Zainea GG, and Thieme ET. Preoperative radiation therapy for locally advanced carcinoma of the rectum. Clinicopathologic correlative review. *Dis. Colon Rectum*, **35(1)** (1992) 16–23.

16. Garcia-Aguilar J, Mellgren A, Sirivongs P, Buie D, Madoff RD, and Rothenberger DA. Local excision of rectal cancer without adjuvant therapy: a word of caution. *Ann. Surg.*, **231(3)** (2000) 345–351.

17. Anderson BO, Hann LE, Enker WE, Dershaw DD, Guillem JG, and Cohen AM. Transrectal ultrasonography and operative selection for early carcinoma of the rectum. *J. Am. Col. Surg.*, **179(5)** (1994) 513–517.

18. Minsky BD, Enker WE, Cohen AM, and Lauwers G. Local excision and postoperative radiation therapy for rectal cancer. *Am. J. Clin. Oncol.*, **17(5)** (1994) 411–416.

19. Steele GD, Jr, Herndon JE, Bleday R, Russell A, Benson A III, Hussain M, et al. Sphincter-sparing treatment for distal rectal adenocarcinoma [see comments]. *Ann. Surg. Oncol.*, **6(5)** (1999) 433–441.

20. Rifkin MD, McGlynn ET, and Marks G. Endorectal sonographic prospective staging of rectal cancer. *Scand. J. Gastroenterol.*, **123(Suppl.)** (1986) 99–103.

21. Saitoh N, Okui K, Sarashina H, Suzuki M, Arai T, and Nunomura M. Evaluation of echographic diagnosis of rectal cancer using intrarectal ultrasonic examination. *Dis. Colon Rectum*, **29(4)** (1986) 234–242.

22. Beynon J, Mortensen NJ, Foy DM, Channer JL, Rigby H, and Virjee J. Preoperative assessment of mesorectal lymph node involvement in rectal cancer. *Br. J. Surg.*, **76(3)** (1989) 276–279.

23. Dworak O. Number and size of lymph nodes and node metastases in rectal carcinomas. *Surgi. Endoscopy*, **3(2)** (1989) 96–99.

24. Hildebrandt U, Klein T, Feifel G, Schwarz HP, Koch B, and Schmitt RM. Endosonography of pararectal lymph nodes. In vitro and in vivo evaluation. *Dis. Colon Rectum*, **33(10)** (1990) 863–868.

25. Habr-Gama A, de Souza PM, Ribeiro U, Jr., Nadalin W, Gansl R, Sousa AH Jr, et al. Low rectal cancer: impact of radiation and chemotherapy on surgical treatment. *Dis. Colon Rectum*, **41(9)** (1998) 1087–1096.

25a. Hiotis SP, Weber SM, Cohen AM, Minsky BD, Paty PB, Guillem JG, et al. Assessing the predictive value of clinical complete response to neoadjuvant therapy for rectal cancer: an analysis of 488 patients *J. Am. Coll. Surg.*, **194(2)** (2002) 131–135.

26. Glaser F, Kuntz C, Schlag P, and Herfarth C. Endorectal ultrasound for control of preoperative radiotherapy of rectal cancer. *Ann. Surg.*, **217(1)** (1993) 64–71.

27. Bernini A, Deen KI, Madoff RD, and Wong WD. Preoperative adjuvant radiation with chemotherapy for rectal cancer: its impact on stage of disease and the role of endorectal ultrasound. *Ann. Surg. Oncol.*, **3(2)** (1996) 131–135.

28. Dershaw DD, Enker WE, Cohen AM, and Sigurdson ER. Transrectal ultrasonography of rectal carcinoma. *Cancer*, **66(11)** (1990) 2336–2340.

29. Beynon J, Mortensen NJ, Foy DM, Channer JL, Rigby H, and Virjee J. The detection and evaluation of locally recurrent rectal cancer with rectal endosonography. *Dis. Colon Rectum*, **32(6)** (1989) 509–517.

30. Mascagni D, Corbellini L, Urciuoli P, and Di Matteo G. Endoluminal ultrasound for early detection of local recurrence of rectal cancer [see comments]. *Br. J. Surg.*, **76(11)** (1989) 1176–1180.

31. Adams DR, Blatchford GJ, Lin KM, Ternent CA, Thorson AG, and Christensen MA. Use of preoperative ultrasound staging for treatment of rectal cancer. *Dis. Colon Rectum*, **42(2)** (1999) 159–166.

32. Glaser F, Schlag P, and Herfarth C. Endorectal ultrasonography for the assessment of invasion of rectal tumours and lymph node involvement. *Br. J. Surg.*, **77(8)** (1990) 883–887.

33. Heneghan JP, Salem RR, Lange RC, Taylor KJ, and Hammers LW. Transrectal sonography in staging rectal carcinoma: the role of gray-scale, color-flow, and Doppler imaging analysis. *Am. J. Roentgenol.*, **169(5)** (1997) 1247–1252.

34. Chan TW, Kressel HY, Milestone B, Tomachefski J, Schnall M, Rosato E, et al. Rectal carcinoma: staging at MR imaging with endorectal surface coil [work in progress]. *Radiology*, **181(2)** (1991) 461–467.

35. Drew PJ, Farouk R, Turnbull LW, Ward SC, Hartley JE, and Monson JR. Preoperative magnetic resonance staging of rectal cancer with an endorectal coil and dynamic gadolinium enhancement. *Br. J. Surg.*, **86(2)** (1999) 250–254.

36. Meyenberger C, Huch Boni RA, Bertschinger P, Zala GF, Klotz HP, and Krestin GP. Endoscopic ultrasound and endorectal magnetic resonance imaging: a prospective, comparative study for preoperative staging and follow-up of rectal cancer. *Endoscopy*, **27(7)** (1995) 469–479.

37. Schnall MD, Furth EE, Rosato EF, and Kressel HY. Rectal tumor stage: correlation of endorectal MR imaging and pathologic findings [see comments]. *Radiology*, **190(3)** (1994) 709–714.

38. Gualdi GF, Casciani E, Guadalaxara A, d'Orta C, Polettini E, and Pappalardo G. Local staging of rectal cancer with transrectal ultrasound and endorectal magnetic resonance imaging: comparison with histologic findings. *Dis. Colon Rectum*, **43(3)** (2000) 338–345.

38a. Murano A, Sasaki F, Kido C, Nakamura T, Kobayashi S, Kato T, et al. Endoscopic MRI using 3D-spoiled GRASS (SPGR) sequence for local staging of rectal carcinoma. *J. Comput. Assist. Tomogr.*, **19(4)** (1995) 586–591.

39. Kim NK, Kim MJ, Yun SH, Sohn SK, and Min JS. Comparative study of transrectal ultrasonography, pelvic computerized tomography, and magnetic resonance imaging in preoperative staging of rectal cancer. *Dis. Colon Rectum*, **42(6)** (1999) 770–775.

40. Maldjian C, Smith R, Kilger A, Schnall M, Ginsberg G, and Kochman M. Endorectal surface coil MR imaging as a staging technique for rectal carcinoma: a comparison study to rectal endosonography. *Abdom. Imaging*, **25(1)** (2000) 75–80.

41. Zagoria RJ, Schlarb CA, Ott DJ, Bechtold RI, Wolfman NT, Scharling ES, et al. Assessment of rectal tumor infiltration utilizing endorectal MR imaging and comparison with endoscopic rectal sonography. *J. Surg. Oncol.*, **64(4)** (1997) 312–317.

42. Brown G, Richards CJ, Newcombe RG, Dallimore NS, Radcliffe AG, Carey DP, et al. Rectal carcinoma: thin-section MR imaging for staging in 28 patients. *Radiology*, **211(1)** (1999) 215–222.

43. de Lange EE, Fechner RE, Edge SB, and Spaulding CA. Preoperative staging of rectal carcinoma with MR imaging: surgical and histopathologic correlation [see comments]. *Radiology*, **176(3)** (1990) 623–628.

44. de Lange EE, Fechner RE, Spaulding CA, and Edge SB. Rectal carcinoma treated by preoperative irradiation: MR imaging and histopathologic correlation. *Am. J. Roentgenol.*, **158(2)** (1992) 287–292.

45. Pema PJ, Bennett WF, Bova JG, and Warman P. CT vs MRI in diagnosis of recurrent rectosigmoid carcinoma. *J. Comput. Assist. Tomogr.*, **18(2)** (1994) 256–261.

46. Blomqvist L, Holm T, Goranson H, Jacobsson H, Ohlsen H, and Larsson SA. MR imaging, CT and CEA scintigraphy in the diagnosis of local recurrence of rectal carcinoma. *Acta Radiol.*, **37(5)** (1996) 779–784.

47. Krestin GP, Steinbrich W, and Friedmann G. Recurrent rectal cancer: diagnosis with MR imaging versus CT. *Radiology*, **168(2)** (1988) 307–311.

48. Huch Boni RA, Meyenberger C, Pok LJ, Trinkler F, Lutolf U, and Krestin GP. Value of endorectal coil versus body coil MRI for diagnosis of recurrent pelvic malignancies. *Abdom. Imaging*, **21(4)** (1996) 345–352.

49. Markus J, Morrissey B, deGara C, and Tarulli G. MRI of recurrent rectosigmoid carcinoma [see comments]. *Abdom. Imaging*, **22(3)** (1997) 338–342.

50. Ito K, Kato T, Tadokoro M, Ishiguchi T, Oshima M, Ishigaki T, et al. Recurrent rectal cancer and scar: differentiation with PET and MR imaging. *Radiology*, **182(2)** (1992) 549–552.

10 Nuclear Medicine in the Diagnosis and Management of Colorectal Cancer

Stanley J. Goldsmith and Lale Kostakoglu

CONTENTS

INTRODUCTION
TECHNICAL BACKGROUND
CLINICAL APPLICATIONS
CONCLUSION
REFERENCES

1. INTRODUCTION

The initial challenge in the care of colorectal cancer patients is accurate staging (i.e., determining the extent of disease in order to select therapy most beneficial for the patient). In one-third of patients, unresectable lesions are unexpectedly found during surgery *(1,2)*. The frequency of "recurrence" indicates that tumor cells had been left at the primary site or had already disseminated but were undetected at the time of initial evaluation despite the exquisite resolution available with contemporary diagnostic imaging such as computed tomography (CT) and magnetic resonance imaging (MRI). When colorectal carcinoma (CRC) does recur, it is necessary to restage the patient to identify if there are additional metastatic sites that would impact on the choice and effectiveness of therapy.

With appropriate radiopharmaceuticals, nuclear medicine imaging, despite its limited anatomic resolution, has the potential to recognize viable tumor based on alterations in tissue metabolism or the expression of surface markers in malignant tissue. Recent advances in nuclear imaging and detection instrumentation and the development of unique radiopharmaceuticals have made it possible to identify these functional differences between tumor and normal tissue. These functional images have been confirmed to have greater sensitivity and specificity for tumor detection in initial and follow-up evaluations of patients with CRC.

At the present time, three tracers are of demonstrated value in the management of patients with CRC. A radiolabeled analog of glucose, F-18 fluorodeoxyglucose (FDG), previously only available at research centers, is now approved by the Food and Drug Administration (FDA) and produced commercially throughout the United States for distribution to nuclear medicine imaging facilities serving most population centers. Two radiolabeled monoclonal antibodies to antigens expressed on CRC, Oncoscint CR/OV® and CEA-Scan®, have also been approved as diagnostic agents by the FDA. They are available in kit form to all licensed

From: *Colorectal Cancer: Multimodality Management*
Edited by: L. Saltz © Humana Press Inc., Totowa, NJ

nuclear medicine facilities. The use of these radiopharmaceuticals has been optimized by parallel advances in nuclear medicine tomographic imaging, either single photon-emission computed tomography (SPECT) for radiolabeled antibody imaging or positron-emission tomography (PET) for FDG imaging.

In addition to the above currently available advances, a number of promising radiolabeled agents and techniques are currently being evaluated in clinical trials. Radiation detecting probe devices have been developed for use during surgery. This device is still experimental in patients with colorectal carcinoma but is likely to become a part of clinical management within the next few years. With these handheld devices and appropriate radiopharmaceuticals, the surgeon is able to detect and localize tumor beyond simple visual observation or external imaging.

2. TECHNICAL BACKGROUND

2.1. F-18 Fluorodeoxyglucose and PET Imaging

F-18 fluorodeoxy glucose (FDG) is an F-18 glucose analog that enters cells via glucose transporter proteins in proportion to blood flow and glucose metabolism. Following entry and phosphorylation to F-18 fluorodeoxyglucose-6-phosphate, there is no further metabolism. The F-18 transported across the cell membrane is thus an indicator of the glucose utilization up to that point. As tumors generally have increased metabolic rates and increased anaerobic glucose metabolism, there is increased glucose membrane transport and intracellular trapping of the F-18 FDG tracer in malignant tissues to a greater degree than that of the surrounding tissue. F-18 FDG is filtered in the renal glomerulus but, unlike glucose, it is not effectively reabsorbed by the renal tubules. Hence, there is rapid clearance of blood and interstitial background activity and good contrast images can be obtained at 1 h after tracer injection. Patients should be fasting for at least 4 h prior to tracer injection so as to assure that blood glucose levels are not elevated. Generally, satisfactory images can be obtained if blood glucose is no greater than 200 mg/dL. If insulin is necessary to lower or maintain blood glucose, tracer administration should be delayed until after stabilization of blood glucose levels to assure that the FDG does not preferentially enter muscle and liver following injection.

F-18 decays by positron emission with a 2-h half-life, providing a coincident emission of two 511-keV photons in 180° opposition to each other. Coincident detection of these two simultaneously emitted photons by either a dual-detector system or a ring detector permits localization of the emission without collimation. Hence, coincidence detection is much more efficient in detecting the signal emitted following positron decay. Furthermore, the technique is inherently tomographic, as the coincident data are used to generate a transaxial map following back-projection or other image-formating techniques. These computer-generated transaxial images can be reformated to create volume displays as well as coronal and sagittal tomographic slices. Imaging must be performed on devices that detect and process the coincident signal produced by positron decay. This can be achieved with either the widely available dual-detector modified gamma camera systems or a so-called dedicated ring-detector PET system. Modified gamma camera systems cost approximately an additional $200,000–250,000 above the cost of the dual-detector gamma camera system ($350,000–450,000). The ring-detector systems cost $1–2 million. The ring-detector systems have better count sensitivity and resolution and, consequently, they provide greater clinical sensitivity for the detection of small lesions. Nevertheless, the dual-detector coincident systems are capable of detecting disease. The positive predictive value and specificity of the two systems are likely to be equivalent, although the ring-detector system would be expected to have better negative predictive value.

2.2. Radiolabeled Antibody Imaging

Two radiolabeled monoclonal antibodies, Oncoscint CR/OV and CEA-Scan, are currently available for the detection of colorectal carcinoma. Both agents have high affinity for specific epitopes expressed on CRC. In separate studies, these agents have shown statistical utility for disease staging and detection of occult lesions. CEA-Scan is a second-generation radiolabeled monoclonal antibody that has several advantages that make it the current radioimmunodetection agent of choice in the evaluation of patients with CRC.

Oncoscint CR/OV was the first radiolabeled monoclonal antibody approved by the FDA for diagnostic purposes. It is an intact IgG that recognizes a high-molecular-weight tumor-associated antigen (TAG-72) that is expressed on a variety of neoplasms. The CR/OV designation indicates approval for use in patients with either CRC or ovarian carcinoma. As an intact IgG, Oncoscint has a relatively long plasma half-life so that tumor-to-background-contrast satisfactory for imaging is not achieved for several days. Patients are usually imaged at 72–96 h after injection. This longer interval between injection and imaging necessitates labeling with In-111. The 5.0–6.0-mCi In-111 dose provides a lower photon flux than is generally available with Tc-99m-labeled agents. In addition, as an intact monoclonal antibody, Oncoscint regularly results in the production by the patient of antibodies to the murine immunoglobulin. These antibodies are known as human antimurine antibodies (HAMA). Although it is possible to repeat studies in patients with HAMA, the presence of HAMA presents an additional patient risk and usually will adversely alter the pharmacokinetics of subsequent antibody injections as well as interfere with in vitro laboratory assays that use murine sera reagents.

CEA-Scan is a Tc-99m-labeled Fab' fragment of a murine IgG that has a high affinity for membrane-expressed CEA (carcino-embryonic antigen). As a Fab' fragment, CEA-Scan is less immunogenic than an intact IgG and usually does not produce a HAMA response. Moreover, it clears rapidly from the circulation. Hence, satisfactory tumor-to-background contrast is obtained at 3–4 h after injection compatible with labeling with the 6-h half-life radionuclide, Tc-99m. A 25-mCi Tc-99m diagnostic dose can be used and there is greater photon flux resulting in images with greater information content than are available when lower doses of In-111 are used. The Fab' fragment has little nonspecific hepatic uptake and, therefore, hepatic metastases can be detected (unlike Oncoscint). CEA-Scan differentiates between the membrane and shed (circulating) CEA and is thus effective regardless of whether serum CEA is elevated or not (i.e., it is not consumed by circulating CEA).

Although both CEA-Scan and Oncoscint CR/OV can be imaged with traditional (noncoincident) imaging equipment, radiolabeled antibody imaging should be performed and interpreted as a SPECT study using a dual-head gamma camera and tomographic processing software capable of producing coronal, sagittal, and transverse slices as well as volume displays. The recent introduction of devices capable of fusing SPECT images on simultaneously acquired CT images may further improve interpretation of these functional images.

2.3. Intraoperative Radiation Probes

Over the past several years, the use of the surgical probe to identify concentrations of radiotracer intraoperatively has found application in the identification of sentinel lymph nodes in patients with melanoma and breast carcinoma. In those instances, a radiocolloid is injected around the primary lesion or at the site of the resected lesion. The radiocolloid infiltrates and identifies the lymphatic drainage from the site. Sentinel and other lymph nodes are identified by gamma camera imaging (lymphoscintigraphy) and/or by the use of a handheld probe device during the operative procedure. In this application, only lymphatic drainage is identified so as to allow removal of sentinel lymph nodes for subsequent histopathologic identification of tumor if present. This technique has had minimal experimental evaluation in CRC. There has been greater interest, however, in the use of the surgical probe to identify tumor-specific radiolabeled antibody injected intravenously prior to surgery. Although this is an area of active investigation, none of the radioimmunodiagnostic agents used experimentally have been approved for this application at this time.

3. CLINICAL APPLICATIONS

In evaluating the utility of the recently available nuclear medicine procedures, the various clinical situations associated with the management of patients with neoplasms should be considered. This includes comparison to conventional imaging in the initial staging of the patient (extent of disease), in determining the response to therapy (differentiating between effects of therapy and persistent tumor), in possibly predicting long-term outcome, and in the detection of recurrence. The sensitivity of detection determines the reliability of identifying the extent of disease at initial diagnosis as well as when a recurrence is suspected or identified. Both sensitivity and specificity determine the reliability in differentiating between changes produced by therapy vs persistent tumor viability. Other issues that have importance at the present time include clinical efficacy, the influence on decision-making and effect on outcome, and cost-effectiveness in terms of possible savings vs incremental costs.

3.1. FDG-PET in Colorectal Cancer

3.1.1. INITIAL STAGING OF COLORECTAL CARCINOMA (EXTENT OF DISEASE)

Whereas some patients present with symptoms related to the primary tumor (obstruction or perforation), CRC is usually detected by one of the various screening procedures currently available leading to direct surgical biopsy by colonoscopy. The next step in patient management involves evaluation of the extent of disease (i.e., identifying if there are local or distal metastases in order to adequately plan therapy). Until recently, this had involved conventional imaging preoperatively and manual and/or visual assessment of the abdominal contents at surgery.

In December 2000, Health Care Financing Administration (HCFA) and Medicare expanded coverage to include reimbursement for FDG studies performed on dedicated ring-detector PET imaging devices for the evaluation of the extent of disease in the initial workup of patients with CRC (3) (see Fig. 1). Previously, reimbursement had been approved only to evaluate previously treated patients with rising CEA or other evidence of disease recurrence. This is based on the highly regarded study of Abdel-Nabi et al. who evaluated the diagnostic usefulness of FDG-PET and correlated the results with CT, surgical and histopathologic findings in 48 patients with primary CRC (4). They found FDG-PET superior to CT in the staging of CRC. At the primary site, the negative predictive value for FDG-PET was higher than the positive predictive value (100% vs 90%), as there were false-positive findings in patients with acute diverticulosis (three patients) and at a recent polypectomy site (one patient). No increased FDG accumulation was noted in hyperplastic polyps. FDG-PET sensitivity, specificity, and positive and negative predictive values for intraluminal primary lesions were 100%, 43%, 90%, and 100%, respectively. FDG-PET was superior to CT in identification of hepatic metastases with a sensitivity of 88% vs 38% and a specificity of 100% vs 97%. For nodal metastases, the sensitivity for both FDG-PET and CT was rather low (29%), although the specificity for FDG-PET was higher than for CT (96% vs 85%).

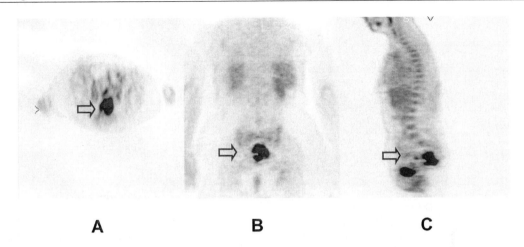

A   **B**   **C**

Fig. 1. F-18 FDG-PET images from a 44-yr-old woman with a 4-mo history of change in bowel habits. Colonoscopy demonstrated a large rectal mass. Tomographic slice images: (**A**—transaxial slice; **B**—coronal slice; **C**—sagittal slice) demonstrate the large rectal carcinoma. An involved lymph node is identified anterior to the bulky primary mass in the transaxial and sagittal images. Activity is also seen in the bladder (sagittal slice). (Image courtesy of Henry Yeung, MD, Nuclear Medicine Service, Memorial Sloan-Kettering Cancer Center, New York.)

Mukai et al. found a sensitivity of 96% for FDG-PET in the detection of the primary tumor and 22% for detection of lymph node metastases *(5)*. Fifteen patients who had histopathologically confirmed negative lymph nodes; two (13%) had false-positive lymph nodes on FDG-PET.

Falk et al. compared FDG-PET with CT for the detection of primary as well as recurrent colorectal tumors in a group of 16 patients *(6)*. In this study also, FDG-PET was found to be more sensitive but less specific than CT in the preoperative detection of the extent of disease in colorectal carcinoma (sensitivity: 90% vs 60%; specificity: 66% vs 100%) *(6)*. The predictive accuracy for the detection of CRC by FDG-PET was 83% and 56% by CT. These studies support the conclusion that at the time of initial diagnosis, preoperative FDG-PET imaging is of value to detect hepatic and extrahepatic metastases and thus improve the selection of surgical candidates. The primary lesion and some loco-regional lymph nodes are also identified, but no incremental value over conventional imaging methods has been reported.

3.1.2. RECURRENT COLORECTAL CANCER

Loco-regional pelvic recurrence and hepatic metastases are the major sites of relapse after resection of colorectal cancer, predominantly within 3 yr of initial diagnosis and surgery *(7,8)*. The recurrence rate after what was believed to be a curative resection of colorectal carcinoma is 10–40%. Approximately 25% of first recurrences are isolated loco-regional failures that can be cured by a second procedure, but recurrence is frequent and considerable mortality and morbidity are observed *(3,7,9)*.

Proper selection of patients for surgical resection is essential, as only 25% of patients with recurrent disease (loco-regional and metastatic) are subsequently cured by surgery. The 5-yr disease-free survival rate after attempted curative resection of the recurrent tumor is only 20–40% *(3)*. These results represent an improvement over what was achieved prior to

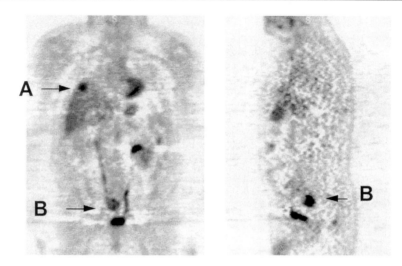

Fig. 2. F-18 FDG images (coronal and sagittal slices) from a 62-yr-old man postresection for a primary coloncarcinoma. During follow-up, a CT scan demonstrated a solitary hepatic metastasis. FDG-PET scan confirmed a finding (**A**) and demonstrated an additional tumor site in the pelvis (**B**). The patient was explored and both sites were resected. Histopathology confirmed tumor. In the coronal slice, the crescent shaped activity in the left chest represents myocardial glucose metabolism. F-18 FDG activity is seen in urine in the left renal pelvis and both ureters, as FDG, unlike glucose, is not reabsorbed in the renal tubules. (Image courtesy of Henry Yeung, MD, Nuclear Medicine Service, Memorial Sloan-Kettering Cancer Center, New York.)

availability of CT and MRI. The detection rates of local recurrence by CT have ranged from 69% to 95% in various studies *(8,10–18)*. The ability to distinguish recurrent tumor from scar tissue on T2-weighted images has been variable *(10–12,15–18)*. The role of dynamic MRI with contrast is still unclear *(17–19)*. In many cases, needle biopsy is required for definitive diagnosis. Nonetheless, false-negative biopsies may result from sampling errors.

The recently approved use of FDG-PET to monitor patients suspected of having recurrent disease (rising CEA or suspicious findings on CT/MRI) provides an opportunity for greater accuracy in the detection and staging of recurrent disease (*see* Fig. 2). For several years, investigators have reported the use of FDG-PET in this setting to detect both for intrahepatic and extrahepatic recurrent CRC *(20–39)* (Tables 1 and 2). Despite the limited number of patients reported to date, FDG-PET consistently demonstrates sensitivity and specificity greater than all other conventional imaging modalities.

3.1.2.1. Local/Pelvic Recurrence. One of the main applications of FDG-PET in recurrent CRC has been the differentiation of pelvic recurrence from postoperative fibrosis in patients with indeterminate results with anatomic imaging procedures (Table 1). In a study by Shiepers et al., FDG-PET provided the correct diagnosis in all patients referred, specifically by differentiating pelvic recurrence from fibrosis *(22)*. FDG-PET was superior to CT in the detection of loco-regional metastases with a sensitivity of 93% vs 60%, specificity of 97% vs 72% and an overall accuracy of 95% vs 65% (Table 1).

In a meta-analysis of 366 patients, FDG-PET had 94.7% sensitivity and 97.3% specificity for the detection of local/pelvic recurrences *(26)*. In another study of 103 patients with loco-regional recurrences, FDG-PET provided additional diagnostic information in 14%. Takeuchi et al. used FDG-PET to confirm the appropriateness of planned surgery. CT or MRI failed to detect 25% of lesions, whereas FDG-PET was more sensitive and accurate,

Table 1
Evaluation of FDG-PET in Loco-regional and Distant Metastases in Recurrent CRC

Authors	Site	No. of patients	PET Sensitivity (%)	PET Specificity (%)	CT Sensitivity (%)	CT Specificity (%)	Rx change
Schiepers et al. *(22)*	Local/pelvic	83	93	97	60	72	NA[a]
Vitola et al. *(24)*	Whole body	24	95	80	NA	NA	25
Delbeke et al. *(20)*	Whole body	61[b]	98	NA	74	NA	33
Keogan et al. *(27)*	Local/pelvic	18	92	80	NA	NA	NA
Ogunbiyi et al. *(28)*	Local/pelvic	47	91	100	52	80	44
Ruhlmann et al. *(36)*	Whole body	59	100	69	NA	NA	NA
Flanagan et al. *(38)*	Whole body	22	100	71	NA	NA	NA
Valk et al. *(35)*	Whole body	115	95	79	78	50	31
Flamen et al. *(29)*	Local/pelvic	103	94	100	NA	NA	20

[a]NA = not studied.
[b]Number of studies.

Table 2
Evaluation of FDG-PET in Hepatic Metastases in Recurrent Colorectal Carcinoma

Authors	No. of patients	PET Sensitivity (%)	PET Specificity (%)	CT Sensitivity (%)	CT Specificity (%)
Schiepers et al. *(22)*	83	94	100	85[a]	98[a]
Vitola et al. *(24)*	55[b]	90	100	86	58
Lai et al. *(21)*	34	100	67	NA[c]	NA
Delbeke et al. *(20)*	127[b]	91	96	81	60
Keogan et al. *(27)*	58	96	100	NA	NA
Ogunbiyi et al. *(28)*	58	95	100	74	85
Valk et al. *(35)*	115	95	100	84	95
Flamen et al. *(29)*	103	98	100	NA	NA
Boykin et al. *(33)*	14	100	NA	50	NA

[a]Combination of CT and Ultrasonography.
[b]Number of lesions.
[c]NA = not studied.

resulting in changes in patient management *(31)*. Although FDG-PET accurately identifies recurrent colorectal cancer in patients who have indeterminate findings on CT or MRI, inflammatory lesions and physiologic bladder activity can produce false-positive FDG PET findings *(40–43)*. The specificity of FDG imaging in evaluation of the pelvis can be improved by removing urinary bladder radioactivity, either by catheterizing the patient or diluting urine and encouraging the patient to void with hydration and diuretics.

3.1.2.2. Hepatic and Abdominal Metastases. In contemporary surgical practice, it is possible to resect hepatic metastases as a potentially curative procedure. Extrahepatic disease, however, precludes the likelihood that such a procedure will be successful. Accordingly, detection of hepatic metastases and accurate detection of disease extent is essential in the selection of patients most likely to benefit from this aggressive surgical approach.

Several studies confirm the value of FDG PET for this purpose. Vitola et al. compared FDG-PET findings with those of CT for the detection of hepatic metastases in 24 patients *(24)*. For hepatic lesions, the sensitivity of FDG-PET vs CT was 90% vs 86% and the specificity was 100% vs 58%. When lesions of <1 cm were excluded, sensitivity improved to 94% (FDG) vs 89% (CT); specificity of FDG remained 100% vs 70% for CT. FDG-PET was accurate in differentiating postsurgical changes from malignant recurrence in the abdomen in seven patients. Flamen et al. found that FDG-PET provided additional diagnostic information in evaluation of hepatic lesions in 6% of 103 recurrent colorectal cancer patients *(29)*. All patients with inconclusive findings on conventional imaging of the liver were correctly classified by FDG-PET. There were no false-positive FDG cases but one false negative in a patient with multiple small (<1 cm) metastases (determined by laparoscopy). In 7% of patients, extrahepatic abdominal metastases were identified by FDG-PET and subsequently confirmed despite (false) negative conventional imaging. Boykin et al. reported more dramatic comparative results than other investigators for FDG-PET vs conventional imaging in the detection of hepatic metastases *(33)*. They found a sensitivity of 85% for FDG-PET and 20% for CT for histologically confirmed intrahepatic metastases. In this series, FDG-PET changed patient management in 49% of patients.

A meta-analysis of 393 patients demonstrated overall weighted averages of FDG-PET to detect liver recurrences as 96.0% sensitivity and 97% specificity *(26)*. FDG-PET had greater sensitivity and specificity than conventional imaging methods, including CT, MRI, and ultrasonography in depicting both hepatic or intraabdominal extrahepatic recurrent colorectal cancer *(20–26,28,29,32–39)* (*see* Table 2 and Fig. 2).

In one of these studies, FDG-PET correctly identified hepatic metastases in 92.5% of patients evaluated *(20)*. There were two false-positive FDG-PET results in patients with hepatic cysts *(32)*. In another study, Ogunbiyi et al. also demonstrated superior sensitivity and specificity for FDG-PET compared to CT, resulting in a change in clinical management in 43% of patients with suspected recurrent or metastatic colorectal cancer *(28)* (Tables 1 and 2). Similarly, FDG-PET revealed unexpected extrahepatic metastases in 18% of patients *(22)*. In this study, false-negative FDG-PET results occurred in patients with lesions smaller than 1 cm. Most false-positive findings were the result of inflammatory disease in the lungs.

3.1.2.3. Distant Metastases and Whole-Body Evaluation. Whole-body FDG-PET was found to be superior to conventional staging techniques in the evaluation of distant metastasis in patients with resected colorectal carcinoma (*see* Tables 1 and 2 and Fig. 3). Valk et al. found whole-body FDG-PET to be more sensitive than CT (93% vs 69%) and slightly more specific than CT (98% vs 96%) at all sites except the retroperitoneum (at which specificity was 100% for both techniques) *(39)*.

In another study investigating the accuracy of FDG-PET in hepatic metastases, extrahepatic abdominal and distant (lung) metastases were serendipitously detected using whole-body FDG-PET, altering surgical decision-making in 25% of patients *(22)*. Ruhlman et al. also confirmed that whole-body FDG-PET located metastatic lesions that would have been otherwise undetected. They found an overall sensitivity of 100%, a specificity of 67%, and positive and negative predictive values of 92% and 100%, respectively *(36)* (*see* Table 1).

Although the number of false-positive studies has been limited, clearly the studies to date have been on relatively selected patient populations even when consecutive patients have been studied. Flamen et al. reported one false-positive FDG-PET in a patient who had focal colitis *(29)*. False-positive unsuspected extra-abdominal lesions have been observed in the abdomen (focal colitis, diverticulitis) and thorax (inflammatory lung disease) *(30)*. When

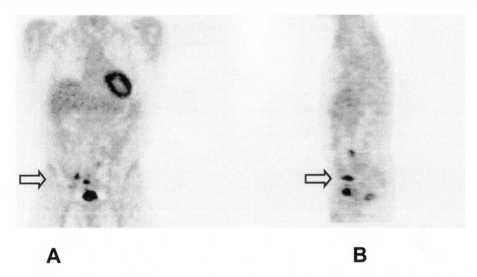

A   B

Fig. 3. F-18 FDG images ([**A**] coronal and [**B**] sagittal) from a 64-yr-old man with CRC, status postresection. The patient was found to have a rising CEA on a follow-up visit. MRI (3 wk earlier) was negative. The FDG-PET images reveal multiple foci in the pelvis and lower para-aortic region consistent with nodal recurrence. The findings were subsequently confirmed at surgery. (Image courtesy of Henry Yeung, MD, Nuclear Medicine Service, Memorial Sloan-Kettering Cancer Center, New York.)

larger populations are studied, additional false-positive, nonspecific findings will likely be observed. Accordingly, despite the great value of FDG-PET imaging in assessing tumor status in patients with CRC and the appropriate approval by HCFA and Medicare for more extensive use of this extraordinary modality, there are inevitable instances of nonspecific positive findings. F-18 FDG is a marker of glucose utilization. Although not totally tumor-specific, it is a valuable addition to the diagnostic armamentarium in the staging and monitoring patients with CRC.

3.1.3. RISING CARCINOEMBRYONIC ANTIGEN LEVELS

Tumor recurrence in the asymptomatic patient may be suspected by detecting rising CEA levels, despite negative or indeterminate conventional imaging studies. Several studies report the high accuracy of FDG-PET for detection of tumor foci in occult disease and to determine resectability in patients with elevation of this tumor marker *(21,29,36,38,39)* (Fig. 3).

Fluorodeoxyglucose (FDG)-PET was true positive in 70% of 22 patients with elevated CEA and negative conventional imaging studies *(38)*. Of these patients with positive FDG-PET, 88% had metastatic disease proven by follow-up surgery or clinical and radiological follow-up. There were two false-positive FDG-PET. Overall positive and negative predictive values for whole-body FDG-PET were found to be 89% and 100%, respectively.

Valk et al. reported positive scan findings on FDG-PET in 29 of 44 (66%) patients with rising CEA *(39)*. FDG-PET was true positive in 19 patients. There were two false-positive FDG-PET: one in the lung and one in the pelvis. Of the 15 patients with negative FDG-PET, two were subsequently found to be false negative by tissue diagnosis during the follow-up period.

In a 1999 study, 8 of 57 (14%) patients had a normal conventional workup associated with rising CEA levels *(29)*. FDG-PET correctly localized metastatic sites in two patients with one false positive. In a separate study of 51 patients with elevated CEA, FDG-PET detected disease in the liver in two patients not detected by CT. The presence of recurrent tumor in these cases was histologically proven *(38)*. In still another group, FDG-PET correctly identified pelvic recurrence in 2 of 35 patients with negative CT and rising CEA. Clinical management changed in 6 of 11 patients (54%) suspected of local recurrence *(39)*.

These findings support the conclusion that whole-body FDG-PET is useful for the evaluation of presumed resectable local recurrence or distant metastases in patients with elevated CEA and normal anatomic imaging findings.

3.1.4. MONITORING RESPONSE TO THERAPY

Although CT is an integral part of the evaluation of extent of disease in colorectal carcinoma, it is deficient in the assessment of residual abnormalities after therapy. FDG-PET provides metabolic information that could be used to monitor tumor response to therapy. It has been shown, however, that up to 25% of FDG uptake can occur in nontumor cells and tissues such as macrophages, neutrophils, fibroblasts, and granulation tissue *(40)*. In vitro studies demonstrated that irradiated tumor cells might have a 10-fold increase in FDG uptake. Large metabolic differences were observed in humans in vivo with FDG after therapy *(41,42)*. Haberkorn et al. has recommended postponing FDG-PET studies for 60 d after radiation therapy to assess therapy response in colorectal cancer *(41)*.

Findlay et al. examined 27 metastatic lesions in 20 patients before and 1–2 wk and 4–5 wk after initiation of 5-fluorouracil (5-FU) chemotherapy *(42)*. They noted a clear correlation between reduction of the tumor metabolism 5 wk after systemic 5-FU treatment and long-term outcome. The tumor-to-liver ratios and standardized uptake values (SUVs) at 4–5 wk discriminated between responders and nonresponders on a lesion-by-lesion and overall patient response assessment (100% and 75%, respectively). There was no correlation, however, between the changes in tumor metabolism at 1–2 wk and therapy outcome. This study confirmed some limitations of the FDG-PET follow-up studies, such as the so-called "flare phenomenon," a marked increase in FDG metabolism in lesions responding to therapy shortly after initiation of chemotherapy.

Guillem et al. assessed response to preoperative radiation and FU-based chemotherapy in a pilot study of 15 patients *(43)*. FDG-PET studies were obtained prior to therapy and at 4–5 wk after in 100% of the patients by FDG-PET compared with 78% by CT.

3.1.5. LIMITATIONS OF FDG-PET IN COLORECTAL CANCER

Fluorodeoxyglucose (FDG)-PET detects tumor recurrences in surgical patients who are otherwise difficult to assess by CT, as well as in patients with distant metastases and small malignant nodes that are not identified by other imaging modalities. FDG is not a tumor-specific substance, however. Leukocytes and macrophages of inflammatory processes also accumulate the tracer. Inflammatory bowel diseases and recent surgical interventions may yield false-positive FDG-PET results *(44)*.

3.1.6. COST-EFFECTIVENESS OF FDG-PET IN COLORECTAL CANCER

Valk et al. *(45)* reported that when FDG-PET was considered as an additional procedure, the savings-to-cost ratio was 2.5 to 1; when FDG-PET was considered as replacing CT of the abdomen and pelvis, the ratio was greater than 4 to 1. The incremental cost of FDG-PET is $1000/patient if CT is replaced and the cost of procedures avoided would be approx $4400/patient. The assumption that the decision for surgery would be based on a positive FDG-PET scan without the association of other tests such as CT portography or diagnostic laparoscopy may not be a realistic option in the clinical setting. Therefore, the cost of these additional confirmatory investigations should be factored into the cost analyses.

3.1.7. Summary: FDG Imaging in Colorectal Carcinoma

FDG-PET (using ring-detector systems) is now available (and approved by HCFA) for the preoperative staging of CRC, evaluation of patients suspected of having recurrent disease, the restaging of patients who have known disease recurrence, and long-term follow-up to exclude recurrence. Dual-detector systems are capable of identifying tumor activity in bulky disease and, hence, may be useful in situations when doubt exists as to the nature of a known mass. The negative predictive value of imaging with dual-detector systems, however, is uncertain. Acceptance of ring-detector FDG imaging is based on demonstrated greater sensitivity in the detection of CRC and greater specificity in excluding disease than CT or MRI regardless of whether it is a loco-regional, hepatic, or extrahepatic site of involvement. The use of FDG-PET in the selection of patients for a second attempt at curative surgery differentiates between patients who will benefit from the procedure and those who will not, thus avoiding the additional financial cost and morbidity of unnecessary surgery. Hence, despite the incremental costs associated with FDG-PET imaging, it is both clinically efficacious and cost-effective.

3.2. Radiolabeled Monoclonal Antibodies in Colorectal Carcinoma

In 1965, Gold and Freedman identified the carcinoembryonic antigen (CEA), a fetal antigen that is overexpressed on certain tumors. This finding became the prototype for tumor-associated antigens, portions of the cell membrane that are expressed on tumor cells to a greater degree than normal tissue. Over time, antibodies, developed to this and other antigens, have become useful as reagents for in vitro diagnosis and, more recently, in vivo application as radiodiagnostic agents *(46–49)*.

The role of monoclonal antibodies in the diagnosis and management of the patient with CRC is similar to other diagnostic imaging techniques: staging at the time of diagnosis, detection of recurrence (including confirmation of sites revealed by other imaging modalities at initial staging and recurrence as well as detection of occult tumors in CT-negative patients) and restaging when the disease has recurred, evaluating the response to treatment, including differentiation between effects of therapy and residual viable tumor, and prediction of outcome (prognosis).

The most significant contribution of radioimmunodiagnosis has been in the evaluation of patients after surgery, radiotherapy, and chemotherapy *(49–64)*. Whereas radioimmunodetection has an advantage over anatomic imaging in the detection of recurrent disease, there have been no direct comparisons with FDG-PET imaging in this group of patients. Based on the mechanism of localization, it would be expected that radiolabeled antibody imaging would be more specific than FDG imaging, as there is no basis for accumulation of tracer in inflammatory or granulation tissue. Furthermore, a tumor may be rendered hypometabolic as a consequence of chemotherapy or radiation but might continue to express the specific epitope recognized by an appropriate radiolabeled antibody or fragment *(see* Fig. 4).

Issues involved in the selection of one or another antibody for clinical use include safety (HAMA), sensitivity, and specificity *(65)*. In general, intact antibodies are more likely to be immunogenic than antibody fragments. Moreover, intact antibodies clear slowly from the circulation so that it may be several days before adequate tumor-to-background contrast permits detection of the tumor by external imaging. The longer biologic half-life of an intact immunoglobulin requires labeling with a radionuclide with a longer physical half-life. This is unfavorable for a diagnostic agent, as both the longer biologic and physical half-lives limit the amount of radioactivity that can be used. Ironically, if the radiolabeled antibody

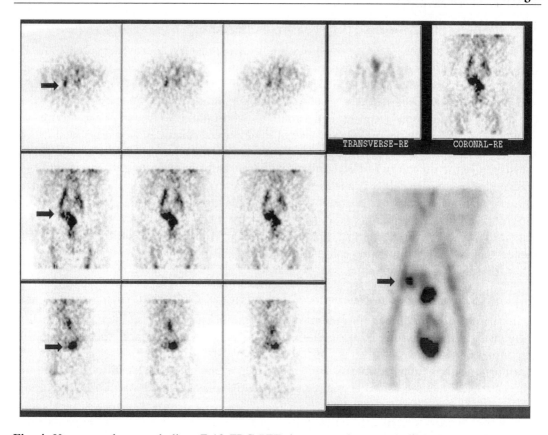

Fig. 4. Upper panel: coronal slices F-18 FDG-PET; lower panel: coronal slices Tc-99m CEA-Scan. Both studies are from a woman with a history of colon carcinoma, ascending colon, resected. She had been receiving postoperative chemotherapy for 10 mo and was observed to have an elevated CEA level (38 ng/mL). The F-18 FDG images are negative in this instance, whereas the Tc-99m anti-CEA images reveal a focal area of accumulation to the right of the bladder (arrows). This was confirmed at surgery to be metastatic adenocarcinoma of the colon. (Image courtesy of Josef Machac, M.D. Division of Nuclear Medicine, Mt. Sinai Medical Center, New York; reproduced with permission.)

were used as a therapeutic agent, a longer effective half-life (representing both the physical and biologic half-lives) would be advantageous in terms of delivering a greater radiation absorbed dose to tumor.

There is extensive literature describing antibodies to epitopes associated with colorectal carcinoma *(47–63)*. Several have been developed and evaluated in research settings *(66,67)*.

Currently, two radiolabeled monoclonal antibodies, CEA-Scan (Tc-99m anti-CEA) and Oncoscint (In-111 anti-TAG-72), have been approved by the FDA for the detection and staging of patients with CRC.

3.2.1. CEA and CEA-Scan

CEA is the prototype of a group of oncofetal antigens. This glycoprotein was isolated from human adult colon cancer and fetal colon epithelium. Preoperative CEA levels reflect the tumor burden. CEA expression is observed in 95% of hyperplastic polyps, adenomas, and adenocarcinomas of the colorectum. There is an increase in CEA expression as colonic lesions progress in aggressiveness from hyperplastic polyps and adenomas to carcinomas *(46)*. CEA-Scan (arcitumomab, IMMU-4; Immunomedics, Inc., Morris Plains, NJ) is the

Coronal PET images

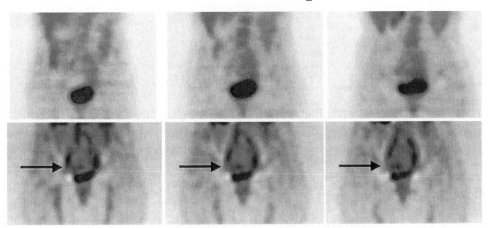

Coronal CEA-Scan images

Fig. 5. SPECT (transaxial, coronal, and sagittal) slices and anterior volume display (lower right) obtained 3 h after injection of 25-mCi Tc-99m anti-CEA Fab′ fragment (CEA-Scan) in a patient with elevated serum CEA not identified on contemporaneous CT scan. Labeled antibody fragment identifies lesion in the pelvis medial to the right iliac vessels and to the right and cephalad to the urinary bladder (containing excreted activity). There is some contamination of external genitalia. (Image courtesy of Division of Nuclear Medicine, Department of Radiology, New York Presbyterian Hospital-Weill Cornell Medical Center, New York.)

second radioimmunoscintigraphy agent to receive FDA approval as an antibody for the detection of recurrent or metastatic colorectal carcinoma *(47–55)*. CEA-Scan is a murine Fab′ fragment developed against CEA, labeled with 25 mCi of technetium-99m pertechnetate (Tc-99m). Imaging is performed at 3–5 h and 18–24 h of antibody administration. As the excretion pattern of antibody fragments is predominantly renal, CEA-Scan has less nonspecific hepatic accumulation and thus has better potential to detect hepatic metastases than Oncoscint (the first approved radiolabeled diagnostic antibody for detection of CRC; *see* Section 3.2.2.). The ability to detect lesions with CEA-Scan is not affected by circulating CEA levels as the antibody fragment apparently preferentially binds to cell surface CEA. No antigen–antibody complexes are detected at CEA levels of 250 ng/mL. Even at levels as high as 2000 ng/mL, less than 50% of the injected antibody is complex associated and metastatic sites are regularly identified.

Moffat et al. reported that CEA-Scan was statistically more sensitive than conventional imaging methods to image occult colorectal tumor sites not identified by other methods *(53)* CEA-Scan detected at least one lesion that had been missed by conventional imaging methods in 34% of the patients studied. The sensitivity of CEA-Scan to detect liver metastases was found to be equivalent to that of conventional modalities (63% vs 64%). CEA-Scan sensitivity was superior elsewhere in the abdomen (55% vs 32%) and pelvis (69% vs 48%) (Fig. 5). More importantly, when conventional imaging modalities were complemented by CEA-Scan, the positive predictive value was 98% compared to 66% for conventional diagnostic tests alone. Less than 1% of patients showed an increase in HAMA titer after receiving CEA-Scan *(51)*.

Hughes et al. compared the accuracy of CT alone with CEA-Scan alone, as well as combined with CT for predicting abdomino-pelvic tumor resectability *(54)*. CEA-Scan was more accurate than CT to assess resectability of locally recurrent or metastatic colorectal cancer (57% vs 47%) both in patients undergoing evaluation for curative abdomino-pelvic resection and in a subset of patients with suspected or proven liver metastases. In conjunction with CT, CEA-Scan identified twice the number of patients who could avoid unnecessary surgery and to increase detection of patients who are most likely to benefit from curative resection by 40%. This study indicates that when both imaging modalities indicate resectability, surgery should follow. Conversely, when both techniques indicate nonresectable tumor, surgery is unnecessary.

The additional use of CEA-Scan with CT thus decreases cost, morbidity, and mortality by avoiding unnecessary abdomino-pelvic surgery. The combined techniques increase resectability by 40% compared to CT alone and identify nonresectability in twice as many patients as CT alone. Concordant CT and CEA-Scan results were accurate in identifying resectability in 67% of the resectable abdomino-pelvic recurrent tumors and nonresectability in 100% of those patients who cannot be cured by current surgical techniques. The study was negative in 64% of the patients without disease. When the two tests were discordant, CEA-Scan was correct substantially more often than CT *(54)*.

In patients with elevated CEA levels but no evidence of recurrent tumor using CT, MRI, or other conventional imaging techniques, the sensitivity, specificity, accuracy, and positive predictive value for CEA-Scan were 100%, 67%, 93%, and 92%, respectively *(55–57)*.

3.2.2. Oncoscint CR/OV

Oncoscint (satumomab pendetide, CYT-103; Cytogen Corporation, Princeton, NJ) was the first antibody agent approved by the FDA for cancer imaging. The monoclonal antibody component of Oncoscint CR/OV is B72.3, a murine IgG1 that recognizes a high-molecular-weight mucin, tumor-associated glycoprotein-72 (TAG-72), which is expressed by more than 80% of colorectal and 95% of common epithelial ovarian carcinomas *(58)*. Oncoscint CR/OV is labeled with 5.0 mCi of indium-111 (In-111) and imaging is performed at ~approx 72 h–120 h after the blood pool background has cleared. Liver metastases are difficult to detect because of accretion of In-111 in the liver, consequently, Oncoscint CR/OV is inferior to conventional imaging to detect hepatic metastases (41% vs 84%). The indications to use this radiolabeled antibody as an imaging agent include the presence of rising CEA level despite an otherwise negative workup, known solitary disease in patients under consideration for curative resection, and equivocal lesions by conventional imaging, particularly in differentiating postoperative changes from recurrent tumor *(59)*. Oncoscint CR/OV has been approved for repeat administration in HAMA-negative patients.

In a retrospective study to determine the diagnostic value of Oncoscint CR/OV immunoscintigraphy in assessing patients with suspected recurrence of carcinoma of the colon and ovary, the combined sensitivity and accuracy of immunoscintigraphy in the detection of extrahepatic disease was found to be significantly higher than that of cross-sectional radiological imaging (87% sensitivity and 83% accuracy for FDG-PET vs 44% and 53% for CT) with an equivalent specificity of 74%. Scintigraphy identified 36% of extrahepatic malignant lesions not diagnosed by conventional radiological techniques and influenced therapeutic planning in 26% of patients. In the liver, conventional imaging had a significantly higher detection rate for metastatic disease than immunoscintigraphy (sensitivity 93% vs 28%) *(60)*.

In a multicenter trial, Oncoscint CR/OV immunoscintigraphy was helpful in the medical and/or surgical management in 44% of patients and provided information unavailable from other diagnostic modalities. In this trial, in 17% of patients, Oncoscint CR/OV immunoscintigraphy revealed occult metastases *(61)*. In another study however, Oncoscint CR/OV was beneficial in only a small group of patients. When the contribution of the scan to diagnosis and management was graded by the surgeon, beneficial effects were observed in only 13% *(62)*. There was no effect in 67%. This issue suggests a need for standardization and refinement of the technical aspects of imaging as well as potential bias in evaluating the contribution of an imaging technique to clinical management. SPECT is strongly recommended in all patients because it was found to identify tumors missed on planar scans in 35% of patients and provided additional information regarding tumor burden in 23% of patients *(63)*.

3.2.3. SUMMARY: RADIOLABELED ANTIBODY IMAGING

At the present time, CEA-Scan, a Tc-99m-labeled antibody fragment, and Oncoscint, an In-111-labeled intact murine antibody, are both available for imaging in staging and evaluating patients suspected of having recurrent CRC. Both agents seem to perform better when used with contemporary dual-head gamma cameras in the SPECT mode. Data derived from comparing the agents to CT or MRI imaging demonstrate greater accuracy for these agents compared to CT or MRI in the detection or exclusion of loco-regional recurrences or the extrahepatic abdomen and distal sites. Because CT is a sensitive modality to image hepatic lesions, antibody imaging of the liver is recommended only as a complementary technique. Although both antibody agents have limited utility vs CT in the evaluation of the liver for metastatic sites, CEA-Scan outperforms Oncoscint in this application. There has been no direct comparison between the two agents; the several advantages of CEA-Scan (less frequent appearance of HAMA, advantages of Tc-99m as a label including better image quality, and same-day imaging) make it the radiolabeled antibody imaging agent of choice for the evaluation of patient with CRC.

3.3. Radioimmunoguided Surgery in Colorectal Carcinoma

As stated, approx 50% of patients undergoing potentially curative surgery for colorectal carcinoma have a recurrence of disease. This high rate of recurrence is a consequence of incomplete excision of microscopic disease. The detection and resection of disease is the principal goal of initial oncologic surgery.

Intraoperative localization and decision-making are surgeon-dependent variables. Radioimmunoguided surgery (RIGS) has been employed as an investigational procedure to improve the accuracy of staging. RIGS employs radiolabeled monoclonal antibodies directed against tumor-associated antigens and a gamma-detection probe to discriminate between normal and abnormal tissue. To date, it has been reported using In-111 labeled antibodies (Oncoscint) at 48–72 h after injection *(68)* and at 18–24 h with Tc-99m-labeled antibodies (OncoSPECT) *(69–72)* as well as at 2–3 wk with I-125 labeled antibodies (B72.3 or CC49) *(73–79)*. OncoSPECT and I-125-labeled CC49 have been used in investigational settings only; neither agent has been approved for use in diagnosis. Currently, investigational studies are in progress evaluating CEA-Scan (Tc-99m-labeled anti-CEA Fab' fragment approved by the FDA as a scanning agent) in combination with surgical probes to guide the surgeon in terms of extent of resection and detection of loco-regional tumor sites.

During surgery, the abdominal cavity is examined with selective radioactivity emissions from tumor tissue. In several reports, RIGS with I-125 CC49 provided immediate staging information that impacted on therapeutic interventions, challenging the adequacy of traditional procedures alone for primary colorectal cancer exploration *(73–76)*. Positive antibody localization was observed in 83% of patients at surgery. Of those patients with localization, additional information was obtained at the time of surgery in 80%. In 34% of patients, staging changes were made as a result of RIGS evaluation. New findings resulted in operative changes in 25%. Thirty percent of the original 36 patients became eligible for adjuvant chemotherapy based on current recommendations because of RIGS findings *(73–76)*. When cases were evaluated separately for those with primary tumor and those with recurrent colorectal cancer, RIGS using I-125 CC49 antibody localized 86% of primary and 97% of recurrent tumors. RIGS altered the planned operative procedure in 50% of cases with primary tumors and in 47% with recurrent tumors *(73)*.

The results of several studies suggest that use of the RIGS identifies patterns of disease dissemination different from those identified by traditional staging techniques. Removal of additional RIGS-positive tissues in nontraditional areas may improve survival through accurate assessment of the extent of disease and the selection of appropriate therapy *(74)*. In a group of colorectal cancer patients who underwent RIGS using I-125 CC49, with a median follow-up of 37 mo, survival in the RIGS-negative group was found to be 100%. In the RIGS-positive group, there was a mortality incidence of 87.5% *(75)*.

Radioimmunoguided surgery can change the surgical procedure in cases with tumor deposits that are not detected by any other imaging modality. RIGS using I-125 CC49 antibody was found to be a highly sensitive method and, thus, may guide therapeutic interventions. In studies performed thus far, RIGS has been more sensitive than clinical or histopathologic examination in detecting the regional spread of a tumor. Routine histologic analysis was able to identify tumor in only 63%, whereas the intraoperative probe signaled the presence of tumor in 89% of cases. In lymph nodes with no evidence of tumor by routine histopathologic examination, a positive RIGS reading was associated with the subsequent confirmation of occult metastases in 33% of cases *(76)*. In a similar study, radioimmunoscintigraphy and RIGS using In-111 B72.3 were evaluated for its usefulness in detecting clinically occult regional lymph node involvement. The overall sensitivity for radioimmunoscintigraphy and RIGS was 71.4% (55.6% in primary tumors and 100% in recurrences) and 82.1% (83.3% in primary tumors and 80% in recurrences), respectively *(68)*.

In investigational settings, the RIGS system has been used to predict patient outcome. In a study using I-125 B72.3 and I-125 CC49, 37.4% of patients underwent a curative resection based on RIGS findings. Among this group, 55% were alive 2–8 yr after operation. In the group with nonresectable tumors, only 2% of patients were alive. There were no survivors in the group in which cancers were found to be traditionally resectable but unresectable with RIGS *(77)*. Likewise, in another study, survival of stage I or II patients was found to be longer than that of stage III or IV patients *(78)*.

Radioimmunoguided surgery has been performed using a Tc-99m-labeled OncoSPECT in patients with newly diagnosed, recurrent, or metastatic CRC. Overall sensitivity for CT, RIGS, and surgery was reported as 43%, 91%, and 96%, respectively. RIGS detected all liver and extrahepatic abdominal tumor sites and correctly predicted histological tumor-free margins and tumor beds in all cases. RIGS did not identify tumor deposits that the surgeon could neither see nor feel *(79)*. It is important that RIGS be utilized by an experienced surgeon.

3.3.1. SUMMARY: RADIOIMMUNOGUIDED SURGERY

Although surgical probes are not yet approved for use in combination with radiolabeled antibodies, the technique appears to be promising in the hands of experienced surgeons. This is a likely area for a future role of nuclear medicine in the management of the patient with CRC.

4. CONCLUSION

At the present time, nuclear medicine offers several imaging techniques for the improved detection of CRC at the various stages of diagnosis and management of the patient with this clinical problem: FDG-PET and a Tc-99m labeled anti-CEA antibody fragment (*CEA-Scan*) specific for CRC. Fluorodeoxyglucose (FDG) PET imaging is revolutionizing the practice of oncology, as it provides high-quality images with greater sensitivity for the detection of viable tumor than conventional imaging modalities. Although the frequency of the nonspecific FDG-PET findings will increase as the technique is used more frequently, it is likely to maintain its advantage in terms of accuracy over CT/MRI. Other positron-emitting radiotracers such as amino acids to characterize protein synthesis or nucleotides to identify foci of increased DNA or RNA synthesis are currently under investigation. Eventually, these tracers may augment FDG-PET in the evaluation of oncology patients in general.

Practitioners and patients not having access to ring-detector FDG-PET imaging are well served with the use of CEA-Scan SPECT imaging, provided that this latter technique is properly performed on well-maintained state-of-the-art equipment.

The data comparing FDG-PET and CEA-Scan to traditional imaging (CT/MRI) demonstrate that both nuclear medicine imaging techniques outperform conventional imaging in the pelvis and abdomen and in the evaluation of the total body. FDG-PET appears to outperform CT even in the liver, whereas the results with CEA-Scan indicate near equivalence. To date, there is only a single comparison of the accuracy of the two nuclear medicine techniques in patients with colorectal carcinoma. In a recent publication, Willkomm et al. performed both FDG-PET and CEA-Scan planar and SPECT imaging in 28 patients in whom the recurrence of CRC was suspected based on either elevated CEA (13 patients), CT findings (9 patients), sonography (4 patients), or severe constipation (2 patients) *(80)*. Although SPECT imaging of the pelvis was performed in all 28 patients, abdominal SPECT was performed in only 15 of the 28 patients. CEA-Scan detected eight of nine local recurrences, whereas FDG-PET detected nine of nine. In addition, there was a false-positive FDG-PET scan. Liver metastases were detected in nine patients by FDG-PET imaging compared to only one with CEA-Scan (only planar imaging of the liver in 13 of the 28 patients). Consequently, the sensitivity of FDG-PET exceeded the sensitivity of CEA-Scan (100% vs 89%), but the lesions missed had no effect on patient management. In this small series, the specificity of FDG-PET was less than that of CEA-Scan (95% vs 100%). The overall accuracy of both techniques was 96%, with FDG having a 90% positive predictive value (PPV) and 100% negative predictive value (NPV), whereas CEA-Scan had a PPV of 100% and a NPV of 95% in this series *(80)*. As indicated, the number of direct comparisons between these two valuable techniques are few in number. It remains to be evaluated whether radiation or chemotherapy interferes with the sensitivity or specificity of one or the other techniques (*see* Fig. 4). These data suggest that both techniques provide greater detectability of colorectal recurrences than traditional imaging methods alone.

The use of radiolabeled antibodies and intraoperative probes for the detection of residual tumor foci remains investigational. Finally, investigations are also underway to evaluate the potential for radiolabeled antibodies as agents to deliver targeted radiotherapy for use either as adjuvant therapy or treatment of otherwise unresectable disseminated disease unresponsive to traditional chemotherapy. These applications have not been discussed in this chapter, as many issues remain before they would be available for clinical use.

Nuclear medicine imaging techniques are no longer a merely interesting additional procedure that can be performed in patients with colorectal carcinoma. Technical advances in radiopharmaceutical and instrument development have made available imaging techniques that have withstood the rigors of clinical investigation, regulatory review, and the challenging cost-effective criteria of the current medical environment.

FDG-PET imaging and CEA-Scan should be viewed as essential elements in the contemporary management of patients with colorectal carcinoma.

REFERENCES

1. Steele G Jr. Follow-up plans after treatment of primary colon and rectum cancer. *World J. Surg.*, **15** (1991) 583–588.
2. Fortner JG, Silva JS, Golbey RB, Cox EB, and Maclean BJ. Multivariate analysis of a personal series of 247 consecutive patients with liver metastases from colorectal cancer. I. Treatment by hepatic resection, *Ann. Surg.*, **199** (1984) 306–316.
3. Tunis S, Stojak M, Richardson S, Burken M, Londner M, Ulrich M, et al. *FDG Positron Emission Tomography (PET)*. HCFA Decision Memorandum CAG-00065, 2000.
4. Abdel-Nabi H, Doerr RJ, Lamonica DM, Cronin VR, Galantowicz PJ, Carbone GM, et al. Staging of primary colorectal carcinomas with fluorine-18 fluorodeoxyglucose whole-body PET: correlation with histopathologic and CT findings. *Radiology*, **206** (1998) 755–760.
5. Mukai M, Sadahiro S, Yasuda S, Ishida H, Tokunaga N, Tajima T, et al. Preoperative evaluation by whole-body 18F-fluorodeoxyglucose positron emission tomography in patients with primary colorectal cancer. *Oncol. Rep.*, **7** (2000) 85–87.
6. Falk PM, Gupta NC, Thorson AG, Frick MP, Boman BM, Christensen MA, et al. Positron emission tomography for preoperative staging of colorectal carcinoma. *Dis. Colon Rectum*, **37** (1994) 153–156.
7. August DA, Ottow RT, and Sugarbaker PH. Clinical perspective of human colorectal cancer metastasis. *Cancer Metastasis Rev.*, **3** (1984) 303–324.
8. Mendez RJ, Rodriguez R, Kovacevich T, Martinez S, Moreno G, and Cerdan J. CT in local recurrence of rectal carcinoma. *J. Comput. Assist. Tomogr.*, **17** (1993) 741–744.
9. Cohen A, Minsky BD, and Schilsky RL. Cancer of the colon. In *Cancer. Principles and Practice of Oncology*. DeVita VT Jr, Hellman S, and Rosenberg SA (eds.), 5th ed. Lippincott, Philadelphia, 1997, pp. 1144–1184.
10. Muller-Schimpflr M, Brix G, Layer G, Schlag P, Engenhart R, Frohmuller S, et al. Recurrent rectal cancer: diagnosis with dynamic MR imaging. *Radiology*, **189** (1993) 881–889.
11. Moss AA. Imaging of colorectal carcinoma. *Radiology*, **170** (1989) 308–310.
12. Ito K, Kato T, Tadokoro M, et al. Recurrent rectal cancer and scar: differentiation with PET and MR imaging. *Radiology*, **182** (1992) 549–552.
13. Freeney PC, Marks WM, Ryan JA, et al. Colorectal carcinoma evaluation with CT: preoperative staging and detection of post-operative recurrence. *Radiology*, **158** (1986) 347–353.
14. Moss AA, Thoeni RF, Schnyder P, et al. Value of computed tomography in the detection and staging of recurrent rectal carcinomas. *J. Comput. Assist. Tomogr.*, **5** (1981) 870–874.
15. de Lange EE, Fecher RE, and Wanebo HJ. Suspected recurrent rectosigmoid carcinoma after abdominoperineal resection: MR imaging and histopathologic findings. *Radiology*, **170** (1989) 323–328.
16. Krestin GP, Steinbrich W, and Friedmann G. Recurrent rectal cancer:diagnosis with MR imaging versus CT. *Radiology*, **168** (1988) 307–311.
17. Balzarini L, Ceglia E, D'Ippolito G, et al. Recurrent recurrence of rectosigmoid cancer: what about the choice of MRI for diagnosis? *Gastrointest. Radiol.*, **15** (1990) 338–342.
18. Dicle O, Obuz F, and Cakmakci H. Differentiation of recurrent rectal, cancer and scarring with dynamic MR imaging. *Br. J. Radiol.*, **72** (1999) 1155–1159.
19. Krestin GP, Steinbrich W, and Friedman G. Recurrent rectal cancer diagnosis with MR imaging versus CT. *Radiology*, **168** (1988) 307–311.
20. Delbeke D, Vitola JV, Sandler MP, et al. Staging recurrent metastatic colorectal carcinoma with PET. *J. Nucl. Med.*, **38** (1997) 1196–1201.
21. Lai DT, Fulham M, Stephen MS, Chu KM, Solomon M, Thompson JF, et al. The role of whole-body positron emission tomography with F18-fluorodeoxyglucose in identifying operable colorectal cancer metastases to the liver. *Arch. Surg.*, **131** (1996) 703–707.

22. Schiepers C, Pennninckx F, De Vadder N , et al. Contribution of PET in the diagnosis of recurrent colorectal cancer: comparison with conventional imaging. *Eur. J. Surg. Oncol.*, **21** (1995) 517–522.

23. Beets G, Penninckx F, Schiepers C, Filez L, Mortelmans L, Kerremans R, et al. Clinical value of whole-body positron emission tomography with (18F) fluorodeoxyglucose in recurrent colorectal cancer. *Br. J. Surg.*, **81** (1994) 1666–1670.

24. Vitola JV, Delbeke D, Sandler MP, et al. Positron emission tomography to stage suspected metastatic colorectal carcinoma to the liver. *Am. J. Surg.*, **171** (1996) 21–26.

25. Strauss LG, Corius JH, Schlag P, et al. Recurrence of colorectal tumors: PET evaluation. *Radiology*, **170** (1989) 329–332.

26. Huebner RF, Park KC, Shepherd JE, Schwimmer J, and Czernin J. A meta-analysis of the literature for whole-body FDG-PET detection of recurrent colorectal cancer. *J. Nucl. Med.*, **41** (2000) 1177–1189.

27. Keogan MT, Lowe VJ, Baker ME, McDermott VG, Lyerly HK, and Coleman RE. Local recurrence of rectal cancer: evaluation with F-18 fluorodeoxyglucose PET imaging. *Abdom. Imaging*, **22** (1997) 332–337.

28. Ogunbiyi OA, Flanagan FL, Dehdashti F, et al. Detection of recurrent and metastatic colorectal cancer: comparison of positron emission tomography and computed tomography. *Ann. Surg. Oncol.*, **4** (1997) 613–620.

29. Flamen P, Stroobants S, Van Cutsem E, et al. Additional value of whole-body positron emission tomography with fluorine-18-2-deoxy-D-glucose in recurrent colorectal cancer. *J. Clin. Oncol.*, **17** (1999) 894–901.

30. Hustinx R, Paulus P, Daenen F, Detroz B, Honore P, Jacquet N, et al. Clinical value of positron emission tomography in the detection and staging of recurrent colorectal cancer. *Gastroenterol. Clin. Biol.*, **23** (1999) 323–329.

31. Takeuchi O, Saito N, Koda K, Sarashina H, and Nakajima N. Clinical assessment of positron emission tomography for the diagnosis of local recurrence in colorectal cancer. *Br. J. Surg.*, **86** (1999) 932–937.

32. Yasuda S, Makuuchi Y, Sadahiro S, Mukai M, Takunaga N, Tajima T, et al. Colorectal cancer recurrence in the liver: detection by PET. *Tokai J. Exp. Clin. Med.*, **23** (1998) 167–171.

33. Boykin KN, Zibari GB, Lilien DL, McMillan RW, Aultman DF, and McDonald JC. The use of FDG-positron emission tomography for the evaluation of colorectal metastases of the liver. *Am. Surg.*, **65** (1999) 1183–1185.

34. Lowe VJ, Delong DM, Hoffman JM, et al. Optimum scanning protocol for FDG PET evaluation of pulmonary malignancy. *J. Nucl. Med.*, **36** (1995) 883–887.

35. Valk PE, Abella-Columna E, Haseman MK, Pounds TR, Tesar RD, Myers RW, et al. Whole-body PET imaging with (18F) fluorodeoxyglucose in management of recurrent colorectal cancer. *Arch. Surg.*, **134** (1999) 503–511; discussion 511–513.

36. Ruhlmann J, Schomburg A, Bender H, et al. Fluorodeoxyglucose whole-body positron emission tomography in colorectal cancer patients studied in routine daily practice. *Dis. Colon Rectum*, **40** (1997) 1195–1204.

37. Cohen AM. Comparison of positron emission tomography and computed tomography in the detection of recurrent and metastatic colorectal cancer. *Ann. Surg. Oncol.*, **4** (1997) 610.

38. Flanagan FL, Dehdashti F, Ogunbiyi OA, Kodner IJ, and Siegel BA. Utility of FDG-PET for investigating unexplained plasma CEA elevation in patients with colorectal cancer. *Ann. Surg.*, **227** (1998) 319–323.

39. Valk PE, Abella-Columna E, Tesar RD, et al. Detection of recurrent colorectal cancer by FDG-PET in patients with serum CEA elevation. *J. Nucl. Med.*, **39(Suppl.)** (1998) 136 p.

40. Kubota R, Yamada S, Kubota K, Ishiwata K, Tamahushi N, Ido T, et al. Intratumoral distribution of F18-fluoro-deoxyglucose in vivo: high accumulation in macrophages and granulation tissues studied by micro-autoradiography. *J. Nucl. Med.*, **33** (1992) 1972–1980.

41. Haberkorn U, Strauss LG, Dimitrakopoulou A, et al. PET studies for Fluorodeoxyglucose metabolism in patients with recurrent colorectal tumors receiving radiotherapy. *J. Nucl. Med.*, **32** (1991) 1485–1490.

42. Findlay M, Young H, Cunningham D, et al. Noninvasive monitoring of tumor metabolism using fluorodeoxyglucose and positron emission tomography in colorectal cancer liver metastases: correlation with tumor response to fluorouracil NTS. *J. Clin. Oncol.*, **14** (1996) 700–708.

43. Guillem JG, Puig-La Calle J Jr, Akhurst T, et al. Prospective assessment of primary rectal cancer response to preoperative radiation and chemotherapy using 18-fluorodeoxyglucose positron emission tomography. *Dis. Colon Rectum*, **43** (2000) 18–24.

44. Miraldi F, Vesselle H, Faulhaber PF, Adler LP, Leisure GP. Elimination of artifactual accumulation of FDG in PET imaging of colorectal cancer. *Clin. Nucl. Med.*, **23** (1998) 3–7.

45. Valk PE, Pounds TR, Tesar RD, Hopkins DM, and Haseman MK. Cost-effectiveness of PET imaging in clinical oncology. *Nucl. Med. Biol.*, **23** (1996) 737–743.

46. Trauner M, Grygar S, Stauber RE, Brodatsch-Hausler E, and Klimpfinger M. Carcinoembryonic antigen, cytokeratin expression and mucin composition in hyperplastic and neoplastic polyps of the colorectum. *Gastroenterology*, **32** (1994) 626–631.

47. Behr TM, Sharkey RM, Juweid ME, et al. Factors influencing the pharmacokinetics, dosimetry and diagnostic accuracy of radioimmunodetection and radioimmunotherapy of carcinoembryonic antigen-expressing tumors. *Cancer Res.*, **56** (1996) 1805–1816.

48. Sharkey RM, Blumenthal RD, Behr TM, et al. Selection of radioimmunoconjugates for the therapy of well-established or micrometastatic colon carcinoma. *Int. J. Cancer*, **29** (1997) 477–485.

49. Goldenberg DM, Goldenberg H, Sharkey RM, et al. Imaging of colorectal carcinoma with radiolabeled antibodies. *Semin. Nucl. Med.*, **19** (1989) 262–281.

50. Goldenberg DM, Deland FH, Bennett SJ, and Primus FJ. Radioimmunodetection of cancer with radioactive antibodies to carcinoembryonic antigen. *Cancer Res.*, **40** (1980) 2984–2992.

51. Goldenberg DM, Kim EE, Bennett SJ, et al. Carcinoembryonic antigen radioimmunodetection in the evaluation of colorectal cancer and in the detection of occult neoplasms. *Gastroenterology*, **84** (1983) 524–532.

52. Lechner P, Lind P, Binter G, and Cesnik H. Anticarcinoembryonic antigen immunoscintigraphy with a Tc-99m-Fab′ fragment (Immu-4™) in primary and recurrent colorectal cancer. A prospective study. *Dis. Colon Rectum*, **36** (1993) 930–935.

53. Moffat FL Jr, Pinsky CM, Hammershaimb L, Petrelli NJ, Patt YZ, Whaley FS, et al. Clinical utility of external immunoscintigraphy with the IMMU-4 technetium-99m Fab′ antibody fragment in patients undergoing surgery for carcinoma of the colon and rectum: results of a pivotal Phase III trial. *J. Clin. Oncol.*, **14** (1996) 2295–2305.

54. Hughes K, Pinsky CM, Petrelli NJ, Moffat FL, Patt YZ, Hammershaimb L, et al. Use of carcinoembryonic antigen radioimmunodetection and computed tomography for predicting the resectability of recurrent colorectal cancer. *Ann. Surg.*, **226** (1997) 621–631.

55. Serafini AN, Klein JL, Wolff BG, et al. Radioimmunoscintigraphy of recurrent, metastatic, or occult colorectal cancer with technetium 99m-labeled totally human monoclonal antibody 88BV59: results of pivotal, phase III multicenter studies [published erratum in *J. Clin. Oncol.*, **16** (1998) 2575]. *J. Clin. Oncol.*, **16(5)** (1998) 1777–1787.

56. Lind P, Lechner P, Arian-Schad K, et al. Anti-carcinoembryonic antigen immunoscintigraphy (technetium-99m-monoclonal antibody BW 431/26) and serum CEA levels in patients with suspected primary and recurrent colorectal carcinoma. *J. Nucl. Med.*, **32** (1991) 1319–1325.

57. Patt YZ, Podoloff DA, Curley S, Kasi L, Smith R, Bhadkamkar V, et al. Technetium 99m-labeled IMMU-4, a monoclonal antibody against carcinoembryonic antigen, for imaging of occult recurrent colorectal cancer in patients with rising serum carcinoembryonic antigen levels. *J. Clin. Oncol.*, **12** (1994) 489–495.

58. LeDoussal J-M, Chetanneau A, Gruaz-Guyon A, et al. Bispecific monoclonal antibody-mediated targeting of an indium-111-labeled DTPA dimer to primary colorectal tumors: pharmacokinetics, biodistribution, scintigraphy and immune response. *J. Nucl. Med.*, **34** (1993) 1662–1671.

59. Markowitz A, Saleemi K, and Freeman LM. Role of In-111 labeled CYT-103 immunoscintigraphy in the evaluation of patients with recurrent colorectal carcinoma. *Clin. Nucl. Med.*, **18** (1993) 685–700.

60. Collier BD, Nabi H, Doerr RJ, et al. Immunoscintigraphy performed with In-111 labeled CYT-103 in the management of colorectal cancer. Comparison with CT. *Radiology*, **185** (1992) 179–186.

61. Dominguez JM, Wolff BG, Nelson H, Forstrom LA, and Mullan BP. ^{111}In-CYT-103 scanning in recurrent colorectal cancer—does it affect standard management? *Dis. Colon Rectum*, **39** (1996) 514–519.

62. Doerr RJ, Abdel-Nabi H, Krag D, and Mitchell EP. Radiolabeled antibody imaging in the management of colorectal cancer: Results of a multicenter clinical study. *Ann. Surg.*, **214** (1991) 118–124.

63. DeJager R, Abdel-Nabi H, Serafini A, et al. Current status of cancer immunodetection with radiolabeled human monoclonal antibodies. *Semin. Nucl. Med.*, **23** (1993) 165–179.

64. Nabi HA, Erb DA, and Cronin VR. Superiority of SPET to planar imaging in the detection of colorectal carcinomas with ^{111}In monoclonal antibodies. *Nucl. Med. Commun.*, **16** (1995) 631–639.

65. Hansen HJ, Sullivan CL, Sharkey RM, et al. HAMA interference with murine monoclonal antibody-based immunoassays. *J. Clin. Immunoassays*, **16** (1993) 294–299.

66. Divgi CR, Scott AM, McDermott K, et al. Clinical comparison of radiolocalization of two monoclonal antibodies (mAbs) against the TAG-72 antigen. *Nucl. Med. Biol.*, **21** (1994) 9–15.

67. Larson SM, El-Shirbiny AM, Divgi CR, Sgouros G, Finn RD, Tschmelitsch J, et al. Single chain antigen binding protein (sFv CC49): first human studies in colorectal carcinoma metastatic to liver. *Cancer*, **80(Suppl.)** (1997) 2458–2468.

68. Muxi A, Pons F, Vidal-Sicart S, Setoain FJ, Herranz R, Novell F, et al. Radioimmunoguided surgery of colorectal carcinoma with an ^{111}In-labelled anti-TAG72 monoclonal antibody. *Nucl. Med. Commun.*, **20** (1999) 123–130.

69. Moffat FL, Vargas-Cuba R, Serafini AN, et al. Preoperative scintigraphy and operative probe scintimetry of colorectal carcinoma using technetium-99m-88BV59. *J. Nucl. Med.*, **36** (1995) 738–745.

70. Gulec SA, Serafini AN, Moffat FL, et al. Radioimmunoscintigraphy of colorectal carcinoma using technetium-99m-labeled, totally human monoclonal antibody 88BV59H21-2. *Cancer Res.*, **55(Suppl.)** (1995) 5774s–5776s.
71. Krause BJ, Baum RP, Staib-Sebler E, Lorenz M, Niesen A, and Hor G. Human monoclonal antibody 99mTc-88BV59: detection of colorectal cancer, recurrent or metastatic disease and immunogenicity assessment. *Eur. J. Nucl. Med.*, **24** (1997) 72–75.
72. Wolff BG, Bolton J, Baum R, et al. Radioimmunoscintigraphy of recurrent, metastatic, or occult colorectal cancer with technetium Tc 99m 88BV59H21-2V67-66 (HumaSPECT-Tc), a totally human monoclonal antibody. *Dis. Colon Rectum*, **41** (1998) 953–962.
73. Arnold MW, Schneebaum S, Berens A, Petty L, Mojzisik C, Hinkle G, et al. Intraoperative detection of colorectal cancer with radioimmunoguided surgery and CC49, a second-generation monoclonal antibody. *Ann. Surg.*, **216** (1992) 627–632.
74. Arnold MW, Schneebaum S, and Martin EW Jr. Radioimmunoguided surgery in the treatment and evaluation of rectal cancer patients. *Cancer Control*, **3** (1996) 42–45.
75. Bertsch DJ, Burak WE Jr, Young DC, Arnold MW, and Martin EW Jr. Radioimmunoguided surgery for colorectal cancer. *Ann. Surg. Oncol.*, **3** (1996) 310–316.
76. Cote RJ, Houchens DP, Hitchcock CL, Saad AD, Nines RG, Greenson JK, et al. Intraoperative detection of occult colon cancer micrometastases using ^{125}I-radiolabeled monoclonal antibody CC49. *Cancer*, **77** (1996) 613–620.
77. Bertsch DJ, Burak WE Jr, Young DC, Arnold MW, and Martin EW Jr. Radioimmunoguided surgery system improves survival for patients with recurrent colorectal cancer. *Surgery*, **118** (1995) 634–638; discussion 638–639.
78. Arnold MW, Young DC, Hitchcock CL, Schneebaum S, and Martin EW Jr. Radioimmunoguided surgery in primary colorectal carcinoma: an intraoperative prognostic tool and adjuvant to traditional staging. *Am. J. Surg.*, **170** (1995) 315–318.
79. Di Carlo V, Stella M, De Nardi P, and Fazio F. Radioimmunoguided surgery: clinical experience with different monoclonal antibodies and methods. *Tumori*, **81(3,Suppl.)** (1995) 98–102.
80. Willkomm P, Bender H, Bangard M, Decker P, Grunwald F, and Biersack H-J. FDG PET and immunoscintigraphy with 99mTc-labeled antibody fragments for the detection of the recurrence of colo-rectal carcinoma. *J. Nucl. Med.*, **41** (2000) 1657–1663.

11 Radiation Therapy of Resectable Rectal Cancer

Nora A. Janjan, Matthew Ballo, Christopher Crane, and Marc Delclos

CONTENTS

INTRODUCTION
RADIATION THERAPY
CONCLUSION
REFERENCES

1. INTRODUCTION

Diagnostic evaluations are critical to determining the location and volume of rectal disease. It is particularly important to identify occult metastatic disease. All of these factors determine whether a course of treatment is designated as curative or palliative. Specific clinical presentations also can influence the sequence of combined modality therapy.

The benefit of adjuvant radiation and chemotherapy for locally advanced disease, defined as having stage T3/T4 primary tumors or positive regional lymph nodes, was clearly observed in several prospective randomized trials *(1–5)*. With surgery alone, the overall 5-yr disease-free survival rate is 55% for patients with rectal cancer. The addition of postoperative radiation therapy has been shown to reduce the local relapse rate among locally advanced rectal cancers. The local failure rate with surgery alone ranges from 35% to 50% and is decreased to 10–20% with the addition of postoperative radiation *(6,7)*. However, the risk of distant metastases without the addition of systemic therapy is approx 20% for stage II disease and 40–60% for stage III disease. Without chemotherapy, the 5-yr survival rates are approx 70–90% for stage II disease, 40% for T3N1 tumors, and 15–20% for T4N1 lesions.

A number of prospective randomized studies have specifically evaluated these issues. The National Surgical Adjuvant Breast and Bowel Project (NSABP) in a three-arm trial compared (1) surgery alone, (2) surgery plus postoperative radiation, and (3) surgery plus postoperative chemotherapy *(5)*. The radiation dose was 46 Gy in 25 fractions; however, only 86% of the patients received the total prescribed dose of radiation. The surgery-plus-postoperative-radiation arm had a decrease in the rate of local recurrence, but this did not affect survival (Table 1). The addition of adjuvant chemotherapy significantly improved

From: *Colorectal Cancer: Multimodality Management*
Edited by: L. Saltz © Humana Press Inc., Totowa, NJ

179

Table 1
Results from the NSABP-RO1 Trial That Randomized Therapy Among
528 Patients Among Surgery (S) Alone, Surgery and Chemotherapy (S + CTX),
and Surgery and Postoperative Radiation Therapy (S + XRT)

	S	S+CTX	S+XRT
Overall survival	38%	46%	39%
Disease-free survival	30%	37%	34%
Local failure	16%	12%	10%

Note: Radiation therapy totaled 40 Gy to 47 Gy. Chemotherapy consisted of 5-fluorouracil/methyl-CCNU/vincristine.

disease-free survival and overall survival, but the rates of local failure and distant metastases were not significantly different compared with those for surgery alone.

Two other randomized studies, the Gastrointestinal Tumor Study Group (GITSG) and the Mayo/North Central Cancer Treatment Group (NCCTG), also showed reductions in local recurrence rates and improvements in disease-free and overall survival when postoperative radiation and chemotherapy were administered to patients with stages B2 and C rectal cancer. The GITSG randomized trial included four treatment arms: (1) surgery alone, (2) surgery and postoperative radiation (40–48 Gy), (3) surgery plus postoperative 5-fluorouracil chemotherapy, and (4) surgery plus postoperative radiation (40–48 Gy) and 5-fluorouracil chemotherapy. Compared to surgery alone, all the arms that included some form of adjuvant therapy resulted in improvements in local control, disease-free, and overall survival *(3,4)*. The addition of radiation therapy decreased the incidence of local failure as the initial form of disease recurrence and reduced the risk of local failure to 10% in the combined modality arm of the trial. With a local failure rate of 27%, postoperative chemotherapy was not shown to reduce the risk of local recurrence (Table 2). These results showed a statistically significant recurrence-free survival and overall survival advantage for combined modality therapy with radiation therapy and chemotherapy over surgery alone.

The advantage of combined-modality therapy was also demonstrated in the Mayo/NCCTG trial that compared outcomes for postoperative radiation alone to the results achieved with postoperative radiation and 5-fluorouracil chemotherapy. In this trial, higher radiation doses were administered: 50.4 Gy in 28 fractions. The addition of chemotherapy lowered the rate of local failure from 25% to 13.5% and the rate of distant metastases from 46% to 29%. These factors improved the disease-free survival rate from 37% to 59% and the overall survival rate from 48% to 58% *(1)*. The combined-modality trial with radiation therapy and chemotherapy reduced local and distant recurrences by 34%, and the overall death rate was reduced by 29%.

Because of these findings, a clinical announcement in 1991 by the National Cancer Institute confirmed that adjuvant radiation and chemotherapy was the standard of care for locally advanced rectal cancer *(8)*. These prospective randomized trials demonstrated that radiation therapy significantly decreases the risk for local recurrence and that adjuvant chemotherapy had a systemic benefit that resulted in improvements in disease-free and overall survival, especially when combined with radiation.

The National Cancer Data-Base found four trends in the patterns of care for rectal cancer between 1985 and 1995. First, stage I disease was found in only one-third of cases. Second, local excision was performed with increasing frequency for stage I disease. Third, stage for stage, there was a decline in the used of abdomino-perineal resections (APRs). Finally,

Table 2
Results from the GITSG-7175 Trial That Randomized Therapy Among 202 Patients
Among Surgery (S) Alone, Surgery and Chemotherapy (S + CTX), Surgery
and Postoperative Radiation Therapy (S + XRT), and Combined Modality Therapy
with Surgery, Radiation Therapy, and Chemotherapy (S + CTX + XRT)

	S	S+CTX	S+XRT	S+CTX+XRT
10-yr overall survival	26%	41%	33%	45%
10-yr disease-free survival	44%	51%	50%	65%
Recurrence	55%	46%	46%	35%
Local failure	25%	27%	20%	10%

Note: Radiation therapy totaled 40–48 Gy. Chemotherapy consisted of 5-FU/methyl-CCNU.

multimodal treatments were used with greater frequency, especially in stage II and III disease *(9)*. Radiation, chemotherapy, and surgery were applied in <1% of stage I, 6% of stage II, 13% of stage III, and 8% of stage IV disease in 1985; by 1995, these values had increased to 11%, 40%, 52%, and 15%, respectively. Survival rates at 5 yr were 62% for chemotherapy and surgery, with or without radiation, as compared to 55% with surgery alone or in combination with radiation for stage II rectal cancer. For stage III rectal cancer, 5-yr survival rates were 31% with surgery alone, 39% with surgery and radiation, and 42% with radiation, chemotherapy, and surgery.

The influence of the National Cancer Institute (NCI) statement was evident in the Patterns of Care study that evaluated the treatment of rectal cancer in the United States between 1992 and 1994 among 507 patients at 57 different institutions. Among these patients, 243 had T3 and/or N1-2 M0 disease. Postoperative radiation was administered to 75%, 22% were treated with preoperative radiation, and 2% received both preoperative and postoperative radiation. Although only 7% were on a clinical trial, 90% received chemotherapy for a median of 21 wk. In this group of 243 patients, 54% underwent a low anterior resection and 46% had an APR. Modern radiation techniques with high-energy photons were administered in the majority of patients, and 93% were treated with three or four radiation portals *(10)*. The prone position was used by 83%, but only 37% used small bowel contrast at simulation, 16% treated patients with a full bladder, and only 11% used a belly board to displace the small bowel. Most patients received 45 Gy to the pelvis and a boost dose of 9 Gy to the primary site, for a total of 54 Gy with conventional fractionation. Overall, the NCI guidelines had a profound influence in that 90% of patients were receiving combined-modality therapy.

The long-term results of a previous Patterns of Care Study, performed between 1988 and 1989, confirmed that only the stage of disease and use of chemotherapy were significant to survival. The 5-yr survival rate with chemoradiation was 69% as compared to 50% with radiation alone. Preoperative radiation resulted in a higher survival rate, 69% at 5 yr, when compared to postoperative radiation alone but not when it was compared to postoperative chemoradiation. Survival was stage dependent; 5-yr overall survival rates were 85% for stage I, 69% for stage II, and 54% for stage III *(11)*. The 5-yr survival rate also dropped from 89% with stage C1 disease to 48% with stage C2/C3 disease.

The concurrent administration of chemotherapy during radiation for rectal cancers has been shown to improve the therapeutic ratio over radiation alone. These sentinel studies provided a model for combined-modality therapy in other sites. Radiosensitization by 5-fluorouracil (5-FU) is thought to occur by effecting the G1–S phase of the cell cycle through the inhibition of thymidylate synthetase. Another metabolite of 5-FU, fluorodeoxyuridine monophosphate, is incorporated into RNA and affects RNA synthesis. When 5-FU is given, the early-S-phase population in the tumor expands and results in enhanced radiosensitivity that is more than that seen with cell synchronization alone *(12–14)*. Correlated with this are the relationships between radiation repair and the molecular sensors at the G_1–S checkpoint, like p53 and cyclin-dependent kinases. In general, radiosensitization is accomplished by limiting tumor repopulation and reducing the efficiency of radiation repair during treatment. When combined with radiation, the effects of 5-FU are additive or supra-additive. The potentiation of radiation response is greatest when 5-FU is present for about 1 d prior to radiation.

Clinical trials with radiation and chemotherapy have been divided into four generic types that depend on how radiation and drugs interact. The first involves spatial cooperation in which each modality treats a different site, such as adjuvant chemotherapy that treats sites outside of the radiation portal or radiation to an area where chemotherapy does not penetrate well. The second relationship involves the ability to give maximum doses of each modality because toxicities do not overlap. The third relates to the protection of normal tissues. The fourth is enhancement of tumor response by the chemotherapy and radiation interaction *(15–18)*. Because of this, the dose and timing of the administration of each agent is critical.

These concepts were demonstrated in two clinical trials for locally advanced rectal cancer. The initial trials combined 5-FU and methyl-CCNU as the systemic agents, but methyl-CCNU was later found to have no benefit. An evaluation was then performed of 1696 patients who received 2 cycles of bolus 5-FU chemotherapy followed by pelvic radiation with chemotherapy and 2 more cycles of 5-FU chemotherapy. The issue was whether biomodulation, with either leucovorin or levamisole, was of benefit *(19)*. Chemotherapy consisted of bolus 5-FU alone, 5-FU with leucovorin, 5-FU with levamisole, or 5-FU with leucovorin and levamisole. Compared to 5-FU alone, no advantage was seen with biomodulation after a median follow-up duration of 48 mo. However, more gastrointestinal toxicity was seen with the three-drug arm compared to bolus 5-FU alone.

The difference between bolus and infusional 5-FU was evaluated among 660 patients with stage II and stage III rectal cancer. Adjuvant 5-FU was given at a dose of 500 mg/m^2 on d 1–5 and d 36–40, and 450 mg/m^2 were given on d 134–138 and d 169–173. During pelvic radiation, which began on d 64, patients received either a 500-mg/m^2 bolus of 5-FU given for three consecutive days during wk 1 and 5 of radiation therapy or infusional 5-FU given at a rate of 225 mg/m^2, 7 d/wk *(20)*. This trial showed significant improvements in the time to relapse and overall survival with infusional 5-FU. Local control rates, however, were similar. These improvements in time to relapse and overall survival were attributed to the systemic effect of 5-FU during radiation therapy. The average dose of 5-FU during radiation was 6546 mg/m^2 when given by infusion and 2499 mg/m^2 when given by bolus technique. It was considered that the higher total doses and the more prolonged exposure to 5-FU enhanced cytotoxicty. The toxicity profiles were also different; bolus 5-FU was associated with more hematological toxicity and infusional 5-FU was associated with more gastrointestinal toxicity.

Combined-modality therapy has significantly improved local and distant rates of disease control and is now the standard of care for locally advanced rectal cancer. However, the challenge is how to best optimize these combined components of therapy.

2. RADIATION THERAPY

Radiation therapy has three general roles in rectal cancer management. First, radiation therapy is used to enhance local–regional control by eliminating microscopic residual disease around the primary tumor and in the draining lymphatics. Second, significant tumor regression can result when radiation is administered preoperatively to locally advanced primary tumors. In these cases, an inoperable lesion can become resectable or amenable to a more conservative surgical approach with sphincter preservation. Third, radiation therapy can be used to palliate symptoms resulting from infiltration of pelvic structures or metastatic disease.

The identified prognostic factors after surgery alone reflect the risk of residual microscopic disease and include stage, tumor location, and serosal, lymphatic, and neurovascular invasion. In addition, the risk of local failure after surgery alone has been shown to increase as the tumor approaches the anus and because of the limited radial *(presacral)* surgical margin *(21,22)*. Adjuvant radiation eradicates microscopic residual tumor and eliminates the risk for local recurrence in approx 90% of patients with these adverse prognostic factors. Extension of tumor into the perirectal fat or adjacent viscera (stage II; T3/T4, N0) can increase the rate of local recurrence to approx 30% with surgery alone (Fig. 1). Tumor in the regional lymphatics (stage III) can also be effectively treated with radiation, reducing the more than 50% rate of local recurrence after surgery alone.

Adjuvant radiation can be administered either preoperatively or postoperatively. Regardless of the sequencing of surgery and radiation, the primary goal is to improve local–regional control by eradicating microscopic residual disease. Each approach has specific advantages and disadvantages. Prospective randomized assessment of these approaches has been attempted, but, because of low patient accrual, the studies had to be closed before they were completed. Emphasis has now been placed on other issues, like the combination of newer systemic agents with radiation and radiation fractionation *(13)*.

2.1. Radiation Field Arrangement and Management of Treatment-Related Side Effects

Careful attention to the technique used for radiation is important with either preoperative or postoperative therapy. Whenever possible, the small bowel should be displaced from the treatment portal. The volume of small bowel in the radiation portal has been shown to directly correlate with radiation toxicity *(23)*.

Observed clinical effects have been correlated with biological evaluations. Using either a single 5-Gy dose of radiation or a continuous dose of 20 cGy/d for a total dose of 5 Gy over 25 d, significant differences were seen in the epithelial ultrastructure *(24)*. With the protracted radiation schedule, the changes in the villous enterocytes, goblet cells, and lamina propria returned to normal within 3 d of completing radiation. Mast cell hyperplasia is a characteristic feature of both the inflammatory and fibrotic component of intestinal radiation injury. It was found that mast cells allow transforming growth factor-β to stimulate a fibrotic reaction *(25)*. Serving to protect the intestinal mucosa during the early phase of radiation enteropathy, mast cells promote intestinal fibrosis after breakdown of the mucosal barrier.

In addition to the effects on the small bowel, changes also occur in the colon with radiation. A radiation-dose-dependent decrease in absorption of water and sodium/chloride ions and a twofold secretion of potassium was noted 4 d after exposure *(26)*. The acute effects of radiation on the bowel wall have been evaluated. Reductions of 40–70% in tensile strength were reported 3 d after surgery when radiation, ranging between 10 and 25 Gy, was given to a colonic anastomosis in the rate model *(27)*. Although the anastomosis remained patent 7 d after surgery, the adjacent area of colon was at risk for perforation. Therefore, the anastomotic region acutely is at risk after intraoperative radiation.

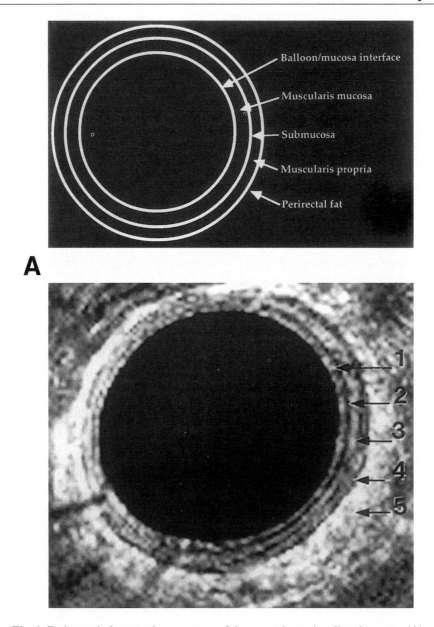

Balloon/mucosa interface

Muscularis mucosa

Submucosa

Muscularis propria

Perirectal fat

A

1
2
3
4
5

Fig. 1. Endorectal ultrasound appearance of the normal rectal wall and a tumor (**A**).

Late radiation effects on the colon have also been evaluated. When various lengths of the colorectum were radiated, a threshold effect was observed between 10 and 15 mm after 32 Gy had been administered in the mouse model *(28)*. Re-epithelization, resulting from the proliferation of epithelial cells outside the crypt on the mucosal surface, was complete after 32 Gy when the irradiated length of colorectum was less than 20 mm. When the radiated length was more than 20 mm, consequential obstruction as a result of secondary fibrosis occurred. A single dose of 10–20 Gy, administered as an intraoperative dose of radiation to the distal limb of a bowel anastomosis, did not threaten anastomotic integrity or bowel function. However, dose-related changes, like fibrosis, were observed between 6 and 12 mo after surgery *(29)*.

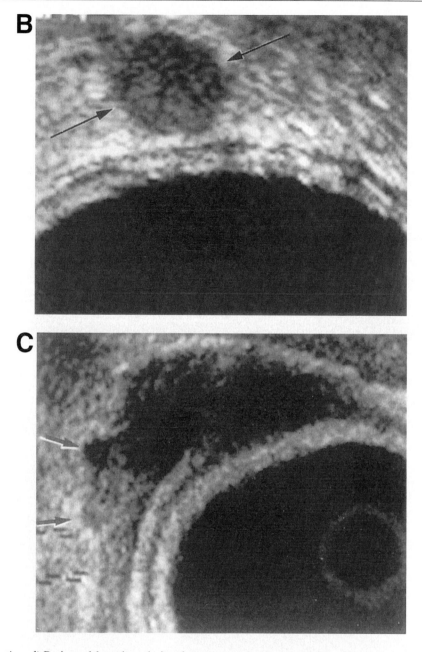

Fig. 1. *(continued)* Perirectal lymph node involvement can be detected with a hypoechoic lesion outside the rectal wall in **(B)**. **(C)** shows tumor extension through the bowel wall into the perirectal fat.

Radiation techniques such as the use of a belly board to displace the small bowel from the radiation portal also help to reduce gastrointestinal side effects (Fig. 2). Based on computed tomography (CT) treatment planning in the supine position and in the prone position with the belly board, the median volume of small bowel was reduced by 54% *(30)*. The median dose to the small bowel was 15 Gy with the belly board technique and 24 Gy in the supine position. The median volume of the bladder was also reduced 62% with the belly board technique. When it is not possible to use a belly board because of patient size or extension

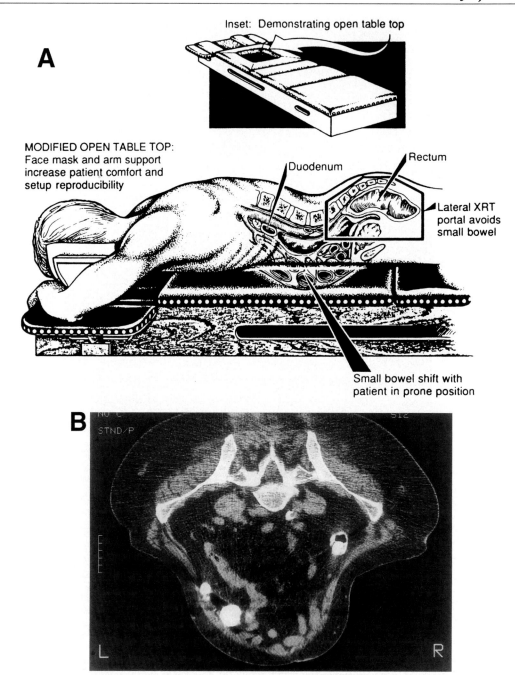

Fig. 2. The belly board technique places the patient in the prone position and allows the small bowel to fall outside of the radiation fields **(A)**. The treatment planning computed tomography scan shown in **(B)** demonstrates bowel displacement with the belly board technique.

of the tumor to anterior structures, treatment in the prone position is preferred. Another study showed a 70% reduction of small bowel in the radiation field that was independent of patient weight, age, gender, or whether preoperative or postoperative radiation was administered *(31)*.

Exclusion of the small bowel is particularly important because the risk for treatment-related diarrhea results from both radiation and chemotherapy. Both of the chemotherapeutic agents used in the treatment of rectal cancer, 5-FU and irinotecan (CPT-11) cause diarrhea. In order to administer the maximum doses of radiation and chemotherapy without interruption, radiation techniques must exclude as much small bowel as possible and an aggressive supportive care approach is needed during treatment.

For most cases, the radiation treatment portals encompass the entire pelvis through a posterior, and right and left lateral treatment portals. High-energy photons, like 18 mV-X, should be used to reduce integral dose. Unlike the treatment of other pelvic malignancies, the external iliac lymph node chain does not need to be routinely included in the treatment portal *(32)*. Anterior fields should be considered when there is anterior extension of disease to the urogenital regions. In some cases, anterior–posterior fields or a four-field arrangement may prove necessary based on tumor extension and/or anatomical constraints. Adequate coverage of the tumor volume should be confirmed with treatment planning imaging. If an anterior portal is used, there also needs to be careful accounting of the dose administered to the small bowel. The volume of small bowel in the field can be determined either with contrast used at the time of simulation and/or CT-based treatment planning.

Even with distal rectal involvement, including infiltration of the anal canal, the risk for inguinal node involvement is limited and radiation treatment portals do not need to include the inguinal region. The risk for recurrence in the inguinal region among distal rectal tumors is less than 5% *(33)*. However, radiation techniques should be modified if inguinal lymph nodes are clinically evident and pathologically confirmed to be involved with metastatic disease. Metastatic involvement in the inguinal nodes portends an especially poor prognosis for dissemination of disease *(34)*.

The superior border of the radiation field, in general, should be placed at the L5–S1 interspace. However, if the rectosigmoid is involved, individual anatomy may dictate that the superior border be placed at the L4–L5 interspace. The inferior border of the field is dictated by the inferior extent of the tumor; generally the inferior aspect of the field should be placed 2 cm inferior to the lowest aspect of the tumor. The anus may need to be included in the treatment field in some cases when the tumor is located in the distal rectum (Fig. 3A). Whenever possible, however, the anus should be blocked from the radiation portal to reduce treatment-related morbidity. For tumors located in the mid and proximal rectum, the inferior border of the radiation field is placed at the bottom of the obturator foramen. The lateral border should include the sacroiliac joints and a 2-cm margin should be placed around the pelvic brim to include the internal iliac lymph node chains in the posterior treatment portal.

For the lateral treatment fields, the superior and inferior borders should be consistent with the posterior portal. With routine simulation, contrast should be placed in the rectum to ensure an adequate margin on the primary tumor. The anterior aspect of the field should be placed 2 cm in front of the most anterior aspect of the sacral promontory and be placed anterior to the femoral heads to include the obterator nodes (Fig. 3B). Every effort should be made to exclude small bowel. To reduce morbidity to the genitalia, a block should be placed anterior to the femur. Posteriorly, the entire sacrum should be included. This is important to avoid the penumbra of the beam and ensure adequate radiation dose to the radial margin of resection in the presacral region. Like the effects on other mechanical devices, care should be taken to exclude chemotherapy infusion pumps from the radiation field *(35)*.

Approaches have also been taken to minimize side effects related to chemotherapy, like hematological and gastrointestinal toxicities. Using a protracted infusion of 5-FU, a higher

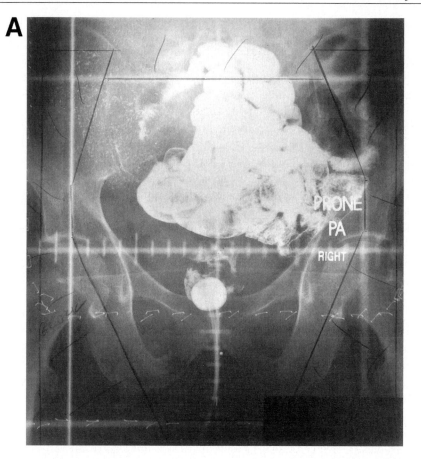

Fig. 3. (A) Routine radiation portals for rectal cancer. The posterior field is shown.

total dose of chemotherapy can be administered with fewer hematological side effects *(20)*. Although the protracted infusion decreased hematological side effects and allowed a higher total dose of chemotherapy, which resulted in improved rates of disease-free and overall survival, gastrointestinal side effects, like diarrhea, increased. Other chemotherapy agents, like CPT-11, also can result in profound diarrhea *(36)*.

Besides gastrointestinal and hematological side effects, other toxicities of chemotherapy must also be monitored during a course of chemoradiation. Specifically, mucositis and hand–foot syndrome can occur. Superinfection, especially with candida, must be closely monitored in the oral and perineal regions. Generally, the treatment is symptomatic with the use of salt and soda oral rinses and emollients in the perineal region. Occasionally, mild nausea due to chemotherapy can occur, so nutritional and fluid balance must be evaluated.

Because radiation effects are well defined, gastrointestinal toxicities that occur in the first 2 wk of radiation generally are attributable to chemotherapy. Regardless of whether it is related to the radiation, the chemotherapy, or both, the management of treatment-related diarrhea is generally the same. Etiologies, like infection, should be considered if the symptoms are not typical or if they are refractory to usual supportive care strategies. Possible infection with *C. difficile* should always be considered, especially with clinical signs, like fever and blood in the stool *(36)*.

A three-step bowel management program has been instituted at The University of Texas M.D. Anderson Cancer Center *(37)*. Results of this bowel management program were

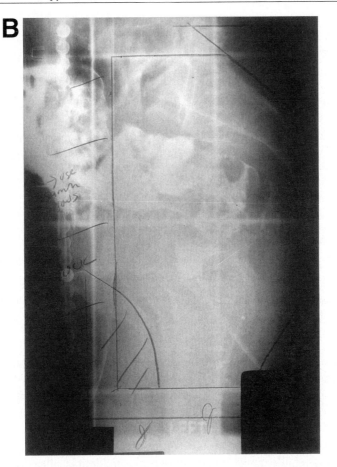

Fig. 3. (B) The lateral fields are represented showing displacement of the bowel.

prospectively evaluated using a validated bowel assessment survey. With a 95% compliance rate for completion of the survey each week during the course of chemoradiation, no significant differences were documented between the presenting symptoms and the symptoms that were reported at the completion of chemoradiation.

At the time of simulation, all patients receive written instructions in bowel management and a prescription for antidiarrheal (loperamide) and an antiemetic agent to be used if necessary. The three-step program anticipates the development of treatment-related toxicity (Table 3). The strategy is proactive; at the first sign of symptoms, the patient should proceed to the next step of management *(37)*. Under this program, the patient should not have more than three bowel movements in a day; it is important to recognize that the patient does not need to have watery or loose stools to follow the bowel management guidelines. The goal is to prevent, rather than treat, symptoms like frequent stooling, fluid and electrolyte imbalance, and skin irritation.

In this bowel management program, Step 1 uses loperamide as needed and Step 2 begins a scheduled administration of loperamide to prevent symptoms of frequent stooling. In Step 3, opioid analgesics are added to the loperamide to relieve the symptoms of abdominal cramping and to exploit the constipating effects of opioid analgesics. Established principles for pain management, that titrate the dose to effect, are used. Unlike loperamide, there is no dose limit with opioid analgesics and usually the doses of opioids that are required in

Table 3
The University of Texas M.D. Anderson Cancer Center Three-Step Bowel Management Program

	Strategy
Step 1	Loperamide prn (1–2 tablets)
Step 2	Loperamide (1–2 tablets) qid on a scheduled basis 1/2 h before meals and before bedtime

Step 3	• Continue loperamide (1–2 tablets) qid and begin opioid analgesics.
	• Add a sustained release analgesic (like morphine or oxycodone) and an immediate release analgesic for breakthrough abdominal cramping/stooling.
	  • The analgesics are titrated to effect using the same principles that are used in pain management.
	    • Because of difficulties in titration and changing needs over the course of radiation, refrain from the use of a fentanyl patch unless used for primary pain management.
	  • The goal is to give sufficient medications to consistently control frequent stooling and abdominal cramping.

Note: If one step is ineffective, the next step is used. Medications are titrated to effect. The goal is to maintain three or fewer stools per day.

Step 3 are modest. Because the treatment-related changes in the bowel do not resolve during therapy, a sustained-release analgesic is preferred in Step 3 to avoid the need for multiple doses of medications during the day *(37)*. Medications that have a 3-hr duration of effect, like tincture of opium or short-acting analgesics, can result in cycles of symptoms if a strict schedule of administration is not followed; because of this, sleep is often also disrupted. Fentanyl patches are often avoided because of the difficulty in titration and because analgesic needs are not always stable as the patient undergoes the course of radiation.

Generally, skin care is restricted to the perianal region because of the bolus effect in this area. With the first signs of dry desquamation, an emollient that also acts as a barrier for the skin, like lantiseptic, is constantly placed on the skin, except during the time of radiation. Routine use of tissues can result in further irritation of the skin. In addition to the discomfort, small regions of moist desquamation in the perianal area can place the patient at risk for a secondary infection and cellulitus resulting from bacteria in the stool. This is of particular concern when chemotherapy is also administered. An emollient that acts as a barrier helps to prevent infection. Among patients who develop a candida infection in the perianal region, a compound with nystatin, desitin, and xylocaine is often of significant benefit. Patients with distal rectal tumors who develop localized moist desquamation in the perianal area should maintain hygiene and derive symptomatic relief with sitz baths or warm compresses and Domboro's powder.

Similar approaches have been used for the treatment of chemotherapy-induced diarrhea. Alternative strategies for the control of diarrhea include the use of loperamide with enkephalinase inhibitors, like acetorphan, to treat the secretory diarrhea induced by CPT-11. The synthetic octapeptide octreotide also is effective with secretory diarrhea. Octreotide prolongs intestinal transit time, promotes absorption of electrolytes in the intestine, decreases mesenteric blood flow, and decreases the secretion of fluids and electrolytes. Octreotide has primarily been used in the treatment of other conditions like carcinoid syndrome, vasoactive intestinal polypeptide (VIP)-secreting tumors, short bowel (ileostomy) syndrome, and dumping syndrome. Also, octreotide has been used to treat diarrhea associated with the use of 5-FU and in the bone marrow transplant setting *(36,38)*. Complete response rates of more than 90% were observed after 3 d of treatment in two pilot trials with 5-FU-based chemotherapy regimens. Given subcutaneously, 100 µg bid to 500 µg tid of octreotide is injected. In other studies, octreotide has been given as a continuous intravenous infusion. The optimal dose and route of administration of octreotide is currently unknown and has been indexed to the clinical presentation *(36)*. The cost-effectiveness of the use of octreotide or alternative strategies is dependent on the cost of preventing hospitalization or infusional therapies for treatment-related complications.

The success of sphincter-preserving strategies must be determined by the late treatment-related complications. Late radiation proctitis may represent a continuum of symptoms. Although there is a radiobiological dissociation between acute and late toxicities, one clinical trial linked acute proctitis to three late symptoms (tenesmus, frequency, and diarrhea) and the EORTC/RTOG score for late effects. There appeared to be five subgroups of patients with different levels of rectal symptoms. One group had minimal symptoms; the second group only had an increased number of bowel movements in a day. Group 3 had tenesmus and bleeding, Group 4 had tenesmus and increased frequency, and Group 5 had all symptoms. Although rectal bleeding and discharge had a significant influence on the EORTC/RTOG scores, tenesmus and bleeding had the most impact on daily living *(39)*. A low concordance was also found between the patient's assessment of their symptoms and the EORTC/RTOG score.

A relationship was also observed between the development of symptomatic acute enteritis and chronic bowel injury in another study of 386 patients. Only 13 patients developed acute radiation-induced enteritis; 3 of these cases also experienced chronic bowel injury. A total of 18 patients developed chronic treatment-related symptoms and reoperation was required in 17 cases *(40)*. The risk for reoperation was 5%, but chronic proctitis developed in 19% at 5 yr. Factors related to an increased risk for complications included transanal excision, increased radiation dose, and increased age.

Other quality-of-life issues relate to fertility. Among men, preoperative sperm preservation is an option given the risk for surgery-induced sexual dysfunction, like retrograde ejaculation *(41)*. If radiation therapy is necessary, sperm preservation should also be considered because the prostate gland is included in the radiation portal.

To determine the health-related quality-of-life, two factors must be considered. The first is the effect of the intervention on survival. The second is the effect of the intervention on the health-related quality of life. By combining these two factors, the quality-adjusted life-years are determined. Determining the quality of life requires analysis of all of the utilities involved *(42)*. These can include the risk of local recurrence, the utility of living with a permanent colostomy, the acute and late side effects of treatment, and the costs associated with the recommended therapies.

Long-term follow-up is required to determine quality of life. With combined modality therapy, patients with locally advanced rectal cancer undergo 1–2 mo of radiation, approximately 1 mo between radiation and surgery, and about 4 mo of adjuvant chemotherapy. A second surgical procedure is added, for takedown of the temporary ileostomy, if a sphincter-preserving surgery is performed. The total length of time under treatment can range from 8 to 12 mo. Quality-of-life ratings predictably improve after 3 yr of follow-up and bowel function is closely linked to quality of life *(43–46)*.

2.2. Postoperative Radiation

The advantages of administering radiation postoperatively include the ability to plan treatment based on complete pathological staging of the primary tumor and a theoretical reduction in perioperative morbidity because surgery is performed in an unirradiated field. Pathological tumor staging assures that adjuvant radiation is indicated and it allows more precision in defining the regions that are to be included in the radiation portal (47). For tumors located in the mid to proximal rectum, postoperative radiation is often used because sphincter-preserving surgery can routinely be performed in these cases without the need for tumor downstaging. In addition, prompt surgical intervention and postoperative radiation are indicated in cases in which there is significant bleeding or risk of obstruction.

The disadvantages of postoperative radiation include relative hypoxia within the operative bed and potential tumor repopulation from microscopic residual disease during postoperative healing. Hypoxia enhances resistance to radiation; approximately three times the radiation dose is required to kill hypoxic tumor cells as to kill the same number of well-oxygenated cells. Therefore, higher total doses of radiation are generally administered postoperatively than preoperatively. In comparison to the 45–50 Gy generally prescribed with preoperative radiation, 53–55 Gy is usually administered postoperatively. However, the risk of radiation-related short- and long-term gastrointestinal toxicity increases precipitously as the total dose of radiation increases (48). The potential risk of radiation morbidity also increases with postoperative radiation because the small bowel is less mobile because of adhesions.

2.3. Trials with Preoperative and Postoperative Radiation: Effects on Local Control and Survival

The impact of radiation alone on local control and survival were evaluated in the Uppsala and the Swedish Rectal Trial. First, the addition of radiation decreased the risk for local failure over surgery alone (49–51). Second, radiation alone was found to improve survival rates over surgery alone (50). Third, preoperative and postoperative radiation was compared (52,53). However, these comparisons between preoperative and postoperative are difficult to interpret because of the significant differences in the fractionation schedules used. Furthermore, issues regarding sphincter preservation with preoperative radiation were not addressed because not enough time was allowed for downstaging between the completion of radiation and surgery.

A prospective randomized trial by the Stockholm Colorectal Cancer Study Group compared preoperative radiation plus surgery to surgery alone. The study involved 285 patients with all stages of disease (49,51). Local recurrence occurred in 16% of the group who received preoperative radiation and in 30% who underwent surgery alone ($p < 0.001$). The advantage was confined to patients with Dukes' B disease, although a trend ($p = 0.068$) for an advantage with radiation therapy was also observed in Dukes' C patients. With a median follow-up of 50 mo, the rate of distant metastases was 19% after preoperative radiation and surgery as compared to 26% after surgery alone ($p = 0.02$), and this translated to a survival advantage for irradiated patients ($p = 0.02$). Although the disease-free interval was initially longer in the preoperative radiation group, the lower rate of distant metastases and overall survival advantage after preoperative radiation were not durable with longer follow-up totaling 107 mo. The loss in the survival advantage, however, was accounted for by the higher perioperative mortality rate in the preoperative radiation group because the disease-specific survival rate continued to show an advantage when radiation was administered ($p < 0.01$).

The advantages of preoperative radiation were then shown in the Swedish Rectal Trial that randomized patients to surgery alone or preoperative radiation. Consistent with the previously reported Stockholm experience, preoperative therapy totaled 25Gy/5 fractions over 1 wk followed by surgery within 1 wk *(50,51)*. After 5 yr of follow-up, the local recurrence rate was 11% in the preoperative radiation group and 27% with surgery alone ($p < 0.001$). Improvements in local control were observed among all stages of disease. The overall survival rate at 5 yr was also significantly improved and totaled 58% in the preoperative radiation group as compared to 48% in the surgery alone group ($p = 0.004$). The cancer-specific survival rates at 9 yr was 74% with preoperative radiation and 65% with surgery alone ($p = 0.002$).

The outcomes and toxicities of preoperative and postoperative radiation were compared in the Uppsala Trial. Treatment was randomized between a short course of preoperative radiation or high-dose postoperative radiation among 471 patients with resectable rectal cancer *(52)*. In the preoperative radiation arm, 236 patients received five 5.1 Gy/fraction to a total dose of 25.5 Gy over 5–7 d; surgical resection was performed 1 wk later. In the postoperative radiation arm, radiation was initiated 4–6 wk after surgery in 235 patients. Patients received 40 Gy at 2 Gy/fraction over 4 wk; at this point, radiation was discontinued for 10–14 d, and then an additional 10 Gy was administered to the entire pelvis and another 10 Gy was administered to a reduced treatment volume. With this postoperative regimen, the pelvis received 50 Gy and the tumor bed received 60 Gy. Only patients who had evidence of transmural extension of disease or positive pelvic nodes at resection received postoperative chemotherapy. Although the radiation doses and the effective biological doses were substantially different in this trial, a local control benefit was observed with preoperative radiation over postoperative radiation; local failure rates at 5 yr were 13% vs 22%. There was no difference in the survival rates among the study groups.

Moderate to mild acute radiation effects were observed in virtually all patients receiving postoperative radiation in these trials. Acute radiation effects, like diarrhea and cystitis, were infrequent in the preoperative arm. Perioperative complications included small bowel obstruction, diagnosed radiographically or requiring surgical intervention, in 6% after surgery alone, 5% after preoperative therapy, and 11% after postoperative radiation. However, perioperative complications were more common after preoperative therapy. For example, perineal wound sepsis occurred after abdominoperineal resection in 33% of the preoperative radiation group and in 18% of the postoperative radiation group *(52–54)*. However, because of perioperative complications, half of the patients in the postoperative group could not start radiation therapy within the recommended 6 wk after surgery.

Although the Stockholm trials identified advantages of combined modality therapy, significant late morbidity was also observed. Peripheral nerves are relatively resistant to the late effects of radiation, but lumbosacral plexopathy occurred with the preoperative radiation regimen used in this trial *(52)*. Other late adverse effects of this preoperative radiation regimen included thromboembolism ($p = 0.01$), femoral neck and pelvic fractures ($p = 0.03$), intestinal obstruction ($p = 0.02$), and postoperative fistulae ($p = 0.01$). However, no increase in genitourinary complications was observed.

The radiation techniques that were used significantly influenced the risk for complications and mortality. Complications resulting from small bowel toxicity were higher because the superior border was placed at L2 in many of the studies, rather than at the L5/S1 interspace *(52–54)*. Higher mortality rates were observed among patients treated with anterior–posterior opposed portals as compared to three- or four-field techniques (15% vs 3%; $p < 0.001$). Because of these complications, the overall mortality rates were the same for the surgery alone and the preoperative radiation groups. Although the addition of radiation therapy significantly improved the local control and disease-specific survival rates, the morbidity of radiation therapy was substantial enough to negate the impact of these results.

Another experience with hypofractionated preoperative radiation among 83 patients, however, did not result in significant treatment-related morbidity. Like the Swedish Rectal Trial, 25 Gy was given in 5 fractions over 1 wk, followed by surgery (50,55). However, anterior–posterior portals were avoided and the superior border of the radiation field was limited to the L5–S1 interspace. With a mean follow-up of about 5 yr, the actuarial local control rate is 95% and the disease-specific survival rate is 77%. Only 13% of cases experienced a ≥ grade 3 perioperative or late toxicity; there was a 3.5% incidence of bowel obstruction. No significant difference in the toxicity profile was seen among the 16 patients who also received chemotherapy during radiation.

Although it does not represent a prospective randomized trial, the Patterns of Care Study evaluated survival on the basis of whether radiation was given preoperatively or postoperatively and whether chemotherapy was given during radiation. Local failure rates were approximately 10% for all stages and treatment arms. The Patterns of Care Study also found a significantly higher survival rate with preoperative radiation and with postoperative chemoradiation when compared to postoperative radiation alone. At 5 yr, the overall survival rate with postoperative radiation was 50% and it was 85% with preoperative radiation and 69% with postoperative chemoradiation (11).

These studies demonstrated the benefit of radiation therapy in reducing risk for local failure with possible impact on overall survival. Variations in radiation techniques and administered chemotherapy impact significantly on morbidity and outcomes. It is difficult to interpret outcomes from radiation with planned treatment interruptions. It is recognized that these treatment interruptions were included to improve tolerance to therapy. Some trials included chemotherapy agents that provided no benefit, but may have contributed to overall toxicity of therapy. The routes and schedules of administration of chemotherapy also has a significant impact on patterns of failure. Because no direct comparison between preoperative and postoperative conventional radiation schedules has been performed with standardized chemotherapy, a comparison of the relative advantages and disadvantages of preoperative and postoperative chemoradiation remain theoretical.

2.4. Preoperative Radiation

Preoperative radiation capitalizes on the disadvantages of postoperative radiation. The key advantage of preoperative radiation is the potential reduction in tumor size, allowing a greater chance for a sphincter-preserving surgical procedure. This is especially important for lesions located in the distal rectum. Response to preoperative radiation also results in sterilization of potential sites of microscopic residual disease, such as the radial surgical margin and regional lymphatics (56–60). Because the blood supply has not been disrupted by surgery, the effects of both radiation and chemotherapy are potentially enhanced. This allows administration of a lower total dose of radiation, which also reduces the risk for radiation morbidity. The risk of radiation morbidity also decreases with preoperative radiation because the small bowel is more mobile before surgery and can be displaced from the radiation field (61,62). The ability to assess response to chemotherapy and radiation also may have prognostic importance.

The disadvantages of preoperative radiation include the lack of pathological tumor staging (56,57). Surgical expertise is needed to minimize perioperative morbidity because surgical resection is performed in an irradiated field (50,63). Additionally, a two-stage surgical approach that initially involves resection with fecal diversion followed by re-establishment of intestinal continuity is generally necessary to allow adequate healing of the anastomosis.

A meta-analysis was performed among 6426 patients with resectable rectal cancer in 14 randomized controlled trials who received preoperative radiotherapy or surgery alone. Even though higher rates of morbidity were reported in some studies, no overall increase in post-operative mortality was reported with radiation *(64)*. Preoperative radiation was found to reduce the 5-yr overall mortality rate, cancer-related mortality rate, and local recurrence rate.

Sphincter preservation is a major goal of preoperative radiation therapy. The current application of preoperative chemoradiation builds upon the experience with postoperative combined-modality therapy and the data that demonstrate the efficacy of preoperative radiation alone *(48,62,65)*. Tumors located <6 cm from the anal verge would generally require an APR. However, variation exists in surgical practices, whether or not preoperative radiation is used. Among 18,695 cases of operable rectal cancer in Ontario, a wide variation was demonstrated in APR rates and referral for postoperative radiation relative to geographic location *(66)*. Sphincter-preservation rates after preoperative radiation or chemoradiation also vary but are reported to range between 65% and 85% *(56,57,67)*. The variation among these results can probably be related to the details of the clinical presentation, including invasion of the sphincter muscles by the tumor and tumor size and circumference. However, the interim analysis of the NASBP trial showed that only 27% of patients were converted from an APR to a sphincter-preserving procedure *(68)*. The reasons for this were considered to be unclear.

Based on sphincter preservation and the other considerations, like lower total radiation dose and tumor oxygenation, many centers have evaluated the use of preoperative radiation therapy. The more recent series have administered chemotherapy with preoperative radiation. The results of these reports are summarized in Table 4. With preoperative radiation alone, the pathological complete response rate is about 15%. With bolus or infusional 5-FU during the first and last week of radiation, the pathologic complete response rates are about 20%. Using a continuous infusion of 5-FU throughout the course of preoperative radiation, the pathological complete response rate increased to 27% *(63)*. Tumor regression or downstaging is evident in about 65% of cases. Sphincter preservation after preoperative chemoradiation is possible in more than two-thirds of patients with low rectal cancers.

Factors that can increase tumor regression and the possibility of performing a sphincter-sparing surgery include allowing an appropriate interval between completion of radiation therapy and surgery to maximize tumor regression, administration of higher radiation doses, and the administration of chemotherapy. Issues specific to chemotherapy during preoperative radiation include the type of agent and the schedule of infusion.

The interval between completion of preoperative radiation and surgery is critical to allow maximal tumor regression. When the interval between preoperative radiation alone, totaling 39 Gy in 3 wk, and surgery increased from 2 wk to 6–8 wk, the downstaging rate was also increased from 10% to 26% *(69)*. Although it was intended that surgery be performed within 10 d of completion of radiation in the Swedish Rectal Cancer Trial, a wide range (5–155 d) of time occurred radiation and surgery *(50)*. It was found that the downstaging rate was only 4% among patient who were resected within 10 d of completing therapy. By comparison, the downstaging rate was 45% when more than 10 d elapsed between completion of radiation and surgery. Another trial specifically evaluated the interval between completion of 39 Gy in 13 fractions and pathologic downstaging after surgery among 201 patients *(70)*.

The possible disadvantage of attempts to increase the total dose given during preoperative radiation is the possible increase in treatment-related toxicity. Although this was not reported in one dose-escalation trial that used an intermittent infusion of 5-FU during radiation, no

Table 4
Results of Published Series with Preoperative Radiation Therapy

Study	No. resected	Preop XRT dose	CTX during XRT	Interval between XRT and resection	Complete response rate	Downstaging rate	SP rate
Janjan et al. *(72)*	42	45 Gy pelvis + CB (7.5 Gy)	CI 5-FU 300 mg/m²; d/wk during pelvic XRT	4–6 wk	31%	86%	79%
Bosset et al. 2000	60	45 Gy	Bolus 5-FU Wk 1: 350–450 mg/m² wk 5 370–350 mg/m²	3 wk (range 13–111 d)	15.6%	30%	58%
Pucciarelli et al. 2000	51	45 Gy	5-d infusion 5-FU 350 mg/m² d 1–5 and 29–33	4–5 wk (range 19–53 d)	15.7%	59%	84%
Valentini et al. 1999	40	45 Gy to the pelvis + 5.4 Gy boost	5-d infusion 5-FU 1000 mg/m² d 1–4 and 29–32 CDDP 60 mg/m² d 1+29	6–8 wk	23%	68%	85%
Movsas et al. *(71)*	23	45 Gy to pelvis + hyperfx boost to total doses of 54.6, 57, or 61.8 Gy	5-d infusion 5-FU 1000 mg/m² d 1–4 and 29–32	4–6 wk	17.4%	57%	30%
Janjan et al. *(63)*	117	45 Gy to pelvis	CI 5-FU 300 mg/m²; d/wk during pelvic XRT	4–6 wk	27%	62%	59%
Wagman et al. 1998	35	46.8 Gy to pelvis + 3.6 Gy boost	No	4–5 wk	14%	63%	77%
Mohiuddin et al. 1998	70	40 to 45 Gy + 10–15 Gy boost	No	5–10 wk	NR	30%	86%

Note: Included are reported rates of sphincter preservation, pathological complete response and tumor downstaging. XRT = radiation therapy; CTX = chemotherapy; SP = sphincter preservation; NR = not reported; hyperfx = hyperfractionated; CI = continuous infusion; CB = concomitant boost.

significant improvements in response parameters, like the rates of pathological complete response, downstaging, or sphincter preservation, were observed *(71)*. A dose-response relationship for downstaging with preoperative radiation alone was identified at 44 Gy with conventional fractionation *(69)*. This relationship held for Duke's stage A and B, but not in stage C disease.

Reports have demonstrated the benefit when 5-FU is administered as a continuous infusion during radiation. This was confirmed in the experience with postoperative chemoradiation where disease-free and overall survival benefit was observed with the administration of 5-FU as a continuous infusion *(20)*. This is also inferred from the results with preoperative radiation using conventional fractionation and from the preliminary results with the concomitant boost experience *(59,60,63,72)*. Using lower total doses of preoperative radiation, 45 Gy, downstaging parameters with a continuous infusion of 5-FU were comparable to series that administered higher total radiation doses. When accelerated fractionation (concomitant boost) was used to deliver a total radiation dose of 52.5 Gy with a continuous infusion of 5-FU, the pathological complete response rates were nearly twice that of other series using the same or higher doses of radiation and bolus/intermittent infusion of 5-FU. The pathological downstaging rates were approximately 20% higher than those achieved with other series that used bolus/intermittent infusion of 5-FU.

In addition to its potential influence on sphincter preservation, tumor downstaging may also have prognostic importance. The level of response to preoperative radiation for locally advanced rectal cancers also has been reported to influence survival rates. Improved survival rates were observed among patients who had pathologic evidence of downstaging after preoperative radiation *(69)*. The 5-yr overall survival after preoperative radiation was 92% for patients whose tumors were downstaged to a Dukes' stage 0-A lesion; these 5-yr survival rates decreased to 67% and 26% when the pathologic stage was Dukes' B and C, respectively. The corresponding disease-free survival rates were 87%, 56%, and 28% for pathologic Dukes' stage 0-A, B, and C tumors, respectively.

Another trial showed that higher cancer-specific survival rates, 100% versus 45% at 5 yr, were observed among patients who had pathologic evidence of tumor downstaging after preoperative radiation and bolus 5-FU. The 5-yr recurrence-free survival rate was 94% with downstaging as compared to 50% without downstaging *(73)*. A similar relationship was seen with 5-FU given as a continuous infusion with preoperative radiation *(74)*. Any response to preoperative chemoradiation resulted in a reduced risk for distant metastases and improved disease-free survival.

Higher rates of tumor regression have been correlated among smaller tumors, with high Ki-67 levels, and mitotic activity, and elevated posttumor proliferative activity strongly correlated with improved survival *(75)*. Because fluorodeoxyglucose–positron-emission tomography (FDG-PET) provides functional imaging of tumors, PET scans are now being used in the investigational setting to evaluate response to preoperative chemoradiation *(76)*.

The risk for pelvic relapse was evaluated as a function of total radiation dose and overall treatment time. Accounting for the overall duration of radiation, the dose-response curve was found to be steep *(77)*. The time-related displacement of the dose-response curve showed a median tumor doubling time of about 4–5 d. This doubling time was more rapid than that of the primary tumor at diagnosis. It was considered that acceleration of growth among subclinical deposits of tumor in the pelvis was rapid during preoperative radiation. Strategies that shorten overall treatment time or that provide uninterrupted administration of antineoplastic therapy should be targeted to improve tumor response with preoperative radiation for rectal cancer. This is consistent with the clinical approach that uses a continuous infusion of 5-FU and with accelerated fractionation.

2.5. Oral Administration of 5-FU Analogs

A variety of oral fluoropyrimidine analogs are becoming available. Most of the data relate to their use as chemotherapeutic agents alone. Data are extremely limited at this point regarding their administration during either preoperative or postoperative radiation *(78–84)*. Although the use of oral fluoropyrimidines has many theoretical advantages, they must be compared to the intravenous administration of 5-FU in order to optimize dose administration for efficacy and to minimize associated toxicity.

Early experience during preoperative radiation involved a dose-escalation trial to establish the maximum tolerated dose (MTD). It was determined that the MTD of oral uracil and tegafur was 350 mg/m^2/d with 90 mg/d of leucovorin when given 5 d/wk concurrent with radiation *(78)*. Results were comparable to those with infusional 5-FU with a sphincter-preserving surgery performed in 12 of 14 patients and a pathologic complete response in 3 cases.

Several advantages exist for the use of an oral route of chemotherapy administration. Among these are the ease of administration and avoidance of the inconvenience, discomfort, and cost associated with either bolus or continuous infusion of 5-FU *(79–81)*. Some of the newer agents also may concentrate to a greater degree within tumor cells as compared to infusional 5-FU. Importantly, though, severe diarrhea is the dose-limiting toxicity in most of these oral agents *(82,83)*. When compared to infusional 5-FU, the incidence of mucositis, neutropenia, and hand–foot syndrome is small *(84)*.

With oral agents, however, come concerns regarding patient compliance in taking the medications. The pharmacokinetics of drug administration also must be assured, especially when taken in lower doses during radiation. A variety of oral fluoropyrimidines have been developed and each has its own metabolic characteristics *(85,86)*. Some result in complete inactivation of dihydropyrimidine dehydrogenase (DPD) activity *(87)*. Because of this it is unclear if the agent should be taken at a specific time relative to the administration of radiation.

Many issues need to be resolved before oral fluoropyrimidines become the new standard of care during radiation therapy. Because of the differences among the agents, each will require clinical assessment with radiation therapy. The activity of other agents, like CPT-11 and oxaliplatin, will need to be considered relative to the use of oral fluoropyrimides as well *(88)*.

2.6. Local Excision

As part of the trend to maintain sphincter function, radiation therapy has been used with local excision among early-stage tumors that involve the distal rectum. A Radiation Therapy Oncology Group trial was among the first reports using this approach. Based on tumor size and stage, grade, and surgical margin, 65 patients were either observed or underwent adjuvant treatment with 5-FU and one of two radiation dose levels *(89)*. A total of 14 patients were followed with observation because they had microscopic confirmation of a total excision, a well/moderately well differentiated stage T1 tumor that was <3 cm in size, and no evidence of vascular or lymphatic permeation on pathology. With a median follow-up of 5 yr, 11 patients had recurrent tumor. Local failure correlated with T stage; 4% T1, 16% T2, and 23% T3 tumors recurred. Other factors that influenced local failure rates were degree of circumferential involvement; 6% of tumors with less than 20% circumferential involvement as compared to an 18% local failure rate when 20–40% of the circumference was involved.

Patient selection is extremely important in performing a local excision. Because lymph nodes are not resected with a local excision, it is contraindicated to perform a local excision on a patient with evident lymph node metastases *(90)*. The depth of tumor penetration and the tumor grade are directly related to the risk for perirectal nodal involvement. The risk for lymph node involvement in a low-grade T2 tumor is about 12% in contrast to the 55%

risk of nodal involvement with a high-grade T2 tumor. Other studies have shown that tumor ulceration and histologic evidence of lymphatic, vascular, or perineural invasion are also associated with an increased risk of nodal metastases *(90,91)*. Tumors should be 3 cm or less in size and involve less than one-half of the rectal circumference. Fewer complications are associated with a transanal rather than a Kraske approach to local excision and postoperative radiation *(92)*.

Radiation therapy after local excision is unnecessary in T1 tumors that have favorable characteristics because the risk for local failure is less than 10%. Postoperative radiation is recommended among T1 tumors with unfavorable characteristics or T2 tumors because the risk for local failure is about 20% *(66,91–93)*. A complete surgical resection with mesorectal excision is recommended among patients with T3 tumors because of the risk for tumor cut-through and inadequate lymph node resection with local excision. The local recurrence rate was approximately 30% among patients with T3 tumors that were treated with local excision and chemoradiation because they refused or were unfit to undergo a radical resection.

Radiation techniques are similar to those with postoperative therapy. The entire pelvis is treated to 45 Gy, with the boost volume receiving a total dose of 54–65 Gy depending on the margins of resection and/or aggressive histologic features *(91)*. It is critical to avoid small bowel in the radiation boost volume.

The use of preoperative chemoradiation followed by local excision is controversial because of the lack of pathologic data. This is especially critical to avoid radiation among T1 cases with favorable characteristics. However, it is less controversial for T2 and T3 tumors. Traditionally, preoperative chemoradiation or radiation alone followed by local excision has been used among patients who refuse or who are medically unfit for a radical resection *(94)*. Because of pathologic downstaging and the theoretical advantages with preoperative chemoradiation, this approach has judiciously applied.

2.7. Endocavitary Radiation and Brachytherapy

Brachytherapy and endocavitary radiation can be used alone or, more commonly, in conjunction with external beam radiation. Administering highly localized doses of radiation can provide high doses of radiation directly to well-defined volumes to achieve local control with definitive radiation. Most often, these approaches are used among patients who are unable or unwilling to undergo surgical resection (*see* Chapter 12).

Contact or endocavitary radiation is another approach in the conservative management of rectal tumors. Soft 50-kV X-rays are produced by a generator that delivers radiation through a tube that contains an anode and ring filament *(95)*. Two aluminum filters can be used and the 0.5-cm filter is used for most applications. With the 0.5-cm aluminum filter and a focal distance of 4 cm, with a 20-cGy/min output, and a 3-cm circular field, the percentage depth dose is 100% at 0 mm, 44% at 5 mm, 23% at 10 mm, and 9% at 20 mm depth. Because of this, highly infiltrative tumors are not amenable to contact therapy. The tumor must be within 12 cm of the anal verge and accessible; on occasion, posterior wall tumors are difficult to localize with the cone.

The dose of the first contact treatment is between 30 and 40 Gy in 2–4 min with a 0.5-mm aluminum filter. One to two weeks later a second, application of contact radiation is administered. Three weeks after the initiation of therapy, the third contact application is performed; at this time, a smaller (2 cm) cone is generally used to account for tumor regression. For 3-cm tumors, 90–120 Gy is given in 4–5 fractions over 5–8 wk. For tumors less than 2 cm that regress completely after two sessions, a total dose of 80 Gy in 4 fractions

(30 Gy on d 1; 20 Gy on d 7; 15 Gy on d 21, and 15 Gy on d 36) is sufficient *(95)*. The normal mucosa of the rectal wall should not receive more than 15–20 Gy.

Like the use of local excision, patient selection is critical to the success of contact therapy. For the same reasons, any patient with lymph node involvement is not a candidate for contact therapy *(95)*. Factors that increase risk for lymph node involvement, like high histologic grade, perineural or lymphvascular invasion, or ulceration, are generally contraindications for contact therapy. The response to contact therapy also is predictive of therapeutic success. The chance for local control is good if the tumor regresses by more than 80% of its original volume by 2 wk after the second contact session.

Complete response was achieved in over 90% of patients with endocavitary therapy in one series. Local failure occurred in 28%, but the addition of external beam radiation in cases with poor prognostic factors improved local control. Local failure was more common with tumor size (>3 cm) and partially fixed tumors. Accounting for salvage therapy, sphincter preservation was accomplished in 84% and local control was accomplished in 82% *(96)*. Severe late effects occurred in 4% of those treated.

The techniques used for brachytherapy depend on anatomic constraints. Four techniques have been described and include the use of metallic needles through a perineal template, an iridium fork, a plastic loop technique, and the use of a remote after-loading device *(95)*. In order to localize the radiation dose to the lesion and avoid treatment of the opposite rectal wall, obturators are often used in conjunction with the implant to distend the rectum.

Patients with lesions <3 cm in size can be treated with brachytherapy alone, but external beam radiation should be added for larger size tumors. Using this approach, 90% rates of local control are obtained without significant complication *(97)*. Although continuous low-dose-rate brachytherapy is usually used, a pulsed low dose rate can give similar late effects and be considered as an alternative approach *(98)*.

Both endocavitary therapy and brachytherapy offer alternative and effective means of administering localized radiation, especially among patients with limited treatment options. Further integration of these techniques should be considered, as therapy is optimized to use more conservative surgical approaches to the treatment of rectal cancer.

2.8. Recurrent Rectal Cancer

Recurrent rectal cancer can vary significantly in its clinical presentation and it requires a broad range of therapeutic approaches. When the recurrence is identified early, the patient is usually asymptomatic and resection is possible. Regrettably, many patients are diagnosed with recurrent rectal cancer only after diagnostic evaluations are performed to evaluate progressive symptoms and they are often found to be inoperable. Because the morbidity of recurrent disease is so profound, aggressive therapeutic attempts are frequently undertaken to secure local–regional control.

Recurrent disease among patients who have previously been treated with radiation poses significant challenges. Approaches have included reirradiation with external beam therapy and intraoperative radiation therapy (IORT). The dose of external beam radiation has varied when given to patients who have been previously been treated with radiation, especially when given in conjunction with IORT. Bleeding, pain, and mass effect were palliated with reirradiation among 100%, 65%, and 24% of cases, respectively; 80%, 33%, and 20%, respectively, were palliated until the time of death *(99,100)*. The acute grade 3 toxicity rate was 31%, and the late grade 3 and grade 4 toxicity rates were 23% and 10%, respectively, including a 17% rate of small bowel obstruction. The only factor that reduced the toxicity rates was hyperfractionation. However, the factors that influenced median survival were

Karnofsky Performance Status (KPS), the initial stage of disease, and the radiation dose given at the time of reirradiation ($\leq$30.6 Gy = 22 mo vs >30.6 Gy = 9.5 mo median survival).

The risk for and outcomes after the diagnosis of recurrent rectal cancer is the same among patients initially treated with an APR or low-anterior resection (18% and 24%, respectively). Of the 175 patients evaluated in one study of recurrent rectal cancer, 25 had an isolated pelvic recurrence *(101)*. The survival rate among the patients with an isolated pelvic recurrence of disease who received radiotherapy was significantly greater (16 mo) as compared to those who were treated with palliative operations or analgesics (2.4 mo).

One study evaluated 519 patients with locally recurrent rectal cancer at The Princess Margaret Hospital. Relapse of disease occurred after an APR among 326 patients, after a low anterior resection among 151 patients, and in 42 after a local excision. No patients had previously been treated with radiation *(102)*. The mean time between the initial surgery and radiation therapy was 18 mo (3–138 mo). The relapse was confined to the pelvis among 355 cases, but distant metastases were found in 32% (164 cases) at the time that the local recurrence was also discovered. A total dose of $\geq$ 35 Gy was given to 214 patients with 1.8- to 2.5-Gy fractions. The median survival was 14 mo and the median time to local disease progression was 5 mo. The pelvic disease progression-free rate was 7% and the 5-yr survival was 5%. Multivariate analysis showed that overall survival was correlated to the ECOG performance status, absence of extrapelvic metastases, long intervals between the initial surgery and radiotherapy, total radiation dose, and absence of obstructive uropathy.

No dose-response relationship was found to exist for recurrent rectal cancer on a review of the available retrospective series in the literature. No significant differences were observed in the initial response or the durability of the response to therapy *(103)*. The significance of persistent pelvic disease is seen in the dose-response relationship when patients with primary untreated cancers were compared to those with postoperative residual disease.

Three dose regimens were used at the Peter MacCallum Cancer Institute for incompletely resected, locally recurrent rectal cancer. These regimens included 50–60 Gy (designated as radical radiation) or 45 Gy (high-dose radiation) with conventional fractionation; palliative radiation of <45 Gy was given to others. No significant difference was observed between the radical or high-dose radiation groups with regard to symptomatic relief (about 80%); only 33% of those receiving palliative therapy, however, achieved partial symptomatic relief *(104)*. The estimated median survival was 16 mo for all patients; for patients with radical radiation, the median survival was 26 mo compared to 16 mo with high-dose radiation. Survival was compromised when macroscopic residual disease was present, with a median survival of 14 mo vs 31 mo with only microscopic residual tumor.

Intraoperative radiation has been used as a supplement to external beam radiation or as the only therapy when further external beam radiation is not possible. The outcomes were evaluated among 73 patients with recurrent rectal cancer; 86% of the patients studied had locally recurrent disease without metastases *(105)*. External beam radiation had been previously administered in 52% and the recurrences were located in the presacral region (radial margin) in 55% of cases. Surgical resection allowed for complete macroscopic resection of disease in 57%, partial resection with gross residual disease in 29%, and no resection in 14% of the recurrences. Intraoperative radiation was given ranging from 10 to 25 Gy; 30 patients received either preoperative or postoperative external beam radiation. Actuarial overall survival equaled 72% at 1 yr, 45% at 2 yr, and 31% at 3 yr; the actuarial local control rate was 71%, 48%, and 31%, respectively. The actuarial disease-free survival was 58%, 27%, and 18%. Therefore, controlling symptoms of recurrent disease was a critical factor for quality of life, given the relatively extended survival among these patients.

Actuarial survival was improved with complete or partial resection. Among the 21 cases of local failure, 8 were in the IORT field, 8 were in the external beam radiation field, and 3 occurred in areas that received both IORT and external beam radiation. In the IORT field, local control was 87% at 1 yr, 72% at 2 yr, and 65% at 3 yr. Actuarial local control in the IORT field was better without rather than with gross residual disease (77% vs 51% at 3 yr). Among patients with an isolated local recurrence and with a partial or complete resection, the local control rates with IORT plus external beam radiation was 61% at 3 yr and 0% with IORT alone. Four patients had long-term morbidity. These included one case of sciatic plexopathy that resolved with further follow-up (12 Gy IORT + 45 Gy postoperatively). Two cases of sacral necrosis occurred at 6 mo (39 Gy preoperatively + 25 Gy IORT) and at 13 mo (40 Gy preoperatively + 20 Gy IORT). There was one case of necrosis of L5 (28 Gy preoperatively + 15 Gy IORT) after 51 mo of follow-up.

The previous study showed an advantage when external beam radiation was added over IORT alone *(105)*. A phase I/II study of IORT for locally advanced or recurrent rectal cancer that was performed by the Radiation Therapy Oncology Group showed an advantage when IORT was added over external beam radiation alone *(106)*. Again, local control was dependent on the amount of residual disease; for all patients, the 2-yr actuarial local control rates were 77% (64% among the recurrent disease group) if no gross disease remained versus 10% if there was gross residual disease after surgery. For all patients and among the recurrent group, the overall survival was improved (88%) if there was no gross residual disease after surgery vs a 46% survival if gross residual disease was present. The 2-yr actuarial risk for major complications attributable to IORT was 16%. In virtually all clinical settings, IORT is feasible and adds less than 1 h to the surgical procedure *(107)*.

Combined-modality therapy, which includes chemoradiation and surgical resection, improved resectability, local control, and survival. In one study of 47 patients who received a preoperative dose of 45 Gy with concomitant 5-FU and mitomycin chemotherapy *(108)*, an objective response to therapy occurred in over 50% of cases and 45% underwent a radical resection. Pain relief was accomplished in 86% and higher radiation doses correlated with better pain control. Radical resection resulted in better local control and survival. The overall 5-yr survival and local control rates were 22% and 32%, respectively; when IORT was given, the 5-yr rates were 79% and 41%, respectively. The modified Suzuki classification was found to be prognostic. In this classification, the recurrent tumor has no contact with the pelvic side wall in the F0 group. In the F1 group, less than 1/4 of the pelvic side wall is involved, and between 1/4 and 1/2 of the circumference of the pelvic side wall is involved in F2 disease. More than 1/2 of the circumference of the pelvic side wall is involved in F3 disease. Infiltration of the bone or small bowel occurs in F4 disease. This classification correlated closely with the level of pain, disease-free survival, and overall survival.

No significant difference was seen among three different intraoperative radiation approaches for recurrent colorectal cancer that included IORT, high-dose-rate brachytherapy, and intraoperative placement of iodine-125 seeds. The overall 5-yr local control rate was 26% *(109)*. Tumors in the para-aortic region had better rates of local control than tumors located in the pelvis (65% vs 19% at 5 yr), but this did not translate into an improvement in overall survival rates. The 5-yr overall survival rate was 4%; only the presence of residual disease (30% for microscopic and 7% for macroscopic at 3-yr) and administration of postoperative external beam radiation (48% vs 12% at 3 yr and 24% and 0% at 5 yr) influenced overall survival rates. Identifying residual disease may also be difficult. Radioimmunoguided surgery has been advocated to identify occult tumor deposits that may result in failure to completely resect the disease *(110)*.

Combined-modality therapy that includes IORT for recurrent colorectal cancer can result in wound-healing problems. With primary closure, one series reported a 46–65% rate of wound-healing problems *(111)*. However, introduction of unirradiated tissue via myocutaneous flap reconstruction reduces the risk for major complications to 12% *(112)*.

Irrespective of the use of IORT, resection of recurrent disease often requires an extensive surgical procedure for tumor clearance. This is often complicated by a prior history of radiation or reirradiation. Resection of recurrent disease was possible among 79% of patients (103 of 131 cases) and this resulted in a 31% 5-yr survival rate. Favorable prognostic factors included a normal preoperative carcinoembryonic antigen (CEA) level and recurrent tumor that is limited to the bowel wall *(113)*. Aggressive surgical resection, including abdominosacral resection for fixed tumors, also can result in a 31% long-term survival rate *(114)*. These aggressive surgical approaches are possible with reconstruction procedures that include placement of a myocutaneous graft.

In summary, long-term survival is possible among patients with recurrent disease if it is found early and total surgical resection is possible. Radiation therapy is needed to clear potential nests of residual microscopic tumor. Because of prior therapies, like surgery and radiation, these tumor cells may be in hypoxic regions that require higher radiation doses. Reirradiation, especially with hyperfractionated treatment schedules, is well tolerated.

3. CONCLUSION

There has been substantial progress in the therapy of rectal cancer, especially with the advent of combined-modality therapy. Each modality contributes to local and systemic control of disease, and they have allowed the development of function-preserving surgical approaches. These combined-modality approaches also are effective in cases of recurrent disease and some patients may be rendered disease-free. Radiation therapy remains an integral aspect in the treatment of all clinical presentations of rectal cancer.

REFERENCES

1. Krook JE, Moertel CG, Gunderson LL, Wieand HS, Collins RT, Beart RW, et al. Effective surgical adjuvant therapy for high-risk rectal carcinoma. *N. Engl. J. Med.*, **324** (1991) 709–715.
2. Douglas HO, Moertel CG, Mayer RJ, et al. Survival after postoperative combination treatment of rectal cancer. *N. Engl. J. Med.*, **315** (1986) 1294–1295.
3. Gastrointestinal Tumor Study Group. Prolongation of the disease-free interval in surgically treated rectal carcinoma. *N. Engl. J. Med.*, **312** (1985) 1465–1472.
4. Gastrointestinal Tumor Study Group. Survival after postoperative combination treatment of rectal cancer. *N. Engl. J. Med.*, **315** (1986) 1294–1295.
5. Fisher B, Wolmark N, Rockette H, Redmond C, Deutsch M, Wickerham DL, et al. other NSABP Investigators. Postoperative adjuvant chemotherapy or radiation therapy for rectal cancer: results from NSABP R-01. *J. Natl. Cancer. Inst.*, **80** (1988) 21–29.
6. Freedman GM and Coia LR. Adjuvant and neoadjuvant treatment of rectal cancer. *Semin. Oncol.*, **22** (1995) 611–624.
7. Gunderson LL and Martenson JA. Postoperative adjuvant irradiation with or without chemotherapy for rectal carcinoma. *Semin. Radiat. Oncol.*, **3** (1993) 55–63.
8. *Adjuvant Therapy of Rectal Cancer.* National Cancer Institute, Bethesda, MD, 1991.
9. Jessup JM, Stewart AK, and Menck HR. The National Cancer Data Base Report on Patterns of Care for Adenocarcinoma of the Rectum, 1985–1995. *Cancer*, **83** (1998) 2408–2418.
10. Minsky BD, Coia L, Haller DG, Hoffman J, John M, Landry J, et al. Radiation therapy for rectosigmoid and rectal cancer: results of the 1992–1994 Patterns of Care Process Survey. *J. Clin. Oncol.*, **16** (1998) 2542–2547.
11. Coia LR, Gunderson LL, Haller D, Hoffman J, Mohiuddin M, Tepper JE, et al. Outcomes of patients receiving radiation for carcinoma of the rectum. *Cancer*, **86** (1999) 1952–1958.

12. Kinsella TJ. An approach to the radiosensitization of human tumors. *Cancer J.*, **2** (1996) 184–193.
13. Milas L. Chemoradiation interactions: potential of newer chemotherapeutic agents. In *American Society of Clinical Oncology Educational Handbook*, American Society of Clinical Oncology, Washington, DC, 2000, pp. 207–213.
14. Koutcher JA, Alfieri AA, Thaler H, Matei C, and Martin DS. Radiation enhancement by biochemical modulation and 5-fluorouracil. *Int. J. Radiat. Oncol. Biol. Phys.*, **39** (1997) 1145–1152.
15. Coleman CN. Clinical radiosensitization: why it does and does not work. *J. Clin. Oncol.*, **17** (1999) 1–3.
16. Coleman CN. Radiation and chemotherapy sensitizers and protectors. In *Cancer Chemotherapy and Biotherapy*, Chabner BA and Longo DL (eds.), 1996, pp. 553–583.
17. Steele GG and Peckham MJ. Exploitable mechanisms in combined radiotherapy-chemotherapy: the concept of additivity. *Int. J. Radiat. Oncol. Biol. Phys.*, **5** (1979) 85–91.
18. Steele GG. The search for therapeutic gain in the combination of radiotherapy and chemotherapy. *Radiother. Oncol.*, **11** (1988) 31–53.
19. Tepper JE, O'Connell MJ, Petroni GR, Hollis D, Cooke E, Benson AB, et al. Adjuvant postoperative fluorouracil modulated chemotherapy combined with pelvic radiation therapy for rectal cancer: initial results of intergroup 0114. *J. Clin. Oncol.*, **15** (1997) 2030–2039.
20. O'Connell MJ, Martenson JA, Wieand HS, Krook JE, Macdonald JS, Haller DG, et al. Improving adjuvant therapy for rectal cancer by combining protracted-infusion fluorouracil with radiation therapy after curative surgery. *N. Engl. J. Med.*, **331** (1994) 502–507.
21. Tominaga T, Sakabe T, Koyama Y, Hamano K, Yasutomi M, Takahashi T, et al. for the Steering Committee of the Colorectal Cancer Chemotherapy Study Group Japan. Prognostic factors for patients with colon or rectal carcinoma treated with resection only-five year followup report. *Cancer*, **78** (1996) 403–408.
22. Phillips RKS, Hittinger R, Blesovsky L, et al. Local recurrence following "curative" surgery for large bowel cancer. 1. The overall picture. *Br. J. Surg.*, **71** (1984) 12–16.
23. Minsky BD, Conti JA, Huang Y, and Knopf K. Relationship of acute gastrointestinal toxicity and the volume of irradiated small bowel in patients receiving combined modality therapy for rectal cancer. *J. Clin. Oncol.*, **13** (1995) 1409–1416.
24. Brennan PC, Carr KE, Seed T, and McCullough JS. Acute and protracted radiation effects on small intestinal morphological parameters. *Int. J. Radiat. Biol.*, **73** (1998) 691–698.
25. Zheng H, Wang J, and Hauer-Jensen M. Role of mast cells in early and delayed radiation injury in rat intestine. *Radiat. Res.*, **153** (2000) 533–539.
26. Dublineau I, Ksas B, and Griffiths NM. Functional changes in the rat distal colon after whole-body irradiation: dose-response and temporal relationships. *Radiat. Res.*, **154** (2000) 187–195.
27. Hendricks T, Wobbes T, deMan BM, Hoogenhout J, and Seifert WF. Moderate doses of intraoperative radiation severely suppress early strength of anatomoses in the rat colon. *Radiat. Res.*, **150** (1998) 431–435.
28. Skwarchuk MW and Travis EL. Volume effects and epithelial regeneration in irradiated mouse colorectum. *Radiat. Res.*, **149** (1998) 1–10.
29. Seifert WF, Biert J, Wobbes T, Verhofstad AAJ, Hoogenhout J, and Hendriks. Late effects of intraoperative radiation therapy in anastomotic rat colon. *Int. J. Radiat. Oncol. Biol. Phys.*, **42** (1998) 623–629.
30. Koelbl O, Richter S, and Flentje M. Influence of patient positioning on dose-volume histogram and normal tissue complication probability for small bowel and bladder in patients receiving pelvic irradiation: a prospective study using a 3D planning system and a radiobiological model. *Int. J. Radiat. Oncol. Biol. Phys.*, **45** (1999) 1193–1198.
31. Das IJ, Lanciano RM, Movsas B, Kagawa K, and Barnes SJ. Efficacy of a belly board device with CT-simulation in reducing small bowel volume within pelvic irradiation fields. *Int. J. Radiat. Oncol. Biol. Phys.*, **39** (1997) 67–76.
32. Chun M, Timmerman RD, Mayer R, Ling MN, Sheldon J, and Fishman EK. Radiation therapy of external iliac lymph nodes with lateral pelvic portals: identification of patients at risk for inadequate regional coverage. *Radiology*, **194** (1995) 147–150.
33. Taylor N, Crane C, Skibber J, Feig B, Ellis L, Vauthey JN, et al. Elective groin irradiation is not indicated among patients with adenocarcinoma of the rectum extending to the anal canal. *Radiology*, **628(Suppl.)** (2000) 352 (abstract).
34. Tocchi A, Lepre L, Costa G, Liotta G, Mazzoni G, Agostini N, et al. Rectal cancer and inguinal metastases—prognostic role and therapeutic indications. *Dis. Colon Rectum*, **42** (1999) 1464–1466.
35. Lacerna MD, Sharpe MB, and Robertson JM. The effect of radiation on an ambulatory chemotherapy infusion pump. *Cancer*, **86** (1999) 2150–2153.
36. Wadler S, Benson AB, Engelking C, Catalano R, Field M, Kornblau SM, et al. Recommended guidelines for the treatment of chemotherapy-induced diarrhea. *J. Clin. Oncol.*, **16** (1998) 3169–3178.

37. Callister M, Janjan N, Crane C, Bisanz A, Evetts P, Allen P, et al. Effective management of symptoms during preoperative chemoradiation for locally advanced rectal cancer. *Int. J. Radiat. Oncol. Biol. Phys.*, **48(Suppl.)** (2000) 177 (abstract).

38. Kornblau S, Benson AB, Catalano R, Champlin RE, Engelking C, Field M, et al. Management of cancer treatment related diarrhea: issues and therapeutic strategies. *J. Pain Symptom Manage.*, **19** (2000) 118–129.

39. Denham JW, O'Brien PC, Dunstan RH, Johansen J, See A, Hamilton CS, et al. Is there more than one late radiation proctitis syndrome? *Radiother. Oncol.*, **51** (1999) 43–53.

40. Miller AR, Martenson JA, Nelson H, Schleck CD, Ilstrup DM, Gunderson LL, et al. The incidence and clinical consequences of treatment-related bowel injury. *Int. J. Radiat. Oncol. Biol. Phys.*, **43** (1999) 817–825.

41. Van Duijvendijk P, Slors JFM, Taat CW, van Lochem LT, Bonsel GJ, deVries JWA, et al. What is the benefit of preoperative sperm preservation for patients who undergo restorative proctocolectomy for benign disease? *Dis. Colon Rectum*, **43** (2000) 838–842.

42. Porter GA and Skibber JM. Outcomes research in surgical oncology. *Ann. Surg. Oncol.*, **7** (2000) 367–375.

43. Ramsey SD, Andersen MR, Etzioni R, Moinpour C, Peacock S, Potosky A, et al. Urban N. Quality of life in survivors of colorectal carcinoma. *Cancer*, **88** (2000) 1294–1303.

44. Ko CY, Rusin LC, Schoetz DJ, Moreau L, Coller JA, Murray JJ, et al. Does better functional result equate with better quality of life? Implications for surgical treatment in familial adenomatous polyposis. *Dis. Colon Rectum*, **43** (2000) 829–837.

45. Soffer EE and Hull T. Fecal incontinence: a practical approach to evaluation and treatment. *Am. J. Gastroenterol.*, **95** (2000) 1873–1880.

46. Ulander K, Jeppsson B, and Grahn G. Quality of life and independence in activities of daily living preoperatively and at follow-up in patients with colorectal cancer. *Support. Care Cancer*, **8** (1997) 402–409.

47. Minsky BD. Multidisciplinary management of resectable rectal cancer. *Oncology*, **10** (1996) 1701–1714.

48. Minsky BD, Cohen AM, Enker WE, and Paty P. Sphincter preservation with preoperative radiation therapy and coloanal anastomosis. *Int. J. Radiat. Oncol. Biol. Phys.*, **31** (1995) 553–559.

49. Cedermark B, Johansson H, Rutqvist LE, Wilking N, for the Stockholm Colorectal Cancer Study Group. The Stockholm I trial of preoperative short term radiotherapy in operable rectal carcinoma: a prospective randomized trial. *Cancer*, **75** (1995) 2269–2275.

50. Swedish Rectal Cancer Trial. Improved survival with preoperative radiotherapy in resectable rectal cancer. *N. Engl. J. Med.*, **336** (1997) 980–987.

51. Stockholm Colorectal Cancer Study Group. Randomized study on preoperative radiotherapy in rectal carcinoma. *Ann. Surg. Oncol.*, **3** (1996) 423–430.

52. Frykholm GJ, Glimelius B, and Pahlman L. Preoperative or postoperative irradiation in adenocarcinoma of the rectum: final treatment results of a randomized trial and an evaluation of late secondary effects. *Dis. Colon Rectum*, **36** (1993) 564–572.

53. Pahlman L and Glimelius B. Pre- or postoperative radiotherapy in rectal and rectosigmoid carcinoma: a report from a randomized multicenter trial. *Ann. Surg.*, **211** (1990) 187–195.

54. Frykholm GJ, Isacsson U, Nygard K, Montelius A, Jung B, Pahlman L, et al. Preoperative radiotherapy in rectal carcinoma—aspects of acute adverse effects and radiation technique. *Int. J. Radiat. Oncol. Biol. Phys.*, **35** (1996) 1039–1048.

55. Myerson RJ, Genovesi D, Lockett MA, Birnbaum E, Fleshman J, Fry R, et al. Five fractions of preoperative radiotherapy for selected cases of rectal carcinoma: long-term tumor control and tolerance to treatment. *Int. J. Radiat. Oncol. Biol. Phys.*, **43** (1999) 537–543.

56. Minsky BD. Adjuvant therapy of rectal cancer. *Semin. Oncol.*, **26** (1999) 540–544.

57. Minsky BD. Preoperative radiation therapy followed by low anterior resection with coloanal anastomosis. *Semin. Radiat. Oncol.*, **8** (1998) 30–35.

58. Bosset JF, Pelissier EP, Manion G, Pavy JJ, Horiot JC, Hamers HP, et al. Plea for a preoperative adjuvant approach in the management of rectal cancer. *Int. J. Radiat. Oncol. Biol. Phys.*, **29** (1994) 205–208.

59. Rich TA. Adjuvant radiotherapy for rectal cancer: more on pre- or postoperative therapy. *Int. J. Radiat. Oncol. Biol. Phys.*, **32** (1995) 547–548.

60. Rich TA, Skibber JM, Ajani JA, Buchholz DJ, Cleary KR, Dubrow RA, et al. Preoperative infusional chemoradiation therapy for stage T3 rectal cancer. *Int. J. Radiat. Oncol. Biol. Phys.*, **32** (1995) 1025–1029.

61. Coucke PA, Sartorelli B, Cuttat JF, Jeanneret W, Gillet M, and Mirimanoff RO. The rationale to switch from postoperative hyperfractionated accelerated radiotherapy to preoperative hyperfractionated accelerated radiotherapy in rectal cancer. *Int. J. Radiat. Oncol. Biol. Phys.*, **32** (1995) 181–188.

62. Minsky BD, Cohen AM, Enker WE, Kelsen DP, Kemeny N, and Frankel J. Efficacy of postoperative 5-FU, high-dose leucovorin, and sequential radiation therapy for clinically resectable rectal cancer. *Cancer Invest.*, **13** (1995) 1–7.

63. Janjan NA, Khoo VS, Rich TA, Evetts PA, Goswitz MS, Allen PK, et al. Locally advanced rectal cancer: surgical complications after infusional chemotherapy and radiation therapy. *Radiology*, **206** (1998) 131–136.

64. Camma C, Giunta M, Fiorica F, Pagliaro L, Craxi A, and Cottone M. Preoperative radiotherapy for resectable rectal cancer—a meta-analysis. *JAMA*, **284** (2000) 1008–1015.

65. Marks G, Mohiuddin M, Masoni L, and Montori A. High-dose preoperative radiation therapy as the key to extending sphincter-preservation surgery for cancer of the distal rectum. *Surg. Oncol. Clin. North. Am.*, **1** (1992) 71–86.

66. Paszat LF, Brundage MD, Groome PA, Schulze K, and Mackillop WJ. A population-based study of rectal cancer: permanent colostomy as an outcome. *Int. J. Radiat. Oncol. Biol. Phys.*, **45** (1999) 1185–1191.

67. Ng AK, Recht A, and Busse PM. Sphincter preservation therapy for distal rectal carcinoma—a review. *Cancer*, **79** (1997) 671–683.

68. Hyams DM, Mamounas EP, Petrelli N, et. al. A clinical trial to evaluate the worth of preoperative multimodal therapy in patients with operable carcinoma of the rectum: a progress report of the National Surgical Adjuvant Breast and Bowel Project protocol R-03. *Dis. Colon Rectum*, **40** (1997) 131–139.

69. Berger C, deMuret A, Garaud P, Chapet S, Bourlier P, Reynaud-Bougnoux A, et al. Preoperative radiotherapy *(RT)* for rectal cancer: predictive factors of tumor downstaging and residual tumor cell density [RTCD]: prognostic implications. *Int. J. Radiat. Oncol. Biol. Phys.*, **37** (1997) 619–627.

70. Francois Y, Nemoz CJ, Baulieux J, Vignal J, Grandjean JP, Partensky C, et al. Influence of the interval between preoperative radiation therapy and surgery on downstaging and on the rate of sphincter-sparing surgery for rectal cancer: the Lyon R90-01 randomized trial. *J. Clin. Oncol.*, **17** (1999) 2396–2402.

71. Movsas J, Hanlon AL, Lanciano R, Scher RM, Weiner LM, Sigurdson ER, et al. Phase I dose escalating trial of hyperfractionated pre-operative chemoradiation for locally advanced rectal cancer. *Int. J. Radiat. Oncol. Biol. Phys.*, **42** (1998) 43–50.

72. Janjan NA, Crane CH, Feig BW, Cleary K, Dubrow R, Curley S, et al. Prospective trial of preoperative concomitant boost radiotherapy with continuous infusion 5-fluorouracil for locally advanced rectal cancer. *Int. J. Radiat. Oncol. Biol. Phys.*, **47** (2000) 713–718.

73. Kaminsky-Forrett MC, Conroy T, Luporsi E, Peiffert D, Lapeyre M, Boissel P, et al. Prognostic implications of downstaging following preoperative radiation therapy for operable T3-T4 rectal cancer. *Int. J. Radiat. Oncol. Biol. Phys.*, **42** (1998) 935–941.

74. Janjan NA, Abbruzzese J, Pazdur R, Khoo VS, Cleary K, Dubrow R, et al. Prognostic implications of response to preoperative infusional chemoradiation in locally advanced rectal cancer. *Radiother. Oncol.*, **51** (1999) 153–160.

75. Willett CG, Warland G, Hagan MP, Daly WJ, Coen J, Shellito PC, et al. Tumor proliferation in rectal cancer following preoperative irradiation. *J. Clin. Oncol.*, **13** (1995) 1417–1424.

76. Guillem JG, Puig-La Calle J, Akhurst T, Tickoo S, Ruo L, Minsky BD, et al. Prospective assessment of primary rectal cancer response to preoperative radiation and chemotherapy using 18-fluorodeoxyglucose positron emission tomography. *Dis. Colon Rectum*, **43** (2000) 18–24.

77. Suwinski R, Taylor JMG, and Withers HR. Rapid growth of microscopic rectal cancer as a determinant of response to preoperative radiation therapy. *Int. J. Radiat. Oncol. Biol. Phys.*, **42** (1998) 943–951.

78. Hoff PM, Janjan NA, Saad ED, Skibber J, Crane C, Lassere Y, et al. Phase I study of preoperative oral UFT/leucovorin and radiation therapy in rectal cancer. *J. Clin. Oncol.*, **18** (2000) 3529–3534.

79. Hoff PM, Lassere Y, Pazdur R, Janjan NA, Crane C, and Skibber J. Preoperative UFT and calcium folinate and radiotherapy in rectal cancer. *Oncology*, **13 (Suppl. 3)** (1999) 129–131.

80. DeMario MD and Ratain MJ. Oral chemotherapy: rationale and future directions. *J. Clin. Oncol.*, **16(7)** (1998) 2557–2567.

81. Sharma S and Saltz LB. Oral chemotherapeutic agents for colorectal cancer. *Oncologist*, **5** (2000) 99–107.

82. Mani S, Hochster H, Beck T, Chevlen EM, O'Rourke MA, Weaver CH, et al. Multicenter phase II study to evaluate a 28-day regimen of oral fluorouracil plus eniluracil in the treatment of patients with previously untreated metastatic colorectal cancer. *J. Clin. Oncol.*, **18(15)** (2000) 2894–2901.

83. Van Cutsem E, Findlay M, Osterwalder B, Kocha W, Dalley D, Pazdur R, et al. Capecitabine, an oral fluoropyrimidine carbamate with substantial activity in advanced colorectal cancer: results of a randomized phase II study. *J. Clin. Oncol.*, **18(6)** (2000) 1337–1345.

84. Pazdur R, Lassere Y, Diaz-Canton E, and Ho DH. Phase I trial of uracil-tegafur (UFT) plus oral leucovorin: 28-day schedule. *Cancer Invest.*, **16(3)** (1998) 145–151.

85. Budman DR, Meropol NJ, Reigner B, Creaven PJ, Lichtman SM, Berghorn E, et al. Preliminary studies of a novel oral fluoropyrimidine carbamate: capecitabine. *J. Clin. Oncol.*, **16(5)** (1998) 1795–1802.

86. Macdonald JS. Carcinoembryonic antigen screening: pros and cons. *Semin. Oncol.*, **26** (1999) 556–560.

87. Ahmed FY, Johnston SJ, Cassidy J, O'Kelly T, Binnie N, Murray GI, et al. Eniluracil treatment completely inactiviates dihydropyrimidine dehydrogenase in colorectal tumors. *J. Clin. Oncol.*, **17(8)** (1999) 2439–2445.

88. Punt CJA. New drugs in the treatment of colorectal carcinoma. *Cancer*, **83** (1998) 679–689.

89. Russell AH, Harris J, Rosenberg PJ, Sause WT, Fisher BJ, Hoffman JP, et al. Anal sphincter conservation for patients with adenocarcinoma of the distal rectum: long-term results of Radiation Therapy Oncology Group Protocol 89-02. *Int. J. Radiat. Oncol. Biol. Phys.*, **46** (2000) 313–322.

90. Johnson DE and Hoffman JP. Surgical considerations for local excision. *Semin. Radiat. Oncol.*, **8** (1998) 39–47.

91. Willett CG. Local excision followed by postoperative radiation therapy. *Semin. Radiat. Oncol.*, **8** (1998) 24–29.

92. Bouvet M, Milas M, Giacco GG, Cleary KR, Janjan NA, and Skibber JM. Predictors of recurrence after local excision and postoperative chemoradiation therapy of adenocarcinoma of the rectum. *Ann. Surg. Oncol.*, **6** (1999) 26–32.

93. Jessup JM, Loda M, and Bleday R. Clinical and molecular prognostic factors in sphincter-preserving surgery for rectal cancer. *Semin. Radiat. Oncol.*, **8** (1998) 54–69.

94. Ahmad NR and Nagle DA. Preoperative radiation therapy followed by local excision. *Semin. Radiat. Oncol.*, **8** (1998) 36–38.

95. Gerard JP, Romestaing P, Ardiet JM, and Mornex F. Endocavitary radiation therapy. *Semin. Radiat. Oncol.*, **8** (1998) 13–23.

96. Maingon P, Guerif S, Darsouni R, Salas S, Barillot I, d'Hombres A, et al. Conservative management of rectal adenocarcinoma by radiotherapy. *Int. J. Radiat. Oncol. Biol. Phys.*, **40** (1998) 1077–1085.

97. Salembier C and Battermann JJ. Interstitial brachytherapy in the conservative treatment of anal and rectal cancers. *Endocuriether./Hyperthermia Oncol.*, **12** (1996) 183–189.

98. Armour EP, White, JR, Armin AR, Corry PM, Coffey M, DeWitt C, et al. Pulsed low dose rate brachytherapy in a rat model: dependence of late rectal injury on radiation pulse size. *Int. J. Radiat. Oncol. Biol. Phys.*, **38** (1997) 825–834.

99. Lingareddy V, Ahmad NR, and Mohiuddin M. Palliative reirradiation for recurrent rectal cancer. *Int. J. Radiat. Oncol. Biol. Phys.*, **38** (1997) 785–790.

100. Mohiuddin M, Marks GM, Lingareddy V, and Marks J. Curative surgical resection following reirradiation for recurrent rectal cancer. *Int. J. Radiat. Oncol. Biol. Phys.*, **39** (1997) 643–649.

101. Nymann T, Jess P, and Christiansen J. Rate and treatment of pelvic recurrence after abdominoperineal resection and low anterior resection for rectal cancer. *Dis. Colon Rectum*, **38** (1995) 799–802.

102. Wong CS, Cummings BJ, Brierley JD, Catton CN, McLean M, Catton P, et al. Treatment of locally recurrent rectal carcinoma-results and prognostic factors. *Int. J. Radiat. Oncol. Biol. Phys.*, **40** (1998) 427–435.

103. Wong R, Thomas G, Cummings B, Froud P, Shelley W, Withers R, et al. In search of a dose-response relationship with radiotherapy in the management of recurrent rectal carcinoma in the pelvis: a systematic review. *Int. J. Radiat. Oncol. Biol. Phys.*, **40** (1998) 437–446.

104. Guiney MJ, Smith JG, Worotniuk V, and Ngan S. Results of external beam radiotherapy alone for incompletely resected carcinoma of rectosigmoid or rectum: Peter MacCallum Cancer Institute Experience 1981–1990. *Int. J. Radiat. Oncol. Biol. Phys.*, **43** (1999) 531–536.

105. Bussieres E, Gilly FN, Rouanet P, Mahe MA, Roussel A, Delannes M, et al. Recurrences of rectal cancers: results of a multimodal approach with intraoperative radiation therapy. *Int. J. Radiat. Oncol. Biol. Phys.*, **34** (1996) 49–56.

106. Lanciano RM, Calkins AR, Wolkov HB, Buzydlowski I, Noyes RD, Sause W, et al. A phase I/II study of intraoperative radiotherapy in advanced unresectable or recurrent carcinoma of the rectum: a Radiation Therapy Oncology Group (RTOG) study. *J. Surg. Oncol.*, **53** (1993) 20–29.

107. Sofo L, Ratto C, Doglietto GB, Valentini V, Trodella L, Ippoliti M, et al. Intraoperative radiation therapy in integrated treatment of rectal cancers—results of a phase II study. *Dis. Colon Rectum*, **39** (1996) 1396–1403.

108. Valentini V, Morganti AG, De Franco A, Coco C, Ratto C, Doglietto GB, et al. Chemoradiation with or without intraoperative radiation therapy in patients with locally recurrent rectal carcinoma-prognostic factors and long term outcome. *Cancer*, **86** (1999) 2612–2624.

109. Martinez-Monge R, Nag S, and Martin EW. Three different intraoperative radiation modalities [electron beam, high-dose-rate brachytherapy, and iodine-125 brachytherapy] in the adjuvant treatment of patients with recurrent colorectal adenocarcinoma. *Cancer*, **86** (1999) 66–71.

110. Schneebaum S, Papo J, Fraif M, Baratz M, Baron J, and Skornik Y. Radioimmunoguided surgery benefits for recurrent colorectal cancer. *Ann. Surg. Oncol.*, **4** (1997) 371–376.

111. Kim HK, Jessup JM, Beard CJ, Bornstein B, Cady B, Stone MD, et al. Locally advanced rectal carcinoma: pelvic control and morbidity following preoperative radiation therapy, resection, and intraoperative radiation therapy. *Int. J. Radiat. Oncol. Biol. Phys.*, **38** (1997) 777–783.
112. Shibata D, Hyland W, Busse P, Kim HK, Sentovich SM, Stelle G, et al. Immediate reconstruction of the perineal wound with gracilis muscle flaps following abdominoperineal resections and intraoperative radiation therapy for recurrent carcinoma of the rectum. *Ann. Surg. Oncol.*, **6** (1999) 33–37.
113. Salo JC, Paty PB, Guillem J, Minsky BD, Harrison LB, and Cohen AM. Surgical salvage of recurrent rectal carcinoma after curative resection: a 10-year experience. *Ann. Surg. Oncol.*, **6** (1999) 171–177.
114. Wanebo HJ, Antoniuk P, Koness RJ, Levy A, Vezeridis M, Cohen SI, et al. Pelvic resection of recurrent rectal cancer—technical considerations and outcomes. *Dis. Colon Rectum*, **42** (1999) 1438–1448.

12   Management of Locally Unresectable Rectal Cancer

Bruce D. Minsky

1. INTRODUCTION

The use of postoperative combined-modality therapy (5-fluorouracil [5-FU]-based chemotherapy plus concurrent pelvic radiation therapy) significantly improves local control and survival for patients with clinically resectable, transmural (T3) rectal cancer (1–4). For patients with unresectable disease (T4), it is more difficult to obtain these results.

In contrast to resectable rectal cancer, unresectable rectal cancer is a heterogeneous disease. For example, there is no uniform definition of resectability. It can vary from a tethered or "marginally resectable" cancer to a fixed cancer with adherence to or direct invasion of adjacent organs or vital structures. This broad definition has prognostic implications because patients with gross invasion of tumor into vital pelvic structures are commonly approached in a palliative rather than a curative fashion. The definition of resectability also depends on whether the assessment is made clinically during an office or radiological exam or at the time of an examination under anesthesia or surgery. For example, tumors thought to be unresectable at the time of clinical or radiographic examination may be found to be more mobile when the patient is relaxed under anesthesia. There are also prognostic differences between primary and recurrent tumors, and many series do not report the results separately. The heterogeneity of the disease and absence of a uniform definition of resectability may explain, in part, the variation in results seen among the series.

Radical surgery alone such as a pelvic exenteration may be curative in selected patients with unresectable disease. These include tumors invading pelvic organs, including the prostate, base of bladder, or uterus where the disease can be resected en bloc with negative margins. Some midline posterior tumors adherent to or invading the distal sacrum may be resectable for cure with an extended abdomino-perineal resection (APR) that includes

From: *Colorectal Cancer: Multimodality Management*
Edited by: L. Saltz © Humana Press Inc., Totowa, NJ

the sacrum. However, despite achieving a complete resection with negative margins, these patients still require combined-modality therapy for local control. In the subset of patients with recurrent unresectable disease, the tumor is commonly more locally extensive than indicated by physical and radiographic examination. With the exception of a limited suture line recurrence, initial surgery in this group of patients will likely leave microscopic or gross residual disease. Therefore, preoperative combined-modality therapy should be used routinely in patients with primary or recurrent unresectable disease.

2. STAGING

Physical examination, computed tomography (CT) scan, magnetic resonance imaging (MRI), and cystoscopy are helpful in staging these patients. The involvement of the sciatic notch as indicated by neurologic symptoms or pelvic imaging suggests a situation unlikely to be helped by surgery. With CT or MRI imaging, recurrent pelvic tumor, especially following an APR, is difficult to differentiate from scar. Positron-emission tomography (PET) may offer a more accurate assessment *(5,6)*.

3. THERAPEUTIC APPROACHES

3.1. Preoperative Radiation Therapy

The primary goals of preoperative therapy are to convert an unresectable cancer to a resectable status and decrease the incidence of local failure. Because surgery commonly leaves residual disease in the pelvis in patients with unresectable disease, the standard approach until recently has been preoperative pelvic radiation therapy. Even when negative margins are achieved, the incidence of local failure is 30% or greater *(7)*.

The only randomized trial is from the British Medical Research Council. A total of 279 patients with clinical T4 primary rectal cancer were randomized to preoperative radiation therapy, albeit with a suboptimal dose of 40 Gy in 20 fractions, versus surgery alone *(8)*. Patients who received preoperative radiation had a significant decrease in local failure (36% vs 46%, $p = 0.04$) and distant failure (35% vs 48%, $p = 0.02$). There was an improvement in median survival (31 mo vs 24 mo, $p = NS$) but no difference in survival (32% vs 28%).

As would be predicted, the results seen in patients with primary disease are more favorable than those with recurrent disease. In the series from the Massachusetts General Hospital (MGH), the rate of complete resection with negative margins was 59% for patients with primary cancers *(9)* compared with 44% of those with recurrent cancers *(10)*. Limiting the analysis to the most favorable group of patients (primary cancers and negative margins), the 5-yr actuarial local failure rate was 29% and disease-free survival was 60%. Therefore, even in the most favorable group of patients, local failure is still almost 30%. At the University of Florida, in the 48% of patients who were able to undergo a complete resection with negative margins, the local failure rate was 55% and the 5-yr determinate survival was 20% *(11,12)*. Tobin and colleagues reported a local failure rate of 20% and 5-yr survival of 60% in 85 patients treated with preoperative radiation *(13)*. At Memorial Sloan-Kettering, 58% of patients underwent a complete resection with negative margins following preoperative radiation and the local failure rate was 25% *(14)*. Similar results are reported from the University of Kentucky *(15)*.

The most favorable outcome of patients with clinical T4 disease are the subset with tethered cancers. In a separate series from the MGH, 28 patients with tethered rectal cancers were treated with preoperative radiation *(16)*. Tethered was defined as the sensation on the examining finger of partial tumor mobility consistent with extensive perirectal spread and adherence but without fixation to unresectable structures. Although a complete resection with negative margins was possible in 93%, the local failure rate was 24%. A local failure rate of 14% and 5-yr survival of 68% in 49 patients with tethered cancers treated with preoperative radiation was reported by Tobin and associates *(13)*.

In conclusion, most series report that over 90% of patients with tethered disease and 48–64% of patients with unresectable disease will be converted to a resectable status following standard doses of preoperative radiation therapy. However, despite a complete resection and negative margins, the local failure rate will vary, depending on the degree of tumor fixation, from 24% to 55%. Because retrospective data suggest an increase in both the response *(17)* and resection *(18)* rates when 5-FU-based chemotherapy is added to preoperative radiation and prospective randomized data reveal an improvement in local control with postoperative combined-modality therapy *(3)*, most patients with unresectable disease receive preoperative combined-modality therapy.

3.2. Improving the Results of Preoperative Radiation Therapy

The dose of radiation required to achieve an adequate level of local control in many cases of unresectable rectal cancer exceeds the tolerance of the surrounding normal tissues. A number of approaches have been used to address this limitation of preoperative radiation. The most promising have included intraoperative radiation therapy (IORT) and the addition of systemic chemotherapy.

3.3. Intraoperative Radiation Therapy

The primary advantage of IORT is that radiation can be delivered at the time of surgery to the site with the highest risk of local failure (the tumor bed) while decreasing the dose to the surrounding normal tissues. IORT is delivered by two techniques: electron beam and brachytherapy. With the electron beam technique, the radiation is delivered by a linear accelerator and, with the use of a cone, is directed to the tumor bed.

Techniques of brachytherapy include low-dose and high-dose radiation. The low-dose method involves implantation of radioactive sources with either removable iridium-192 afterloading catheters or iodine-125 or palladium-103 permanent seeds *(19)* . If needed, the permanent seeds can be sutured or implanted directly into the tumor. As an alternative, they can be placed in a dexon mesh, which is then sutured to the tumor bed *(20)*. Most of the experience with low-dose brachytherapy has been in patients with gross residual disease. It has also been used as an alternative to electron beam IORT in patients with negative margins *(21,22)*. High-dose-rate (HDR) brachytherapy utilizes a flexible multichannel applicator that conforms to the tumor bed. The applicator is positioned and an iridium-192 source and is programmed to deliver a uniform dose to the area at risk using a dose rate similar to electron beam IORT *(22,23)*.

One technical advantage of brachytherapy compared to electron beam is there are virtually no clinical situations when, because of anatomic or technical constraints, that IORT cannot be delivered *(22)*. In contrast, electron beam IORT was not able to be delivered because of anatomic or technical constraints in 10% of patients in the M.D. Anderson series *(24)* and in 9% of patients in both the MGH recurrent *(25)* and primary unresectable *(26)* series.

The results of treatment depend on whether the patient has primary unresectable or recurrent disease as well as the margins of resection (negative vs microscopic vs gross residual). The discussion will be limited to patients who, in general, receive preoperative pelvic radiation with or without 5-FU-based chemotherapy. Most receive 45–50.4 Gy to the pelvis and 10–20 Gy IORT with either electrons or HDR brachytherapy. In general, patients with negative margins have received lower IORT doses (10–15 Gy), whereas those with microscopic or gross residual disease have received higher doses (15–20 Gy).

3.3.1. PRIMARY UNRESECTABLE DISEASE

The most extensive experience with preoperative therapy followed by IORT has been reported from MGH *(26)*. As seen in Table 1, for patients with negative margins, local failure is decreased from 18% without IORT to 11% with IORT. In patients with positive margins, local failure is decreased from 83% without IORT to 43% with IORT if there is gross residual, and to 32% with IORT if there is microscopic residual disease. For the total patient group (with or without IORT), the 5-yr disease-free survival was 63% for patients with negative margins and 32% for patients with positive margins. These results underscore the importance of delivering preoperative therapy in order to help achieve the most complete resection as possible. If negative margins cannot be obtained, then microscopic residual is still preferable to gross residual. Series from the Mayo Clinic *(27)* and Memorial Sloan-Kettering *(22)* report similar local failure rates in patients with negative margins (7% and 8%, respectively). The results of other selected series from Munich *(23)*, Heidelberg *(28)*, and the NE Deaconess Hospital *(20)* are seen in Table 1.

3.3.2. RECURRENT DISEASE

The largest experience with IORT in patients with recurrent disease is from the Mayo Clinic *(30)*. In contrast with the series of patients treated for primary unresectable disease, those with recurrent disease have less uniform treatment programs. For example, some have received prior pelvic radiation *(25,30,31)* and others were treated with IORT alone *(22,34)*. Selected series in which all patients received IORT are seen in Table 2.

In a report from the Mayo Clinic, 119 patients received, in general, 50.4–54 Gy preoperatively followed by a 7.5- to 20-Gy electron beam IORT *(30)*. The higher IORT doses were used for patients with residual disease. For patients with negative margins, the crude local failure rate was 6% and increased to 18% for microscopic and 25% for gross residual disease. The 5-yr actuarial local failure rates were 27% for microscopic disease and 45% for gross residual disease. For the total patient group, overall 5-yr survival was 20%. The M.D. Anderson *(24)*, Memorial Sloan-Kettering *(22)*, and the French IORT groups *(33)* reported similar local failure rates for the total patient group (36%, 37%, and 31%, respectively). In the series by Hashiguchi et al. of 25 patients selected to receive IORT, the 5-yr survival was 21% *(36)*.

Other series have not reported such favorable results. In a series from MGH, the 5-yr actuarial local failure rate for patients with gross residual was 89%, and for the total patient group, it was 70% *(25)*. The 5-yr disease-free survival was 21% for patients with negative margins and only 7% for those with positive margins. Investigators from Eindhoven also reported that patients with gross residual disease had a significantly lower rate of 3-yr actuarial local control (21% vs 79%, $p = 0.01$), disease-free survival (11% vs 54%, $p = 0.0008$), and overall survival (35% vs 74%, $p < 0.05$) compared with those with negative or microscopic positive margins *(34)*. At Memorial Sloan-Kettering there were no survivors at 2 yr with positive margins *(22)*, whereas in the Heidelberg series, the 4-yr disease free survival was 29% *(35)*. In contrast to patients with recurrent disease who have negative or microscopic positive margins, it is unclear if those with positive margins benefit from aggressive therapy.

3.4. Complications of Electron Beam IORT

Complications such as neuropathy, vasculitis, bone necrosis, and ureteral injury in canines who received IORT have been described by Gillette et al. *(37,38)*. In two series, hyperthermia

Table 1
Primary Locally Advanced/Unresectable Rectal Cancer ± IORT (Selected Series)

Series	No. of patients	Months (follow-up)	Preoperative treatment[a]	IORT	Local failure					Survival		
					Margins				Total	Margins		Total
					Negative		Positive			Negative	Positive	
					No.	Negative	No.	Positive				
Mayo (27)	61	18 9 (minimum)	45–55 Gy ± 5-FU 10–20 Gy IORT	Yes	18	6% crude 7% 5 yr	19 (micro) 16 (gross)	5% crude 14% 5 yr 25% crude 27% 5 yr	13% crude 16% 5 yr		Gross 21% 5 yr	46% 5 yr
MGH (26)	145	41 (median)	45–50.4 Gy ± 5-FU ± 10–20 Gy IORT	Yes	45	11% 5 yr	21 (micro) 7 (gross) 28 total	32% 5 yr 43% 5 yr 35% 5 yr		63% 5 yr DFS	32% 5 yr DFS	
Heidelberg (28)	40	18 (median)	41.4 Gy + 5-FU 10–18 Gy IORT	No Yes	66	18% 5 yr	6 total	83% 5 yr		91% DFS		
Memorial Sloan-Kettering (22)	18	18 (median)	50.4 Gy + 5-FU/LV 10–20 Gy HDR IORT	Yes		8% 2 yr		62% 2 yr	19% 2 yr	77% 2 yr DFS	38% 2 yr DFS	69% 2 yr
NE Deaconess Hospital (29)	27	24 (median)	50.4 Gy ± 5-FU 12.5–17 Gy Orthovoltage IORT	Yes					27% crude			41% NED
Munich (23)	19	—	39.6 Gy BID + 5-FU 15 Gy HDR IORT	Yes					10% crude			

[a]In most patients. *Note:* BID = twice-a-day radiation; HDR = high-dose-rate intraoperative radiation; NED = no evidence of disease; DFS = disease-free survival.

Table 2
Recurrent Rectal Cancer: Intraoperative Radiation ± Preoperative or Postoperative Therapy (Selected Series)

Series	No. of patients	Months (follow-up)	Preoperative treatment[a]	Local failure — Margins — Negative No.	Local failure — Margins — Negative	Local failure — Margins — Positive No.	Local failure — Margins — Positive	Local failure — Total	Survival — Margins — Negative	Survival — Margins — Positive	Survival — Total
Mayo (30)	119	—	50.4–54 Gy / 7.5–20 Gy IORT / Some postop EBRT	17	6% crude	40 (micro) / 65 (gross)	18% crude / 27% 5 yr / 40% 5 yr (gross)	20% crude / 37% 5 yr / 25% crude			20% 5 yr
MGH (25)	41	31 (median)	50.4 Gy ± 5-FU / 10–20 Gy IORT / Some prior EBRT	27	58% 5 yr (or micro+)	14	89% 5 yr (gross)	70% 5 yr	21% 5 yr DFS	7% 5 yr DFS	16% 5 yr
Heidelberg (35)	31	28 (median)	41.4 Gy (22 preop) / Mean 13.7 Gy IORT	14	21% crude / 22% 4 yr	9 (micro) / 8 (gross)	33% crude / 39% 4 yr / 37% crude / 40% 4 yr	29% crude	71% 4 yr DFS	29% 4 yr DFS	48% 4 yr (DFS) / 58% 4 yr
Memorial Sloan-Kettering (22)	46	18 (median)	(16) 50.4 Gy ± 5-FU/LV / 10–20 Gy HDR IORT / (25) 10–20 Gy IORT alone		18% 2 yr		81% 2 yr	37% 2 yr	71% 2 yr DFS	0% 2 yr DFS	47% 2 yr
NE Deaconess Hospital (29)	13	24 (median)	50.4 Gy ± 5-FU / 12.5–17 Gy / Orthovoltage IORT					73%			27% NED
French IORT Group (33)	73	30 (median)	(30) 39 Gy ± 5-FU / 10–15 Gy IORT / (43) 10–15 Gy IORT alone					31% 3 yr (57% margins−)			31% 3 yr
M.D. Anderson (24)	43[b]	26 (median)	45 Gy + 5-FU ± CDDP / 10–20 Gy IORT					36%			37% 5 yr (DFS)
Eindhoven (34)	37	37 (mean)	(17) 50.4 Gy preop / 10 Gy IORT / (5) 30 Gy reirradiation / 15 Gy IORT / (15) 17.5 Gy IORT	15	13% crude	8 (micro) / 14 (gross)	13% crude / 43% crude	24% crude / 40% 3 yr			58% 5 yr / 32% 3 yr (DFS) / 58% 3 yr
Catholic University Rome (31)	11	80 (median)	45–46.8 Gy preop / ± 5-FU/MMC					20% crude			41% 5 yr

[a] In most patients. *Note*: EBRT = external beam pelvic radiation therapy; HDR = high-dose-rate intraoperative radiation; DFS = disease-free survival.
[b] Excluding 10 patients with multifocal or extrapelvic disease.

increased the neurological complications of IORT *(39,40)*. In canines, IORT induced secondary malignancies are seen in 15%, with most occurring at doses >25 Gy *(44)*.

In series with longer follow-up, similar morbidity has been reported in humans. The incidence of toxicity depends on whether the patient has primary or recurrent cancer. In the MGH IORT series, the incidence of complications were higher in those with recurrent disease (10% soft tissue or sacral injury and 10% pelvic neuropathy) compared with primary disease (2% sacral necrosis or ureteral obstruction) *(9,10)*. In the Eindhoven series, 16% of patients developed neuropathy; however, it was grade 3 in only 3% *(34)*.

Investigators at the Mayo Clinic have reported higher complication rates *(42)*. In patients with primary or recurrent colorectal cancer, the incidence of peripheral neuropathy was 32%. The symptoms of pain, numbness, and tingling resolved in 40% of patients; however, only 13% had resolution of weakness. Ureteral obstruction or hydronephrosis were seen in 63% of patients who did not have evidence of ureteral obstruction at presentation. Although there was no relationship between the incidence of complications and the external beam dose, the incidence of complications increased with the IORT dose.

It is difficult to clearly separate treatment-related complications from disease-related complications. The total incidence ranges from 15% to 50% in most series and is highest in patients with recurrent, unresectable disease. Complications such as delayed healing, infection, fistula, and neuropathy may be the result of recurrent tumor, aggressive surgery, radiation, or, more likely, a combination of these. In the RTOG 85-08 trial, the 2-yr actuarial risk of significant complications in the 42 patients with advanced or recurrent rectal cancer who received IORT as a component of their therapy was 16% *(43)*. However, compared with a nonrandomized group who underwent surgery without IORT, there was no significant increase in acute surgical complications in the IORT patients *(44)*.

In conclusion, the phase I/II data suggested that the addition of IORT improved local control compared with preoperative therapy alone. The results in the subset of patients with recurrent cancer and/or residual disease are still not optimal. Unfortunately, there are no phase III trials of IORT.

3.5. Preoperative Combined-Modality Therapy

Based on the positive results seen in patients with resectable rectal cancer who receive adjuvant postoperative combined-modality therapy *(1–3)*, there has been a shift to preoperative combined-modality therapy.

As seen in Tables 1 and 2, there are a number of phase I/II trials of preoperative combined-modality therapy for patients with unresectable disease. In most series, patients received 45–50.4 Gy of pelvic radiation at 1.8–2.0 Gy/fraction plus two cycles of concurrent 5-FU based chemotherapy with bolus 5-FU/leucovorin or continuous-infusion 5-FU, followed by surgery (± IORT) and an additional four cycles of postoperative chemotherapy. Some have used methotrexate *(45)* or interferon *(46)*. Marsh et al. have combined chronobiologically shaped 5-FU infusion with preoperative radiation therapy *(12)*. Phase I/II trials examining the use of newer chemotherapeutic agents such as Tomudex *(47–50)*, UFT/leucovorin *(51,52)*, CPT-11 *(53–55)*, oxaliplatin *(56–58)*, eniluracil *(59)*, and capecitabine *(60)* with preoperative radiation therapy are in progress.

The presence of unresectable disease is, by itself, not a contraindication to sphincter preservation. Sphincter-preservation rates following preoperative therapy in patients with primary unresectable disease range from 24% to 50% *(15,24,26,31,61)*. However, data from Shibata et al. from Memorial Sloan-Kettering Cancer Center (MSKCC) revealed that in 18 patients who underwent IORT as a component of their therapy and had sphincter preservation, 56% reported fair to poor functional outcome and 56% were dissatisfied with their quality of life (62). For this patient group who are considered for a coloanal anastomosis or a very low anterior resection, they may be better served by a permanent diversion.

3.6. Relationship Between Response Rate and Survival

It is unclear if the response rate predicts outcome. Furthermore, because most studies that examine this issue do not report the results of patients with clinically resectable and unresectable disease separately, the data are difficult to interpret.

The pathologic complete response rate after combined-modality therapy varies from 10% to 30%. In a retrospective series of 33 patients from the study by Mohiuddin and associates, the pathologic complete response rate was higher in patients who received 55–60 Gy vs 45–50 Gy (44% vs 13%, $p < 0.05$) (15). The highest pathologic complete response rate was seen in the subset of 12 patients who received both continuous infusion 5-FU and the higher radiation dose of 55–60 Gy (67%). However, these differences did not translate into a significant local control or survival advantage.

Other series suggest that there is an advantage in outcome with increased downstaging. In an analysis by Kaminsky-Forrett et al. of 88 patients with clinical T3–4 rectal cancers who received preoperative radiation with or without 5-FU/leucovorin, there was a decrease in local failure (4% vs 15%) and a significant increase in 5-yr cancer-specific survival (100% vs 45%, $p = 0.01$) in patients who achieved a complete or near-complete response (pathologic stage T0-2N0 disease) compared with those with less of a response (pathologic stage T3–4 and/or N1-2) (63). Ahmad and colleagues reported a 5-yr actuarial local control rate of 96% and a 91% survival rate in the subset of 49 of a total of 315 patients with clinical T3–4 disease who achieved a complete response following preoperative radiation (64).

3.7. Predictive Tumor Markers

A variety of tumor markers have been identified that may help predict tumors that respond favorably to preoperative therapy (Table 3). Based on the experience that rapidly dividing cells are more sensitive to radiation, Willett et al. analyzed the proliferative index in patients with unresectable disease who received preoperative radiation therapy with or without 5-FU (74). Tumors with a higher proliferation index had a higher response rate to preoperative therapy, and following radiation, there was a corresponding reduction in the proliferative index (75). In a follow-up study, the authors reported that the addition of 5-FU to pre-operative radiation decreased three markers of proliferation (mitotic counts, Ki-67, and PCNA) compared with radiation therapy alone (66).

Tumors with a low spontaneous apoptosis index and positive BCL-2 staining had lower rates of downstaging in a series of 50 patients who received preoperative combined modality therapy reported by Rich and associates (76). In 167 patients treated with preoperative radiation, there was a significant increase in downstaging in well-differentiated cancers (77). Using residual tumor cell density rather than stage as a measure, this difference did not reach statistical significance. By univariate analysis, patients who achieved a pathologic complete response had a nonsignificant improvement in survival. Berger and associates found that well-differentiated tumors had a greater degree of downstaging compared with moderately or poorly differentiated tumors (78).

Desai and colleagues reported a higher incidence of recurrence but less downstaging in PCNA-positive rectal cancers (79). By multivariate analysis, Neoptolemos and associates showed that this index did not add to the prognostic value of the Dukes' staging system (80).

Table 3
Molecular Predictors of Response to Preoperative Therapy in Rectal Cancer

Series	No. of patients	Clinical stage	Preoperative therapy	% CR	Findings
Desai et al. (65)	23	T3–4	RT	9	↑ downstaging with normal *p53* and/or PCNA negative
Fu et al. (67)	49	T1–3	RT	4	↑ downstaging, ↑ local failure, and ↓ survival with mutated *p53* and normal p21
Sakakura et al. (68)	28	T3–4	CMT + hyperthermia	—	↑ downstaging with ↑ apoptotic index—highest correlation with wild-type *p53*
Scott et al. (69)	24	T3–4	CMT	25	apoptotic index with ↑ CR. No relationship to *p53* or *bcl-2*
Tannapfel et al. (70)	32	T3–4	CMT	—	apoptotic index following pre-op CMT. ↓ proliferative capacity ([Ki67, PCNA] following CMT but did not predict the CR rate).
Luna-Perez et al. (71)	26	T3–4	CMT	15	↑ CR with normal *p53* versus mutated *p53*
Willett et al. (66)	153	T3–4	RT ± CMT	12	↑ downstaging with ↑ growth fraction (↑ mitotic count and Ki-67 and PCNA)
Nehls et al. (72)	100	T1–3	RT	—	No change in *p53* expression pre-RT vs post-RT
Adell et al. (73)	148	T1–4	RT	—	In *p53* negative patients, preoperative RT decreased local failure, whereas *p53* positive patients had no benefit from preoperative RT.

Note: All analysis were performed by immunohistochemistry on paraffin fixed tissues.
CR = pathologic complete response; CMT = combined-modality therapy (radiation plus chemotherapy).

The proliferative index may be useful in predicting the response to preoperative therapy however, given the conflicting data, additional experience is needed.

Although some tumor markers may be predictive of response, the decision to use preoperative therapy should not be made solely on their presence or absence. The development of tumor markers to predict response and prognosis remains an active area of investigation *(81)*.

3.8. Intraoperative or Postoperative Radiation Therapy for Residual Disease

For a variety of reasons, some patients with unresectable cancer do not receive preoperative therapy or, despite a preoperative assessment of resectability are not able to undergo a complete resection. In this setting, does IORT and/or postoperative pelvic radiation therapy have any benefit? As previously discussed, the interpretation of treatment results is complicated because many studies combine patients with primary and recurrent cancers as well as those with gross and microscopic residual disease. Patients are randomly selected to receive chemotherapy and some series include patients with metastatic disease. The discussion will be limited to those series in which patients have disease limited to the pelvis.

Therapeutic options are limited for patients who have failed prior pelvic radiation. The standard therapy is usually palliative surgery or systemic chemotherapy. Furthermore, the response rate with chemotherapy may be reduced in a pelvis that has received full-dose radiation.

There are a variety of aggressive options for patients who have failed prior pelvic radiation (Table 4). Although these are investigational approaches, they may offer an improvement in local control in selected patients.

3.9. Subtotal Resection and Postoperative Radiation Therapy

In a report from the Mayo Clinic, 17 patients with rectal cancer received postoperative radiation therapy (40–60 Gy) ± 5-FU *(86)*. The overall local failure rate was 76% and the 5-yr actuarial survival was 24%. The 7 patients with gross residual disease had a higher incidence of local failure (86% vs 70%) and lower survival (14% vs 30%) compared to the 10 patients with microscopic residual disease. There was no clear dose-response curve; however, only one patient received ≥ 56 Gy.

In a separate report from the Mayo Clinic, the results of 106 patients who underwent a palliative (subtotal) resection for locally recurrent rectal cancer were presented *(87)*. 5-FU was delivered in 48%. In the subset of 34 patients with gross residual disease who received IORT and postoperative therapy, the 3-yr survival was 44%. However, despite the encouraging survival rate, 40% developed local failure and 60% developed distant failure. Univariate analysis revealed a significant improvement in survival in those patients with microscopic compared with gross residual disease, the use of IORT, a limited number of sites of tumor fixation, and higher performance status. These data suggest that even in patients with locally recurrent residual disease, an aggressive approach should be considered.

Other reports have included patients with both rectal and colon cancers as well as patients with both primary and recurrent disease. At MGH, patients received higher doses of radiation (60–70 Gy) compared with the Mayo Clinic external beam alone series *(88)*. Seven patients received electron beam IORT. For the total group, local failure was 42% and 5-yr disease-free survival was 18%. The 23 patients with gross residual disease had a higher local failure rate (57% vs 30%) and a significant decrease in survival (4% vs 42%) compared with the 30 patients with microscopic residual disease. The improvement in local control when compared with the Mayo Clinic external beam alone series may have been related

Table 4
Aggressive Surgical Plus Radiotherapeutic Salvage Techniques

Series	No. of patients	Treatment	Median[a] follow-up	Margins	% Local failure	Survival
USC/Mayo (82)	30	Surgery and brachytherapy	27	(20) Gross+	62%	23% NED
				(8) Micro +	34%	
				(2) Negative	0%	
Mayo (83)	16	Sacral resection + IORT	18	—	25%	48% 2 yr
Thomas Jefferson Univ. (84)	39	Preoperative 36 Gy (reirradiation) + surgery	36	—	55% 5 yr	24% 5 yr / 45 mo median
Ohio State (85)	26[b]	Surgery and IORT	28	—	77% 4 yr	36% 4 yr / 23 mo median
Memorial Sloan-Kettering (19)	36	Surgery and brachytherapy	24	Gross+	44%	25% 4 yr
Memorial Sloan-Kettering (22)	46	HDR IORT[c] plus surgery	17.5	—	37% 2 yr	47% 2 yr
Catholic University, Rome (31)	13	Preoperative 23.4 Gy (reirradiation) ± surgery ± brachytherapy	80	—	59% 5 yr	30% 5 yr

Note: NED = no evidence of disease; IORT = intraoperative radiation therapy, EBRT = external beam radiation therapy; HDR = high-dose-rate intraoperative radiation.

[a]Months.
[b]Only 69% with prior EBRT.
[c]Includes 16 patients who received preoperative radiation who did not receive prior pelvic radiation.

to the higher radiation doses. There was no clear dose-response curve in patients with gross disease; however, patients with microscopic residual disease who received <60 Gy did have a higher incidence of local failure compared with those who received ≥60 Gy (38% vs 26%).

The volume of gross residual disease may also have an impact on the local failure rate. As seen in Tables 1 and 2, this is consistent with the reports from MGH *(25,26)* and the Mayo Clinic *(27,30)* IORT series where patients with gross residual disease had lower survival and higher local failure rates compared with patients with microscopic residual disease.

In patients who undergo a complete resection and have potential microscopic disease, 45–50.4 Gy is the recommended dose, which is within the tolerance of the surrounding normal tissues. However, when microscopic or gross biopsy-proven residual disease is present (i.e., following a subtotal resection), the dose of radiation required is higher. Even in situations where the small bowel can be excluded from the external beam radiation field, other surrounding normal tissues in the pelvis limit the dose to 60–65 Gy, which may be inadequate for controlling large volumes of gross residual tumor. Therefore, it is not surprising that the results for patients with residual disease who receive postoperative radiation therapy are disappointing. The obvious advantage of preoperative therapy is that it increases the ability to achieve negative margins thereby allowing maximum surgery and IORT.

3.10. Reirradiation with External Beam Followed by Surgery

Mohiuddin et al. reported the use of reirradiation in a selected group of 39 patients with a local recurrence who received prior pelvic radiation (Table 4) *(84)*. They were retreated with a median dose of 36 Gy using limited lateral fields plus continuous infusion 5-FU. A partial pelvic field was used and the bladder and small bowel were excluded as much as possible from the radiation field. With a median follow-up of 3 yr, the 5-yr actuarial local failure rate was 55% and survival was 24%. Valentini and colleagues treated 13 patients in a similar fashion (however, four underwent surgery ± brachytherapy) and reported a 5-yr local control and survival rate of 41% and 30%, respectively *(31)*. Although retreatment with limited radiation fields may be an option in highly selected patients, this approach should be considered experimental.

3.11. Palliative Radiation Therapy Without Surgery

The most favorable results are reported for patients who are able to undergo surgery as a component of their therapy. There are, however, a subset of patients who are unable to undergo surgery because they are medically inoperable, present with extensive unresectable disease grossly invading bone, have received prior pelvic radiation, or refuse surgery. In general, they have been treated with external beam with or without chemotherapy *(14,84,89–94)*.

As seen in Table 5, in a series of 519 patients treated with radiation therapy alone at the Princess Margaret Hospital, the median survival was 14 mo and the 5-yr survival rate was 5% *(92)*. In the subset of patients who received conventional doses of radiation (≥ 50 Gy), the median survival was 24 mo and the 5-yr survival was 13%. Other selected series reviewed in Table 5 report similar results (14% at 3 yr *(84)* and 31% at 2 yr) *(93)* however, they have shorter follow-up and a smaller number of patients. In a subset of patients without metastatic disease who received >46 Gy, Overgaard et al. reported a 30% 2 yr survival *(95)*. A 30% 3-yr survival was reported by Minsky and associates *(14)*.

The data from Princess Margaret Hospital also suggest that pelvic radiation provides very effective palliation. In the subset of 84 patients who received >45 Gy, the following

Table 5
Nonsurgical Palliative Radiotherapeutic Options

Series	Treatment	No. of patients	Subset	Median[a] (follow-up)	% LF	% Survival	Definition of palliation	% Palliation of those patients with symptoms at presentation					
								Pain	Bleeding	Neuro	Mass	Discharge	Total
Princess Margaret Hospital (92)	20–60 Gy ± 5-FU	519	Total	—	93% 5 yr	5% 5 yr	6–8 wk s/p EBRT	78	68	27	53	44	
	>45 Gy ± 5-FU	84		—	—	—	6–8 wk s/p EBRT	89	79	52	71	50	
	≥50 Gy ± 5-FU	74	Resectable, but refused	—	85% 5 yr	13% 5 yr							
	≥50Gy ± 5-FU	42		—		21% 5 yr							
Thomas Jefferson Univ. (84)	Reirradiation with 30.6 Gy ± 5-FU (failed EBRT)	52	Total	16	—	14% 3 yr	Complete	65	100		24		
							Partial	28	—		64		
							Total	93	100		88		
							Duration	9 mo	10 mo		8 mo		
							Until death	33	100		20		
Centre Hospitalier Lyon Sud (94)	Intracavitary + 39 Gy accelerated EBRT ± brachytherapy	29	Total	46	38%	68% 5 yr							
Peter McCallum Cancer Institute (93)	50–60 Gy	39	Radically treated	49	—	31% 2 yr	Complete						33
							Partial						52
							Total						85

Note: EBRT = external beam radiation therapy; LF = local failure; s/p = following.
[a]Months.

presenting symptoms were palliated by 6–8 wk following the completion of radiation: pain, 89%; bleeding, 79%; neurologic, 52%; mass effect, 71%; discharge, 50%; urologic, 22%; and other, 42% *(92)*. In the series from Thomas Jefferson University, complete plus partial symptomatic relief was achieved in the following categories: pain (65% + 28%), bleeding (100%), and mass effect (24% + 64%) *(84)*. The duration of palliation was 8–10 mo.

The palliative benefits of pelvic radiation are also seen in elderly patients. Valentini et al. delivered combined modality therapy (38–45 Gy plus mitomycin-C and continuous infusion 5-FU) to a group of 17 patients with a median age of 79 (range: 75–90) *(96)*. Symptomatic relief was obtained in four of four patients with pelvic pain and five of six patients with rectal bleeding. The 18% incidence of grade 3+ toxicity was similar to that reported for the general population who receive preoperative combined-modality therapy.

In summary, the data suggest that patients with advanced rectal cancers who are medically inoperable should be treated aggressively with pelvic radiation therapy as a component of their therapy. It offers not only a defined cure rate but a high degree of palliation of symptoms.

3.12. Treatment of Gross Residual Disease with IORT Alone

There is a subset of patients with recurrent rectal cancer who have clinically unresectable gross residual pelvic disease and, because of prior full-dose pelvic radiation therapy, would require an attempt at resection without the benefit of preoperative and/or postoperative radiation therapy. Furthermore, when IORT is not available, this group of patients is commonly approached in a palliative fashion because surgery alone will not control gross residual disease.

As seen in Table 4, the limited data suggest that IORT with either electrons or brachytherapy does not improve the ultimate survival rate in this group of patients. However, it does offer reasonable local control (56–60%) with acceptable morbidity. Because local control alone is an important end point in the treatment of rectal cancer, it is appropriate to continue to evaluate IORT as part of an overall aggressive approach in patients in this clinical setting.

3.13. Postoperative Combined-Modality Therapy

Although most patients now receive preoperative therapy, there are two randomized trials comparing postoperative combined-modality therapy with radiation alone. The first trial was reported from the Radiation Therapy Oncology Group (RTOG) and included 129 patients with residual, primary unresectable, or recurrent rectal cancers who were randomized to radiation therapy plus concurrent 5-FU followed by maintenance 5-FU methyl CCNU (MeCCNU) vs radiation therapy alone *(97)*. Some patients received IORT. There was no significant difference in the estimated actuarial 2-yr survival rate in patients who received combined-modality therapy compared with radiation therapy alone (44% vs 36%). Of the patients with gross residual disease (in either arm), 25% were without evidence of disease, 6% were locally controlled, and 50% died with a component of local failure.

In the second trial, the Eastern Cooperative Oncology Group (ECOG) randomized 30 patients with recurrent, residual, or primary inoperable rectal cancer to postoperative continuous-course radiation therapy versus split-course radiation therapy plus 5-FU followed by maintenance 5-FU/MeCCNU *(98)*. The median survival in both arms was 17 mo. The five patients with primary inoperable cancer (defined as gross residual disease) had the shortest 2-yr survival (0%) compared with the 16 with recurrent (25%) or the 9 with residual disease (54%).

In conclusion, postoperative combined-modality therapy, as designed and delivered in these two randomized trials, did not have a significant impact on survival compared with postoperative radiation therapy alone in this subset of patients. Other chemotherapeutic agents and schedules are being investigated.

3.14. Hyperthermia

There is an in vitro synergistic interaction of radiation and hyperthermia. Hyperthermia, in conjunction with radiation, has been mostly used as a palliative modality in rectal cancer *(99–104)*. The results of this combination in patients with various pelvic and abdominal malignancies has been reported in a phase I/II trial by the RTOG *(105)*. The acute and long-term toxicities were acceptable in 68% of the patients; however, hyperthermia had to be discontinued because of discomfort. Final results of this trial are pending. Hyperthermia has also been reported to increase the neurological complications of patients receiving IORT *(39,40)*.

3.15. Neutron Beam Radiation Therapy

The theoretical advantages of neutrons compared with more conventional photon radiation include increased sensitivity of hypoxic cells and more advantageous radiation repair and sensitivity characteristics of normal tissues. The results of two randomized trials that compared neutrons and photons in patients with unresectable and recurrent rectal cancers were reported by Duncan et al. *(106)*. A total of 35 patients received neutrons using a variety of techniques and doses. Not only were there were no significant differences in local control or survival, but patients who received neutrons experienced higher acute and late grade 3+ skin toxicity. The preferential absorption in fat of neutrons may have contributed to the increased incidence of complications. Similar severe and fatal complications were reported in a series of 25 patients with advanced rectal cancer treated by Batterman and colleagues *(107)*. Despite the theoretical advantages, there is little interest in the treatment of rectal cancer with neutrons.

3.16. Radiosensitizers

Various mechanisms for 5-FU-mediated radiosensitization have been proposed however, none alone explain all of the interactions *(108)*. Randomized clinical trials in rectal cancer have clearly shown that 5-FU is a radiosensitizer. When combined with adjuvant postoperative radiation therapy, it significantly decreases local failure compared with radiation therapy alone in patients with resectable disease *(1–3)*. Nonrandomized data from Rhomberg et al. suggest that razoxane may improve local control and median survival in patients who receive radiation for inoperable recurrent rectal cancer *(109)*. Trials of other radiosensitizers have not revealed a clear benefit.

3.17. Radioprotectors

The benefit of radioprotectors is controversial. There are six randomized trials examining the efficacy of various compounds to decrease bowel toxicity. These trials have included such compounds as butyric acid to decrease chronic radiation proctitis *(110)*, sucralfate enemas *(111)*, and oral preparations *(112)* to decrease acute radiation proctitis, olsalazine to decrease acute enteritis *(113)*, and mesalazine to decrease acute radiation enteritis *(114)*. All of these randomized trials have been negative. In a randomized trial of 73 patients with pelvic malignancies, the addition of 5-aminosalicylic acid increased rather than decreased acute radiation toxicity. Diarrhea was more frequent with the radiation plus 5-aminosalicylic acid arm compared with radiation alone (91% vs 74%, $p = 0.07$) *(115)*.

Liu et al. performed a randomized trial of pelvic radiation therapy (2.25 Gy/fraction to 45 Gy) with or without the radioprotector WR-2721 in patients with inoperable or unresectable rectal cancer *(116)*. The incidence of RTOG long-term grade 3+ gastrointestinal, genitourinary, and skin toxicity was 3% in the radiation-therapy-alone arm compared with 0% in the radiation-therapy-plus WR-2721 arm. A separate trial by Montana and colleagues showed no benefit with a topical application of WR-2721 to the rectal mucosa *(117)*. Based on these data, WR-2721 does not offer radioprotection in patients with rectal cancer who receive pelvic radiation therapy.

3.18. Altered Radiation Fractionation Approaches

Various fractionation programs have evolved with the goal of enhancing tumor cell damage by radiation without increasing normal tissue injury *(118)*. The repair of subcellular injury, regeneration, cell-cycle redistribution, and reoxygenation are all factors at the cellular level contributing to differences in how various normal tissues and tumors respond to fractionated radiation. The use of hyperfractionation and accelerated fractionation schemes take advantage of some of these factors. The late effects should be the same as or, more likely, less than conventional fractionation schemes. A phase I trial from Lausanne of postoperative accelerated hyperfractionation (1.6 Gy twice a day [bid] to 48 Gy) reported acceptable acute toxicity *(119)*. Recent data from this group suggests that bid radiation is better tolerated when delivered preoperatively as compared with postoperatively *(120)*. Bozzetti et al. reported a pathologic complete response rate of only 9% in 59 patients with ultrasound stage T2–3 disease who preoperatively received 1.5 Gy bid to 45 Gy *(121)*.

The major limitation of accelerated hyperfractionation is acute normal tissue toxicity. Because it is unlikely that these altered fractionation schemes can be combined with adequate doses of systemic chemotherapy, Movsas and colleagues have limited the hyperfractionated portion to the boost. In their phase I trial of preoperative combined-modality therapy patients receive conventional pelvic radiation plus continuous infusion 5-FU followed by a boost with escalating doses of hyperfractionated radiation (1.2 Gy bid) *(122)*. Providing the small bowel was excluded after 52.3 Gy, the recommended dose level with this approach was 61.8 Gy.

In a randomized trial of patients receiving radiation therapy for pelvic malignancies, three-dimensional conformal radiation therapy decreased the volume of normal tissue in the field however, it did not decrease acute toxicity *(123)*.

3.19. Three-Dimensional Radiation Treatment Planning

Innovative techniques using three-dimensional (3D) treatment planning are being investigated. In a report from the Photon Treatment Planning Collaborative Working Group, it was found that the most important contribution of 3D treatment planning in rectal cancer was the ability to plan and localize the target and normal tissues at all levels of the treatment volume rather than using the traditional method of planning with only a single central transverse slice and simulation films *(124)*. There was also a slight improvement when there were no constraints on the type of plans (i.e., when non-coplanar beams were used). A randomized trial of conformal versus conventional radiation therapy in 266 evaluable patients with pelvic malignancies has been reported by Tait et al. *(123)*. Although there was a decrease in the volume of normal tissue volumes in the radiation field with conformal versus conventional treatment (689 vs 792 cm^3), there was no difference in the level of symptoms or in medication prescribed.

Investigators in Uppsala examined six patients with rectal cancer who underwent both proton and conventional photon treatment planning *(125)*. By dose-volume histogram analysis, protons offered only a marginal benefit in sparing normal tissues.

3.20. Approach to Patients with Synchronous Metastatic Disease

There are a subset of patients who present with unresectable disease and synchronous extrapelvic disease. Because the natural history of these patients is dependent on a variety of factors such as the volume and site(s) of metastatic disease and the disease-free interval in those with recurrent disease, treatment recommendations are individualized. There is no standard of care. The management of these patients is discussed in greater detail in the chapter on metastatic disease. At Memorial Sloan-Kettering, the general approach is often to deliver preoperative combined-modality therapy both as a therapeutic measure and to help identify those who may benefit from an aggressive surgical approach. If in following the completion of therapy, there has been a response in both the primary and metastatic site(s), then the patient is evaluated, on a case-by-case basis, for resection of the primary and metastasis.

4. CONCLUSIONS

In summary, unresectable rectal cancer is a heterogeneous disease and it is difficult to accurately compare different series because of this selection bias. However, in patients who have not received prior external beam radiation, the data suggest that the best results are obtained with preoperative combined-modality therapy, followed by maximum surgical resection plus IORT. Combined-modality therapy regimens with newer chemotherapeutic regimens are being actively investigated.

REFERENCES

1. Gastrointestinal Tumor Study Group. Prolongation of the disease-free interval in surgically treated rectal carcinoma. *N. Engl. J. Med.*, **312** (1985) 1465–1472.
2. Gastrointestinal Tumor Study Group. Adjuvant therapy of colon cancer: results of a prospectively randomized trial. *N. Engl. J. Med.*, **310** (1984) 737–743.
3. Krook JE, Moertel CG, Gunderson LL, Wieand HS, Collins RT, Beart RW, et al. Effective surgical adjuvant therapy for high-risk rectal carcinoma. *N. Engl. J. Med.*, **324** (1991) 709–715.
4. Wolmark N, Weiand HS, Hyams DM, Colangelo L, Dimitrov N, Romond EH, et al. Randomized trial of postoperative adjuvant chemotherapy with or without radiotherapy for carcinoma of the rectum: National Surgical Adjuvant Breast and Bowel Project protocol R-02. *J. Natl. Cancer Inst.*, **92** (2000) 388–396.
5. Guillem JG, Puig-La Calle J, Akhurst T, Tickoo S, Ruo L, Minsky BD, et al. Prospective assessment of primary rectal cancer response to preoperative radiation and chemotherapy using 18-fluorodeoxyglucose positron emission tomography. *Dis. Colon Rectum*, **43** (2000) 18–24.
6. Whiteford MH, Whiteford HM, Yee LF, Ogunbiyi OA, Dehdashti F, Siegel BA, et al. Usefulness of FDG-PET scan in the assessment of suspected metastatic or recurrent adenocarcinoma of the colon and rectum. *Dis. Colon Rectum*, **53** (2000) 759–770.
7. Dosoretz DE, Gunderson LL, Hedberg S, Hoskins B, Blitzer PH, Shipley W, et al. Preoperative irradiation for unresectable rectal and rectosigmoid carcinomas. *Cancer*, **52** (1983) 814–818.
8. Medical Research Council Rectal Cancer Working Party. Randomized trial of surgery alone versus radiotherapy followed by surgery for potentially operable, locally advanced rectal cancer. *Lancet*, **348** (1996) 1605–1609.
9. Willett CG, Shellito PC, Tepper JE, Eliseo R, Convery K, and Wood WC. Intraoperative electron beam radiation therapy for primary locally advanced rectal and rectosigmoid carcinoma. *J. Clin. Oncol.*, **9** (1991) 843–849.

10. Willett CG, Shellito PC, Tepper JE, Eliseo R, Convery K, and Wood WC. Intraoperative electron beam radiation therapy for recurrent locally advanced rectal or rectosigmoid carcinoma. *Cancer*, **67** (1991) 1504–1508.

11. Mendenhall WM, Bland KI, Pfaff WW, Million RR, and Copeland EM III. Initially unresectable rectal adenocarcinoma treated with preoperative irradiation and surgery. *Ann. Surg.*, **205** (1986) 41–44.

12. Marsh RW, Chu NM, Vauthey JN, Mendenhall WM, Lauwers GY, Bewsher C, et al. Preoperative treatment of patients with locally advanced unresectable rectal adenocarcinoma utilizing continuous chronobiologically shaped 5-fluorouracil infusion and radiation therapy. *Cancer*, **78** (1996) 217–225.

13. Tobin RL, Mohiuddin M, and Marks G. Preoperative irradiation for cancer of the rectum with extrarectal fixation. *Int. J. Radiat. Oncol. Biol. Phys.*, **21** (1991) 1127–1132.

14. Minsky BD, Cohen AM, Enker WE, Harrison LB, and Sigurdson E. Radiation therapy for unresectable rectal cancer. *Int. J. Radiat. Oncol. Biol. Phys.*, **21** (1991) 1283–1289.

15. Mohiuddin M, Regine WF, John WJ, Hagihara PF, McGrath PC, Kenady DE, et al. Preoperative chemoradiation in fixed distal rectal cancer: dose time factors for pathological complete response. *Int. J. Radiat. Oncol. Biol. Phys.*, **46** (2000) 883–888.

16. Willett CG, Shellito PC, Rodkey GV, and Wood WC. Preoperative irradiation for tethered rectal carcinoma. *Radiother. Oncol.*, **21** (1991) 141–142.

17. Minsky BD, Cohen AM, Kemeny N, Enker WE, Kelsen D, Reichman B, et al. Enhancement of radiation induced downstaging of rectal cancer by 5-FU and high dose leucovorin chemotherapy. *J. Clin. Oncol.*, **10** (1992) 79–84.

18. Minsky BD, Cohen A, Enker W, Kelsen D, Kemeny N, Ilson D, et al. Pre-operative 5-FU, low dose leucovorin, and concurrent radiation therapy for rectal cancer. *Cancer*, **73** (1994) 273–278.

19. Minsky BD, Cohen AM, Enker WE, Harrison LB, Fass D, and Sigurdson E. Intraoperative brachytherapy alone in incompletely resected recurrent rectal cancer. *Radiother. Oncol.*, **21** (1991) 115–120.

20. Dibiase SJ, Rosenstock JG, Shabason L, and Corn BW. Tumor bed brachytherapy with a mesh template: an accessible alternative to intraoperative radiotherapy. *J. Surg. Oncol.*, **66** (1997) 104–109.

21. Minsky BD, Kemeny N, Cohen AM, Enker WE, Kelsen DP, Reichman B, et al. Preoperative high-dose leucovorin/5-fluorouracil and radiation therapy for unresectable rectal cancer. *Cancer*, **67** (1991) 2859–2866.

22. Harrison LB, Minsky BD, Enker WE, Mychalczak B, Guillem J, Paty PB, et al. High dose rate intraoperative radiation therapy (HDR-IORT) as part of the management strategy for locally advanced primary and recurrent rectal cancer. *Int. J. Radiat. Oncol. Biol. Phys.*, **42** (1998) 325–330.

23. Huber FT, Stepan R, Zimmermann F, Fink U, Molls M, and Siewert JR. Locally advanced rectal cancer: resection and intraoperative radiotherapy using the flab method combined with preoperative or postoperative radiochemotherapy. *Dis. Colon Rectum*, **39** (1996) 774–779.

24. Lowy AM, Rich TA, Skibber JM, Dubrow RA, and Curley SA. Preoperative infusional chemoradiation, selective intraoperative radiation, and resection for locally advanced pelvic recurrence of colorectal adenocarcinoma. *Ann. Surg.*, **223** (1996) 177–185.

25. Wallace JH, Willett CG, Shellito PC, Coen JJ, and Hoover HC. Intraoperative radiation therapy for locally advanced recurrent rectal or rectosigmoid cancer. *J. Surg. Oncol.*, **60** (1995) 122–127.

26. Nakfoor BM, Willett CG, Shellito PC, Kaufman DS, and Daly WJ. The impact of 5-fluorouracil and intraoperative electron beam radiation therapy on the outcome of patients with locally advanced primary rectal and rectosigmoid cancer. *Ann. Surg.*, **228** (1998) 194–200.

27. Gunderson LL, Nelson H, Martenson JA, Cha S, Haddock M, Devine R, et al. Locally advanced primary colorectal cancer: intraoperative electron and external beam irradiation + 5-FU. *Int. J. Radiat. Oncol. Biol. Phys.*, **37** (1997) 601–614.

28. Kallinowski F, Eble MJ, Buhr HJ, Wannenmacher M, an Herfarth CH. Intraoperative radiotherapy for primary and recurrent rectal cancers. *Eur. J. Surg. Oncol.*, **21** (1995) 191–194.

29. Kim HK, Jessup JM, Beard CJ, Bornstein B, Cady B, Stone MD, et al. Locally advanced rectal carcinoma: pelvic control and morbidity following preoperative radiation therapy, resection, and intraoperative radiation therapy. *Int. J. Radiat. Oncol. Biol. Phys.*, **38** (1997) 777–783.

30. Gunderson LL, Nelson H, Martenson JA, Cha S, Haddock M, Devine R, et al. Intraoperative electron and external beam irradiation with or without 5-fluorouracil and maximum surgical resection for previously unirradiated, locally recurrent colorectal cancer. *Dis. Colon Rectum*, **39** (1996) 1379–1395.

31. Valentini V, Morganti AG, De Franco A, Coco C, Ratto C, Doglietto GB, et al. Chemoradiation with or without intraoperative radiation therapy in patients with locally recurrent rectal carcinoma. Prognostic factors and long term outcome. *Cancer*, **86** (1999) 2612–2624.

32. Grinnell RS. The lymphatic and venous spread of carcinoma of the rectum. *Ann. Surg.*, **116** (1942) 200–215.

33. Bussieres E, Gilly FN, Rouanet P, Mahe MA, Roussel A, Delannes M, et al. Recurrences of rectal cancers: results of a multimodal approach with intraoperative radiation therapy. *Int. J. Radiat. Oncol. Biol. Phys.*, **34** (1995) 49–56.

34. Mannaerts GHH, Martijn H, Crommelin MA, Stultiens GNM, Dries W, Repelaraer van Driel OJ, et al. Intraoperative electron beam radiation therapy for locally recurrent rectal carcinoma. *Int. J. Radiat. Oncol. Biol. Phys.*, **45** (1999) 297–308.

35. Eble MJ, Lehnert T, Treiber M, Latz D, Herfarth C, and Wannenmacher M. Moderate dose intraoperative and external beam radiotherapy for locally recurrent rectal carcinoma. *Radiother. Oncol.*, **49** (1998) 169–174.

36. Hashiguchi Y, Sekine T, Sakamoto H, Tanaka Y, Kazumoto T, Kato S, et al. Intraoperative irradiation after surgery for locally recurrent rectal cancer. *Dis. Colon Rectum*, **42** (1999) 886–895.

37. LeCouteur RA, Gillette EL, Powers BE, Child G, McChesney SL, Ingram JT. Peripheral neuropathies following experimental intraoperative radiation therapy. *Int. J. Radiat. Oncol. Biol. Phys.*, **17** (1989) 583–590.

38. Powers BE, Gillette EL, McChesney SL, LeCouteur RA, and Withrow SJ. Bone necrosis and tumor induction following experimental intraoperative irradiation. *Int. J. Radiat. Oncol. Biol. Phys.*, **17** (1989) 559–567.

39. Vujaskovic Z, Gillette SM, Powers BE, Stukel TA, LaRue SM, Gillette EL, et al. Effects of intraoperative irradiation and intraoperative hyperthermia on canine sciatic nerve: neurologic and electrophysiologic study. *Int. J. Radiat. Oncol. Biol. Phys.*, **34** (1995) 125–131.

40. Vujaskovic Z, Powers BE, Paardekoper G, Gillette SM, Gillette EL, and Colaacchio TA. Effects of intraoperative irradiation (IORT) and intraoperative hyperthermia (IOHT) on canine sciatic nerve: histopathological and morphometric studies. *Int. J. Radiat. Oncol. Biol. Phys.*, **43** (1999) 1103–1109.

41. Johnstone PAS, Laskin WB, DeLuca AM, Barnes M, Kinsella TJ, and Sindelar WF. Tumors in dogs exposed to experimental intraoperative radiotherapy. *Int. J. Radiat. Oncol. Biol. Phys.*, **34** (1996) 853–857.

42. Gunderson LL, O'Connell MJ, and Dozois RR. The role of intraoperative irradiation in locally advanced primary and recurrent rectal adenocarcinoma. *World J. Surg.*, **16** (1992) 495–501.

43. Lanciano RM, Calkins AR, Wolkov HB, Buzydlowski J, Noyes RD, Sause W, et al. A phase I/II study of intraoperative radiotherapy in advanced unresectable or recurrent carcinoma of the rectum: a radiation therapy oncology group (RTOG) study. *J. Surg. Oncol.*, **53** (1993) 20–29.

44. Noyes RD, Weiss SM, Krall JM, Sause WT, Owens JR, Wolkov HB, et al. Surgical complications of intraoperative radiation therapy: the Radiation Therapy Oncology Group experience. *J. Surg. Oncol.*, **50** (1993) 209–215.

45. Minsky BD, Conti J, Cohen AM, Kelsen DP, Saltz L, Guillem J, et al. Acute toxicity of neoadjuvant bolus 5-FU/methotrexate and leucovorin rescue followed by continuous infusion 5-FU plus pre-operative radiation therapy for rectal cancer. *Radiat. Oncol. Invest.*, **4** (1996) 90–97.

46. Perera F, Fisher B, Kocha W, Plewes E, Taylor M, and Vincent M. A phase I pilot study of pelvic radiation and alpha-2A interferon in patients with locally advanced or recurrent rectal cancer. *Int. J. Radiat. Oncol. Biol. Phys.*, **37** (1997) 297–303.

47. Botwood N, James R, Vernon C, and Price P. A phase I study of "Tomudex" (raltitrexed) with radiotherapy (RT) as adjuvant treatment in patients (pt) with operable rectal cancer. *Proc. ASCO*, **17** (1998) 277a (abstract).

48. James RD, Price P, and Valentini V. Raltitrexed (Tomudex) concomitant with radiotherapy as adjuvant treatment for patients with rectal cancer: preliminary results of phase I studies. *Eur. J. Cancer*, **35** (1999) s19–s22.

49. Valentini V, Morganti AG, Fiorentino G, Luzi S, Smaniotto D, Turriziani A, et al. Chemoradiation with raltitrexed (Tomudex) and concomitant preoperative radiotherapy has potential in the treatment of stage II/III resectable rectal cancer. *Proc ASCO*, **18** (1999) 257a (abstract).

50. James RD, Price P and Smith M. Raltitrexed (Tomudex) plus radiotherapy is well tolerated and warrants further investigation in patients with advanced inoperable/recurrent rectal cancer. *Proc. ASCO*, **18** (1999) 288a (abstract).

51. Feliu J, Calvillo J, Escribano A, De Castro J, Espinosa A, Ordonez A, et al. Neoadjuvant therapy of rectal carcinoma with UFT-folinic acid (LV) plus radiotherapy. *Proc. ASCO*, **18** (1999) 239a (abstract).

52. Pfeiffer P. Concurrent UFT/L-leucovorin and curative intended radiotherapy (60 Gy) in patients with locally advanced rectal cancer (LARC): a phase I/II trial. *Proc. ASCO*, **19** (2000) 255a (abstract).

53. Mitchell E, Ahmad N, Fry RD, Anne PR, Rakanic J, Goldstein SD, et al. Combined modality therapy of locally advanced or recurrent adenocarcinoma of the rectum: preliminary report of a phase I trial of chemotherapy (CT) with CPT-11, 5-FU, and concomitant irradiation (RT). *Proc. ASCO*, **18** (1999) 247a (abstract).

54. Minsky BD, O'Reilly E, Wong D, Sharma S, Paty P, Guillem J, et al. Daily low-dose irinotecan (CPT-11) plus pelvic irradiation as preoperative treatment of locally advanced rectal cancer. *Proc. ASCO*, **18** (1999) 266a (abstract).

55. Anne P, Mitchell EP, Ahmad N, Fry RD, Rakinic J, Goldstein SD, et al. Radiosensitization in locally advanced adenocarcinoma of the rectum using combined modality therapy (CMT) with CPT-11, 5-fluorouracil, concomitant irradiation. *Proc ASCO*, **19** (2000) 250 (abstract).

56. Carraro S, Roca E, Cartelli C, Rafailovici L, Lougedo M, Wasserman E, et al. Oxaliplatin (OXA), 5-florouracil (5-FU) and leucovorin (LV) plus radiotherapy in unresectable rectal cancer (URC): preliminary results. *Proc. ASCO*, **19** (2000) 291a (abstract).

57. Freyer G, Bossard N, Romestaing P, Mornex F, Trillet-Lenoir V, and Gerard JP. Oxaliplatin (OXA), 5-fluorouracil (5-FU), L-folinic acid (FA) and concomitant irradiation in patients with rectal cancer; a phase I study. *Proc. ASCO*, **19** (2000) 260a (abstract).

58. Glynne-Jones R, Falk S, Maughan T, Sebag-Montefiore D, Meadows HM, and Das-Gupta A. Results of preoperative radiation and oxaliplatin in combination with 5-fluorouracil (5-FU) and leucovorin (LV). *Proc. ASCO*, **19** (2000) 310a (abstract).

59. Cohen DP, Lee CG, Anscher MS, Ludwig KA, Tyler DS, Seigler HF, et al. Phase I study of chemoradiation therapy with oral Eniluracil (776C85)/5-fluorouracil in patients with rectal adenocarcinoma. *Proc. ASCO*, **19** (2000) 261a (abstract).

60. Dunst J, Reese T, and Frings S. Phase I study of Capecitabine combined with standard radiotherapy in patients with rectal cancer. *Proc. ASCO*, **19** (2000) 256a (abstract).

61. Minsky BD, Cohen A, Enker W, Kelsen D, Kemeny N, Ilson D, et al. Pre-operative 5-FU, low dose leucovorin, and radiation therapy for locally advanced/unresectable rectal cancer. *Int. J. Radiat. Oncol. Biol. Phys.*, **37** (1997) 289–295.

62. Shibata D, Guillem JG, Lanouette NM, Paty P, Minsky B, Harrison L, et al. Functional and quality of life outcomes in patients with rectal cancer after combined modality therapy, intraoperative radiation therapy, and sphincter preservation. *Dis. Colon Rectum*, **43** (2000) 752–758.

63. Kaminsky-Forrett MC, Conroy T, Luporsi E, Peiffert D, Lapeyre M, Boissel P, et al. Prognostic implications of downstaging following preoperative radiation therapy for operable T3-T4 rectal cancer. *Int. J. Radiat. Oncol. Biol. Phys.*, **42** (1998) 935–941.

64. Ahmad NR, Nagle DA, and Topham A. Pathologic complete response predicts long-term survival following preoperative radiation therapy for rectal cancer. *Int. J. Radiat. Oncol. Biol. Phys.*, **39** (1997) 284 (abstract).

65. Gama AH, Gansl RC, Souza PMB, Simon SD, Costa FO, Aquilar PB, et al. Primary treatment of low rectal cancer with combined chemotherapy and radiation therapy (C+RT): results of a pilot study. *Proc. ASCO*, **12** (1993) 215 (abstract).

66. Willett CG, Hagan M, Daley W, Warland G, Shellito PC, and Compton CC. Changes in tumor proliferation of rectal cancer induced by preoperative 5-fluorouracil and irradiation. *Dis. Colon Rectum*, **41** (1998) 62–67.

67. Fu CG, Tominaga O, Nagawa H, Nita ME, Masaki T, Ishimaru G, et al. Role of p53 and p21/WAF1 detection in patient selection for preoperative radiotherapy in rectal cancer patients. *Dis. Colon Rectum*, **41** (1988) 58–74.

68. Sakakura C, Koide KI, Kimura A, Taniguchi H, Hagiwara A, Yamaguchi T, et al. Analysis of histologic therapeutic effect, apoptosis rate and p53 status after combined treatment with radiation, hyperthermia, and 5-fluorouracil suppositories for advanced rectal cancers. *Br. J. Cancer*, **77** (1998) 159–166.

69. Scott N, Hale A, Deakin M, Hand P, Adab FA, Hall C, et al. A histopathological assessment of the response of rectal adenocarcinoma to combination chemo-radiotherapy: relationship to apoptotic activity, p53, and bcl-2 expression. *Eur. J. Surg. Oncol.*, **24** (1998) 169–173.

70. Tannapfel A, Nusslein S, Fietkau R, Katalinic A, Kockerling F, and Wittekind C. Apoptosis, proliferation, bax, bcl-2, and p53 status prior to and after preoperative radiochemotherapy for locally advanced rectal cancer. *Int. J. Radiat. Oncol. Biol. Phys.*, **41** (1998) 585–591.

71. Luna-Perez P, Arriola EL, Cuadra Y, Alvarado I, and Quintero A. p53 Protein overexpression and response to induction chemoradiation therapy in patients with locally advanced rectal adenocarcinoma. *Ann. Surg. Oncol.*, **5** (1998) 203–208.

72. Nehls O, Klump B, Holzmann K, Lammering G, Borchard F, Gruenagel HH, et al. Influence of p53 status on prognosis in preoperatively irradiated rectal carcinoma. *Cancer*, **85** (1999) 2541–2548.

73. Adell G, Sun XF, Olle S, Klintenberg C, Sjodahl R, and Nordenskjold B. p53 Status: an indicator for the effect of preoperative radiotherapy of rectal cancer. *Radiother. Oncol.*, **51** (1999) 169–174.

74. Willett CG, Warland G, Coen J, Shellito PC, and Compton CC. Rectal cancer: the influence of tumor proliferation on response to preoperative irradiation. *Int. J. Radiat. Oncol. Biol. Phys.*, **32** (1995) 57–61.

75. Willett CG, Warland G, Hagan MP, Daly WJ, Coen J, Shellito PC, et al. Tumor proliferation in rectal cancer following preoperative irradiation. *J. Clin. Oncol.*, **13** (1995) 1417–1424.

76. Rich TA. Infusional chemoradiation for operable rectal cancer: post-, pre-, or nonoperative management? *Oncology*, **11** (1997) 295–315.

77. Rich TA, Sinicrope F, Stephens C, Myen R, Terry N, Meistrich M, et al. Downstaging of T3 rectal cancer after preoperative infusional chemoradiation is correlated with spontaneous apoptosis index and BCL-2 staining. *Int. J. Radiat. Oncol. Biol. Phys.*, **36** (1996) 259 (abstract).

78. Berger C, de Muret A, Garaud P, Chapet S, Bourlier P, Reynaud-Bougnoux A, et al. Preoperative radiotherapy (RT) for rectal cancer: predictive factors of tumor downstaging and residual tumor density (RTCD): prognostic implications. *Int. J. Radiat. Oncol. Biol. Phys.*, **37** (1997) 619–627.

79. Desai GR, Meyerson RJ, Higashikubo R, Birnbaum E, Fleshman J, Fry R, et al. Carcinoma of the rectum: possible cellular predictors of metastatic potential and response to radiation therapy. *Dis. Colon Rectum*, **39** (1996) 1090–1096.

80. Neoptolemos JP, Oates GD, Newbold KM, Robson AM, McConkey C, and Powell J. Cyclin/proliferation cell nuclear antigen immunohistochemistry does not improve the prognostic power of Dukes' or Jass' classifications for colorectal cancer. *Br. J. Surg.*, **82** (1995) 184–187.

81. Nicholl ID and Dunlop MG. Molecular markers of prognosis in colorectal cancer. *J. Natl. Cancer Inst.*, **91** (1999) 1267–1269.

82. Goes RN, Beart RW, Simons AJ, Gunderson LL, Grado G, and Streeter O. Use of brachytherapy in management of locally recurrent rectal cancer. *Dis. Colon Rectum*, **40** (1997) 1177–1179.

83. Magrini S, Nelson H, Gunderson L, and Sim FH. Sacropelvic resection and intraoperative electron irradiation in the management of recurrent anorectal cancer. *Dis. Colon Rectum*, **39** (1996) 1–9.

84. Lingareddy V, Ahmad NR, and Mohiuddin M. Palliative reirradiation for recurrent rectal cancer. *Int. J. Radiat. Oncol. Biol. Phys.*, **38** (1997) 785–790.

85. Nag S, Martinez-Monge R, Mills J, Bauer C, Grecula J, Nieroda C, et al. Intraoperative high dose rate brachytherapy in recurrent metastatic colorectal carcinoma. *Ann. Surg. Oncol.*, **5** (1998) 16–22.

86. Schild SE, Martenson JA, Gunderson LL, and Dozois RR. Long-term survival and patterns of failure after postoperative radiation therapy for subtotally resected rectal adenocarcinoma. *Int. J. Radiat. Oncol. Biol. Phys.*, **16** (1989) 459–463.

87. Suzuki K, Gunderson LL, Devine RM, Weaver AM, Dozois RR, Ilstrup DM, et al. Intraoperative irradiation after palliative surgery for locally recurrent rectal cancer. *Cancer*, **75** (1995) 939–952.

88. Allee PE, Tepper JE, Gunderson LL, and Munzenrider JE. Postoperative radiation therapy for incompletely resected colorectal carcinoma. *Int. J. Radiat. Oncol. Biol. Phys.*, **17** (1989) 1171–1176.

89. Papillon J and Berard PH. Endocavitary irradiation in the conservative treatment of adenocarcinoma of the low rectum. *World J. Surg.*, **16** (1992) 451–457.

90. Kodner IJ and Shemesh EI. Radiation therapy as definitive treatment for adenocarcinoma of the rectum. *Surgery*, **114** (1993) 850–860.

91. Brierley JD, Cummings BJ, Wong CS, Keane TJ, O'Sullivan B, Catton CN, et al. Adenocarcinoma of the rectum treated by radical external radiation therapy. *Int. J. Radiat. Oncol. Biol. Phys.*, **31** (1995) 255–259.

92. Wong CS, Cummings BJ, Brierley JD, Catton CN, McLean M, Catton P, et al. Treatment of locally recurrent rectal carcinoma—results and prognostic factors. *Int. J. Radiat. Oncol. Biol. Phys.*, **40** (1998) 427–435.

93. Guiney MJ, Smith JG, Worotniuk V, Ngan S, and Blakey D. Radiotherapy treatment for isolated loco-regional recurrence of rectosigmoid cancer following definitive surgery: Peter McCallum Cancer Institute experience: 1981–1990. *Int. J. Radiat. Oncol. Biol. Phys.*, **38** (1997) 1019–1025.

94. Gerard JP, Roy P, Coquard R, Barbet N, Romestaing P, Ayzac L, et al. Combined curative radiation therapy alone in (T1) T2-3 rectal adenocarcinoma: a pilot study of 29 patients. *Radiother. Oncol.*, **38** (1996) 131–137.

95. Overgaard M, Overgaard J, and Sell A. Dose-response relationship for radiation therapy of recurrent, residual, and primarily inoperable colorectal cancer. *Radiother. Oncol.*, **1** (1984) 217–225.

96. Valentini V, Morganti AG, Luzi S, Mantello G, Mantini G, Salvi G, et al. Is chemoradiation feasible in elderly patients? A study of 17 patients with anorectal carcinoma. *Cancer*, **80** (1997) 1387–1392.

97. Rominger CJ, Gelber RD, Gunderson LL, and Conner N. Radiation therapy alone or in combination with chemotherapy in the treatment of residual or inoperable carcinoma of the rectum and rectosigmoid or pelvic recurrence following colorectal surgery. Radiation Therapy Oncology Group study (76–16). *Am. J. Clin. Oncol.*, **8** (1985) 118–127.

98. Danjoux CE, Gelber RD, Catton GE, and Klaassen DJ. Combination chemo-radiotherapy for residual, recurrent, or inoperable carcinoma of the rectum: ECOG Study (EST 3276). *Int. J. Radiat. Oncol. Biol. Phys.*, **11** (1985) 765–771.

99. Nishimura Y, Hiraoka M, Akuta K, Jo S, Nagata Y, Masunaga SI, et al. Hyperthermia combined with radiation therapy for primarily unresectable and recurrent colorectal cancer. *Int. J. Radiat. Oncol. Biol. Phys.*, **23** (1992) 759–768.

100. Graf R, Wust P, Gellermann J, Mohr B, Gogler H, Riess H, et al. Phase II trial of radiation therapy with 45 Gy, 5-fluorouracil (5-FU), and mitomycin-C (MMC) in patients with anal cancer—a rationale to add regional hyperthermia. *Int. J. Radiat. Oncol. Biol. Phys.*, **36** (1996) 296 (abstract).

101. Furuta K, Konishi F, Kanazawa K, Saito K, and Sugawara T. Synergistic effects of hyperthermia in preoperative radiochemotherapy for rectal carcinoma. *Dis. Colon Rectum*, **40** (1997) 1303–1312.

102. Ohno S, Tomoda M, Tomisaki S, Kitamura K, Mori M, Maehara Y, et al. Improved surgical results after combining preoperative hyperthermia with chemotherapy and radiotherapy for patients with carcinoma of the rectum. *Dis. Colon Rectum*, **40** (1997) 401–406.

103. Ichikawa D, Yamaguchi T, Yoshioka Y, Sawai K, and Takahashi T. Prognostic evaluation of preoperative combined treatment for advanced cancer in the lower rectum with radiation, intraluminal hyperthermia, and 5-fluorouracil suppository. *Am. J. Surg.*, **171** (1996) 346–350.

104. Anscher MS, Lee C, Hurwitz HI, Tyler DS, Prosnitz LR, Jowell P, et al. A pilot study of preoperative continuous infusion 5-fluorouracil, external microwave hyperthermia, and external beam radiotherapy for treatment of locally advanced, unresectable, or recurrent rectal cancer. *Int. J. Radiat. Oncol. Biol. Phys.*, **47** (2000) 719–724.

105. Emami B, Myerson RJ, Scott C, Gibbs F, Lee C, and Perez CA. Phase I/II study, combination of radiotherapy and hyperthermia in patients with deep-seated malignant tumors: report of a pilot study by the Radiation Therapy Oncology Group. *Int. J. Radiat. Oncol. Biol. Phys.*, **20** (1991) 73–79.

106. Duncan W, Arnott SJ, Jack WJL, Orr JA, Kerr GR, and Williams JR. Results of two randomized trials of neutron therapy in rectal adenocarcinoma. *Radiother. Oncol.*, **8** (1987) 191–198.

107. Battermann JJ. Results of d+T fast neutron irradiation on advanced tumors of the bladder and rectum. *Int. J. Radiat. Oncol. Biol. Phys.*, **8** (1982) 2159–2164.

108. Pu AT, Robertson JM, and Lawrence TS. Current status of radiation sensitization by fluoropyrimidines. *Oncology*, **9** (1995) 707–714.

109. Rhomberg W, Eiter H, Hergan K, and Schneider B. Inoperable recurrent rectal cancer: results of a prospective trial with radiation therapy and razoxane. *Int. J. Radiat. Oncol. Biol. Phys.*, **30** (1994) 419–425.

110. Talley NA, Chen F, King D, Jones M, and Talley NJ. Short-chain fatty acids in the treatment of radiation proctitis. A randomized, double-blind, placebo-controlled, cross-over pilot trial. *Dis. Colon Rectum*, **40** (1997) 1046–1050.

111. O'Brien PC, Franklin CI, Dear KBG, Hamilton CC, Poulsen M, Joseph DJ, et al. A phase III double-blind randomised study of rectal sufralfate suspension in the prevention of acute radiation proctitis. *Radiother. Oncol.*, **45** (1997) 117–123.

112. Martenson JA Jr, Bollinger JW, Sloan JA, Novotny PJ, Utias RE, Michalak JC, et al. Sucralfate in the prevention of treatment-induced diarrhea in patients receiving pelvic radiation therapy: a North Central Cancer Treatment Group Phase III double-blind placebo-controlled trial. *J. Clin. Oncol.*, **18** (2000) 1239–1245.

113. Martenson JA, Hyland G, Moertel CG, Mailliard JA, O'Fallon JR, Collins RT, et al. Olsalizine is contraindicated during pelvic radiation therapy: results of a double-blind randomized clinical trial. *Int. J. Radiat. Oncol. Biol. Phys.*, **35** (1996) 299–303.

114. Resbeut M, Marteau P, Cowen D, Richaud P, Bourdin S, Dubois JB, et al. A randomized double blind placebo controlled multicenter study of mesalazine for the prevention of acute radiation enteritis. *Radiother. Oncol.*, **44** (1997) 59–63.

115. Baughan CA, Canney PA, Buchanan RB, and Pickering RM. A randomized trial to assess the efficacy of 5-aminosalicylic acid for the prevention of radiation enteritis. *Clin. Oncol.*, **5** (1993) 19–24.

116. Liu T, Liu Y, He S, Zhang Z, and Kligerman MM. Use of radiation with or without WR-2721 in advanced rectal cancer. *Cancer*, **69** (1992) 2820–2825.

117. Montana GS, Anscher MS, Mansbach CM II, Daly N, Delannes M, Clarke-Pearson D, et al. Topical application of WR-2721 to prevent radiation-induced proctosigmoiditis. *Cancer*, **69** (1992) 2826–2830.

118. Withers HR. Biological basis for altered fractionation schemes. *Cancer*, **55** (1985) 2086–2095.

119. Coucke PA, Cuttat JF, and Mirimanoff RO. Adjuvant postoperative accelerated hyperfractionated radiotherapy in rectal cancer: a feasibility study. *Int. J. Radiat. Oncol. Biol. Phys.*, **27** (1993) 885–889.

120. Coucke PA, Sartorelli B, Cuttat JF, Jeanneret W, Gillet M, and Mirimanoff RO. The rationale to switch from postoperative hyperfractionated accelerated radiotherapy to preoperative hyperfractionated accelerated radiotherapy in rectal cancer. *Int. J. Radiat. Oncol. Biol. Phys.*, **32** (1995) 181–188.

121. Bozzetti F, Baratti D, Andreola S, Zucali R, Schiavo M, Spinelli P, et al. Preoperative radiation therapy for patients with T2-T3 carcinoma of the middle-to-lower rectum. *Cancer*, **86** (1999) 398–404.

122. Movsas B, Hanlon A, Lanciano R, Scher RM, Weiner LM, Sigurdson ER, et al. Phase I dose escalating trial of hyperfractionated pre-operative chemoradiation for locally advanced rectal cancer. *Int. J. Radiat. Oncol. Biol. Phys.*, **42** (1998) 43–50.

123. Tait DM, Nahum AE, Meyer LC, Law M, Dearnaley DP, Horwich A, et al. Acute toxicity in pelvic radiotherapy; a randomised trial of conformal versus conventional treatment. *Radiother. Oncol.*, **42** (1997) 121–136.
124. Shank B, LoSasso T, Brewster L, Burman C, Cheng E, Chu JCH, et al. Three-dimensional treatment planning for post-operative treatment of rectal carcinoma. *Int. J. Radiat. Oncol. Biol. Phys.*, **21** (1991) 253–265.
125. Isacsson U, Montelius A, Jung B, and Glimelius B. Comparative treatment planning between proton and X-ray therapy in locally advanced rectal cancer. *Radiother. Oncol.*, **41** (1997) 263–272.

13   Radiation Therapy for Hepatic Metastases

John M. Robertson

CONTENTS

1. INTRODUCTION

In the mid-1960s, it was reported that only a modest dose of external beam radiation therapy (RT) given to the whole liver could produce clinically significant hepatic dysfunction *(1)*. Because this dose was well below that required for the primary treatment of a number of solid tumors, RT was generally only considered for palliation, and research efforts were directed toward determining the degree of symptomatic benefit. Additional attempts were made to increase the relative effect of whole-liver RT by adding radiation sensitizers or chemotherapy. Other efforts avoided irradiation of the whole liver by using radiopharmaceuticals, either placed directly in the liver or administered via vascular infusion.

In the last decade, there have been tremendous improvements in the ability to plan RT treatment *(2)*. Prior to these developments, RT was typically planned using a single contour of the external surface of the patient at the center of the treatment region. Target volumes to be irradiated and normal tissues to be avoided were then outlined on the contour using bone landmarks, contrast on plain X-rays, and/or the physician's best guess at transferring anatomy from a diagnostic computed tomography (CT) scan. With the recent advances in radiographic imaging, computer graphics, and computational speed, a complete three-dimensional representation of the patient's external shape and internal anatomy is possible. This has allowed the routine use of radiation beams that are not confined to the axial plane, potentially sparing a maximal volume of liver from the radiation *(3)*. Three-dimensional treatment planning has also allowed the radiation oncologist to have an accurate measurement of the distribution of dose within the normal tissues. These developments led to a resurgence

From: *Colorectal Cancer: Multimodality Management*
Edited by: L. Saltz © Humana Press Inc., Totowa, NJ

Table 1
Development of Radiation-Induced Liver Disease
in Patients Irradiated to the Whole Liver

Dose (Gy)	No. of patients with RILD / No. treated
<30	0 / 5
30–35	1 / 8
35–40	5 / 9 (1 fatal)
40–51	7 / 18 (2 fatal)

Source: Modified from ref. 1.

of interest in the use of external beam RT. Indeed, recent studies have shown that a hepatic radiation dose of over three times the whole-liver tolerance dose can be given safely if enough normal liver is spared (4).

2. RADIATION-INDUCED LIVER DISEASE

The typical symptoms of radiation-induced liver disease (RILD) occur 1–2 mo after the end of RT (for review, see ref. 5). The clinical appearance is similar to suprahepatic vein obstruction or Budd–Chiari syndrome, with fatigue, rapid weight gain, and increased girth. Although ascites and hepatomegaly may be present on physical exam, jaundice is usually absent. Blood tests reveal moderate elevations of aspartate transaminase and alanine transaminase and a normal or slightly increased bilirubin, but an alkaline phosphatase that is 3–10 times normal. Radiographic studies are useful for ruling out progressive hepatic disease as the cause of dysfunction, but it cannot rule in RILD, as reversible changes resulting from RT are frequently observed (6). Biopsy of the liver will show the typical pattern of veno-occlusive disease, with severe congestion of the sinusoids in the central lobules and atrophy of the inner portion of the liver plates (5). However, in contrast to Budd–Chiari syndrome, there are no changes in the larger veins of the liver.

The risk of developing RILD is dependent on both the dose of radiation given and the volume of liver irradiated. In the original description of RILD, 40 patients with lymphoma or ovarian cancer were treated with 13–51 Gy (median: 39 Gy) to the whole liver (1). Thirteen developed RILD, which was lethal in three patients and had an obvious relationship with the dose administered (Table 1). A later, prospective study by the Radiation Therapy Oncology Group (RTOG) tested four different dose and fractionation combinations for whole-liver RT, from as short as 21 Gy in 7 treatments to as long as 30 Gy in 15 treatments and found no evidence of RILD in over 100 patients treated (7). The safety of the 21 Gy in the 7-treatment schedule was redemonstrated in a prospective trial in which 81 patients were treated without RILD (8). The RTOG also performed the only phase I study of RT dose, administering 27 Gy, 30 Gy, and 33 Gy at 1.5 Gy twice a day (9). None of the 122 patients treated to 27 and 30 Gy experienced RILD, however, 5 of 51 patients entered at the 33-Gy level revealed clinical or biochemical evidence of RILD but no grade ≥4 toxicity. Overall, through this and other reports (10), it seems fairly certain that the whole liver can tolerate 30–35 Gy in standard fractionation or hyperfractionation, but above this amount, the risk of RILD rises steeply (11).

There is considerable evidence that a portion of the liver can be irradiated to a very high dose as long as other volumes of the liver have not been irradiated directly. Although this observation has been recognized for decades (1), quantification of the relationship has been

Table 2
Results of Palliative Whole-Liver RT

Author (ref.)	Dose (Gy)	No. of patients	Symptomatic improvement (% Any improvement / % complete resolution)						
			Pain	Hepatomeg	Fever/NS	Anorexia	Fatigue	N/V	Jaundice
Phillips et al. *(22)*	20–37.5	36	87 / 87	—	61 / 61	65 / 65	55 / 55	44 / 44	—
Sherman et al. *(23)*	15–30	55	90 / 54	93 / 62	—	—	—	—	—
Borgelt et al. *(7)*	20–30.4	103	55 / 24	—	45 / 27	28 / 9	19 / 7	49 / 34	27 / 17
Leibel et al. *(8)*	21	187	80 / 54	—	—	—	—	—	—
Mohuiddin et al. *(20)*	8–31	33	71 / —	59 / —	67 / —	35 / —	17 / —	25 / —	25 / —
	33–59.39	12	100 / —	89 / —	*	*	*	*	*

Note: Hepatomeg = hepatomegaly; NS = night sweats; N/V = nausea and vomiting; — = not reported; * = less than 5 patients with complaint.

described only recently *(12,13)*. Using three-dimensional treatment planning techniques, investigators have found that a dose of RT as high as 90 Gy can be given safely to liver abnormalities as long as a minimum volume of normal liver was not irradiated *(4)*.

The risk of developing RILD may be increased by the coadministration of chemotherapeutic agents and RT, resulting from both direct hepatotoxicity *(14)* and radiosensitization *(15)*. The largest experience with combined chemotherapy and hepatic RT is with the fluoropyrimidines, which have little hepatotoxicity but are mild radiation sensitizers. The combination of either systemic or hepatic arterial fluoropyrimidines with whole-liver RT to approximately 30 Gy has been tested in multiple studies, without evidence that the whole-liver tolerance dose was reduced *(16–18)*. Hematologic toxicity may be affected as one trial of concurrent 5-fluorouracil (5-FU) and whole-liver RT required a major chemotherapy dose reduction during the study *(19)*; however, other studies using a similar combination have not reported undue toxicity *(16–18,20)*. Severe or fatal liver dysfunction has been reported with other chemotherapeutic agents. One phase II trial combined hepatic arterial 5-FU and mitomycin C with whole-liver RT and found 11 of 13 patients with significant persistent liver enzyme elevations and one death as a result of hepatic dysfunction with an RT dose of only 19.5 Gy at 1.5 Gy/d *(21)*. This experience suggests that the combination of whole-liver RT with any new drug will require a phase I study to determine the safe dose of either modality.

3. PALLIATIVE TREATMENT

Whole-liver RT in symptomatic patients has resulted in excellent palliation (Table 2), with pain improvement in 55–89% of patients *(7,8,17,20,22,23)* and complete relief in about 50% *(8)*. Symptomatic improvement in pain was prompt and occurred within a median of about 2 wk from the beginning of treatment *(7,8)*. Patients with more severe symptoms experienced the greatest degree of improvement in one prospective trial, with 70% of those in severe pain but only 27% of patients with mild pain reporting improvement *(7)*. Other symptoms, such as nausea, vomiting, fever, jaundice and anorexia, have also been reported to improve in 25–50% of patients *(7,20,22)*. The duration of palliative benefit has been variable, with one study reporting an average of only 1.2 mo of improved symptoms *(22)*, but others finding that pain relief lasted for most of the patients remaining median 4.5-mo lifetime *(23)*. In the largest prospective series *(8)*, symptomatic patients experienced a median duration of response of 13 wk and 52% of those surviving 3 mo remained improved. Retrospective studies have suggested no additional palliative benefit with combined liver RT and concurrent chemotherapy *(22,23)*; however, there are no randomized trials available.

The RTOG tested a number of different dose and fractionation regimens in a prospective, nonrandomized pilot study *(7)*. A total of 103 evaluable patients with liver metastases, including 55 from the gastrointestinal tract, were treated with 1 of 6 different RT schedules, ranging from 21 Gy in 7 fractions to 30.4 Gy in 19 fractions. Approximately one-quarter of patients were unable to complete the treatment, primarily the result of declining performance status. Of the 78 patients with abdominal pain, 55% experienced some improvement in pain, with complete relief in 24%. There was no relationship among the frequency of pain relief and the primary tumor, extent of metastases, or treatment regimen. The toxicity was acceptable, with 16% of patients compaining of nausea and vomiting, which led to an early termination of therapy in only 3%.

The RTOG also performed the largest randomized prospective trial of palliative liver RT, testing 21 Gy in seven fractions alone vs combined with the hypoxic cell sensitizer misonidazole *(8)*. There were 187 evaluable patients, including 60% with metastatic colon cancer, and patients were stratified according to the primary site of disease. The addition of misonidazole was associated with an 87% rate of improvement in pain with complete relief in 63% vs 74% improvement, with complete relief in 47% of patients treated with RT alone ($p = 0.08$ and $p = 0.20$, respectively). Patients with metastatic colon cancer had a significantly greater frequency of palliative benefit than other primary sites ($p = 0.02$). Symptoms other than pain were not reported. The objective response was assessed by CT scan in 164 patients and included 1 complete and 11 partial responses with no difference between the treatment arms. Although responses were rare and there was no survival benefit with misonidazole, this study did demonstrate the palliative benefit of short-course whole-liver RT in a prospective multicenter setting.

A higher dose of RT may be associated with an increased rate of palliation. One study reported 45 patients treated for metastatic colorectal cancer and found that the palliation rates were substantially better in 12 patients who were treated with whole-liver RT plus a boost to a total dose of 33–60 Gy, compared to 33 historical controls treated with whole-liver RT alone *(20)*. This finding has not been tested in randomized prospective trials.

4. PRIMARY TREATMENT

The surgical results with liver resection suggest that control of hepatic metastases may be associated with long-term survival. Typically, resection has been limited to patients without involved hepatic lymph nodes, unresectable extrahepatic disease, or more than three metastatic deposits *(24)*. Even with these criteria, approx 50% of patients explored were found to be unresectable in a prospective multi-institutional study, usually resulting from the presence of bilobar disease found at exploration *(25)*. Nonresection therapies, such as RT, are not impaired by vascular considerations or lobar location and offer the possibility of successful treatment in a larger group of patients, ideally approaching the success rate reported for resection.

Because of the wide variety of prognostic factors, it is very difficult to compare treatments in the absence of randomized trials. For example, a review of 1568 patients with resected liver metastases found seven variables with an independent prognostic value: age, extension of the primary tumor to the serosa, lymphatic spread of the primary tumor, time interval from the primary tumor to metastases, size of the largest metastasis, number of metastases,

Table 3
Response and Survival Rates of Whole-Liver Radiation Therapy

Author (ref.)	No. of patients	Dose RT (Gy)	Chemo	Response rate (%)	Median survival (mo)
Herbsman et al. (30)	13	25–30	HA FUdR	—	16.2
Friedman et al. (31)	22 (19 C)	13.5–21	HA 5-FU	47.6 55% C	See article
Rotman et al. (17)	23	22–32	IV 5-FU	65	6.5
Leibel et al. (8)	94 (57 C)	21	None	4	See article
	93 (55 C)	21	Misonidazole	10	See article
Wiley et al. (29)	19	25.5	HA 5-FU	37	6
Lawrence et al. (18)	20 (? C)	33	HA FUdR	39	8[a]
Russell et al. (9)	173 (130 C)	27–33	None	—	4.2
Mohiuddin et al. (20)	33	8–31	IV/HA	—	4

Note: Chemo = chemotherapy administered concurrently with RT; C = colorectal cancer; — = not available; HA = hepatic arterial; FUdR = fluorodeoxyuridine; IV = intravenous.
[a]Includes patients treated with focal liver RT.

and margins of the hepatic resection (26). Patients with none to two of these variables had a 2-yr survival of 79%, whereas those with five to seven of the variables had a 2-yr survival of 43%. Prognostic factors for patients with unresectable disease have also been identified and include performance status and the presence of extrahepatic disease (17,27).

4.1. Whole Liver Treatment

The success of whole-liver RT alone has been reported by the RTOG in the above-mentioned prospective randomized study testing the addition of the radiosensitizer misonidazole (8). In the control arm, 94 patients with hepatic metastases, including 57 with metastatic colorectal cancer, were treated with 21 Gy in 7 fractions and had an objective response rate of 4%. Patients with metastatic colorectal cancer and a Karnofsky performance status ≥80 had a median survival of 6 mo. Modifying the RT by using hyperfractionation, which administered a slightly higher dose of RT (up to 33 Gy), produced no recognizable survival benefit (9).

There are two randomized studies of whole-liver RT combined with chemotherapy or radiosensitizers. One was a trial that randomized whole-liver RT to 25.5 Gy in 17 fractions given 2 wk after completion of a course of hepatic arterial 5-FU (28). The study involved 37 patients with metastatic colorectal cancer and found no benefit in response rate (37%) or survival (median 6 mo) with the addition of RT. The other randomized study was the previously mentioned trial of concurrent liver RT and misonidazole that found a nonsignificant increase in the response rate to 10% and no survival benefit (8).

A number of nonrandomized studies have successfully combined intravenous or hepatic arterial fluoropyrimidine chemotherapy with whole-liver RT without evidence of severe toxicity. The reported response rates have varied from 39% to 65%, with median survival rates ranging from 4 to 16.2 mo (17,18,20,29,30). In general, these studies reported higher response rates but similar median survival rates to that of whole-liver RT alone (Table 3). One study (29) reported a median survival that was more than double the whole-liver RT alone rates, however, only 13 patients were treated in this trial and this finding probably reflects the selection bias inherent in any nonrandomized study.

4.2. Focal Liver Treatment

There is a considerable amount of experience demonstrating that a higher dose of RT may be given safely to the liver if a sufficient volume of normal liver remained untreated. One example of this principle is the use of radiopharmaceuticals, which achieve selectivity by direct placement in the tumor using brachytherapy techniques or infusion via the hepatic artery or by systemic administration with targeted monoclonal antibodies (for a thorough review, *see* ref. *31*). Brachytherapy techniques have included remote afterloading interstitial iridium-192 *(32,33)*, which delivered 30 Gy in a single treatment, and permanent iodine-125 *(34–36)*, which delivered a 160-Gy minimum peripheral dose over the lifetime of the isotope. The primary disadvantage of brachytherapy is the need for an open abdomen in order to place the catheters used to direct the radioactive material. On the other hand, the abdominal exploration may have allowed both the optimal selection of patients without extrahepatic disease and the best available definition of the target volume for RT. Indeed, there has been pathologic verification of a complete response in patients treated with brachytherapy *(33)*. In the largest experience with brachytherapy, 56 patients with unresectable or residual disease after surgical resection of liver metastases were treated with permanent iodine-125 and had a 23% 5-yr actuarial control of liver disease and an 8% 5-yr actuarial survival *(36)*. Other methods using radiopharmaceuticals, such as yttrium-90 microspheres via direct injection *(37)* or the hepatic artery *(38)*, or radiolabeled anticarcinoembryonic antigen monoclonal antibody *(39)* have also been reported.

Focal liver RT using external beam treatment has been studied with the use of sophisticated three-dimensional radiation therapy treatment planning *(18)*. In a report of 22 patients with unresectable colorectal liver metastases, 14 of whom had progressed after previous chemotherapy, external beam RT to a total dose of 48–72.6 Gy was combined with hepatic arterial fluorodeoxyuridine *(40)*. An objective response was found in 11 patients with an overall median survival of 20 mo, which compared favorably to other modalities. However, the responses were not durable and hepatic progression was frequent (Fig. 1). Further studies at the same institution have used modeling of the risk of RILD *(41)* to safely administer 40.5–81 Gy (median: 54 Gy) combined with hepatic arterial fluorodeoxyuridine to 16 patients with colorectal liver metastases *(4)* and found an 86% response rate and an 18-mo median survival. In this trial, the maximum tolerable dose of focal liver RT has not been reached and further improvements may be achieved. Overall, the use of focal liver RT to escalate the dose of radiation has been demonstrated to be safe when three-dimensional treatment planning was used, with excellent response rates, even in patients with chemotherapeutic failure, and encouraging median survival rates (Table 4). Another method using three-dimensional treatment planning to treat focal portions of the liver is extracranial stereotactic RT *(42)*. This technique was based on the successful use of stereotactic RT for brain tumors and administered a single large dose of external beam RT. Preliminary results of response rates and survival have not yet been reported.

5. ADJUVANT THERAPY

The possible role of adjuvant whole-liver RT combined with systemic 5-FU for the prevention of liver metastases was tested by the Gastrointestinal Tumor Study Group *(19)*. A total of 300 participants with resected Dukes' stage B2 and C colon cancer were randomized to either observation or combined concurrent liver RT with 21 Gy at 3 Gy per fraction combined with 350–500 mg/m^2 intravenous 5-FU and followed by two further courses of 5-FU chemotherapy. The study found no delay in the development of liver metastases or a

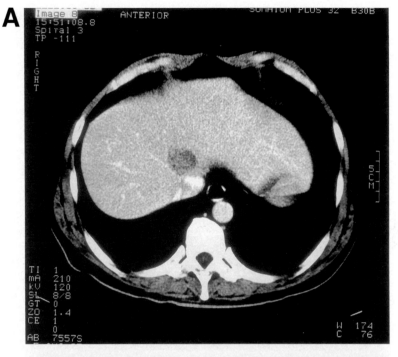

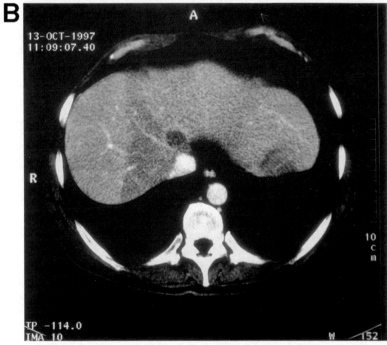

Fig. 1. CT scan of patient prior to RT (**A**) and after 50 Gy RT using three-dimensional treatment planning techniques at 1 mo (**B**) and 3 mo (**C**) after treatment *(continued)*.

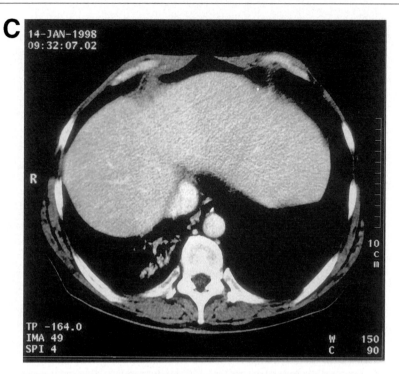

Fig. 1. *(continued).*

survival benefit and did encounter significant hematologic toxicity in about 60% of patients treated with 500 mg/m^2, prompting a reduction in the chemotherapy dose.

After a partial hepatectomy for liver metastases, the presence of a positive resection margin is a well-recognized risk factor for recurrence *(26,43)*. Despite this finding, the possible role of adjuvant whole-liver RT or RT directed only to the resection margin to prevent a recurrence has not been tested. The surgical experience, however, has suggested that the margin itself was not at any particular increased risk *(44)*, implying that adjuvant RT directed only to the positive margin would not be of benefit.

6. FUTURE DIRECTIONS

There are several possible directions for the development of improved therapies using RT. Because the safe dose of external beam RT is highly dependent on the volume of normal liver irradiated and higher doses of RT may lead to improved therapeutic results, the techniques to reduce the volume of liver irradiated may be helpful. One such avenue relates to the volume of liver included as a result of breathing motion. In current applications, the motion of the liver resulting from breathing has been added to the superior and inferior dimensions of the target volume to ensure that the tumor was always within the irradiated volume. If this volume could be reduced or eliminated, then the safe dose of RT could be increased accordingly *(45,46)*.

Another area of exploration is the combination of aggressive focal liver RT with long-term administration of hepatic arterial chemotherapy. Considering that a randomized trial has demonstrated the benefit of six cycles of hepatic arterial flourodeoxyuridine with intravenous 5-FU vs intravenous 5-FU alone for patients with resected liver metastases *(47)*, it is possible that a similar benefit could be achieved after focal high-dose hepatic RT.

Table 4
Response and Survival Rates of Focal Liver RT

Author (ref.)	No. of patients	Dose RT (Gy)	Chemo	Response rate	Median survival
Lawrence et al. (18)	13 (? C)	45–60	HA FUdR	64%	8[a]
Thomas et al. (33)	22	20–30 HDR	None	—	14
Armstrong et al. (35)	12	160 I-125	None	—	18
Robertson et al. (40)	22	48–72.6	HA FUdR	50%	20
Mohiuddin et al. (20)	12	33–60	IV/HA	—	14
Martinez-Monge et al. (36)	56	160 I-125	None	—	20
Dawson et al. (4)	43 (16 C)	28.5–90	HA FUdR	86%	18

Note: C = colorectal cancer; HA = hepatic arterial; FUdR = fluorodeoxyuridine; HDR = high-dose-rate brachytherapy; — = not available; I-125 = permanent iodine-125.
[a]Includes patients with whole-liver RT.

The dual blood supply of the liver suggests that studies of radiation sensitizers infused via the hepatic artery or radioprotectors given intravenously or by means of the portal vein may be successful. Aside from the fluoropyrimidines, other sensitizers such as the thymidine analogs bromodeoxyuridine (48) and iododeoxyuridine, and other nucleosides such as gemcitabine (15) and cisplatin may be considered for study.

The mechanism of the development of RILD may also provide avenues for research. Recent evidence has suggested that cytokines such as transforming growth factor-β may at least participate in the process leading to RILD (49). Thus, aggressive thrombolytic therapy, as is currently under study for bone marrow transplantation patients (50), may be able to prevent the development of RILD.

REFERENCES

1. Ingold JA, Reed GB, Kaplan HS, and Bagshaw MA. Radiation hepatitis. *Am. J. Roentgenol.*, **93** (1965) 200–208.
2. Robertson JM, Kessler ML, and Lawrence TS. Clinical results of three-dimensional conformal irradiation. *J. Natl. Cancer Inst.*, **86** (1994) 968–974.
3. Ten Haken RK, Lawrence TS, McShan DL, Tesser RJ, Fraass, BA, and Lichter AS. Technical considerations in the use of 3-D beam arrangements in the abdomen. *Radiother. Oncol.*, **22** (1991) 19–28.
4. Dawson LA, McGinn CJ, Normolle D, et al. Escalated focal liver radiation and concurrent hepatic artery fluorodeoxyuridine for unresectable intrahepatic malignancies. *J. Clin. Oncol.*, **18** (2000) 2210–2218.
5. Lawrence TS, Robertson JM, Anscher MS, Jirtle RL, Ensminger WD, and Fajardo LF. Hepatic toxicity resulting from cancer treatment. *Int. J. Radiat. Oncol. Biol. Phys.*, **31** (1995) 1237–1248.
6. Yamasaki SA, Marn CS, Francis IR, Robertson JM, and Lawrence TS. High-dose localized radiation therapy for treatment of hepatic malignant tumors: CT findings and their relation to radiation hepatitis. *Am. J. Roentgenol.*, **165** (1995) 79–84.
7. Borgelt BB, Gelber R, Brady LW, Griffin T, and Hendrickson FR. The palliation of hepatic metastases: results of the Radiation Therapy Oncology Group pilot study. *Int. J. Radiat. Oncol. Biol. Phys.*, **7** (1981) 587–591.
8. Leibel SA, Pajak TF, Massullo V, et al. A comparison of misonidazole sensitized radiation therapy to radiation therapy alone for the palliation of hepatic metastases: results of a Radiation Therapy Oncology Group randomized prospective trial. *Int. J. Radiat. Oncol. Biol. Phys.*, **13** (1987) 1057–1064.
9. Russell AH, Clyde C, Wasserman TH, Turner SS, and Rotman M. Accelerated hyperfractionated hepatic irradiation in the management of patients with liver metastases: Results of the RTOG dose escalating protocol. *Int. J. Radiat. Oncol. Biol. Phys.*, **27** (1993) 117–123.
10. Kim TH, Panahon AM, Friedman M, and Webster JH. Acute transient radiation hepatitis following whole abdominal irradiation. *Clin. Radiol.*, **27** (1976) 449–454.

11. Emami B, Lyman J, Brown A, et al. Tolerance of normal tissue to therapeutic irradiation. *Int. J. Radiat. Oncol. Biol. Phys.*, **21** (1991) 109–122.

12. Lawrence TS, Ten Haken RK, Kessler ML, et al. The use of 3-D dose volume analysis to predict radiation hepatitis. *Int. J. Radiat. Oncol. Biol. Phys.*, **23** (1992) 781–788.

13. Jackson A, Ten Haken RK, Robertson JM, Kessler ML, Kutcher GJ, and Lawrence TS. Analysis of clinical complication data for radiation hepatitis using a parallel architecture model. *Int. J. Radiat. Oncol. Biol. Phys.*, **31** (1995) 883–891.

14. Menard DB, Gisselbrecht C, Marty M, Reyes F, and Dhumeaux D. Antineoplastic agents and the liver. *Gastroenterology*, **78** (1980) 142–164.

15. McGinn CJ, Shewach DS, and Lawrence TS. Radiosensitizing nucleosides. *J. Natl. Cancer Inst.*, **88** (1996) 1193–1203.

16. Byfield JE, Barone RM, Frankel SS, and Sharp TR. Treatment with combined intra-arterial 5-FUdR infusion and whole-liver radiation for colon carcinoma metastatic to the liver. *Am. J. Clin. Oncol. (CCT)*, **7** (1984) 319–325.

17. Rotman M, Kuruvilla AM, Choi K, et al. Response of colo-rectal hepatic metastases to concomitant radiotherapy and intravenous infusion 5 fluorouracil. *Int. J. Radiat. Oncol. Biol. Phys.*, **12** (1986) 2179–2187.

18. Lawrence TS, Dworzanin LM, Walker-Andrews SC, et al. Treatment of cancers involving the liver and porta hepatis with external beam irradiation and intraarterial hepatic fluorodeoxyuridine. *Int. J. Radiat. Oncol. Biol. Phys.*, **20** (1991) 555–561.

19. Nauta R, Smith FP, and Stablein DM. Adjuvant therapy with hepatic irradiation plus fluorouracil in colon carcinoma. *Int. J. Radiat. Oncol. Biol. Phys.*, **21** (1991) 1151–1156.

20. Mohiuddin M, Chen E-T, and Ahmad N. Combined liver radiation and chemotherapy for palliation of hepatic metastases from colorectal cancer. *J. Clin. Oncol.*, **14** (1996) 722–728.

21. McCracken JD, Weatherall TJ, Oishi N, Janaki L, and Boyer C. Adjuvant intrahepatic chemotherapy with mitomycin and 5-FU combined with hepatic irradiation in high-risk patients with carcinoma of the colon: a Southwest Oncology Group phase II pilot study. *Cancer Treat. Rep.*, **69** (1985) 129–131.

22. Phillips R, Karnofsky DA, Hamilton LD, and Nickson JJ. Roentgen therapy of hepatic metastases. *Am. J. Roentgenol.*, **71** (1954) 826–834.

23. Sherman DM, Weichselbaum R, Order SE, Cloud L, Trey C, and Piro AJ. Palliation of hepatic metastasis. *Cancer*, **41** (1978) 2013–2017.

24. Hughes KS, Simon R, Songhorabodi S, et al. Resection of the liver for colorectal carcinoma metastases: a multi-institutional study of indications for resection. *Surgery*, **103** (1988) 278–288.

25. Steele G Jr, Bleday R, Mayer RJ, Lindblad A, Petrelli N, and Weaver D. A prospective evaluation of hepatic resection for colorectal carcinoma metastases to the liver: Gastrointestinal Tumor Study Group protocol 6584. *J. Clin. Oncol.*, **9** (1991) 1105–1112.

26. Nordlinger B, Guiguet M, Vaillant J-C, et al. Surgical resection of colorectal carcinoma metastases to the liver. A prognostic scoring system to improve case selection, based on 1568 patients. *Cancer*, **77** (1996) 1254–1262.

27. Leibel SA, Guse C, Order SE, et al. Accelerated fractionation radiation therapy for liver metastases: selection of an optimal patient population for the evaluation of late hepatic injury in RTOG studies. *Int. J. Radiat. Oncol. Biol. Phys.*, **18** (1990) 523–528.

28. Wiley AL, Wirtanen GW, Stephenson JA, Ramirez G, Demets D, and Lee JW. Combined hepatic artery 5-fluorouracil and irradiation of liver metastases. A randomized study. *Cancer*, **64** (1989) 1783–1789.

29. Herbsman H, Hassan A, Gardner B, et al. Treatment of hepatic metastases with a combination of hepatic artery infusion chemotherapy and external radiotherapy. *Surg. Gynecol. Obstet.*, **147** (1978) 13–17.

30. Friedman M, Cassidy M, Levine M, Phillips T, Spivack S, and Resser KJ. Combined modality therapy of hepatic metastasis. *Cancer*, **44** (1979) 906–913.

31. Ho S, Lau WY, Leung TWT, and Johnson PJ. Internal radiation therapy for patients with primary or metastatic hepatic cancer. A review. *Cancer*, **83** (1998) 1894–1907.

32. Dritschilo A, Harter KW, Thomas D, et al. Intraoperative radiation therapy of hepatic metastases: technical aspects and report of a pilot study. *Int. J. Radiat. Oncol. Biol. Phys.*, **14** (1988) 1007–1011.

33. Thomas DS, Nauta RJ, Rodgers JE, et al. Intraoperative high-dose rate interstitial irradiation of hepatic metastases from colorectal carcinoma. Results of a Phase I–II trial. *Cancer*, **71** (1993) 1977–1981.

34. Donath D, Nori D, Turnbull A, Kaufman N, and Fortner JG. Brachytherapy in the treatment of solitary colorectal metastases to the liver. *J. Surg. Oncol.*, **44** (1990) 55–61.

35. Armstrong JG, Anderson LL, and Harrison LB. Treatment of liver metastases from colorectal cancer with radioactive implants. *Cancer*, **73** (1994) 1800–1804.

36. Martinez-Monge R, Nag S, Neiroda CA, and Martin EW. Iodine-125 brachytherapy in the treatment of colorectal adenocarcinoma metastatic to the liver. *Cancer*, **85** (1999) 1218–1225.

37. Tian JH, Xu BX, Zhang JM, Dong BW, Liang P, and Wang XD. Ultrasound-guided internal radiotherapy using yttrium-90-glass microspheres for liver malignancies. *J. Nucl. Med.*, **37** (1996) 958–963.
38. Gray BN, Anderson JE, Burton MA, et al. Regression of liver metastases following treatment with yttrium-90 microspheres. *Aust. NZ J. Surg.*, **62** (1992) 105–110.
39. Mittal BB, Zimmer MA, Sathiaseelan V, et al. Phase I/II trial of combined 131I anti-CEA monoclonal antibody and hyperthermia in patients with advanced colorectal adenocarcinoma. *Cancer*, **78** (1996) 1861–1870.
40. Robertson JM, Lawrence TS, Walker S, Kessler ML, Andrews JC, and Ensminger WD. The treatment of colorectal liver metastases with conformal radiation therapy and regional chemotherapy. *Int. J. Radiat. Oncol. Biol. Phys.*, **32** (1995) 445–450.
41. McGinn CJ, Ten Haken RK, Ensminger WD, Walker S, Wang S, and Lawrence TS. Treatment of intrahepatic cancers with radiation doses based on a normal tissue complication probability model. *J. Clin. Oncol.*, **16** (1998) 2246–2252.
42. Herfarth KK, Debus J, Lohr F, et al. Extracranial stereotactic radiation therapy: set-up accuracy of patients treated for liver metastases. *Int. J. Radiat. Oncol. Biol. Phys.*, **46** (2000) 329–335.
43. Fong Y, Cohen AM, Fortner JG, et al. Liver resection for colorectal metastases. *J. Clin. Oncol.*, **15** (1997) 938–946.
44. Nordlinger B, Vaillant J-C, Guiguet M, et al. Survival benefit of repeat liver resections for recurrent colorectal metastasis: 143 cases. *J. Clin. Oncol.*, **12** (1994) 1491–1496.
45. Ten Haken RK, Balter JM, Marsh LH, Robertson JM, and Lawrence TS. Potential benefits of eliminating planning target volume expansions for patient breathing in the treatment of liver tumors. *Int. J. Radiat. Oncol. Biol. Phys.*, **38** (1997) 613–617.
46. Wong JW, Sharpe MB, Jaffray DA, et al. The use of active breathing control (ABC) to reduce margin for breathing motion. *Int. J. Radiat. Oncol. Biol. Phys.*, **44** (1999) 911–919.
47. Kemeny N, Huang Y, Cohen AM, et al. Hepatic arterial infusion of chemotherapy after resection of hepatic metastases from colorectal cancer. *N. Engl. J. Med.*, **341** (1999) 2039–2048.
48. Robertson JM, Ensminger WD, Walker S, and Lawrence TS. A Phase I trial of intravenous bromodeoxyuridine and radiation therapy for pancreatic cancer. *Int. J. Radiat. Oncol. Biol. Phys.*, **37** (1997) 331–336.
49. Anscher MS, Peters WP, Reisenbichler H, Petros WP, and Jirtle RL. Transforming growth factor beta as a predictor of liver and lung fibrosis after autologous bone marrow transplantation for advanced breast cancer. *N. Engl. J. Med.*, **328** (1993) 1592–1598.
50. Bearman SI. The syndrome of hepatic veno-occlusive disease after marrow transplantation. *Blood*, **85** (1995) 3005–3020.

III   Surgery of Colorectal Cancer

14 Surgical Pathology of Colorectal Cancer

Carolyn C. Compton

CONTENTS

1. INTRODUCTION

From initial diagnosis through definitive treatment, pathologic evaluation plays a central role in the care of patients with colorectal cancer. The pathologic stage of a surgically resected colorectal carcinoma is widely recognized as the most accurate predictor of survival and it typically determines the appropriateness of adjuvant treatment as well. Numerous additional pathologic factors have been shown by multivariate analyses to have prognostic significance that is independent of stage, and these may help to further substratify tumors. In this chapter, the pathologic features of colorectal cancers that predict outcome after surgical resection and have direct bearing on patient care are reviewed.

2. DIAGNOSTIC BIOPSY IN COLORECTAL CANCER

Masses or ulcers discovered by rectal examination, imaging, or endoscopic studies that are suspicious for colorectal carcinoma typically require biopsy confirmation as carcinomas before initiating treatment. Although clinical diagnosis of established colon carcinomas is usually accurate, a number of benign and malignant conditions that may mimic colonic carcinoma grossly require exclusion on biopsy. For example, other tumors that may resemble colorectal carcinoma include colorectal lymphomas, carcinoid tumors, gastrointestinal stromal tumors (mural sarcomas), metastatic tumors that exhibit tropism for the gastrointestinal tract (e.g., malignant melanoma), and malignancies of adjacent organs that directly invade the colorectum (e.g., cancers of the ovary, endometrium, bladder, or prostate). Benign lesions that may mimic colorectal cancer include adenomas, hamartomas, solitary rectal ulcers, stercoral ulcers, endometriomas, and Crohn's disease or diverticular disease with mural stricturing. In acquiring biopsies from a colonic lesion, the diagnostic yield is maximized

From: *Colorectal Cancer: Multimodality Management*
Edited by: L. Saltz © Humana Press Inc., Totowa, NJ

when multiple samples are taken from the edges and base of an ulcerating mass or from the intact surface of a polypoid mass. However, when stricturing is present, endoscopic access to diagnostic tissue may be compromised, and in this situation, brush cytology may be a useful alternative approach. Even when direct and targeted access to the lesion is possible, biopsies may fail to reveal a definitive diagnosis if the tumor is extensively ulcerated or otherwise necrotic. In these cases, elevated serum carcinoembryonic antigen (CEA) levels and/or the presence of associated adenomatous epithelium from the edge of the lesion increase the certainty that the mass is a carcinoma.

The type and amount of information that can be derived from a diagnostic biopsy is limited. Even if the biopsy successfully demonstrates the presence of carcinoma, an accurate determination of the histologic type or tumor grade is limited by sampling error. In some cases, the presence of stromal invasion also may be difficult to diagnose definitively, and even if the presence of tissue invasion can be identified with certainty, it is never possible to determine the depth of invasion from biopsy material.

3. PATHOLOGIC EVALUATION OF A MALIGNANT POLYP

The diagnosis and treatment of colorectal cancers by endoscopic polypectomy has become commonplace. The cancer may be unsuspected at endoscopy and revealed only on microscopic examination of the polypectomy specimen. "Malignant polyps" are adenomas that contain any amount of "invasive" carcinoma, which is defined as tumor that penetrates through the muscularis mucosae into the submucosa. They also encompass polypoid carcinomas, in which the entire polyp head is replaced by carcinoma. By definition, malignant polyps exclude adenomas containing intraepithelial carcinoma or intramucosal carcinoma because these polyps possess no biological potential for metastasis (see Section 4.6.). Polyps containing invasive carcinoma represent about 5% of all adenomas (1,2). The chance that any given adenoma will contain invasive malignancy increases with polyp size, and the incidence of invasive carcinoma in adenomas greater than 2 cm in greatest dimension ranges from 35% to 53% (3). Therefore, any polyp greater than 2 cm in diameter should be approached with the suspicion that it might harbor an invasive cancer. If technically possible, it is recommended that these polyps be removed intact rather than piecemeal, with as great a margin as possible at the base or stalk. Only when the polypectomy specimen is unfragmented can the true resection margin be identified with certainty on pathological examination. Identification of the resection margin is necessary for determining both the adequacy of the excision and the closest approach of the tumor, a parameter that predicts the risk of tumor recurrence (see below).

Malignant polyps constitute a form of early carcinoma that may be cured by endoscopic polypectomy alone (4–6). However, the incidence of an unfavorable outcome (i.e., lymph node metastasis or local recurrence from residual malignancy) for malignant polyps treated by polypectomy alone varies from about 10% to 20% (7,8). Pathologic evaluation is critical in defining polyps with an increased risk of residual or recurrent disease, and the subsequent clinical management of the patient may be based, in part, on the findings (4). The histopathologic parameters that are known to be associated with a significantly increased risk of adverse outcome are as follows (9–18):

1. High tumor grade (poorly differentiated adenocarcinoma, signet-ring-cell carcinoma, small-cell carcinoma, or undifferentiated carcinoma)
2. Tumor at or less than 1 mm from the resection margin
3. Small (thin-walled) vessel (lymphatic or venular) involvement by tumor

In the presence of one or more of these features, the risk of an adverse outcome following polypectomy is estimated to be about 10–25% *(10,19–22)*. Therefore, if one or more of these high-risk features are found on pathologic examination, further therapy may be indicated. Optimal management is decided on an individual case basis *(23)*, but segmental resection of the involved colonic segment, local excision (e.g., transanal disk excision for a low rectal lesion), or radiation therapy may be considered. In the absence of high-risk features, the chance of adverse outcome is extremely small, and polypectomy alone is considered curative.

In the pathologic evaluation of malignant polyps, assessment of small vessel invasion can be difficult and, not surprisingly, is associated with the greatest degree of interobserver variability *(8)*. In fact, small vessel invasion may be impossible to diagnose definitively in some cases and ultimately may be judged as being indeterminate. An absolute diagnosis of vessel invasion is dependent on finding carcinoma cells within an endothelial-lined space. Contraction artifact in the tissue, tumor-induced stromal sclerosis, and extracellular pools of mucin secreted by tumor cells may all complicate the evaluation of vessel invasion. Examination of additional tissue levels of the specimen, review by a second observer, and/or immunohistochemical staining for endothelial markers (e.g., factor VIII or CD34) may or may not help to resolve the dilemma. In published cases in which the malignant polyps have lacked definitive evidence of high-risk features but the patients have gone on to die of their disease, lymphatic invasion had been judged (on blinded review) as indeterminate because of a lack of interobserver agreement *(8)*. This suggests that even the suspicion of small vessel invasion on pathologic examination should be considered as potentially important.

4. PATHOLOGIC EVALUATION AND STAGING OF SURGICALLY RESECTED COLORECTAL CANCER

The pathology report of a colorectal cancer resection specimen typically documents the anatomic site of the malignancy, the histologic type, the parameters that determine the local tumor stage, and the histopathologic confirmation of distant metastasis, if applicable. Other reported features include those having additional prognostic or predictive value as well as those that may be important for clinicopathologic correlation or quality control (e.g., actual tumor size vs size measurement by imaging techniques). The essential pathologic features of a colorectal cancer and the clinical significance of these findings are reviewed individually in the following subsections.

4.1. The Anatomic Site of the Tumor

Documentation of the exact anatomic location of a colorectal carcinoma is typically part of the "gross" or "macroscopic" examination of the specimen. Because of distortion of the anatomy by tumor and/or lack of clear-cut anatomic landmarks in the resected segment, orientation of the specimen may be difficult in some cases, and the assistance of the surgeon may be required.

The anatomic site of the tumor is often documented by measurement from known landmarks according to general guidelines defining colonic topography. In general, four major anatomic divisions of the colon are recognized: the right (ascending) colon, the middle (transverse) colon, the left (descending) colon, and the sigmoid colon. The right colon is subdivided into the cecum (peritoneally located and measuring about 6 × 9 cm) and the ascending colon (retroperitoneally located and measuring 15–20 cm long). The descending colon, also located retroperitoneally, is 10–15 cm in length. The descending colon becomes the sigmoid colon at the origin of the mesosigmoid, and the sigmoid colon becomes the rectum at the termination of the mesosigmoid. The upper third of the rectosigmoid segment is covered by peritoneum on the front and both sides. The middle third is covered by peritoneum only on the anterior surface. The lower third (also known as the rectum or rectal ampulla) has no peritoneal covering *(24)*. Clinically, the rectum is defined as commencing opposite the sacral promontory and ending at the upper border of the anal canal. When measuring below with a rigid sigmoidoscope, it extends 16 cm from the anal verge. A tumor is classified as rectal if its inferior margin lies less than 16 cm from the anal verge or if any part of the tumor is located at least partly within the supply of the superior rectal artery *(25)*.

Additional guidelines for assigning a tumor site have been established by the American Joint Committee on Cancer (AJCC) *(24)*. Tumors located at the border between two subsites of the colon (e.g., cecum and ascending colon) are registered as tumors of the subsite that is more involved. If two subsites are involved to the same extent, the tumor is classified as an "overlapping" lesion. Tumors may also be classified as overlapping when the anatomic distinction between two subsites according to above guidelines is precluded because of tumor distortion *(26)*.

4.2. Tumor Size

Measurement on the gross pathologic examination is considered the definitive determination of tumor size. Although it is recorded for purposes of documentation and may be important for quality control (e.g., comparisons with dimensions derived via imaging modalities), tumor size is not related to outcome. Eight separate studies have shown that tumor size is of no prognostic significance in colorectal cancer *(27–34)*.

4.3. Tumor Configuration

Tumor configuration is usually classified as exophytic (fungating), endophytic (ulcerative), diffusely infiltrative (linitis plastica), or annular. Exophytic growth may be subclassified as either pedunculated or sessile. Overlap among these types is common. The clinical significance of tumor configuration is moot. Although most studies have failed to demonstrate an independent influence of gross tumor configuration on prognosis *(32,35,36)*, exophytic growth has proven to be an adverse prognostic factor in some multivariate analyses *(37–39)*. The uncommon linitis plastica configuration has been linked with an unfavorable prognosis *(40)*, but the prognostic import may be related primarily to the histologic type (signet-ring-cell carcinoma) and high grade of carcinomas that typically exhibit this gross morphology.

4.4. Histologic Type

For consistency and uniformity in pathologic reporting, the internationally accepted histologic classification of colorectal carcinomas proposed by the World Health Organization (Table 1) is recommended by the College of American Pathologists *(41,42)*. It should be noted, however, that medullary carcinoma has been added to the newly revised WHO classification *(42)*. Medullary carcinoma is a distinctive type of nongland-forming carcinoma that previously would have been classified as "undifferentiated carcinoma." It is composed of uniform polygonal tumor cells that exhibit solid growth in nested, organoid, or trabecular patterns and are characteristically infiltrated by lymphocytes (tumor-infiltrating lymphocytes). The importance of this unique type is its strong association with microsatellite instability and DNA repair gene dysfunction.

Table 1
World Health Organization Classification of Colorectal Carcinoma

Adenocarcinoma
Mucinous adenocarcinoma (>50% mucinous)
Signet-ring-cell carcinoma (>50% signet-ring cells)
Squamous cell carcinoma
Adenosquamous carcinoma
Small-cell (oat-cell) carcinoma
Medullary carcinoma
Undifferentiated carcinoma
Other (e.g., papillary carcinoma)

Note: The term "carcinoma, NOS" (not otherwise specified) is not part of the WHO classification.

Histologic type is always designated in the pathology report, but aside from a few notable exceptions, it has no independent prognostic significance *(32,33,35,38,39,43–50)*. The exceptions include rare types such as signet-ring-cell carcinoma and small-cell carcinoma, which are prognostically unfavorable, and medullary carcinoma, which is prognostically favorable *(51)*. As mentioned earlier, the latter is a histologic type that was not formerly recognized in the WHO classification (and would have been classified as undifferentiated carcinoma) but is now known to be associated with microsatellite instability and/or the hereditary nonpolyposis colon cancer syndrome. By convention, some histologic types are always assigned a specific histologic grade. For example, signet-ring-cell carcinoma, small-cell carcinoma, and undifferentiated carcinoma (histologic type) are all defined as high-grade, itself an adverse prognostic factor overall (*see* Section 4.5.).

To date, no large studies on prognostic factors in colorectal cancer have considered the relationship between the genetic status of the tumor (i.e., with or without microsatellite instability), histologic type, and outcome. This shortfall is particularly relevant to mucinous carcinoma, a histologic type representing a high proportion of microsatellite unstable colorectal cancers but, overall, occurring most frequently without microsatellite instability. Thus, it is not surprising that among all of the histologic types of colonic cancer, the prognostic significance of mucinous carcinoma has been the most controversial. A few studies, largely limited to univariate analyses, have indicated that mucinous adenocarcinoma may be an adverse prognostic factor *(50,52–54)*. More specifically, mucinous carcinoma has been linked with adverse outcome only if occurring in specific anatomic regions of the bowel (e.g., the rectosigmoid) *(52,54)* or in a specific subsets of patients (i.e., those less than 45 yr of age) *(55)*. In yet other studies, an association with decreased survival has been demonstrated only when mucinous carcinoma and signet-ring-cell carcinoma have been grouped together and compared to typical adenocarcinoma *(56–58)*. However, data of this type may be merely a reflection of the aggressive biologic behavior of signet-ring-cell tumors. Only one multivariate analysis has shown mucinous carcinoma to be a stage-independent predictor of adverse outcome *(31)*, but the study was limited to tumors presenting with large bowel obstruction, which itself is an adverse prognostic feature.

Signet-ring-cell type of adenocarcinoma and small-cell (oat-cell) carcinoma are the only histologic types of colonic carcinoma that consistently have been found to have an stage-independent adverse effect on prognosis *(59–61)*. Small-cell carcinoma is a malignant neuroendocrine carcinoma that is similar histologically and biologically to small-cell (oat-cell) carcinoma of the lung. Less clear is the general prognostic significance of focal neuroendocrine differentiation that may occur as a variable feature in other histologic types of colorectal cancer. Two studies, the most recent of which included a multivariate analysis of 350 cases *(62)*, have indicated that extensive neuroendocrine differentiation may adversely affect outcome *(62,63)*.

In summary, based on current evidence, it must be concluded that the only histologic types of colorectal cancer that are prognostically significant are signet-ring-cell and small-cell carcinomas (prognostically unfavorable) and medullary carcinoma (prognostically favorable). Mucinous carcinoma, when it is associated with microsatellite instability, is also prognostically favorable.

4.5. Tumor Grade

In general practice, the histologic grading of colorectal cancer is evaluated subjectively to a large degree. Although a number of grading systems have been suggested in the literature, a single widely accepted and employed standard for grading is lacking. Among the suggested grading schemes, both the number of strata as well as the criteria for distinguishing among them vary markedly. In some systems, grade is defined on the basis of a single microscopic feature, such as the degree of gland formation, and in other systems, a large number of features are included in the evaluation. Irrespective of the complexity of the criteria, however, most systems stratify tumors into three or four grades as follows:

Grade 1: well differentiated
Grade 2: moderately differentiated
Grade 3: poorly differentiated
Grade 4: undifferentiated

However, variation in the appearance of individual histologic features may be extensive enough to make implementation of the even the simplest grading systems problematic and, ultimately, subjective. Thus, a significant degree of interobserver variability in colorectal cancer grading exists *(64)*. Despite the variability in its assessment, histologic grade has been shown by numerous multivariate analyses to be a stage-independent prognostic factor *(27,28,30–32,36,37,45,48,65–71)*. Specifically, high tumor grade has been shown to be an adverse prognostic factor. In the vast majority of studies documenting the prognostic power of tumor grade, the subclassifications of the grading scheme have been collapsed to produce a two-tiered stratification for data analysis as follows:

Low-grade: well differentiated and moderately differentiated
High-grade: poorly differentiated and undifferentiated

In general practice, the pathologic diagnosis of poorly differentiated or undifferentiated tumors is relatively consistent and the associated interobserver variability is small *(64)*. However, differentiation between well differentiated and moderately differentiated carcinomas is less reproducible and is associated with significant interobserver variability *(64)*. A two-tiered grading system that eliminated this distinction might be expected to greatly improve diagnostic consistency. Given its proven prognostic value, relative simplicity, and reproducibility, a two-tiered grading system for colorectal carcinoma (i.e., low-grade and high-grade) has been recommended by a multidisciplinary colorectal working group of a consensus conference sponsored by the College of American Pathologists *(72)*. In the proposed system, stratification is based solely on the proportion of gland formation by the tumor (e.g., greater or less than 50% gland formation).

4.6. Pathologic Stage

The best estimation of prognosis in colorectal cancer is related to the anatomic extent of disease determined on pathologic examination of the resection specimen *(40)*. Although a large number of staging systems have been developed for colorectal cancer over the years, use of the TNM (Tumor, Nodes, Metastasis) Staging System of the AJCC and the International Union Against Cancer (UICC) is recommended by the College of American Pathologists *(24,41)*. The TNM system is widely used by national, regional, and local tumor registries in the United States, and it is internationally accepted.

In the TNM system, the designation "T" refers to the local extent of the primary tumor at the time of diagnosis. The designation "N" refers to the status of the regional lymph nodes, and "M" refers to distant metastatic disease. The symbol "p" used as a prescript refers to the pathologic determination of the TNM (e.g., pT1), as opposed to the clinical determination (designated by the prescript "c"). Pathologic classification is based on gross and microscopic examination of the resection specimen of a previously untreated primary tumor. Assignment of pT requires a resection of the primary tumor or biopsy adequate to evaluate the highest pT category; pN entails removal of nodes adequate to validate lymph node metastasis; and pM implies microscopic examination of distant lesions. Clinical classification (cTMN) is usually determined by imaging techniques carried out before treatment during the initial evaluation of the patient or when pathologic classification is not possible *(24)*. It is the *grouping* of a T, an N, and an M parameter that determines the stage of the tumor and relates to prognosis. A TNM stage grouping can be constructed using a combination of clinically derived and pathologically derived data (e.g., pT1, cN0, cM0). However, when pathologic data become available (following surgical resection of the tumor, for example), it typically replaces the corresponding clinically determined parameter. This convention is based on the presumption that pathologically derived data are more accurate.

The definitions of the individual TNM categories and stage groupings for colorectal carcinoma are shown in Table 2. TNM stage-related survival is shown in Table 3 *(73,74)*. It is considered the responsibility of the pathologist to assign a pTNM stage grouping when reporting on a colorectal cancer resection specimen. Thus, the pathologically determined T and N categories of the tumor should be explicitly assigned and included in the pathology report. However, the pathologist often lacks knowledge of the status of distant metastatic disease, and assignment of pMX is appropriate in this circumstance. It also may be appropriate to use other staging systems (e.g., Dukes' or Modified Astler–Coller classifications) in pathology reporting, depending on institutional tradition, but it is suggested that these be used in addition to (not in place of) the TNM stage grouping.

Specific issues related to the assignment of pathologic TNM are discussed in detail in the following subsections.

4.6.1. DEFINITION OF pTIS

For colorectal carcinomas, the staging category pTis (carcinoma *in situ*) includes both malignant cells that are confined within the glandular basement membrane (intraepithelial carcinoma) and those that are invasive into the mucosal lamina propria (intramucosal carcinoma). Intramucosal carcinoma that extends into but not through the muscularis mucosae also is included in the pTis category. Penetration of the muscularis mucosae

Table 2
AJCC/UICC TNM Definitions and Stage Groupings

Primary Tumor (T)
  TX   Primary tumor cannot be assessed
  TO   No evidence of primary tumor
  Tis Carcinoma *in situ* (intraepithelial or intramucosal carcinoma)
  T1   Tumor invades the submucosa
  T2   Tumor invades the muscularis propria
  T3   Tumor invades through the muscularis propria into the subserosa or into the nonperitonealized
       pericolic or perirectal tissues
           pT3a—minimal invasion: <1 mm beyond the border of the muscularis propria
           pT3b—slight invasion: 1–5 mm beyond the border of the muscularis propria
           pT3c—moderate invasion: >5–15 mm beyond the border of the muscularis propria
           pT3d—extensive invasion: >15 mm beyond the border of the muscularis propria
  T4   Tumor directly invades other organs or structures (T4a) or perforates the visceral
       peritoneum (T4b)

Regional Lymph Nodes (N)
  NX   Regional lymph nodes cannot be assessed
  NO   No regional lymph node metastasis
  N1   Metastasis in one to three lymph nodes
  N2   Metastasis in four or more lymph nodes

Distant Metastasis (M)
  MX   Presence of distant metastasis cannot be assessed
  M0   No distant metastasis
  M1   Distant metastasis

TNM Stage Groupings				Modified Astler–Coller Stage
Stage 0	Tis	N0	M0	N/A
Stage I	T1	N0	M0	Stage A
	T2	N0	M0	Stage B1
Stage II	T3	N0	M0	Stage B2
	T4	N0	M0	Stage B3
Stage III	Any T	N1	M0	Stage C1 (T2); C2 (T3); C3 (T4)
	Any T	N2	M0	Stage C1 (T2); C2 (T3); C3 (T4)
Stage IV	Any T	Any N	M1	Stage D

and invasion of the submucosa is classified as pT1. High-grade (severe) dysplasia and intraepithelial carcinoma sometimes may be used synonymously, especially in cases of inflammatory bowel disease *(75)*.

It is noteworthy that for all organ systems other than the large intestine, "carcinoma *in situ*" refers exclusively to malignancy that has not yet penetrated the basement membrane of the epithelium from which it arose, and "invasive carcinoma" encompasses all tumors that penetrate the underlying stroma. Stromal invasion of any degree is a feature of extreme importance in all noncolorectal sites because of the possible access of tumor cells to stromal lymphatics or blood vessels and the consequent risk of metastasis. In colorectal cancer, however, the designation "pTis" (i.e., carcinoma *in situ*) is used to refer to both intraepithelial malignancies and cancers that have invaded the mucosal stroma (intramucosal carcinomas) because the colonic mucosa is biologically unique. In contrast to the mucosa elsewhere in the gastrointestinal tract (or, indeed, in the entire body), tumor invasion of the lamina propria

Table 3
Correlations Between TNM Stage and Survival
in Colorectal Carcinoma

TNM stage	5-yr survival
Stage 0, I (Tis, T1; N0; M0)	>90%
Stage I (T2; N0; M0)	80–85%
Stage II (T3, T4; N0; M0)	70–75%
Stage III (T2; N1-3; M0)	70–75%
Stage III (T3; N1-3; M0)	50–65%
Stage III (T4; N1-3; M0)	25–45%
Stage IV (M1)	<3%

has no associated risk of regional nodal metastasis. Therefore, for the colon and rectum, inclusion of intramucosal carcinoma in the pTis category is justified. Nevertheless, the term "carcinoma *in situ*" in reference to colorectal cancer can be confusing, depending on whether it is used to refer to the T category of the TNM staging system or to intraepithelial tumor only, as it does in all other epithelial systems. Therefore, the terms "intraepithelial carcinoma" and "intramucosal carcinoma" may be preferred descriptive terms for colorectal tumors in the pTis category *(72,76)*.

4.6.2. OPTIONAL EXPANSION OF pT3

The T3 category refers to all transmurally invasive tumors that are confined to the perimuscular soft tissue (i.e., that have neither violated the serosal surface nor infiltrated an adjacent structure). However, all T3 tumors may not be equivalent. The extent of extramural soft tissue invasion has been reported to influence prognosis *(26)*. The deeper the tumor invades into the perimuscular tissues, the worse the prognosis. This adverse effect is observed whether or not regional lymph node metastasis is present. In recognition of the prognostic importance of this phenomenon, it has been proposed that pT3 be substratified as shown in Table 2. However, because extramural extension of >5 mm appears to be the critical level of invasion linked to adverse outcome in most studies, a simpler (two-tiered) subdivision, such as pT3a/b and pT3c/d, may be justified *(26)*. In either case, substratification of T3 is currently optional. Extramural extension of the tumor within lymphatics or veins does not count as local spread of tumor as defined by T3 *(26)*.

4.6.3. SUBCLASSIFICATION OF pT4

The highest category of local extent is pT4, which includes both extension into adjacent organs or structures (pT4a) and penetration of the parietal peritoneum with or without involvement of an adjacent structure (pT4b). A free perforation of a colorectal carcinoma into the peritoneal cavity is also classified as T4b *(26)*. Among the features that define T4 tumors, serosal penetration is clearly the most dire. A number of large studies have evaluated serosal penetration as a separate pathologic variable and have demonstrated by multivariate analysis that it has independent adverse prognostic significance *(27,32,77,78)*. As shown in Table 4, the median survival time following surgical resection for cure is significantly shorter for pT4 tumors that penetrate the visceral peritoneum compared to pT4 tumors without serosal involvement, with or without distant metastasis *(26)*. A careful pathologic study of

Table 4
Prognostic Significance of Serosal Involvement by Tumor in Colorectal Carcinoma

	5-yr survival rate	Median survival time (mo)
pT4a,M0	49%	58.2
pT4b,M0	43%	46.2
pT4a,M1	12%	22.7
pT4b,M1	0%	15.5

local peritoneal involvement by Shepherd et al. *(77)* has suggested that the prognostic power of this feature may supersede that of regional lymph node status (N category).

Despite its biologic importance, serosal involvement is often underdiagnosed by pathologists. Documentation of peritoneal involvement by tumor demands meticulous pathologic analysis and may require extensive sampling and/or serial sectioning. Thus, it can be missed on routine histopathologic examination. In fact, it has been shown that cytologic examination of serosal scrapings reveals malignant cells in as many as 26% of tumor specimens categorized as pT3 by histologic examination alone *(77,79)*. In addition, the histopathologic findings associated with peritoneal penetration are heterogeneous and standard guidelines for their diagnostic interpretation are lacking. These problems lead both to a high degree of interobserver variability and to underdiagnosis of peritoneal involvement, because most pathologists tend to err on the side of conservative interpretation.

In the pathologic study by Shepherd et al. *(77)*, the spectrum of microscopic features that may be seen with local peritoneal involvement by tumor was specifically addressed. Three types of local peritoneal involvement were defined: (1) a mesothelial inflammatory and/or hyperplastic reaction with tumor close to, but not at, the serosal surface; (2) tumor present at the serosal surface with inflammatory reaction, mesothelial hyperplasia, and/or erosion/ulceration; and (3) free tumor cells on the serosal surface (in the peritoneum) with underlying ulceration of the visceral peritoneum. All three types of local peritoneal involvement were associated with decreased survival, whereas tumor well clear of the serosal had no independent adverse effect on prognosis *(77)*. Therefore, it has been recommended that the definition of T4b be modified to encompass the three types of reactions outlined *(76)*.

For T4a, it should be noted that direct invasion of other organs or structures includes invasion of other segments of the colorectum by way of the serosa or mesocolon (e.g., invasion of the sigmoid colon by carcinoma of the cecum). In contrast, intramural extension of tumor from one subsite (segment) of the large intestine into an adjacent subsite or into the ileum (e.g., for a cecal carcinoma) or anal canal (e.g., for a rectal carcinoma) does *not* affect the pT classification *(26)*.

4.6.4. EVALUATION OF REGIONAL LYMPH NODES

Stage-related outcome data are derived from studies in which the pathologic evaluation of the regional lymph nodes has been performed by conventional histologic staining of macroscopically identified lymph nodes. Because it has been shown that many nodal metastases in colorectal cancer are found in small lymph nodes (less than 5 mm in diameter) *(80)*, diligent search for lymph nodes in resection specimens is essential. However, universally accepted standards for acceptable lymph node harvests and for handling of the recovered lymph nodes are lacking in general pathology practice. Typically, all lymph nodes found are submitted either in part (e.g., half of a bisected node) or *in toto* for microscopic examination,

Table 5

Definitions of Regional Lymph Node Groups in Anatomic Subsites of the Colorectum

Cecum: anterior cecal, posterior cecal, ileocolic, right colic

Ascending colon: ileocolic, right colic, middle colic

Hepatic flexure: middle colic, right colic

Transverse colon: middle colic

Splenic flexure: middle colic, left colic, inferior mesenteric

Descending colon: left colic, inferior mesenteric, sigmoid

Sigmoid colon: inferior mesenteric, superior rectal sigmoidal, sigmoid mesenteric[a]

Rectosigmoid colon: perirectal,[a] left colic, sigmoid mesenteric, sigmoidal, inferior mesenteric, superior rectal, middle rectal

Rectum: perirectal,[a] sigmoid mesenteric, inferior mesenteric, lateral sacral, presacral, internal iliac, sacral promontory, superior rectal, middle rectal, inferior rectal

---

[a]Lymph nodes along the sigmoid arteries are considered pericolic nodes and their involvement is classified as pN1 or pN2 according to the number involved. Perirectal lymph nodes include the mesorectal (paraproctal), lateral sacral, presacral, sacral promontory (Gerota), middle rectal (hemorrhoidal), and inferior rectal (hemorrhoidal) nodes. Metastasis in the external iliac or common iliac nodes is classified as pM1 *(26)*.

---

and wide variation in the numbers of lymph nodes recovered from resection specimens exists. In truth, the actual number of lymph nodes present in any given resection specimen may be limited by anatomic variation, surgical technique, or both. However, it has been shown that a minimum of 12–15 lymph nodes must be examined in order to accurately predict regional node negativity *(64,72,81)*. For this reason, it has been suggested that 12 lymph nodes be considered the minimum acceptable harvest from a careful specimen dissection and that if fewer than 12 nodes are found after careful gross examination, additional techniques (i.e., visual enhancement techniques such as fat clearing) be considered *(72)*. It has been further recommended that all grossly negative or equivocal lymph nodes be submitted entirely for microscopic examination *(72)* and that involvement of grossly positive lymph nodes be confirmed by either complete or partial microscopic examination.

Regional lymph nodes must be examined separately from lymph nodes outside of the anatomic site of the tumor because metastasis in any lymph node in the regional nodal group is classified as pN disease, whereas all other nodal metastases are classified as pM1. The regional lymph node groups of the anatomic subsites of the colorectum are listed in Table 5. On microscopic examination, tumor in a regional lymph node, whether arriving there via afferent lymphatics or direct invasion through the capsule, is regarded as metastatic disease. In addition, microscopic examination of the extramural adipose tissue may reveal discrete nodules of tumor that may represent lymph nodes that have been replaced by metastatic tumor but cannot be identified as such with certainty. In order to eliminate arbitrary decisions by different pathologists as to whether or not such nodules were to be interpreted as nodal metastasis, the AJCC/UICC had established a guideline known as the 3-mm rule. Any extramural tumor nodule within the regional lymph node distribution of the tumor that measured > 3 mm in diameter but lacked histologic evidence of residual lymph node tissue was classified as pN disease, whereas tumor nodules measuring ≤ 3 mm in diameter were classified in the pT3 category as discontinuous extramural extension of tumor *(26)*. Multiple nodules > 3 mm in size were considered as metastasis in a single lymph node for purposes of classification *(24)*. Recently, this approach has been called into question by evidence suggesting that pericolonic tumor deposits of any size correlate with shorter survival independently of lymph node metastasis *(82)*. The evidence also indicates that the number of pericolonic tumor correlates inversely with disease-free survival *(82)*. Thus, the 3-mm rule has been abandoned by the AJCC/UICC, and the 6th editions of their TNM staging manuals will recommend that smooth-bordered extramural tumor nodules of any size be regarded as replaced lymph nodes and be classified in the N category as regional nodal metastasis.

The detection of regional lymph node metastasis has long been limited to the use of conventional pathologic techniques (either gross or histologic) and straightforward morphologic diagnosis. Recently, however, attention is being focused on alternative methods of detection of metastatic cells. Tumor detected only by special techniques or a minute amount of tumor (measuring ≤ 0.2 mm) detected histologically is known as micrometastasis. At present, the clinical significance of micrometastatic disease is unproven and the data are insufficient to recommend either the routine examination of multiple tissue levels of paraffin blocks or the use of special/ancillary techniques such as immunohistochemistry for epithelial and/or tumor-associated antigens (e.g., cytokeratin, carcinoembryonic antigen, etc.) or polymerase chain reaction (PCR) techniques to identify tumor RNA/DNA. Furthermore all of these approaches are costly and some can be difficult to quality control.

In one recent study of stage II colorectal cancers ($N = 26$), more than 50% of cases showed evidence of micrometastatic disease in "negative" regional lymph nodes analyzed by reverse transcription (RT)-PCR for CEA *(83)*. The 5-yr survival rate was 50% for patients with micrometastatic disease and 91% for patients without micrometastasis. However, in a larger study ($N = 77$) using immunohistochemistry to identify micrometastasis (found in 25% of cases), no difference in the 10-yr survival was observed among patients with and without micrometastasis *(84)*. Clearly, larger statistically robust studies with careful quality control of methodology are required to further define the biological significance of minute amounts of metastatic tumor in regional nodes and its impact on outcome. Pending definitive studies, it is recommended that any histologically identified focus of tumor that measures ≤ 2.0 mm but > 0.2 mm be classified as N1 by the pathologist but be accompanied by a note stating that the biologic significance is unknown *(72,85)*. Isolated tumor cells, cell clusters that measures ≤0.2 mm on hematoxylin and eosin (H&E) stains, or micrometastasis detected only by special studies (immunohistochemical or molecular) should be reported but classified as N0.

4.6.5. Definition of Distant Metastasis

As stated earlier, metastasis to any nonregional lymph node or metastasis to any distant organ or tissue is classified as M1 disease. Peritoneal seeding of abdominal organs is also considered M1 disease, as is positive peritoneal fluid cytology. Isolated tumor cells found in the bone marrow are classified as distant micrometastasis, but, like nodal micrometastasis (*see* Section 4.6.4.), their significance is as yet unproven *(26)*.

Multiple tumor foci in the mucosa or submucosa of adjacent bowel ("satellite lesions" or "skip metastasis") are not classified as distant metastasis. However, "satellite" lesions must be distinguished from additional primary tumors in which obvious evidence of origin from an overlying adenoma exists.

4.6.6. Pathologic Staging of Residual Carcinoma

By definition, the TNM categories describe the anatomic extent of malignant tumors that have not been previously treated, and the predictive value of the corresponding TNM stage groupings is based solely on data derived from outcome studies of such tumors following complete surgical resection. Tumor that remains in a resection specimen after previous (neoadjuvant) treatment of any type (radiation therapy alone, chemotherapy therapy alone, or any combined-modality treatment) is codified by the TNM using a prescript "y" to indicate the posttreatment status of the tumor *(24)*. For many therapies, the classification of residual disease has been shown to be a strong predictor of posttreatment outcome. In addition, the ypTNM classification provides a standardized framework for the collection of data needed to accurately evaluate new therapies.

In contrast, tumor remaining in the patient after primary surgical resection (e.g., corresponding to a proximal, distal, or radial resection margin (*see* Section 4.7.) that is shown to be involved by tumor on pathologic examination) is categorized by a system known as the R classification as follows *(24)*.

RX   Presence of residual tumor cannot be assessed
R0   No residual tumor
R1   Microscopic residual tumor
R2   Macroscopic residual tumor

4.6.7. Pathologic Staging of Recurrent Colorectal Carcinoma

In contrast to residual disease, tumor that is locally recurrent after a documented disease-free interval following surgical resection should be classified according to the TNM categories and modified with the prefix "r" (e.g., rpT1). By convention, the recurrent tumor topographically assigned to the proximal segment of the anastomosis unless the proximal segment is the small intestine *(24,26)*.

4.7. Status of Surgical Resection Margins
(Proximal, Distal, Circumferential (Radial), and Mesenteric)

The pertinent margins of a colorectal cancer resection specimen include the proximal- and distal transverse margins, the mesenteric margin, and, when appropriate, the circumferential (radial) margin. The circumferential resection margin (CRM) represents the retroperitoneal or perineal adventitial soft-tissue margin closest to the deepest penetration of tumor. For all segments of the large intestine that are either incompletely encased (ascending colon, descending colon, upper rectum) or not encased (lower rectum) by peritoneum, the CRM is created by blunt dissection of the retroperitoneal or subperitoneal aspect, respectively, at operation.

When the distance between the tumor and the nearest transverse margin is 5 cm or more, anastomotic recurrences are very rare. Therefore, it may be justified to forego histologic examination of the proximal and/or distal margin if they are 5 cm or more from the tumor *(86)*. It has even been suggested (in guidelines from the Royal College of Pathologists in the UK) that donuts from stapling devices, which are the true margins of resection, need not be examined histologically of the tumor is > 30 mm from the cut end of the main specimen *(87)*. In low anterior rectal resection specimens of rectal cancers, however, distal margins are often critical since 5-cm cuffs of normal mucosa may be hard to achieve. A margin of 2 cm of normal tissue is accepted as adequate to prevent local recurrence, and in many cases, distal margins of 1 cm or less also prove sufficient *(88)*. Thus, on pathologic examination, the distance of the tumor from the transverse margins is always recorded, but microscopic examination may be considered optional if those distances are greater than 5 cm.

The CRM has been demonstrated to be of importance in relation to the risk of local recurrence after surgical resection of the rectal carcinomas *(89–92)*. Multivariate analysis has suggested that tumor involvement of the CRM is the most critical factor in predicting local recurrence in rectal cancer *(91,92)*. For this reason, routine assessment of the radial margin is recommended in all applicable colorectal cancers, and measurement of the distance from the tumor to the CRM, representing the "surgical clearance" around the tumor, is also suggested

(41,90). It is recommended that the CRM be considered involved if tumor is present 1 mm or less from the nonperitonealized surface of the resection specimen. For segments of the colon that are completely encased by a peritonealized (serosal) surface (e.g., transverse and sigmoid colon), the mesenteric resection margin may be relevant because tumors may extend to this margin with (pT4) or without (pT3) penetrating the serosal surface. It should be examined when the point of deepest penetration of the tumor is on the mesenteric aspect of the colon. For those tumors limited to an antimesenteric peritonealized aspect of the bowel, the mesenteric margin is not relevant.

Because of its association with local recurrence, involvement of the CRM or the mesenteric margin has implications for adjuvant therapy. Whether the primary tumor is classified as pT3 (without serosal penetration) or pT4b (with serosal penetration), resection is considered complete only if all surgical margins are negative, including the CRM. That is, whether or not the tumor penetrates a serosal surface, resection is considered complete if the resection margins are free of tumor. If a CRM or mesenteric margin is involved by tumor, however, adjuvant therapy (e.g., local radiation) may be appropriate irrespective of the T category of the tumor.

4.8. Venous, Lymphatic, or Perineural Invasion by Tumor

In at least 10 different studies, venous invasion by tumor has been demonstrated by multivariate analysis to have an independent adverse impact on outcome *(27,31,32,37–39,55,56,71,93)* and by univariate analysis in several additional studies *(43,94–96).* However, some studies identifying venous invasion as an adverse prognostic factor on univariate analysis have failed to confirm its independent impact on prognosis on multivariate analysis *(34,96).* Similarly disparate results have also been reported for lymphatic invasion *(34,38,39,45,93,95,97–99).* In several studies, vascular invasion as a general feature was found to be prognostically significant by multivariate analysis, but no distinction between lymphatic and venous vessels was made. Yet, in other studies, the location of the vascular involvement (e.g., invasion of extramural veins) has been a strong determinate of prognostic significance *(56,64).* Overall, therefore, data from existing studies are difficult to amalgamate. Nevertheless, the importance of venous and lymphatic invasion by tumor is strongly suggested and largely confirmed by the literature.

It is likely that the disparities among existing studies on vessel invasion are directly related to inherent problems related to the pathologic analysis of this feature. Definitive diagnosis of vessel invasion requires the identification of tumor within an endothelial-lined channel. However, assessment of vessel invasion may be difficult and may be complicated by tumor-induced fibrosis and fixation artifact. Interobserver variability may be substantial in the interpretation of small vessel (i.e., lymphatic or postcapillary venule) invasion, and large vessel (i.e., muscular vein) invasion with tumor infiltration of the vessel wall and destruction of the vascular architecture may also be difficult to recognize. Special techniques such as immunohistochemical staining of endothelium or elastic tissue stains of venous walls may increase the ease and accuracy of evaluation. However, because these techniques are labor-intensive, time-consuming, and expensive, they are not routinely performed. Additional limitations in the detection of vessel invasion are related to specimen sampling. For example, it has been shown that the reproducibility of the detection of extramural venous invasion increases proportionally from 59% with examination of two blocks of tissue at the tumor periphery to 96% with examination of five blocks *(64).* At present, however, no widely accepted standards or guidelines for the pathologic evaluation of vessel invasion exist, and pathology sampling practices may vary widely on both individual and institutional levels.

Complicating this issue is the impact of cost containment on surgical pathology practice, which, in general, has tended to reduce overall sampling of resection specimens. The College of American Pathologists is recommending that at least three blocks (optimally five blocks) of tumor at its point of deepest extent be submitted for microscopic examination *(72)*. By AJCC/UICC convention, lymphovascular invasion and venous invasion are classified as L1 and V1, respectively. Conversely L0 and V0 indicate the absence of lymphovascular and venous invasion, respectively.

4.9. Tumor Border Configuration and Perineural Invasion

For colorectal cancer, the growth pattern of the tumor at the advancing edge (tumor border) has been shown to have prognostic significance that is independent of stage and may predict liver metastasis. Specifically, an irregular, infiltrating pattern of growth as opposed to a pushing border has been demonstrated to be an independent adverse prognostic factor by several univariate *(43,56,100,101)* and multivariate analyses *(33,46,47,59,77,102,103)*. Defined as microscopic clusters of undifferentiated cancer cells just ahead of the invasive front of the tumor, irregular growth at the tumor periphery has also been referred to as "focal dedifferentiation" *(99)* and "tumor budding" *(102)*. It is recommended that pathologic assessment of tumor border configuration be routinely reported in transmurally invasive colorectal tumors.

Jass et al. *(46)* assessed interobserver variability among pathologists evaluating tumor border configuration in general practice (no specific definition provided) and found only a 70% (fair) agreement in diagnosis of infiltrating growth pattern. However, concordance was found to improve to 90% when the following diagnostic criteria for defining infiltrating growth were employed *(46)*:

Naked-Eye Examination of a Microscopic Slide of the Tumor Border
- Inability to define limits of invasive border of tumor
- Inability to resolve host tissue from malignant tissue

Microscopic Examination of the Tumor Border
- "Streaming dissection" of muscularis propria (dissection of tumor through the full thickness of the muscularis propria without stromal response)
- Dissection of mesenteric adipose tissue by small glands or irregular clusters or cords of cells
- Perineural invasion (several studies have shown perineural invasion alone to be an independent indicator of poor prognosis by multivariate analysis) *(18,27,31,39,45,93)*.

4.10. Host Lymphoid Response to Tumor

Lymphocytic infiltration of tumor or peritumoral tissue is indicative of a host immunologic response to the invasive malignancy and has been shown by multivariate analysis in several studies to be a favorable prognostic factor *(36,46,56,59)*. In contrast, other studies have either failed to confirm the prognostic significance of a peritumoral lymphoid reaction *(33,103)* or demonstrated its significance only by univariate analysis *(43,104–107)*. The results of these studies are difficult to compare because the histologic criteria for qualitative and quantitative evaluation differ from study to study. Some of the specific features that have been studied include perivascular lymphocytic cuffing in the muscularis propria, perivascular lymphocytic cuffing in the pericolonic fat or subserosa, lymphocytic infiltration at the tumor edge, and a transmural "Crohn's-like" lymphoid reaction. However, in some reports, little if any explanation of the criteria used for evaluation of this parameter have been offered. Therefore, although this feature appears promising as a favorable prognostic factor, further studies using comparable criteria are needed for confirmation.

Agreement has emerged, however, that large numbers of tumor infiltrating lymphocytes (TILs) are uniquely associated with microsatellite instability in colorectal cancers *(108)* and, for that reason, may be a favorable prognostic factor. Indeed, large numbers of TILs are one of the diagnostic features of medullary carcinomas of the colorectum but they may be found in other histologic types of tumors with microsatellite instability. Therefore, it is recommended that TILs be distinguished from peritumoral lymphocytic infiltrates and that moderate to high densities of TILs (approx 4 per high-power field) be reported *(72)*.

REFERENCES

1. Sherlock P and Winawer SJ. Are there markers for the risk of colorectal cancer? *N. Engl. J. Med.*, **311** (1984) 118–119.
2. Itzkowitz SH. Gastrointestinal adenomatous polyps. *Semin. Gastrointest. Dis.*, **7** (1996) 105–116.
3. Muto T, Bussey HJR, and Morson BC. The evolution of cancer of the colon and rectum. *Cancer*, **36** (1975) 2251–2270.
4. Jass JR. Malignant colorectal polyps. *Gastroenterology*, **109** (1995) 2034–2035.
5. Morson BC, Whiteway JE, Jones EA, et al. Histopathology and prognosis of malignant colorectal polyps treated by endoscopic polypectomy. *Gut*, **25** (1984) 437–444.
6. Wolff WI and Shinya H. Definitive treatment of "malignant" polyps of the colon. *Ann. Surg.*, **182** (1975) 516–525.
7. Wilcox GM, Anderson PB, and Colacchio TA. Early invasive carcinoma in colonic polyps: a review of the literature with emphasis on the assessment of the risk of metastasis. *Cancer*, **57** (1986) 160–171.
8. Cooper HS, Deppisch LM, Gourley WK, et al. Endoscopically removed malignant colorectal polyps: clinicopathologic correlations. *Gastroenterology*, **108** (1995) 1657–1665.
9. Cranley JP, Petras RE, Carey WD, et al. When is endoscopic polypectomy adequate therapy for colonic polyps containing invasive carcinoma? *Gastroenterology*, **91** (1986) 419–427.
10. Cooper HS. Surgical pathology of endoscopically removed malignant polyps of the colon and rectum. *Am. J. Surg. Pathol.*, **7** (1983) 613–623.
11. Cooper HS. The role of the pathologist in the management of patients with endoscopically removed malignant colorectal polyps. *Pathol. Annu.*, **23** (1988) 25–43.
12. Cooper HS, Deppisch LM, Kahn EI, et al. Pathology of the malignant colorectal polyp. *Hum. Pathol.*, **29** (1998) 15–26.
13. Cunningham KN, Mills LR, Schuman BM, et al. Long-term prognosis of well-differentiated adenocarcinoma in endoscopically removed colorectal adenomas. *Dig. Dis. Sci.*, **39** (1994) 2034–2037.
14. Haggitt RC, Glotzbach RE, Soffer EE, et al. Prognostic factors in colorectal carcinomas arising in adenomas: implications for lesions removed by endoscopic polypectomy. *Gastroenterology*, **89** (1985) 328–336.
15. Lipper S, Kahn LB, and Ackerman LV. The significance of microscopic invasive cancer in endoscopically removed polyps of the large bowel. A clinicopathologic study of 51 cases. *Cancer*, **52** (1983) 1691–1699.
16. Kyzer S, Begin LR, Gordan PH, et al. The care of patients with colorectal polyps that contain invasive adenocarcinoma. *Cancer*, **70** (1992) 2044–2050.
17. Muller S, Chesner IM, Egan MJ, et al. Significance of venous and lymphatic invasion in malignant polyps of the colon and rectum. *Gut*, **30** (1989) 1385–1391.
18. Volk EE, Goldblum JR, Petras RE, et al. Management and outcome of patients with invasive carcinoma arising in colorectal polyps. *Gastroenterology*, **109** (1995) 1801–1807.
19. Coverlizza S, Risio M, Ferrari A, et al. Colorectal adenomas containing invasive carcinoma: pathologic assessment of lymph node metastatic potential. *Cancer*, **64** (1989) 1937–1947.
20. Nivatvongs S and Goldberg SM. Management of patients who have polyps containing invasive carcinoma removed via colonoscope. *Dis. Colon Rectum*, **21** (1978) 8–11.
21. Nivatvongs S, Rojanasakul A, Reiman HM, et al. The risk of lymph node metastasis in colorectal polyps with invasive adenocarcinoma. *Dis. Colon Rectum*, **34** (1991) 323–328.
22. Wilcox GM, Anderson PB, and Colacchio TA. Early invasive carcinoma in colonic polyps: a review of the literature with emphasis on the assessment of the risk of metastasis. *Cancer*, **57** (1986) 160–171.
23. Wilcox GM and Beck JR. Early invasive cancer in adenomatous colonic polyps ("malignant polyps"). Evaluation of the therapeutic options by decision analysis. *Gastroenterology*, **92** (1987) 1159–1168.

24. Fleming ID, Cooper JS, Henson DE, et al. (eds.). *AJCC Manual for Staging of Cancer.* 5th ed. Philadelphia, Lippincott–Raven, 1997.

25. Fielding LP, Arsenault PA, Chapuis PH, et al. Clinicopathological staging for colorectal cancer: an International Documentation System (IDS) and an International Comprehensive Terminology (ICAT). *J. Gastroenterol. Hepatol.*, **6** (1991) 325–344.

26. Wittekind C, Henson DE, Hutter RVP, Sobin LH, eds. TNM Supplement. *A Commentary on Uniform Use.* 2nd ed. Wiley-Liss, New York, 2001.

27. Chapuis PH, Dent OF, Fisher R, et al. A multivariate analysis of clinical and pathological variables in prognosis after resection of large bowel cancer. *Br. J. Surg.*, **72** (1985) 698–702.

28. D'Eredita G, Serio G, Neri V, et al. A survival regression analysis of prognostic factors in colorectal cancer. *Aust. NZ J. Surg.*, **66** (1996) 445–451.

29. Frank R, Saclarides T, Leurgans S, et al. Tumor angiogenesis as a predictor of recurrence and survival in patients with node-negative colon cancer. *Ann. Surg.*, **222** 695–699.

30. Griffin M, Bergstralh E, Coffey R, et al. Predictors of survival after curative resection of carcinoma of the colon and rectum. *Cancer*, **60** (1987) 2318–2324.

31. Mulcahy HE, Skelly MM, Husain A, et al. Long-term outcome following curative surgery for malignant large bowel obstruction. *Br. J. Surg.*, **83** (1996) 46–50.

32. Newland R, Dent O, Lyttle M, et al. Pathologic determinants of survival associated with colorectal cancer with lymph node metastases. A multivariate analysis of 579 patients. *Cancer*, **73** (1994) 2076–2082.

33. Roncucci L, Fante R, Losi L, et al. Survival for colon and rectal cancer in a population-based cancer registry. *Eur. J. Cancer*, **32A** (1996) 295–302.

34. Takebayashi Y, Akiyama S, Yamada K, et al. Angiogenesis as an unfavorable prognostic factor in human colorectal carcinoma. *Cancer*, **78** (1996) 226–231.

35. Crucitti F, Sofo L, Doglietto G, et al. Prognostic factors in colorectal cancer: current status and new trends. *J. Surg. Oncol.*, **2** (1991) 76–82.

36. Deans G, Heatley M, Anderson N, et al. Jass' Classification revisited. *J. Am. Coll. Surg.*, **179** (1994) 11–17.

37. Freedman L, Macaskill P, and Smith A. Multivariate analysis of prognostic factors for operable rectal cancer. *Lancet*, **II** (1984) 733–736.

38. Michelassi F, Ayala J, Balestracci T, et al. Verification of a new clinicopathologic staging system for colorectal adenocarcinoma. *Ann. Surg.*, **214** (1991) 11–18.

39. Michelassi F, Block GE, Vannucci L, et al. A 5- to 21-year follow-up and analysis of 250 patients with rectal adenocarcinoma. *Ann. Surg.*, **208** (1988) 379–387.

40. Hobday TJ and Erlichman C. Colorectal cancer. In *Prognostic Factors in Cancer.* Gospodarowicz MK, Henson DE, Hutter RVP, O'Sullivan B, Sobin LH, Wittekind C, eds. Wiley-Liss, New York, 2001, pp. 311–332.

41. Compton CC. Updated protocol for the examination of specimens removed from patients with carcinomas of the colon and rectum excluding carcinoid tmors, lymphomas, sarcomas, and tumors of the vermiform appendix. A basis for checklists. *Arch. Pathol. Lab. Med.*, **124** (2000) 1016–1025.

42. Hamilton SR, Rubio CA, Vogelstein B, et al. Carcinoma of the colon and rectum. In *World Health Organization Classification of Tumours. Tumours of the Digestive System.* IARC Press, Lyon France, 2000, pp. 101–119.

43. Carlon C, Fabris G, Arslan-Pagnini C, et al. Prognostic correlations of operable carcinoma of the rectum. *Dis. Colon Rectum*, **28** (1985) 47–50.

44. Green J, Timmcke A, Mitchell W, et al. Mucinous carcinoma—just another colon cancer? *Dis. Colon Rectum*, **36** (1993) 49–54.

45. Hermanek P, Guggenmoos-Holzmann I, and Gall FP. Prognostic factors in rectal carcinoma. A contribution to the further development of tumor classification. *Dis. Colon Rectum*, **32** (1989) 593–599.

46. Jass J, Atkin W, Cuzick J, et al. The grading of rectal cancer: historical perspectives and a multivariate analysis of 447 cases. *Histopathology*, **10** (1986) 437–459.

47. Jass J, Love S, and Northover J. A new prognostic classification of rectal cancer. *Lancet*, **I** (1987) 1303–1306.

48. Robey-Cafferty SS, el-Naggar AK, Grignon DJ, et al. Histologic parameters and DNA ploidy as predictors of survival in stage B adenocarcinoma of colon and rectum. *Mod. Pathol.*, **3** (1990) 261–266.

49. Spratt J and Spjut H. Prevalence and prognosis of individual clinical and pathologic variables associated with colorectal carcinoma. *Cancer*, **20** (1967) 1976–1985.

50. Umpleby HC and Williamson RC. Carcinoma of the large bowel in the first four decades. *Br. J. Surg.*, **71** (1984) 272–277.

51. Jesserun J, Romero-Guadarrama M, and Manivel JC. Medullary adenocarcinoma of the colon: clinicopathologic study of 11 cases. *Hum. Pathol.*, **30** (1999) 843–848.

52. Minsky B, Mies C, Rich T, et al. Colloid carcinoma of the colon and rectum. *Cancer*, **60** (1987) 3103–3112.
53. Secco G, Fardelli R, Campora E, et al. Primary mucinous adenocarcinomas and signet-ring cell carcinomas of colon and rectum. *Oncology*, **51** (1994) 30–34.
54. Symonds D and Vickery A. Mucinous carcinoma of the colon and rectum. *Cancer*, **37** (1976) 1891–1900.
55. Heys S, Sherif A, Bagley J, et al. Prognostic factors and survival of patients aged less than 45 years with colorectal cancer. *Br. J. Surg.*, **81** (1994) 685–688.
56. Harrison J, Dean P, El-Zeky F, et al. From Dukes through Jass: pathological prognostic indicators in rectal cancer. *Hum. Pathol.*, **25** (1994) 498–505.
57. Sasaki O, Atkin WS, and Jass JR. Mucinous carcinoma of the rectum. *Histopathology*, **11** (1987) 259–272.
58. Shepherd N, Saraga E, Love S, et al. Prognostic factors in colonic cancer. *Histopathology*, **14** (1989) 613–620.
59. Halvorsen T and Seim E. Association between invasiveness, inflammatory reaction, desmoplasia and survival in colorectal cancer. *J. Clin. Pathol.*, **42** (1989) 162–166.
60. Öfner D, Riedmann B, Maier H, et al. Standardized staining and analysis of argyrophilic nucleolar organizer region associated proteins (AgNORs) in radically resected colorectal adenocarcinoma-correlation with tumour stage and long-term survival. *J. Pathol.*, **75** (1995) 441–448.
61. Staren ED, Gould VE, Warren WH, et al. Neuroendocrine carcinomas of the colon and rectum: a clinico-pathologic correlation. *Surgery*, **104** (1988) 1080–1089.
62. DeBruine A, Wiggers T, Beek C, et al. Endocrine cells in colorectal adenocarcinomas: incidence, hormone profile and prognostic relevance. *Int. J. Cancer*, **54** (1993) 765–771.
63. Gaffey M, Mills S, and Lack E. Neuroendocrine carcinoma of the colon and rectum. A clinicopathologic, ultrastructural, and immunohistochemical study of 24 cases. *Am. J. Surg. Pathol.*, **14** (1990) 1010–1023.
64. Blenkinsopp WK, Stewart-Brown S, Blesovsky L, et al. Histopathology reporting in large bowel cancer. *J. Clin. Pathol.*, **34** (1981) 509–513.
65. Böttger TC, Potratz D, Stöckle M, et al. Prognostic value of DNA analysis in colorectal carcinoma. *Cancer*, **72** (1993) 3579–3587.
66. Fisher E, Sass R, Palekar A, et al. Dukes' classification revisited. Findings from the National Surgical Adjuvant Breast and Bowel Projects. *Cancer*, **64** (1989) 2354–2360.
67. Jessup JM, Lavin PT, Andrews CW, et al. Sucrase-isomaltase is an independent prognostic marker for colorectal carcinoma. *Dis. Colon Rectum*, **38** (1995) 1257–1264.
68. Jessup J, McGinnis L, Steele G, et al. The National Cancer Data Base Report on Colon Cancer. *Cancer*, **78** (1996) 918–926.
69. Ruschoff J, Bittinger A, Neumann K, et al. Prognostic significance of nucleolar organizing regions (NORs) in carcinomas of the sigmoid colon and rectum. *Pathol. Res. Pract.*, **186** (1990) 85–91.
70. Scott NA, Wieand HS, Moertel CG, et al. Colorectal cancer. Dukes' stage, tumor site, preoperative plasma CEA level, and patient prognosis related to tumor DNA ploidy pattern. *Arch. Surg.*, **122** (1987) 1375–1379.
71. Wiggers T, Arends J, Volovics A. Regression analysis of prognostic factors in colorectal cancer after curative resections. *Dis. Colon Rectum*, **31** (1988) 33–41.
72. Compton CC, Fielding LP, Burgart LJ, et al. Prognostic factors in colorectal cancer: College of American Pathologists consensus statement 1999. *Arch. Pathol. Lab. Med.*, **124** (2000) 979–994.
73. Steele G Jr, Mayer RJ, Podolsky DK, et al. Cancer of the colon, rectum, and anus. In *Cancer Manual*. 9th ed. Osteen RT (ed.). American Cancer Society, Farmington, MA, pp. 399–410.
74. Stower M and Hardcastle J. The results of 1115 patients with colorectal cancer treated over an 8-year period in a single hospital. *Eur. J. Surg. Oncol.*, **11** (1985) 119–123.
75. Sobin LH and Wittekind C (eds.). *TNM Classification of Malignant Tumours: International Union Against Cancer*. 5th ed. Wiley, New York, 1997.
76. Compton CC, Fenoglio-Preiser CM, Pettigrew N, et al. American Joint Committee on Cancer Prognostic Factors consensus conference: Colorectal Working Group. *Cancer*, **88** (2000) 1739–1757.
77. Shepherd N, Baxter K, and Love S. The prognostic importance of peritoneal involvement in colonic cancer: A prospective evaluation. *Gastroenterology*, **112** (1997) 1096–1102.
78. Tominaga T, Sakabe T, Koyama Y, et al. Prognostic factors for patients with colon or rectal carcinoma treated with resection only. Five-year follow-up report. *Cancer*, **78** (1996) 403–408.
79. Zeng Z, Cohen AM, Hajdu S, et al. Serosal cytologic study to determine free mesothelial penetration of intraperitoneal colon cancer. *Cancer*, **70** (1992) 737–740.
80. Herrera-Ornelas L, Justiniano J, Castillo N, et al. Metastases in small lymph nodes from colon cancer. *Arch. Surg.*, **122** (1987) 1253–1256.
81. Scott KWM and Grace RH. Detection of lymph node metastases in colorectal carcinoma before and after fat clearance. *Br. J. Surg.*, **76** (1989) 1165–1167.

82. Goldstein NS and Turner JR. Pericolonic tumor deposits in patients with T3N+M0 colon adenocarcinomas. Markers of reduced disease free survival and intra-abdominal metastases and their implications for TNM classification. *Cancer*, **88** (2000) 2228–2238.

83. Liefers G-J, Cleton-Jansen A-M, van de Velde CJ, et al. Micrometastases and survival in stage II colorectal cancer. *N. Engl. J. Med.*, **339** (1998) 223–228.

84. Jeffers MD, O'Dowd GM, Mulcahy H, et al. The prognostic significance of immunohistochemically detected lymph node micrometastases in colorectal carcinoma. *J. Pathol.*, **172** (1994) 183–187.

85. Hermanek P, Hutter RVP, Sobin LH, et al. Classification of isolated tumor cells and micrometastasis. *Cancer*, **86** (1999) 2668–2673.

86. Cross SS, Bull AD, and Smith JHF. Is there any justification for the routine examination of bowel resection margins in colorectal adenocarcinoma? *J. Clin. Pathol.* **42** (1989) 1040–1042.

87. Sloane JP, Ansell ID, Quirke P, and Underwood JCE. Standards and Minimum Datasets for Reporting Common Cancers. Minimum Dataset for Colorectal Cancer Histopathology Reports. The Royal College of Pathologists, London, UK, 1998.

88. Quirke P. Limitations of existing systems of staging for rectal cancer: the forgotten margin. In *Rectal Cancer Research*. Rajagopalan NT, ed. Springer-Verlag, New York, NY, 2001, pp. 63–81.

89. Adam IJ, Mohamdee MO, Martin IG, et al. Role of the circumferential margin involvement in the local recurrence of rectal cancer. *Lancet*, **344** (1994) 707–711.

90. Chan K, Boey J, and Wong S. A method of reporting radial invasion and surgical clearance of rectal carcinoma. *Histopathology*, **9** (1985) 1319–1327.

91. Quirke P and Scott N. The pathologist's role in the assessment of local recurrence in rectal carcinoma. *Surg. Oncol. Clin. N. Amer.*, **3** (1992) 1–17.

92. Quirke P, Durdy P, Dixon MF, et al. Local recurrence of rectal adenocarcinoma due to inadequate surgical resection. *Lancet*, **II** (1986) 996–999.

93. Knudsen JB, Nilsson T, Sprechler M, et al. Venous and nerve invasion as prognostic factors in postoperative survival of patients with resectable cancer of the rectum. *Dis. Colon Rectum*, **26** (1983) 613–617.

94. Horn A, Dahl O and Morild I. Venous and neural invasion as predictors of recurrence in rectal adenocarcinoma. *Dis. Colon Rectum*, **34** (1991) 798–804.

95. Lee Y. Local and regional recurrence of carcinoma of the colon and rectum: I. Tumour-host factors and adjuvant therapy. *Surg. Oncol.*, **4** (1995) 283–293.

96. Talbot I, Ritchie S, Leighton MH, et al. The clinical significance of invasion of veins by rectal cancer. *Br. J. Surg.*, **67** (1980) 439–442.

97. Takahashi Y, Tucker S, Kitadai Y, et al. Vessel counts and expression of vascular endothelial growth factor as prognostic factors in node-negative colon cancer. *Arch. Surg.*, **132** (1997) 541–546.

98. Minsky B, Mies C, Recht A, et al. Resectable adenocarcinoma of the rectosigmoid and rectum. II. The influence of blood vessel invasion. *Cancer*, **61** (1988) 1417–1424.

99. Minsky B, Mies C, Rich T, et al. Lymphatic vessel invasion in an independent prognostic factor for survival in colorectal cancer. *Int. J. Radiat. Oncol. Biol. Phys.*, **17** (1989) 311–318.

100. Ono M, Sakamoto M, Ino Y, et al. Cancer cell morphology at the invasive front and expression of cell adhesion-related carbohydrate in the primary lesion of patients with colorectal carcinoma with liver metastasis. *Cancer*, **78** (1996) 1179–1186.

101. Sinicrope F, Hart J, Brasitus T, et al. Relationship of P-glycoprotein and carcinoembryonic antigen expression in human colon carcinoma to local invasion, DNA ploidy, and disease relapse. *Cancer*, **74** (1994) 2908–2917.

102. Hase K, Shatney C, Johnson D, et al. Prognostic value of tumor "budding" in patients with colorectal cancer. *Dis. Colon Rectum*, **36** (1993) 627–635.

103. Thynne GS, Weiland LH, Moertel CG, et al. Correlation of histopathologic characteristics of primary tumor and uninvolved regional lymph nodes in Dukes' C colonic carcinoma with prognosis. *Mayo Clin. Proc.*, **55** (1980) 243–245.

104. Shirouzu K, Isomoto H, and Kakegawa T. Prognostic evaluation of perineural invasion in rectal cancer. *Am. J. Surg.*, **165** (1993) 233–237.

105. Pihl E, Malahy MA, Khankhanian N, et al. Immunomorphological features of prognostic significance in Dukes' class B colorectal carcinoma. *Cancer Res.*, **37** (1977) 4145–4149.

106. Svennevig JL, Lunde OC, Holter J, et al. Lymphoid infiltration and prognosis in colorectal carcinoma. *Br. J. Cancer*, **49** (1984) 375–377.

107. Zhou XG, Yu BM, and Shen YX. Surgical treatment and late results in 1226 cases of colorectal cancer. *Dis. Colon Rectum*, **26** (1983) 250–256.

108. Jass JR, Do KA, Simms LA, et al. Morphology of sporadic colorectal cancer with DNA replication errors. *Gut,* **42** (1998) 673–679.

15 Surgery of Colon Cancer

Alfred T. Culliford IV and Philip B. Paty

CONTENTS

1. PREOPERATIVE ASSESSMENT

1.1. Clinical Presentation

Colon cancers typically develop slowly and silently, and most patients present with few or subtle symptoms. Brief episodes of rectal bleeding, constipation, diarrhea, or abdominal discomfort may be the only indication of disease, even among patients with advanced, incurable cancer. Severe or long-standing symptoms generally indicate extensive disease but do not necessarily preclude curative treatment. Asymptomatic patients are frequently first identified because of anemia or fecal occult blood or they are diagnosed by endoscopic screening.

1.2. Diagnosis

A definitive diagnosis of colon cancer is achieved by endoscopic visualization and biopsy of the malignant lesion. Nearly all colon cancers present as a mass lesion, typically with friability and ulceration. Because of tumor heterogeneity, biopsies may reveal only adenomatous or inflammatory tissue and thus fail to document invasive adenocarcinoma. Repeat biopsies are rarely necessary, as the presence of a malignant-appearing lesion that is too large for endoscopic removal is a clear indication for surgical resection. The use of endoscopic digital imaging for instant photodocumentation of tumors has significantly enhanced endoscopic reporting *(1,2)*. Anatomic localization of the tumor within the colon is another important aspect of diagnosis. Colonoscopy is not always reliable for localization, and in selected cases, it should be supplemented with barium enema *(3)*.

From: *Colorectal Cancer: Multimodality Management*
Edited by: L. Saltz © Humana Press Inc., Totowa, NJ

1.3. Evaluation of the Colon

Synchronous colonic cancers and synchronous colonic polyps are present in 2–7% and 25–40% of patients, respectively *(4,5)*. Complete colonoscopy to the cecum is the preferred method of clearing the colon prior to surgery, as it is the most sensitive test and also allows for either removal or tattooing of secondary lesions *(6,7)*. Air-contrast barium enema and virtual colonoscopy are alternative methods of polyp identification when complete colonoscopy is not possible for technical reasons or patient refusal *(3,8,9)*.

1.4. Extent of Disease

Preoperative imaging of the chest, abdomen, and pelvis to evaluate the extent of local and metastatic cancer is necessary for optimal treatment planning. Approximately 20% of patients present with established metastases and up to 5% have locally advanced tumors with invasion of adjacent organs *(5)*. Preoperative imaging allows better preparation for the surgical procedure and will, in some cases, alter surgical management. For example, bulky local–regional disease may prepare the surgeon for extended lymphadenectomy and adjacent organ resection. Limited metastatic disease in the liver may suggest the feasibility of combined colon–liver resection and influence the choice of abdominal incision. The presence of small, indeterminant nodules in the liver, retroperitoneum, or pelvis can guide the surgeon's abdominal exploration and may call for intraoperative ultrasound and biopsy. Lung or mediastinal nodules may prompt bronchoscopy, mediastinoscopy, or thoracoscopic biopsy. Detection of extensive or multiorgan metastatic disease may be an indication for initial systemic chemotherapy. In addition to its influence on cancer management, preoperative imaging of abdominal aortic aneurysm, portal hypertension, or other pathology may affect the nature and timing of colon surgery.

Spiral technology has improved the speed and resolution of computed tomography (CT) imaging in the chest, abdomen, and pelvis and is the emerging standard for preoperative anatomic imaging *(10)*. For patients with indeterminate liver lesions on CT scan, magnetic resonance imaging (MRI) can discriminate small hepatic metastases from benign cysts and hemangiomas with a high degree of accuracy *(11)*. Tumor imaging with fluorodeoxyglucose (FDG)-18–positron-emitting tomography provides additional information and will alter the management of a small subset of high-risk cases *(12)*.

1.5. Colon Cancer Syndromes

Colon cancer may arise in the setting of a familial cancer syndrome or in the presence of inflammatory bowel disease. It is essential for the surgeon to recognize such cases and take appropriate steps to assure proper diagnosis and management *(5,13–18)*. Table 1 summarizes the most common syndromes, their clinical features, and surgical considerations.

1.6. Inflammatory Bowel Disease

There is a well-documented increased risk of colon cancer among patients with inflammatory bowel disease *(19,20)*. Two clear independent risk factors for the development of colon cancer are duration and extent of the colitis *(21,22)*. For ulcerative colitis, the risk of developing carcinoma is estimated to be 1–2% per annum for each year after the first decade of disease *(23–25)*.

Regular colonoscopic evaluations are advocated to detect early or precancerous lesions *(26)*. At present, debate exists as to how often colonoscopy should be performed. Several studies have indicated that biennial colonoscopy is probably inadequate in preventing

Table 1
Colon Cancer Syndromes

Syndrome	Clinical features	Surgical considerations
FAP	No family history in 20%	TAC + ileorectal anastomosis
	Presentation in teens, 20s, 30s, 40s	TPC + ileal J-pouch anal
	Hundreds of colonic polyps	anastomosis
Attenuated FAP	Presentation in 40s, 50s, 60s	TAC + ileorectal anastomosis
	0-100 colonic polyps	TPC + ileal J-pouch anal
		anastomosis
HNPCC	Strong family history of cancer (colon,	Standard hemicolectomy
	endometrial, and other types)	Subtotal colectomy
	Synchronous and metachronous colon cancers	Prophylactic TAH/BSO
Ulcerative colitis	Distal or pan colitis	TPC + end ileostomy
	Autoimmune cholangitis in 10%	TPC + ileal J-pouch anal
		anastomosis
		Liver biopsy
Crohn's disease	Segmental or pan colitis	Standard hemicolectomy
	Anal fistulas	TPC + end ileostomy
	Terminal ileitis	
	Small bowel cancer	

FAP, familial autosomal polyposis; TAC, total abdominal colectomy; TPC, total proctocolectomy; HNPCC, Hereditary Nonpolyposis Colorectal Cancer; TAH/BSO, total abdominal hysterectomy and bilateral salpingoopherorectomy.

patients from developing carcinoma *(23,27,28)*. Consequently, annual colonoscopy is recommended *(10)*.

An alternative to a surveillance program for colon cancer prevention is elective total proctocolectomy *(29)*. For patients who have pan-colitis, disease greater than 10 yr, or age of onset of 15 yr or less, a total proctcolectomy with ileoanal anastomosis is indicated. The presence of pan-colitis increases the relative risk of developing carcinoma 15-fold over matched normal controls *(29)*. Crohn's colitis also confers an increased risk for colon cancer; the risk is highest in patients diagnosed with Crohn's disease before age 30 *(5,30)*.

1.7. Comorbidity and Operative Risk

An elective colon resection is a well-tolerated procedure with an overall operative mortality of less than 1%. Patients' suitability for general anesthesia and an abdominal exploration must be considered. Angina pectoris, severe cardiac valvular disease, congestive heart failure, chronic respiratory failure, large aortic aneurysm, recent venous thromboembolism, severe neurologic impairment, second cancers, and severely compromised performance status are the most common reasons to defer or withhold surgical treatment. Given the nature of colon cancer and the consequences of no surgery, it is uncommon not to proceed with colon resection for patients with localized tumors. When possible, medical comorbidities are addressed in the preoperative period to minimize operative risk.

1.8. Preoperative Evaluation

The usual components of the preoperative evaluation for patients with colon cancer are listed in Table 2. Additional studies and consultations may be required for patients with advanced disease or significant comorbidities.

Table 2
Preoperative Evaluation of Patients with Colon Cancer

- Informed consent
- History and physical
- Complete colonoscopy with biopsy
- CT scan of abdomen/pelvis
- Chest X-ray
- Electrocardiogram
- Blood tests
  - Complete blood count
  - Electrolytes
  - Liver function tests
  - Coagulation profile
  - Type and screen
- Bowel preparation

2. SURGICAL MANAGEMENT

2.1. Bowel Preparation

Adequate preoperative bowel preparation is important to minimize the risk of postoperative wound and intra-abdominal infections. A thorough mechanical bowel cleansing is advocated to minimize the fecal load within the colon. There are several regimens for bowel preparation in use today; each with relative advantages and disadvantages in regard to patient compliance, efficiency, influence on fluid and electrolyte balance, and effect on fecal micro-organisms *(31–36)*. A 1-d outpatient preparation with poly(ethylene glycol) solutions or phosphasoda has proven safe and effective. Patients with partially obstructing tumors may require a longer preparation or hospital admission.

2.2. Antibiotic Prophylaxis

For optimal risk reduction, antibiotic prophylaxis is added to mechanical bowel preparation. In the absence of perioperative antibiotics, the overall infection rate for colon surgery is between 30% and 60% *(37,38)*. Preoperative administration of oral antibiotics reduces the bacterial colonization of the large bowel and is effective in reducing infectious complications by 60–80% compared to untreated controls *(39)*. Neomycin plus metronidazole and neomycin plus erythromycin are popular regimens. Systemic antibiotics are recommended just prior to operation, so adequate tissue levels are present at the time of contamination. A prospective double-blind study reported a reduction of wound infections from 28% to 14% when systemic antibiotics were added to an oral antibiotic preparation *(40)*.

2.3. Venous Thromboembolism Prophylaxis

Patients with malignancy are at increased risk of thromboembolic complications, and all patients having a colectomy require prophylaxis *(41)*. The most common measures are intermittent pneumatic compression devices and subcutaneous heparin. Oral anticoagulants or dextran are also effective. Prophylaxis with anticoagulant drugs does produce a slight increase in risk of hemorrhagic complications *(42–44)*.

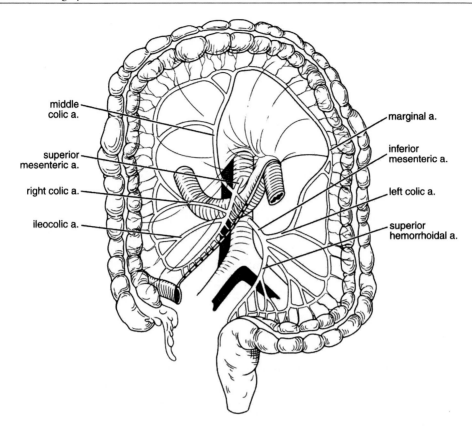

middle colic a.

superior mesenteric a.

right colic a.

ileocolic a.

marginal a.

inferior mesenteric a.

left colic a.

superior hemorrhoidal a.

Fig. 1. Anatomic segments and vascular supply of the colon.

2.4. Anatomy and General Principles

The colon can be divided into an intraperitoneal portion and a retroperitoneal portion. The cecum, transverse colon, and sigmoid colon are mobile structures that lie free within the peritoneal cavity and are completely covered with serosa. On the other hand, the dorsal aspects of the ascending colon, hepatic flexure, splenic flexure, and descending colon lack a serosa, and these retroperitoneal segments are relatively fixed. Local treatment failures of cancers within the intraperitoneal colon generally involve peritoneal seeding; local failures in the retroperitoneal colon may present as local recurrence involving the retroperitoneal soft tissues, kidney, ureter, and pancreas.

The arterial blood supply to the right colon, derived from the mid-gut, is from the ileocolic, right, and middle colic branches of the superior mesenteric artery (Fig. 1). The left colon, derived from the hindgut, receives its blood supply from the left colic and sigmoid branches of the inferior mesenteric artery. Collateral blood supply is provided by the marginal artery of Drummond, which courses near the colon and connects the superior and inferior mesenteric arteries. The venous drainage of the colon parallels its arterial supply, with drainage into the portal venous system.

The lymphatic drainage of the colon flows sequentially through epicolic, paracolic, intermediate, and principal nodes. Lymphatic vessels originate in the bowel wall as a plexus within the submucosa and drain into the intramuscular lymphatics, which course radially through the bowel wall and into the subserosa. The subserosal lymphatics drain into the epicolic nodes, which lie in close proximity to the colon along the arterial arcades. The epicolic nodes drain into the paracolic nodes, which lie along the marginal arteries. The paracolic nodes then drain into the intermediate nodes, which course along the major colic vessels. Ultimately, the intermediate nodes drain into the principal nodes, which lie at the origins of the superior and inferior mesenteric arteries and are contiguous with the para-aortic nodes.

2.5. General Surgical Principles

Colon cancers are treated by wide resection of the bowel and adjacent mesentery. Surgical lymphadenectomy is considered both a therapeutic and staging procedure (*see* Table 3). The paracolic nodes along the vascular arcade are the most numerous and are a significant site for metastatic disease. Because the route of lymphatic flow follows the arterial and venous anatomy, tumors that lie in close proximity to a large vascular pedicle have a relatively uniform lymphatic drainage. However, for tumors that lie between two vascular pedicles, lymphatic flow may course in either or both directions (Fig. 2). Based on the location, vascular anatomy, and clinical features of the primary tumor, the surgeon determines the lymph node stations at risk, which in turn determines the extent of lymphadenectomy and subsequent colon resection.

Besides the hematogenous and lymphatic routes, another potential route of dissemination is intraluminal spread. Tumor cells can exfoliate and implant themselves at the anastomosis, producing a suture line recurrence. For colon cancer, this phenomenon is infrequent, occurring in less than 1% of cases. It is important to avoid unnecessary manipulation of the tumor *(10)*.

The "no touch" technique, popularized by Turnbull et al. *(45)*, requires ligation of the regional arterial and venous blood supply before mobilization of the colon and mesentery. The rationale is that intraoperative manipulation of the tumor during dissection may dislodge cancer cells into regional veins with the potential for spread to distant organs. This theory arose from the observation that cancer cells are detectable in the portal vein during intraoperative manipulation of the tumor *(45,46)*. In 1988, a prospective randomized study by Wiggers et al. *(47)* did not show a statistical difference in survival between initial mesenteric vascular ligation vs initial tumor mobilization. Nevertheless, early identification and ligation of vascular pedicles and avoidance of unnecessary tumor manipulation are still advisable.

2.6. Abdominal Exploration

Primary colon resections are generally performed through a midline laparotomy incision. This incision provides good exposure to the entire contents of the abdominal cavity and may easily be extended superiorly or inferiorly. For hemicolectomy, a right or left transverse incision is also effective. Upon entering the abdomen, an initial exploration is performed by gentle palpation and inspection. The examination includes the primary tumor site, the mesentery and omentum, the stomach and pancreas, the liver and hepatoduodenal ligament, peritoneal surfaces, including both hemidiaphragms, the small intestine, the appendix and remaining colon, the para-aortic lymph nodes, and the pelvic structures. Palpable abnormalities are visualized and, if appropriate, biopsied. In the absence of intraoperative findings that change the planned procedure, the surgeon then proceeds with the resection.

Table 3
TNM Classification of Colon Cancer/AJCC/UICC Stage Grouping

Primary tumor (T)

T×	Primary tumor cannot be assessed
T0	No evidence of primary tumor
Tis	Carcinoma *in situ:* intraepithelial or invasion of lamina propria
T1	Tumor invades submucosa
T2	Tumor invades muscularis mucosa
T3	Tumor invades through the muscularis propria into the subserosa, or into nonperitonealized pericolic tissues
T4	Tumor directly invades other organs or structures, and/or perforates visceral peritoneum

Regional lymph nodes (N)

N×	Regional lymph nodes cannot be assessed.
N0	No regional lymph node metastasis.
N1	Metastasis in 1–3 regional lymph nodes.
N2	Metastasis in 4 or more regional lymph nodes.

Distant metastis (M)

M×	Distant metastasis cannot be assessed.
M0	No distant metastasis.
M1	Distant metastasis.

Stage grouping—AJCC/UICC

Stage 0	Tis	N0	M0
Stage I	T1 or T2	N0	M0
Stage II	T3 or T4	N0	M0
Stage III	Any T	N1 or N2	M0
Stage IV	Any T	Any N	M1

2.7. Colon Resection

The goals of resection are (1) complete removal of the colonic tumor and regional lymph nodes and (2) re-establishment of bowel continuity. The extent of mesenteric and bowel resection is based primarily on the regional vascular anatomy. The preferred approach is initial ligation of the major regional arterial branches at their origin, followed by a wide en-bloc surgical resection of the mesentery and colon. Only in a small minority of patients with minimally invasive polypoid cancers is segmental colectomy with limited lymphadenectomy appropriate. The site of bowel transection is generally determined by the adequacy of arterial blood supply following mesenteric resection. Removal of at least 5–10 cm of colon both proximal and distal to the tumor is desirable. The lateral margins of resection are often the bowel serosa and fascia propria of the mesentery. If the tumor invades deep into the retroperitoneum or is attached to adjacent viscera or parietes, an in-continuity resection of the involved tissues is performed. For elective operations, bowel continuity is routinely restored by primary anastomosis.

There remains debate as to the therapeutic benefit of routinely extending regional lymphadenectomy to include the central/principal lymph nodes in addition to the paracolic and intermediate lymph nodes. Enker and colleagues reported excellent results for treatment of colon cancer with extensive lymphadenectomy *(48)*. Studies by Gabriel and by Nicholls suggest a survival benefit for high ligation, especially when intermediate lymph nodes are involved. However, a more recent study did not demonstrate a survival benefit for high ligation of the inferior mesenteric artery for sigmoid cancers *(5)*. Despite uncertainty about

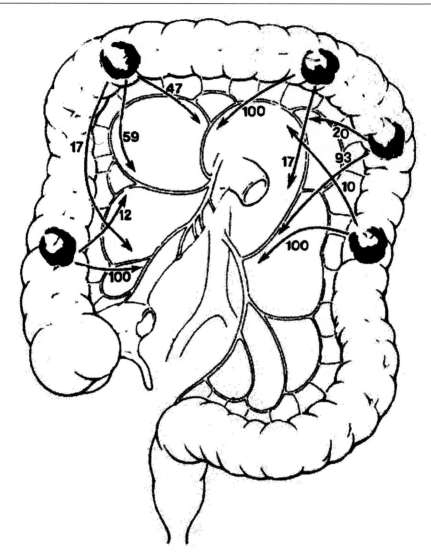

Fig. 2. For tumors that lie between two vascular pedicles, lymphatic flow may drain in either or both directions. From a study of cleared specimens, it was possible to determine the preferential route by the location of hepatic metastases. The numbers in the figure signify the percentage of metastasizing carcinomas in the above locations that have demonstrated positive nodes along a given vascular route. For example, node positive tumors lying between the ileocoloc and right colic arcades metastasize along the ileocolic arcade in 100% of cases and along the right colon in 12% of cases *(47a)*.

its optimal extent in the individual patient, lymphadenectomy should be regarded as an essential component of surgical therapy for colon cancer. Unlike other solid tumors such as lung, bladder, and cervix cancer in which surgical cure of node positive cancers is rare, approx 50% of node-positive (stage III) colon cancers can be cured by surgery alone *(49)*. Because of the safety of wide lymphadenectomy and the impossibility of predicting the extent of mesenteric lymph node spread by palpation and inspection, routine use of wide lymphatic resection is recommended. Less extensive lymphadenectomy may be acceptable when there is unresectable metastatic disease. Removal of at least 12 regional lymph nodes is considered necessary for accurate pathologic staging *(50)*. Standard resections for primary

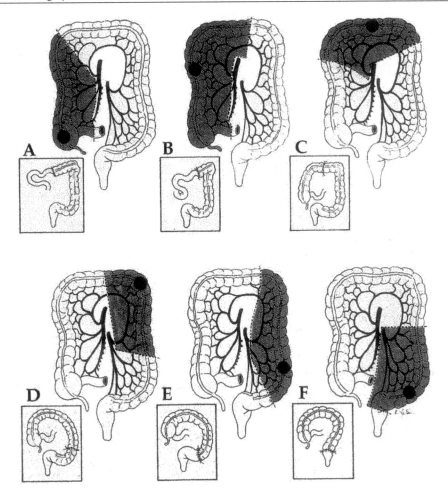

Fig. 3. Extent of surgical resection for cancer of the colon at various sites. The cancer is represented by a black disk. Anastomosis of the bowel remaining after resection is shown in the insets. Panel **A** represents treatment of a cecal lesion, Panel **B** an ascending colon lesion, Panel **C** a transverse colon lesion, Panel **D** a splenic flexure lesion, Panel **E** a descending colon lesion, and Panel **F** a sigmoid colon lesion *(50a).*

colon cancer are shown in Fig 3. The survival of over 1800 patients surgically treated for colon cancer at Memorial Sloan-Kettering Cancer Center is presented in Fig. 4.

2.7.1. RIGHT COLON

Patients with tumors of the cecum, ascending colon, and hepatic flexure are treated by right hemicolectomy. The terminal ileum (10–15 cm length), cecum, ascending colon, and proximal transverse colon are removed. Vascular structures ligated include the ileocolic, right colic, and the right branch of the middle colic arteries. If mesenteric lymph nodes near the origin of the middle colic artery are clinically suspicious, then an extended right hemicolectomy should be performed. The subsequent anastomosis (Fig. 3, panel A) is between the ileum and transverse colon.

2.7.2. TRANSVERSE COLON

Patients with tumors of the transverse colon may undergo an extended right hemicolectomy (Fig. 3, panel B) or a transverse colectomy (panel C). In a transverse colectomy, the middle

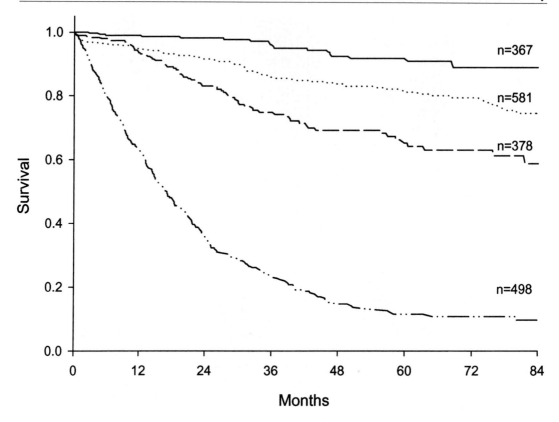

Fig. 4. Kaplan-Meier Survival Curves for 1824 patients operated on for colon cancer at Memorial Sloan Kettering Cancer Center. Top solid line represents stage I patients; dotted line, stage II; dashed line, stage III; and the bottom dashed/dotted line, stage IV.

colic artery is ligated at or near its origin. After removal of an adequate segment of transverse colon, the right colon and left colon are joined near the midline. Because both the hepatic and splenic flexures are fixed, this operation requires extensive mobilization of the colon to avoid tension on the anastomosis. It can be a difficult procedure unless the transverse colon is long and redundant. Extended right hemicolectomy is generally preferable. The procedure entails a right colectomy plus transverse colectomy with high ligation of the left branch of the middle colic artery. The terminal ileum, cecum, ascending colon, and transverse colon are removed. The anastomosis is performed between ileum and descending colon, which is perfused by the ascending branch of the left colic artery. This procedure achieves a maximal lymphadenectomy along the middle colic vessels and is preferred for high-risk cancers of the transverse colon.

2.7.3. DESCENDING COLON

Cancers arising at the splenic flexure or within the descending colon are treated with left hemicolectomy (Fig. 3, panel D). The left colic artery is ligated at its origin and the splenic flexure and descending colon are removed. The remaining transverse colon may then be stapled or hand-sewn to the sigmoid colon. For more distal lesions, a portion or all of the sigmoid colon may also be resected with high ligation of one or more of the sigmoidal arterial branches. The anastomosis of the transverse colon is made to the distal sigmoid or upper rectum (Fig. 3, panel E).

2.7.4. Sigmoid Colon

For sigmoid tumors, a sigmoid colectomy is the standard resection. The patient is positioned in dorsal lithotomy with the legs supported in stirrups to allow transanal stapling. For proximal or advanced sigmoid cancers, the inferior mesenteric artery (IMA) is ligated at its origin; the left colic artery is then ligated proximal to its bifurcation into ascending and descending branches. For more distal or early sigmoid cancers, the arterial ligation may be done at the origin of the superior rectal artery with preservation of the inflow through the IMA into the left colic artery (Fig. 3, panel F). In both cases, the lymph nodes along the sigmoidal arteries and the superior rectal artery are removed. High ligation of the IMA allows removal of lymph nodes along the IMA; it may also require removal of some of the descending colon. Because of the potential for injury to the preaortic sympathetic nerve plexus, many surgeons reserve high ligation of the inferior mesenteric artery for those cases judged to be at high risk for nodal dissemination.

2.8. Colon Anastomosis

There are three basic techniques for performing an entero-enteric anastomosis: suturing, stapling, or placing an anastomotic ring device. There are no large, definitive, randomized clinical trials comparing all three techniques, but the available randomized data indicate that there is no difference in complication rates or recovery time *(51)*. The choice of technique is made according to the surgeon's preference. Meticulous care must be given when performing colonic anastomoses, as the morbidity and mortality of dehiscence are significant *(52)*. It is up to the surgeon to achieve a mechanically secure anastomosis while maintaining optimal blood supply and minimizing tension, inflammation, and infection *(53,54)*.

Hand-sewn colonic anastomoses are frequently performed in two layers: an inner layer of absorbable suture material to approximate the mucosa and bowel wall, and an outer layer of nonabsorbable suture material to secure the serosal edges together while incorporating the submucosa for strength. This represents Czerney's modification of the Lembert anastomosis (originally a single-layer technique) *(55,56)*. A one-layer anastomosis is preferred by many surgeons, and large clinical studies and experimental data from animal models support the safety of one-layer suturing. A retrospective analysis *(57)* of single-layer anastomoses in 1000 patients over a 9-yr period observed that anastomotic leakage (1%), obstruction (2%), wound complication rate (2%), and mortality (1%) are comparable or better than other series reporting outcomes using two layer technique *(51,58)*.

Advocates of stapled anastomoses cite shorter time to completion and equal safety and functional results compared to the hand-sewn technique. A prospective trial with 652 patients comparing stapled and hand-sewn techniques found no statistical difference in clinical leak rates (4.5% vs 4.4%) *(59)*. Another prospective randomized trial of 250 patients found no difference in clinical or radiographic leak rate *(60)*. Concern that stapled anastomoses might yield a higher incidence of anastomotic recurrence has been dispelled by prospective trials showing equivalence to sutured anastomoses *(59)*. A variety of linear and circular staplers are in widespread use for colonic surgery.

Anastomotic devices that compress the proximal and distal bowel walls between two or three rings have been in use for more than a century. At present, the biofragmentable anastomosis ring (Valtrac BAR) is commercially available. The Valtrac device *(61)* is made of polyglycolic acid with barium sulfate added for radiographic visualization. The device snaps together and rapidly creates an end-to-end anastomosis. Several experimental and clinical studies have validated the safety of the Valtrac device compared to hand-sewn and stapled anastomosis *(51,61–66)*.

2.9. Adjunct Techniques

2.9.1. Intraoperative Ultrasound

Intraoperative ultrasound (IOUS) has been touted as the most sensitive method for detection of hepatic metastases. A comparison of IOUS, CT scan, and preoperative ultrasound published in 1987 reported that each modality had a specificity of approx 90% for detection of hepatic metastases from colon cancer. However, sensitivity of IOUS was superior at 98%, vs 48% and 41% for CT scan and preoperative ultrasound, respectively *(67)*. Consequently, a subset of patients will have hepatic involvement detectable only by IOUS. In a study of 55 patients undergoing resection for colorectal cancer, occult hepatic metastases were detected by IOUS alone in 5% of cases. When analysis was restricted to patients with T3 or T4 lesions and patients operated on for recurrence, the yield from IOUS increased to 10% of patients *(68)*. However, the authors concluded that routine use of IOUS is not warranted in patients with colon cancer who have had a good quality preoperative CT scan. With the availability of spiral CT scans, the diagnostic yield of intraoperative ultrasound is likely to be even lower. At present, its most useful roles are for the characterization of indeterminant liver lesions and as an aide in defining liver anatomy during liver resection.

2.9.2. Radioimmunoguided Surgery

Radioisotope-labeled monoclonal antibodies that recognize specific tumor surface antigens can be used for intraoperative localization of tumor deposits. Several days or weeks prior to surgery, patients are intravenously administered the labeled antibody. Intraoperatively, a handheld gamma detection probe is used to identify tissues with high levels of antibody uptake. In a study of 36 patients, there was 83% positive antibody localization. In patients who localized, staging changes were made in 34% and operative changes were made in 25% *(69)*. Despite some success in identifying occult sites of disease, nonspecific uptake of signal remains problematic. Use of radiolabeled antibodies remains investigational.

2.9.3. Sentinel Node Evaluation

Sentinel lymph node identification has played a significant role in the evaluation of patients with melanoma and breast cancer. The success of this technique in these two diseases has sparked enthusiasm in the treatment of other malignancies, notably colon cancer. A recent review *(70)* summarized the experience of intraoperative sentinel lymph node identification in 85 patients. At the time of operation, the surgeon injects lymphazurin 1% dye subserosally around the tumor. The dye will quickly travel through the lymphatics into the draining lymph nodes, turning pale to deep blue (Fig. 5). The first four such lymph nodes are identified and marked with a suture as sentinel lymph nodes. The standard resection then proceeds. These sentinel lymph nodes are then analyzed pathologically, as are the other lymph nodes in the specimen. A theoretical advantage is that the pathologist may then focus on the sentinel nodes, potentially identifying micrometastatic disease that may upstage the patient, who may then benefit from further adjuvant therapy. More prospective analysis of this technique is required, but the early experience is encouraging.

2.10. Prophylactic Resections

2.10.1. Gallbladder

Patients with gallstones detected on preoperative imaging studies may be safely treated with cholecystectomy at the time of elective colon resection. Initial laparoscopic cholecystectomy followed by open colectomy may be advantageous for patients with sigmoid or rectal

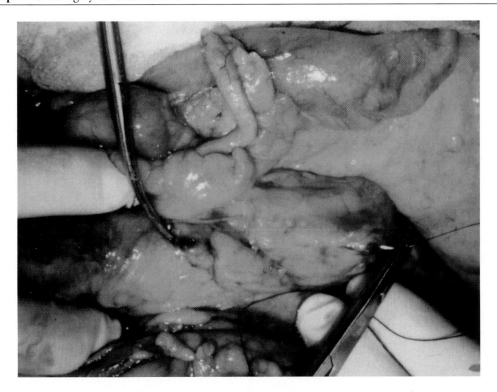

Fig. 5. A sentinel lymph node being marked with a suture after a cecal lesion (top of photograph) has been injected with lymphazurin 1%. Note tracking of blue dye between two lymph nodes. (Personal correspondence, used with permission, S. Saha, MD, Michigan State University.)

cancers. Prophylactic cholecystectomy for asymptomatic gallstones detected intraoperatively is not necessary and is generally not advisable.

2.10.2. APPENDIX

When a mass in the appendix is encountered intraoperatively, appendectomy with frozen-section analysis of the mass lesion is appropriate treatment. Most of these lesions will prove to be mucoceles or small carcinoid tumors, and no further treatment is required. Right colectomy is indicated for carcinoid tumors larger than 1.5 cm and for appendiceal adenocarcinomas *(71–73)*. Prophylactic removal of a normal appendix is not recommended.

2.10.3. OVARIES

Careful intraoperative assessment of the ovaries in a woman with colon cancer is essential. Metastatic spread to the ovaries may be present at the time of initial colonic resection or may develop subsequently and, in some cases, require reoperation. Consequently, prophylactic oophorectomy at the time of colon surgery has been advocated. No definitive randomized study to assess the impact of prophylactic oophorectomy on cancer recurrence or survival has been performed. Some justification for prophylactic oophorectomy can be found in retrospective studies *(74–77)*. In one large study, in which 201 women received prophylactic oophorectomy at time of large bowel surgery, there was a 2% incidence of ovarian involvement by metastatic colon carcinoma. In the control arm (134 patients), 2.2% of patients developed subsequent ovarian disease (2 primary ovarian carcinoma and 1 metastatic breast carcinoma) *(77)*. A randomized study comparing prophylactic oophorectomy vs no oophorectomy in stage II and III colon cancer demonstrated a benefit in 5-yr disease-free survival for the oophorectomy group (80%) compared to no oophorectomy (65%) *(78)*. Further patient accrual is necessary in this trial of 155 patients in order to achieve more statistical power; however, the possibility of a recurrence-free survival advantage emphasizes the need to continue this preliminary work. Based on the available data, offering prophylactic adjuvant oophorectomy to postmenopausal women with colon cancer is reasonable. For premenopausal women, only those patients with a clearly increased risk of developing ovarian carcinoma (strong family history, known carrier of breast cancer (BRCA) or hereditary nonpolyposis colorectal cancer [HNPCC] mutation) or those with established metastatic (stage IV) colon cancer are considered for prophylactic oophorectomy. Preoperative consultation with a gynecologist to discuss ovarian cancer risk and postoperative hormone replacement is advisable.

3. SPECIAL SITUATIONS

3.1. Small Colon Tumors

In a minority of cases, the colon tumor may be too small to be identified intraoperatively by palpation. When this is recognized preoperatively, the best solution is tattooing of the tumor site by endoscopic injection of India ink. Another preoperative solution is air-contrast barium enema, which is often successful in localizing small tumors. Alternatively, the tumor may be identified at the time of surgery by intraoperative colonoscopy.

3.2. Obstructing Colon Carcinomas

Obstructing colon carcinomas frequently occur in the descending colon and sigmoid colon, but they may also occur in the cecum when cancer invades the ileocecal valve. Malignant obstruction can progress insidiously for months and then present to the surgeon as an acutely ill, undiagnosed patient with a dilated, unprepped, and often ischemic colon. In this setting, urgent hemicolectomy has significantly increased risks of anastomotic leak, infection, colostomy, and death *(52,79)*.

Following fluid resuscitation and enemas, the site and severity of colon obstruction is documented by single-column gastrograffin enema. Passage of contrast through the obstructing lesion suggests that clinical improvement may be possible. Stable patients should be given a chance to resolve the obstruction and convert to an elective operation. Further workup with CT scan and colonoscopy is desirable. However, patients with unremitting colon obstruction may require urgent abdominal exploration.

For obstructing tumors of the right and transverse colon, the preferred management for clinically stable patients is resection and primary anastomosis *(79)*. The obstructed colon is resected, and anastomosis between ileum and distal colon can be performed safely.

Surgical management for obstructing left-sided colon carcinoma may be done in one, two, or three stages. One-stage operations with resection and primary anastomosis have significant benefit. Temporary colostomy and the complications associated with reoperation for colostomy reversal are avoided. There are two options for one-stage operation: standard colectomy with on-table colonic lavage or subtotal colectomy. The safety of the colonic lavage technique has been well documented, with a mortality rate of less than 10% and an anastomotic leakage rate of 5% *(79–82)*. A prospective, randomized trial comparing subtotal colectomy with standard colectomy with colonic lavage showed that the two techniques have similar rates of complication and mortality *(83)*. However, the colonic lavage group had significantly better bowel function with fewer bowel movements and less diarrhea.

Standard colectomy plus colonic lavage is the preferred method of one-stage resection for most patients with acutely obstructing cancers of the left colon. Subtotal colectomy may be preferable for patients with synchronous tumors, prior colectomy, cecal ischemia, or cecal perforation.

Resection of the obstructing left-sided cancer with proximal colostomy is reserved for cases in which primary anastomosis is felt to be unsafe: poor nutrition, immunosuppression, peritonitis, and shock. Proximal diversion (i.e., a three-stage approach) does not often have any safety advantage over resection plus diversion and is reserved for acutely unstable patients *(84–86)*.

3.3. Perforating Cancers

Colonic perforation is a surgical emergency. The differential diagnosis includes perforated diverticulitis, perforated gastroduodenal ulcer, and appendicitis. Colonic perforation may occur at the site of an ulcerated carcinoma or, more commonly, proximal to an obstructing carcinoma. The primary goals of treatment are to save the patient's life and to control the infection. After resection of the perforated segment, the surgeon may create an ileostomy or colostomy proximally and oversew the distal colon (Hartmann procedure) or create a mucous fistula. If there is a left-sided colon lesion causing right-sided perforation, a subtotal colectomy should be performed.

3.4. Contiguous Organ Involvement

Direct invasion of adjacent organs by colon carcinoma occurs in approx 10% of patients *(87,88)*. At operation, the colon may be adherent either because of inflammation with dense adhesions or actual cancer invasion. Pathologically, approximately half of clinically adherent viscera are the result of inflammatory adhesions only *(88)*. Invasion of a hollow viscus such as bladder or bowel may create a malignant fistula. The goal of resection is to obtain a tumor-free margin; all or part of the adherent organ is removed in continuity with the diseased segment of colon. Carcinomas in the cecum or sigmoid may directly invade the ovaries, fallopian tubes, uterus, or small bowel. Bulky carcinomas of the hepatic flexure, transverse colon, or splenic flexure may invade the gallbladder, duodenum, stomach, pancreas, or spleen. High-quality preoperative CT scanning will prepare the surgeon for the possibility of multivisceral resection. Figure 6 shows the preoperative CT scan of a patient who presented with a large splenic flexure tumor and was treated with in-continuity left colectomy, distal pancreatectomy, splenectomy, and partial gastrectomy. Final pathology revealed a T4N0 adenocarcinoma with invasion of the pancreas and inflammatory adhesions to spleen and stomach. For colon cancer invading the abdominal wall, the colon must often be resected together with abdominal fascia. Primary closure is preferred, but use of synthetic mesh is acceptable if contamination has been minimal. Aggressive surgery in locally advanced cases will result in cure rates between 20% and 50% *(88,89)*. Marking the resection field with metallic surgical clips is helpful if postoperative adjuvant radiotherapy may be required.

3.5. Synchronous Primary Tumors

Synchronous colon cancers occur in 2–5% of patients *(4.90)*. One-third of patients will have associated benign polyps. Consequently, it is recommended to clear the colon preoperatively, either with air-contrast barium enema or, preferably, colonoscopy. For patients who require resection of two colonic lesions, most are managed with subtotal colectomy. Patients with carcinomas in the same anatomic region may be treated with a conventional hemi-colectomy.

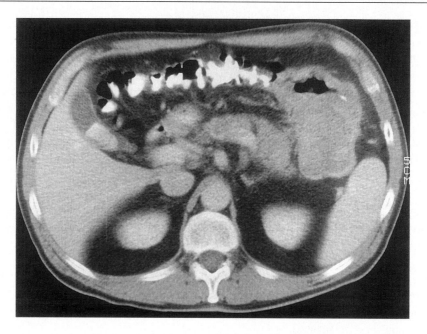

Fig. 6. Preoperative abdominal CT scan of 64-yr-old male who was operated on at Memorial Sloan Kettering Cancer Center for a locally invasive splenic flexure lesion. Operative treatment included a left hemicolectomy, distal pancreatectomy, splenectomy, and partial gastrectomy. The tumor measured 13 cm by 10 cm and was 5 cm in maximal thickness; it was adherent to the distal pancreas, posterior wall of stomach, and splenic hilum. Pathologically, the spleen, stomach, and pancreas were not involved by tumor.

3.6. Synchronous Liver Metastases

Synchronous hepatic involvement in colon cancer is reported to occur in 8–25% of patients at initial presentation *(91–95)*. The majority of patients have diffuse hepatic parenchymal disease that is not amenable to surgical resection. However, about one-fourth of patients with hepatic involvement at presentation may have lesions that are solitary or few in number and may be potentially resectable *(92,96–98)*. The surgeon may elect to perform a combined colon and hepatic resection, or do a staged procedure in which the colon is resected and then the hepatic resection is performed at a later date (*see* Chapter 20).

In retrospective analysis, survival appears to be equivalent between synchronous colon and hepatic resection and delayed hepatic resection. In fact, a staged procedure may allow the biologic behavior and metastatic phenotype of the tumor to declare itself, theoretically enhancing the ability to select patients who are most likely to benefit from resection *(99)*. In a recent retrospective review of the Memorial Sloan-Kettering experience in 132 patients looking at combined vs staged resection for colorectal cancer with hepatic involvement, the two groups had similar complication rates when matched for extent of surgery. Median survival was not different in the two groups (44 vs 43 mo) (Grace et al., unpublished data).

3.7. Metachronous Colon Cancer

Estimates of the incidence of metachronous colon cancer vary between 2% and 26% *(100–103)*. These data emphasize the importance of close endoscopic surveillance following initial surgery. Subtotal colectomy is generally the procedure of choice for management of metachronous carcinoma. This procedure reduces the risk of a second recurrence. Subtotal colectomy also minimizes the risk of devascularizing a colonic segment related to prior surgical ligation of vascular pedicles.

3.8. Rising CEA

Postoperative surveillance involves serial serum carcinoembryonic antigen (CEA) levels. A rise in CEA in the asymptomatic patient may represent a new primary cancer, recurrent colon cancer, or an unrelated condition such as bronchitis or cholecystitis. When endoscopic evaluation and CT scanning fail to detect a recurrent cancer, it is controversial whether such patients should be subjected to exploratory laparoscopy or open surgery. The most recent data suggest CEA-directed surgery for recurrent colon cancer has at best a minimal impact on survival *(5)*. Recent work with FDG-18–PET scanning has shown that it may be more sensitive and specific than CT scan for detection of recurrent colon cancer, but it remains unestablished as to whether FDG-18–PET scanning alters outcome or management in this setting *(104)*.

4. COMPLICATIONS

4.1. Anastomotic Leak

The published rates of anastomotic leak following colectomy vary between 4% and 18%, depending on anatomic location and method of detection. Subclinical leaks may occur in as many as 35% of patients *(105)*. The smaller leaks may often be treated conservatively, but larger leaks with associate abscess or with symptoms require intervention. Surgical options to treat anastomotic leaks include closure of the leak, proximal diversion, and resection of the anastomosis with proximal colostomy. Each of these operations may be performed with or without a drainage procedure. Certain leaks may be treated successfully by percutaneous drainage alone. Patients with gross anastomotic dehiscence, associated bowel obstruction, or peritonitis generally require surgical treatment.

4.2. Anastomotic Stricture

In contradistinction to leaks, anastomotic strictures are generally late complications of colon surgery, with an incidence of 2–5% *(106)*. Patients are diagnosed with bowel obstruction or during follow-up surveillance with barium enema or colonoscopy. Treatment is through endoscopic or operative approaches. Endoscopically, patients may have the stricture forcefully dilated (using balloons or bouginage) or ablated (using laser or electrocautery). Dilation incurs a small risk of perforation. Ablation techniques are used more often when there is a suture line recurrence rather than with a benign stricture. Operative treatment involves resection of the involved segment and reanastomosis. Although this technique is possible, repeated operation may be technically challenging and carries an increased morbidity and mortality with it, especially in patients with significant coexisting illnesses.

4.3. Small Bowel Obstruction

Postoperative ileus is a normal phenomenon following abdominal operations and generally represents a temporary motor dysfunction of the peristaltic mechanism. It is most prevalent in the left colon, with return to normal motor function generally within 3–5 d. In elective colon surgery, routine postoperative nasogastric decompression is not necessary. An ileus that persists longer than 1 wk may be a sign of an underlying pathologic condition, such as electrolyte imbalance, excessive narcotic use, an intra-abdominal fluid abscess, peritonitis, or a mechanical small bowel obstruction. Mechanical obstructions will usually resolve with conservative treatment using nasogastric decompression and parenteral nutrition.

4.4. Wound Complications

The risk of a postoperative wound infection depends on the bacterial contamination of the wound, the condition of the wound when the abdomen is closed, and the host's systemic defense. Colon resections for malignancy incur a risk of wound infection between 3% and 16% (107). This range includes cases in which there was frank contamination of the operative field or preoperative perforation. For the majority of elective colon resections, the wound infection rate is 3–5%. In the presence of a grossly contaminated operative field with a high risk of wound infection, the surgeon may elect not to close the skin, allowing for delayed wound closure.

5. UNCOMMON COLON TUMORS

5.1. Lymphoma

Colonic lymphoma is a rare tumor, accounting for less than 1% of all cancers affecting the large bowel (108). Of all lymphomas arising in the gastrointestinal tract, the colon is the primary site in approx 15% of cases (109). A pathologically confirmed large bowel lymphoma may be considered primary if the following criteria are met: if there is no radiologic evidence of lymphoma in the chest, if the peripheral blood smear and bone marrow aspiration are within normal limits, and if there is no hepatosplenomegaly or palpable peripheral adenopathy (5). The majority are B-cell lymphomas of intermediate to high grade.

Clinical presentation is indistinguishable from that of colonic adenocarcinoma (110,111). Although surgical resection is often technically feasible, optimal therapy for gastrointestinal lymphoma has not yet been identified. Historically, surgical resection has been the initial treatment, with complete resection achieved in 50–80% (108,111–114). However, primary therapy with systemic chemotherapy can be successful, with surgery reserved for chemotherapy failures. Available retrospective data regarding surgery, radiation therapy, and chemotherapy are difficult to interpret because of small series size and lack of uniformly accepted regimens. Overall, 5-yr survival rates for colonic lymphoma are approx 50% (109,111,112,115).

5.2. Gastrointestinal Stromal Tumors (GIST)

Gastrointestinal stromal tumors (GISTs) arise from intestinal pacemaker cells within the muscularis propria of the intestine. GIST accounts for most of the cases formerly characterized as leiomyosarcoma of the colon. These stromal tumors account for less than 1% of large bowel malignancies. Most present as large intraluminal masses and may have significant local invasion. GISTs are treated with wide surgical resection along with the associated mesentery. Lymphatic spread is extremely rare, and extensive lymphadenectomy is not indicated. Prognosis for patients with GISTs depends on tumor size, histologic grade, and contiguous organ involvement (116–118). Recurrences most commonly arise in the peritoneal cavity or liver; these patients have a poor prognosis. Traditional chemotherapy and radiation had little benefit. The discovery of STI571 (an inhibitor of tyrosine kinase activity of the protooncogene c-kit) as an active agent for treatment of GISTs is an exciting advance that may lead to improved outcomes for colonic GISTs (119).

5.3. Carcinoid

Gastrointestinal sites account for nearly 95% of all carcinoids, with the colon being involved in about 6% of cases (half of these involve the cecum) (120,121). The appendix is the most common site (35% of cases) and will be discussed in the next section (121). Patients with carcinoid of the colon almost never present with the traditional carcinoid syndrome; usually, the clinical presentation is indistinguishable from adenocarcinoma (121,122). Lesions tend to be advanced, with nodal involvement in 60% and liver metastases in 40% (120,122,123). Surgical treatment is by standard colon resection. Five-year survival of early-stage carcinoid is nearly 80% (120); overall patient survival, however, is between 25% and 35%, owing to the preponderance of advanced cases at presentation (120,122). Synchronous or metachronous lesions are reported in 15–40% of patients with gastrointestinal carcinoids (120,121,124–126), with nearly two-thirds of these occurring in the gastrointestinal tract.

6. APPENDIX TUMORS

Neoplasms of the appendix are rare, with an incidence of approx 1% in all appendectomy specimens (127). Carcinoids account for between 70% and 90% of all appendiceal tumors. The remainder are benign mucoceles, mucinous cyst–adenocarcinoma, adenocarcinoma, lymphosarcoma, paraganglioma, and granular cell tumors (128). Recognition is rare prior to surgery; initial preoperative diagnosis is often appendicitis or a gynecologic disease process. Because of this, patients often undergo a second operation as definitive therapy.

In one series of appendiceal carcinoids, 54% of patients presented with signs/symptoms of appendicitis, and in 46% of patients, the diagnosis was made incidentally (73). Appropriate treatment is based on size: Carcinoids that are less than 1 cm in size may be treated by appendectomy alone, whereas those that are greater than 2 cm require a right hemicolectomy. Controversy exists for tumors that measure 1–2 cm (73,128). Prognosis is generally favorable, with 5-yr survival varying from 90% to 100% (121,129–132). The most significant prognostic indicator is presence or absence of hepatic metastasis at time of surgery. It is rare for appendiceal carcinoids to metastasize to the liver (73). In one study, carcinoids less than 1.5 cm never metastasized, those between 1.5 and 2.0 cm had minimal metastatic potential, and those larger than 2.0 cm (only 1% of all appendiceal carcinoids) metastasized frequently (127).

Primary adenocarcinoma of the appendix, similar to appendiceal carcinoid, often presents as acute appendicitis. Treatment is right hemicolectomy, ideally at initial operation. Patients treated with appendectomy alone have been shown to have a worse 5-yr survival than those treated with right hemicolectomy: 50–68% vs 25–30%, respectively (72,128). In the small number of cases reported, prognosis is the same as for other colon adenocarcinomas (128).

Mucoceles of the appendix may be benign or malignant, and both are characterized by an obstructed, mucin-filled appendix. Most benign lesions are small and are cured by simple appendectomy. Cystadenocarcinoma, by definition, has invaded the appendiceal wall and possibly spread to other peritoneal sites. Treatment requires wide resection of the primary disease, right hemicolectomy, and debulking of peritoneal implants. Five-year survival in patients with metastatic cystadenocarcinoma of the appendix may approach 50%, in part due to the indolent nature of metastatic progression *(127)*.

REFERENCES

1. Epstein M. Fiber optics in medicine. *Critical Reviews in Biomedical Engineering,* **7** (1982) 79–120.
2. Eusebio EB. A practical aid in colonoscopy. *Dis. Colon Rectum,* **32** (1989) 996–997.
3. Gollub MJ and Flaherty F. Barium enema following incomplete colonoscopy. *Clin. Imaging,* **23** (1999) 367–374.
4. Langevin JM and Nivatvongs S. The true incidence of synchronous cancer of the large bowel. A prospective study. *Am. J. Surg.,* **147** (1984) 330–333.
5. Hellman S, DeVita VT, and Rosenberg SA. *Cancer: Principles and Practice of Oncology.* Lippincott–Raven, Philadelphia, 1997, pp. lxviii, 92, 3125.
6. Isler JT, Brown PC, Lewis FG, and Billingham RP. The role of preoperative colonoscopy in colorectal cancer. *Dis. Colon Rectum,* **30** (1987) 435–439.
7. Pagana TJ, Ledesma EJ, Mittelman A, and Nava HR. The use of colonoscopy in the study of synchronous colorectal neoplasms. *Cancer,* **53** (1984) 356–359.
8. Pescatore P, Glucker T, Delarive J, et al. Diagnostic accuracy and interobserver agreement of CT colonography (virtual colonoscopy). *Gut,* **47** (2000) 126–130.
9. Vining DJ. Virtual colonoscopy. *Gastrointest. Endoscopy Clin. North Am.,* **7** (1997) 285–291.
10. Cohen AM and Winawer SJ. *Cancer of the Colon, Rectum, and Anus.* McGraw-Hill, New York, 1995, pp. xxii, 1154, [8] of plates.
11. Laing AD and Gibson RN. MRI of the liver. *J. Magn. Reson. Imaging,* **8** (1998) 337–345.
12. Yasuda S, Makuuchi Y, Sadahiro S, et al. Colorectal cancer recurrence in the liver: detection by PET. *Tokai J. Exp. Clin. Med.,* **23** (1998) 167–171.
13. Bodmer WF, Bailey CJ, Bodmer J, et al. Localization of the gene for familial adenomatous polyposis on chromosome 5. *Nature,* **328** (1987) 614–616.
14. Arvanitis ML, Jagelman DG, Fazio VW, Lavery IC, and McGannon E. Mortality in patients with familial adenomatous polyposis. *Dis. Colon Rectum,* **33** (1990) 639–642.
15. Lynch HT, Smyrk T, Watson P, et al. Hereditary colorectal cancer. *Semin. Oncol.,* **18** (1991) 337–366.
16. Lynch HT, Smyrk TC, Watson P, et al. Genetics, natural history, tumor spectrum, and pathology of hereditary nonpolyposis colorectal cancer: an updated review. *Gastroenterology,* **104** (1993) 1535–1549.
17. Fitzgibbons RJ Jr, Lynch HT, Stanislav GV, et al. Recognition and treatment of patients with hereditary nonpolyposis colon cancer (Lynch syndromes I and II). *Ann. Surg.,* **206** (1987) 289–295.
18. Lin KM, Shashidharan M, Ternent CA, et al. Colorectal and extracolonic cancer variations in MLH1/MSH2 hereditary nonpolyposis colorectal cancer kindreds and the general population. *Dis. Colon Rectum,* **41** (1998) 428–433.
19. Levin B. Inflammatory bowel disease and colon cancer. *Cancer,* **70** (1992) 1313–1316.
20. Levin B. Ulcerative colitis and colon cancer: biology and surveillance. *J. Cell. Biochem.,* **16G(Suppl.)** (1992) 47–50.
21. Jain SK and Peppercorn MA. Inflammatory bowel disease and colon cancer: a review. *Dig. Dis.,* **15** (1997) 243–252.
22. Willenbucher RF. Inflammatory bowel disease. *Semin. Gastrointest. Dis.,* **7** (1996) 94–104.
23. Lennard-Jones JE, Melville DM, Morson BC, Ritchie JK, and Williams CB. Precancer and cancer in extensive ulcerative colitis: findings among 401 patients over 22 years. *Gut,* **31** (1990) 800–806.
24. Greenstein AJ, Sachar DB, Smith H, et al. Cancer in universal and left-sided ulcerative colitis: factors determining risk. *Gastroenterology,* **77** (1979) 290–294.
25. Schottenfeld D, Sherlock P, and Winawer SJ. Colorectal cancer: prevention, epidemiology, and screening. *Progress in Cancer Research and Therapy.* Raven, New York, 1980, Vol. 13, pp. xxii, 410.
26. Axon ATR. Screening and surveillance of ulcerative colitis. *Gastrointest. Endoscopy Clin. North Am.,* **7** (1997) 129–145.
27. Leidenius M, Kellokumpu I, Husa A, Riihela M, and Sipponen P. Dysplasia and carcinoma in long-standing ulcerative colitis: an endoscopic and histological surveillance programme. *Gut,* **32** (1991) 1521–1525.
28. Nugent FW, Haggitt RC, and Gilpin PA. Cancer surveillance in ulcerative colitis [see comments]. *Gastroenterology,* **100** (1991) 1241–1248.
29. Ekbom A, Helmick C, Zack M, and Adami HO. Ulcerative colitis and colorectal cancer. A population-based study. *N. Engl. J. Med.,* **323** (1990) 1228–1233.

30. Ekbom A, Helmick C, Zack M, and Adami HO. Increased risk of large-bowel cancer in Crohn's disease with colonic involvement. *Lancet*, **336** (1990) 357–359.

31. Keighley MR. A clinical and physiological evaluation of bowel preparation for elective colorectal surgery. *World J. Surg.*, **6** (1982) 464–470.

32. DiPalma JA, Brady CED, Stewart DL, et al. Comparison of colon cleansing methods in preparation for colonoscopy. *Gastroenterology*, **86** (1984) 856–860.

33. Beck DE and Fazio VW. Current preoperative bowel cleansing methods. Results of a survey. *Dis. Colon Rectum*, **33** (1990) 12–15.

34. Hares MM and Alexander-Williams J. The effect of bowel preparation on clonic surgery. *World J. Surg.*, **6** (1982) 175–181.

35. Hares MM, Nevah E, Minervini S, Bentley S, Keighley M, and Alexander-Williams J. An attempt to reduce the side effects of mannitol bowel preparation by intravenous infusion. *Dis. Colon Rectum*, **25** (1982) 289–291.

36. Beck DE, Fazio VW, and Jagelman DG. Comparison of oral lavage methods for preoperative colonic cleansing. *Dis. Colon Rectum*, **29** (1986) 699–703.

37. Burton RC. Postoperative wound infection in colonic and rectal surgery. *Br. J. Surg.*, **60** (1973) 363–365.

38. Clarke JS, Condon RE, Bartlett JG, Gorbach SL, Nichols RL, and Ochi S. Preoperative oral antibiotics reduce septic complications of colon operations: results of prospective, randomized, double-blind clinical study. *Ann. Surg.*, **186** (1977) 251–259.

39. Matheson DM, Arabi Y, Baxter-Smith D, Alexander-Williams J, and Keighley MR. Randomized multicentre trial of oral bowel preparation and antimicrobials for elective colorectal operations. *Br. J. Surg.*, **65** (1978) 597–600.

40. Condon RE, Bartlett JG, Greenlee H, et al. Efficacy of oral and systemic antibiotic prophylaxis in colorectal operations. *Arch. Surg.*, **118** (1985) 496–502.

41. Greenfield LJ and Mulholland MW. *Surgery: Scientific Principles and Practice*. Lippincott–Raven, Philadelphia, 1997, pp. xxxi, 2363, [11] of plates.

42. Kakkar VV and De Lorenzo F. Prevention of venous thromboembolism in general surgery. *Baillieres Clin. Haematol.*, **11** (1998) 605–619.

43. Stratton MA, Anderson FA, Bussey HI, et al. Prevention of venous thromboembolism: adherence to the 1995 American College of Chest Physicians consensus guidelines for surgical patients. *Arch. Intern. Med.*, **160** (2000) 334–340.

44. Wheeler HB and Anderson FA Jr. Prophylaxis against venous thromboembolism in surgical patients. *Am. J. Surg.*, **161** (1991) 507–511.

45. Turnbull RB Jr, Kyle K, Watson FR, and Spratt J. Cancer of the colon: the influence of the no-touch isolation technic on survival rates. *Ann. Surg.*, **166** (1967) 420–427.

46. Cole WH, Roberts SS, and Strehl FW. Modern concepts in cancer of the colon and rectum. *Cancer*, **19** (1966) 1347–1358.

47. Wiggers T, Jeekel J, Arends JW, et al. No-touch isolation technique in colon cancer: a controlled prospective trial. *Br. J. Surg.*, **75** (1988) 409–415.

47a. Hertzer FP and Slanetz CA. Patterns and significance of lymphatic spread from cancer of the colon and rectum, in *Lymphatic System Metastasis* (Weiss L, Gilbert HA, and Ballon SC, eds.), GK Hall, Boston, MA, (1980) p. 283.

48. Enker WE, Laffer UT, and Block GE. Enhanced survival of patients with colon and rectal cancer is based upon wide anatomic resection. *Ann. Surg.*, **190** (1979) 350–360.

49. Jessup JM, McGinnis LS, Steele GD Jr, Menck HR, and Winchester DP. The National Cancer Data Base. Report on colon cancer. *Cancer*, **78** (1996) 918–926.

50a. Schrock, TR. Large Intestine, in *Current Surgical Diagnosis and Treatment* (Way LW, ed.), Appleton and Lange, Norwalk, CT, (1994) p. 659.

50. Compton CC. Pathology report in colon cancer: what is prognostically important? [see comments]. *Dig. Dis.*, **17** (1999) 67–79.

51. Corman ML, Prager ED, Hardy TG Jr, and Bubrick MP. Comparison of the Valtrac biofragmentable anastomosis ring with conventional suture and stapled anastomosis in colon surgery. Results of a prospective, randomized clinical trial. *Dis. Colon Rectum*, **32** (1989) 183–187.

52. Schrock TR, Deveney CW, and Dunphy JE. Factor contributing to leakage of colonic anastomoses. *Ann. Surg.*, **177** (1973) 513–518.

53. Van Winkle W Jr and Hastings JC. Considerations in the choice of suture material for various tissues. *Surg. Gynecol. Obstet.*, **135** (1972) 113–126.

54. Ballantyne GH. The experimental basis of intestinal suturing. Effect of surgical technique, inflammation, and infection on enteric wound healing. *Dis. Colon Rectum*, **27** (1984) 61–71.

55. Ballantyne GH. Intestinal suturing. Review of the experimental foundations for traditional doctrines. *Dis. Colon Rectum*, **26** (1983) 836–843.

56. Getzen LC. Intestinal suturing. I. The development of intestinal sutures. *Curr. Probl. Surg.*, (1969) 3–48.

57. Max E, Sweeney WB, Bailey HR, et al. Results of 1,000 single-layer continuous polypropylene intestinal anastomoses. *Am. J. Surg.*, **162** (1991) 461–467.

58. Debas HT and Thomson FB. A critical review of colectomy with anastomosis. *Surg. Gynecol. Obstet.*, **135** (1972) 747–752.

59. Docherty JG, McGregor JR, Akyol AM, Murray GD, and Galloway DJ. Comparison of manually constructed and stapled anastomoses in colorectal surgery. West of Scotland and Highland Anastomosis Study Group [see comments]. *Ann. Surg.*, **221** (1995) 176–184.

60. Friend PJ, Scott R, Everett WG, and Scott IH. Stapling or suturing for anastomoses of the left side of the large intestine. *Surg. Gynecol. Obstet.*, **171** (1990) 373–376.

61. Hardy TG Jr, Pace WG, Maney JW, Katz AR, and Kaganov AL. A biofragmentable ring for sutureless bowel anastomosis. An experimental study. *Dis. Colon Rectum*, **28** (1985) 484–490.

62. Maney JW, Katz AR, Li LK, Pace WG, and Hardy TG. Biofragmentable bowel anastomosis ring: comparative efficacy studies in dogs. *Surgery*, **103** (1988) 56–62.

63. Hardy TG Jr, Aguilar PS, Stewart WR, et al. Initial clinical experience with a biofragmentable ring for sutureless bowel anastomosis. *Dis. Colon Rectum*, **30** (1987) 55–61.

64. Bubrick MP, Corman ML, Cahill CJ, Hardy TG Jr, Nance FC, and Shatney CH. Prospective, randomized trial of the biofragmentable anastomosis ring. The BAR Investigational Group. *Am. J. Surg.*, **161** (1991) 136–142; discussion 142–143.

65. Cahill CJ, Betzler M, Gruwez JA, Jeekel J, Patel JC, and Zederfeldt B. Sutureless large bowel anastomosis: European experience with the biofragmentable anastomosis ring. *Br. J. Surg.*, **76** (1989) 344–347.

66. Forde KA, McLarty AJ, Tsai J, Ghalili K, and Delany HM. Murphy's Button revisited. Clinical experience with the biofragmentable anastomotic ring. *Ann. Surg.*, **217** (1993) 78–81.

67. Machi J, Isomoto H, Yamashita Y, Kurohiji T, Shirouzu K, and Kakegawa T. Intraoperative ultrasonography in screening for liver metastases from colorectal cancer: comparative accuracy with traditional procedures. *Surgery*, **101** (1987) 678–684.

68. Stone MD, Kane R, Bothe A Jr, Jessup JM, Cady B, and Steele GD Jr. Intraoperative ultrasound imaging of the liver at the time of colorectal cancer resection. *Arch. Surg.*, **129** (1994) 431–435; discussion 435–436.

69. Arnold MW, Schneebaum S, Berens A, Mojzisik C, Hinkle G, and Martin EW Jr. Radioimmunoguided surgery challenges traditional decision making in patients with primary colorectal cancer. *Surgery*, **112** (1992) 624–629; discussion 629–630.

70. Saha S, Wiese D, Badin J, et al. Technical details of sentinel lymph node mapping in colorectal cancer and its impact on staging [see comments]. *Ann. Surg. Oncol.*, **7** (2000) 120–124.

71. Nitecki SS, Wolff BG, Schlinkert R, and Sarr MG. The natural history of surgically treated primary adenocarcinoma of the appendix [see comments]. *Ann. Surg.*, **219** (1994) 51–57.

72. Conte CC, Petrelli NJ, Stulc J, Herrera L, and Mittelman A. Adenocarcinoma of the appendix. *Surg. Gynecol. Obstet.*, **166** (1988) 451–453.

73. Roggo A, Wood WC, and Ottinger LW. Carcinoid tumors of the appendix. *Ann. Surg.*, **217** (1993) 385–390.

74. O'Brien PH, Newton BB, Metcalf JS, and Rittenbury MS. Oophorectomy in women with carcinoma of the colon and rectum. *Surg. Gynecol. Obstet.*, **153** (1981) 827–830.

75. Ballantyne GH, Reigel MM, Wolff BG, and Ilstrup DM. Oophorectomy and colon cancer. Impact on survival. *Ann. Surg.*, **202** (1985) 209–214.

76. Birnkrant A, Sampson J, and Sugarbaker PH. Ovarian metastasis from colorectal cancer. *Dis. Colon Rectum*, **29** (1986) 767–771.

77. Cutait R, Lesser ML, and Enker WE. Prophylactic oophorectomy in surgery for large-bowel cancer. *Dis. Colon Rectum*, **26** (1983) 6–11.

78. Young-Fadok TM, Wolff BG, Nivatvongs S, Metzger PP, and Ilstrup DM. Prophylactic oophorectomy in colorectal carcinoma: preliminary results of a randomized, prospective trial. *Dis. Colon Rectum*, **41** (1998) 277–283; discussion 283–285.

79. Phillips RK, Hittinger R, Fry JS, and Fielding LP. Malignant large bowel obstruction. *Br. J. Surg.*, **72** (1985) 296–302.

80. Thomson WH and Carter SS. On-table lavage to achieve safe restorative rectal and emergency left colonic resection without covering colostomy. *Br. J. Surg.*, **73** (1986) 61–63.

81. Foster ME, Johnson CD, Billings PJ, Davies PW, and Leaper DJ. Intraoperative antegrade lavage and anastomotic healing in acute colonic obstruction. *Dis. Colon Rectum*, **29** (1986) 255–259.

82. Tan SG, Nambiar R, Rauff A, Ngoi SS, and Goh HS. Primary resection and anastomosis in obstructed descending colon due to cancer. *Arch. Surg.*, **126** (1991) 748–751.

83. Anonymous. Single-stage treatment for malignant left-sided colonic obstruction: a prospective randomized clinical trial comparing subtotal colectomy with segmental resection following intraoperative irrigation. The SCOTIA Study Group. Subtotal Colectomy versus On-table Irrigation and Anastomosis [see comments]. *Br. J. Surg.*, **82** (1995) 1622–1627.

84. Welch JP and Donaldson GA. Management of severe obstruction of the large bowel due to malignant disease. *Am. J. Surg.*, **127** (1974) 492–499.

85. Deans GT, Krukowski ZH, and Irwin ST. Malignant obstruction of the left colon. *Br. J. Surg.*, **81** (1994) 1270–1276.

86. MacKenzie S, Thomson SR, and Baker LW. Management options in malignant obstruction of the left colon. *Surg. Gynecol. Obstet.*, **174** (1992) 337–345.

87. Kelley WE Jr, Brown PW, Lawrence W Jr, and Terz JJ. Penetrating, obstructing, and perforating carcinomas of the colon and rectum. *Arch. Surg.*, **116** (1981) 381–384.

88. Gall FP, Tonak J, and Altendorf A. Multivisceral resections in colorectal cancer. *Dis. Colon Rectum*, **30** (1987) 337–341.

89. Welch JP and Donaldson GA. Perforative carcinoma of colon and rectum. *Ann. Surg.*, **180** (1974) 734–740.

90. Enker WE and Dragacevic S. Multiple carcinomas of the large bowel: a natural experiment in etiology and pathogenesis. *Ann. Surg.*, **187** (1978) 8–11.

91. Wood CB, Gillis CR, and Blumgart LH. A retrospective study of the natural history of patients with liver metastases from colorectal cancer. *Clin. Oncol.*, **2** (1976) 285–288.

92. Greenway B. Hepatic metastases from colorectal cancer: resection or not. *Br. J. Surg.*, **75** (1988) 513–519.

93. Ridge JA and Daly JM. Treatment of colorectal hepatic metastases. *Surg. Gynecol. Obstet.*, **161** (1985) 597–607.

94. Bengtsson G, Carlsson G, Hafstrom L, and Jonsson PE. Natural history of patients with untreated liver metastases from colorectal cancer. *Am. J. Surg.*, **141** (1981) 586–589.

95. Bengmark S and Hafstrom L. The natural history of primary and secondary malignant tumors of the liver. I. The prognosis for patients with hepatic metastases from colonic and rectal carcinoma by laparotomy. *Cancer*, **23** (1969) 198–202.

96. Scheele J, Stangl R, Altendorf-Hofmann A, and Gall FP. Indicators of prognosis after hepatic resection for colorectal secondaries. *Surgery*, **110** (1991) 13–29.

97. Taylor B, Langer B, Falk RE, and Ambus U. Role of resection in the management of metastases to the liver. *Can. J. Surg.*, **26** (1983) 215–217.

98. Adson MA. Resection of liver metastases—when is it worthwhile? *World J. Surg.*, **11** (1987) 511–520.

99. Cady B and Stone MD. The role of surgical resection of liver metastases in colorectal carcinoma. *Semin. Oncol.*, **18** (1991) 399–406.

100. Nava H, Carlsson G, Petrelli NJ, Herrera L, and Mittelman A. Follow-up colonoscopy in patients with colorectal adenomatous polyps. *Dis. Colon Rectum*, **30** (1987) 465–468.

101. Carlsson G, Petrelli NJ, Nava H, Herrera L, and Mittelman A. The value of colonoscopic surveillance after curative resection for colorectal cancer or synchronous adenomatous polyps. *Arch. Surg.*, **122** (1987) 1261–1263.

102. Evers BM, Mullins RJ, Matthews TH, Broghamer WL, and Polk HC Jr. Multiple adenocarcinomas of the colon and rectum. An analysis of incidences and current trends. *Dis. Colon Rectum*, **31** (1988) 518–522.

103. Reilly JC, Rusin LC, and Theuerkauf FJ Jr. Colonoscopy: its role in cancer of the colon and rectum. *Dis. Colon Rectum*, **25** (1982) 532–538.

104. Valk PE, Abella-Columna E, Haseman MK, et al. Whole-body PET imaging with [18F]fluorodeoxyglucose in management of recurrent colorectal cancer. *Arch. Surg.*, **134** (1999) 503–511; discussion 511–513.

105. Daly JM and DeCosse JJ. Complications in surgery of the colon and rectum. *Surg. Clin. North Am.*, **63** (1983) 1215–1231.

106. Thies E, Lange V, and Miersch WD. Peranal dilatation of a postsurgical colonic stenosis by means of a flexible endoscope. *Endoscopy*, **15** (1983) 327–328.

107. Mehigan D, Zuidema GD, and Cameron JL. The role of systemic antibiotics in operations upon the colon. *Surg. Gynecol. Obstet.*, **153** (1981) 573–576.

108. Contreary K, Nance FC, and Becker WF. Primary lymphoma of the gastrointestinal tract. *Ann. Surg.*, **191** (1980) 593–598.

109. Rao AR, Kagan AR, Potyk D, et al. Management of gastrointestinal lymphoma. *Am. J. Clin. Oncol.*, **7** (1984) 213–219.

110. Shepherd NA, Hall PA, Coates PJ, and Levison DA. Primary malignant lymphoma of the colon and rectum. A histopathological and immunohistochemical analysis of 45 cases with clinicopathological correlations. *Histopathology*, **12** (1988) 235–252.

111. Wychulis AR, Beahrs OH, and Woolner LB. Malignant lymphoma of the colon. A study of 69 cases. *Arch. Surg.*, **93** (1966) 215–225.

112. Auger MJ and Allan NC. Primary ileocecal lymphoma. A study of 22 patients. *Cancer*, **65** (1990) 358–361.

113. Naqvi MS, Burrows L, and Kark AE. Lymphoma of the gastrointestinal tract: prognostic guides based on 162 cases. *Ann. Surg.*, **170** (1969) 221–231.

114. Hwang WS, Yao JC, Cheng SS, and Tseng HH. Primary colorectal lymphoma in Taiwan. *Cancer*, **70** (1992) 575–580.

115. Blackledge G, Bush H, Dodge OG, and Crowther D. A study of gastro-intestinal lymphoma. *Clin. Oncol.*, **5** (1979) 209–219.

116. DeMatteo RP, Lewis JJ, Leung D, Mudan SS, Woodruff JM, and Brennan MF. Two hundred gastrointestinal stromal tumors: recurrence patterns and prognostic factors for survival. *Ann. Surg.*, **231** (2000) 51–58.

117. Akwari OE, Dozois RR, Weiland LH, and Beahrs OH. Leiomyosarcoma of the small and large bowel. *Cancer*, **42** (1978) 1375–1384.

118. McGrath PC, Neifeld JP, Lawrence W Jr, Kay S, Horsley JS 3rd, and Parker GA. Gastrointestinal sarcomas. Analysis of prognostic factors. *Ann. Surg.*, **206** (1987) 706–710.

119. Weisberg E and Griffin JD. Mechanism of resistance to the ABL tyrosine kinase inhibitor STI571 in BCR/ABL-transformed hematopoietic cell lines. *Blood*, **95** (2000) 3498–3505.

120. Ballantyne GH, Savoca PE, Flannery JT, Ahlman MH, and Modlin IM. Incidence and mortality of carcinoids of the colon. Data from the Connecticut Tumor Registry. *Cancer*, **69** (1992) 2400–2405.

121. Godwin JD 2nd. Carcinoid tumors. An analysis of 2,837 cases. *Cancer*, **36** (1975) 560–569.

122. Rosenberg JM and Welch JP. Carcinoid tumors of the colon. A study of 72 patients. *Am. J. Surg.*, **149** (1985) 775–779.

123. Staren ED, Gould VE, Warren WH, et al. Neuroendocrine carcinomas of the colon and rectum: a clinicopathologic evaluation. *Surgery*, **104** (1988) 1080–1089.

124. Greenberg RS, Baumgarten DA, Clark WS, Isacson P, and McKeen K. Prognostic factors for gastrointestinal and bronchopulmonary carcinoid tumors. *Cancer*, **60** (1987) 2476–2483.

125. Sauven P, Ridge JA, Quan SH, and Sigurdson ER. Anorectal carcinoid tumors. Is aggressive surgery warranted? [see comments]. *Ann. Surg.*, **211** (1990) 67–71.

126. Thompson GB, van Heerden JA, Martin JK Jr, Schutt AJ, Ilstrup DM, and Carney JA. Carcinoid tumors of the gastrointestinal tract: presentation, management, and prognosis. *Surgery*, **98** (1985) 1054–1063.

127. Lyss AP. Appendiceal malignancies. *Semin. Oncol.*, **15** (1988) 129–137.

128. Rutledge RH and Alexander JW. Primary appendiceal malignancies: rare but important [see comments]. *Surgery*, **111** (1992) 244–250.

129. Olney JR, Urdaneta LF, Al-Jurf AS, Jochimsen PR, and Shirazi SS. Carcinoid tumors of the gastrointestinal tract. *Am. Surg.*, **51** (1985) 37–41.

130. Andaker L, Lamke LO, and Smeds S. Follow-up of 102 patients operated on for gastrointestinal carcinoid. *Acta Chir. Scand.*, **151** (1985) 469–473.

131. Brookes VS, Waterhouse JA, and Powell DJ. Malignant lesions of the small intestine: a ten-year survey. *Br. J. Surg.*, **55** (1968) 405–410.

132. Moertel CG, Dockerty MB, and Judd ES. Carciniod tumors of the veriform appendix. *Cancer*, **21** (1968) 270–278.

16 Laparoscopy in Colorectal Cancer Management

Heidi Nelson and Bernardo Tisminezky

CONTENTS

1. INTRODUCTION

1.1. Historical Review

The successful removal of the gallbladder with minimally invasive surgery in the late 1980s and the demonstration of initial benefits of less morbidity and shorter recovery times with laparoscopic cholecystectomy *(1,2)* encouraged other surgeons to apply this new method in their field of expertise. In the case of colon and rectal surgery, the next logical step was the development laparoscopic bowel resection. The reasons for the initial use in colonic surgery were the avoidance of a long and often painful incision and a more rapid postoperative recovery. Aspiring to these goals, surgeons began performing laparoscopic colectomy as early as 1990. The first laparoscopic-assisted colonic resection was a right hemicolectomy, which was accomplished by Moises Jacobs in Miami, FL, in June 1990 *(3)*. Joseph Udo performed a laparoscopic colostomy closure on November 1990 *(4)*. The anastomosis was constructed with a circular stapling device. The introduction of laparoscopic intestinal staplers allowed intraperitoneal transection of the bowel. Using this instrument for ligation of the mesentery and transection of the colon, Dennis Fowler performed the first laparoscopic-assisted sigmoid resection in October 1990 *(5)*. Using a similar technique described by Fowler, Patrick Leahy performed the first laparoscopic-assisted low anterior resection for a proximal rectal cancer in November 1990 *(4)*. The first series of 20 patients who underwent laparoscopic-assisted colectomy was published in 1991 by Jacobs et al. *(3)*. The authors provided a detailed description of their technique. Although limited by the lack of

From: *Colorectal Cancer: Multimodality Management*
Edited by: L. Saltz © Humana Press Inc., Totowa, NJ

appropriate instruments, these surgeons were able to perform right and sigmoid colectomies. Other investigators were then stimulated to follow this accomplishment. Subsequently, the literature has been replete with reports of series of varying sizes, innovative techniques for virtually every colorectal operation, and the results, complications, and consequences associated with the new technology.

The application of minimally invasive techniques in the treatment of different intra-abdominal pathologies has lead to the evolution and progression of therapeutic laparoscopy surgical techniques into more complex operations. Currently, organs such as the bile duct, appendix, kidney, liver, lymph nodes, esophagus, stomach, and spleen have been successfully treated using laparoscopic techniques (6–12).

1.2. Oncological Issues Pertinent to the Application of Laparoscopic Surgery in Colorectal Cancer

Whether laparoscopic colectomy proves merely to be a new technology or to truly represent a singular advance in the management of patients with colorectal disease remains to be proven.

Several issues still concern the many of surgeons when laparoscopic techniques are used for the treatment of colorectal malignant disease. Controversies exist regarding the fulfillment of oncological surgical principles by this new method. The adequacy of intraperitoneal staging, extent of resection, and the problem of port site recurrences are three of the main issues that deserve discussion. Although visual inspection of the peritoneal cavity and both surfaces of the liver can clearly be achieved using laparoscopic inspection, the fact that organ palpation is not possible with minimally invasive surgery generates the concern of whether a complete intraperitoneal staging can be performed with this technology. Traditionally, palpation of peritoneal surfaces and of intra-abdominal organs has been a requirement for complete staging of colorectal cancer. Liver palpation allows the surgeon to detect deep hepatic parenchymal lesions; to compensate for this limitation, a preoperative computed tomography (CT) scan or abdominal ultrasound give useful information on abnormalities within the hepatic parenchyma and appear to complement laparoscopic visualization. It is likely that this combination will be as accurate as intraoperative bimanual palpation; however, this remains to be proven in controlled trials. New approaches such as laparoscopic ultrasonography have been tested in several studies (13,14), demonstrating that laparoscopic ultrasound probes can detect intrahepatic lesions with high accuracy rates. Laparoscopic ultrasonography staging, however, is not widely practiced and has yet to be proven in a controlled trial.

Other concerns have regarded whether the extent of resection is adequate with laparoscopic colectomy. A curative laparoscopic oncologic resection should include resection of suitable margins of normal bowel wall and excision of draining regional lymph nodes accompanying the major vascular pedicle of the involved bowel. Fortunately, current data suggest that the same bowel resection can be accomplished with laparoscopic surgery as with open surgery. A number of studies have demonstrated that the number of lymph nodes in a specimen resected laparoscopically is similar to that of a conventional open procedure (Table 1) (15–28). Because of the ease and reproducibility of counting lymph nodes in a resected specimen, it has become a factor by which surgeons measured the adequacy of an oncologic resection. However, more important than the actual number of nodes is the anatomical dissection. An appropriate oncologic resected specimen should contain not only paracolic nodes but also the deep central nodes. This anatomical dissection is accomplished when a high pedicle ligation is performed. Several clinical studies have shown that such an anatomical dissection is feasible with laparoscopic colectomy (29–31).

Table 1
Comparison of Lymph Node Harvest for LAC vs OS

Author, year	No. of lymph nodes	
	Laparoscopic	Open
Tate, 1993 *(15)*	10.0	13.0
Peters, 1993 *(16)*	9.0	8.5
Musser, 1994 *(17)*	10.6	7.9
Ota, 1994 *(18)*	8.8	18.8
Hoffman, 1994 *(19)*	8.0	6.1
Darzi, 1995 *(20)*	9.5	6.0
Lacy, 1995 *(21)*	12.7	12.8
Saba, 1995 *(22)*	6.0	10.0
Fine, 1995 *(23)*	9.0	10.0
Lord, 1996 *(24)*	7.8	8.9
Stage, 1997 *(25)*	7.0	8.0
Wu, 1997 *(26)*	13.0	—
Goh, 1997 *(27)*	20.0	19.0
Khalili, 1998 *(28)*	12.0	16.0

The greatest criticism of the laparoscopic approach in treating malignant colorectal disease has come from the issue of abdominal wall or port site recurrences. Despite all of the current discussion, this form of recurrence is not a totally new phenomena. In 1913, Dr. William Mayo reported a case of adenocarcinoma recurrence in a colostomy site proximal to the original tumor *(32)*. Similarly, in 1928, an abdominal wall recurrence was published after a colon resection when a Mikulicz procedure was performed *(33)*. The rate of incisional recurrence after open surgery for colorectal cancer varies from 7.6% *(34)* to 0.8% *(35)* to 0.6% *(36)*. Similar reports of trocar site recurrence after laparoscopic colectomies have been published. Although earlier articles suggested that the rate was anywhere between 2.5% and 21% *(37–39)*, more recent large studies have demonstrated that it is possible to reproducibly have a 0% implantation rate, or at least a rate of 1% or less (Table 2) *(28,30,37–45)*. However, the reported presence of viable exfoliated tumor cells in the abdominal cavity after laparoscopic colectomy *(46)* and the high incidence of trocar site recurrence in the earlier years of laparoscopic colectomy prompted concerns and recommendations that laparoscopic colectomy for colorectal cancer should preferably be performed only in the context of prospective randomized trials *(47)*.

Animal models and clinical trials have been used to try to understand the possible etiology for implantation of tumor cells into the trocar sites. It seems that the main cause of this problem is direct contact, direct inoculation from surgical instruments, or unprotected extraction of the surgical specimen, resulting in port site tissue trauma and implantation *(46,48)*. The role of pneumoperitoneum in tumor cells seeding appears to be secondary. Although many animal models have shown that a pneumoperitoneum increases the risk of incisional and port site recurrence *(49)*, this risk appears to be related to the size of the inoculum *(50)*, the number of manipulations required through each port site *(51)*, and port site leakage *(52)*. The single most important factor to avoid altered patterns of spread is surgical technique. The surgeon's contribution to the seeding of tumor cells is based on traumatic manipulation of the tumor, tumor perforation, replacement of trocars, and failure to use wound protection during extraction. The fact that wound implants are absent in newer

Table 2
Wound Implant Recurrence After LAC for Colon Cancer

Author, year	No./total	%	Stage of disease (Duke)	Interval to recurrence (months)	Location of recurrence
Guillou, 1993 (37)	1/57	1.8	C	3	Port site
Berends, 1994 (38)	3/14	21	B,C,D	NS	Paraumbilical (2) Port site
Ramos, 1994 (40)	3/208	1.5	C,C,C	6,8,21	Port site (2) Extration site
Lumley, 1996 (41)	1/103	0.9	D	NS	Port site
Boulez, 1996 (39)	3/117	2.5	B,C	NS	Port site (3)
Fleshman, 1996 (42)	4/372	1.1	D,C,B,A	NS	Midline incision Port site (2) Subcutaneous fat
Franklin, 1996 (30)	0/191	0			
Fielding, 1997 (43)	2/149	1.3	C,D	NS	Port site (2)
Bouvet, 1998 (44)	0/91	0			
Khalili, 1998 (28)	0/80	0			
Leung, 1999 (45)	1/179	0.5	D	NS	Port site

NS, not stated.

series suggest that once the learning curve is achieved, careful techniques with attention to detail in tumor manipulation minimizes the risk of port site recurrence.

2. DESCRIPTION OF PRACTICAL APPLICATION

2.1. Preoperative Management

In general, indications for laparoscopic surgery do not differ from those of laparotomy for colorectal malignancy; however, patient selection and tumor-related factors are critical variables for obtaining good results and benefits from this technology (Table 3).

Pulmonary and hemodynamic changes that may be caused by pneumoperitoneum (53–56) influence the selection of patients to be operated on with laparoscopic surgery. Patients suffering from heart disease with marginal cardiac reserve, major vascular disease, or severe respiratory pathologies have an absolute contraindication to this type of procedure.

Patient selection may be also be contraindicated if certain conditions are present, such as portal hypertension, coagulopathy, pregnancy, previous surgery with multiple incisions, or obese body habitus. Pregnancy has been considered a contraindication for laparoscopic surgery; however, a number of articles describing emergency laparoscopic cholecystectomy and appendectomy during pregnancy have been published (57,58). All reports have had successful results and all patients delivered full-term, healthy babies, with technical modifications including a direct technique to establish pneumoperitoneum, lower insufflation pressures (between 8 and 10 mm Hg), or access through a gasless approach, and cannulas placed higher than usual because of the enlarged uterus.

Patients who have had multiple prior laparotomies, especially if these procedures have been performed in the same region of planned surgery, may have significant intra-abdominal adhesions. The risk of perforation or incidental bowel insufflation during establishment of pneumoperitoneum is increased as a result of bowel adhesions to the anterior abdominal wall (59). Also, extensive adhesions increased the time of the procedure, as well the chance

Table 3
Contraindications

Absolute
    Patient-related
        Major cardiac disease
        Severe pulmonary disease
        Liver disease with portal hypertension
        Coagulopathy
        Pregnancy
        Tumor-related
        Tumor infiltration into adjacent structures (T4)
        Acute complications: Obstruction, perforation, and ileus
Relative
    Patient-related
        Morbid obesity
        Multiple previous abdominal surgeries
        Same site scars
        "Prohibitive adhesions"
    Tumor-related
        Large mass (>8–10 cm)
        Primary tumor with resectable liver metastasis
        Transverse colon cancer
        Carcinomatosis

of conversion because of the unclear anatomy and/or possible organ injuries sustained during dissection. However, laparoscopic enterolysis is feasible, making adhesions a relative contraindication.

Morbid obesity is probably the most common relative contraindication to laparoscopic colectomy. Major obstacles can arise with morbid obese patients, including proper and stable positioning on the operating table, adverse effects of steep positional changes, proper reach of laparoscopic instruments, and exposure of the viscera. Under these circumstances, the chance of converting a laparoscopic into an open surgery are high; the policy in our institution is to counsel obese patients on an increased risk of conversion and proceed with at least laparoscopic exploration.

Certain features of the colonic tumor, including size, location, stage, and presence of local complications may mitigate against laparoscopic resection. Neoplasms larger than 8 cm in diameter are often technically difficult to dissect laparoscopically, increasing the risk of bowel injury and intraperitoneal spillage of tumor cell. More importantly, removing a mass of this magnitude would require an incision larger than 6 cm; therefore, no cosmetic benefit will be obtained from the procedure. In this instance, a conventional laparotomy should be performed.

Lesions located in the transverse colon are more difficult to dissect because of omental attachments and the need to dissect two flexures. Tumors of the right, left, and sigmoid are generally amenable to the laparoscopic approach. Tumors 15 cm above the anal verge are readily resected with laparoscopic techniques; however, those located less than 15 cm from the anal verge are more challenging. The technical limit of a laparoscopic anterior resection is the distal anastomosis. Because of anatomical (narrow pelvis) and instrument (laparoscopic intestinal staplers) limitations, the stapled suture line is easiest when it is 10–12 cm from the anal verge. Therefore, the colonic lesion must be at least 14–15 cm or greater from the anal verge in order to achieve an adequate distal margin. Tumors less than 14 cm from the anal verge often require an assisted approach to place a stapler or clamp below the tumor.

Any tumor involving contiguous structures requires an en-bloc multivisceral resection. Whether en-bloc resection is truly feasible with laparoscopic techniques remains to be proven; therefore, T4 lesions should be operated with a conventional laparotomy. Other lesion factors that contraindicate a minimally invasive approach are acute tumor complications such as obstruction, ileus, and perforation with diffuse peritoneal contamination. An obstructing tumor resulting in dilated bowel increases the risk of perforation during pneumoperitoneum and port access. Further visualization of the abdominal cavity is reduced.

In laparoscopic colectomy, identification of the tumor site is often difficult. Marking the precise site of the pathology is essential to avoiding resection of the wrong bowel segment (60,61). Several methods have been described for identifying the lesion site. The topical injection of India ink or blue dye by preoperative colonoscopy is the most prevalent method to mark the tumor site; however, such a procedure has the risk of injecting the dye into the peritoneal cavity or causing fat necrosis (62,63). In addition, the injected marker may also spread so widely that the intended site margins may increase in size or the dye may diffuse into the retroperitoneal portion, making laparoscopic tumor localization difficult (64).

Intraoperative colonoscopy is another widely performed technique to locate lesions. Apart from requiring an experienced endoscopist and specific instruments in the operating room, intraoperative colonoscopy can pose problems resulting from bowel distention by air insufflated during the procedure, which may interfere with operative exposure. Clamping of the proximal bowel by the surgeon should avoid this complication.

An alternative approach consists of the use of mucosal clipping during preoperative colonoscopy. Several methods of exposing the clip-marked site have been described. Intraoperative fluoroscopy is one method used for identifying the clips, but this requires X-ray equipment and a technician in the operating room. Other techniques utilize intraoperative ultrasound (65) or a metallic detection probe (66) to localize the clips. Both methods seem to be accurate in localizing the clip-marked site; however, training and expensive equipment are required to successfully apply these two alternatives. A simpler approach is to take an X-ray during a diagnostic colonoscopy, with the tip of the endoscope adjacent to the tumor. The developed film can be used as a reference to locate the site to be excised.

Preparation of the patient for surgery is the same for laparoscopic as for standard colectomy. Bowel cleansing is performed the day before surgery. Prophylaxis against deep venous thrombosis and thrombophlebitis is provided by the application of pressure stockings and sequential compression devices (67). Systemic prophylactic antibiotics are administered at induction of anesthesia (68,69). To avoid the risk of injury of the stomach and bladder at surgery, a nasogastric tube and urinary catheter are inserted. Patients who are likely to need a temporary or permanent stoma are marked prior to surgery by a stoma therapist.

Once a patient has been selected for laparoscopic colon surgery, he or she must be counseled regarding potential risks, benefits, and the possible need for conversion to an open surgical procedure.

2.2. Intraoperative Procedure

The following items are the basic equipment needed to perform a laparoscopic colectomy (Fig. 1): (1) video imaging set including; a video-camera unit, the laparoscope, a light source, monitoring and recording devices, (2) the insufflator unit or abdominal-wall-elevating

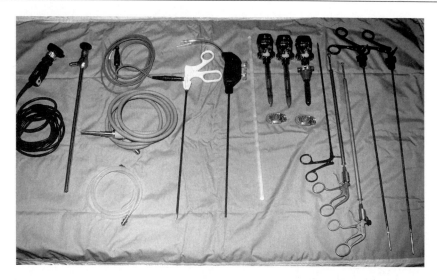

Fig. 1. Basic equipment and instruments used for laparoscopic colon surgery. From left to right: video-camera cord, 30° laparoscope, electrocautery cord, light cord, CO_2-insufflator tubing, dissecting scissors, suction and irrigating system, exchange rod, three 10- to 12-mm trocars with 5-mm adaptors, blunt dissectors, and Babcock and alligator clamps. When combined with a general laparoscopic pan, these instruments create a full complement of the required equipment. Reprinted with permission of Mosby and Mayo Foundation *(69a)*.

instrument, (3) suction and irrigating device, (4) hemostasis source, and (5) laparoscopic instruments. This last item should include not only the standard general laparoscopic surgery equipment but also instruments specific for colorectal surgery. Simple modifications in the general-surgery laparoscopic instrument pan should include reusable grasping instruments such as Babcock and alligator clamps. The instrument length should be at least 38–40 cm in order to reach the pelvis and abdominal cavity from any port site. Trocars and cannulas of 10 or 12 mm with stability threads plus adaptors for 5-mm instruments are preferable. To reduce costs, reusable instruments are used routinely. Disposable instruments are kept in the operating room and opened only as needed. All available instruments and equipment should be checked and calibrated for efficiency, with replacements immediately available in case of malfunction during the procedure.

The patient should be secured to the operating table such that multiple steep positions can be accomplished. Positioning of the patient depends on the anatomic position of the tumor and the location of the proposed anastomosis. The supine position for right and left hemicolectomies and modified lithotomy for sigmoid and abdominoperineal resection are preferred. The patient legs are fitted with pneumatic athrombotic stockings before placing them in Allen or Lloyd–Davies stirrups. Ankle straps or beanbags are used to secure the patient during steep table positioning. Once the patient is positioned on the operating room table, the cords from the video camera, light source, insufflator, and cautery should be placed in a convenient configuration, so as not to interfere with the operative field (Fig. 2).

The video monitor and patient's tumor should be placed in direct linear alignment with the surgeon's hands and eyes in order to avoid reverse images. To achieve this position, the surgeon and assistant are on the side opposite to the tumor, the monitor is on the side of the tumor, and the working ports are directly in between.

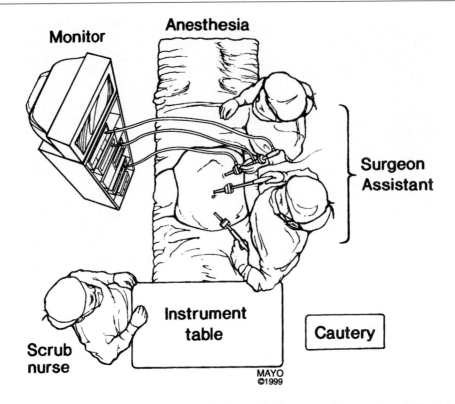

Fig. 2. Position of the equipment and the surgical team for laparoscopic resection of the right colon. With the patient supine, the monitor and the nurse are positioned on the same side and the surgeon and assistant on the side opposite of the pathology; this minimizes reverse-image problems. The cords are placed along the lateral aspects of the sterile field, so as not to interfere with the working field. Reprinted with permission of Mosby and Mayo Foundation *(69a)*.

3. RESECTION OF RIGHT COLON

The resection of the right colon starts by placing the first port in a supraumbilical site, if no previous midline incision exists (Fig. 3). In the case of a patient with a midline scar, the first port should be placed in the left upper quadrant, to avoid possible adhesions. Once the port is inserted with a Hasson technique, a pneumoperitoneum of 12–14 mm Hg is created by insufflating carbon dioxide into the abdominal cavity. The next two ports are positioned under direct vision: one in the suprapubic midline 8 cm caudad to the first trocar and the third cannula is inserted in the left upper quadrant below the rib cage in the mid-clavicular line.

Once all of the ports are positioned, the exploratory–early-conversion phase begins. Massive adhesions, small bowel fixed pelvis, extensive right upper or lower quadrant scarring, bulky or extended tumor or disseminated disease could compromise a laparoscopic colectomy, indicating an early conversion to an open procedure. Although a brief attempt at adhesiolysis is reasonable, prolonged attempts should be discouraged.

The next step involves mobilization of the cecum (Fig. 4). To facilitate the procedure, the operating room table is placed in Trendelenburg, with the right side inclined upward. This displaces the small bowel out of the operative field. The dissection is begun by cephalad and medial retraction of the ileocecal area. Countertraction of the ileocecal junction toward the left shoulder raises the cecum, achieving transperitoneal visualization of ureter and

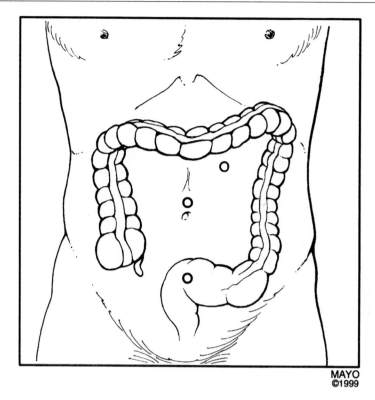

Fig. 3. Position of the cannulas for laparoscopic right hemicolectomy. Two cannulas are inserted in the midline, the first supraumbilical and the second a handbreadth or about 8 cm below the first trocar. A third cannula is inserted at the left upper quadrant below the rib cage in the mid-clavicular line. Reprinted with permission of Mosby and Mayo Foundation *(69a)*.

iliacs (Fig. 5). Dissection is then continued by grasping the cut edge of the peritoneum, not the bowel. The direction of excision starts around the base of the cecum toward the lateral peritoneal attachments (white line of Toldt) and ends at the hepatic flexure.

As dissection continues up the right pericolic gutter, the retraction on the edge of the colon is changed to a caudad and medial direction, and reverse Trendelenburg is instituted to better visualize the peritoneal attachments toward the hepatic flexure and duodenum (Fig. 6). As the hepatic flexure is approached, the hepatocolic ligament and small vessels in the gastrocolic ligament should be pinched closed with a grasper, cauterized twice, and then divided; as an alternative, vascular clips can be applied. In order to obtain adequate mobilization, the dissection of the transverse colon should extend as far as the right branch of the middle colic vessel. At this point in the dissection, the ileum, right colon, and hepatic flexure are usually extremely mobile and several choices are available for identification and control of the mesenteric vessels. Usually, an extracorporeal division of mesenteric vessels is performed. This allows for a quicker and easier identification and proximal ligation of the right colic and right branch of the middle colic vessels. However, in obese patients with significant mesenteric fat or thick abdominal wall that precludes adequate exteriorization, intracorporeal ligation is indicated (Fig. 7). The colon is elevated to expose the mesentery of the superior mesenteric, ileocolic, right colic, and middle colic vessels, all of which can be visualized. Applying moderate tension on the junction of the ileum and cecum readily displays the ileocolic vessels and facilitates intracorporeal ligation. Mesenteric windows are created within the avascular planes, and the vascular pedicle is then secured by using

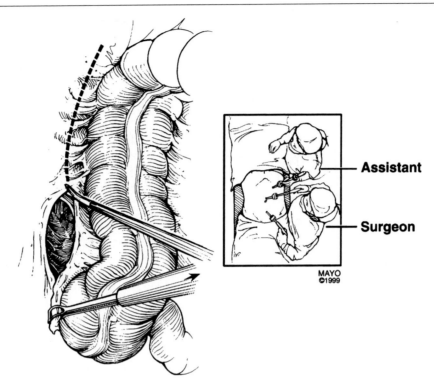

Fig. 4. Cecal dissection. The distal ileum and cecum are mobilized by using a grasping instrument and scissors, dissecting the path of the white line of Toldt. Note that traction is exerted on the peritoneal attachments, not on the bowel. As depicted in the inset, every attempt should be made to have the retracting instrument in the nondominant hand and the dissecting instrument in the dominant hand of the surgeon. Reprinted with permission of Mosby and Mayo Foundation *(69a)*.

hemoclips, endoloops, or a linear vascular stapler. Once the major vascular pedicle is ligated, the bowel should be fully mobile and ready for exteriorization.

The next technical step involves the exteriorization, resection, and anastomosis (Fig. 8). The incision at the supraumbilical port is extended vertically to 4–6 cm depending on the size of the patient and specimen. This incision is much smaller than a laparotomy and the evisceration of the pathological segment must be carefully done, to avoid injury of the tumor and to minimize the risk of spreading malignant cells to local and distant sites. A simple extension may be adequate to relieve the resistance and allow effortless removal of the segment. In addition, the wound must be protected with gauze or a plastic drape, to avoid direct contact of wound with the tumor. It is important to maintain mesenteric orientation at all times for proper creation to the anastomosis. As mentioned earlier, a proximal vascular ligation is carried out and the resection of the specimen is performed in a standard manner, respecting appropriate proximal and distal margins. Then, an anastomosis is performed according to the surgeon's preference, with proper mesenteric orientation. The mesenteric defect is closed if necessary. The bowel is returned to the peritoneal cavity. The wound and abdomen are irrigated, with further closure of the incision in two layers. The camera is then reinserted, insufflation is re-established, and irrigation of the peritoneal cavity is then performed with saline solution to wash and evaluate for residual hemorrhage. Once hemostasis is assured, the trocars are removed and the puncture sites are closed at the fascial level to prevent hernias. In many cases, this last step can be obviated by direct visualization

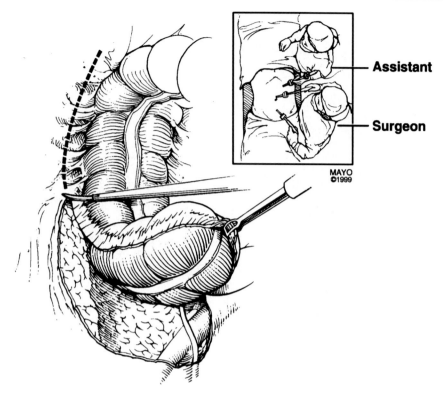

Fig. 5. Mobilization of the cecum. Countertraction of the ileocecal junction toward the left shoulder raises the cecum, achieving transperitoneal visualization of ureter and iliacs and facilitating retroperitoneal dissection. Reprinted with permission of Mosby and Mayo Foundation *(69a)*.

of the port sites after removal of the cannulas using a lift technique. If the procedure has gone smoothly, the surgical field has been dry (clean, nonbloody irrigant effluant) and all anatomic structures well visualized (such as ureter), then it is reasonable to inspect the port sites directly through the periumbilical wound using angled retractors to lift the abdominal wall. Suture closure of the 10/12-cannula sites can be accomplished from the peritoneal and skin sides.

4. RESECTION OF LEFT COLON

For left-sided pathology, the same technical principles applied for a right colectomy are performed but in a mirror image. The same five-step approach can be applied to the descending colon excision. The surgeon stands on the right side of the patient, aligned facing a monitor. The assistant (camera operator) stands on the same side as the surgeon in the more cephalad position, the scrub nurse stands on the patient's left side, at the foot, with the instruments on a Mayo stand over the foot of the operating table.

Typically, three trocars are used during the left-sided procedure. A supraumbilical cannula is inserted first for insufflation of the peritoneal cavity. After the exploratory phase is concluded as described earlier, the other two cannulas are placed as follows: One is inserted in the lower abdominal midline and the second one is introduced in the middle right upper quadrant, below the rib cage. Next, the patient is placed in a steep head-down positioning, and the table is rotated to the right, causing the small bowel to fall away from the left lower quadrant. The videolaparoscope is positioned at the umbilical port during most of

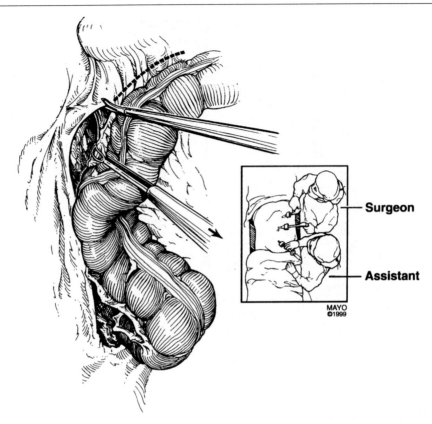

Fig. 6. Mobilization of the hepatic flexure. The ascending colon is retracted caudally using a Babcock or alligator clamp applied to the peritoneal attachment. The hepatocolic ligament is divided and hemostasis is obtained by electrocautery or clips. The hepatic flexure is approached by reversing the Trendelenburg as well as the surgeon, assistant, and camera positions. Reprinted with permission of Mosby and Mayo Foundation (69a).

the procedure but can be moved to the right upper quadrant port, if necessary, to improve exposure. The surgeon's assistant holds the videolaparoscope through the umbilical port while the surgeon operates using the other two port sites.

The descending-sigmoid junction is retracted cephalad-medially using atraumatic grasping forceps such as a Babcock or alligator clamp placed on the left lateral peritoneal reflection. The left colon is then mobilized along the white line of Toldt using cautery scissors dissection or the ultrasonic scalpel. As the dissection develops, the left ureter is identified crossing the iliac artery. Direct visualization of the left ureter to avoid its injury must be achieved at this point in the procedure. In addition, cautery should never be used in the vicinity of the ureter. If the ureter cannot be identified, the case should be converted to an open technique. The ureter is followed cephalad as the mobilization of the left colon continues toward the peritoneal reflection.

Once the splenic flexure is reached, the table is changed to the reverse Trendelenburg (head-up) position to improve exposure. The videolaparoscope is changed to the inferior midline port and the surgeon and assistant switch positions. In order to dissect the left transverse colon, the surgeon retracts the descending and transverse colon inferomedially by grasping the cephalad part of the splenic flexure. Traction on the splenic flexure exposes the attachments to the side wall, spleen, and stomach. Care must be taken to avoid pulling on the spleen and causing a capsular tear and hemorrhage. A linear stapler or harmonic

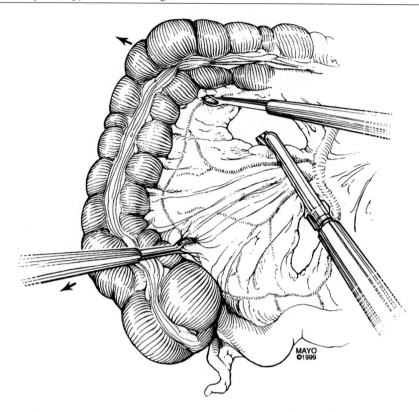

Fig. 7. Intracorporeal vascular ligation. Vascular pedicle ligation of the ileocolic and right colic arteries can be accomplished using a 30-mm linear stapler. The vascular structures should be swept free of critical retroperitoneal structures, such as the ureter, before they are ligated. Full cecal and hepatic flexure mobilization followed by intracorporeal vascular pedicle ligation facilitates the extracorporeal delivery of the right colon. Reprinted with permission of Mosby and Mayo Foundation *(69a)*.

scalpel are very helpful in completing the dissection at the ileocolic ligament. Applying a countertraction and upward force on the flexure toward the abdominal wall and toward the right hip creates an operative field that enables the surgeon to free the greater omentum from the transverse colon. The omentum is dissected free in the avascular plane using cautery scissors dissection, vascular clips, or the ultrasonic scalpel. The omentum should be taken with the colon if the tumor is in this location. In this case, the omentum is mobilized at the level planned for transection of the transverse colon.

After the splenic flexure has been dissected, the descending and left transverse colon is then reflected caudad and toward the right hip. The dissection continues on the posterior surface of the mesocolon, exposing the psoas and quadratus muscles as well the left ureter. In addition, the origin of the left colic artery can be exposed, and the inferior mesenteric artery can be identified and isolated. If needed, intracorporeal vessel ligation of the sigmoidal and left colic vascular pedicles can be accomplished using clips, endoloops, or a vascular linear stapler.

Exteriorization, resection, and anastomosis are performed as described for resection of the right colon.

5. RESECTION OF SIGMOID

Patient positioning for sigmoid colon resection includes placing the patient in a Lloyd–Davies position using Allen stirrups (Fig. 9). The angle between the thigh and the abdomen

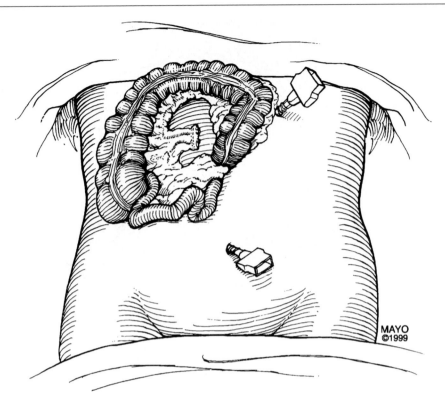

Fig. 8. Bowel exteriorization for resection and anastomosis. Once the bowel is fully mobilized, it is delivered out through a small (4–6 cm) incision made by enlarging the supraumbilical cannula site. A standard bowel resection and anastomosis (maintaining proper bowel orientation) is performed. Then, the bowel is returned to the abdominal cavity. If necessary, cannulas are left in place for one final laparoscopic inspection prior to completion. Reprinted with permission of Mosby and Mayo Foundation *(69a)*.

must be flat to minimize the likelihood of leg interference during instrument manipulation, especially from the lower ports. The left arm is positioned alongside the patient's flank. The surgeon stands on the right side of the patient; the camera operator and surgeon's assistant stand on the left side. The scrub nurse stands on the cephalad-left side, and the monitor is placed between the two legs of the patient.

Three to four ports are usually sufficient to complete a laparoscopic sigmoidectomy (Fig. 10). Two 10- to 12-mm cannulas located at the supraumbilical and right lower quadrant are the most reproducible sites. An additional third or fourth port can be placed in the left lower quadrant and/or inferior midline, depending on the planed location of exteriorization. If a transverse lower left quadrant incision is required, a third port on the left lower quadrant site is introduced. On the contrary, if a midline incision is planned, then a third port should be moved to the inferior lower midline site. The cannula location should be adjusted for each patient to maximize the ability to reach multiple fields and minimize cross-field interference.

Once a pneumoperitoneum is insufflated and feasibility of the procedure is explored, the operating table is placed in a steep Trendelenburg, right-side-down position, to displace the small bowel toward the right upper quadrant leaving the sigmoid mesentery exposed (Fig. 11). The cephalad assistant operates the laparoscope, and the caudad assistant, using a grasping instrument introduced through the lower quadrant cannula, grasps the pericolic mesentery and retracts it toward the right side of the patient. The surgeon raises the left peritoneal reflection and incises the peritoneal attachment with the use of scissors or cautery.

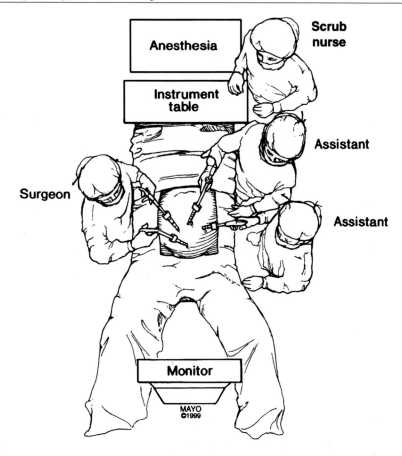

Fig. 9. Position of the equipment and the surgical team for laparoscopic resection of the sigmoid colon. With the patient in legs-up position, a monitor is placed between the legs. Two assistants and the nurse stand on the patient's left side and the surgeon stand on the patient's right side. Reprinted with permission of Mosby and Mayo Foundation *(69a).*

With this technique, the left gutter can be readily entered and the ureter and pelvic vessels can be identified. Conversion to an open surgical procedure is necessary if the ureter is not confidently identified. The incision is extended cephalad to the descending colon, following the line of Toldt and caudad to left side of the distal rectum. The dissection of the root of mesentery is extended toward the midline of the sacral promontory. Care should be taken to ensure that the ureter is swept down and away from the mesenteric structures so that it is not inadvertently injured during ligation of the vascular pedicle. With the sigmoid colon retracted to the left, the medial leaf of the mesosigmoid is incised at the root of the mesentery. A lifting traction on the medial mesenteric attachment at the sigmoid–rectum junction by an atraumatic grasper allows the dissection to continue cephalad. The dissection in the avascular plane is extended cephalad to the origin of the inferior mesenteric artery. The superior hemorrhoidal and sigmoid vessels are then visualized, as the sigmoid colon and proximal rectum are brought under tension.

Elevating the dissected colon exposes the mesenteric vessels; two incisions are made in the avascular planes on both sides of the vessels. The superior hemorrhoidal vessels and sigmoid arteries are isolated; vascular pedicle ligation at the level of aortic bifurcation is executed employing vascular staplers, clips, or endoloops (Fig. 12). After ligation is achieved, the

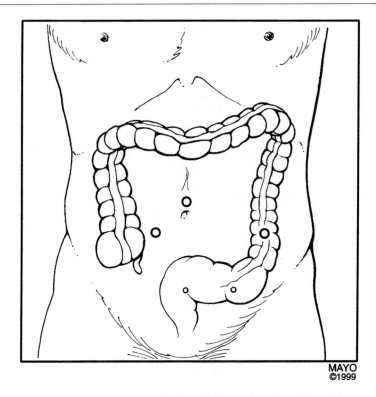

MAYO
©1999

Fig. 10. Position of the cannulas for laparoscopic sigmoid resection. Two 10- to 12-mm cannulas located at the supraumbilical and right lower quadrant are the most reproducible sites. An additional third or fourth port can be placed in the left lower quadrant and/or inferior midline, depending on the planned location of exteriorization. If a transverse lower left quadrant incision is required, a third port on the left lower quadrant site is introduced. On the contrary, if a midline incision is planned, then a third port should be moved to the inferior lower midline site. Cannula location and size (5 mm vs 10 mm) should be adjusted for each patient to maximize the ability to reach multiple fields and minimize cross-field interference. Reprinted with permission of Mosby and Mayo Foundation (69a).

sigmoid should become more mobile for anastomotic purposes. If necessary, the descending colon can be dissected further cephalad, including the splenic flexure.

Once the bowel is mobilized and the vascular pedicles are ligated, a plane at a level that allows an adequate safety margin is developed between the upper rectum and its mesorectum. With the sigmoid colon held up, the upper rectum is transected using an Endo GIA #30 fired once or twice or using the harmonic scalpel or clips. Next, the mesorectum can be transected similarly at the same level with an Endo GIA or dissected with cautery scissors (Fig. 13A,B).

The exteriorization phase of the procedure begins by extending the left lower port site incision to the estimated cross-sectional diameter of the tumor approx 6–8 cm (Fig. 14). The proximal bowel is then exteriorized and resected. The anvil of a circular stapler is secured within the bowel with a purse-string suture. The bowel with anvil is returned to the abdominal cavity and the wound closed and pneumoperitoneum reinsufflated. The shaft of the circular stapler is then introduced gently per anus, and once the mesentery of the proximal bowel is properly oriented with the distal rectum, both bowels ends are approximated and the stapler fired (Fig. 15). Next, the anastomosis is inspected by proctoscopy and leaks and hemostasis are checked. All cannulas are removed under direct visualization and the fascial defects and skin closed.

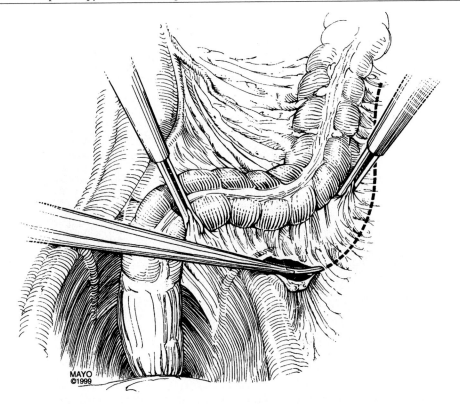

Fig. 11. Sigmoid dissection. The assistant's grasper and the surgeon's Babcock achieve a two-point traction on the sigmoid lateral peritoneal attachment. The surgeon utilizes a scissors to incise the peritoneal attachment. The dissection is continued cephalad following the white line of Toldt. Mobilizing the sigmoid colon should allow visualization of the left ureter. Reprinted with permission of Mosby and Mayo Foundation *(69a)*.

5.1. Operative Complications

Operative complications can be divided into intraoperative and postoperative categories. Because postoperative complications of laparoscopic right and left colon and sigmoidectomy are not unlike postoperative complications of their similar open procedures, only intraoperative complications will be discussed here (Table 4). Recognition and management of intraoperative laparoscopic complications are two essential factors to minimize serious postoperative morbidities. A surgeon should know what type of corrective measure must be taken and whether the complication can be treated laparoscopically or rapid conversion is necessary. The latter depends on the severity of the lesion and the surgeon's laparoscopic experience.

Intraoperative laparoscopic complications can occur at different stages of the procedure and, generally, they can be divided into patient positioning-related, Veress needle and trocar insertion-related, pneumoperitoneum-related, or colectomy technique-related complications.

Patient positioning on the operating table is critical to the success of laparoscopic procedures but has potential problems. The lithotomy position may cause femoral or peroneal neuropathy or contribute to an exarcebation of lower extremity ischemia. The Trendelenburg position may reduce pulmonary reserve, increase airway pressure, and cause gastroesophageal reflux. Careful patient positioning with padding of pressure points is imperative, as is securing the patient to the table. Sequential compression devices should be used to minimize the incidence of deep venous thrombosis.

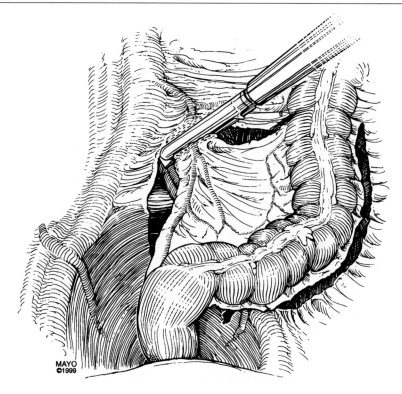

Fig. 12. Intracorporeal vascular ligation. Mesenteric windows are developed in an avascular plane and then vascular pedicle ligation at the level of aortic bifurcation is executed employing a vascular linear 30-mm stapler. After ligation, the sigmoid should become more mobile for anastomotic purposes. Reprinted with permission of Mosby and Mayo Foundation *(69a)*.

Veress needle and trocar insertions are relatively safe procedures, and although the incidence of reported injury is low, dangerous complications can occur. Several injuries have been reported during the blind insertion of these instruments, such as puncturing and/or perforation of intra-abdominal organs and vessels. Published series have reported major hemorrhage or large retroperitoneal hematomas occurring as a result of puncture of great vessels or solid organs, especially in thin patients. Damage to hollow organs resulting in superficial trauma, serosal tears, or perforation may happen. In order to reduce the risk of injury caused by blind insertion of the Veress needle and the first trocar, many surgeons prefer the open technique of Hasson *(70)*. This procedure enables the surgeon direct visualization of the peritoneal cavity; therefore, port placement has minimal risks of perforating or damaging an organ or vessel. The increased operative time for the cut-down technique is made up by the reduced time required for insufflation.

Pneumoperitoneum-related complications occur as a result of the physiologic or traumatic changes produced by an increase of intra-abdominal pressure, type and temperature of gas selected for insufflation, or insufflation of a misplaced Veress needle. Increased intra-abdominal pressure affects pulmonary mechanics, cardiopulmonary physiology, peripheral vascular resistance, as well as renal function *(54–56,71–73)*. Low-temperature CO_2 insufflation may cause hypercarbia, acidemia, and hypothermia *(74,75)*. Misplacement of the insufflating Veress needle can lead to subcutaneous emphysema or to a more rare complication but potentially lethal gas embolism *(76–78)*.

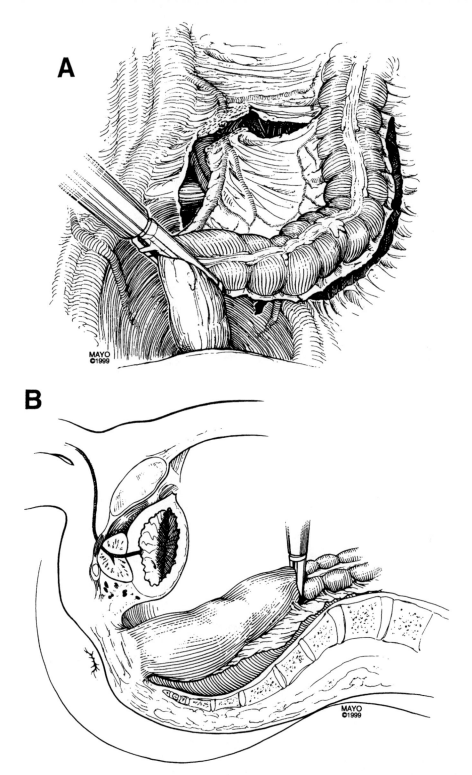

Fig. 13. Intracorporeal rectal transection. (**A**) After pedicle ligation, the sigmoid and proximal rectum becomes fully mobilized. Next, a linear stapler is positioned at the distal margin of the mobilized rectum and then fired to divide it. (**B**) A sagittal cross-section of the same procedure. Note that the mesorectum is separated from the rectum, prior to division. After the rectum is divided, the mesorectum is exposed, it can then be divided with another linear stapler or using the harmonic scalpel. Reprinted with permission of Mosby and Mayo Foundation *(69a)*.

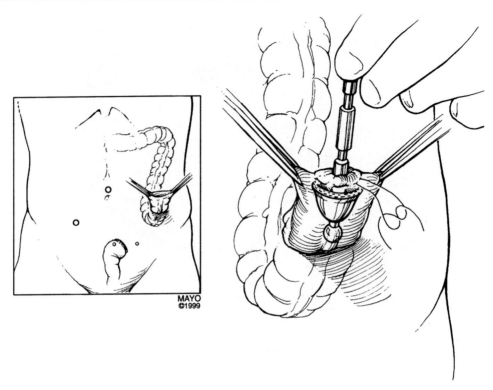

Fig. 14. Laparoscopic-assisted sigmoidectomy. The left inferior quadrant cannula site is extended into a 4-cm transverse incision (inset). The specimen is delivered extracorporeally and the proximal margin identified. The bowel is resected and a purse-string suture is placed in order to secure the anvil of a circular stapler. Next, the bowel is returned to abdominal cavity. The wound is closed to re-establish the pneumoperitoneum. Reprinted with permission of Mosby and Mayo Foundation *(69a)*.

Technique-related complications include bleeding and visceral injury. Bleeding can occur during a variety of maneuvers. During the division of the omentum, especially in the region of the splenic flexure the risk of bleeding is increased because of shearing of it. If the omentum is thickened and foreshortened in the splenic flexure, it may be wise to use the linear cutting stapler with vascular staples to transect the omentum. Significant bleeding may occur during dissection of the sigmoid mesentery. Most often, the vessel involved can be grasped and clipped, and hemostasis can be achieved. A surgeon should never apply clips or sutures blindly. If the surgeon is unable to stop the bleeding or is not able to get appropriate exposure, the decision to convert to an open procedure should be made.

Bowel trauma resulting from excessive traction can result in inadvertent enterotomy. This problem can be avoided by using atraumatic bowel graspers when feasible and retracting the colon by the peritoneal reflection edge. Depending on the degree of perforation, intraperitoneal contamination, and technical ability, the enterotomy or colotomy can be repaired intracorporeally by an assisted technique or, if necessary, by conversion to an open procedure.

Ureteral injury can be caused by inadvertent energy transfer from the electrocautery unit or the Harmonic Scalpel or from inclusion in the stapling device during transection of the mesenteric pedicle. This combination can be manifest by postoperative fever or ileus or excessive drainage from drains that is high in creatinine. Because delayed recognition of ureteral injury increases the rate of nephrectomy, immediate recognition is important.

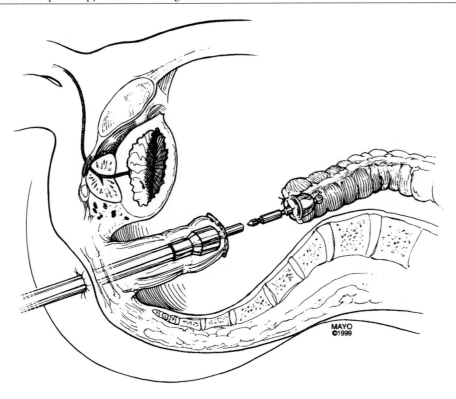

Fig. 15. Intracorporeal colorectal anastomosis. Sagittal cross-sectional view demonstrating the shaft of the stapler in the rectum (distal end) and the circular anvil in the descending colon. Both ends are connected, maintaining proper mesentery orientation, and the stapler is then fired. The donuts are inspected for integrity. Reprinted with permission of Mosby and Mayo Foundation *(69a)*.

Recognition of a ureteral injury usually mandates conversion to an open procedure for repair. Clearly, identifying the ureter during dissection and conversion to an open procedure if this is not possible can minimize the risk of this complication.

5.2. Postoperative Management

Postoperative management and treatment after laparoscopy colectomy is similar to that for open surgery. Early removal of the nasogastric tube and Foley catheter is practiced in the recovery room or the day following surgery. Ambulation is started as early as the day of surgery, with minimal discomfort. Dietary intake is rapidly offered with clear liquids on the day of surgery or as soon after surgery as the patient reports hunger. The diet is progressively advanced as tolerated. Antibiotic therapy is the same as for conventional colectomy. Patients are dismissed when food and orally administered analgesics can be tolerated, usually between 3 and 6 d postoperatively. Typically, patients undergoing right colectomy are ready for dismissal at 3 d, but sigmoid colectomy patients are often not dismissed until d 5.

6. REVIEW OF RESULTS

6.1. Learning Curve

The learning curve is most typically described within the context of operative times, rates of conversion, and rates of complications. Operative times are experience dependent. It can

Table 4
Intraoperative Laparoscopic Complications

Patient positioning-related
    Lower extremity ischemia
        Femoral neuropathy
        Peroneal neuropathy
        Decrease arterial and venous flow
        Pressure points
    Increase intraabdominal pressure
        Reduce pulmonary reserve
        Increase airway pressure
        Gastroesophageal reflux
Veress needle and trocar insertion-related
    Hemorrhage
        Puncture of major vessels
        Transection of abdominal wall vessels
        Injury of solid organs
    Hollow organ perforation
        Stomach
        Small and large bowel
        Bladder
Pneumoperitoneum-related
    Increase intraabdominal pressure
        Hypoxia
        Hypercarbia and acidemia
        Cardiac arrhythmias
        Decreased cardiac output
        Higher risk of DVT
    Type and temperature of gas selected
        Hypothermia
        Hypercarbia and acidemia
    Insufflation of misplaced veress needle
        Subcutaneous emphysema
        Bowel insufflation
        Gas embolism
Technique-related
    Hemorrhage
        Excessive traction of tissues
        Poor identification of vessels
    Organ injury
        Excessive direct traction of bowel
        Poor identification of ureter
        Cauterization inadvertent injuries
        Anastomosis of a rotated bowel

be assumed that early in the surgeon's experience, laparoscopic colectomies will require longer operative times. This has been well documented for laparoscopic-assisted colectomies (LACs). The average operative time was 189 min. Early-phase cases presented an average of 246 min vs 155 min for the late phases, with an average time reduction of 35% (Table 5) *(19,28,31,41,44,45,67,79–86)*. Small reductions in operative time may be accomplished within the first 11–15 cases *(82)*. Significant reductions require an experience between 35 and

Table 5
Operative Times (min): Laparoscopic-Assisted Colectomy (LAC) vs Open Surgery

Author, year	No. of patients	LAC Completed Early-cases	LAC Completed Late-cases	Average time	Time reduction(%)	Converted	Open
Senagore, 1993 (79)	38	–	–	174	–	204	126
Dean, 1994 (67)	122	–	–	129	–	114	–
Hoffman, 1994 (19)	80	258	185	–	28	244	183
Jansen, 1994 (80)	51	294	186	–	37	–	–
Van Ye, 1994 (81)	14	348	160	–	54	–	–
Simons, 1995 (82)	144	160	130	–	19	–	–
Wishner, 1995 (83)	150	250	140	–	44	–	–
Lumley, 1996 (41)	240	–	–	186	–	–	–
Wexner, 1996 (84)	140	–	–	168	–	–	–
Stitz, 1996 (85)	80	210	140	–	33	–	–
Agachan, 1996 (86)	175	201	141	–	30	–	–
Khalili, 1998 (28)	90	–	–	161	–	–	163
Milsom, 1998 (31)	55	–	–	200	–	–	125
Bouvet, 1998 (44)	53	–	–	240	–	270	150
Leung, 1999 (45)	201	–	–	203	–	–	–

70 cases (81,83,86,87). Once a breakpoint is reached, the surgeon's technical efficiency and proficiency are increased; therefore, the difference in operative times between open and laparoscopic surgery drops to a minimum (average of 4 min) during late phases of the learning curve (19,82,83,85,86).

The conversion rate is another form of measuring the learning curve. The trend for conversion rates is similar to the trend for operative times, as experience is gained conversion rates decrease (Table 6) (19,24,28,30,31,40,41,45,67,83–86,88,96). However, the more experience surgeons have with a new technique, the more they are likely to feel capable of completing more difficult and challenging cases; therefore, acceptable rates of conversion will prevail (91). Efforts have been made to predict risk factors for conversion. The only factor that significantly predicted a high rate of conversion in 75% of the cases was weight exceeding 90 kg (67). Schwandner and colleagues concluded that risk factors contributing to the possibility of conversion in LACs included male gender, ages between 55 and 64 yr, extreme body habitus, and inflammatory disease (96). Similarly, the location of the tumor will affect the degree of technical difficulty; therefore, the percentage of converted cases will vary depending on the type of resection. A multicenter study by the American Society of Colon and Rectal Surgery (ASCRS) had an overall conversion rate of 22.8%. Rectal cases had a conversion rate of 33.5%; right hemicolectomies presented only a 16% rate of conversion (87).

As the surgeon's experience with LAC has grown, intraoperative technical complications have become infrequent (61,67,86,91). Data have shown great variability on the number of cases required to achieve a plateau. As low as 20 cases (91) to a maximum of 100 cases (85), with an average of 40–50 cases (43,83,97), are needed to significantly reduce the rate of morbidities. Surgical experience and patient selection are the most critical factors by which a surgeon can prevent complications.

Table 6
LAC: Conversion Rates

Author, year	No. of patients	Early cases (%)	Late cases (%)	Overall converstion rate (%)
Ambroze, 1994 (88)	110	–	–	12
Dean, 1994 (67)	122	–	–	48
Mathis, 1994 (89)	359	–	–	14.8
Hoffman, 1994 (19)	80	30	15	23
Zucker, 1994 (90)	65	–	–	3
Senagore, 1995 (91)	60	20	10	–
Ortega, 1995 (92)	1027	–	–	24
Ramos, 1995 (40)	95	–	–	34.7
Wishner, 1995 (83)	150	30	20	23.3
Reissman, 1996 (93)	100	9	9	7
Agachan, 1996 (86)	167	–	–	22.7
Fleshman, 1996 (94)	372	–	–	15.6
Kwok, 1996 (95)	83	33	8.9	16.9
Lord, 1996 (24)	76	32	8	25
Wexner, 1996 (84)	140	–	–	11
Lumley, 1996 (41)	240	–	–	7.9
Franklin, 1996 (30)	192	–	–	4.1
Stitz, 1996 (85)	320	10	5	8.1
Khalili, 1998 (28)	80	–	–	7.5
Milsom, 1998 (31)	55	–	–	7.2
Leung, 1999 (45)	179	25.4	14.8	17.7
Schwandner, 1999 (96)	298	–	–	7.4

6.2. Morbidity and Mortality Rates

Published data suggest that morbidity and mortality rates are similar to those for open procedures (Table 7) (19,28,30,41,44,45,67,68,84,95,98,99). The specific contribution of laparoscopic procedures to morbidity is difficult to quantify. One study reported a 14% incidence of laparoscopic-related complications (61). A reduction in morbidity rates in the short term and long term for certain types of postoperative complication favoring patients treated with LAC have been reported. A matched control study of the elderly found a significant reduction in postoperative complications, from 30% in open controls to 14% in those undergoing laparoscopy (100). A diminished incidence in wound infection by up to 50% with LAC has been an unexpected finding but has been shown in several studies (30,41,101). In addition, decreased rates of reoperated surgery because of symptomatic adhesions after LAC has been published (97). Animal studies have demonstrated reduced risks of adhesions following laparoscopic surgery compared to open laparotomy (102). Similar results have been obtained in humans treated with minimally invasive surgery in the abdomen (103,104). In a randomized study of 40 patients, a second laparoscopy performed 3 mo after the primary procedure (laparoscopic vs open appendectomy) revealed the presence of significant adhesions in 80% of patients treated with laparotomy compared to only 10% in the laparoscopic group (104).

Table 7
Laparoscopic-Assisted Colectomy vs Open Surgery: Morbidity and Mortality Rates

	LAC			*Open*		
Author, year	*No. of patients*	*Morbidity (%)*	*Mortality (%)*	*No. of patients*	*Morbidity (%)*	*Mortality (%)*
Dean, 1994 *(67)*	122.0	11.0	0.0	–	–	–
Hoffman, 1994 *(19)*	80.0	23.0	0.0	–	–	–
Tucker, 1995 *(98)*	114.0	6.0	0.0	–	–	–
Kwok, 1996 *(95)*	83.0	12.0	0.0	–	–	–
Wexner, 1996 *(84)*	140.0	22.0	0.0	–	–	–
Lumley, 1996 *(41)*	221.0	7.2	1.6	280.0	7.9	–
Franklin, 1996 *(30)*	191.0	17.0	0.4	224.0	23.8	0.0
Bouvet, 1998 *(44)*	53.0	24.0	1.0	57.0	21.0	0.0
Khalili, 1998 *(28)*	80.0	19.0	1.2	90.0	22.0	0.0
Milsom, 1998 *(99)*	55.0	15.0	1.8	54.0	15.0	1.8
Psaila, 1998 *(68)*	25.0	4.0	4.0	29.0	6.0	6.0
Leung, 1999 *(45)*	201.0	13.8	1.7	–	–	–

6.3. Benefits

Several outcomes in different clinical trials have repeatedly demonstrated significant benefits achieved by LAC when compared to open surgery *(16,19,21,101,105)*. Short-term patient-related benefits are those that occur during the perioperative period. They include diminished incisional pain with reduced use of parenteral narcotics, a shorter period of postoperative ileus, and reduced length of hospital stay, as well as fewer wound infections. Another postoperative parameter that has been showed to benefit from LAC is the rapid recovery of immunologic defenses.

Minimal-sized incisions associated with laparoscopic procedures seem to result in diminished incisional pain and postoperative discomfort *(106)*. In order to verify this assumption, as a measure to quantify differences in pain tolerance between patients treated with open vs laparoscopic procedures many authors have used the number of doses or numbers of days with narcotic usage required during the postoperative period *(30,101,107–110)*. The majority showed a decrease in narcotic requirements by the laparoscopic group, although this was not universal. Of more significance is the report by Stage et al. *(25)*, who, using a visual analog scale, demonstrated a decrease in pain scores with LAC in a randomized control trial.

Another potential benefit that can be achieved from small incisions is the cosmesis factor. Such benefits may make laparoscopic colonic resection a favorite procedure in certain types of patient, especially the younger population. Obviously, this benefit can be considered of lesser importance. However, many patients view cosmesis as a vital consideration. The importance of cosmesis and self-image to quality of life in patients recently diagnosed with malignancy is intangible but should not be ignored.

Reduction in the period of ileus is perhaps the most important factor that allows for shorter length of stay (LOS). Lesser surgical trauma to the abdominal wall and to intra-abdominal organs during LAC is probably the main reason contributing to a shorter postoperative ileus.

Table 8
Comparison in Time to Return of Bowel Function (days) Between LAC vs Open Surgery

Author, year	No. of patients (LAC/OS)	Laparoscopic	Converted	Open	Indicators
Senagore, 1993 (79)	38/102	3	4.3	4.9	Oral intake
Peters, 1993 (16)	28/–	2.3	–	4.6	Flatus
Ambroze, 1994 (88)	110/–	3	–	–	Oral intake
Dean, 1994 (67)	122/–	2.3	4.8	–	Oral intake
Hoffman, 1994 (19)	80/53	2	3	4	Flatus
Bokey, 1996 (101)	28/33	4.5	–	4.4	Flatus
Milsom, 1998 (31)	54/53	3	–	4	Flatus
Khalili, 1998 (28)	80/90	3.9	–	4.9	Oral intake
Leung, 1999 (45)	179/–	4	–	–	Oral intake
Delgado, 1999 (111)	27/–	3	–	–	Oral intake

The reduction in size of incisions in addition to a decreased manipulation of the bowel results in less visceral and parietal edema. Consequently, less pain is felt by the patient, allowing for an earlier ambulation, passage of flatus, oral intake, and less narcotic consumption. The effect on ileus has been documented in terms of times to first bowel movement, times to flatus, or oral intake (Table 8) (16,19,28,31,45,67,79,88,101,111). The outcomes from these matched series benefit patients treated with LAC when compared to open cases. In general, a reduction of LOS has been repeatedly observed when studies comparing LAC and open surgery have been analyzed (Table 9) (17,19,24,28,30,31,44,68,79,81,101,112–114). However, most trial designs do not stand up to critical evaluation. Highly subjective parameters such as pain or tiredness can only be assessed objectively in comparative trials, when the patient is blinded as to the actual treatment received. If patients are aware of the access route, open or laparoscopically, their personal expectations are likely to influence the results of the trials. Animal models reproducibly demonstrate a shorter postoperative ileus for LAC compared with open surgery (102,115). To avoid psychological conditioning and anticipation bias, Reissmann and colleagues designed a prospective randomized trial of early diet after traditional open surgery to study the possibility that earlier feeding rather than laparoscopic surgery was responsible for reduced length of ileus (116). Patients in the early-feeding arm tolerated diet earlier than in the conventional arm, where diet was introduced after passage of flatus. The outcomes obtained challenged the belief that evidence of resolution of ileus was required before oral feeding could be tolerated, however, in spite of these results the hospital stay was not reduced.

In addition to lowering the LOS in those patients treated with LAC, the ability of patients to return more quickly to their daily activities after LAC has been assessed. A nonrandomized case-control-led study in the elderly found that in addition to a faster postoperative recovery, elderly patients treated with LAC preserved a greater postoperative independence. Ninety-five percent of those patients treated with LAC remained independent and were able to return to their homes instead of a nursing home after discharge, versus 76% of those patients treated with open surgery (117).

The effects and potential benefits of the immune response to surgical trauma during laparoscopic surgery have been studied, with conflicting results. Cell-mediated immune function, serum markers of physiologic stress, and tumor growth rates are the principal parameters of immune response studied. Potential benefits have been demonstrated to exist

Table 9
Analysis of Length of Hospital Stay (LOS) and Costs for LAC vs OS or Converted Colectomy

Author, year	No. of patients (laparoscopic/open)	Length of stay (days)			Costs (in US dollars)		
		Laparoscopic	Open	Converted	Laparoscopic	Open	Converted
Falk, 1993 (112)	34/–	5	8	8	12,500	13,000	15,000
Senagore, 1993 (79)	38/102	6	9.9	9.3	12,131	14,449	17,583
Van Ye, 1994 (81)	14/20	9.1	10.3	–	18,300	18,200	–
Musser, 1994 (17)	18/24	8.5	9.9	–	9811	11,207	–
Hoffman, 1994 (19)	80/53	5.2	7.8	6.5	12,464	10,213	13,956
Pfeifer, 1995 (113)	53/53	7.28	8.41	5.71	29,626	26,903	19,702
Bokey, 1995 (101)	28/33	12	12.2	–	9064[a]	7881[a]	–
Franklin, 1996 (30)	191/224	5.7	9.7	–	–	–	–
Liberman, 1996 (114)	14/14	–	–	–	11,500	13,400	–
Lord, 1996 (24)	55/30	5.3	8.6	8.2	–	–	–
Psaila, 1998 (68)	25/20	10.7	17.8	–	2900	3300	–
Milsom, 1998 (31)	55/54	6	7	–	–	–	–
Khalili, 1998 (28)	80/90	7.7	8.2	11.1	14,800	14,200	–
Bouvet, 1998 (44)	91/57	6	7	8	12,000	11,000	15,000

[a]Australian dollars.

in favor of minimally invasive surgery in some studies. The immune response experiments resulted in better preservation of delayed-type hypersensitivity, decreased level of interleukin 6 (IL-6, a serum marker of stress), and less tumor growth *(118–120)*. Other investigators have found that both laparoscopic colectomy and open surgery affect the immune response, with no advantage for either procedure *(121)*. Fukushima et al. concluded that stress responses for both operations resulted in same levels of IL-6 *(122)*. Therefore, the benefits of minimally invasive surgery with regard to the immune system and its consequences require further clarification *(100)*. In addition to the benefits already mentioned, HIV-positive patients could possibly benefit from LAC procedure. Some authors suggest that laparoscopic surgery is less likely to worsen the patient's already compromised immune system and that the surgical team theoretically benefits from better protection, with reduced risk of contamination from direct tissue manipulation *(123)*.

Long-term related benefits with minimally invasive techniques have been associated in nonrelated trials with a reduction in the incidence and extent of adhesions *(104,124)*. This has two potentially important implications: The incidence of small bowel obstruction may be reduced, as has been noted in some series *(30,43,61,100,101)* and additional abdominal procedures during reoperation may be made easier by decreasing intraoperative times and risks of complications.

6.4. Cost Issues

Despite a trend toward a reduced LOS, the overall cost of laparoscopic resections has historically been higher (Table 9) *(17,19,24,28,30,31,44,68,79,81,101,112–114)*. This has been related in part to both longer operative times and higher equipment costs, inflating the overall operative charges, not being balanced fully by savings postoperatively because of earlier discharge and reduced analgesic requirement. With experience, operating times become more closely approximate to those of open bowel surgery, reducing the costs. Further savings are expected as more reusable equipment becomes available. In the future, a faster recovery and potentially lower risks of both short- and long-term complications could offset some of the total health care cost of laparoscopic surgery *(125)*. In addition, the cost saving to the community at large of an earlier return to full preoperative activity and employment may considerably influence the economics of LAC. Future prospective randomized clinical trials will clarify some of these issues.

6.5. Prospective Randomized Trials

The majority of the literature on laparoscopic surgery for colorectal malignancy has been in the form of prospective nonrandomized trials with or without historical controls *(15,24,30,41,95,126,127)*. Most of these studies are composed of a small number of patients and are influenced by several types of bias. These kinds of analysis have insufficient statistical power to detect differences between LAC and open surgery regarding survival, safety, and cost-effectiveness. Large multi-institutional prospective randomized trials of sufficient size to detect small but clinically relevant differences in outcomes will be necessary to prove whether or not laparoscopic colectomy for cancer is safe and effective as an oncologic procedure and whether or not it offers real and significant benefits.

In order to test whether this new medical technology is superior to the standard open colectomy procedure, a randomized prospective trial comparing the two procedures is necessary. The primary goal of this randomized trial is to evaluate whether laparoscopic colectomy is equivalent to open colectomy in terms of disease-free and overall survival rates.

However, the long-term results relative to recurrence and survival will take a minimum of 8 yr of follow-up. As mentioned in the previous sections, LAC observes the basic surgical principles of a standard open colectomy performed for curable disease and we therefore feel that it is unlikely to compromise patient survival. If this proves to be true, then the choice between the two procedures will be determined by an assessment of their effects on secondary issues such as cost and quality of life.

A cost-effective analysis of laparoscopic colectomy is an essential part of evaluating this new surgical procedure. The cost-effective ratio is defined as improvement in survival (increased years) per extra dollars required to achieve this benefit. If laparoscopic colectomy results in equivalent survival rates and is less expensive than the standard approach, it would be considered the optimal procedure; however, if laparoscopic colectomy costs are equivalent to standard open colectomy and there are no differences in survival rates, then the effect of the new procedure on issues such as quality of life should be taken into account. Quality of life can be measured using parameters such as pain control, time to return to normal activity, and hospital length of stay. LAC is likely to improve all of these parameters. In addition, by attempting to lower operating-room costs by reducing operative time with gained experience and using more reusable instruments, the cost-effective ratio may well favor the laparoscopic procedure over the open conventional colectomy.

A US phase III trial comparing laparoscopic-assisted colectomy to open colectomy for cancer began in 1994 *(47)*. This multi-institutional trial proposes to study 1200 patients with colon cancer of the right, left, and sigmoid colon to undergo laparoscopic or open colectomy for curable colon cancer. Patients are stratified according to tumor site, primary surgeon, and ASA classification. In order to avoid the steep part of the learning curve, only surgeons that have performed at least 20 documented laparoscopic colorectal procedures are considered for participation in the trial. In addition, for quality assurance purposes, video documentation of certain key facets of the operation are being reviewed for credentialing and for auditing of the trial. This clinical trial will attempt to test if similar disease-free survival and overall survival rates are achieved. Also, aspects such as safety, including early and late morbidities and operative mortality will be compared and analyzed. Issues with regard to cost-effectiveness and quality of life will also be considered between both groups of patients. Preliminary results from the ongoing NIH-supported Laparoscopic Versus Open Colectomy for Cancer Trial *(100)* have been reported as of September 1998. Sixty-five surgeons representing 45 centers in the United States and Canada have accrued 530 patients *(128)*. Total bowel length, proximal and distal margins, mesenteric length, and number of lymph nodes harvest are similar between the two techniques and are consistent with the above-mentioned studies.

Numerous other national and international trials are underway. Some of these trials have varied the eligibility criteria from that of the NIH trial *(47)*. The increased number of prospective randomized trials around the world demonstrates the degree of enthusiasm for this new technological surgical approach and the fact that there is great interest in discovering the true potential of the procedure.

7. CONCLUDING REMARKS

In spite of the fact that early results of laparoscopic colectomy for cancer have repeatedly demonstrated this approach to be feasible, safe, and reasonable, the fate of this procedure rests on the analysis of the large multicenter prospective randomized trials currently under way, particularly with regard to oncological issues such as the long-term recurrence and survival rates. The success or failure of laparoscopic surgery in the treatment of colorectal malignancy will be decided by assessment of its oncological safety. It is likely that results will confirm the validity of the laparoscopic approach for colon cancer. Until such time as these data are available, however, it is recommended that patients undergoing laparoscopic colectomy for carcinoma be enrolled in prospective randomized trials.

REFERENCES

1. Cuschieri A, Berci G, and McSherry CK. Laparoscopic cholecystectomy [editorial]. *Am. J. Surg.*, **159(3)** (1990) 273.
2. Berci G and Sackier JM. The Los Angeles experience with laparoscopic cholecystectomy. *Am. J. Surg.*, **161(3)** (1991) 382–384.
3. Jacobs M, Verdeja JC, and Goldstein HS. Minimally invasive colon resection (laparoscopic colectomy). *Surg. Laparoscopy Endoscopy*, **1(3)** (1991) 144–150.
4. Sgambati SA and Ballantyne GH. History of minimally invasive colorectal surgery. In *Laparoscopic Colorectal Surgery*. Jager RM and Wexner SD (eds.), Churchill Livingstone, New York, 1996.
5. Fowler DL and White SA. Laparoscopy-assisted sigmoid resection. *Surg. Laparoscopy Endoscopy*, **1(3)** (1991) 183–188.
6. Huscher CG, Anastasi A, Crafa F, Recher A, and Lirici MM. Laparoscopic gastric resections. *Semin. Laparosc. Surg.*, **7(1)** (2000) 26–54.
7. Memon MA, Hassaballa H, and Memon MI. Laparoscopic common bile duct exploration: the past, the present, and the future. *Am. J. Surg.*, **179(4)** (2000) 309–315.
8. Ozmen MM, Zulfikaroglu B, Tanik A, and Kale IT. Laparoscopic versus open appendectomy: prospective randomized trial. *Surg. Laparoscopy Endoscopy Percutan. Tech.*, **9(3)** (1999) 187–189.
9. Rassweiler J, Fornara P, Weber M, Janetschek G, Fahlenkamp D, Henkel T, et al. Laparoscopic nephrectomy: the experience of the laparoscopy working group of the German Urologic Association [see comments]. *J. Urol.*, **160(1)** (1998) 18–21.
10. Janetschek G, Hobisch A, Peschel R, and Bartsch G. Laparoscopic retroperitoneal lymph node dissection. *Urology*, **55(1)** (2000) 136–140.
11. Luketich JD, Nguyen NT, Weigel T, Ferson P, Keenan R, and Schauer P. Minimally invasive approach to esophagectomy. *J. Soc. Laparoendosc. Surg.*, **2(3)** (1998) 243–247.
12. Donini A, Baccarani U, Terrosu G, Corno V, Ermacora A, Pasqualucci A, et al. Laparoscopic vs open splenectomy in the management of hematologic diseases. *Surg Endosc.*, **13(12)**, (1999) 1220–1225.
13. Foley EF, Kolecki RV, and Schirmer BD. The accuracy of laparoscopic ultrasound in the detection of colorectal cancer liver metastases. *Am. J. Surg.*, **176(3)** (1998) 262–264.
14. Marchesa P, Milsom JW, Hale JC, O'Malley CM, and Fazio VW. Intraoperative laparoscopic liver ultrasonography for staging of colorectal cancer. Initial experience. *Dis. Colon Rectum*, **39(10 Suppl.)** (1996) S73–S78.
15. Tate JJ, Kwok S, Dawson JW, Lau WY, and Li AK. Prospective comparison of laparoscopic and conventional anterior resection [see comments]. *Br. J. Surg.*, **80(11)** (1993) 1396–1398.
16. Peters WR and Bartels TL. Minimally invasive colectomy: are the potential benefits realized? *Dis. Colon Rectum*, **36(8)** (1993) 751–756.
17. Musser DJ, Boorse RC, Madera F, and Reed JF III. Laparoscopic colectomy: at what cost? *Surg. Laparoscopy Endoscopy*, **4(1)** (1994) 1–5.
18. Ota DM, Nelson H, and Weeks JC. Controversies regarding laparoscopic colectomy for malignant diseases. *Curr. Opin. Gen. Surg.*, (1994) 208–213.
19. Hoffman GC, Baker JW, Fitchett CW, and Vansant JH. Laparoscopic-assisted colectomy. Initial experience. *Ann. Surg.*, **219(6)** (1994) 732–740.
20. Darzi A, Lewis C, Menzies-Gow N, Guillou PJ, and Monson JR. Laparoscopic abdominoperineal excision of the rectum. *Surg. Endoscopy*, **9(4)** (1995) 414–417.
21. Lacy AM, Garcia-Valdecasas JC, Pique JM, Delgado S, Campo E, Bordas JM, et al. Short-term outcome analysis of a randomized study comparing laparoscopic vs open colectomy for colon cancer. *Surg. Endoscopy*, **9(10)** (1995) 1101–1105.
22. Saba AK, Kerlakian GM, Kasper GC, and Hearn AT. Laparoscopic assisted colectomies versus open colectomy. *J. Laparoendosc. Surg.*, **5(1)** (1995) 1–6.
23. Fine AP, Lanasa S, Gannon MP, Cline CW, and James R. Laparoscopic colon surgery: report of a series. *Am. Surg.*, **61(5)** (1995) 412–416.

24. Lord SA, Larach SW, Ferrara A, Williamson PR, Lago CP, and Lube MW. Laparoscopic resections for colorectal carcinoma. A three-year experience. *Dis. Colon Rectum*, **39(2)** (1996) 148–154.
25. Stage JG, Schulze S, Moller P, Overgaard H, Andersen M, Rebsdorf-Pedersen VB, et al. Prospective randomized study of laparoscopic versus open colonic resection for adenocarcinoma [see comments]. *Br. J. Surg.*, **84(3)** (1997) 391–396.
26. Wu JS, Birnbaum EH, and Fleshman JW. Early experience with laparoscopic abdominoperineal resection. *Surg. Endosc.*, **11(5)** (1997) 449–455.
27. Goh YC, Eu KW, and Seow-Choen F. Early postoperative results of a prospective series of laparoscopic vs. open anterior resections for rectosigmoid cancers. *Dis. Colon Rectum*, **40(7)** (1997) 776–780.
28. Khalili TM, Fleshner PR, Hiatt JR, Sokol TP, Manookian C, Tsushima G et al. Colorectal cancer: comparison of laparoscopic with open approaches. *Dis. Colon Rectum*, **41(7)** (1998) 832–838.
29. Moore JW, Bokey EL, Newland RC, and Chapuis PH. Lymphovascular clearance in laparoscopically assisted right hemicolectomy is similar to open surgery. *Aust. NZ J. Surg.*, **66(9)** (1996) 605–607.
30. Franklin ME Jr, Rosenthal D, Abrego-Medina D, Dorman JP, Glass JL, Norem R, et al. Prospective comparison of open vs. laparoscopic colon surgery for carcinoma. Five-year results. *Dis. Colon Rectum*, **39(10 Suppl.)** (1996) S35–S46.
31. Milsom JW and Kim SH. Laparoscopic versus open surgery for colorectal cancer. *World J. Surg.*, **21(7)** (1997) 702–705.
32. Mayo W. Grafting and traumatic dissemination of carcinoma in the course of operations for malignant diseases. *JAMA*, **60** (1913) 512–514.
33. Sistrunk W. The Mikulicz operation for resection of the colon: its advantages and dangers. *Ann. Surg.*, **88** (1928) 597–606.
34. Welch JP and Donaldson GA. The clinical correlation of an autopsy study of recurrent colorectal cancer. *Ann. Surg.*, **189(4)** (1979) 496–502.
35. Hughes ES, McDermott FT, Polglase AL, and Johnson WR. Tumor recurrence in the abdominal wall scar tissue after large-bowel cancer surgery. *Dis. Colon Rectum*, **26(9)** (1983) 571–572.
36. Reilly WT, Nelson H, Schroeder G, Wieand HS, Bolton J, and O'Connell MJ. Wound recurrence following conventional treatment of colorectal cancer. A rare but perhaps underestimated problem. *Dis. Colon Rectum*, **39(2)** (1996) 200–207.
37. Guillou PJ, Darzi A, and Monson JR. Experience with laparoscopic colorectal surgery for malignant disease. *Surg. Oncol.*, **2(Suppl. 1)** (1993) 43–49.
38. Berends FJ, Kazemier G, Bonjer HJ, and Lange JF. Subcutaneous metastases after laparoscopic colectomy [letter] [see comments]. *Lancet*, **344(8914)** (1994) 58.
39. Boulez J. Surgery of colorectal cancer by laparoscopic approach. *Ann. Chir.*, **50(3)** (1996) 219–230.
40. Ramos JM, Gupta S, Anthone GJ, Ortega AE, Simons AJ, and Beart RW Jr. Laparoscopy and colon cancer. Is the port site at risk? A preliminary report. *Arch. Surg.*, **129(9)** (1994) 897–899.
41. Lumley JW, Fielding GA, Rhodes M, Nathanson LK, Siu S, and Stitz RW. Laparoscopic-assisted colorectal surgery. Lessons learned from 240 consecutive patients. *Dis. Colon Rectum*, **39(2)** (1996) 155–159.
42. Fleshman JW, Fry RD, Birnbaum EH, and Kodner IJ. Laparoscopic-assisted and minilaparotomy approaches to colorectal diseases are similar in early outcome. *Dis. Colon Rectum*, **39(1)** (1996) 15–22.
43. Fielding GA, Lumley J, Nathanson L, Hewitt P, Rhodes M, and Stitz R. Laparoscopic colectomy. *Surg. Endoscopy*, **11(7)** (1997) 745–749.
44. Bouvet M, Mansfield PF, Skibber JM, Curley SA, Ellis LM, Giacco GG, et al. Clinical, pathologic, and economic parameters of laparoscopic colon resection for cancer. *Am. J. Surg.*, **176(6)** (1998) 554–558.
45. Leung KL, Meng WC, Lee JF, Thung KH, Lai PB, and Lau WY. Laparoscopic-assisted resection of right-sided colonic carcinoma: a case-control study. *J. Surg. Oncol.*, **71(2)** (1999) 97–100.
46. Mathew G, Watson DI, Ellis T, De Young N, Rofe AM, and Jamieson GG. The effect of laparoscopy on the movement of tumor cells and metastasis to surgical wounds. *Surg. Endoscopy*, **11(12)** (1997) 1163–1166.
47. Nelson H, Weeks JC, and Wieand HS. Proposed phase III trial comparing laparoscopic-assisted colectomy versus open colectomy for colon cancer. *J. Natl. Cancer Inst. Monogr.*, **(19)** (1995) 51–56.
48. Weiss EG and Wexner SD. Laparoscopic port site recurrences in oncologic surgery—a review. *Ann. Acad. Med. Singapore*, **25(5)** (1996) 694–698.
49. Jones DB, Guo LW, Reinhard MK, Soper NJ, Philpott GW, Connett J, et al. Impact of pneumoperitoneum on trocar site implantation of colon cancer in hamster model. *Dis. Colon Rectum*, **38(11)** (1995) 1182–1188.
50. Wu JS, Jones DB, Guo LW, Brasfield EB, Ruiz MB, Connett JM, et al. Effects of pneumoperitoneum on tumor implantation with decreasing tumor inoculum. *Dis. Colon Rectum*, **41(2)** (1998) 141–146.
51. Hewett PJ, Thomas WM, King G, and Eaton M. Intraperitoneal cell movement during abdominal carbon dioxide insufflation and laparoscopy. An in vivo model. *Dis. Colon Rectum*, **39(10 Suppl.)** (1996) S62–S66.

52. Allardyce RA, Morreau P and Bagshaw PF. Operative factors affecting tumor cell distribution following laparoscopic colectomy in a porcine model. *Dis. Colon Rectum*, **40(8)** (1997) 939–945.

53. Wittgen CM, Naunheim KS, Andrus CH, and Kaminski DL. Preoperative pulmonary function evaluation for laparoscopic cholecystectomy. *Arch. Surg.*, **128(8)** (1993) 880–885.

54. Johannsen G, Andersen M, and Juhl B. The effect of general anaesthesia on the haemodynamic events during laparoscopy with CO_2-insufflation. *Acta Anaesthesiol. Scand.*, **33(2)** (1989) 132–136.

55. Luz CM, Polarz H, Bohrer H, Hundt G, Dorsam J, and Martin E. Hemodynamic and respiratory effects of pneumoperitoneum and PEEP during laparoscopic pelvic lymphadenectomy in dogs. *Surg. Endoscopy*, **8(1)** (1994) 25–27.

56. Safran DB and Orlando R III. Physiologic effects of pneumoperitoneum. *Am. J. Surg.*, **167(2)** (1994) 281–286.

57. Sungler P, Heinerman PM, Steiner H, Waclawiczek HW, Holzinger J, Mayer F, et al. Laparoscopic cholecystectomy and interventional endoscopy for gallstone complications during pregnancy. *Surg. Endosc.*, **14(3)** (2000) 267–271.

58. Andreoli M, Servakov M, Meyers P, and Mann WJ Jr. Laparoscopic surgery during pregnancy. *J. Am. Assoc. Gynecol. Laparoscopy*, **6(2)** (1999) 229–233.

59. Reich H. Laparoscopic bowel injury. *Surg. Laparoscopy Endoscopy*, **2(1)** (1992) 74–78.

60. Wexner SD, Cohen SM, Ulrich A, and Reissman P. Laparoscopic colorectal surgery—are we being honest with our patients? *Dis. Colon Rectum*, **38(7)** (1995) 723–727.

61. Larach SW, Patankar SK, Ferrara A, Williamson PR, Perozo SE, and Lord AS. Complications of laparoscopic colorectal surgery. Analysis and comparison of early vs. latter experience. *Dis. Colon Rectum*, **40(5)** (1997) 592–596.

62. Park SI, Genta RS, Romeo DP, and Weesner RE. Colonic abscess and focal peritonitis secondary to india ink tattooing of the colon [see comments]. *Gastrointest. Endoscopy*, **37(1)** (1991) 68–71.

63. Coman E, Brandt LJ, Brenner S, Frank M, Sablay B, and Bennett B. Fat necrosis and inflammatory pseudotumor due to endoscopic tattooing of the colon with india ink [see comments]. *Gastrointest. Endoscopy*, **37(1)** (1991) 65–68.

64. Kim SH, Milsom JW, Church JM, Ludwig KA, Garcia-Ruiz A, Okuda J, et al. Perioperative tumor localization for laparoscopic colorectal surgery. *Surg. Endoscopy*, **11(10)** (1997) 1013–1016.

65. Montorsi M, Opocher E, Santambrogio R, Bianchi P, Faranda C, Arcidiacono P, et al. Original technique for small colorectal tumor localization during laparoscopic surgery. *Dis. Colon Rectum*, **42(6)** (1999) 819–822.

66. Ohdaira T, Konishi F, Nagai H, Kashiwagi H, Shito K, Togashi K, et al. Intraoperative localization of colorectal tumors in the early stages using a marking clip detector system. *Dis. Colon Rectum*, **42(10)** (1999) 1353–1355.

67. Dean PA, Beart RW Jr., Nelson H, Elftmann TD, and Schlinkert RT. Laparoscopic-assisted segmental colectomy: early Mayo Clinic experience. *Mayo Clin. Proc.*, **69(9)** (1994) 834–840.

68. Psaila J, Bulley SH, Ewings P, Sheffield JP, and Kennedy RH. Outcome following laparoscopic resection for colorectal cancer [see comments]. *Br. J. Surg.*, **85(5)** (1998) 662–664.

69. Lacy AM, Garcia-Valdecasas JC, Delgado S, Grande L, Fuster J, Tabet J, et al. Postoperative complications of laparoscopic-assisted colectomy. *Surg. Endoscopy*, **11(2)** (1997) 119–122.

69a. Tisminezky B and Nelson H. Laparoscopic approach to colon cancer, in *Advances in Surgery, vol. 34* (Cameron JL, Balch CM, and Langer B, eds.), Mosby, St. Louis, 2000, pp. 67–119.

70. Hasson HM. Window for open laparoscopy [letter]. *Am. J. Obstet. Gynecol.*, **137(7)** (1980) 869–870.

71. Caldwell CB and Ricotta JJ. Changes in visceral blood flow with elevated intraabdominal pressure. *J. Surg. Res.*, **43(1)** (1987) 14–20.

72. Breton G, Poulin E, Fortin C, Mamazza J, and Robert J. Clinical and hemodynamic evaluation of cholecystectomies performed under laparoscopy. *Ann. Chir.*, **45(9)** (1991) 783–790.

73. Wittgen CM, Andrus CH, Fitzgerald SD, Baudendistel LJ, Dahms TE, and Kaminski DL. Analysis of the hemodynamic and ventilatory effects of laparoscopic cholecystectomy. *Arch. Surg.*, **126(8)** (1991) 997–1000.

74. Kent RB III. Subcutaneous emphysema and hypercarbia following laparoscopic cholecystectomy. *Arch. Surg.*, **126(9)** (1991) 1154–1156.

75. Jacobs VR, Morrison JE Jr., Mettler L, Mundhenke C, and Jonat W. Measurement of CO(2) hypothermia during laparoscopy and pelviscopy: how cold it gets and how to prevent it. *J. Am. Assoc. Gynecol. Laparoscopy*, **6(3)** (1999) 289–295.

76. Derrien P, Lavenac G, Chaillou M, Lebois E, Milon D, and Mambrini A. Gas embolism during laparoscopy for cholecystectomy. *Cah. Anesthesiol.*, **44(3)** (1996) 215–218.

77. Beck DH and McQuillan PJ. Fatal carbon dioxide embolism and severe haemorrhage during laparoscopic salpingectomy. *Br. J. Anaesth.*, **72(2)** (1994) 243–245.

78. Cottin V, Delafosse B, and Viale JP. Gas embolism during laparoscopy: a report of seven cases in patients with previous abdominal surgical history. *Surg. Endoscopy*, **10(2)** (1996) 166–169.

79. Senagore AJ, Luchtefeld MA, Mackeigan JM, and Mazier WP. Open colectomy versus laparoscopic colectomy: are there differences? *Am. Surg.*, **59(8)** (1993) 549–553.

80. Jansen A. Laparoscopic-assisted colon resection. Evolution from an experimental technique to a standardized surgical procedure. *Ann. Chir. Gynaecol.*, **83(2)** (1994) 86–91.

81. Van Ye TM, Cattey RP, and Henry LG. Laparoscopically assisted colon resections compare favorably with open technique. *Surg. Laparoscopy Endoscopy*, **4(1)** (1994) 25–31.

82. Simons AJ, Anthone GJ, Ortega AE, Franklin M, Fleshman J, Geis WP, et al. Laparoscopic-assisted colectomy learning curve. *Dis. Colon Rectum*, **38(6)** (1995) 600–603.

83. Wishner JD, Baker JW Jr, Hoffman GC, Hubbard GW, Gould RJ, Wohlgemuth SD, et al. Laparoscopic-assisted colectomy. The learning curve. *Surg. Endoscopy*, **9(11)** (1995) 1179–1183.

84. Wexner SD, Reissman P, Pfeifer J, Bernstein M, and Geron N. Laparoscopic colorectal surgery: analysis of 140 cases. *Surg. Endoscopy*, **10(2)** (1996) 133–136.

85. Stitz RW and Lumley JW. Laparoscopic colorectal surgery—new advances and techniques. *Ann. Acad. Med. Singapore*, **25(5)** (1996) 653–656.

86. Agachan F, Joo JS, Weiss EG, and Wexner SD. Intraoperative laparoscopic complications. Are we getting better? *Dis. Colon Rectum*, **39(10 Suppl.)** (1996) S14–S19.

87. Bennett CL, Stryker SJ, Ferreira MR, Adams J, and Beart RW Jr. The learning curve for laparoscopic colorectal surgery. Preliminary results from a prospective analysis of 1194 laparoscopic-assisted colectomies [published erratum appears in *Arch. Surg.* (1997) **(7)** 781] [see comments]. *Arch. Surg.*, **132(1)** (1997) 41–44.

88. Ambroze WL Jr, Orangio GR, Armstrong D, Schertzer M, and Lucas G. Laparoscopic surgery for colorectal neoplasms. *Semin. Surg. Oncol.*, **10(6)** (1994) 398–403.

89. Mathis CR and MacFadyen BV Jr. Laparoscopic colorectal resection: a review of the current experience. *Int. Surg.*, **79(3)** (1994) 221–225.

90. Zucker KA, Pitcher DE, Martin DT, and Ford RS. Laparoscopic-assisted colon resection. *Surg. Endoscopy*, **8(1)** (1994) 12–17.

91. Senagore AJ, Luchtefeld MA, and Mackeigan JM. What is the learning curve for laparoscopic colectomy? *Am. Surg.*, **61(8)** (1995) 681–685.

92. Ortega AE, Beart RW Jr, Steele GD Jr, Winchester DP, and Greene FL. Laparoscopic Bowel Surgery Registry. Preliminary results. *Dis. Colon Rectum*, **38(7)** (1995) 681–685.

93. Reissman P, Cohen S, Weiss EG, and Wexner SD. Laparoscopic colorectal surgery: ascending the learning curve. *World J. Surg.*, **20(3)** (1996) 277–281.

94. Fleshman JW, Nelson H, Peters WR, Kim HC, Larach S, Boorse RR, et al. Early results of laparoscopic surgery for colorectal cancer. Retrospective analysis of 372 patients treated by Clinical Outcomes of Surgical Therapy (COST) Study Group. *Dis. Colon Rectum*, **39(10 Suppl.)** (1996) S53–S58.

95. Kwok SP, Lau WY, Carey PD, Kelly SB, Leung KL, and Li AK. Prospective evaluation of laparoscopic-assisted large bowel excision for cancer. *Ann. Surg.*, **223(2)** (1996) 170–176.

96. Schwandner O, Schiedeck TH, and Bruch H. The role of conversion in laparoscopic colorectal surgery: Do predictive factors exist? *Surg. Endoscopy*, **13(2)** (1999) 151–156.

97. Hoffman GC, Baker JW, Doxey JB, Hubbard GW, Ruffin WK, and Wishner JA. Minimally invasive surgery for colorectal cancer. Initial follow-up. *Ann. Surg.*, **223(6)** (1996) 790–796.

98. Tucker JG, Ambroze WL, Orangio GR, Duncan TD, Mason EM, and Lucas GW. Laparoscopically assisted bowel surgery. Analysis of 114 cases. *Surg. Endoscopy*, **9(3)** (1995) 297–300.

99. Milsom JW, Bohm B, Hammerhofer KA, Fazio V, Steiger E, and Elson P. A prospective, randomized trial comparing laparoscopic versus conventional techniques in colorectal cancer surgery: a preliminary report [see comments]. *J. Am. Coll. Surg.*, **187(1)** (1998) 46–54.

100. Stocchi L and Nelson H. Laparoscopic colectomy for colon cancer: trial update. *J. Surg. Oncol.*, **68(4)** (1998) 255–267.

101. Bokey EL, Moore JW, Chapuis PH, and Newland RC. Morbidity and mortality following laparoscopic-assisted right hemicolectomy for cancer. *Dis. Colon Rectum*, **39(10 Suppl.)** (1996) S24–S28.

102. Bessler M, Whelan RL, Halverson A, Allendorf JDF, Nowygrod R, and Treat MR. Controlled trial of laparoscopic-assisted vs open colon resection in a porcine model. *Surg. Endoscopy*, **10(7)** (1996) 732–735.

103. Jacobi CA, Krahenbuhl L, Blochle C, Bonjer HJ, and Gutt CN. Peritonitis and adhesions in laparoscopic surgery. First workshop on experimental laparoscopic surgery, Frankfurt 1997. *Surg. Endoscopy*, **12(8)** (1998) 1099–1101.

104. de Wilde RL. Goodbye to late bowel obstruction after appendicectomy [letter]. *Lancet*, **338(8773)** (1991) 1012.

105. Ramos JM, Beart RW Jr, Goes R, Ortega AE, and Schlinkert RT. Role of laparoscopy in colorectal surgery. A prospective evaluation of 200 cases [see comments]. *Dis. Colon Rectum*, **38(5)** (1995) 494–501.

106. Schwenk W, Bohm B, and Muller JM. Postoperative pain and fatigue after laparoscopic or conventional colorectal resections. A prospective randomized trial. *Surg. Endoscopy*, **12(9)** (1998) 1131–1136.

107. Young-Fadok TM, Smith CD, and Sarr MG. Laparoscopic minimal-access surgery: where are we now? Where are we going? *Gastroenterology*, **118(2 Suppl. 1)** (2000) S148–S165.

108. Bauer JJ, Harris MT, Grumbach NM, and Gorfine SR. Laparoscopic-assisted intestinal resection for Crohn's disease. *Dis. Colon Rectum*, **38(7)** (1995) 712–715.

109. Begos DG, Arsenault J, and Ballantyne GH. Laparoscopic colon and rectal surgery at a VA hospital. Analysis of the first 50 cases. *Surg. Endoscopy*, **10(11)** (1996) 1050–1056.

110. Plasencia G, Jacobs M, Verdeja JC, and Viamonte M III. Laparoscopic-assisted sigmoid colectomy and low anterior resection. *Dis. Colon Rectum*, **37(8)** (1994) 829–833.

111. Delgado GF, Garcia LA, Domingo dP, Grau CE, and Martin DJ. Laparoscopic reconstruction of intestinal continuity following Hartmann's procedure. Rev. Esp. Enferm. Dig., **90(7)** (1998) 499–502.

112. Falk PM, Beart RW Jr, Wexner SD, Thorson AG, Jagelman DG, Lavery IC, et al. Laparoscopic colectomy: a critical appraisal. *Dis. Colon Rectum*, **36(1)** (1993) 28–34.

113. Pfeifer J, Wexner SD, Reissman P, Bernstein M, Nogueras JJ, Singh S et al. Laparoscopic vs open colon surgery. Costs and outcome. *Surg. Endoscopy*, **9(12)** (1995) 1322–1326.

114. Liberman MA, Phillips EH, Carroll BJ, Fallas MJ, Rosenthal R, and Hiatt J. Cost-effective management of complicated choledocholithiasis: laparoscopic transcystic duct exploration or endoscopic sphincterotomy. *J. Am. Coll. Surg.*, **182(6)** (1996) 488–494.

115. Davies W, Kollmorgen CF, Tu QM, Donohue JH, Thompson GB, Nelson H, et al. Laparoscopic colectomy shortens postoperative ileus in a canine model. *Surgery*, **121(5)** (1997) 550–555.

116. Reissman P, Teoh TA, Cohen SM, Weiss EG, Nogueras JJ, and Wexner SD. Is early oral feeding safe after elective colorectal surgery? A prospective randomized trial. *Ann. Surg.*, **222(1)** (1995) 73–77.

117. Stocchi L, Nelson H, Young-Fadok TM, Larson DR, and Ilstrup DM. Safety and advantages of laparoscopic vs. open colectomy in the elderly: matched-control study. *Dis. Colon Rectum*, **43(3)** (2000) 326–332.

118. Allendorf JD, Bessler M, Whelan RL, Trokel M, Laird DA, Terry MB, et al. Postoperative immune function varies inversely with the degree of surgical trauma in a murine model. *Surg. Endoscopy*, **11(5)** (1997) 427–430.

119. Bessler M, Whelan RL, Halverson A, Treat MR, and Nowygrod R. Is immune function better preserved after laparoscopic versus open colon resection? *Surg. Endoscopy*, **8(8)** (1994) 881–883.

120. Bouvy ND, Marquet RL, Jeekel J, and Bonjer HJ. Laparoscopic surgery is associated with less tumour growth stimulation than conventional surgery: an experimental study [see comments]. *Br. J. Surg.*, **84(3)** (1997) 358–361.

121. Hewitt PM, Ip SM, Kwok SP, Somers SS, Li K, Leung KL, et al. Laparoscopic-assisted vs. open surgery for colorectal cancer: comparative study of immune effects. *Dis. Colon Rectum*, **41(7)** (1998) 901–909.

122. Fukushima R, Kawamura YJ, Saito H, Saito Y, Hashiguchi Y, Sawada T, et al. Interleukin-6 and stress hormone responses after uncomplicated gasless laparoscopic-assisted and open sigmoid colectomy. *Dis. Colon Rectum*, **39(10 Suppl.)** (1996) S29–S34.

123. Oliveira L, Reissman P, and Wexner SD. Can laparoscopic surgery improve the immune response to surgery in an HIV-positive patient? [letter]. *Surg. Endoscopy*, **10(7)** (1996) 779.

124. Reissman P, Teoh TA, Skinner K, Burns JW, and Wexner SD. Adhesion formation after laparoscopic anterior resection in a porcine model: a pilot study. *Surg Laparoscopy Endoscopy*, **6(2)** (1996) 136–139.

125. Ota DM. Laparoscopic colon resection for cancer—a favorable view. *Adv. Surg.*, **29** (1996) 141–153.

126. Kockerling F, Reymond MA, Schneider C, Wittekind C, Scheidbach H, Konradt J, et al. Prospective multicenter study of the quality of oncologic resections in patients undergoing laparoscopic colorectal surgery for cancer. The Laparoscopic Colorectal Surgery Study Group. *Dis. Colon Rectum*, **41(8)** (1998) 963–970.

127. Guillou PJ and Murchan PM. Laparoscopic colorectal surgery. *Eur. J. Gastroenterol. Hepatol.*, **9(8)** (1997) 766–772.

128. Young-Fadok TM. Minimally invasive techniques for colorectal cancer. *Surg. Oncol.*, **7(3–4)** (1998) 165–173.

17 Management of Cancer in a Polyp

David A. Rothenberger and Julio Garcia-Aguilar

CONTENTS

1. INTRODUCTION

As screening colonoscopy becomes more commonplace, the diagnosis of cancer in a polyp will undoubtedly be made more often. Thus, the subject matter of this chapter—the appropriate management of patients with such a lesion—will become increasingly important.

Management of cancer in a polyp is controversial for many reasons, including confusing terminology, conflicting and imprecise data, and the necessity to predict and balance the risks of residual or metastatic cancer after polypectomy with the morbidity, mortality, and effectiveness of more extensive treatment in each patient. For management of colon polyps with cancer, the alternative to polypectomy and observation is colectomy. For rectal polyps with cancer, appropriate management is more complex because diagnostic tests may provide more precise staging information that can be useful in decision-making. The natural history of distal rectal polyps with cancer may differ from that observed in colon polyps, and alternative therapies varying from local treatment to radical abdominoperineal resection are available.

The endoscopist who undertakes polypectomy must assume responsibility for accurate localization of the lesion and proper handling of the resected polyp specimen. The pathologist has the responsibility of thoroughly assessing and classifying cancer in a polyp and clearly communicating the interpretation to the clinician. The clinician-surgeon has the ultimate responsibility of reviewing and interpreting the available information and individualizing management and follow-up based on discussions with the patient.

From: *Colorectal Cancer: Multimodality Management*
Edited by: L. Saltz © Humana Press Inc., Totowa, NJ

2. DEFINITIONS

Nonstandardized terminology regarding malignancy in a polyp creates confusion, fosters miscommunication, and makes it difficult to compare the results of one series with those of another. As a consequence, patient care is often adversely impacted. Routine use of the TNM nomenclature would avoid much of the terminology confusion. Physicians should understand the definitions and implications of the following terms.

Cancer in a polyp is an imprecise term used variably to describe a broad spectrum of polypoid neoplasms ranging from a single tubular adenoma with a small focus of high-grade dysplasia, to an early, invasive adenocarcinoma arising in a tubular, tubulovillous, or villous adenoma, to a more advanced adenocarcinoma with only a small focus of residual benign adenomatous tissue.

Noninvasive adenocarcinoma. Colorectal adenocarcinomas are considered noninvasive when cancer cells are confined to the mucosa *(1)*. Because there is no lymphatic drainage of the lamina propria (the mucosal tissue superficial to the muscularis mucosa), there is no potential for recurrence or metastasis if such lesions are removed in their entirety. They are totally benign. Terms used synonymously to describe such lesions include high-grade dysplasia, severe dysplasia, carcinoma *in situ*, and intramucosal carcinoma. The latter two terms are easily misinterpreted and can result in overtreatment. Using the TNM system, such lesions are classified as $T_{is}N_xM_x$.

Invasive adenocarcinoma. A colorectal adenocarcinoma is considered invasive when cancer cells penetrate through the muscularis mucosa into the submucosa, thus gaining access to lymphovascular channels and acquiring the potential to recur locally or metastasize distantly *(1)*.

A malignant polyp is an adenoma that contains an invasive, so-called "early" adenocarcinoma in which the cancer extends directly from the mucosa through the muscularis mucosa into but not beyond the submucosa *(2)*. Using the TNM classification, these lesions are $T_1N_xM_x$.

A polypoid carcinoma is a descriptive term applied to an invasive adenocarcinoma with the gross morphology of a polyp but without residual adenoma on histology *(1)*.

Sessile vs pedunculated polyp. Macroscopically, polyps are described as sessile or pedunculated. This is an important distinction because the submucosa in a pedunculated polyp is found in the head, neck, and stalk, whereas in a sessile polyp, it is a flat continuation of the adjacent normal bowel *(3)* (*see* Fig. 1).

3. BACKGROUND

Adenomas are the most common neoplasms of the large bowel and are found in approx 60% of men and 40% of women by the age of 50 yr *(4)*. They are classified by histologic appearance as tubular (75%), tubulovillous (15%), or villous adenomas (10%) *(5)*. Although most adenocarcinomas of the colorectum begin as benign polyps, the majority of adenomas do not become malignant *(2,4)*.

Both the size of the adenoma and the proportion of the adenoma, which has villous histology, are correlated positively with the probability of cancer developing in a polyp *(1)*. In large colonoscopic polypectomy series, 1.5–12% of resected adenomas contain invasive adenocarcinoma *(2,4,6–10)*. This wide variance is dependent on the mix and size of polyps included in the analysis. O'Brien et al. *(9)* reported that 1.1% of adenomas less than 0.5 cm in diameter, 4.6% of adenomas 0.5–0.9 cm in diameter, and 20.6% of those ≥1.0 cm in diameter had high-grade dysplasia. A recent study of polyps removed endoscopically or by

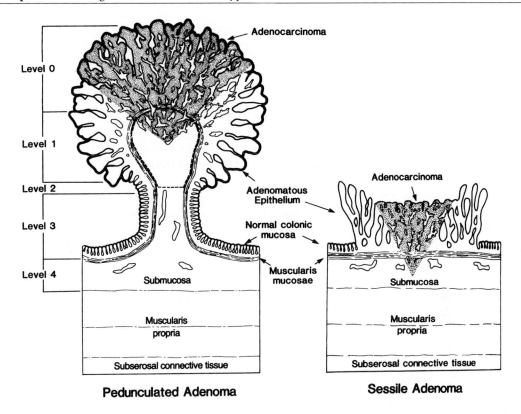

Fig. 1. Levels of invasion in a pedunculated adenoma (left) and a sessile adenoma (right). The stippled areas represent zones of carcinoma. Note that any invasion below the muscularis mucosae in a sessile lesion represents level-4 invasion (i.e., invasion into the submucosa of the bowel wall). In contrast, invasive carcinoma in a pedunculated adenoma (left) must traverse a considerable distance before it reaches the submucosa of the underlying bowel wall. The dotted line in the head of the pedunculated adenoma represents the zone of level-1 invasion. Although more pedunculated adenomas have a tubular pattern and most sessile adenomas are villous, exceptions to this generalization occur *(3)*. (Copyright 1985 by the American Gastroenterological Association; reprinted by permission of W.B. Saunders Company.)

surgery showed no cases of invasive cancer in 5027 adenomas less than 0.6 cm in diameter *(8)*. Other studies report the risk of invasive cancer arising in an adenoma is approx 0.1% for a polyp less than 0.6 cm in diameter, 1% for a polyp 1.0 cm in diameter, and as high as 40% in villous adenomas over 3.0 cm in diameter *(11–13)*. Fortunately, most polyps are identified and removed endoscopically when they are relatively small with little or no villous component. Thus, the National Polyp Study reported an incidence of cancer in 1.5% of polyps in patients undergoing polypectomy for the first time *(9)*.

4. ENDOSCOPY ASSESSMENT

When a colonoscopist identifies a polyp, its morphology, gross appearance, location, and likelihood of being safely and completely removed by endoscopic techniques must be determined to decide whether polypectomy is a reasonable initial treatment option. A second decision is then necessary to determine whether the polypectomy has provided optimal therapy. Because definitive treatment recommendations are based on histologic assessment of the polyp, the endoscopist should strive to provide the pathologist with a single, properly oriented specimen whenever possible.

Most polyps with a small focus of invasive cancer appear grossly identical to benign polyps and are safely snare-excised in a routine manner. At the opposite end of the spectrum, there are polypoid lesions that are obvious invasive cancers. Polypectomy for such lesions should be discouraged because it risks complications such as bleeding or perforation and rarely provides adequate treatment. In between these two extremes are polyps that should raise the suspicion of harboring invasive cancer but are potentially amenable to curative endoscopic resection. Polyps that are large, sessile, and/or villous in appearance or those with an irregular surface contour, ulceration, a "gritty" consistency, or firmness noted as the snare or biopsy forceps is pushed into the head of the polyp should be considered at high risk for invasive cancer.

Such high-risk-for-cancer polyps are optimally managed slightly differently from routine adenomas, especially if the lesion is in the rectum. For pedunculated polyps, the snare is placed closer to the bowel to provide an extra margin of stalk for pathology assessment because stalk margin is the most important parameter used to recommend further therapy. For broad-based colon polyps, the endoscopist must first determine whether the entire lesion can be removed safely. This often requires submucosal injection, piecemeal snare excision, and occasionally more than one endoscopic session. If the entire lesion cannot be safely resected, colectomy is indicated, except for high-operative-risk patients. If polypectomy is performed, the endoscopist should try to recover all of the fragments for histopathology evaluation. Because a short stalk may retract into the head of the polyp and because tissue tends to curl up in formalin, it is wise to identify the resection site of suspicious polyps by marking it with India ink or pinning the polyp through the resection site before placing the specimen in fixative.

It is especially critical to distinguish rectal from colonic polyps. In our experience, a disproportionate number of rectal polyps are sessile compared to colonic polyps. The rectum is accessible to diagnostic studies such as endorectal ultrasonography (ERUS) and to therapeutic interventions such as full-thickness excision or endocavitary radiation. If the gross morphology and size of a rectal polyp suggest the possibility of invasive cancer, it is best to defer polypectomy and perform a staging ERUS. The accuracy for identifying benign T_0 rectal lesions was 93% in our series (14). Depending on the size of the lesion and technical considerations, an ultrasound stage T_0 lesion can be managed by either endoscopic snare polypectomy or operative excision. If endoscopic snare polypectomy cannot remove a rectal lesion in a single specimen, operative excision is performed because it provides a better specimen for histopathology. Ultrasound stage T_2 lesions or any node-positive lesions are best not treated by local excision alone and are not the subject of this chapter (15).

Sessile ultrasound stage T_1 lesions are optimally managed by full-thickness operative excision by a traditional endoanal approach or by transanal endoscopic microsurgery rather than by endoscopic polypectomy. This provides the pathologist with a specimen that can be pinned out and oriented for fixation and accurate histologic assessment. This approach avoids the frustrating and not-uncommon scenario in which a well-intentioned endoscopist performs a piecemeal excision of a rectal polyp. The pieces cannot be oriented properly and, thus, a subsequent histologic finding of cancer creates a management dilemma. Often, it is impossible to determine whether the cancer is invasive or *in situ* and, if invasive, how deep it extends and whether it has been removed completely. It is impossible to predict the risk of residual cancer in the bowel wall or adjacent lymphatics. "To be safe," radical surgery may be undertaken often subjecting the patient to unnecessary morbidity and operative mortality. Conversely, if the radical resection option is proctectomy, there will be pressure to observe and follow such a patient. This may be inappropriate and unnecessarily subject the patient to development of an incurable cancer.

The localization of any suspicious polyp is critical to planning subsequent operative intervention should the histologic criteria be present to recommend radical surgery *(16)*. The endoscopist should use anatomic terms when describing a colon polyp's location (i.e., ascending colon near the ileocecal valve or left transverse colon near the splenic flexure) rather than using a centimeter level. Rectal polyps should be localized by the quadrant of the rectum involved and the level in centimeters from the anal verge. These parameters are most accurately measured by rigid proctoscopy. Flexible endoscopes can be partly coiled within the rectum, and if used to measure the level of a lesion, they can give erroneous and misleading information to the surgeon contemplating removal of a segment of bowel without an endoscopically visible or palpable lesion to guide the extent of resection. Similarly, it is important to remember that endoscope markings visualized at the edge of the buttocks during colonoscopy may be up to 10–20 cm or more from the anal verge. This is not an unimportant issue because the technical challenges and morbidity are much greater for a low anterior resection than for a rectosigmoid resection. Ideally, the site of any polyp thought likely to harbor malignancy should be marked at the time of polypectomy by endoscopic injection of either India ink, which is permanent, or by indocyanine green, which lasts up to 7 d *(11,17–20)*. If the finding of invasive cancer is a surprise on pathology assessment, the patient should be recalled promptly to measure and mark the site of the polypectomy ulcer before it heals and is impossible to localize. If the polypectomy site is localized in the rectum, staging ERUS is recommended. Although ERUS following endoscopic polypectomy of a T_1 rectal lesion cannot reliably distinguish cautery artifact from residual tumor in the rectal wall, it may identify metastatic lymph nodes in the perirectal tissue. Such a finding would usually argue for radical treatment. In the absence of ultrasound-identified lymph node metastasis, it is probably best to perform a full-thickness transanal excision of the polypectomy site, especially if the histologic margin was doubtful. Histologic review will determine the completeness of the excision and provide information necessary to make definitive treatment recommendations.

5. PATHOLOGY ASSESSMENT

Following polypectomy, histologic assessment of the resected lesion is performed to predict the stage and prognosis of cancer arising in a polyp. The estimated probability of residual tumor in the bowel wall or regional lymph nodes is the basis for recommending definitive treatment and subsequent surveillance.

Haggitt et al. *(3)* classified cancers arising in polyps based on their level of invasiveness (Fig. 1). A noninvasive carcinoma confined to the mucosa is Level 0, whereas invasive carcinomas invading into the head, neck, and stalk of a pedunculated polyp are Levels 1, 2, and 3, respectively. Haggitt Level 4 defines a cancer invading into submucosa at the base of the stalk of a pedunculated polyp or in any sessile polyp. If invasion is into the muscularis propria, the cancer is T_2, and the Haggitt classification does not apply. Haggitt et al. reported the level of invasiveness for T_1 colorectal cancers correlated with the incidence of metastasis to regional lymph nodes *(3)*. Level-0 lesions are benign and the incidence of metastasis is 0% after complete removal of such polyps. The incidence of residual cancer in the bowel wall or regional lymph nodes or the risk of recurrent or metastatic disease on long-term follow-up after polypectomy has been reported to be 0.7% for Level 1, 5% for Level 2,

12.9% for Level 3, and 15–25% for Level 4 *(3,21–23)*. Thus, the Haggitt classification was thought to be useful in predicting prognosis and of great value in decision-making regarding the necessity of colectomy.

Additional histologic risk factors have been described and are thought by some authors to be more reliable predictors of greater risk of residual malignancy or metastatic disease than depth of invasiveness *(1)*. These factors include tumor within 2 mm of the resection line, unfavorable histology (poorly differentiated, signet-ring or mucinous adenocarcinoma), and lymphatic or venous invasion.

Intuitively, it would seem that cancer at or near the margin of polyp resection would result in recurrence. However, the definition of an adequate margin is controversial. Cooper et al. *(24,25)* reported that there were no local recurrences of cancer if the tumor-free margin was 3 mm or more, but if the tumor was at or near (2 mm) the margin, there was a local recurrence in 18.3% and lymph node metastasis in 11.5%. Morson et al. *(26)* reviewed the experience with snare polypectomy of malignant polyps at St. Mark's Hospital, London, England. They classified histologic local clearance as complete, doubtful, or incomplete. On the basis of the assessment, 14 of 60 patients underwent surgical resection, but residual tumor was only found in 2 patients, 1 of whom died of metastatic disease and 1 of whom survived long term. No recurrent cancer developed in the 46 patients treated by polypectomy only. Thus, the cancer-specific death rate was only 1.7%. Morson et al. *(26)* speculated that cases in which the excision was doubtfully complete were, in fact, complete, as a result of the use of diathermy, which destroyed tissue at the margin of excision during polypectomy.

Poorly differentiated histology and lymphatic or vascular invasion have been reported to predict a high rate of residual tumor and/or local lymph node metasasis *(1,27)*. Cooper et al. *(25)* used the histopathologic criteria of lymphatic or venous invasion and an incomplete margin of clearance as criteria to predict failure in 140 patients who had undergone removal of a polyp with invasive cancer. Cancer-specific failure occurred in 14 of 71 patients (20%) with such criteria; in 2 of 23 patients (9%) when the assessment was uncertain, and in none of 46 patients when these factors were not present. A resection margin of <1 mm correlated with treatment failure.

Volk et al. *(28)* reported no treatment failures in 16 of 47 patients with malignant adenoma if the resection margin was ≥2 mm and the tumor was not poorly differentiated. In contrast, 10 of 30 patients with poorly differentiated cancer experienced tumor recurrence after local excision.

A Mayo Clinic study of 151 patients who underwent resection for cancer in a polyp found a 0% incidence of lymph node metastasis in Haggitt Level-1, -2, and -3 polyps in the absence of other histologic risk factors *(29)*. This raised doubt as to the necessity of distinguishing four levels of invasiveness because only tumors invading the submucosa at the base of the polyp, whether pedunculated or sessile (Haggitt Level 4), were those with positive lymph nodes, which could potentially benefit from radical bowel resection. Indeed, Haggitt et al. *(3)* reported that Level-4 invasion was present in 7 of 8 adverse outcomes in their series of 64 malignant polyps. Although the presence of unfavorable histologic features is associated with an increased risk of lymph node metastasis in early colorectal cancers, it remains unclear whether these histologic features have a variable or uniform influence at each level of invasiveness in the Haggitt classification. Despite this, almost all articles now agree that the most reliable predictor of risk of residual or metastatic carcinoma other than a positive margin after polypectomy is Haggitt Level-4 submucosal invasion. The overall risk of regional lymph node metastasis is approx 10% when Haggitt Level-4 submucosal invasion has occurred *(7)*. The presence of one or more histologic risk factors plus Haggitt Level-4 submucosal invasion increases the incidence of residual malignancy after polypectomy to as high as 25% *(29,30)*.

Whereas Haggitt Level-4 submucosal invasion is clearly important in predicting prognosis, one must remember that 75–90% of cases with such invasion do *not* have regional lymph node metastasis. Thus, a more precise staging system to predict adverse outcomes would clearly be of value, especially for high-operative-risk patients or for those with distal rectal polyps, for which the radical surgery option would be proctectomy. Thus, it is not surprising that a new classification system based on the extent of submucosal invasion has been developed to assess T_1 cancers *(31,32)*. Invasive lesions extending through the muscularis mucosa into the submucosa but not into the muscularis propria were classified as follows:

Sm_1: slight submucosal invasion (upper third)
Sm_2: intermediate submucosal invasion (middle third)
Sm_3: invasion near the muscularis propria (lower third)

Using this classification scheme, Haggitt Level-1, -2, and -3 polyps would all be Sm_1 lesions, and Haggitt Level-4 polyps, whether sessile or pedunculated, could be Sm_1, Sm_2, or Sm_3 depending on the depth of submucosal invasion. A recent series from Japan showed that for 182 Haggitt Level-4 lesions classified as Sm_1 ($n = 64$), Sm_2 ($n = 82$), or Sm_3 ($n = 36$), local recurrence developed in 0, 4 (5%), and 0 patients, respectively, and lymph node metastasis developed in 0, 4 (5%), and 9 (25%) patients, respectively *(31)*. Although lymphovascular invasion was present in 30% of Sm_1 polyps and 12.5% were poorly differentiated, none of the 64 patients with Sm_1 tumors developed a local recurrence or lymph node metastasis. The authors concluded that postpolypectomy assessment of submucosal level of invasion could decrease the incidence of unnecessary surgery for Sm_1 and possibly Sm_2 lesions. Additionally, they concluded that lymphovascular invasion, histologic grade, and diameter were not risk factors.

Nivatvongs and colleagues used this classification to reclassify 344 T_1 sessile colorectal lesions in patients who underwent colorectal radical resections at the Mayo Clinic *(30)*. There were 70 Sm_1 lesions, 120 Sm_2 lesions, and 154 Sm_3 lesions. A multivariate analysis showed that there were three independent risk factors predictive of lymph node metastasis in T_1 colorectal cancers: (1) level Sm_3 invasion, (2) lymphovascular invasion, and (3) origin in the distal third of the rectum. The latter factor, if confirmed by others, has significant implications for therapy because it is precisely for such distal-third rectal lesions that conservative alternatives to radical resection, usually requiring proctectomy and colostomy, are sought by patients and surgeons alike. This series from the Mayo Clinic has a significant selection bias because these lesions were judged not to be amenable to local therapy.

6. DEFINITIVE TREATMENT

The clinician-surgeon has the ultimate responsibility of deciding whether polypectomy alone is adequate treatment or whether radical resection is necessary. One must balance the risk of residual cancer at the excision site, in regional nodes, or in distant sites such as liver or lungs with the morbidity and mortality of alternative treatment (usually radical surgery) and the effectiveness of that treatment.

The first obligation is to accurately understand the facts of each case. Following complete polypectomy, only the T stage of the lesion can be accurately defined and the N stage and

M stage can only be inferred. If the surgeon was not the colonoscopist, a careful review of the colonoscopy notes and discussion with the endoscopist is a first step. How confident is the endoscopist that the entire polyp has been removed? Was a residual stalk left *in situ*? How did the endoscopist localize the lesion and how confident is he that the localization is accurate?

The next step is to personally review the histology slides with a competent gastrointestinal pathologist. It is not uncommon that this step has resulted in a revision of the initial pathology report or altered the clinician's understanding of the pathology report in a way that completely changes the choice of definitive therapy. The surgeon must understand the depth of invasion of cancer, the margin of resection, and the presence of other histologic risk factors such as lymphovascular involvement or other unfavorable features. By direct review of the histology, the surgeon quickly learns how large the focus of cancer is and whether there are problems with accurate interpretation of the specimen. Often, polyps are oriented and cut in such a way that accurate assessment is impossible. The importance of this personal review with a gastrointestinal pathologist cannot be overemphasized.

Based on the clinical and pathological information, the surgeon can make a recommendation regarding definitive treatment. If additional therapy is being considered, the surgeon must assess the patient's operative risks. Today, mortality for normal-risk individuals should be less than 1% following colectomy and less than 2–3% following proctectomy. For rectal polyps, the surgeon must consider whether other operative approaches in addition to radical resection are feasible and, if so, whether they can be effective. In some instances, one may simply want to re-resect the base of the polyp site by transanal approach to be sure that the wall margin is clear. In other cases, one may consider adjuvant chemoradiation therapy. Most often, the alternative is radical resection. For most rectal lesions, this requires a low or extended low anterior resection following the principles of total mesorectal excision and providing restorative anastomosis for all but the most distal lesions. For those with involvement of the distal anal canal, abdominoperineal resection is usually necessary. Before embarking on a specific radical operation, the surgeon should remember that only a portion of node-positive patients, perhaps 30–60%, will be cured by radical surgery. For presumed T_1 lesions thought to be best treated by radical surgery, no adjuvant therapy is given preoperatively. Only if nodal metastasis are identified would this be recommended.

At this point, the surgeon has the obligation to educate the patient by discussing the nature of the cancer in the polyp, the inferred risk of residual cancer or lymph node metastasis based on histologic criteria, and the recommended definitive therapy. A realistic review of morbidity and mortality of that therapy, as well as its anticipated effectiveness, is mandatory. Many authors have recommended treatment algorithms, but, ultimately, the patient must help decide which option suits his situation best *(33–38)*.

The authors' general approach is presented, but it must be remembered that each case is unique, and considerable judgment is required to achieve optimal management of a patient with cancer in a polyp (Tables 1 and 2). Polypectomy and observation should be considered definitive treatment for all patients with pedunculated polyps of the colon and rectum with invasive cancer classified as Haggitt Levels 1, 2, or 3 if the following favorable criteria are present: (1) the lesion has been totally removed and the resection margin is clear of cancer by ≥2 mm, (2) the histology is well or moderately differentiated, and (3) there is no lymphovascular invasion. The risk of residual cancer or lymph node metastasis in such polyps is probably less than 0.3%, which is less than the operative mortality for a radical colorectal resection. Whether the presence of a poorly differentiated histologic pattern and/or lymphovascular invasion in such pedunculated polyps should tip the scale to advising

Table 1
Suggested Criteria for Polypectomy and Observation for Cancer in a Polyp

- Complete excision of lesion
- ≥2 mm clear margins
- Well or moderately differentiated
- No lymphovascular invasion
- Haggitt Levels 1, 2, or 3 in pedunculated polyps
- Haggitt Level 4 (pedunculated or sessile polyp) with Sm_1 invasion

Table 2
Suggested Criteria for Radical Colorectal Resection for Cancer in a Polyp

Strong indicators
- Incomplete excision of lesion
- Microscopic cancer at resection margin
- Haggitt Level 4 (pedunculated or sessile polyp) with Sm_3 invasion

Relative indicators
- Poorly differentiated
- Lymphovascular invasion
- Excision doubtfully complete
- Haggitt Level 4 (pedunculated or sessile polyp) with Sm_2 invasion

radical surgery is controversial. The trend seems to be to follow such patients carefully after polypectomy, but data are lacking to make such a policy mandatory.

For any Haggitt Level-4 polyp, whether pedunculated or sessile, the risk of residual cancer or nodal metastasis is higher and correlates with the degree of invasion into the submucosa. For Sm_1-level cancers with the above-described favorable features, the risk is probably 1–2%, which is equivalent to the operative mortality of radical surgery. Thus, polypectomy can be considered definitive therapy for virtually all patients with such lesions. For Sm_2 lesions with otherwise favorable features, the risk of residual cancer or nodal metastasis is increased to 2–10%, making radical resection the likely best option for good-risk patients. Whether and how the presence of poorly differentiated histology or lymphovascular invasion should alter this algorithm is unclear from available data. Such features may independently increase the cancer risk, thus making radical resection more appealing. For good-risk patients, the presence of such adverse histologic features usually leads to the recommendation that radical surgery be performed. However, such features predict a poorer prognosis regardless of treatment, and one must remember that radical surgery for cancers that are poorly differentiated and have lymphatic and vascular invasion is *not* uniformly curative even if submucosa invasion is limited to Sm_1 or Sm_2. For Sm_3 invasive cancers, the risk of residual cancer or nodal metastases is high enough that colorectal resection is indicated for most such patients regardless of histologic features.

Malignant polyps in the distal rectum require special consideration. They are generally sessile, and as noted by Nivatvongs *(30)*, they may be more aggressive. Radical resection generally requires permanent colostomy or an ultralow anastomosis which often produces less-than-ideal functional results. Alternative treatment techniques are available for such distal lesions, including full-thickness local excision, endocavitary radiation, or adjuvant chemoradiation. A discussion of pros and cons of these alternatives is beyond the scope of this chapter but has been recently reviewed *(39)*.

7. FOLLOW-UP

If polypectomy is considered definitive therapy, long-term follow-up should be established to search for any local recurrence and to remove metachronous polyps. The endoscopist must first accurately localize the site of resection of a malignant polyp and must be certain that the entire lesion has been removed. For sessile colon polyps removed in piecemeal fashion, this can be difficult. Subsequent examinations are often necessary to perform additional, small, "touch-up" polypectomies of residual adenomatous tissue at the periphery of the original lesion. The endoscopist should repeat such examinations every 1–3 mo until there is no residual adenoma and the polypectomy site has totally healed. It is not necessary to do a total colonoscopy; endoscopy to the site of the malignant polyp is sufficient, assuming that the index colonoscopy was complete to the cecum. After local control is achieved, surveillance colonoscopy examinations can be scheduled generally 1 yr after the index examination, and if no abnormalities are noted, again 3 yr later. More frequent limited endoscopies to the polyp site may be justified if the risk of local recurrence is judged to be high. This is rarely the case, however, because most such patients should have been referred for radical colectomy.

Follow-up of rectal lesions is unique. Our protocol is to follow patients after local excision of T_1 lesions from the rectum with rigid proctoscopy and endorectal ultrasonography every 4 mo for the first 3 yr and then every 6 mo for the subsequent 2 yr. Using this protocol, we have identified local recurrences in the mucosa or adjacent lymph nodes while they were amenable to radical salvage surgery. The estimated 5-yr overall survival rate in our series was 72% after local excision of 69 T_1 cancers vs 80% after radical surgery of 30 T_1 lesions (not statistically significant) *(40)*. Whether survival is compromised on longer follow-up remains open to study.

8. CONCLUDING COMMENTS

The many controversies surrounding management of the patient with cancer in a polyp are unlikely to be resolved by single-investigator or single-institution studies. The need for a national registry, standardized definitions, expert review of resected speciments, and long-term follow-up is apparent.

REFERENCES

1. Mitros FA. Polyps: the pathologist's perspective. *Semin. Surg. Oncol.*, **11** (1995) 379–385.
2. Morson BC and Bussey HJR. *Predisposing Causes of Intestinal Cancer.* Current Problems in Surgery. Yearbook Medical, Chicago, 1970, pp. 3–50.
3. Haggitt RC, Glotzbach RE, Soffer EE, et al. Prognostic factors in colorectal carcinomas arising in adenomas: implications for lesions removed by endoscopic polypectomy. *Gastroenterology*, **89** (1985) 328–336.
4. Winawer SJ, Fletcher RH, Miller L, et al. Colorectal cancer screening: clinical guidelines and rationale. *Gastroenterology*, **112** (1997) 594–642.
5. Morson BC. The polyp–cancer sequence in the large bowel. *Proc. R. Soc. Med.*, **67** (1974) 451–457.
6. Hermanek P and Gall FP. Early (microinvasive) colorectal carcinoma. Pathology, diagnosis, surgical treatment. *Int. J. Colorect. Dis.*, **1** (1986) 79–84.
7. Nivatvongs S. Complications in colonoscopic polypectomy. An experience with 1555 polypectomies. *Dis. Colon Rectum*, **29** (1986) 825–830.
8. Nusko G, Mansmann W, Partzsch W, et al. Invasive carcinoma in colorectal adenomas: multivariate analysis of patient and adenoma characteristics. *Endoscopy*, **29** (1997) 626–631.

9. O'Brien MJ, Winawer SJ, Zauber AG, et al. The national polyp study. *Gastroenterology*, **98** (1990) 371–379.
10. Shinya H and Wolff WI. Morphology, anatomic distribution, and cancer potential of colonic polyps: an analysis of 7000 polyps endoscopically removed. *Ann. Surg.*, **190** (1979) 679–683.
11. Cohen LB and Waye JD. Treatment of colonic ployps—practical considerations. *Clin. Gastroenterol.*, **15** (1986) 359–376.
12. Morson BC. Precancerous conditions of the large bowel. *Proc. R. Soc. Med.*, **64** (1971) 959–962.
13. Simon JB. Colonic polyps, cancer and fecal occult blood [editorial]. *Ann. Intern. Med.*, **118** (1993) 71–72.
14. Pollack J, Mellgren A, Wong W, et al. How accurate is endorectal ultrasonograpy in the staging of rectal tumors? [podium abstract]. *Dis. Colon Rectum*, **43** (2000) A26.
15. Garcia-Aguilar J, Mellgren A, Sirivongs P, et al. Local excision of rectal cancer without adjuvant therapy: a word of caution. *Ann. Surg.*, **3** (2000) 345–351.
16. Hilliard G, Ramming K, Thompson J Jr, et al. The elusive colonic malignancy: a need for definitive preoperative localization. *Am. Surg.*, **56** (1990) 742–744.
17. Hammond DC, Lane FR, MacKeigan JM, et al. Endoscopic tattooing of the colon: clinical experience. *Am. Surg.*, **59** (1993) 205–210.
18. Hyman N and Waye JD. Endoscopic four quadrant tattoo for the identification of colonic lesions at surgery. *Gastrointest. Endoscopy*, **37** (1991) 56–58.
19. Lightdale CJ. India ink colonic tattoo: blots on the record. *Gastrointest. Endoscopy*, **37** (1991) 99–100.
20. Ponsky JL and King JF. Encoscopic marking of colon lesions. *Gastrointest. Endoscopy*, **22** (1975) 42–43.
21. Coverlizza S, Risio M, Ferrari A, et al. Colorectal adenomas containing invasive carcinoma: pathologic assessment of lymph node metastatic potential. *Cancer*, **64** (1989) 1937–1947.
22. Pollard C, Nivatvongs S, Rojanasakul A, et al. The fate of patients following polypectomy alone for polyps containing invasive carcinoma. *Dis. Colon Rectum*, **35** (1992) 933–937.
23. Stein B and Coller J. Management of malignant colorectal polyps. *Surg. Clin. North Am.*, **73** (1993) 47–66.
24. Cooper HS. Surgical pathology of endoscopically removed malignant polyps of the colon and rectum. *Am. J. Surg. Pathol.*, **7** (1983) 613–623.
25. Cooper HS, Deppish LM, Gourley WK, et al. Endoscopically removed malignant colorectal polyps clinicopathological correlations. *Gastroenterology*, **108** (1995) 1657–1665.
26. Morson BC, Whiteway JE, Jones FA, et al. Histopathology and prognosis of malignant colorectal polyps treated by endoscopic polypectomy. *Gut*, **25** (1984) 437–444.
27. Bond JH. Colon polyps and cancer. *Endoscopy*, **31** (1999) 60–65.
28. Volk EE, Goldblum JR, Petras RE, et al. Management and outcome of patients with invasive carcinoma arising in colorectal polyps. *Gastroenterology*, **109** (1995) 1801–1807.
29. Nivatvongs S, Rojanasakul A, Reiman HM, et al. The risk of lymph node metastasis in colorectal polyps with invasive adenocarcinoma. *Dis Colon Rectum*, **34** (1991) 323–328.
30. Nivatvongs S. "The malignant polyp: When is enough enough?" The William C. Bernstein, M.D. Memorial Lecture. Colon and Rectal Surgery: Principles and Practice 2000, Minneapolis, MN, 2000.
31. Kikuchi R, Takano M, Takagi K, et al. Management of early invasive colorectal cancer. Risk of recurrence and clinical guidelines. *Dis. Colon Rectum*, **38** (1995) 1286–1295.
32. Kudo S. Endoscopic mucosal resection of flat and depressed types of early colorectal cancer. *Endoscopy*, **25** (1993) 455–461.
33. Cohen LB and Waye JD. Colonoscopic polypectomy of polyps with adenocarcinoma: When is it curative? In *Difficult Decisions in Digestive Diseases*. Barkin JS and Rogers AI (eds.), Yearbook Medical, Boca Raton, 1989, pp. 528–535.
34. Haggitt RC. Controversies, dilemmas, and dialogues: when is colonoscopic resection of an adenomatous polyp containing a "malignancy" sufficient? *Am. J. Gastroenterol.*, **85** (1990) 1564–1568.
35. Koretz RL. Malignant polyps: Are they sheep in wolves' clothing? *Ann. Intern. Med.*, **118** (1993) 63–68.
36. Kryzer S, Begin LR, Gordon PH, et al. The care of patients with colorectal polyps that contain invasive adenocarcinoma: Endoscopic polypectomy or colectomy? *Cancer*, **70** (1992) 2044–2050.
37. Russell JB, Chu DZ, Russell MP, et al. When is polypectomy sufficient treatment for colorectal cancer in a polyp? *Am. J. Surg.*, **160** (1990) 665–668.
38. Sitzler PJ, Seow-Choen F, Ho YH, et al. Lymph node involvement and tumor depth in rectal cancers. An analysis of 805 patients. *Dis. Colon Rectum*, **40** (1997) 172–176.
39. Finne CO and Garcia-Aguilar J. Local treatment of rectal cancer. In *Colon and Rectal Cancer*. Edelstein PS (ed.), Wiley–Liss, New York, 2000, pp. 259–309.
40. Mellgren A, Sirivongs P, Rothenberger DA, et al. Is local excision adequate therapy for early rectal cancer? *Dis. Colon Rectum*, **43** (2000) 1064–1074.

18 Surgery of Rectal Cancer

Aaron R. Sasson and Elin R. Sigurdson

CONTENTS

1. HISTORICAL PERSPECTIVES

The first successful operation for rectal cancer was performed by Lisfranc in 1826 *(1)*. This consisted of excising the anus and rectum via the perineum, which resulted in the functional equivalent of a perineal colostomy. As surgical techniques improved and general anesthesia developed, more extensive resections were undertaken. However exposure to the upper rectum was limited, and in an attempt to improve access, Verneuil (1873) and Kocher (1876) excised the coccyx and portion of the sacrum. It was Kraske (1885), after whom the procedure was named, who introduced the posterior approach of resecting the rectum through the sacrum while preserving the anus and sphincter muscles *(2)*.

The first reported combined abdominal and perineal resection was performed by Czerny (1884). This occurred after Czerny was unsuccessful at excising the rectum via a perineal approach and completed the resection via the abdomen. Sir Ernest Miles, in 1908, described his modification of Czerny's operation. Miles emphasized the importance of including the surrounding regional lymphatics with complete extirpation of the rectum and anus too; principles that apply today *(1)*.

In 1921, a technique to treat upper-rectal tumors via an anterior resection (abdominal incision only) was proposed by Henri Hartmann *(3)*. This was initially described as a two-stage operation with performance of an end colostomy followed by a resection at a later time. During the early 20th century, improvements in surgical technique allowed for one-stage

From: *Colorectal Cancer: Multimodality Management*
Edited by: L. Saltz © Humana Press Inc., Totowa, NJ

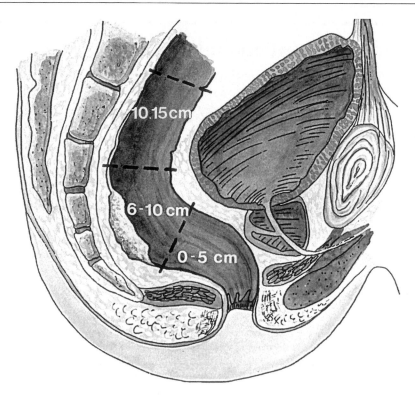

Fig. 1. View of the rectum in its anatomical position in the pelvis. The rectum has been "divided" into thirds, with a lesion depicted in the mid rectum.

procedures and restoration of intestinal continuity. With the advent of stapling devices and a better understanding of rectal anatomy, the possibilities of anterior resection and sphincter preservation has increased in the last several decades.

2. ANATOMY

The performance of rectal surgery is based on a thorough understanding of rectal and anal anatomy. The exact proximal and distal boundaries of the rectum are not well defined, with surgeons and anatomists in disagreement. The length of the rectum is typically 12–15 cm and lies between the sigmoid colon and the anal canal. The distinction between the distal sigmoid colon and the proximal rectum can be difficult, although, morphologically, the rectum can be differentiated by the absence of haustrations, taeniae, or epiploic appendices. In the presence of a bulky tumor or significant inflammation, these anatomical features may be obscured and this area is often referred to as the rectosigmoid junction.

Conceptually, the rectum is often divided into three segments, upper, middle, and lower, with each segment approx 5 cm long (Fig. 1). The upper third of the rectum is covered by the pelvic peritoneum anteriorly and laterally. The middle third is covered by peritoneum only anteriorly, and the lower third is completely extraperitoneal. This peritoneal coverage is commonly described by surgeons as the anterior and posterior peritoneal reflection, with the anterior reflection extending deeper into the pelvis than the posterior reflection. In clinical trials, most authors use 12 cm from the anal verge, by rigid sigmoidoscopy, as the upper limit of the rectum.

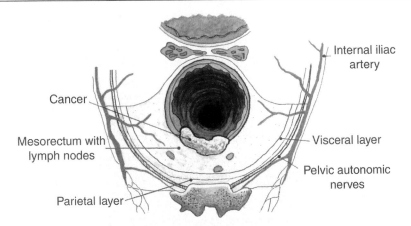

Fig. 2. The mesorectum containing the draining lymphatics of the rectum is surrounded by the visceral layer of the pelvic fascia.

2.1. FASCIAL RELATIONSHIPS

The anatomical fascial layers of the pelvis is a complex subject. However, identifying the proper plane of dissection is crucial for surgical extirpation of a rectal tumor. The rectum, along with its blood supply, nerves, fat, and lymph nodal bearing tissue is enveloped by the fascia propria of the rectum (also known as the visceral layer of the pelvic fascia) *(4)*. The surrounding fatty tissue covered by this fascial layer, which contains the lymphatic drainage, is referred to as the mesorectum (Fig. 2). This tissue contains the regional lymph nodes draining the rectum and may harbor metastatic disease. Complete surgical removal of the mesorectum may be an important factor in decreasing the rate of local recurrences.

2.2. Arterial Supply

The blood supply for the rectum is derived from the superior, middle, and inferior rectal arteries with contribution from the median sacral artery (direct branch from the aorta). The superior rectal artery is the terminal branch of the inferior mesenteric artery and supplies the upper third of the rectum, as well as providing collateral blood flow to the middle and lower rectum. The middle rectal arteries originate from the internal iliac arteries, however, the number (paired or unpaired) as well as the vessel caliber are highly variable. They course through the pelvis and enter the mesorectum, occasionally giving branches that enter via the lateral ligaments (band of connective tissue containing autonomic nerves from the pelvic plexus) *(4,5)*. The presence of a discrete middle rectal artery is infrequent, and when present, it is often distal to the lateral ligaments *(5)*. The internal pudendal arteries (terminal branches of the internal iliac arteries) give rise to the inferior rectal arteries and provide blood supply to the lower rectum and anal canal.

2.3. VENOUS AND LYMPHATIC DRAINAGE

Venous drainage of the rectum is by submucosal venous plexuses and closely follows the arterial supply. The inferior and middle rectal veins drain into the systemic circulation, whereas the superior rectal vein drains into the portal system. The lymphatic drainage of the rectum resembles the arterial and venous distribution. The first draining nodes are contained within the mesorectum. Depending on the tumor location, secondary lymph node

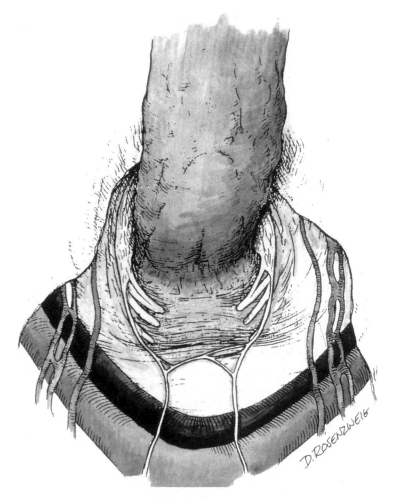

Fig. 3. The parietal layer of the pelvic fascia has been removed, exposing the autonomic nerves in the pelvis.

involvement may occur in the para-aortic nodes, the internal iliac nodes, or in the superficial inguinal lymph nodes.

2.4. Pelvic Nerves

There is an extensive network of autonomic nerves supplying the pelvic organs (Fig. 3). An understanding of these nerves and their anatomical relation with the rectum is important in minimizing postoperative genitourinary complications. The network is comprised of neural tissue from the superior hypogastric plexus, hypogastric nerves, the pelvic splanchnic nerves, and the pelvic plexus. This network is invested in the parietal fascia and lies outside the fascia propria *(4)*. The superior hypogastric plexus receives sympathetic fibers from low thoracic and upper lumbar nerve roots. This plexus is located along the inferior mesenteric artery and courses caudally to give rise to the hypogastric nerves at the level of the sacral promontory. Injury to either the superior hypogastric plexus or the hypogastric nerves will result in ejaculatory dysfunction in men. Pelvic splanchnic nerves provide a parasympathetic supply and originate from the second, third, and fourth sacral nerve roots. These nerves

Table 1
Surgical Procedures for Excising the Rectum for Rectal Cancer

Low anterior resection (sphincter preservation)
    Colorectal anastomosis
    Coloanal anastomosis
Abdominal perineal resection

course laterally and caudally and overlie the piriformis muscle. The pelvic splanchnic nerves, along with the hypogastric nerves, coalesce to the pelvic plexus. Branches from the pelvic plexus supplying the rectum are contained in the lateral ligaments, whereas branches to the genitourinary organs course anteriorly. Awareness of the location of these neural structures during pelvic dissection is important in preventing postoperative sexual and urinary dysfunction.

3. CHOICE OF OPERATION

Surgical resection is the mainstay of treatment for rectal cancer. The operative options available are local resection or radical surgery. Radical surgery includes low anterior resection (LAR) (with colorectal or coloanal anastomosis) or abdomino-perineal resection (APR) (Table 1). Determining which procedure is suitable is dependent on a thorough preoperative evaluation. Factors such as tumor stage, tumor distance from the anal verge, circumferential involvement, and tumor differentiation are important when selecting operative intervention (local resection vs radical surgery). Further information regarding local excision of rectal tumors including patient selection criteria and surgical technique can be found in Chapter 19.

The term "low anterior resection" is used to describe a surgical procedure in which a portion of the rectum is excised through an abdominal incision with preservation of the anal sphincters, allowing for restoration of gastrointestinal continuity. In comparison, abdomino-perineal resection includes performing a LAR in combination with removing the distal rectum and anus via a perineal incision. The key determinant in deciding if an LAR is possible is the distance of the tumor from the anal verge. An accurate assessment is accomplished with a digital rectal examination and rigid proctoscopy. For patients with associated rectal pain or after completion of preoperative radiation therapy, inspection of the rectum typically may require general anesthesia. Patients with tumors fixed in the pelvis should be treated with preoperative chemoradiotherapy. Occasionally, for very distal rectal cancers, the ability to perform a sphincter-preserving procedure can only be determined intraoperatively. Contraindications to sphincter preservation include tumor involvement of the sphincter muscles, preexisting fecal incontinence or dysfunction, and tumor invasion of the prostate or distal aspect of the vagina. Patient characteristics that can limit the ability to perform a LAR include a narrow pelvis (more common in males) and obesity (Table 2). Additionally, comorbid conditions such as chronic obstructive pulmonary disease, coronary artery disease, diabetes mellitus, cirrhosis, and renal insufficiency have been identified as predictive factors of postoperative morbidity *(6)*.

3.1. PREOPERATIVE STAGING

Accurate staging of rectal cancer is essential for proper management, and several imaging modalities are currently available. Although the accuracy of computed tomography (CT)

Table 2
Contraindications to Sphincter Preservation

Absolute
    Tumor involvement of sphincter muscles
    Pre-existing fecal incontinence or dysfunction
    Invasion of the prostate or distal vagina
Relative
    Narrow pelvis
    Obesity
    Confounding comorbid conditions

ranges from 55% to 72% for primary rectal cancer, CT can provide useful information regarding the presence of metastatic disease *(7,8)*. Computed tomography is helpful in detecting and evaluating locally recurrent rectal cancer as well as locally advanced disease. The two imaging methods that can accurately, greater than 80%, determine the depth of tumor invasion include endoscopic ultrasound (EUS) and endorectal magnetic resonance imaging (EMRI). Both modalities are capable of identifying discrete layers of the rectal wall. Although EUS and EMRI can detect the presence of perirectal lymph nodes, their major limitation is the inability to adequately predict lymph node involvement *(7)*. Radiographic evaluation of tumor response to preoperative therapy is difficult because EUS and EMRI cannot differentiate perirectal edema, fibrosis, or inflammation from tumor. Additional limitations of these modalities include operator dependence for EUS and cost and availability for EMRI.

3.2. Comparison of Outcome

Abdomino-perineal resection is considered the "gold standard" operation for distal rectal tumors. The rationale use of LAR vs APR must be based on equivalent oncologic results. Sphincter-preserving operations must achieve equal local control and survival rates as abdomino-perineal resections. Although there are many retrospective reviews, there have been no prospective randomized trials comparing the two operations. Several large retrospective reviews have not been able to identify a significant difference in the rate of local failure or overall survival *(9–12)*. Patient selection bias and the different treatment modalities utilized prevent any meaningful comparisons between these trials. However, two studies reviewed data obtained from large prospective trials studying the effects of adjuvant therapy *(9,10)*. Investigators reviewing the NSABP R-01 trial identified a local recurrence of 13% for sphincter-preserving operations compared to 5% for APR, although no statistical difference in survival was detected. An analysis of two randomized trials from Sweden (1292 patients) reported similar conclusions *(10)*. Despite the lack of a prospective randomized trial, LAR and APR appear to have equivalent tumor control.

4. TECHNIQUE

For either a LAR or APR, a mechanical bowel preparation is given the day prior to surgery. An enterostomal nurse should be consulted for preoperative marking of a stoma site and for counseling in the event that sphincter preservation is not possible. An epidural catheter, for control of postoperative pain, can be placed just prior to the operation. Appropriate antibiotic and antithrombotic prophylaxis is instituted. After the administration of general anesthesia, the patient is placed in a modified lithotomy position. At this point, a digital and proctoscopic examination should be performed. Tumor distance from the anal verge, mobility from the pelvic side walls, and involvement of anterior organs can be assessed and may influence the choice of operation.

4.1. Low Anterior Resection

After a midline incision is made, the abdominal cavity is thoroughly inspected. Particular attention is paid to the peritoneal surface and liver, and any suspicious abnormality is biopsied and documented. The attachments of the sigmoid and descending colon to the lateral wall of the abdomen are transected. During this dissection, the left ureter is identified and protected from injury. The terminal branch of the inferior mesenteric artery (sigmoid and superior rectal arteries) is divided distal to the left colic artery, which preserves the blood supply to the descending colon. In some instances, the left colic artery must be divided so that the left colon can reach into the pelvis. In these instances, mobilization of the splenic flexure is mandatory, so a tension-free anastomosis is possible.

Next, the presacral space (the area between the sacrum and the rectum) is developed sharply and this can be dissected down to the level of the coccyx. After completing the posterior dissection, anterior dissection of the rectum begins in the midline in the rectovesical pouch in males and in the rectouterine pouch in females. In men, care is taken to avoid injury to the bladder, prostate, or seminal vesicles, whereas in women, the posterior aspect of the vagina is in close proximity to the anterior wall of the rectum. Exposure of the lateral aspects of the rectum can be difficult, but it is facilitated by first performing the posterior and anterior dissection. Once the rectum has been fully mobilized, the distance of the tumor from the sphincter muscles should be reassessed, as an additional 4–5 cm of length can be achieved after the rectum has been dissected free and straightened. This may allow sphincter preservation for very distal rectal cancers. The rectum is then transected distal to the lesion and the specimen examined to ascertain the length of distal margin (the adequate margin length needed will be discussed in a later section). After gastrointestinal continuity is established, the patient's abdomen is closed.

4.2. Abdomino-Perineal Resection

The abdominal portion of an APR is similar to the LAR, with the notable exception that the rectum is not divided. The perineal portion of the operation is performed after the abdominal portion when the rectum has been completely mobilized. When two teams of operating surgeons are employed, the perineal portion can be performed simultaneously.

An elliptical incision around the anus is made to incorporate the sphincter muscles. The ischiorectal fossa is entered, and dissection is carried out posteriorly to the level of the coccyx. The anococcygeal ligament is transected and the pelvis is entered. Laterally, the levator muscles are divided. Anterior dissection is the most intricate portion of the perineal phase of the operation and is reserved until after completing the posterior and lateral dissection. In males, the prostatic urethra and seminal vesicles are in close proximity to the rectum at this level. In women, an anteriorly located cancer may require a limited resection of the posterior vaginal wall. After completing the anterior dissection, the entire specimen can be extracted through the perineal incision. The perineal wound is closed primarily and drains are placed in the pelvis. The colostomy is placed at a site marked preoperatively and the abdomen is closed.

5. OPERATIVE CONSIDERATIONS

5.1. Margins

Resection of cancers of the upper rectum can be accomplished easily with generous distal margins (i.e., 4–5 cm). The amount of rectum that can be sacrificed during surgery for low rectal cancers is limited. The ability to perform sphincter preservation is often dictated by the extent of distal tumor spread, and the exact length of distal rectal margin needed has not been definitively determined. A prospective pathologic analysis of microscopic intramural tumor spread demonstrated the need for 12 mm of distal margin clearance *(13)*. An important concept that was also emphasized in this report was the degree of contraction that occurs in the fixed specimen. Several retrospective studies have concluded that a 2-cm distal margin was sufficient for control of local failure *(11,14)*. Subsequent analyses have suggested that even a smaller distal margin may be adequate. Shirouzu et al. observed distal spread in less than 4% of the 505 specimens of patients who underwent "curative surgery" *(15)*. Incidence of distal spread in stage II disease was 1.2% and never exceeded 1 cm. In stage III disease, 10% of specimens had distal spread, with half of them limited to less than 1 cm. A prospective study from the University of Minnesota concluded that a distal margin of 1 cm is adequate for most rectal cancers *(16)*. However, two pathologic tumor characteristics that may warrant more extensive distal clearance include poorly differentiated and mucinous neoplasms *(14)*.

Extramural spread into the mesorectum is more frequent than intramural spread and the distance of spread is much greater. Pathologic assessment of the mesorectum requires detailed examination and serial sectioning of the specimen *(17)*. In two recent reports, tumor deposits in the mesorectum were identified in 20–25% of the specimens *(18,19)*. The maximum distal spread encountered was 4–5 cm. Hida and associates examined 198 specimens and found no distal extramural spread in T1 or T2 tumors. However, T3 and T4 tumors had distal tumor deposits in 22% and 50%, respectively *(19)*. The presence of distal mesorectal spread has been associated with increased frequency of local recurrence and possibly with decreased overall survival *(20,21)*.

In addition to examining the mesorectum, serial transverse sectioning of the specimen permits assessment of the radial margins *(17)*. Involvement of the radial margins is associated with a significantly increased local recurrence rate *(17,22,23)*. In addition, multivariate analyses have demonstrated positive radial margins as an independent prognosticator for local recurrence and overall survival *(22,24)*. Theoretically, complete resection of perirectal tissue as occurs in total mesorectal excision (TME) should decrease the number of positive circumferential margins and minimize the risk of residual disease in the mesorectum. However, in bulky tumors, a positive radial margin may not be an indicator of inadequate surgery, but rather a marker of advanced disease *(25)*.

5.2. Total Mesorectal Excision

In an effort to decrease local recurrence by extirpating the regional lymphatics, Heald and colleagues, in 1982, introduced the concept of TME *(26)*. A recent update of Heald's experience with TME documented a local recurrence rate of 3% in patients undergoing "curative resections" *(27)*. This low rate of regional failure is remarkable considering the infrequent utilization of adjuvant therapy. The use of TME has been adopted by many centers, with a local recurrence rate ranging from 7% to 13% *(28–32)*. Although Heald is credited with promoting a standardized surgical technique as a means of improving

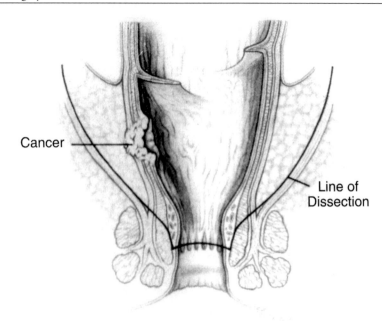

Fig. 4. Figure depicting excision of the entire mesorectum with amputation of the rectum at the dentate line for a distal rectal cancer. (From Daly JM and Cady B [eds.]. *Atlas of Surgical Oncology.* Mosby Yearbook, St. Louis, MO, 1993, p. 577. Reproduced with permission.)

outcome, the benefits of "wide anatomical resection" was also described by Enker and associates *(33).*

From a technical standpoint, TME involves resection of the rectum with its surrounding envelope, the fascia propria. This compartment, known as the mesorectum, contains the perirectal fat and draining lymphatic tissue. Heald has described the space between the fascia propria and the parietal fascia (the tissue investing the pelvic walls and nerves) as the "holy plane" of rectal surgery *(34).* Anatomically, the mesorectum is thin anteriorly and separating it from the genitourinary structures in males and the posterior vaginal wall in females can be challenging. The space between the fascia propria and parietal fascia is often dissected sharply (with use of electrocautery or scissors) to prevent disruption of the fascia propria and violation of the mesorectum.

Despite the many advocates of TME, there have been no prospective randomized trials comparing conventional resection with TME. However, comparison of the outcome after TME with historical controls suggests superior local control with TME *(30,35).* Havenga and colleagues recently reported results of an international review of TME and conventional surgery *(36).* Data from five active rectal cancer institutions were collected and reviewed (total of 1411 patients), with each center contributing over 200 patients. A local recurrence rate of 32–35% was reported after conventional surgery. Performance of TME was associated with a markedly reduced local recurrence rate (4–9%). Also of significance was a 30% absolute increase in the overall and cancer-specific survival in the TME group.

The removal of the entire mesorectum is controversial, and critics of TME have questioned the need for routine resection of the entire mesorectum for all rectal cancers (Fig. 4). For middle and low rectal lesions, the entire mesorectum is excised, as opposed to transecting the mesorectum at an appropriate distal margin. Excising the entire mesorectum results in

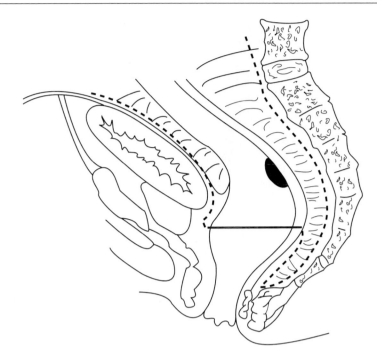

Fig. 5. Excision of the entire mesorectum (dashed lines) with transection of the rectum (solid lines). Note that the mesorectum is not divided at the same level as the rectum, this ensures complete removal of potential spread in the distal mesorectum. However, this also results in a denuded rectum distally.

a denuded rectum, which can then be amputated at the desired level (Fig. 5). For cancers located at the upper rectum, total mesorectal excision would produce an excessively long avascular rectum and compromise the integrity of an anastomosis. Several investigators have recently examined the need for routine TME for upper rectal tumors *(31,32,37,38)*. Although these studies are nonrandomized, no compromise in the local recurrence rate was identified when a selective approach of TME was applied to upper rectal cancers. However, the surgical technique utilized in these reports included excising the mesorectum 4–5 cm distal to the rectal tumor; this ensures an adequate resection of the surrounding lymphatic tissue.

The dramatic reduction in local recurrence after TME, as originally reported by Heald, was accomplished without the use of adjuvant therapy *(26)*. A retrospective review from the Mayo Clinic analyzed 514 patients who were treated without any adjuvant therapy *(28)*. An overall local control rate of 7% was reported, however, more than half of the patients had stage I disease. Of note, distant metastases predominated as the site of failure in these selected patients not receiving adjuvant therapy. Bokey et al. performed a similar analysis (*n* = 596), in which nearly 40% of the patients had nodal involvement *(31)*. The overall 5-yr actuarial local recurrence rate was 11%. Multivariate analysis identified positive nodes and venous invasion as pathologic features that were independent predictive factors for local recurrence. Merchant and associates reviewed their experience of TME without adjuvant treatment in 95 patients with T3N0M0 (stage II). The overall local recurrence rate was 9% and the only histopathologic feature significant for predicting local failure was lymphatic invasion (Table 3) *(39)*. Currently, a prospective randomized trial is in progress to evaluate TME with and without preoperative radiotherapy *(40)*.

Table 3
Pathologic Factors Affecting Outcome After TME

1. Lymph node metastasis
2. Vascular invasion
3. Lymphatic invasion
4. Positive radial margin
5. Distal mesorectal spread

Although the oncologic results of TME seem promising, critical analysis of Heald's data is warranted. In his most recent update, Heald summarized his experience with TME in 519 patients during the last two decades *(27)*. Nearly 10% of patients received preoperative therapy for tumor fixation and "unresectability," and information regarding adjuvant chemotherapy is lacking. Of the 465 patients undergoing LAR, only 80% were deemed to have had a "curative" resection; however, the criteria used to determine a "curative" resection are not clearly stated. Also lacking is detailed data correlating the local recurrence rates with the tumor stage. For the entire series, the local recurrence rate of 6% at 5 yr and 8% at 10 yr was reported. Of concern was the difference in rate of local recurrence between LAR and APR; 5% vs 17% at 5 yr. This dramatic difference between the two operations is not easily explainable, although the possibility of poor pathologic prognostic factors or implantation of tumor cells during the operation in the APR group have been proposed *(41)*. Regardless of these limitations, the merits of TME are obvious and more studies are needed to define the appropriate use of this surgical technique.

5.3. Nerve Preservation

Urinary and sexual dysfunction are recognized complication of surgery for rectal cancer. These complications are a result of injury to the sympathetic and parasympathetic nerves that are present in the pelvis. With the use of sharp mesorectal excision and greater awareness of the autonomic nerves, genitourinary complications can be minimized *(42)*.

Sexual dysfunction after rectal surgery is characterized by impotence and ejaculatory dysfunction *(see* Chapter 37). Although physical injury to the autonomic nerves may play a role in the development of these dysfunctions, the cause is likely to be multifactorial. Comorbid conditions such as diabetes, vascular disease, and aging, as well as psychological factors may contribute. The incidence of permanent impotence varies widely in the literature because of variations in definition, evaluation, and surgical technique. A recent review of 6 prospective and 12 retrospective studies identified a 51% rate of impotence after APR vs 29% after LAR *(43)*. The increased rate of impotence after APR may reflect selection bias, as patients requiring APR may have more advanced disease and adverse pathologic features *(44)*. Havenga and colleagues observed that in male patients, with normal preoperative sexual function, 57% of patients having an APR had retained sexual function, in comparison to 86% of patients having a LAR *(45)*. Additionally, they identified age >60 as a significant predictor of poor outcome. Postoperative sexual dysfunction in women is less well understood and studied; however, they reported that 85% of female patients evaluated had preserved sexual function.

Urinary dysfunction after surgery for rectal cancer is often temporary. The incidence of permanent bladder dysfunction ranges from 0% to 19%, and the incidence may be greater after APR than LAR *(43)*. A recent report utilizing urodynamic studies after TME

Table 4
Potential Sites of Nerve Injury During Rectal Surgery

Location	Nerve
Origin of inferior mesenteric artery	Superior hypogastric plexus
Sacral promontory	Hypogastric nerves
Lateral ligaments	Pelvic plexus
Behind prostate and seminal vesicles	Parasympathetic nerves

documented bladder denervation in 2 of the 49 patients studied *(46)*. Denervation was characterized by a weak detrusor pressure, decreased flow, and increased residual volume.

Anatomical studies of the pelvic autonomic nerves have identified several sites during rectal surgery that are vulnerable to injury (Table 4) *(4,42,43)*.

1. Origin of inferior mesenteric artery. The superior hypogastric plexus is located posterior to the artery near its origin from the aorta. Proximal ligation of the artery at its origin may injure the plexus, and injury at this level may result in ejaculatory dysfunction *(47)*.
2. Posterior pelvic dissection. Fibers from the superior hypogastric plexus course caudally over the sacral promontory to form the hypogastric nerves, and they lie 1–2 cm medial and parallel to the ureters. Failure to identify the appropriate plane posteriorly places these nerves at risk of injury and also result in ejaculatory dysfunction *(47)*. Staying in the fascial plane just posterior to the superior rectal artery will help identify the fascia propria. If the hypogastric nerves are encountered during the dissection, the surgeon is in the wrong plane.
3. Lateral dissection. Medial traction of the distal rectum reveals the lateral ligaments, which are a band of connective tissue containing autonomic fibers from the pelvic plexus to the rectum. Excessive lateral dissection low in the pelvis may damage this plexus. The lack of any significant vascular structure in the lateral ligaments allows division without the need to clamp and ligate the ligaments, thus minimizing the chance of injury to the plexus.
4. Anterior dissection. The narrow space between the rectum and prostate and seminal vesicles makes the anterior rectal dissection precarious. During this portion of the operation, parasympathetic nerves lying posterior to the prostate and seminal vesicles may be damaged, resulting in impotence. Furthermore, obtaining hemostasis in this difficult to access area also places these nerves in jeopardy. These anatomical factors may help explain why sexual dysfunction occurs more commonly in APR than in LAR.

6. RECONSTRUCTION

After LAR, intestinal continuity can be restored using a variety of techniques and can be performed with either a hand-sewn or stapled anastomosis. During the last 20 yr, the ability to safely perform resections of the distal rectum has been enhanced by the increasing use of intestinal stapling devices. The rational use of either method, hand-sewn or stapled, must result in equivalent oncologic and functional outcome. A large, 732 patients, prospective randomized trial comparing hand-sewn versus staple anastomosis failed to detect any difference in the local recurrence rates between these two techniques *(48)*. This confirms the findings of previous studies *(49)*. A commonly used method of reconstruction employs a double-stapled technique, in which the rectum is transected with one stapler and continuity is restored with use of a circular stapler. Multiple studies have demonstrated the safety and low recurrence rate using this technique *(50–52)*.

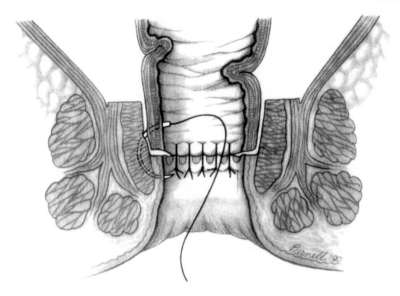

Fig. 6. Depiction of a hand-sewn coloanal anastomosis. (From Daly JM and Cady B [eds.]. *Atlas of Surgical Oncology.* Mosby Yearbook, St. Louis, MO, 1993, p. 583. Reproduced with permission.)

Restoration of gastrointestinal continuity after resection of very distal rectal cancers can be accomplished with a coloanal anastomosis (Fig. 6). The procedure involves excising the distal rectal mucosa (via a perineal approach) and performing a transanal anastomosis. However, an "ultralow" resection combined with a straight coloanal anastomosis has a significant impact on postoperative bowel function. Contributing factors include excision of the rectal reservoir and alteration in the physiologic pathways, resulting in increased stool frequency, decreased urgency threshold, and varying degrees of fecal incontinence *(53)*. The range of postoperative dysfunction has been directly related to the level of the anastomosis *(54)*. With decreasing length of residual rectum, the degree of incontinence and altered defecation increase. Despite these drawbacks, the application of coloanal anastomosis in carefully selected patients can be accomplished without compromising the oncologic result *(55,56)*.

In an effort to reduce the physiologic impact and improve postoperative function, Parc et al. and Lazorthes et al. in 1986 described their initial experience with the colonic J-pouch (Fig. 7) *(57,58)*. The pouch functions as a neorectal reservoir, providing an increase in capacity and compliance. Multiple prospective randomized trials have demonstrated better functional outcome with a colonic J-pouch compared to a straight coloanal anastomosis *(59,60)*. The improvement in function, decreased frequency, decreased "clustering" of stools, and decreased use of antidiarrhea agents has been reported in long-term studies to be present even after 2 yr postoperatively *(61,62)*.

There are several standardized technical factors regarding the creation of a pouch and include complete mobilization of the splenic flexure, high ligation of the inferior mesenteric vessels, and use of a well-vascularized diverticular-free colon. However, the optimal length of the pouch has been controversial, either 5 cm or 10 cm. Two prospective randomized trials comparing small vs large colonic J-pouches demonstrated equal continence rates, defecation frequency, and urgency *(63,64)*. However, patients with large (10 cm) J-pouches had difficulty evacuating their bowels and often needed enemas. The cause of the evacuation

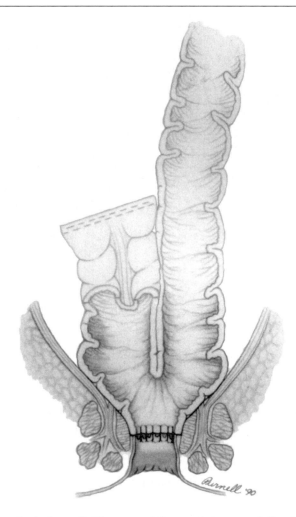

Fig. 7. Illustration of a colonic J-pouch. The apex of the pouch is secured (hand-sewn or stapled) to the dentate line. The ideal length of the pouch is 5 cm. (From Daly JM and Cady B [eds.]. *Atlas of Surgical Oncology.* Mosby Yearbook, St. Louis, MO, 1993, p. 587. Modified with permission).

difficulty was recently examined by Hida and colleagues with serial pouchograms and they concluded that excessive pouch enlargement resulted in a deterioration in function *(65)*.

The minimum length of residual rectum required to achieve acceptable functional result has not been clearly determined. A study recently concluded that a colonic J-pouch reconstruction should be utilized when the level of anastomosis is less than 4 cm *(66)*. Additionally, they recommended that formation of a pouch when the anastomosis level is between 4–8 cm may be beneficial. Acceptable bowel function after straight colorectal reconstruction was observed when the anastomosis level was greater than 8 cm from the anal verge.

7. COMPLICATIONS

Postoperative morbidity from rectal cancer surgery includes all of the potential complications of major surgery. A review of outcome after surgery for rectal cancer from the Veteran

Table 5
Factors Associated with Increased Risk of Anastomotic Leak

Height of the anastomosis from the anal verge (<7 cm)
Total mesorectal excision (TME)
Male sex
Obesity
Lack of diverting stoma in "ultralow" resection

Administration database identified prolonged ileus, urinary tract infection, pneumonia, and deep-wound infection as the most common postoperative complications (67). Overall, 30-d postoperative mortality was 3.2% but was significantly higher in patients with complications. Complications that were associated with a mortality of over 50% included deep venous thrombosis, pulmonary embolism, acute renal failure, and cerebral vascular accident. A review from the Mayo Clinic's experience with carcinoma of the rectum identified increasing age, male sex, and increasing weight as significant risk factors for postoperative complications (68). Additionally, the complication rate after APR was significantly greater than for LAR.

The complication associated with LAR that results in significant morbidity and mortality is anastomotic leak (Table 5). There is a great deal of controversy regarding the superiority of hand-sewn vs stapled anastomosis in preventing anastomotic leaks. A recent meta-analysis was unable to identify a difference in the radiographic leak rate with either technique (69). The single most important factor associated with anastomotic leak is the height of the anastomosis from the anal verge. Vignali and associates reviewed the results of 1014 stapled rectal anastomoses (70). Although univariate analysis identified diabetes mellitus, use of pelvic drainage, and duration of surgery as significant cofactors, multivariate analysis identified the level of anastomosis (<7 cm) as the only variable related to anastomotic leak. The difference in leak rate was 8% when the height was less than 7 cm and 1% when greater than 7 cm. Rullier et al. identified male sex and level of anastomosis as independent risk factors (71). Anastomoses within 5 cm of the anal verge were 6.5 times more likely to leak than those above 5 cm, and the risk for men was nearly 3 times greater than for women.

The performance of TME for mid and low rectal tumors results in a denuded avascular distal rectum and a heightened concern for anastomotic leakage. A review of 219 patients from Heald's group reported an 11% incidence of major leaks after TME (72). An interesting prospective study examined the effects of introducing TME as a new surgical technique (73). Patients treated with TME were compared to consecutive patients who did not have TME. The anastomotic leakage rate was double in the TME group (16%) compared to the non-TME group (8%).

With increasing use of ultralow resections, TME, and coloanal J-pouches, there is renewed interest in the use of temporary diverting stomas. The routine use of a protective stoma in low rectal anastomoses (<5 cm from the anal verge) particularly for men and obese patients has been advocated (71). Law and associates reviewed the results of 196 patients undergoing TME and observed that the presence of a diverting stoma was a significant factor in decreased anastomotic leaks (74). The benefit was particularly evident in male patients. The advantage of a defunctioning stoma in low anastomoses and coloanal pouches has recently been reported (75). Not only did patients with a diverting stoma have a decreased leak rate, but they also had less clinical sequelae (i.e., peritonitis and need for reoperation).

8. SURGEON-RELATED FACTORS

There are a variety of variables influencing outcome in patients with rectal cancer, including stage at presentation, tumor biology, and surgeon-related factors. The impact of the surgeon in patient outcome is currently under scrutiny. A wide range of morbidity and mortality rates, local recurrence rates, and survival rates among different surgeons have been reported *(76,77)*. Whether advanced fellowship training, number of operative procedures performed each year, or a combination of these two factors is responsible has not yet been determined. Harmon et al. examined the Maryland state discharge database and reported that higher-volume surgeons had improved outcomes (mortality rates, length of hospital stay, and cost) *(78)*. Interestingly, median-volume surgeons achieved equivalent results as compared to high-volume surgeons when they operated at high- or medium-volume hospitals. This implies that not only surgical experience but also the number of rectal operations performed at a specific hospital may influence patient outcome. Porter and colleagues analyzed the impact of advanced training on local recurrence and survival *(79)*. They reviewed the results of 52 surgeons performing a total of 683 operations in Edmonton, Canada. Surgeons trained in colorectal surgery had a significantly improved local recurrence rate and disease-specific survival as compared to surgeons without specialized training and less experience. However, an analysis of the Ontario Cancer Registry concluded that neither hospital volume or teaching status (institutions involved with the training of physicians) had an impact on surgical outcomes *(80)*, although there was a suggestion that high-volume hospitals had improved long-term survival. Unfortunately, because of the database design, information regarding local recurrence rates was unavailable.

9. LOCALLY ADVANCED CANCER

An estimated 10% of patients with rectal cancer will present with involvement of contiguous pelvic structures *(81)*. Patients with rectal cancer complaining of urinary symptoms, vaginal bleeding, or neuropathic pain should raise clinical suspicion of a locally advanced tumor. The ability to radiographically assess tumor infiltration of surrounding structures would greatly assist in preoperative patient preparation and operative decision-making. Currently, CT scans appear inadequate. A study recently demonstrated increased sensitivity and specificity of high-resolution magnetic resonance imaging (MRI) compared to conventional CT scans *(82)*.

Surgical management of locally advanced tumors requires en-bloc resection of the malignancy and may require multivisceral resection (prostate and bladder in men and vagina, uterus, and bladder in women). The operative intent should be complete extirpation with negative margins. The presence of either gross residual disease or microscopic margins has a detrimental impact on prognosis *(83)*. The adherence of a large rectal tumor to the surrounding tissue does not always correlate with pathologic evaluation. In fact, only 50% (range: 33–84%) of specimens suspected of tumor involvement actually demonstrated histologic invasion *(81)*. The use of CT scans and intraoperative palpation to assess bladder involvement was found to have an accuracy of only 70%, whereas the presence of bladder symptoms preoperatively was found to be more predictive *(84,85)*.

Pathologic factors associated with poor outcome include S-phase fraction greater than 10% and lymph node metastases *(86,87)*. Hida et al. reviewed their experience with multivisceral resection and observed an 82% 5-yr survival in node-negative patients, in contrast to 55% in node-positive patients *(87)*. There have been several recent reports demonstrating the ability of preoperative chemotherapy and radiotherapy to downstage locally advanced rectal cancer *(88–90)*. Mohiuddin and associates concluded that pathologic downstaging was a significant prognostic factor *(90)*. In addition to preoperative external beam radiation, Kim and associates examined the impact of intraoperative radiation therapy (IORT) *(91)*. They reported a benefit of IORT in the control of microscopic residual disease; however, no benefit was seen when gross residual disease was left, once again emphasizing the importance of complete surgical resection.

10. SUMMARY

There have been many advances during the last several decades in the surgical management of rectal cancer, including mechanical stapling devices and a better understanding of pelvic anatomy. Sphincter preservation can now be accomplished in more patients than in the past without comprising oncologic outcome, although an abdominal perineal resection should be performed when clinically indicated. The surgical technique utilizing wide anatomic resection or, as Heald advocates, TME has potential benefit in reducing local recurrences. In addition, the use of a precise surgical technique can allow for greater nerve preservation and fewer postoperative genitourinary complications.

REFERENCES

1. Breen RE and Garnjobst W. Surgical procedures for carcinoma of the rectum. A historical review. *Dis. Colon Rectum*, **26** (1983) 680–685.
2. Graney MJ and Graney CM. Colorectal surgery from antiquity to the modern era. *Dis. Colon Rectum*, **23** (1980) 432–441.
3. Hartmann H. New procedure for removal of cancers of the distal part of the pelvic colon. *Dis. Colon Rectum*, **27** (1984) 273.
4. Bissett IP and Hill GL. Extrafascial excision of the rectum for cancer: a technique for the avoidance of the complications of rectal mobilization. *Semin. Surg. Oncol.*, **18** (2000) 207–215.
5. Heald RJ and Moran BJ. Embryology and anatomy of the rectum. *Semin. Surg. Oncol.*, **15** (1998) 66–71.
6. Ondrula DP, Nelson RL, Prasad ML, Coyle BW, and Abcarian H. Multifactorial index of preoperative risk factors in colon resections. *Dis. Colon Rectum*, **35** (1992) 117–122.
7. Vining DJ. Rectal imaging and cancer. *Semin. Surg. Oncol.*, **15** (1998) 72–77.
8. Cance WG, Cohen AM, Enker WE, and Sigurdson ER. Predictive value of a negative computed tomographic scan in 100 patients with rectal carcinoma. *Dis. Colon Rectum*, **34** (1991) 748–751.
9. Wolmark N and Fisher B. An analysis of survival and treatment failure following abdominoperineal and sphincter-saving resection in Dukes' B and C rectal carcinoma. A report of the NSABP clinical trials. National Surgical Adjuvant Breast and Bowel Project. *Ann. Surg.*, **204** (1986) 480–489.
10. Holm T, Rutqvist LE, Johansson H, and Cedermark B. Abdominoperineal resection and anterior resection in the treatment of rectal cancer: results in relation to adjuvant preoperative radiotherapy. *Br. J. Surg.*, **82** (1995) 1213–1216.
11. Heimann TM, Szporn A, Bolnick K, and Aufses AH Jr. Local recurrence following surgical treatment of rectal cancer. Comparison of anterior and abdominoperineal resection. *Dis. Colon Rectum*, **29** (1986) 862–864.
12. Lavery IC, Lopez-Kostner F, Fazio VW, Fernandez-Martin M, Milsom JW, and Church JM. Chances of cure are not compromised with sphincter-saving procedures for cancer of the lower third of the rectum. *Surgery*, **122** (1997) 779–784.
13. Kwok SP, Lau WY, Leung KL, Liew CT, and Li AK. Prospective analysis of the distal margin of clearance in anterior resection for rectal carcinoma. *Br. J. Surg.*, **83** (1996) 969–972.
14. Hojo K. Anastomotic recurrence after sphincter-saving resection for rectal cancer. Length of distal clearance of the bowel. *Dis. Colon Rectum*, **29** (1986) 11–14.
15. Shirouzu K, Isomoto H, and Kakegawa T. Distal spread of rectal cancer and optimal distal margin of resection for sphincter-preserving surgery. *Cancer*, **76** (1995) 388–392.
16. Vernava AM III, Moran M, Rothenberger DA, and Wong WD. A prospective evaluation of distal margins in carcinoma of the rectum. *Surg. Gynecol. Obstet.*, **175** (1992) 333–336.
17. Quirke P, Durdey P, Dixon MF, and Williams NS. Local recurrence of rectal adenocarcinoma due to inadequate surgical resection. Histopathological study of lateral tumour spread and surgical excision. *Lancet*, **2** (1986) 996–999.

18. Reynolds JV, Joyce WP, Dolan J, Sheahan K, and Hyland JM. Pathological evidence in support of total mesorectal excision in the management of rectal cancer. *Br. J. Surg.*, **83** (1996) 1112–1115.

19. Hida J, Yasutomi M, Maruyama T, Fujimoto K, Uchida T, and Okuno K. Lymph node metastases detected in the mesorectum distal to carcinoma of the rectum by the clearing method: justification of total mesorectal excision. *J. Am. Coll. Surg.*, **184** (1997) 584–588.

20. Scott N, Jackson P, al-Jaberi T, Dixon MF, Quirke P, and Finan PJ. Total mesorectal excision and local recurrence: a study of tumour spread in the mesorectum distal to rectal cancer. *Br. J. Surg.*, **82** (1995) 1031–1033.

21. Cawthorn SJ, Parums DV, Gibbs NM, et al. Extent of mesorectal spread and involvement of lateral resection margin as prognostic factors after surgery for rectal cancer. *Lancet*, **335** (1990) 1055–1059.

22. Adam IJ, Mohamdee MO, Martin IG, et al. Role of circumferential margin involvement in the local recurrence of rectal cancer. *Lancet*, **344** (1994) 707–711.

23. de Haas-Kock DF, Baeten CG, Jager JJ, et al. Prognostic significance of radial margins of clearance in rectal cancer. *Br. J. Surg.*, **83** (1996) 781–785.

24. Ng IO, Luk IS, Yuen ST, et al. Surgical lateral clearance in resected rectal carcinomas. A multivariate analysis of clinicopathologic features. *Cancer*, **71** (1993) 1972–1976.

25. Hall NR, Finan PJ, al-Jaberi T, et al. Circumferential margin involvement after mesorectal excision of rectal cancer with curative intent. Predictor of survival but not local recurrence? *Dis. Colon Rectum*, **41** (1998) 979–983.

26. Heald RJ, Husband EM, and Ryall RD. The mesorectum in rectal cancer surgery—the clue to pelvic recurrence? *Br. J. Surg.*, **69** (1982) 613–616.

27. Heald RJ, Moran BJ, Ryall RD, Sexton R, and MacFarlane JK. Rectal cancer: the Basingstoke experience of total mesorectal excision, 1978–1997. *Arch. Surg.*, **133** (1998) 894–899.

28. Zaheer S, Pemberton JH, Farouk R, Dozois RR, Wolff BG, and Ilstrup D. Surgical treatment of adenocarcinoma of the rectum. *Ann. Surg.*, **227** (1998) 800–811.

29. Enker WE, Merchant N, Cohen AM, et al. Safety and efficacy of low anterior resection for rectal cancer: 681 consecutive cases from a specialty service. *Ann. Surg.*, **230** (1999) 544–552.

30. Bolognese A, Cardi M, Muttillo IA, Barbarosos A, Bocchetti T, and Valabrega S. Total mesorectal excision for surgical treatment of rectal cancer. *J. Surg. Oncol.*, **74** (2000) 21–23.

31. Bokey EL, Ojerskog B, Chapuis PH, Dent OF, Newland RC, and Sinclair G. Local recurrence after curative excision of the rectum for cancer without adjuvant therapy: role of total anatomical dissection. *Br. J. Surg.*, **86** (1999) 1164–1170.

32. Leong AF. Selective total mesorectal excision for rectal cancer. *Dis. Colon Rectum*, **43** (2000) 1237–1240.

33. Enker WE, Laffer UT, and Block GE. Enhanced survival of patients with colon and rectal cancer is based upon wide anatomic resection. *Ann. Surg.*, **190** (1979) 350–360.

34. Heald RJ. The "Holy Plane" of rectal surgery. *J. R. Soc. Med.*, **81** (1988) 503–508.

35. Bissett IP, McKay GS, Parry BR, and Hill GL. Results of extrafascial excision and conventional surgery for rectal cancer at Auckland Hospital. *Aust. NZ J. Surg.*, **70** (2000) 704–709.

36. Havenga K, Enker WE, Norstein J, et al. Improved survival and local control after total mesorectal excision or D3 lymphadenectomy in the treatment of primary rectal cancer: an international analysis of 1411 patients. *Eur. J. Surg. Oncol.*, **25** (1999) 368–374.

37. Hainsworth PJ, Egan MJ, and Cunliffe WJ. Evaluation of a policy of total mesorectal excision for rectal and rectosigmoid cancers. *Br. J. Surg.*, **84** (1997) 652–656.

38. Lopez-Kostner F, Lavery IC, Hool GR, Rybicki LA, and Fazio VW. Total mesorectal excision is not necessary for cancers of the upper rectum. *Surgery*, **124** (1998) 612–617.

39. Merchant NB, Guillem JG, Paty PB, et al. T3N0 rectal cancer: results following sharp mesorectal excision and no adjuvant therapy. *J. Gastrointest. Surg.*, **3** (1999) 642–647.

40. Kapiteijn E, Kranenbarg EK, Steup WH, et al. Total mesorectal excision (TME) with or without preoperative radiotherapy in the treatment of primary rectal cancer. Prospective randomised trial with standard operative and histopathological techniques. Dutch ColoRectal Cancer Group. *Eur. J. Surg.*, **165** (1999) 410–420.

41. Heald RJ, Smedh RK, Kald A, Sexton R, and Moran BJ Abdominoperineal excision of the rectum—an endangered operation. Norman Nigro Lectureship. *Dis. Colon Rectum*, **40** (1997) 747–751.

42. Havenga K, DeRuiter MC, Enker WE, and Welvaart K. Anatomical basis of autonomic nerve-preserving total mesorectal excision for rectal cancer. *Br. J. Surg.*, **83** (1996) 384–388.

43. Lindsey I, Guy RJ, Warren BF, and Mortensen NJ. Anatomy of Denonvilliers' fascia and pelvic nerves, impotence, and implications for the colorectal surgeon. *Br. J. Surg.*, **87** (2000) 1288–1299.

44. Enker WE, Havenga K, Polyak T, Thaler H, and Cranor M. Abdominoperineal resection via total mesorectal excision and autonomic nerve preservation for low rectal cancer. *World J. Surg.*, **21** (1997) 715–720.

45. Havenga K, Enker WE, McDermott K, Cohen AM, Minsky BD, and Guillem J. Male and female sexual and urinary function after total mesorectal excision with autonomic nerve preservation for carcinoma of the rectum. *J. Am. Coll. Surg.*, **182** (1996) 495–502.

46. Nesbakken A, Nygaard K, Bull-Njaa T, Carlsen E, and Eri LM. Bladder and sexual dysfunction after mesorectal excision for rectal cancer. *Br. J. Surg.*, **87** (2000) 206–210.

47. Maas CP, Moriya Y, Steup WH, Kiebert GM, Kranenbarg WM, and van de Velde CJ. Radical and nerve-preserving surgery for rectal cancer in The Netherlands: a prospective study on morbidity and functional outcome. *Br. J. Surg.*, **85** (1998) 92–97.

48. Docherty JG, McGregor JR, Akyol AM, Murray GD, and Galloway DJ. Comparison of manually constructed and stapled anastomoses in colorectal surgery. West of Scotland and Highland Anastomosis Study Group. *Ann. Surg.*, **221** (1995) 176–184.

49. Wolmark N, Gordon PH, Fisher B, et al. A comparison of stapled and handsewn anastomoses in patients undergoing resection for Dukes' B and C colorectal cancer. An analysis of disease-free survival and survival from the NSABP prospective clinical trials. *Dis. Colon Rectum*, **29** (1986) 344–350.

50. Laxamana A, Solomon MJ, Cohen Z, Feinberg SM, Stern HS, and McLeod RS. Long-term results of anterior resection using the double-stapling technique. *Dis. Colon Rectum*, **38** (1995) 1246–1250.

51. Moore JW, Chapuis PH, and Bokey EL. Morbidity and mortality after single- and double-stapled colorectal anastomoses in patients with carcinoma of the rectum. *Aust. NZ J. Surg.*, **66** (1996) 820–823.

52. Detry RJ, Kartheuser A, Delriviere L, Saba J, and Kestens PJ. Use of the circular stapler in 1000 consecutive colorectal anastomoses: experience of one surgical team. *Surgery*, **117** (1995) 140–145.

53. Otto IC, Ito K, Ye C, et al. Causes of rectal incontinence after sphincter-preserving operations for rectal cancer. *Dis. Colon Rectum*, **39** (1996) 1423–1427.

54. Matzel KE, Stadelmaier U, Muehldorfer S, and Hohenberger W. Continence after colorectal reconstruction following resection: impact of level of anastomosis. *Int. J. Colorect. Dis.*, **12** (1997) 82–87.

55. Cavaliere F, Pemberton JH, Cosimelli M, Fazio VW, and Beart RW Jr. Coloanal anastomosis for rectal cancer. Long-term results at the Mayo and Cleveland Clinics. *Dis. Colon Rectum*, **38** (1995) 807–812.

56. Gamagami RA, Liagre A, Chiotasso P, Istvan G, and Lazorthes F. Coloanal anastomosis for distal third rectal cancer: prospective study of oncologic results. *Dis. Colon Rectum*, **42** (1999) 1272–1275.

57. Parc R, Tiret E, Frileux P, Moszkowski E, and Loygue J. Resection and colo-anal anastomosis with colonic reservoir for rectal carcinoma. *Br. J. Surg.*, **73** (1986) 139–141.

58. Lazorthes F, Fages P, Chiotasso P, Lemozy J, and Bloom E. Resection of the rectum with construction of a colonic reservoir and colo-anal anastomosis for carcinoma of the rectum. *Br. J. Surg.*, **73** (1986) 136–138.

59. Hallbook O, Pahlman L, Krog M, Wexner SD, and Sjodahl R. Randomized comparison of straight and colonic J pouch anastomosis after low anterior resection. *Ann. Surg.*, **224** (1996) 58–65.

60. Seow-Choen F and Goh HS. Prospective randomized trial comparing J colonic pouch-anal anastomosis and straight coloanal reconstruction. *Br. J. Surg.*, **82** (1995) 608–610.

61. Lazorthes F, Chiotasso P, Gamagami RA, Istvan G, and Chevreau P. Late clinical outcome in a randomized prospective comparison of colonic J pouch and straight coloanal anastomosis. *Br. J. Surg.*, **84** (1997) 1449–1451.

62. Dehni N, Tiret E, Singland JD, et al. Long-term functional outcome after low anterior resection: comparison of low colorectal anastomosis and colonic J-pouch-anal anastomosis. *Dis. Colon Rectum*, **41** (1998) 817–822.

63. Hida J, Yasutomi M, Fujimoto K, et al. Functional outcome after low anterior resection with low anastomosis for rectal cancer using the colonic J-pouch. Prospective randomized study for determination of optimum pouch size. *Dis. Colon Rectum*, **39** (1996) 986–991.

64. Lazorthes F, Gamagami R, Chiotasso P, Istvan G, and Muhammad S. Prospective, randomized study comparing clinical results between small and large colonic J-pouch following coloanal anastomosis. *Dis. Colon Rectum*, **40** (1997) 1409–1413.

65. Hida J, Yasutomi M, Maruyama T, Tokoro T, Wakano T, and Uchida T. Enlargement of colonic pouch after proctectomy and coloanal anastomosis: potential cause for evacuation difficulty. *Dis. Colon Rectum*, **42** (1999) 1181–1188.

66. Hida J, Yasutomi M, Maruyama T, et al. Indications for colonic J-pouch reconstruction after anterior resection for rectal cancer: determining the optimum level of anastomosis. *Dis. Colon Rectum*, **41** (1998) 558–563.

67. Longo WE, Virgo KS, Johnson FE, et al. Outcome after proctectomy for rectal cancer in Department of Veterans Affairs Hospitals: a report from the National Surgical Quality Improvement Program. *Ann. Surg.*, **228** (1998) 64–70.

68. Pollard CW, Nivatvongs S, Rojanasakul A, and Ilstrup DM. Carcinoma of the rectum. Profiles of intraoperative and early postoperative complications. *Dis. Colon Rectum*, **37** (1994) 866–874.

69. MacRae HM and McLeod RS. Handsewn vs. stapled anastomoses in colon and rectal surgery: a meta-analysis. *Dis. Colon Rectum*, **41** (1998) 180–189.

70. Vignali A, Fazio VW, Lavery IC, et al. Factors associated with the occurrence of leaks in stapled rectal anastomoses: a review of 1,014 patients. *J. Am. Coll. Surg.*, **185** (1997) 105–113.

71. Rullier E, Laurent C, Garrelon JL, Michel P, Saric J, and Parneix M. Risk factors for anastomotic leakage after resection of rectal cancer. *Br. J. Surg.*, **85** (1998) 355–358.

72. Karanjia ND, Corder AP, Bearn P, and Heald RJ. Leakage from stapled low anastomosis after total mesorectal excision for carcinoma of the rectum. *Br. J. Surg.*, **81** (1994) 1224–1226.

73. Carlsen E, Schlichting E, Guldvog I, Johnson E, and Heald RJ. Effect of the introduction of total mesorectal excision for the treatment of rectal cancer. *Br. J. Surg.*, **85** (1998) 526–529.

74. Law WI, Chu KW, Ho JW, and Chan CW. Risk factors for anastomotic leakage after low anterior resection with total mesorectal excision. *Am. J. Surg.*, **179** (2000) 92–96.

75. Dehni N, Schlegel RD, Cunningham C, Guiguet M, Tiret E, and Parc R. Influence of a defunctioning stoma on leakage rates after low colorectal anastomosis and colonic J pouch-anal anastomosis. *Br. J. Surg.*, **85** (1998) 1114–1117.

76. Phillips RK, Hittinger R, Blesovsky L, Fry JS, and Fielding LP. Local recurrence following 'curative' surgery for large bowel cancer: I. The overall picture. *Br. J. Surg.*, **71** (1984) 12–16.

77. Holm T, Johansson H, Cedermark B, Ekelund G, and Rutqvist LE. Influence of hospital- and surgeon-related factors on outcome after treatment of rectal cancer with or without preoperative radiotherapy. *Br. J. Surg.*, **84** (1997) 657–663.

78. Harmon JW, Tang DG, Gordon TA, et al. Hospital volume can serve as a surrogate for surgeon volume for achieving excellent outcomes in colorectal resection. *Ann. Surg.*, **230** (1999) 404–411.

79. Porter GA, Soskolne CL, Yakimets WW, and Newman SC. Surgeon-related factors and outcome in rectal cancer. *Ann. Surg.*, **227** (1998) 157–167.

80. Simunovic M, To T, Baxter N, et al. Hospital procedure volume and teaching status do not influence treatment and outcome measures of rectal cancer surgery in a large general population. *J. Gastrointest. Surg.*, **4** (2000) 324–330.

81. Lopez MJ and Monafo WW. Role of extended resection in the initial treatment of locally advanced colorectal carcinoma. *Surgery*, **113** (1993) 365–372.

82. Beets-Tan RG, Beets GL, Borstlap AC, et al. Preoperative assessment of local tumor extent in advanced rectal cancer: CT or high-resolution MRI? *Abdom. Imaging*, **25** (2000) 533–541.

83. Izbicki JR, Hosch SB, Knoefel WT, Passlick B, Bloechle C, and Broelsch CE. Extended resections are beneficial for patients with locally advanced colorectal cancer. *Dis. Colon Rectum*, **38** (1995) 1251–1256.

84. Balbay MD, Slaton JW, Trane N, Skibber J, and Dinney CP. Rationale for bladder-sparing surgery in patients with locally advanced colorectal carcinoma. *Cancer*, **86** (1999) 2212–2216.

85. Law WL, Chu KW, and Choi HK. Total pelvic exenteration for locally advanced rectal cancer. *J. Am. Coll. Surg.*, **190** (2000) 78–83.

86. Meterissian SH, Skibber JM, Giacco GG, el-Naggar AK, Hess KR, and Rich TA. Pelvic exenteration for locally advanced rectal carcinoma: factors predicting improved survival. *Surgery*, **121** (1997) 479–487.

87. Hida J, Yasutomi M, Maruyama T, et al. Results from pelvic exenteration for locally advanced colorectal cancer with lymph node metastases. *Dis. Colon Rectum*, **41** (1998) 165–168.

88. Vauthey JN, Marsh RW, Zlotecki RA, et al. Recent advances in the treatment and outcome of locally advanced rectal cancer. *Ann. Surg.*, **229** (1999) 745–752.

89. Janjan NA, Khoo VS, Abbruzzese J, et al. Tumor downstaging and sphincter preservation with preoperative chemoradiation in locally advanced rectal cancer: the M. D. Anderson Cancer Center experience. *Int. J. Radiat. Oncol. Biol. Phys.*, **44** (1999) 1027–1038.

90. Mohiuddin M, Hayne M, Regine WF, et al. Prognostic significance of postchemoradiation stage following preoperative chemotherapy and radiation for advanced/recurrent rectal cancers. *Int. J. Radiat. Oncol. Biol. Phys.*, **48** (2000) 1075–1080.

91. Kim HK, Jessup JM, Beard CJ, et al. Locally advanced rectal carcinoma: pelvic control and morbidity following preoperative radiation therapy, resection, and intraoperative radiation therapy. *Int. J. Radiat. Oncol. Biol. Phys.*, **38** (1997) 777–783.

19   Conservative Management of Early-Stage Rectal Cancer

Mitchell C. Posner and Glenn D. Steele, Jr.

1. INTRODUCTION

Paradigm shifts in the management of cancer patients occur when challenges to existing treatment strategies are proven to be scientifically sound, biologically and clinically appropriate, and improve the quality of life of patients without compromising oncologic principles. The primacy of the Halsted radical mastectomy as the only viable therapeutic option for patients with operable breast cancer was inviolate for almost a century until numerous clinical trials demonstrated that breast-preserving strategies were equivalent to mastectomy in terms of their biologic outcome while maintaining a woman's positive self-image through avoidance of a mutilating procedure *(1–4)*.

Radical resection of rectal cancer, first introduced by Miles in the early 1900s in the form of abdomino-perineal resection (APR) *(5)*, has been the gold standard to which all local–regional approaches are compared. Improvements in surgical technique and instrumentation have enabled low anterior resection with primary colorectal or coloanal anastomosis to be considered an appropriate alternative to APR while avoiding a permanent colostomy. However, the morbidity and mortality of these radical approaches to distal rectal adenocarcinoma (DRA) are considerable and frequently lead to compromised function, with a resultant negative impact on patient quality of life. In a therapeutic scenario that is analogous to the introduction of breast-sparing techniques in breast cancer, considerable

From: *Colorectal Cancer: Multimodality Management*
Edited by: L. Saltz © Humana Press Inc., Totowa, NJ

enthusiasm now exists for employing conservative sphincter-sparing therapeutic approaches for selected patients with "early" rectal cancer.

Defining the patient population for which conservative surgical and nonsurgical techniques would be a viable therapeutic option is critical in determining whether these measures provide equivalent efficacy to their more traditional, radical counterparts. "Early"-stage rectal cancer refers to those tumors confined to the rectal wall with no objective evidence, either clinical, radiographic, or pathologic, of perirectal lymph node involvement. Conservation therapeutic strategies for rectal cancer must target both the primary and insidious regional lymph node disease in order to achieve the following goals: (1) cancer control that is comparable to conventional surgical therapy, (2) equivalent survival compared to radical surgery, taking into account the results of initial treatment and, if necessary, salvage therapy for local recurrence, and (3) sphincter preservation with avoidance of a permanent colostomy.

This review will detail the indications and techniques of a variety of conservative approaches to rectal cancer focusing on sphincter-sparing surgical options. We will summarize the available data, both retrospective and prospective, with regard to the outcome end points of local tumor control, results of salvage therapy, morbidity and mortality, and quality of life. Finally, the authors will offer recommendations for selection and treatment of patients with DRA based on outcome analysis and provide an assessment of relevant issues to be addressed by future clinical trials.

2. RESULTS OF TRADITIONAL RADICAL SURGERY

Transabdominal extirpative procedures, namely abdomino-perineal resection and low anterior resection, are considered the standard of care to which all conservative sphincter-sparing approaches need to be compared. The goals to be achieved with any local regional technique in the management of rectal cancer include the following: (1) optimizing long-term survival (i.e., cure), (2) minimizing local–regional failure, thereby avoiding the profound morbidity associated with local recurrence, and (3) providing patients with an acceptable quality of life posttreatment. The latter goal is a function of multiple variables related to both the disease itself and the treatment applied. No one would argue that minimizing local failure, reducing postoperative morbidity, and avoiding a permanent colostomy would substantially contribute to a patients perception of a satisfactory quality of life.

The rate of local recurrence is associated with the extent of wall penetration, presence and number of involved regional lymph nodes, tumor location and biology, surgical technique, and the use of regional and/or systemic adjuvant therapy. The results of radical surgical approaches are reviewed in detail in Chapter 18. Therefore, we will only briefly summarize treatment outcome (local recurrence, disease-free and overall survival), morbidity, and mortality associated with radical surgical techniques to provide a framework for which to compare the results of conservative management for early-stage rectal cancer. Local recurrence rates rise as the T stage increases. Local recurrence rates for patients with T1 lesions treated with either APR or low anterior resection range from 0% to 10% in reported series *(6–9)*. Rates of local recurrence for similarly treated patients with T2 tumors range from as low as 5% to as high as 20%. It is critical to point out that these recurrence rates are in patients with documented N0 disease by pathologic review. The rate of local recurrence within these subsets will vary depending on the type of pelvic dissection, the location of the tumor within the rectum (i.e., low vs mid/high), and whether adjuvant therapy has been delivered. The lowest rates of local recurrence are documented in reports from either individual investigators or institutions where strict adherence to meticulous pelvic dissection in the form of either total mesorectal excision or tumor-specific (5 cm below the distal edge of the rectal tumor) mesorectal excision is practiced *(10–12)*. Local failure is more likely when tumors are located in the lower (≤5 cm) rectum *(13,14)* and less likely with the addition of radiotherapy with or without systemic therapy *(15,16)*. Stage for stage, there appears to be no difference in local recurrence rates between APR and low anterior resection *(17–19)*.

Radical resection of carcinoma of the rectum is associated with a perioperative mortality ranging from 2% to 5% *(20–25)*. Mortality rates rise with increasing age and comorbid medical conditions. The cost to the patient, in terms of both early and late morbidity associated with radical resection, is substantial and has a significant impact on patient quality of life. Sexual dysfunction in both men and women can occur in as many as 50% of patients with equivalent complication rates reported with regard to urologic function *(26,27)*. Restorative resections (low anterior resection with either colorectal or coloanal anastomosis) have an associated anastomotic leak rate that has been reported to be as high as 20% in patients undergoing total mesorectal excision *(28–31)*. In order to avoid this devastating complication, many surgeons routinely perform a diverting ostomy, which, in the best of circumstances, is a temporary inconvenience. Many patients will forego closure of their ostomy for many months until they have completed adjuvant chemoradiotherapy and some will, unfortunately, be saddled with a permanent ostomy because of unresolved technical complications. Low pelvic anastomosis following low anterior resection, with or without adjuvant therapy, also has functional consequences related to the frequency of bowel movements, soilage, incontinence, and so forth *(32,33)*. Although the most obvious downside of an abdomino-perineal resection is the permanent colostomy, a substantial percentage of patients can have perineal wound complications. In addition, complications related to the stoma are not inconsequential and can occur in as many as 50% of patients *(34)*. Finally, complications are associated with postoperative adjuvant radiotherapy in a surgically dissected pelvis. All of the above can result in a less than satisfactory result in terms of quality of life for patients and have implications both at home and in the workplace. These issues have fueled interest in "conservative" surgical and nonsurgical strategies in the management of early-stage rectal cancer in an attempt to provide local–regional tumor control and cure while minimizing or eliminating the morbidity associated with a radical resection and avoidance of a permanent colostomy.

3. INDICATIONS FOR CONSERVATIVE MANAGEMENT

Selection of patients who are appropriate candidates for conservative approaches to rectal cancer is critical to ensure a successful outcome and to provide a "clean" cohort of patients treated in a uniform manner to determine whether nonradical surgery is a satisfactory alternative to radical surgery and would not compromise the potential for cure. Although this would seem to be a relatively simple task, data from two prospective, multi-institutional trials *(35,36)* to be described in detail later, confirm that the selection process and adherence to technical guidelines is a formidable task. In both of these prospective studies that examined the utility of local excision for rectal cancer, patients were required to have tumors that were less than 4 cm in diameter, involved <40% of the rectal circumference, and the proximal extent of the tumor was no higher than 10 cm from the anal verge. Most surgeons would agree that these guidelines define the very upper limits of what is feasible and, therefore, would only attempt local excision for smaller tumors that involve much less of the surface area of the rectum and are more easily accessible through a transanal approach. For other conservative management approaches such as endocavitary radiation and tumor ablation, the criteria are even more stringent so that these techniques can adequately encompass the tumor volume.

Whereas these anatomic considerations are crucial for appropriate patient selection, histopathologic surrogates for tumor biology may more accurately define those patients best suited to conservative management. Depth of invasion of the rectal wall is an important predictor of outcome following conservative management. Patients with tumors whose invasion is limited to the submucosa (T1) are more likely to have a long-term disease-free state than patients with tumors that either invade into (T2) or through (T3) the muscularis propria. This is most likely a result of the increased risk of perirectal lymph nodes, which correlates with the depth of penetration of the tumor into the rectal wall *(37–41)*. The risk of lymph node metastases is as high as 15% for T1 lesions, 30% for T2, and 60% for T3 rectal cancer.

Techniques that have been used to evaluate and attempt to stage early rectal cancer include digital rectal examination, computed tomography (CT) *(see* Chapter 7), endorectal ultrasound (EUS), and magnetic resonance imaging (MRI) *(see* Chapter 9). Digital examination is moderately accurate in determining the T stage, especially for T3 and greater lesions but is unable to provide any assessment of lymph node involvement and, therefore, is limited in its ability to properly select patients for conservative management. CT scanning is less accurate than either ultrasonography or MRI in determining depth of invasion and/or lymph node metastases *(42,43)*. Both EUS and MRI with an endorectal coil are the most accurate pretreatment methods of staging available with an overall accuracy of 80–90% for establishing depth of invasion and 65–80% for determining the presence of lymph node metastases *(42–46)*. The reproducibility and accuracy of staging via EUS is highly operator dependent and, therefore, the above-mentioned results are not universally applicable. Endorectal coil MRI, although equivalent in terms of its accuracy, is more expensive than EUS but may be justified in select rectal cancers that are very low lying and where the application of EUS may be technically limited if not impossible.

Other routinely available pathologic variables have been described as predictive of a more aggressive tumor biology *(47–49)*. These include poorly differentiated histology, lymphatic and/or vascular invasion, and perineural invasion. Although conclusive evidence is lacking, all of the above have been associated with tumor recurrence following local excision or standard radical surgery and may need to be taken into account in designing future trials of conservative therapy. It is hoped that the explosion in molecular technology will yield molecular and genetic markers that will prove to be useful in biologically predicting which patients are most likely to benefit from nonradical approaches to rectal carcinoma.

4. CONSERVATIVE MANAGEMENT TECHNIQUES

4.1. Nonsurgical Techniques

The alternatives to radical resection of early-stage rectal cancer can be categorized as nonsurgical and surgical conservative approaches. Nonsurgical conservative techniques include endocavitary radiotherapy, electrofulguration, and laser ablation. The therapeutic intent of all of these nonresection procedures is to destroy all viable tumor. Endocavitary radiation first described by Papillon in 1973 *(50)* can effectively control small rectal cancers with limited invasion of the rectal wall (T1) and may result in substantial palliation of more advanced lesions *(51)*. However, the specialized equipment for this technique is not readily available and the major drawbacks include the need for multiple treatments and the lack of

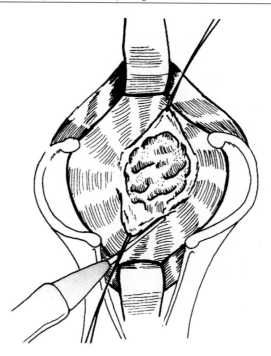

Fig. 1. Full thickness excision of low-lying rectal cancer via transanal approach.

a surgical specimen to determine pathologic stage, prognosis, and indications for additional adjuvant therapy. Fulguration in one form or another has been around for almost 100 yr but is plagued by the same issues related to the lack of pathologic specimen as endocavitary radiation and is less standardized in its application (52,53). Suffice to say that at the present time with no data available from properly controlled prospective series, none of the above techniques should be endorsed as "standard" alternatives to radical resection except in very select circumstances. These select situations would include the very elderly or other patients with substantial comorbidity that would preclude standard resection. However, with advancements in anesthesia and perioperative care, it is difficult to imagine a patient with early-stage rectal cancer who would not be a candidate for a surgical option.

4.2. Surgical Techniques

Conservative surgical approaches to early-stage rectal cancer include transanal excision, transcoccygeal or transsacral excision, and transsphincteric excision. Local excision via a transanal approach is the favored technique for conservative resection of distal rectal adenocarcinoma. Following either general or epidural anesthesia, patients are placed in the lithotomy or prone jackknife position depending on the location of the tumor. The anus is dilated and self-retaining rectal retractors are placed, often supplemented with thin-bladed deaver retractors. Traction sutures of 3-0 dexon are placed proximal to the lesion to deliver the tumor as close to the anus as possible. A full-thickness excision is then commenced with the needle-point cautery with the intent of obtaining at least a 1-cm margin in all directions (Fig. 1). The specimen is then oriented and pinned onto a corkboard for the pathologist. The defect in the rectal wall is closed with interrupted 3-0 absorbable sutures and rigid proctoscopy is performed to ensure that the rectal lumen has not been compromised. More recent advances in minimally invasive surgical equipment offer an alternative approach to

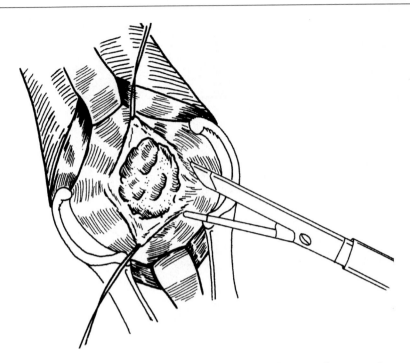

Fig. 2. Endoscopic linear stapler facilitated excision of rectal cancer via transanal approach.

tumors that are the most difficult to excise through a transanal route—those between 5 and 10 cm from the anal verge. After placement of stay sutures proximally and distally, multiple fires of a laparoscopic linear stapler can accomplish a full-thickness excision (Fig. 2).

The transcoccygeal or transsacral (Kraske) approach can be achieved with the patient in the prone jackknife position. The incision is made in the midline overlying the distal sacrum and coccyx. The coccyx is removed, and if necessary for higher lying tumors, the sacrum is partially split. The levator ani muscles are retracted laterally and the mesorectal fat and rectum encountered and mobilized. The rectal tumor is resected with a 1-cm margin and oriented for the pathologist as described previously. The rectal wall is approximated with 3-0 absorbable sutures and the remaining tissues serially closed. For transcoccygeal or transanal approaches, fecal fistula occurs in approx 5–20% of patients, often requiring a temporary proximal diversion.

The transsphincteric or York–Mason approach is similar to the above-described transcoccygeal approach except for the addition of division of the levator ani and external sphincter muscles. This procedure, because it involves division of the sphincteric mechanism, leads to a higher incidence of incontinence and is not recommended.

5. RESULTS OF CONSERVATIVE SURGICAL THERAPY

There are numerous reports that have evaluated conservative surgery for early-stage rectal cancer, the vast majority of which are small, single-institution, retrospective series that attempt to determine the efficacy of this approach. We will briefly touch on the cumulative results of these noncontrolled series of local excision alone or local excision combined with postoperative adjuvant therapy to lay the groundwork for carefully analyzing the study design and outcome of the multi-institutional prospective trials of local excision with or without chemoradiotherapy for distal rectal adenocarcinoma. Finally, we will briefly touch on the role of preoperative radiotherapy and local excision.

5.1. Local Excision Alone

The role of local excision in the treatment of rectal cancer has been explored in a number of single-institution retrospective series that have been summarized in recent reviews on the topic *(54–56)*. A wide range of local recurrence rates and survival rates have been reported that just begins to scratch the surface of the difficulty in interpreting these uncontrolled studies. Local recurrence rates as reported in these series range from 2% to 47% and 5-yr survival rates of 65–100%. The factors that are predictive of survival include depth of rectal wall invasion, poorly differentiated histology, tumor size, and positive resection margins. Separating out variables that are independent predictors of local recurrence is a challenge because of the small number of patients in most of these series. The wide latitude of rates of local recurrence and survival reflect the uncontrolled nature of these series and the heterogeneous population studied. Selection bias and variability within these series are evident when one takes into account patient inclusion criteria based on T stage and tumor size, treatment offered (local excision, ablation, adjuvant chemoradiation), surgical technique and margin status, definition of local recurrence, and survival analysis.

A recent report from the University of Minnesota is illustrative of the difficulties encountered in a retrospective analysis of local excision for early rectal cancer *(6)*. In this review, 108 patients with T1 and T2 adenocarcinoma of the rectum treated by transanal excision were compared to 153 patients with T1,N0 and T2,N0 rectal cancer treated with radical surgery. Local recurrence was significantly higher in patients treated with local excision compared to radical surgery (28% vs 4%, $p < 0.001$). This significant difference in local recurrence rates was evident for both T1 (18% local excision vs 0% radical surgery, $p < 0.03$) and T2 (47% local excision vs 6% radical surgery, $p < 0.001$) tumors. Interestingly, there was no difference between the groups with regard to cancer-specific mortality. The inherent bias and flaws of this type of retrospective review are readily apparent. The authors selected patients with known N0 disease who had undergone radical surgery in the form of low anterior resection and abdomino-perineal resection and compared them to patients with known and similar T stage but with no pathologic information regarding lymph node status who had undergone local excision alone. Because the local excision group will have as high as a 30% risk of lymph node involvement, the comparison between these unmatched groups is invalid and may reflect biologic predetermination as opposed to being a result of the type of surgery performed. In addition, the extremely high local recurrence rate in the T2 patients treated with local excision that approached 50% was substantially higher than what had been reported in the past and suggests that the technique of local excision, pathologic analysis of local excision specimens, and the definition of "local" recurrence was in no way a straightforward proposition and may have led to this unusually high rate of local recurrence. The ability to perform an appropriate full-thickness excision and to obtain an adequate circumferential and deep margin are problems that have even been encountered in well-designed prospective multi-institutional trials where surgical guidelines for excision have been explicitly outlined prior to an attempt at excision *(35,36)*. It is not unreasonable to assume that these same difficulties are encountered but not analyzable in a retrospective review where prospective inclusion and treatment standards are absent. Again, this University of Minnesota report is reflective of the difficulties encountered in all retrospective reviews, even from good groups, and provides an impetus to continue to implement prospective trials in order to determine the appropriateness of the conservative management approach. At the very least, these small uncontrolled series do suggest that select patients with small, distal rectal adenocarcinoma can undergo a sphincter-sparing conservative surgical procedure that is oncologically sound and does not compromise either local–regional control or survival.

5.2. Local Excision Plus Postoperative Adjuvant Therapy

Local recurrence following conservative surgery for rectal cancer is a result of (1) undetected microscopically positive circumferential margins and/or (2) involved regional lymph nodes. The ability of the surgeon to obtain an adequate margin of resection during local excision may be compromised by the technical limitations that are encountered during a local excision. Furthermore, despite obtaining grossly free margins, microscopic disease at the margin of resection may not be evident even following careful pathologic analysis. Most importantly, as the depth of invasion of the primary tumor increases, the risk of occult lymph node metastases substantially increases, as noted earlier. Because these factors likely contribute to local recurrence following more standard radical resections, it seems appropriate to extrapolate from multi-institutional prospective randomized trials that have demonstrated a benefit from the addition of radiation and/or chemoradiation after low anterior resection or APR to the cohort of patients undergoing local excision in attempt to reduce local recurrence.

Numerous small, single-institution retrospective series of local excision followed by either radiotherapy as a single modality or combined chemotherapy and radiation therapy in the adjuvant setting have been conducted and reported (54–56). A cumulative review of these series leads one to conclude that postoperative adjuvant therapy leads to local recurrence rates (range: 0–18%) that appear lower than those observed following local excision alone. These local recurrence rates translate into survival rates in the range 70–100%.

Three single-institution prospective series where surgical technique and the delivery of postoperative adjuvant therapy have been standardized deserve mention (Table 1). Wood and Willett (57) treated 20 patients with conservative surgery and postoperative adjuvant therapy. Utilizing transrectal ultrasound and CT scanning, patients with transmural penetration or perirectal lymph node involvement were encouraged to undergo APR and forego local excision attempts. Of the 20 patients selected for local excision, only 1 patient had a T3 lesion and 3 patients' tumors were declared Tx with no definition of the depth of invasion, with the remainder of patients being either T1 or T2. All patients received postoperative radiotherapy and 15 of the 20 patients received intravenous 500 mg/m^2 5-fluorouracil (5-FU) on the first 3 d and the last 3 d of radiation. At a median follow-up of 47 mo, local control was achieved in all patients and two patients failed at distant sites. Although this was a small series, it punctuated the need for careful selection criteria to achieve optimal local control. Ota et al. (58) at M.D. Anderson Cancer Center treated 46 patients with local excision and postoperative radiotherapy. All patients with T3 lesions and one patient with a T2 lesion and confirmed vascular invasion received 5-fluorouracil as a continuous infusion during radiotherapy. At a median follow up of 36 mo, four patients (8%) had a local recurrence, two of whom had a concurrent systemic recurrence, and four patients had a distant recurrence only. None of the 16 T1 patients had a recurrence, 1 of 15 (7%) T2 patients recurred, and 47% of the 15 T3 patients developed recurrent disease. The overall survival rate was 93% in 3 yr and the local-recurrence-free survival rate was 90%. Finally, Bleday et al. (48) at the New England Deaconess Hospital treated 48 patients with local excision and those patients with T2 or T3 lesions received adjuvant postoperative chemoradiotherapy (5400 cGy with 500 mg/m^2 5-FU delivered on the first and last 3 d concurrent with radiotherapy). At a mean follow-up of 40 mo, four (8%) patients recurred (2/21 T1, 0/21T$_2$, and 2/6 T3). Factors

Table 1
Prospective, Single Institution Series of Local Excision and Postoperative Adjuvant Therapy

Institution/author Follow-up	n Outcome	Treatment
MGH/Wood et al. Median 47 mo	20 LR 0/20 (0%) (5 T_1, 11 T_2, 1 T_3, 3 TX)	4500 cGy 5FU 500 mg/m^2 ×3 d (first and fifth week RT)
MDACC/Ota et al. Median 30 mo	46 (16 T_1, 15 T_2, 15 T_3)	5300 cGy 5FU 300 mg/m^2 for 7 T_3, 1 T_2 M–F × 5 wk
NEDH/Bleday et al. Mean 41 mo	48 (21 T_1, 21 T_2, 6 T_3)	5400 cGy 5FU 500 mg/m^2 d 1–3, 28–30 for all T_2, T_3 tumors

MGH, Massachusetts General Hospital; MCACC, M.D. Anderson Cancer Center; NEDH, New England Deaconess Hospital; 5FU, 5 fluorouracil; RT, radiotherapy; LR, local recurrence; DR, distant recurrence.

that predicted local recurrence were lymphatic invasion and an involved surgical margin. These three small prospective single-institution trials demonstrated that local excision for select patients could achieve excellent local control and that adjuvant postoperative therapy decreased the rate of local occurrence. Single-institution trials like the ones described laid the ground work for multi-institutional cooperative group trials to determine the propriety of conservative management of distal rectal adenocarcinoma.

5.3. Multi-institutional Prospective Trials of Local Excision With or Without Adjuvant Chemoradiotherapy

Two phase II prospective multi-institutional trials designed to determine the efficacy of local excision with or without adjuvant chemoradiotherapy have been completed and initial results reported *(35,36)*. Radiation Therapy Oncology Group (RTOG) Protocol 8902 included patients who were considered unsuitable for low anterior resection and would have required an APR as standard therapy. The primary tumor had to be below the pelvic peritoneal reflection and within 10 cm of the anal verge, clinically mobile, 4 cm or less in greatest diameter, and occupy 40% or less of the rectal circumference. Sixty-five patients underwent en-bloc transmural excision (Fig. 3). Patients with T1 lesions with margins of at least 3 mm, with well-differentiated or moderately differentiated cancers, 3 cm in largest diameter, no lymphatic or vascular invasion, and normal carcinoembryonic antigen (CEA) underwent no further therapy and were observed. Patients with T2 or T3 lesions or T1 lesions that did not fulfill the above criteria were treated with postoperative adjuvant radiotherapy to a total dose of 50–56 Gy with concurrent continuous infusion 5-FU (1000 mg/m^2/24 h) on the first and last 4 d of radiotherapy. Patients assigned to chemoradiotherapy who had less than 3-mm margins received an additional radiotherapy boost to the target volume to a total dose of 59.4–65 Gy. Patients could be registered before or after surgical excision with 12/65 (18%) of eligible patients registered prior to local excision. T1 lesions were histologically confirmed in 27 patients, T2 lesions in 25 patients, and T3 lesions in 13 patients. Two of

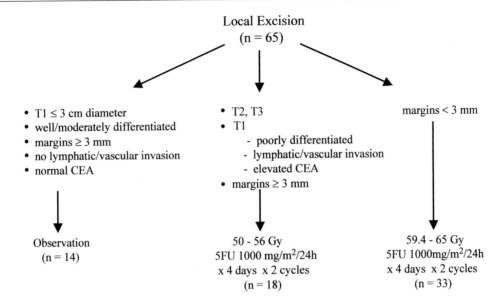

Fig. 3. Radiation Therapy Oncology Group (RTOG) protocol 8902 treatment schema.

the 65 patients were considered unevaluable based on inadequate surgical or pathologic information submitted for review. Interestingly, 60% of patients had *major* deviations in surgical compliance. Major deviations included failure to perform en-bloc transmural excision, failure to adequately assess surgical margins, failure to orient and ink the freshly excised specimen, or failure to provide preoperative measurement of clinical parameters specified in the protocol. These major deviations punctuate the difficulty in performing an adequate excision and appropriate analysis of the resected specimen.

Local and distant failure rates are listed in Table 2. At a median follow-up of 6.1 yr, 2 of 27 T1 patients, 5 of 25 T2 patients, and 4 of 13 T3 patients recurred. Salvage surgery was attempted in five patients who recurred with initial local failure and was successful in achieving local control in all five patients, although four of these five patients developed distant metastases. Actual freedom from pelvic relapse was 88% at 5 yr. RTOG 8902 closed to patient registration when Cancer and Leukemia Group B (CALGB) 8984 was activated as an intergroup study with participation of the Southwest Oncology Group, the Eastern Cooperative Oncology Group, and the RTOG.

CALGB 8984, an intergroup, multi-institutional phase II trial, registered patients with biopsy-proven adenocarcinoma of the rectum ≤10 cm proximal to the dentate line, ≤4 cm diameter, and involving ≤40% of the rectal circumference. Of the 177 patients registered before operation, 161 patients had an attempt at full-thickness complete excision. Fifty-one patients did not meet the eligibility criteria and were excluded based on involved or unclear pathologic margins and tumor stage greater than T2 or less than T1. Of the 110 patients who met all of the postsurgical eligibility requirements, 59 patients had T1 lesions and 51 patients had T2 lesions. As per protocol design, patients with T1 lesions underwent no further treatment following complete excision and were observed for recurrence and survival. Patients with T2 lesions received adjuvant radiotherapy to a total dose of 5400 cGy with concurrent bolus infusion 5-FU (500 mg/m^2) on the first 3 d and the last 3 d of radiotherapy. Recurrence and survival rates are summarized in Tables 3 and 4. At a median follow-up of 48 mo, 4 of 59 T1 patients recurred. Three patients had a local recurrence, two local only, and one with local and distant failure. Both patients with local-only recurrence

Table 2
RTOG 8902 Patterns of Failure

	T stage			
Recurrence	T_1 (n = 27)	T_2 (n = 25)	T_3 (n = 13)	Total (n = 65)
Local alone	1 (4%)	2 (8%)	0	3 (5%)
Distant alone	1 (4%)	1 (4%)	1 (8%)	3 (5%)
Local and distant	0	2 (8%)	3 (23%)	5 (8%)
Total	2 (7%)	5 (20%)	4 (31%)	11 (17%)

Table 3
CALGB 8984 T_1 Failures (48 mo Follow-Up)

Recurrence	n (%)	Outcome
Local only	2 (3%)	APR
	1	– NED
	1	– DOD
Liver Only	1 (2%)	Resect–NED
Local and Distant	1 (2%)	– NED
Total	4 (7%)	
	2	– NED
	2	– DOD

APR, abdominoperineal resection; NED, no evidence of disease; DOD, dead of disease.

Table 4
CALGB 8984 T_2 Failures (48 mo Follow-Up)

Recurrence	n (%)	Outcome
Local only	5 (10%)	APR
	4	– NED
	1	– DOD
Distant Only	3 (6%)	– DOD
Local and Distant	2 (4%)	APR–DOD
Total	10 (20%)	
	4	– NED
	6	– DOD

APR, abdominoperineal resection; NED, no evidence of disease; DOD, dead of disease.

underwent APR as salvage, with one patient disease-free at last follow-up. Ten of 51 (20%) T2 patients had recurrence, 7 of whom had either a local-only recurrence or combined local and distant failure. Of the five patients with local-only recurrence, four remain free of disease following salvage APR and one patient died of distant disease. The two patients with concurrent local and distant failure also underwent APR, both of whom died of distant disease. Overall and failure-free survival at 6 yr for T1 patients was 87% and 83%, respectively, whereas for patients with T2 lesions, overall and failure-free survival was 85% and 71%, respectively. It is interesting to note that the investigators point out that the survival for all eligible patients in this study of local excision, with or without chemoradiation,

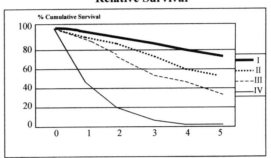

Fig. 4. Survival of patients with stage I rectal cancer treated by local excision in the CALGB 8984 trial and survival of stage I patients registered in the National Cancer Data Base.

almost exactly paralleled the survival of stage I patients registered in the National Cancer Database treated for the most part with radical resection (Fig. 4). These data, like those reported in the RTOG Trial, suggest that carefully selected patients with T1 and T2 distal rectal adenocarcinoma can be approached with conservative surgical techniques that preserve sphincter function and achieve excellent tumor control.

5.4. Preoperative Radiotherapy Plus Local Excision

The theoretical advantage of preoperative radiotherapy is to convert a patient who initially was deemed not a candidate for local excision to one, through downstaging, in whom local excision is now feasible. There is no direct evidence that this outcome can be achieved or whether any detrimental effects would occur by altering the proposed procedure postradiotherapy. Results from a number of small single-institution series *(59,60)* suggest that (1) downstaging can occur and (2) that local control can be achieved. Obviously, this question would need to be addressed in the context of a controlled, prospective, multi-institutional trial to determine whether the goals of preoperative radiotherapy can be realized, evaluate whether this approach provides adequate tumor control, and define a group of patients for whom this technique is appropriate. It is safe to say that in the vast majority of patients, there would not appear to be any clear advantage of preoperative chemoradiotherapy over postoperative chemoradiotherapy and the major disadvantage of preoperative chemoradiotherapy is the lack of a nontreated surgical specimen to accurately stage the primary tumor. This approach in other solid tumors, most notably the breast, has been proven to be effective and it would seem to be most appropriate in patients with T3 lesions with significant comorbid conditions who would not be a candidate for radical resection or patients who refuse the more standard surgical option.

6. SALVAGE SURGERY FOR LOCAL RECURRENCE

The concern regarding the rate of local recurrence in patients treated with conservative management techniques for distal rectal adenocarcinoma would be moot if all such patients could be cured by subsequent radical resection. Of the seven patients in CALGB 8984 who sustained a local failure as their only manifestation of disease recurrence, five were salvaged by APR with no evidence of recurrent disease at last follow-up. However, durability of salvage is still unclear because of an inadequate follow-up interval. In RTOG 8902, five patients who recurred with initial local failure underwent attempted surgical salvage;

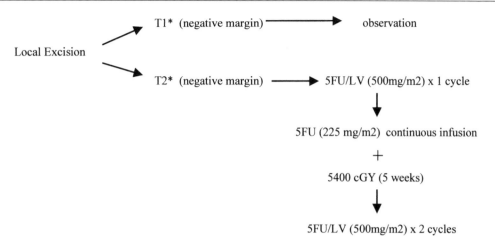

* must have no lymphatic, vascular or perineural invasion

Fig. 5. Proposed schema for next generation CALGB sphincter sparing trial of distal rectal adenocarcinoma.

however, four of these five patients ultimately developed distant disease. At the present time, it is therefore uncertain whether salvage resection provides the same chance of cure as a radical resection performed at the time of primary tumor presentation as the initial procedure. As in earlier studies of breast cancer, the obvious question is whether local recurrence of rectal cancer is a cause of subsequent distant metastases or simply a marker of more aggressive tumor biology. If the situation is analogous to breast cancer in which local recurrence following breast-sparing surgery appears to be a surrogate marker for distant failure, then conservative management approaches for appropriately selected patients with distal rectal adenocarcinoma pose no additional risks. However, because of the small number of local recurrences witnessed to date and the short follow-up time following attempts at salvage radical resection, no definitive conclusion can yet be drawn regarding the efficacy of rescue therapy.

7. AUTHORS' TREATMENT RECOMMENDATIONS

The multi-institutional prospective cooperative group trials have provided important natural history information and a foundation upon which subsequent trials can be built. However, as would be expected, many questions remain unanswered and issues unresolved. These include (1) the ideal pretreatment staging method, (2) defined selection criteria for conservative management of pathologic T1, T2, and even some T3 lesions, (3) optimal therapeutic regimen, and (4) the efficacy of rescue radical resection. Although these issues remain outstanding, it would seem most appropriate to recommend that patients considered candidates for conservative management of their distal rectal adenocarcinoma be treated under the auspices of a clinical trial. The CALGB will be initiating a replacement study for the closed 8984 trial. The schema for this intergroup study is detailed in Fig. 5. Understanding that less than 2% of patients will enter a clinical trial, the authors recommend the following for patients for whom conservative approaches are contemplated. Patients with rectal lesions ≤3 cm in greatest diameter and ≤1/3 of the circumference of the rectal wall should undergo endorectal ultrasound as the most appropriate pretreatment staging tool available at the present time. Following full-thickness, en-bloc excision of the rectal cancer, patients with

T1 lesions with free margins of resection and no evidence of vascular/lymphatic/perineural invasion or with well-differentiated histology require no further treatment and should be placed in a long-term follow-up program. Patients with T1 lesions that do not fit the above criteria or T2 lesions on final histologic review should be treated with postoperative adjuvant chemoradiotherapy. The therapeutic regimen outlined in 8984 is appropriate; however, the authors recognize that continuous infusion 5-FU throughout the course of radiation therapy is now considered standard, following traditional resection of rectal cancer, and although no data regarding its utility following local excision are available, the toxicity profile for this regimen is well described and, therefore, its use may be considered reasonable. Patients with T3 rectal adenocarcinoma should be offered standard radical resection as the best available option for treatment of their cancer. All patients offered a conservative therapeutic option should understand the potential risks involved with increased rates of local recurrence, although the exact implications of local recurrence and the value of salvage resection is not yet fully understood in this setting.

8. FUTURE ISSUES

Future studies will be required to address the pivotal issues related to conservative management approaches to rectal cancer and to define the exact role of nontraditional sphincter-sparing techniques in the management of patients with distal rectal adenocarcinoma. It is hoped that advances and refinements in imaging technology will more accurately stage patients prior to any therapeutic intervention. Combining this with more sophisticated molecular genetic markers in addition to using validated histologic prognosticators of outcome will provide substantive criteria to select patients who are ideally suited to nonradical surgical management. Establishing the optimal therapeutic regimen to control both local and distant failure following local incision will be essential to the success of conservative management of rectal cancer. Extrapolation from phase III trials of adjuvant postoperative chemoradiotherapy following standard, radical resections would seem to be appropriate, and as more novel and efficacious agents are introduced into therapeutic armamentarium, these also should be examined in this setting. Furthermore, the value of induction chemoradiotherapy prior to local excision with or without postoperative adjuvant therapy needs to be examined within the context of a controlled trial. This approach may actually expand the indications and increase the number of patients who are candidates for conservative management approaches. It is imperative that the utility of salvage resection be determined. As mentioned earlier, if salvage radical resection of local recurrence leads to an outcome that is no worse than patients treated initially with standard radical resection, then conservative management techniques become more attractive as a primary therapeutic option and the indications for exercising this option increase.

The only way to answer these questions adequately is to critically analyze patient outcome within the context of a clinical trial. The biologic significance of this issue is paramount and could potentially elevate conservation rectal sparing surgery to the same level as lumpectomy for the management of breast cancer. Finally, the future of clinical trials examining the role of local excision without adjuvant therapy should incorporate quality-of-life instruments in order to determine functional outcome following this sphincter-sparing approach. Although all assume that quality of life is enhanced by the avoidance of a colostomy, function must be carefully scrutinized following sphincter preservation to ensure that the outcome is acceptable.

There is no doubt that conservative management techniques have a role in the management of patients with rectal cancer. It is incumbent on all surgeons and oncologists who care for these patients to delineate the appropriateness of this procedure and, along with our patients, be confident in the outcome from both an oncologic and quality-of-life perspective.

REFERENCES

1. Fisher B, Anderson S, Redmond CK, Wolmark N, Wickerham DL, and Cronin WM. Reanalysis and results after 12 years of follow-up in a randomized clinical trial comparing total mastectomy with lumpectomy with or without irradiation in the treatment of breast cancer. *N. Engl. J. Med.*, **333(22)** (1995) 1456–1461.

2. Blichert-Toft M, Rose C, Andersen JA, Overgaard M, Axelsson CK, Andersen KW, et al. Danish randomized trial comparing breast conservation therapy with mastectomy: six years of life-table analysis. Danish Breast Cancer Cooperative Group. *J. Natl. Cancer Inst. Monogr.*, **11** (1992) 19–25.

3. Jacobson JA, Danforth DN, Cowan KH, d'Angelo T, Steinberg SM, Pierce L, et al. Ten-year results of a comparison of conservation with mastectomy in the treatment of stage I and II breast cancer. *N. Engl. J. Med.*, **332(14)** (1995) 907–911.

4. Veronesi U, Salvadori B, Luini A, Greco M, Saccozzi R, del Vecchio M, et al. Breast conservation is a safe method in patients with small cancer of the breast. Long-term results of three randomised trials on 1,973 patients. *Eur. J. Cancer*, **31A(10)** (1995) 1574–1579.

5. Miles WE. A method of performing abdominoperineal excision for carcinoma of the rectum and the terminal portion of the pelvic colon. *Lancet*, **2** (1908) 1812–1813.

6. Mellgren A, Sirivongs P, Rothenberger D, Madoff RD, and Garcia-Aguilar J. Is local excision adequate therapy for early rectal cancer? *Dis. Colon Rectum*, **43** (2000) 1064–1074.

7. Sticca RP, Rodriguez-Bigas M, Penetrante RB, et al. Curative resection for stage I rectal cancer: natural history, prognostic factors, and recurrence patterns. *Cancer Invest.*, **14(5)** (1996) 491–497.

8. Willet CG, Lewandrowski K, Donnelly S, et al. Are there patients with stage I rectal carcinoma at risk for failure after abdominoperineal resection? *Cancer*, **69** (1992) 1651–1655.

9. McCall, JL, Cox MR, and Wattchow DA. Analysis of local recurrence rates after surgery alone for rectal cancer. *Int. J. Colorect. Dis.*, **10** (1995) 126–132.

10. Heald RJ, Chir M, Moran BJ, Ryall RDH, Sexton R, and MacFarlane JK. Rectal cancer. The Basingstoke experience of total mesorectal excision, 1978–1997. *Arch. Surg.*, **133** (1998) 894–899.

11. Lopez-Kostner F, Lavery IC, Hool GR, Rybicki LA, and Fazio VW. Total mesorectal excision is not necessary for cancers of the upper rectum. *Surgery*, **124** (1998) 612–618.

12. Enker WE, Havenga K, Polyak T, Thaler H, and Cranor M. Abdominoperineal resection via total mesorectal excision and autonomic nerve preservation for low rectal cancer. *World J. Surg.*, **21** (1997) 715–720.

13. McDermott FT, Hughes ESR, Pihl E, et al. Local recurrence after potentially curative resection for rectal cancer in a series of 1008 patients. *Br. J. Surg.*, **72** (1985) 34–47.

14. Moosa AR, Ree PC, Parks JE, et al. Factors influencing local recurrence after abdominoperineal resection for cancer of the rectum and rectosigmoid. *Br. J. Surg.*, **62** (1975) 727–730.

15. Krook JE, Moertel CG, Gunderson LL, et al. Effective surgical adjuvant therapy for high-risk rectal carcinoma. *N. Engl. J. Med.*, **324** (1991) 709–715.

16. Fisher B, Wolmark N, Rockette H, et al. Postoperative adjuvant chemotherapy or radiation therapy for rectal cancer: results from NSABP protocol R-01. *J. Natl. Cancer Inst.*, **80** (1988) 21–29.

17. Wolmark N and Fisher B. An analysis of survival and treatment failure following abdominoperineal and sphincter-saving resection in Dukes' B and C rectal carcinoma. *Ann. Surg.*, **204(4)** (1986) 480–489.

18. Heimann TM, Szporn A, Bolnick K, et al. Local recurrence following surgical treatment of rectal cancer: comparison of anterior and abdominoperineal resection. *Dis. Colon Rectum*, **29** (1986) 862–864.

19. Odou MW and O'Connell TX. Changes in the treatment of rectal carcinoma and effects on local recurrence. *Arch. Surg.*, **121** (1986) 1114–1116.

20. Rothenberger DA and Wong WD. Abdominoperineal resection for adenocarcinoma of the low rectum. *World J. Surg.*, **16** (1992) 478.

21. Arenas RB, Fichera A, Mhoon D, et al. Total mesenteric excision in the surgical treatment of rectal cancer: a prospective study. *Arch. Surg.*, **133** (1998) 608–611.

22. Jatzko GR, Jagoditsch M, Lisborg PH, et al. Long-term results of radical surgery for rectal cancer: multivariate analysis of prognostic factors influencing survival and local recurrence. *Eur. J. Surg. Oncol.*, **25** (1999) 284–291.

23. Enker WE, Thaler HT, Cranor MI, et al. Total mesorectal excision in the operative treatment of carcinoma of the rectum. *J. Am. Coll. Surg.*, **181** (1995) 335–346.

24. Sugihara K, Moriya Y, Akasu T, et al. Pelvic autonomic nerve preservation for patients with rectal carcinoma: oncologic and functional outcome. *Cancer*, **78** (1996) 1871–1880.

25. Zaheer S, Pemberton JH, Farouk R, et al. Surgical treatment of adenocarcinoma of the rectum. *Ann. Surg.*, **227** (1998) 800–811.
26. Pollard CW, Nivatvongs S, Rojanasakul A, et al. Carcinoma of the rectum: profiles of intraoperative and early postoperative complications. *Dis. Colon Rectum*, **25** (1982) 866–874.
27. Rosen L, Veidenheimer MC, Coller JA, et al. Mortality, morbidity and patterns of recurrence after abdominoperineal resection for cancer of the rectum. *Dis. Colon Rectum*, **25** (1994) 202–205.
28. Hojo K, Sawada T, and Moriya Y. An analysis of survival and voiding, sexual function after wide iliopelvic lymphadenectomy in patients with carcinoma of the rectum, compared with conventional lymphadenectomy. *Dis. Colon Rectum*, **32** (1989) 128–133.
29. Heald RJ, Chir M, Smedh RK, Kald A, Sexton R, and Moran BJ. Abdominoperineal excision of the rectum-An endangered operation. *Dis. Colon Rectum*, **40** (1997) 747–751.
30. Hainsworth PJ, Egan MJ, and Cunliff WJ. Evaluation of a policy of total mesorectal excision for rectal and rectosigmoid cancers. *Br. J. Surg.*, **84** (1997) 652–656.
31. Aitken RJ. Mesorectal excision for rectal cancer. *Br. J. Surg.*, **83** (1996) 214–216.
32. Kollmorgen CF, Meagher AP, Wolff BG, Pemberton JH, Martenson JA, and Illstrup DM. The long-term effect of adjuvant postoperative chemoradiotherapy for rectal carcinoma on bowel function. *Ann. Surg.*, **220(5)** (1994) 676–682.
33. Karanjia ND, Schache DJ, and Heald RJ. Function of the distal rectum after low anterior resection for carcinoma. *Br. J. Surg.*, **79** (1992) 114–116.
34. Williams NS and Johnston D. The quality of life after rectal excision for low rectal cancer. *Br. J. Surg.*, **70** (1983) 460–462.
35. Steele GD Jr, Herndon JE, Bleday R, Russell A, Benson A III, Hussain M, et al. Sphincter-sparing treatment for distal rectal adenocarcinoma. *Ann. Surg. Oncol.*, **6(5)** (1999) 433–442.
36. Russell AH, Harris J, Rosenberg PJ, Sause WT, Fisher BJ, Hoffman JP, et al. Anal sphincter conservation for patients with adenocarcinoma of the distal rectum: long-term results of Radiation Therapy Oncology Group protocol 89-02. *Int. J. Radiat. Oncol. Biol. Phys.*, **45(2)** (2000) 313–322.
37. Brodsky JT, Richard GK, Cohen AM, and Minsky BD. Variables correlated with the risk of lymph node metastasis in early rectal cancer. *Cancer*, **69** (1992) 322–326.
38. Morson BC. Factors influencing the prognosis of early cancer of the rectum. *Proc. R. Soc. Med.*, **59** (1966) 607–608.
39. Sitzler PJ, Seow-Choen F, Ho YH, and Leong AP. Lymph node involvement and tumor depth in rectal cancers: an analysis of 805 patients. *Dis. Colon Rectum*, **40** (1997) 1472–1476.
40. Huddy SPJ, Husband EM, Cook MG, et al. Lymph node metastases in early rectal cancer. *Br. J. Surg.*, **80** (1993) 1457–1458.
41. Saclarides TJ, Bhattacharyya AK, Britton-Kuzel C, et al. Predicting lymph node metastases in rectal cancer. *Dis. Colon Rectum*, **37** (1994) 52–57.
42. Kim NK, Kim MJ, Yun SH, Sohn SK, and Min JS. Comparative study of transrectal ultrasonography, pelvic computerized tomography, and magnetic resonance imaging in preoperative staging of rectal cancer. *Dis. Colon Rectum*, **42(6)** (1999) 770–775.
43. Merrick SH. Improving the treatment of colorectal cancer: the role of EUS. *Cancer Invest.*, **16(8)** (1998) 572–581.
44. Massari M, De Simone M, Cioffi U, Rosso L, Chiarelli M, and Gabrielli F. Value and limits of endorectal ultrasonography for preoperative staging of rectal carcinoma. *Surg. Laparoscopy Endoscopy*, **8(6)** (1998) 438–444.
45. Akasu T, Kondo H, Moriya Y, Sugihara K, Gotoda T, Fujita S, et al. Endorectal ultrasonography and treatment of early stage rectal cancer. *World J. Surg.*, **24(9)** (2000) 1061–1068.
46. Gualdi GF, Casciani E, Guadalaxara A, d'Orta C, Polettini E, and Pappalardo G. Local staging of rectal cancer with transrectal ultrasound and endorectal magnetic resonance imaging: comparison with histologic findings. *Dis. Colon Rectum*, **43(3)** (2000) 338–345.
47. D'Eredita G, Serio G, Nrei V, et al. A survival regression analysis of prognostic factors in colorectal cancer. *Aust. NZ J. Surg.*, **66** (1996) 445–451.
48. Bleday R, Breen E, Jessup JM, et al. Prospective evaluation of local excision for small rectal cancers. *Dis Colon Rectum*, **40** (1997) 388–392.
49. Bognel C, Rekacewicz C, Mankarios H, et al. Prognostic value of neural invasion in rectal carcinoma: a multivariate analysis on 339 patients with curative resection. *Eur. J. Cancer*, **45** (1995) 894–898.
50. Papillon J. Endocavitary radiation of early rectal cancers for cure: a series of 123 cases. *Proc. R. Soc. Med.*, **66** (1973) 1179–1183.
51. Gerard JP, Romenstaing P, Ardiet JM, et al. Sphincter preservation in rectal cancer: endocavitary radiation therapy. *Semin. Radiat. Oncol.*, **8** (1998) 13–23.

52. Hughes EP, Veidenheimer MC, Cormal ML, et al. Electrocoagulation of rectal cancer. *Dis. Colon Rectum*, **25** (1982) 215–219.

53. Salvati EP, Rubin RJ, Eisenstat TE, et al. Electrocoagulation of selected carcinoma of the rectum. *Surg. Gynecol. Obstet.*, **166** (1998) 393–397.

54. Weber TK and Petrelli NJ. Local excision for rectal cancer: an uncertain future. *Oncology*, **12(6)** (1998) 933–947.

55. Bleday R. Local excision of rectal cancer. *World J. Surg.*, **21** (1997) 706–714.

56. Bleday R and Steele G Jr. Current protocols and outcomes of local therapy for rectal cancer. *Surg. Oncol. Clin. North Am.*, **9(4)** (2000) 751–758.

57. Wood WC and Willett CG. Update of the Massachusetts General Hospital experience of combined local excision and radiotherapy for rectal cancer. *Surg. Oncol. Clin. North Am.*, **1** (1992) 131–136.

58. Ota DM, Skibber J, and Rich TA. Anderson Cancer Center experience with local excision and multimodality therapy for rectal cancer. *Surg. Oncol. Clin. North Am.*, **1** (1992) 147–152.

59. Otmezguine Y, Grimard L, Calitchi E, et al. A new combined approach in the conservative management of rectal cancer. *Int. J. Radiat. Oncol. Biol. Phys.*, **17(3)** (1989) 539–545.

60. Mohiuddin M, Marks G, and Bannon J. High-dose preoperative radiation and full thickness local excision: a new option for selected T-3 distal rectal cancers. *Int. J. Radiat. Oncol. Biol. Phys.*, **30(4)** (1994) 845–849.

20 Surgical Management of Hepatic Colorectal Metastases

William R. Jarnagin and Yuman Fong

CONTENTS

1. INTRODUCTION

The liver is the most common site for hematogeneous spread of cancers of colorectal origin. Nearly half of all patients with colorectal cancer will develop hepatic involvement at some point. Until recently, patients with hepatic colorectal metastases were given no hope of long-term survival. The mistaken belief that hematogeneous metastases are always widely distributed dictated that therapy directed at hepatic metastases was unlikely to impact the natural history of the disease. Furthermore, hepatic resection was previously associated with a very high mortality and major consumption of hospital resources and was therefore considered impractical as a treatment option. Data over the last three decades, however, have shown that both views are inaccurate. Of the approx 50,000 annual cases of hepatic colorectal metastases (1) encountered in the United States, a large proportion are amenable to potentially curative resection. This observation, combined with the increasing safety of hepatic resection in general, prompted several centers to pursue surgery as possible treatment for this disease.

The current status of resection as the most effective therapy for hepatic colorectal metastases is not the result of carefully planned and executed randomized studies. On the contrary, no randomized trial comparing resection to any other therapy has ever been completed. There are, however, data regarding the natural history of patients with unresected disease, which is rapidly fatal; median survival of 5–10 mo is typically reported in this setting (2–7). It has been argued that the improved results of resection is largely the result

From: *Colorectal Cancer: Multimodality Management*
Edited by: L. Saltz © Humana Press Inc., Totowa, NJ

Table 1
Results of Liver Resection for Metastatic Colorectal Cancer;
Published Series with More Than 200 Patients

Study	n	Operative Mortality (%)	Survival			
			1 yr (%)	5 yr (%)	10 yr (%)	Median (mo)
Hughes et al. 1986 (15)	607[a]	—	—	33	—	—
Scheele et al. 1991 (16)	109	6		39		
Rosen et al. 1992 (17)	280	4		25		
Gayowski et al. 1994 (18)	204	0	91	32	33	
Scheele et al. 1995 (10)	359	4	83	33	20	40
Fong et al. 1997 (19)	577	4	85	35	—	40
Nordlinger et al. 1992 (20)	1568[a]	2		28		
Jamison et al. 1997 (10)	280	4	84	27	20	33
Fong et al. 1999 (11)	1001	3		37		

[a]Multi-institutional reviews.

of patient selection. However, patients with limited hepatic disease, who would now be considered candidates for resection, do poorly when either not treated or treated with systemic therapy alone. In older studies addressing this issue, patients with clinically limited but unresected disease had a 1-yr survival of 77%, a 3-yr survival of 14–23%, and a 5-yr survival of 2–8% (8,9).

Improved survival can be achieved with systemic chemotherapy. It is important to emphasize, however, that complete response and a 5-yr survival with any chemotherapeutic regimen are rare. By contrast, median survival of patients after resection is on the order of 40 mo (10–12), 5-yr survival is 30–40%, and 10-yr survival is approx 20%. These comparative results have made any random-assignment trial of resection vs nonresectional approach unethical. It is generally accepted that surgery is the standard therapy for metastatic disease isolated to the liver.

2. RESULTS OF HEPATIC RESECTION

Hepatic resection for metastatic colorectal cancer was not immediately embraced, even after initial reports had shown its potential utility (13). The first significant study that showed a clear survival benefit of resection was from James Foster. This multicenter series analyzed cases from 99 institutions and demonstrated a 20% 5-yr survival in 168 patients following resection (14). Several studies have since been published confirming these initial favorable results (10,11,15–21). Table 1 lists all published series to date with more than 200 patients. After resection, approximately one-third of the patients survive 5 yr and median survival ranges from 28 to 40 mo. In two series with sufficient follow-up, 10-yr survival is approximately 20% (10,21). The accumulated data show clearly that appropriately selected patients can benefit from hepatic resection and a substantial percentage of patients may be cured. Additionally, the increasing safety of major hepatic resections has become evident from published reports over the past several years. Operative mortality at most major centers is less than 5% (15–18,21–32). The improvement in the safety with which these operations can now be performed coupled with the favorable long-term results have prompted an increasingly aggressive surgical approach and may explain the plateau in operative mortality

Table 2
Selection Criteria for Hepatectomy

General medical condition
    Patient with symptomatic cardiopulmonary disease or asymptomatic patients over
        age 65 are sent for cardiopulmonary evaluation
Extent of disease[a]
    Colonoscopy within 6 mo
    Helical CT of abdomen and pelvis
    Chest X-ray
Adequate residual liver
    Baseline liver function
    CT portography
Biology of disease
    Clinical risk score

[a]Patients should have disease limited to the liver, although patients with colonic recurrence or limited lung metastases are occasionally considered.

at approx. 2–4%. Extended hepatic resection or trisegmentectomies are now routine at many centers. Because of the improved perioperative results, the technical and medical limits have been redefined and continue to evolve.

3. PREOPERATIVE EVALUATION

The favorable results of hepatectomy are results not only of improvements in operative technique and perioperative care but also, in large measure, of refinements in patient selection criteria. In general, three criteria must be met before patients are considered for resection: (1) medically fit for major surgery, (2) disease limited to the liver, and (3) resection that removes all hepatic disease and preserves adequate liver parenchyma for full recovery. In addition to these minimal criteria, disease biology is increasingly recognized as a potent predictor of outcome, although attempts to quantify this in a clinically useful manner have been difficult. Sufficient data now exist, however, to use clinical factors related to the primary lesions and the hepatic metastases to identify patients most likely to benefit from resection (Table 2).

From a general health standpoint, assessing patients for liver resection is no different than for other major operations. Active patients, under age 65, with no history or signs of cardiopulmonary disease tolerate liver resection without undue risk of postoperative cardiopulmonary complications. Patients with a history of cardiopulmonary disease and most patients over age 65 are routinely sent for formal cardiopulmonary evaluation. Pulmonary disease in particular is of concern because the pain associated with a high abdominal incision and the inevitable postoperative pleural effusion combine to limit respiratory effort.

Advanced age was once considered a complete contraindication for major liver resection *(33)*. However, recent data show that age alone should not preclude patients from resection *(10,29,34)*. Older patients, without coexisting major medical problems, have no greater operative morbidity than do younger patients *(35)*.

3.1. Evaluating the Extent of Disease

In assessing the extent of disease, studies should be targeted at the most likely sites of extrahepatic metastases. A colonoscopy showing no evidence of recurrent cancer should be done within 12 mo of the proposed liver resection. This is essential because anastomotic recurrences or second primaries may be treated at the same laparotomy or may defer the liver resection until after the colon resection. A high-quality computed tomography (CT) scan of the abdomen and pelvis within 4–6 wk of operation is also important, allowing evaluation of both hepatic and extrahepatic sites of disease (36). Many surgeons and oncologists would consider a chest CT as a standard preoperative investigation; however, we advocate evaluation of the chest with a posteroanterior (PA) and lateral chest radiograph. This change in philosophy arose from the documented low yield of chest CT in patients with normal chest radiographs (37). Two-thirds of lesions found on chest CT and not visible on plain chest films are benign, but they may, nevertheless, prompt invasive diagnostic maneuvers and anxiety.

[18]F-fluoroxyglucose–whole-body positron-emission tomography (FDG-PET) is an emerging modality that is being used increasingly for disease staging in patients with metastatic colorectal cancer (see Chapter 10). This technique exploits the higher rates of glucose uptake and utilization in malignant cells compared to normal cells. The positron-emitting glucose analog-2 [^{18}F]-fluoro-2-deoxyglucose (FDG) is selectively transported into and retained in tumor cells, and whole-body imaging is performed to assess for glucose avid areas (38,39). To date, four studies have examined the utility of FDG-PET in this patient population, and the results suggest that therapy is changed in up to 25% of patients (40–43). It is important to point out that a positive FDG-PET result does not prove the existence of cancer, as areas of inflammation are also glucose avid. Furthermore, the increased yield of PET scanning will depend on the quality of other imaging studies. Prospective studies are needed and are ongoing to verify these data and to clearly define the role of PET scanning.

A major determinant of resectability is the extent of hepatic parenchyma that must be removed, which is not necessarily a function of hepatic tumor volume only. Indeed, in many patients, the volume of disease is such that even a radical resection will not remove all of the tumors; however, others may have limited disease that is located near major vascular structures such that resection would compromise the vascular integrity of the liver remnant. It is important to emphasize that decisions regarding the technical aspects of resection should be made in conjunction with an experienced hepatic surgeon. Following hepatic resection in the noncirrhotic patient, liver regeneration occurs rapidly, and up to 80% of functional parenchyma can be removed with the expectation of recovery (44). In practical terms, this means that six of eight liver segments can be removed with relative safety; however, the operative mortality is increased somewhat with more extensive resections (10,11). Accurate assessment of hepatic disease extent is imperative for surgical planning, both to avoid unnecessary exploration for those with disease that is not amenable to complete resection and to allow planning of resections to best extirpate disease while preserving the maximal parenchyma for recovery.

Computed tomographic portography (CTAP) remains the most sensitive test for full assessment of hepatic lesions. During CTAP, contrast is injected into the superior mesenteric artery and rapidly reaches the portal circulation. Timed scans are then obtained during the arterial and portal venous phases. This study also provides added information regarding the hepatic arterial supply, which is important in patients who will undergo placement of an hepatic artery infusion pump. Colorectal metastases are mainly supplied by hepatic arterial blood and appear as perfusion defects surrounded by hypervascular liver tissue. Although it is a very sensitive study capable of identifying small lesions that escape detection on other studies, it is expensive and invasive. Helical CT scanning technology continues to improve, however, and may ultimately provide the sensitivity of CTAP with less cost and without the need for angiography. Duplex ultrasonography and magnetic resonance imaging (MRI) are also useful for assessing hepatic tumors, particularly in delineating the relationship of the tumor to major vasculature structures *(45)*. Magnetic resonance imaging (MRI) can also provide diagnostic characterization of liver tumors, such as hemangiomas or adenomas, when there is diagnostic uncertainty. In our practice, helical CT of the abdomen and pelvis, chest X-ray, and CT portography are the studies used in the vast majority of patients.

3.2. Patient Selection

In determining resectability of hepatic metastases, one must assess not only the technical issues associated with the operation but also consider the likelihood of favorable long-term outcome as determined by biologic factors. All cases of hepatic colorectal metastases are, by definition, stage IV disease, and traditional assessment by TMN staging is not very useful in guiding therapy. Molecular markers may ultimately prove to be the most useful determinants of outcome but remain investigational and far removed from clinical utility. On the other hand, a great deal of data now exist that allow the correlation of outcome with factors related to the primary tumor and the hepatic disease. Previously, the number of hepatic metastases was used to guide therapy, as illustrated by the reluctance of some to resect more than solitary lesions. Data from centers have since shown that long-term survival is possible after resection of multiple hepatic tumors, and the absolute number of lesions alone is therefore an inadequate predictor of outcome *(46)*. It is much more likely that adequate assessment of disease biology will require consideration of multiple clinical factors. Indeed, many studies have analyzed long-term outcome after resection of hepatic colorectal metastases in an attempt to better define selection criteria *(10,12,18,47)*. A well-defined and accurate set of selection criteria has obvious practical importance. Such a system would help identify patients most likely to benefit from resection and would better define high-risk patients in clinical trials to allow for more reasonable comparison of results.

Age, gender *(48,49)*, primary tumor grade, or location *(16,24,47,50,51)* have not consistently been demonstrated to affect outcome. In most studies, the most powerful predictors of tumor recurrence and therapeutic failure are tumor at the resection margin *(15,17,22,23,50,52)* and the presence of extrahepatic metastases found at the time of hepatic resection. These two criteria are not terribly helpful for preoperative patient selection, as few surgeons would subject a patient to resection expecting a positive margin or in the setting of extrahepatic disease. Other variables that are prognostically important include regional lymph nodal involvement by the primary tumor *(15,29)*, symptomatic liver tumors *(15)*, a short disease-free interval between presentation of the primary and the metastatic lesion *(15–17)*, a large numbers of tumors *(15,17)*, the presence of satellite nodules *(16,17)*, a high preoperative carcinoembryonic antigen (CEA) level *(10,53)*, and extent of liver involvement of more than 39% *(29,50)*.

In our recent analysis of 1001 consecutive liver resections *(11)*, the following variables were identified as independent predictors of outcome: (1) lymph node positive primary lesion, (2) disease-free interval from diagnosis of the primary to diagnosis of the liver disease <12 mo, (3) number of liver tumors greater than one, (4) size of liver tumors >5 cm, and (5) preoperative CEA level of greater than 200 ng/mL (Table 3). The presence of any one of these adverse clinical factors was still associated with a 5-yr survival of 13–34%; therefore, no one factor can be considered a contraindication to resection. However, as the number of adverse factors increased, there was a progressive increase in the likelihood of recurrence and a corresponding and progressive decrease in survival (Table 4). These variables were used as the basis of a clinical risk score by assigning one point for the presence of each factor and shows promise as a means of improving patient selection for resection. At present, this scoring system is not used to exclude patients from resection, but those with multiple

Table 3
Clinical Risk Score

1 Lymph-node-positive primary
2 Disease-free interval between colon and liver disease <12 mo
3 Size of liver tumors >5 cm
4 Number of liver tumors greater than one
5 Preoperative CEA level of greater than 200 ng/mL

Note: Each of the unfavorable characteristics is assigned one point. The sum of the positive characteristics is the clinical risk score.
Source: Ref. *11.*

adverse risk factors (score of 4 or 5) would be encouraged to enter clinical trials of resection combined with aggressive adjuvant therapy.

4. TECHNICAL ASPECTS OF LIVER RESECTION

A complete description of the technical aspects of hepatic resection is beyond the scope of this review. A more detailed account of operative hepatic surgery can be found in major texts *(54,55)*.

Laparoscopy, either immediately prior to planned open exploration and possible resection or as a separate procedure, should be considered before committing the patient to a laparotomy. Several studies suggest that diagnostic laparoscopy may be useful for patients under evaluation for resection of hepatic colorectal metastases *(56–58)*, with some reporting that up to half of patients may be found to have unresectable disease and spared an unnecessary laparotomy. In a recent study from Memorial Sloan-Kettering Cancer Center (MSKCC) in New York, 104 consecutive patients with potentially resectable hepatic malignancies underwent staging laparoscopy. Sixty-three percent of the patients were eventually treated by resection. Of the 39 patients with unresectable disease, laparoscopy identified 26 (67%) and reduced the hospital stay by an average of 6 d compared to patients who did not have laparoscopy *(58)*. Most of the previous studies in this area have included patients with a variety of hepatobiliary malignancies. However, in a recent analysis of 103 patients with hepatic colorectal metastases, the authors have documented a 75% overall resectability and a 14% yield of laparoscopy *(59)*. Despite the small number of patients who benefited from laparoscopy in this study, likely the result of extensive, high-quality preoperative imaging, laparoscopic identification of unresectable disease significantly reduced hospital stay and hospital charges. Although the utility of laparoscopy for use in metastatic colorectal cancer is not completely proven, these results encourage its use in patients at high risk for occult unresectable disease, such as those with a high clinical risk score. Laparoscopic inspection is most likely to identify peritoneal metastases or additional hepatic lesions that may preclude resection. Lymph node involvement by cancer either in the porta hepatis or in the retroperitoneum is difficult to find laparoscopically *(58)*. Whether whole-body [18]FDG-PET scan results may complement laparoscopic inspection in directing laparoscopic identification and biopsy of cancer-bearing lymph nodes is the subject of current ongoing prospective studies.

If no contraindications to resection are found during laparoscopy, full, open exploration is performed. The peritoneal cavity, pelvis, retroperitoneum and porta hepatis are carefully examined for evidence of extrahepatic disease, and any suspicious findings are biopsied and sent for frozen-section histology. The liver is examined by bimanual palpation and open

Table 4
Relation of CRS and Clinical Outcome

Score	1-yr Survival	3-yr Survival	5-yr Survival	Median survival (mo)
0	93	72	60	74
1	91	66	44	51
2	89	60	40	47
3	86	42	20	33
4	70	38	25	20
5	71	27	14	22

Note: Survival (%) as related to clinical risk score.
Source: Ref. *11*; reprinted with permission.

intraoperative ultrasound. The initial impetus for using intraoperative ultrasound was for the detection of small, deep hepatic lesions that were not palpable *(60)*. Current imaging with contemporary equipment is now sufficiently accurate, however, that the findings on intraoperative ultrasound alone rarely changes the planned operation *(61)*. Nevertheless, intraoperative ultrasound is invaluable for confirming the preoperative impression.

After the liver is mobilized and resectability confirmed, the inflow and outflow vasculature are controlled before parenchymal transection. Classical extrahepatic control of the inflow vessels for a formal lobectomy has changed little since its formal description by Lortat-Jacob in 1952 *(62)*. The hepatic artery and portal vein feeding the side of the liver to be resected is isolated within the portal hepatis, ligated, and divided. This devascularizes the portion of the liver to be removed, demarcating the line of transection.

Important observations by Glisson *(63)*, Cantlie *(64)*, Couinaud *(65)*, and Goldsmith and Woodburne *(66)* have advanced our understanding of hepatic anatomy and have allowed further refinements in hepatic resectional surgery. The surface anatomy of the liver belies a much more complex organ that is composed of eight separate segments, each with its own arterial and portal venous blood supply and biliary drainage. The vascular supply to and biliary drainage from each segment enter the liver as a triad enveloped in the tough fibrous Glisson's sheath, which can be isolated within the liver parenchyma an ligated *en masse* to devascularize each anatomic unit. Understanding these anatomic relationships has allowed for precise, parenchymal-sparing segmental resections. These anatomic resections are particularly important during hepatic resection for malignant disease. In the past, small limited resections of tumor tended to be nonanatomic wedge resections, which have a high risk for a positive resection margin for tumor, as high as 19% in some series *(19)* to 35% *(10)*. The reason for this is that delineating the edge of the tumor by palpation alone is difficult. Furthermore, as traction is placed on the specimen during wedge resection, there is a tendency for the soft liver to fracture along the interface with the hard tumor. Anatomic segmental resections *(54,67)* decrease the likelihood of a positive margin. Indeed, in a recent comparison between wedge and segmental resections in a single institution, the margin positivity rate was 19% and 2%, respectively, which translated into improved long-term survival for those subjected to anatomic segmental resections *(68)*. Additionally, many patients with colorectal metastases have hepatic steatosis as a result of systemic chemotherapy. For these patients, major sacrifice of functional parenchyma is associated with an increased risk of postoperative hepatic insufficiency, and segmental resection would be preferred, if technically possible.

Over the past several years, there has been a trend toward intrahepatic control of inflow vasculature for sectoral resections and lobectomies. The main right or left portal pedicle can be isolated and ligated *en masse* to rapidly devascularize part of or the entire lobe of the liver and reduce the risk of damage to the blood supply or biliary drainage of the liver remnant. If a sublobar resection is planned, the branches of the main pedicle can be identified and individually ligated to delineate the lines of parenchymal transection of the areas of interest. A technological advance that has improved such intraparenchymal vascular control has been the surgical vascular stapler. The major lobar pedicles can be isolated and staple-ligated quickly to completely devascularize the parenchyma to be resected *(69)*. It should be emphasized that the intrahepatic pedicle ligation approach should be used only if the tumor is more than 2 cm away from the pedicle to avoid compromising the resection margin. Furthermore, for a right lobectomy, if tumor is sufficiently far from the hilus, ligation of the anterior and posterior right portal pedicles separately rather than ligating the main right portal pedicle allows for an additional margin of safety against inadvertent damage to left-sided biliary or vascular structures. In addition, before proceeding with pedicle ligation, the liver should be completely mobilized and all retrohepatic veins draining directly into the vena cava must be ligated. This will prevent inadvertent tearing of these veins, which can result in major hemorrhage.

To further reduce blood loss during parenchymal transection, temporary clamping of the gastrohepatic ligament (Pringle maneuver) is used. Studies clearly demonstrate that even cirrhotic livers can tolerate normothermic ischemia for 30–75 min *(70–72)*. We prefer intermittent clamping with 5–10 min of occlusion alternated with 1–2 min of unclamping *(73)*.

Major bleeding during liver resection usually results from injury to the hepatic veins. Ligation of the hepatic veins draining the portion of the liver to be removed before parenchymal transection helps to minimize blood loss. For example, prior to liver transection for a lobectomy, the small hepatic veins draining from the back of the liver directly into the vena cava should be individually ligated, as should the main right or left hepatic vein. Vascular staplers have also greatly facilitated ligation of major hepatic veins and large accessory veins.

An alternative approach to resection utilizes a technique called hepatic vascular isolation *(74,75)*. After inflow occlusion with a Pringle maneuver, vascular clamps are placed on the vena cava above and below the liver, thus excluding it completely from vascular perfusion and drainage. This is an extension of the techniques used for liver transplantation and certainly can reduce blood loss during the parenchymal transection phase of the operation. Vascular isolation is a fundamentally different approach and requires different anesthetic management. The drawbacks to this technique include the additional operative time necessary for dissection and isolation of the retrohepatic cava. Also, interrupting the venous return from the inferior vena cava can produce major, detrimental hemodynamic consequences requiring administration of large fluid volumes to maintain adequate cardiac output. Continuous inflow occlusion is generally required. In a direct comparison of hepatic resection with and without vascular isolation, Belghiti and colleagues found that patients subjected to vascular exclusion had greater blood loss, longer ischemia time, longer operative time, and longer hospital stay *(76)*.

The authors prefer a technique utilizing a low central venous pressure (CVP) to limit hepatic venous bleeding. By keeping the CVP less than 5 cm H_2O, the backflow through the venous tributaries is reduced and bleeding is minimized *(73)*. To improve venous return with such a low CVP and to minimize the accompanying risk of air embolism, the patient is kept in a Trendelenburg position. For transecting the hepatic parenchyma, we use a clamp to crush the liver tissue and occlude intrahepatic vascular and biliary structures with clips, sutures, or in some cases, the vascular stapler. Although specialized instruments have been adapted for dividing the liver, such as the CUSA *(77)*, harmonic scalpel *(78)*, and water-jet dissector *(79)*, we find that the clamp crush technique *(54)* is equally effective and has the additional advantages of speed and low cost.

Special parenchymal transection instruments may be useful in specific situations. For example, for laparoscopic liver resections *(80)*, the harmonic scalpel is invaluable. Although clamp crushing is also possible during laparoscopic resection, the multiple exchanges of instruments required to divide the tissue and ligate the vessels and bile ducts make this approach extremely cumbersome laparoscopically. The harmonic scalpel facilitates laparoscopic resections by allowing transection and ligation of vessels using one instrument. The harmonic scalpel may also find a role for transecting cirrhotic parenchyma. In a normal liver, clamp crushing easily teases away the soft liver parenchyma from the vessels. With cirrhosis, the liver is fibrotic and hard, and vessels often tear during clamp crushing. The harmonic scalpel allows for transecting and sealing of vascular structures in a single move.

Three different studies have demonstrated drains to be unnecessary after liver resection *(81–83)*. In fact, drains may be detrimental by promoting infection or resulting in problems with fluid management by causing ascitic leaks. We use drains when hepatic resection is combined with biliary reconstruction, in the setting of an infected surgical field, when the thoracic cavity has been entered (either transdiaphragmatically or through a thoracoabdominal incision) to prevent biliary pleural fistula or when there is unequivocal leak of bile at the end of the resection.

5. COMPLICATIONS

As surgeons have become better at hepatic resection, there has been a tendency toward increasingly aggressive resections. This appears to explain the high percentage of major resections in recent series *(10,11,20)*; the plateau in perioperative mortality at 2–4%. Liver failure is the most common cause of death, but it is uncommon in patients without underlying hepatic parenchymal disease and occurs in only 1–5% of all major resections for metastatic colorectal cancer *(16,28,29,84,85)*. Major hemorrhage is also a major cause of perioperative mortality, but this complication has become increasingly less common (1–3%).

Nonlethal complications occur in 20–50% of hepatic resections and include biliary leak or fistula *(16,28)* and perihepatic abscess *(16,23,26,28,29)*. These complications once required reoperation to correct, but most are now readily managed by interventional radiologists without the need for a return to the operating room. Cardiopulmonary complications include myocardial infarction (1% in most series) *(16,23,26,29)*, sympathetic pleural effusions that may require tube thoracostomy (5–10%) *(26,86)*, pneumonia (5–22%) *(28,29)*, and pulmonary embolism (1%) *(16,84)*. Most complications do not result in long-term sequela and often do not prolong the hospital stay. Indeed, at high-volume centers, median hospital stay even for the most extensive resection typically less than 2 wk. In a series of 1001 consecutive resections performed at MSKCC, the median hospital stay was 9 d and intensive care unit (ICU) admission was required for only 7% of patients *(34)*. These results show that major liver resections can be performed with sufficiently low mortality and morbidity and result in a sufficiently favorable outcome to be standard treatment for metastatic colorectal cancer.

6. ADJUVANT THERAPY

Because two-thirds of patients will recur after hepatectomy, it seems intuitive that adjuvant therapy should be considered. However, no randomized trial has been completed that evaluates the role of systemic therapy in this patient population. Justifications for using adjuvant systemic chemotherapy after hepatic resection for metastases has been based on the extrapolation of data supporting the use of chemotherapy after resection of lymph-node-involved primary colorectal tumors *(87)*. Furthermore, until very recently, the only drug approved for use for metastatic colorectal cancer was 5-fluorouracil (5-FU), which had been used in many patients before hepatic resection. The common practice was, therefore, to offer adjuvant 5-FU chemotherapy after hepatic resection to patients who had not been previously treated. For the majority of patients who had previously received 5-FU-based chemotherapy and, particularly, if there was no evidence of tumor response, additional treatment was usually not offered. Irinotecan (CPT-11) has been approved for use for nonresectable metastatic colorectal cancer as second-line treatment. Likewise, the use of oxaliplatin in this setting remains to be determined. Future studies may establish these drugs as effective options to treat microscopic residual disease after resection.

The majority of studies examining utility of adjuvant therapy have involved regional hepatic chemotherapy, because the most common site for tumor recurrence after resection of hepatic colorectal metastases is the residual liver *(26,50,88–90)* (*see* Chapter 32).

In a recent report, Bismuth and colleagues evaluated the role of neoadjuvant chemotherapy. The study comprised 330 patients referred for liver resection but were deemed to have unresectable disease and referred for systemic therapy with 5-FU, folinic acid, and oxaliplatin. After treatment, 53 (16%) patients had responded such that they were now considered to be candidates for resection. The 5-yr survival of these resected patients was 40%, comparable to those resected initially *(91)*. Although the likelihood of such a favorable change in the extent of hepatic disease is uncommon with systemic therapy, patients should be periodically re-evaluated for resectability during treatment and reconsidered for resection if appropriate. These data should not, however, be misinterpreted as supporting the routine administration of chemotherapy prior to liver resection; at present, there are no data to support such an approach. It would indeed be interesting to determine if neoadjuvant therapy is useful in selecting among patients at high risk for subsequent recurrence after liver resection. Patients known to be at high risk for recurrence, such as those with multiple synchronous lesions or those with a high clinical risk score, would be ideal for a study investigating this question.

7. PATIENT FOLLOW-UP

After hepatic resection, patients should be followed closely because recurrent disease is common and effective therapies are available. Nearly half of all initial recurrences will involve the residual liver *(15,19,90)* and these are also the most amenable to further treatment. An increasing number of reports have examined the efficacy of multiple hepatic resections as treatment for recurrent liver disease *(24,26,89,92–98)* and have demonstrated long-term survival in up to 41% of patients. The most important predictor of good outcome after re-resection is a long interval between the first and second liver resection. Indeed, in a recent study of 96, 5-yr survivors after liver resection, nearly half had a further liver recurrence in the first 5 yr after the first liver resection that was successfully treated by re-resection *(99)*.

The lungs are the next most common site of recurrence, accounting for up to one-quarter of cases. Patients with limited pulmonary recurrence should also be considered for resection because selected patients will benefit *(100,101)*. Patients with limited pulmonary disease and a long interval between the hepatic resection and appearance of the lung metastasis or metastases are most likely to benefit. Most of the remaining recurrences occur at other intra-abdominal sites. Patients with second colorectal primary tumors or with anastomotic recurrences should also be considered for further surgical therapy. The liver, lung, and colon are, therefore, the primary focus of a follow-up strategy, not only because they are the most common sites of recurrence but because further recurrence may be effectively treated. Recurrences not amenable to resection should be considered for treatment with chemotherapy or, if appropriate, one of the ablative techniques, namely cryoablation and radio-frequency ablation (*see* Chapters 23 and 24). Although cryoablation and radio-frequency ablation can be effective in treating hepatic lesions, proof of a definitive role for these in the setting of recurrent colorectal cancer await prospective clinical trials *(102–112)*.

REFERENCES

1. Wingo PA, Tong T, and Bolden S. Cancer statistics, 1995, CA. *Cancer J. Clin.*, **45** (1995) 8–30.
2. Jaffe BM, Donegan WL, Watson F, et al. Factors influencing survival in patients with untreated hepatic metastases. *Surg. Gynecol. Obstet.*, **127** (1968) 1–11.
3. Bengmark S and Hafstrom L. the natural history of primary and secondary malignant tumors of the liver: I. The prognosis for patients with hepatic metastases from colonic and rectal carcinoma by laparotomy. *Cancer*, **23** (1969) 198–202.
4. Goslin R, Steele G, Zamcheck N, et al. Factors influencing survival in patients with hepatic metastases from adenocarcinoma of the colon and rectum. *Dis. Colon Rectum*, **25** (1982) 749–754.
5. Bengtsson G, Carlsson G, and Hafström L. Natural history of patients with untreated liver metastases from colorectal cancer. *Am. J. Surg.*, **141** (1981) 586–589.
6. Finan PJ, Marshall RJ, Cooper EH, and Giles GR. Factors affecting survival in patients presenting with synchronous hepatic metastases from colorectal cancer: a clinical and computer analysis. *Br. J. Surg.*, **72** (1985) 373–377.
7. De Brauw LM, De Velde CJH, and Bouwhuis-Hoogerwerf ML. Diagnostic evaluation and survival analysis of colorectal cancer patients with liver metastases. *J. Surg. Oncol.*, **34** (1987) 81–86.
8. Wood CB, Gillis CR, and Blumgart LH. A retrospective study of the natural history of patients with liver metastases from colorectal cancer. *Clin. Oncol.*, **2** (1976) 285–288.
9. Wagner JS, Adson MA, Van Heerden JA, Adson MH, and Ilstrup DM. The natural history of hepatic metastases from colorectal cancer. A comparison with resective treatment. *Ann. Surg.*, **199** (1984) 502–508.
10. Scheele J. Liver resection for colorectal metastases. *World J. Surg.*, **19** (1995) 59–71.
11. Fong Y, Fortner JG, Sun R, Brennan MF, and Blumgart LH. Clinical score for predicting recurrence after hepatic resection for metastatic colorectal cancer: analysis of 1001 consecutive cases. *Ann. Surg.*, **230** (1999) 309–321.
12. Nordlinger B, Guiguet M, Vaillant JC, Balladur P, Boudjema K, Bachellier P, et al. Surgical resection of colorectal carcinoma metastases to the liver. A prognostic scoring system to improve case selection, based on 1568 patients. *Assoc. Fr. Chir. Cancer*, **77(7)** (1996) 1254–1262.
13. Silen W. Hepatic resection for metastases from colorectal carcinoma is of dubious value. *Arch. Surg.*, **124** (1989) 1021–1024.
14. Foster JH. Survival after liver resection for secondary tumors. *Am. J. Surg.*, **135** (1978) 389–394.
15. Hughes KS, Simon R, Songhorabodi S, Adson MA, Ilstrup DM, Fortner JG, et al. Resection of the liver for colorectal carcinoma metastases: a multi-institutional study of patterns of recurrence. *Surgery*, **100** (1986) 278–284.
16. Scheele J, Stangl R, Altendorf-Hofmann A, and Gall FP. Indicators of prognosis after hepatic resection for colorectal secondaries. *Surgery*, **110** (1991) 13–29.
17. Rosen CB, Nagorney DM, Taswell HF, Helgeson SL, Ilstrup DM, Van Heerden JA, et al. Perioperative blood transfusion and determinants of survival after liver resection for metastatic colorectal carcinoma. *Ann. Surg.*, **110** (1992) 492–505.
18. Gayowski TJ, Iwatsuki S, Madariaga JR, Selby R, Todo S, Irish W, et al. Experience in hepatic resection for metastatic colorectal cancer: analysis of clinical and pathological risk factors. *Surgery*, **116** (1994) 703–711.
19. Fong Y, Cohen AM, Fortner JG, Morrerro A, Prassad M, Blumgart LH, et al. Liver resection for colorectal metastases. *J. Clin. Oncol.*, **15** (1997) 938–946.
20. Nordlinger B, Jaeck D, Guiget M, et al. In *Surgical Resection of Hepatic Metastases: Multicentric Retrospective Study by the French Association of Surgery.* Nordlinger B (ed.), Springer-Verlag, Paris, 1992, pp. 129–146.

21. Jamison RL, Donohue JH, Nagorney DM, Rosen CB, Harmsen WS, and Ilstrup DM. Hepatic resection for metastatic colorectal cancer results in cure for some patients. *Arch. Surg.*, **132** (1997) 505–511.

22. Adson MA, Van Heerden JA, Adson MH, Wagner JS, and Ilstrup DM. Resection of hepatic metastases from colorectal cancer. *Arch. Surg.*, **119** (1984) 647–651.

23. Fortner JG, Silva JS, Golbey RB, Cox EB, and Maclean BJ. Multivariate analysis of a personal series of 137 consecutive patients with liver metastases from colorectal cancer. I. Treatment by hepatic resection. *Ann. Surg.*, **199** (1984) 306–316.

24. Butler J, Attiyeh FF, and Daly JM. Hepatic resection for metastases of the colon and rectum. *Surg. Gynecol. Obstet.*, **162** (1986) 109–113.

25. Pagana TJ. A new technique for hepatic infusional chemotherapy. *Semin. Surg. Oncol.*, **2** (1986) 99–102.

26. Nordlinger B, Parc R, Delva E, Quilichini M, Hannoun L, and Huguet C. Hepatic resection for colorectal liver metastases. *Ann. Surg.*, **205** (1987) 256–263.

27. Cobourn CS, Makowka L, Langer B, Taylor B, and Falk R. Examination of patient selection and outcome for hepatic resection for metastatic disease. *Surg. Gynecol. Obstet.*, **165** (1987) 239–246.

28. Schlag P, Hohenberger P, and Herfarth Ch. Resection of liver metastases in colorectal cancer—competitive analysis of treatment results in synchronous versus metachronous metastases. *Eur. J. Surg. Oncol.*, **16** (1990) 360–365.

29. Doci R, Gennari L, Bignami P, Montalto F, Morabito A, and Bozzetti F. One hundred patients with hepatic metastases from colorectal cancer treated by resection: analysis of prognostic determinants. *Br. J. Surg.*, **78** (1991) 797–801.

30. Younes RN, Rogatko A, and Brennan MF. The influence of intraoperative hypotension and perioperative blood transfusion on disease-free survival in patients with complete resection of colorectal liver metastases. *Ann. Surg.*, **214** (1991) 107–113.

31. Rees M, Plant G, and Bygrave S. Late results justify resection for multiple hepatic metastases from colorectal cancer. *Br. J. Surg.*, **84** (1997) 1136–1140.

32. Jenkins LT, Millikan KW, Bines SD, Staren ED, and Doolas A. Hepatic resection for metastatic colorectal cancer. *Am. Surg.*, **63** (1997) 605–610.

33. Fortner JG and Lincer RM. Hepatic resection in the elderly. *Ann. Surg.*, **211** (1990) 141–145.

34. Fong Y, Blumgart LH, Fortner JG, and Brennan MF. Pancreatic or liver resection for malignancy is safe and effective for the elderly. *Ann. Surg.*, **222** (1995) 426–437.

35. Fong Y, Blumgart LH, Fortner JG, and Brennan MF. Pancreatic or liver resection for malignancy is safe and effective for the elderly. *Ann. Surg.*, **222(4)** (1995) 426–434; discussion 434–437.

36. Baron RL, Freeny PC, and Moss AA. The liver. In *Computed Tomography of the Body with Magnetic Resonance Imaging.* Moss AA, Gamsu G, and Genant HK (eds.), Saunders, Philadelphia, 1992, pp. 735–821.

37. Povoski SP, Fong Y, Sgouros SC, Kemeny NE, Downey RJ, and Blumgart LH. Role of chest CT in patients with negative chest x-rays referred for hepatic colorectal metastases. *Ann. Surg. Oncol.*, **5(1)** (1998) 9–15.

38. Yonekura Y, Benua RS, Brill AB, Som P, Yeh SDJ, Kemeny NE, et al. Increased accumulation of 2-deoxy-2-[18F]fluoro-D-glucose in liver metastases from colon carcinoma. *J. Nucl. Med.*, **23** (1982) 1133–1137.

39. Dimitrakopoulou A, Strauss LG, Clorius JH, Ostertag H, Schlag P, Heim M, et al. Studies with positron emission tomography after systemic administration of fluorine-18-uracil in patients with liver metastases from colorectal carcinoma. *J. Nucl. Med.*, **34** (1993) 1075–1081.

40. Beets G, Penninckx F, Schiepers C, Filez L, Mortelmans L, Kerremans R, et al. Clinical value of whole-body positron emission tomography with [18F]fluorodeoxyglucose in recurrent colorectal cancer. *Br. J. Surg.*, **81** (1994) 1666–1670.

41. Vitola JV, Delbeke D, Sandler MP, Campbell MG, Powers TA, Wright JK, et al. Positron emission tomography to stage suspected metastatic colorectal carcinoma to the liver. *Am. J. Surg.*, **171** (1996) 21–26.

42. Lai DTM, Fulham M, Stephen MS, Chu KM, Solomon M, Thompson JF, et al. The role of whole-body positron emission tomography with [18F]fluorodeoxyglucose in identifying operable colorectal cancer metastases to the liver. *Arch. Surg.*, **131** (1996) 703–707.

43. Fong Y, Saldinger PF, Akhurst T, Macapinlac H, Yeung H, Finn RD, et al. Utility of 18F-FDG-PET scanning on selection of patients for reseciton of hepatic colorectal metastases. *Am. J. Surg.*, **178** (1999) 282–287.

44. Fausto N. Hepatic regeneration. In *Hepatology.* Zakim D and Boyer TD (eds.), Saunders, Philadelphia, 1996, pp. 32–57.

45. Castaing D, Emond J, Kunstlinger F, and Bismuth H. Utility of operative ultrasound in the surgical management of liver tumors. *Ann. Surg.*, **204** (1986) 600–605.

46. Weber SM, Jarnagin WR, DeMatteo RP, Blumgart LH, and Fong Y. Survival after resection of multiple hepatic colorectal metastases. *Ann. Surg. Oncol.*, **7(9)** (2000) 643–650.

47. Cady B, Stone MD, McDermott WV Jr, Jenkins RL, Bothe A Jr, Lavin PT, et al. Technical and biological factors in disease-free survival after hepatic resection for colorectal cancer metastases. *Arch. Surg.*, **127** (1992) 561–569.
48. Vogt P, Raab R, Ringe B, and Pichlmayr R. Resection of synchronous liver metastases from colorectal cancer. *World J. Surg.*, **15** (1991) 62–67.
49. Nakamura S, Yokoi Y, Suzuki S, Baba S, and Muro H. Results of extensive surgery for liver metastases in colorectal carcinoma. *Br. J. Surg.*, **79(1)** (1992) 35–38.
50. Ekberg H, Tranberg KG, Andersson R, Lundstedt C, Hagerstrand I, Ranstam J, et al. Pattern of recurrence in liver resection for colorectal secondaries. *World J. Surg.*, **11** (1987) 541–547.
51. Hill DL and Grubbs CJ. Retinoids and cancer prevention. *Annu. Rev. Nutr.*, **12** (1992) 161–181.
52. Cady B and McDermott WV. Major hepatic resection for metachronous metastases from colon cancer. *Ann. Surg.*, **201** (1985) 204–209.
53. Hughes KS, Rosenstein RB, Songhorabodi S, Adson MA, Ilstrup DM, Fortner JG, et al. Resection of the liver for colorectal carcinoma metastases. A multi-institutional study of long-term survivors. *Dis. Colon Rectum*, **31** (1988) 1–4.
54. Blumgart LH. Liver resection for benign disease and for liver and biliary tumors. In *Surgery of the Liver and Biliary Tract*. 3rd ed. Blumgart LH and Fong Y (eds.), Churchill Livingstone, Edinburgh, 2000, pp. 1639–1695.
55. Blumgart LH and Fong Y. Surgical options in the treatment of hepatic metastasis from colorectal cancer. *Curr. Probl. Surg.*, **21(5)** (1995) 333–421.
56. Babineau TJ, Lewis WD, Jenkins RL, Bleday R, Steele GD, and Forse RA. Role of staging laparoscopy in the treatment of hepatic malignancy. *Am. J. Surg.*, **167** (1994) 151–155.
57. John T, Grieg JD, Crosbie JL, Miles FA, and Garden OJ. Superior staging of liver tumors with laparoscopy and laparoscopic ultrasound. *Ann. Surg.*, **220** (1994) 711–719.
58. Jarnagin WR, Bodniewicz J, Dougherty E, Conlon K, Blumgart LH, and Fong Y. A prospective analysis of staging laparoscopy in patients with primary and secondary hepatobiliary malignacies. *J. Gastrointest. Surg.*, **4** (2000) 34–43.
59. Jarnagin WR, Conlon K, Bodniewicz J, Dougherty E, DeMatteo R, Blumgart LH, et al. A clinical scoring system predicts the yield of diagnostic laparoscopy in patients with potentially resectable hepatic colorectal metastases. *Cancer*, **91** (2001) 1121–1128.
60. Vassiliades VG, Foley WD, Alarcon J, Lawton T, et al. Hepatic metastases: CT versus MR imaging at 1.5T. *Gastrointest. Radiol.*, **16** (1991) 159–163.
61. Jarnagin WR, Bach AM, Winston CB, Hann LE, Heffernan N, Loumeau T, et al. What is the yield of intraoperative ultrasound during partial hepatectomy for malignant disease? *J. Amer. Coll. Surg.*, (2001), in press.
62. Lortat-Jacob JL and Robert HG. Hepatectomie droite reglee. *Press. Med.*, **60** (1952) 549–556.
63. Glisson F. *Anatomia Hepatis*. Pullein, London, O 1654.
64. Cantlie J. On a new arrangement of the right and left lobes of the liver. *J. Anat. Physiol.*, **32** (1897) iv–ix.
65. Couinaud C. *Surgical Anatomy of the Liver. Revisited*. Paris, 1989.
66. Goldsmith NA and Woodburne RT. The surgical anatomy pertaining to liver resection. *Surg. Gynecol. Obstet.*, **105** (1957) 310–318.
67. Scheele J. Segment oriented resection of the liver: rationale and technique in hepatobiliary and pancreatic malignancies. In Lygidakis NJ and Tytgat GNJ (eds.), Thieme, Stuttgart, 1989.
68. DeMatteo RP, Palese C, Jarnagin WJ, Sun R, Blumgart LH, and Fong Y. Segmental resection is superior to wedge resection for colorectal liver metastases: analysis of 270 cases. *J. Gastrointest. Surg.*, **4** (2000) 178–184.
69. Fong Y and Blumgart LH. Useful stapling techniques in liver surgery. *J. Am. Coll. Surg.*, **185(1)** (1997) 93–100.
70. Kim YI, Nakashima K, Tada I, Kawano K, and Kobayashi M. Prolonged normothermic ischaemia of human cirrhotic liver during hepatectomy: a preliminary report. *Br. J. Surg.*, **80** (1993) 1566–1570.
71. Nagasue N, Uchida M, Kubota H, Hayashi T, Kohno H, and Nakamura T. Cirrhotic livers can tolerate 30 minutes ischaemia at normal environmental temperature. *Eur. J. Surg.*, **161** (1995) 181–186.
72. Man K, Fan ST, Ng IO, Lo CM, Liu CL, and Wong J. Prospective evaluation of Pringle maneuver in hepatectomy for liver tumors by a randomized study. *Ann. Surg.*, **226(6)** (1997) 704–711.
73. Melendez JA, Arslan V, Fischer ME, Wuest D, Jarnagin WR, Fong Y, et al. Perioperative outcomes of major hepatic resections under low central venous pressure anesthesia: blood loss, blood transfusion, and the risk of postoperative renal dysfunction. *J. Am. Coll. Surg.*, **187(6)** (1998) 620–625.
74. Huguet C and Gavelli A. Experience with total vascular isolation of the liver. *Semin. Liver Dis.*, **14** (1994) 115–119.
75. Emre S, Schwartz ME, Katz E, and Miller CM. Liver resection under total vascular isolation. Variations on a theme. *Ann. Surg.*, **217(1)** (1993) 15–19.

76. Belghiti J, Noun R, Zante E, Ballet T, and Sauvanet A. Portal triad clamping or hepatic vascular exclusion for major liver resection. *Ann. Surg.*, **224** (1996) 155–161.

77. Little JM and Hollands MJ. Impact of the CUSA and operative ultrasound on hepatic resection. *HPB Surg.*, **3(4)** (1991) 271–277.

78. Maruta F, Sugiyama A, Matsushita K, Ishida K, Ikeno T, Shimizu F, et al. Use of the Harmonic scalpel in open abdominoperineal surgery for rectal carcinoma. *Dis. Colon Rectum*, **42(4)** (1999) 540–542.

79. Baer HU, Maddern GJ, and Blumgart LH. New water-jet dissector: initial experience in hepatic surgery. *Br. J. Surg.*, **78** (1991) 502–503.

80. Fong Y, Jarnagin W, Conlon KC, DeMatteo R, Dougherty E, and Blumgart LH. Hand-assisted laparosocpic liver resection: lessons from an initial experience. *Arch Surg.*, **135** (2000) 854–859.

81. Franco D, Karaa A, Meakins JL, Borgonovo G, Smadja C, and Grange D. Hepatectomy without abdominal drainage. *Ann. Surg.*, **210** (1989) 748–750.

82. Fong Y, Brennan MF, Brown K, Heffernan N, and Blumgart LH. Drainage is unnecessary after elective liver resection. *Am. J. Surg.*, **171(1)** (1996) 158–162.

83. Belghiti J, Kabbej M, Sauvanet A, Vilgrain V, Panis Y, and Fekete F. Drainage after elective hepatic resection: a randomized trial. *Ann. Surg.*, **218(6)** (1993) 748–753.

84. Cunningham JD, Fong Y, Shriver C, Melendez J, Marx WL, and Blumgart LH. One hundred consecutive hepatic resections: blood loss, transfusion and operative technique. *Arch. Surg.*, **129** (1994) 1050–1056.

85. Doci R, Gennari L, Bignami P, Montalto F, Morabito A, Bozzetti F, et al. Morbidity and mortality after hepatic resection of metastases from colorectal cancer. *Br. J. Surg.*, **82** (1995) 377–381.

86. Coppa GF, Eng K, Ranson JH, Gouge TH, and Localio SA. Hepatic resection for metastatic colon and rectal cancer. An evaluation of preoperative and postoperative factors. *Ann. Surg.*, **202** (1985) 203–208.

87. Moertel CG, Fleming TR, Macdonald JS, et al. Levamisole and fluorouracil for adjuvant therapy of resected colon carcinoma. *N. Engl. J. Med.*, **322** (1990) 352–358.

88. Maeda T, Hasebe Y, Hanawa S, Watanabe M, Nakazaki H, Kuramoto S, et al. Trial of percutaneous hepatic cryotherapy: preliminary report, *Nippon Geka Gakkai Zasshi J. Jpn. Surg. Soc.*, **93** (1992) Issue 6, (in Japanese) p. 666.

89. Hohenberger P, Schlag P, Schwarz V, and Herfarth C. Tumor recurrence and options for further treatment after resection of liver metastases in patients with colorectal cancer. *J. Surg. Oncol.*, **33** (1990) 245–251.

90. Bozzetti F, Bignami P, Morabito A, Doci R, and Gennari L. Patterns of failure following surgical resection of colorectal cancer liver metastases. *Ann. Surg.*, **205** (1987) 264–270.

91. Bismuth H, Adam R, Levi F, et al. Resection of nonresectable liver metastases from colorectal cancer after neoadjuvant chemotherapy. *Ann. Surg.*, **224(4)** (1996) 509–522.

92. Bozetti F, Bignami P, Montalto F, Doci R, and Gennari L. Repeated hepatic resection for recurrent metastases from colorectal cancer. *Br. J. Surg.*, **79** (1992) 146–148.

93. Griffith KD, Sugarbaker PH, and Chang AE. Repeat hepatic resections for colorectal metastases. *Br. J. Surg.*, **77** (1990) 230–233.

94. Fortner JG. Recurrence of colorectal cancer after hepatic resection. *Am. J. Surg.*, **155** (1998) 378–382.

95. Lange JF, Leese T, Castaing D, and Bismuth H. Repeat hepatectomy for recurrent malignant tumors of the liver. *Surg. Gynecol. Obstet.*, **169** (1989) 119–126.

96. Vaillant JC, Balladur P, Nordlinger B, Karaitianos I, Hannoun L, Huguet C, et al. Repeat liver resection for recurrent colorectal metastases. *Br. J. Surg.*, **80** (1993) 340–344.

97. Tuttle TM, Curley SA, and Roh MS. Repeat hepatic resection as effective treatment for recurrent colorectal liver metastases. *Ann. Surg. Oncol.*, **4(2)** (1997) 125–130.

98. Adam R, Bismuth H, Castaing D, et al. Repeat hepatectomy for colorectal liver metastases. *Ann. Surg.*, **104(1)** (1997) 51–62.

99. D'Angelica M, Brennan MF, Fortner JG, Cohen AM, Blumgart LH, and Fong Y. Ninety five year survivors after liver resection for metastatic colorectal cancer. *J. Am. Coll. Surg.*, **185(6)** (1997) 554–559.

100. Smith JW, Fortner JG, and Burt M. Resection of hepatic and pulmonary metastases from colorectal cancer. *Surg. Oncol.*, **1** (1992) 399–404.

101. Minnard E, Fong Y, Weigel T, Fortner JG, Blumgart LH, and Burt M. Surgical resection for hepatic and pulmonary colorectal metastases. *Proc. Am. Soc. Clin. Oncol.*, **15** (1996) 552.

102. Hass GM and Taylor CB. Quantitative hypothermal method for production of local injury of tissue. *Arch. Pathol.*, **45** (1937) 563–580.

103. Ravikumar TS, Steele G Jr, Kane R, and King V. Experimental and clinical observations on hepatic cryosurgery for colorectal metastases. *Cancer Res.*, **51** (1991) 6323–6327.

104. Ravikumar TS, Kane R, Cady B, Jenkins R, Clouse M, and Steele G Jr. A 5-year study of cryosurgery in the treatment of liver tumors. *Arch. Surg.*, **126** (1991) 1520–1523; discussion.

105. Morris DL and Ross WB. Australian experience of cryablation of liver tumors. *Surg. Oncol. Clin. North Am.*, **5** (1996) 391–397.
106. Onik G, Rubinsky B, Zemel R, Weaver L, Diamond D, Cobb C, et al. Ultrasound-guided hepatic cryosurgery in the treatment of metastatic colon carcinoma. *Cancer*, **67** (1991) 901–907.
107. Morris DL, Horton MD, Dilley AV, Warlters A, and Clingan PR. Treatment of hepatic metastases by cryotherapy and regional cytotoxic perfusion. *Gut*, **34** (1993) 1158–1161.
108. Preketes AP, Caplehorn JR, King J, Clingan PR, Ross WB, and Morris DL. Effect of hepatic artery chemotherapy on survival of patients with hepatic metastases from colorectal carcinoma treated with cryotherapy. *World J. Surg.*, **19(5)** (1995) 768–771.
109. Ron IG, Kemeny NE, Tong B, Sullivan D, Fong Y, Saltz L, et al. Phase I/II study of escalating doses of systemic irinotecan (CPT-11) with hepatic arterial infusion of floxuridine (FUDR) and dexamethasone (D), with or without cryosurgery for patients with unresectable hepatic metastases from colorectal cancer. *Proc. Am. Soc. Clin. Oncol.*, **18** (1999) 236a.
110. Siperstein AE, Rogers SJ, Hansen PD, and Gitomirsky A. Laparoscopic thermal ablation of hepatic neuroendocrine tumor metastases. *Surgery*, **122(6)** (1997) 1147–1154.
111. Nagata Y, Hiraoka M, Akuta K, Abe M, Takahashi M, Jo S, et al. Radiofrequency thermotherapy for malignant liver tumors. *Cancer*, **65** (1990) 1730–1736.
112. Buscarini L, Rossi S, Fornari F, Di Stasi M, and Buscarini E. Laparoscopic ablation of liver adenoma by radiofrequency electrocauthery. *Gastrointest. Endoscopy*, **41(1)** (1995) 68–70.

21 Resection of Colorectal Metastases to the Lung

Robert J. Downey

CONTENTS

Pulmonary metastasectomy, or the surgical resection of malignant disease metastatic to the lung, has been performed for a wide variety of malignancies and probably most commonly for metastatic colorectal carcinoma. In this chapter, we will briefly review the history of metastasectomy, then review criteria for patient selection, the conduct of the operation, the results reported both for isolated lung and for liver and lung metastases, and possible areas for further investigation.

1. HISTORICAL BACKGROUND

The management of pulmonary metastatic disease by surgical resection is not a new concept. Published accounts of cases managed by surgery date from the late 19th century and have been recently reviewed by Martini and McCormack (1). A brief summary of the development of the field is as follows. In 1882, Weinlechner (2) published the first description of the resection of discontiguous metastatic disease; while resecting a chest wall sarcoma, he removed two incidentally discovered lung metastases. Unfortunately, the patient only survived for 24 h. Successful isolated attempts at resection of metastases encountered at the time of another planned resection were reported (3), until the first publication describing the resection of a pulmonary metastasis as a separate procedure in 1927 (4).

The first series of patients operated on for solitary lung metastases was published by Alexander and Haight in 1947 (5), and included 8 patients with sarcoma, and 16 with carcinoma. With only 1 postoperative death, 12 of 24 patients were felt to be free of recurrent

From: *Colorectal Cancer: Multimodality Management*
Edited by: L. Saltz © Humana Press Inc., Totowa, NJ

disease 1–12 yr after surgery. Other than a demonstration of feasibility and possible efficacy, this article is important in that Alexander and Haight proposed the first criteria for patient selection for pulmonary metastasectomy. These criteria include that the primary site of disease must be controlled or controllable, there could be no other sites of metastatic disease, and the patient must be medically able to tolerate the planned procedure. Today, we would add only that there be no better alternative nonsurgical therapy.

The first pulmonary metastasectomy at Memorial Sloan-Kettering Cancer Center was performed in 1940. This technique became progressively adopted for a wide range of histologic types. The evidence provided from the MSKCC experience, although retrospective, provides some of the strongest support for the likely efficacy of the procedure. Reports from the physicians treating pediatric patients with osteogenic sarcoma delineated the very poor survival for patients with this disease; 83% of patients with this disease developed pulmonary metastases within 2 yr, and of these, none survived beyond 5 yr. This experience lead to an attempt to resect all pulmonary disease in a group of 29 patients. Complete resection was possible in 22 with a 5-yr survival of 32% and a 20-yr survival of 18% (6). The Memorial Sloan-Kettering Cancer Center experience, by 1976, included 409 patients (7), by 1990 it included over 1100 patients, and now it exceeds 2000 patients.

Since 1965, by Martini's review (1), there have been over 400 publications in the literature addressing the subject of the surgical treatment of pulmonary metastatic disease. Despite the widespread adoption of pulmonary metastasectomy for the treatment of many differing histologies and the extensive literature on the subject, there has never been a prospective randomized study of the efficacy of this modality. Multiple large retrospective studies have been published (8–12). All reports include multiple histologic types with widely differing behaviors, and/or only consider patients undergoing surgical resection, leaving the denominator of all patients treated for the disease unknown and/or fail to specify the varying regimens of preoperative or postoperative chemotherapy or radiation therapy administered.

In addition to survival, most studies have examined possible prognostic indicators such as the number of lesions, tumor-doubling time, disease-free interval from time of resection of the primary lesion, bilaterality of lesions, and need for re-resection for recurrent disease. The results of these small studies were often contradictory and have been supplanted by the publication of a large international study. In 1996, Pastorino et al. (13) published the accumulated results of the International Registry of Lung Metastases, which assessed the results achieved by 5206 metastasectomies performed at 18 centers in Europe and North America. Colorectal malignancies were not examined as a separate histologic type, but placed with all other epithelial malignancies. The median survival after complete resection for all histologies was 35 mo and was 36% at 5 yr and 26% at 10 yr. Multivariate analysis suggested a better prognosis for patients with completely resected disease, metastatic germ cell tumors (but no difference between epithelial malignancies, sarcoma, or melanoma), disease-free intervals of 36 mo or more, and single metastases. Based on this, the authors proposed four distinct prognostic groups for patients with epithelial, sarcomatous, or melanoma metastases:

Group I: resectable, no risk factors (disease-free interval [DFI] ≥ 36 mo and single metastases)
Group II: resectable, one risk factor (DFI < 36 mo or multiple metastases)
Group III: resectable, two risk factors (DFI < 36 mo and multiple metastases)
Group IV: unresectable lesions

The median survival was significantly different among the four groups, with a median survival for group I of 61 mo, for group II of 34 mo, for group III of 24 mo, and for group IV of 14 mo. As prolonged survival was seen in some patients in any group with resectable disease, this stratification is best viewed as defining high-risk groups to be the first target for innovative adjuvant or neoadjuvant or experimental therapies.

2. INCIDENCE

It is estimated that approx 130,000 new cases of colorectal cancer will be diagnosed in the United States per year. Approximately 75% are able to undergo apparently curative resections, but 45–64% *(14,15)* (47,000–67,000 patients in the United States) will experience some form of recurrence within 5 yr. Overall, the most common site of metastatic disease is the liver (33% of patients) *(16)*. The lung is the most common extra-abdominal metastatic site (22% of patients with metastatic disease) *(16)*. Overall, recurrences involving the lung are seen in 9% of patients after apparently curative colorectal operations, of which approx 10% will be resectable *(17)*. Combining these estimates suggests that approx 1000 patients in the United States per year have resectable lung metastases.

3. PATHOLOGY

Spread to the lung is almost certainly hematologic, with the cells embolizing the pulmonary arterial circulation. This means that the most common location of pulmonary metastases is readily amenable to a minimal surgical resection such as a wedge resection, as two-thirds occurring in the outer one-third of the lung.

Colorectal metastases may spread from the lung parenchymal lesions to involve hilar and mediastinal lymph nodes (so-called "metastases metastasizing"). The best current estimate is that this occurs in approx 15% of patients with otherwise resectable lung disease *(13)*, but this should be considered as only a rough estimate, as sampling of mediastinal lymph nodes is only infrequently performed at the time of metastasectomy.

Both direct extension into or submucosal metastases to the tracheobronchial tree are not uncommon with colorectal carcinoma. For all malignancies that spread to the lung, examination of the entire tracheobronchial tree at autopsy will reveal that approximately 18% of patients will have endobronchially disease; however, only 2–3% of patients will have disease visible at bronchoscopy. Prognosis after diagnosis of endobronchial disease is probably limited with an estimated survival of 12 mo *(18,19)*, although figures for colorectal carcinoma alone are not available.

4. PREOPERATIVE EVALUATION OF THE PATIENT FOR METASTASECTOMY

As discussed earlier, the general guidelines for selecting a patient for metastasectomy are as follows:

1. The patient should be medically able to tolerate the planned procedure with an adequate postresection pulmonary reserve.
2. The lung lesions should appear to be amenable to complete resection.
3. There should be no extrapulmonary disease, or any extrapulmonary site should be controllable.
4. There should be no treatment other than surgery that is likely to afford a more favorable outcome.

Selecting a patient to undergo the planned surgical resection with an expected low morbidity and mortality and with adequate postoperative pulmonary reserve is similar to selecting a patient for resection of a primary lung malignancy. The evaluation to ensure that there are no extrapulmonary sites of disease is guided by the histology involved; for metastatic colon cancer, a thoracic, abdominal, and pelvic CT, a CEA level, and a recent colonoscopy probably suffice. A CEA level is of unclear prognostic value, but if elevated preoperatively, it should fall to normal levels if all disease has been resected, and it can then serve as a marker for re-recurrent disease.

The additional benefit of thoracic computed tomograms (CT) performed after a negative chest radiograph (CXR) in the evaluation of patients either at initial presentation or with extrathoracic recurrence is probably limited *(20,21)*. However, when colorectal metastases to the lung are suspected, thoracic CTs will add important additional information in the planning of resection, such as the detection of possible unresectable disease, such as small effusions and enlarged mediastinal lymph nodes. If no signs of unresectable disease are seen, review emphasizes the number and laterality of nodules. As discussed later, because it is not the practice of the Thoracic Surgery Service at Memorial Sloan-Kettering Cancer Center (MSKCC) to perform routine bilateral thoracic explorations in the absence of evidence for bilateral disease, a review of the thoracic CT scan focuses on whether sufficient evidence is present in each hemithorax suggestive of metastases to justify exploration of that side.

The conventional CT scan only approximates the tumor load in the lung. Sixty percent of the time either more or less actual metastases are found by manual palpation of the lung than preoperative CT scans predicted *(22)*; the implications of this are explored further in a subsequent section. The improved accuracy of spiral CT scan is being explored *(23)*; preliminary results suggest that smaller lesions are detected, but the likelihood that these represent metastases diminishes with smaller size (size of lesions/sensitivity of helical CT: <6 mm/69%, 6–10 mm/90%, >10 mm/100%). For this reason, we use the CT scan primarily to evaluate for clearly unresectable disease and to provide evidence for at least one nodule sufficiently worrisome for metastatic disease to justify thoracotomy.

Currently, there is insufficient information available to allow recommendations of the usefulness of positron-emission tomography (PET) scan imaging *(24)*, either to rule out other sites of colorectal metastatic disease or to localize disease within the lung, although this is clearly an area worthy of further investigation.

5. OPERATIVE APPROACH

Bronchoscopy should be performed on all patients undergoing metastasectomy to ensure that there are no endobronchially visible lesions, which can be expected to be found in 2–3% of patients. Endobronchial lesions may be resected with a lobectomy or pneumonectomy; removal by bronchotomy or by extraction through a rigid bronchoscope with laser cauterization of the surrounding tissues is feasible but appears less likely to afford complete removal *(18)*. There is no comprehensive information available on whether the finding of endobronchial disease alters prognosis.

Mediastinoscopy should be considered for any patient with metastatic colorectal cancer and radiographically enlarged mediastinal or hilar lymph nodes or with a hilar metastases *(25)*. Should involved lymph nodes be found at mediastinoscopy, the pulmonary resection is usually aborted, as a complete resection likely to benefit the patient is unlikely to be achieved.

The choice of a thoracic incision is guided by the location of the radiographically apparent disease. At MSKCC, if bilaterally resectable disease is noted, then simultaneous resection by a "hemiclamshell" thoracotomy (bilateral anterior thoracotomies with transverse sternotomy), or bilateral anterior thoracotomies, or, less commonly, median sternotomy is performed. Bilateral posterolateral thoracotomies, either at one sitting or as separate procedures, are usually performed if the patient has a contraindication to an anterior approach (such as prior sternotomy for coronary bypass or other cardiac surgery), or the presence of a breast reconstruction with a rectus flap with a vascular pedicle, or the lesions are either posterior within the lung (particularly in the left lower lobe behind the heart) or an anatomic resection such as a segmentectomy is anticipated. Should bilateral thoracotomies be planned, the choice of the first side could either be based on the probability of finding unresectable disease on one side over the other, or if only a small resection is needed on one side and a lobectomy on the other, the smaller resection could be performed first so that, after recovery, the patient has the maximal amount of contralateral lung during the lobectomy should problems arise in the postoperative period.

The need to palpate radiographically uninvolved lung is the subject of considerable debate. At MSKCC, we routinely perform unilateral thoracotomies if unilateral disease is only apparent radiographically. However, our logic in doing this is certainly open to criticism. First, there are surgeons *(26–28)* who report that they have performed median sternotomies even if the disease appears confined to a hemithorax and have found contralateral disease 30–60% of the time. It is not clear that removing this disease while radiographic inapparent confers a survival advantage.

As was discussed, approx 30% of patients had more disease within a single lung than was predicted by CT scan; if so, and following the same logic as we employ in exploring only chest, it could be argued from this that for the approx 70% of patients without other disease than that radiographically apparent, thoracoscopy may be adequate, with the understanding that reoperation may be necessary should further disease become apparent in that hemithorax. Video-assisted thoracic surgical techniques have been demonstrated to be able to remove all radiographically evident disease *(29)*; a study has been activated through the CALGB to test this prospectively.

At exploration, resection of all palpable abnormalities is undertaken, with removal of as little normal lung parenchyma as possible. Resection is most often removal of a wedge of tissue with the use of staplers or needle cautery resection *(30)*, although segmentectomy, lobectomy, or even pneumonectomy *(31)* may be necessary to incorporate all disease. It is important to note that a new pulmonary lesion in a patient with a prior history of a colon malignancy may represent metastatic colonic disease, or a new malignancy either primary to the lung or metastatic from a site other than the colon or benign. Intraoperative frozen section is usually able to guide the extent of surgical resection by distinguishing metastatic colorectal from primary lung malignancies. Should it be unclear which is present, commonly an operation is performed that "splits the difference"; that is, a generous wide wedge or a segmentectomy, if possible, is performed.

Given the propensity for colon cancer to metastasize to lymph nodes, it is reasonable to perform a mediastinal lymph node sampling at the time of metastasectomy. When lymph node spread is found, it is probable that this represents unresectable disease, and no further resections are usually performed. There is also no information available on the effectiveness of adjuvant therapy for these patients should a complete resection of all disease including lymph node spread be performed.

6. RESULTS OF TREATMENT

6.1. Pulmonary Metastasectomy for Isolated Colorectal Metastases

The early articles on the subject of metastasectomy combined histologies; although colorectal metastases are often included, the majority of the articles present their data in such

Table 1
Results of Series of Pulmonary Metastasectomy for Colorectal Carcinoma

Authors (ref.)	Year	No. of patients	Significant prognostic factors	5-yr Survival (%)
Wilking et al. (32)	1985	27	No. of metastases	9
Goya et al. (41)	1989	62	No. of metastases	42
			Size of metastases	
Mori et al. (33)	1991	35	None	38
McAfee et al. (34)	1992	119	No. of metastases	31
			Serum CEA	
McCormack et al. (35)	1992	144	None	40
Shirouzu et al. (36)	1995	22	No. of metastases	NA[a]
			Size of metastases	
Okumura et al. (37)	1996	159	No. of metastases	40
			Lymph node involvement	
Yano et al. (38)	1997	36	No. of metastases	NA
Zanella et al. (39)	1997	22	None	62

[a]NA = Not available.

a way as to make comments on the specific problem of colorectal metastases impossible. With a few exceptions, the following discussion will be limited to those articles that have appeared over the last decade addressing the specific issue of the surgical management of colorectal carcinoma metastatic to the lung.

The results of the recent series are summarized in Table 1 (32–39). Overall, it appears that it is possible to select patients with a reasonable probability of achieving a 5-yr survival approaching 40% after surgery. Prognostic factors that are repeatedly shown to influence survival include the number of metastases and the size of the largest lesion (the exact cutoff varying between series). Importantly, this is only partially inconsistent with the prognostic groups outlined earlier, as Pastorino's (13) work did not examine the value of the size of the largest lesion; unlike Pastorino's work (13), though, most of the studies specifically reviewing colorectal carcinoma metastases did assess the value of a disease-free interval and did not find it valuable. The major shortcomings of these studies are that they are retrospective and, therefore, patient selection is subject to unclear biases, the frequency and prognostic value of thoracic lymph node metastases are not assessed, and the role of induction and adjuvant treatments is incompletely described.

6.2. Combined Pulmonary and Hepatic Metastasectomy for Colorectal Carcinoma

It is probable that some patients with colorectal malignancies metastatic to the lung benefit from resection; as discussed in Chapter 20, it is also probable that patients with isolated metastases to the liver also benefit from surgical resection (40). There is now a growing body of literature to suggest that patients with either synchronous or metachronous lung and liver metastases may experience long-term benefit from resection.

Initial reported experience with combined resections amounted to little more than case reports (41–43), but suggested that some patients may experience extended disease-free survival with acceptable operative mortality.

The most recent experience is retrospective and summarized in Table 2 (44–47). These data suggest that the institutions reporting results are able to perform the procedures with

Table 2
Resection of Hepatic and Pulmonary Colorectal Metastases

Authors (ref.)	Year	No. of patients	% Op. mortality	Med survival (mo)	5-yr Survival (%)
Ambiru et al. (44)	1998	6	0	32	NA[a]
Murata et al. (45)	1998	30	0	30	44
Regnard et al. (46)	1998	43	0	19	11
Lehnert et al. (47)	1999	17	0	34	<15
Robinson et al. (48)	1999	25	NA	16	9

[a]NA = not available.

a very acceptable mortality, but the benefit achieved varies among institutions, with 5-yr survivals ranging from 9% to 45%. Certainly, patient selection is probably the most important variable. The most detailed analysis of prognostic factors is provided by the Cleveland Clinic Group (48) and suggests that ideal patient characteristics for resection include age < 50 yr, solitary liver metastasis, >4 yr interval from primary colorectal cancer resection to pulmonary resection as the best predictors of extended survival. As always, such criteria are helpful but still only guidelines and it would be difficult to manage a patient with a solitary site of resectable pulmonary 5 yr after initial colectomy disease nonoperatively, for example, because of an age of 55. The criteria are best viewed as delineating the highest-risk group as appropriate subjects for innovative therapies.

7. AREAS OF RESEARCH

It is probable, although not proved, that the resection of colorectal metastases to the lung can provide prolonged survival. The benefit is probably only afforded to a few and further work is necessary to better define the patient likely to benefit, and to better integrate medical and surgical therapies. A short summary of areas for further exploration include the following:

1. Prospective randomized trials comparing metastasectomy to best nonsurgical therapy, beginning with groups of patients with probable poor prognosis (multiple metastases, short disease-free interval)
2. A prospective study of mediastinal lymph node staging at the time of metastasectomy to establish the frequency and the prognosis for a patient with mediastinal nodal disease
3. Investigation on coordinating surgery with adjuvant and neoadjuvant therapies—in particular, new drugs such as CPT-11
4. Investigation into regional intensification of chemotherapy within the lung (49)
5. Trials to establish the possible role for thoracoscopy and routine bilateral explorations
6. Prospective evaluation of the efficacy of resection from metastases to multiple organs (i.e., synchronous liver and lung)
7. Prospective evaluation of the utility of newer imaging modalities, such as PET scan, in delineating the extent of both local and distant recurrent disease

REFERENCES

1. Martini N and McCormack PM. Evolution of the surgical management of pulmonary metastases. *Chest Surg. Clin. North Am.*, **8(1)** (1998) 13–27.
2. Weinlechner JW. Zur Kasuistick der Tumoren an der Brustwand und deren Behandlung. *Wien Med. Wochenschr.*, **32** (1882) 589–591, 624–628.

3. Kronlein RU. Ueber Lungenchirurgie. *Berl. Klin. Wchnschr.*, **21** (1884) 129–132.

4. Divis G. Ein Beitrag Zur Operativen Behandlung der Lungeschwulste. *Acta Chir. Scand.*, **62** (1927) 329–341.

5. Alexander J and Haight C. Pulmonary resection for solitary metastatic sarcomas and carcinomas. *Surg. Gynecol. Obstet.*, **85** (1947) 129–146.

6. Beattie EJ JR, Harvey JC, Marcove R, and Martini N. Results of multiple pulmonary resections for metastatic osteogenic sarcoma after two decades. *J. Surg. Oncol.*, **46** (1991) 154–155.

7. McCormack PM and Martini N. The changing role of surgery for pulmonary metastases. *Ann. Thorac. Surg.*, **28** (1979) 139–145.

8. Patterson GA, Todd TR, Ilves, Pearson FG, and Cooper JD. Surgical management of pulmonary metastases. *Can. J. Surg.*, **25** (1982) 102–105.

9. Takita H, Merrin C, Didolkar MS, Douglass HO, and Edgerton F. The surgical management of multiple lung metastases. *Ann. Thorac. Surg.*, **24(4)** (1977) 359–364.

10. Venn GE, Sarin S, and Goldstraw P. Survival following pulmonary metastasectomy. *Eur. J. Cardiothorac. Surg.*, **3(2)** (1989) 105–109.

11. Mountain CF, McMurtrey MJ, and Hermes KE. Surgery for pulmonary metastasis: a 20-year experience. *Ann. Thorac. Surg.*, **38** (1984) 323–330.

12. Gadd MA, Casper ES, Woodruff JM, McCormack PM, and Brennan MF. Development and treatment of pulmonary metastases in adult patients with extremity soft tissue sarcoma. *Ann. Surg.*, **218** (1993) 705–712

13. Pastorino U, Buyse M, Friedel G, et al. Long-term results of lung metastasectomy: prognostic analyses based on 5206 cases. The International Registry of Lung Metastases. *J. Thorac. Cardiovasc. Surg.*, **113** (1997) 37–49.

14. Wilking N, Petrelli NJ, Herrera L, Regal AM, and Mittelman A. Surgical resection of pulmonary metastases from colorectal carcinoma. *Dis. Colon Rectum*, **28** (1985) 562–564.

15. August DA, Ottow RT, and Sugarbaker PH. Clinical perspectives on human colorectal cancer metastases. *Cancer Metastasis Rev.*, **3** (1984) 303–324.

16. Galandiuk S, Wienand HS, Moertel CG, et al. Pattern of recurrence after curative resection of carcinoma of the colon and rectum. *Surg. Gynecol. Obstet.*, **174** (1992) 27–32.

17. Pihl E, Hughes ES, McDermott FT, Johnson WR, and Katrivessis H. Lung recurrence after curative surgery for colorectal cancer. *Dis. Colon Rectum*, **30** (1987) 417–419.

18. Heitmiller RF, Marasco WJ, Hruban RH, and Marsh BR. Endobronchial metastases. *J. Thorac. Cardiovasc. Surg.*, **106** (1993) 537–542.

19. Argyros GJ and Torrington KG. Fiberoptic bronchoscopy in the evaluation of carcinoma metastatic to the lung. *Chest*, **105** (1994) 454–457.

20. Povoski SP, Fong Y, Sgouros SC, Kemeny NE, Downey RJ, and Blumgart LH. Role of chest CT in patients with negative chest x-rays referred for hepatic colorectal metastases. *Ann. Surg. Oncol.*, **5(1)** (1998) 9–15.

21. Kronawitter U, Kemeny NE, Heelan R, Fata F, and Fong Y. Evaluation of chest computed tomography in the staging of patients with potentially resectable liver metastases from colorectal carcinoma. *Cancer*, **86** (1999) 229–235.

22. McCormack PM, Ginsberg KB, Bains MS, et al. Accuracy of lung imaging in metastases with implications for the role of thoracoscopy. *Ann. Thorac. Surg.*, **56** (1993) 863–866.

23. Diederich S, Semik M, Lentschig MG, Winter F, Scheld HH, Roos N, et al. Helical CT of pulmonary nodules in patients with extrathoracic malignancy: CT–surgical correlation. *Am. J. Roentgenol.*, **172(2)** (1999) 353–360.

24. Ogunbiyi OA, Flanagan FL, Dehdashti F, et al. Detection of recurrent and metastastic colorectal cancer: comparison of positron emission tomography and computed tomography. *Ann. Surg. Oncol.*, **4(8)** (1997) 613–620.

25. Todd TR. Pulmonary metastasectomy. Current indications for removing lung metastases. *Chest*, **103** **(4 Suppl.)** (1993) 401S–403S.

26. Pastorino U, Valente M, Gasparini M, et al. Median sternotomy and multiple lung resections for metastatic sarcomas. *Eur. J. Cardiothorac. Surg.*, **4** (1990) 477–481.

27. Roth JA, Putnum JC, Wesley MN, and Rosenberg SA. Differing determinants of prognosis following resection of pulmonary metastases from osteogenic and soft tissue sarcoma patients. *Cancer*, **55** (1985) 1361–1366.

28. Johnston MR. Median sternotomy for resection of pulmonary metastases. *J. Thorac. Cardiovasc. Surg.*, **85** (1983) 516–522.

29. Rusch VW, Bains MS, Burt ME, McCormack PM, and Ginsberg RJ. Contribution of video thoracoscopy to the management of the cancer patient. *Ann. Surg. Oncol.*, **1(2)** (1995) 94–98.

30. Cooper JD, Perelman M, Todd TR, Ginsberg RJ, Patterson GA, and Pearson FG. Precision cautery excision of pulmonary lesions. *Ann. Thorac. Surg.*, **41** (1986) 51–53.

31. Koong HN, Pastorino U, and Ginsberg RJ. Is there a role for pneumonectomy in pulmonary metastases? International Registry of Lung Metastases. *Ann. Thorac. Surg.*, **68** (1999) 2039–2043.

32. Wilking N, Petrelli NJ, Herrera L, Regal AM, and Mittelman A. Surgical resection of pulmonary metastases from colorectal adenocarcinoma. *Dis. Colon Rectum*, **28** (1985) 562–564.

33. Mori M, Tomoda H, Ishida T, et al. Surgical resection of pulmonary metastases from colorectal adenocarcinoma. Special reference to repeated pulmonary resections. *Arch. Surg.*, **126** (1991) 1297–1301.

34. McAfee MK, Allen MS, Trastek VF, Ilstrup DM, Deschamps C, and Pairolero PC. Colorectal lung metastases: results of surgical excision. *Ann. Thorac. Surg.*, **53** (1992) 780–785.

35. McCormack PM, Burt ME, Bains MS, Martini N, Rusch VW, and Ginsberg RJ. Lung resection for colorectal metastases. 10-year results. *Arch. Surg.*, **127** (1992) 1403–1406.

36. Shirouzu K, Isomoto H, Hayashi A, Nagamatsu Y, and Kakegawa T. Surgical treatment for patients with pulmonary metastases after resection of primary colorectal carcinoma. *Cancer*, **76** (1995) 393–398.

37. Okumura S, Kondo H, Tsuboi M, et al. Pulmonary resection for metastatic colorectal cancer: experiences with 159 patients. *J. Thorac. Cardiovasc. Surg.*, **112** (1996) 867–874.

38. Yano T, Fukuyama Y, Yokoyama H, et al. Failure in resection of multiple pulmonary metastases from colorectal cancer. *J. Am. Coll. Surg.*, **185** (1997) 120–122.

39. Zanella A, Marchet A, Mainente P, Nitti D, and Lise M. Resection of pulmonary metastases from colorectal carcinoma. *Eur. J. Surg. Oncol.*, (1997) 424–427.

40. Fong Y, Cohen AM, Fortner JG, et al. Liver resection for colorectal metastases. *J. Clin. Oncol.*, **15** (1997) 938–946.

41. Goya T, Miyazawa N, Kondo H, Tsuchiya R, Naruke T, and Suemasu K. Surgical resection of pulmonary metastases from colorectal cancer: 10 year follow-up. *Cancer*, **64** (1989) 1418–1421.

42. Gough DB, Donohue JH, Trastek VA, and Nagorney DM. Resection of hepatic and pulmonary metastases in patients with colorectal cancer. *Br. J. Surg.*, **81** (1994) 94–96.

43. Smith JW, Fortner JG, and Burt M. Resection of hepatic and pulmonary metastases from colorectal cancer. *Surg. Oncol.*, **1** (1992) 399–404.

44. Ambiru S, Miyazaki M, Ito H, et al. Resection of hepatic and pulmonary metastases in patients with colorectal carcinoma. *Cancer*, **82** (1998) 274–278.

45. Murata S, Moriya Y, Akasu T, Fujita S, and Sugihara K. Resection of both hepatic and pulmonary metastases in patients with colorectal carcinoma. *Cancer*, **83** (1998) 1086–1093.

46. Regnard JF, Grunenwald D, Spaggiari L, et al. Surgical treatment of hepatic and pulmonary metastases from colorectal cancers. *Ann. Thorac. Surg.*, **66** (1998) 214–218.

47. Lehnert T, Knaebel HP, Duck M, Bulzebruck H, and Herfarth C. Sequential hepatic and pulmonary resections for metastatic colorectal cancer. *Br. J. Surg.*, **86** (1999) 241–243.

48. Robinson BJ, Rice TW, Strong SA, Rybicki LA, and Blackstone EH. Is resection of pulmonary and hepatic metastases warranted in patients with colorectal cancer? *J. Thorac. Cardiovasc. Surg.*, **117** (1999) 66–75.

49. Ratto GB, Toma S, Civalleri D, Passerone GC, Esposito M, Zaccho D, et al. Isolated lung perfusion with platinum in the treatment of pulmonary metastases from soft tissue sarcomas. *J. Thorac. Cardiovasc. Surg.*, **112** (1996) 614–622.

22 Surgical Management of Peritoneal Surface Spread of Colorectal Cancer

Paul H. Sugarbaker

CONTENTS

1. INTRODUCTION

The grim surgical reality that accompanies colorectal cancer resection suggests that approximately 50% of patients who come to the surgeon with a contained malignancy have this cancer converted to a disseminated disease process. Flawed surgical technology causes a surgically induced dissemination of microscopic residual disease in a large percentage of patients. Inadequate exposure, imperfect hemostasis, inadequate lymphadenectomy, and qualitatively poor margins of excision lead to the spillage of cancer cells in 30–50% of patients. Minor technical changes in the surgical approach to this disease can make a great difference in survival. The goal of cancer surgery for large bowel cancer is complete clearance and containment. Surgeons must believe that they are the most important prognostic variables before finding the commitment required to modify the current surgical approach.

2. THE SKILL OF THE SURGEON AS A PROGNOSTIC VARIABLE

The surgical literature contains several early pleas for modifications in surgical technology. Turnbull and associates *(1)* emphasized the "no touch isolation technique." Although the statistical support for these concepts may not be acceptable by modern-day standards, one cannot overlook the remarkably outstanding results achieved by Turnbull.

From: *Colorectal Cancer: Multimodality Management*
Edited by: L. Saltz © Humana Press Inc., Totowa, NJ

Phillips et al. published a report on the local recurrence after curative surgery for large bowel cancer (2). They called attention to the intersurgeon variability with local recurrence for colorectal cancer resections. The incidence of local recurrence was determined for surgeons performing more than 30 resections. Three surgeons had a local recurrence rate of < 5%; seven of 5–10%, three 10–15%, six 15–20%, and one >20% ($p < 0.05$). After stratification by patient's sex and Dukes' classification, the statistical significance remained.

McArdle and Hole in 1991 showed a variability among surgeons in terms of patients' postoperative morbidity and mortality and ultimate survival (3). The proportion of patients undergoing apparently curative resection varied among surgeons from 40% to 76%. These data showed that the intensity of the surgical effort that was exerted in an attempt to achieve a "curative approach" varied greatly within the surgical community. The short-term consequences of surgery (i.e., morbidity and mortality) also varied greatly when individual surgeons rather that institutions were assessed. Most striking was the fact that survival at 10 yr in patients who underwent a curative resection varied from 20% to 63% between the consultant surgeons responsible for managing colorectal patients.

Hermanek and colleagues presented data in 1995 to show that locoregional recurrence varied from >50% to approx 5% among German surgeons (4). There was also a marked correlation between loco-regional recurrence and 5-yr survival rates. A rate of local–regional recurrence ≤5% was associated with an almost 80% 5-yr survival rate. The local recurrence rate of >50% was associated with a low, approx 40% 5-yr survival rate. A difference in the 5-yr survival rate of 40% occurred between the groups of patients operated on by the individual surgeons. Surgeons with a low local recurrence rate have high survival rates and vice versa ($p < 0.005$). Thus, although the TNM status was the predominant prognosticator, the surgeon was an independent prognostic factor by which to determine survival.

In 1997, Holm and colleagues reviewed the influence of preoperative radiation therapy and other variables on the outcome of patients with rectal cancer (5). They found that patients operated on by surgeons who had been certified specialists for at least 10 yr had a lower risk of local recurrence and death from rectal cancer. Patients operated on in university hospitals also had a lower risk of death related to technical factors. They concluded that there was a significant surgeon-related variation in patient outcome, which was probably related to surgical technique.

In 1998, Porter and colleagues compared the outcome of patients treated by trained colorectal surgeons who operated frequently for rectal cancer with surgeons lacking specialized training and performing < 21 procedures over the 8 yr of the study (6). The risk of local recurrence was increased in patients whose surgery was performed by surgeons without colorectal training and by those performing fewer resections. Similarly, a decreased disease-specific survival rate was found to be independently associated with surgeons lacking specialized colorectal training ($p = 0.03$) and surgeons performing occasional rectal resections ($p = 0.005$). The 5-yr survival with trained and frequently operating surgeons was 67.3% and with untrained and infrequently operating surgeons, it was 39.2%.

Anthone et al. asked the question "Does designated surgical interest improve the surgical management of colorectal cancer?" These authors compared survival in patients operated on by members of the American Society of Colon and Rectal Surgery to that for surgeons who were not members (7). The database was comprised of 11,677 patients with colon and rectal cancer. Of the total cases performed by society members, 38% of patients died; of all operations performed by nonmembers of the society, 46% of patients died. Patients operated on by members of the society were more likely to be alive at the time of follow-up than patients operated on by other surgeons (odds ratio of 1.39, 95% confidence interval = 1.15–1.68).

The surgical techniques resulting in differences in surgeon-related survival statistics was reviewed by Averbach et al. in 1995 *(8)*. They concluded that the surgeon's efforts to contain a malignant process during the cancer resection varied greatly. In their view, local recurrence correlated directly with reduced survival. Scott and colleagues suggested that preservation of the mesorectum could reduce the local recurrence rates following surgery for rectal cancer to the 5% level *(9)*. They concluded that incomplete excision of the mesorectum contributes to local recurrence in a large proportion of patients with rectal cancer, particularly those with tumors in the middle and lower third of the rectum *(9)*. Heald and Ryall *(10)* have presented clinical data to strongly suggest that advanced surgical training can result in a great reduction in local rectal cancer recurrence and an improvement in survival.

3. FAILURE ANALYSIS OF PRIMARY COLORECTAL CANCER OPERATIONS

The reoperative data provided by Gunderson and Sosin provide information regarding anatomic sites of first recurrence of large bowel cancer *(11)*. These sites of first recurrence are of great value in establishing the technical flaws in surgery that allow cancer spread. However, even though cancer spread on abdominal or pelvic surfaces is related to faulty surgical technique, surgeons cannot be held responsible for dissemination via portal blood or in distant lymph nodes, lungs, or other systemic sites. Liver metastases will occur prior to death in approx 30% of patients according to Pikren and colleagues *(12)*. Systemic sites of disease progression may occur. Systemic disease results from metastases from metastases. In other words, implants of cancer throughout the body arise from metastases located within the liver or from lymph node metastases that seed via the thoracic duct. Surgery cannot reduce the incidence of cancer metastases to liver, lymph nodes, and distant sites but should eliminate the spread to the resection site and to peritoneal surfaces.

Although the presence versus absence of lymph node metastases is a strong prognostic indicator for resected colorectal cancer, cancer progression within lymph nodes after colon or rectal resection is unusual. Lofgren and co-workers reported that the pattern of local recurrence was identical in patients with and without positive lymph nodes *(13)*. A dissemination of cancer along lymph node chains was an unusual finding. These authors concluded that local recurrence was from cancerous tissue broken into and disseminated at the time of removal of the primary lesion. If the surgeon removes the lymph nodes en bloc down to the origins of the major blood vessels (right colic, middle colic, or inferior mesenteric) of the colon or rectum, further disease progression along lymph node chains rarely, if ever, occurs.

If colorectal cancer fails within abdominal lymph nodes, on peritoneal surfaces, or at the resection site, one must interpret this as "iatrogenic recurrence" *(14)*. These sites of recurrence testify to the fact that the surgeon's resection did not provide adequate clearance and containment of the primary malignancy. The surgeon should take full responsibility for all local–regional failures with large bowel cancer (Fig. 1).

The incidence of failure with liver metastases, metastases at systemic sites, or loco-regional spread on the peritoneal surfaces will be observed in direct proportion to the aggressive nature of the malignancy. The most aggressive tumors may show surgical treatment failure within liver and systemic sites as well as locoregional failure. The least aggressive tumors would be expected to have isolated loco-regional failures. Iatrogenic recurrence is related to a faulty surgical technique. Advanced treatment strategies are necessary to eradicate loco-

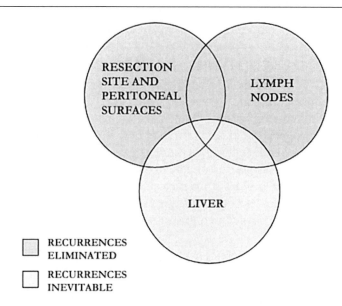

Fig. 1. Sites of treatment failure for large bowel cancer. The surgeon should accept responsibility for recurrence at the anatomic sites represented in the shaded areas.

regional recurrence in some patients, especially those whose malignancy demonstrates an aggressive behavior. The causes of iatrogenic recurrence involve the following:

1. Insufficient lymphadenectomy
2. Traumatized margins of excision immediately adjacent to the primary cancer resulting in microscopic residual disease
3. Blood loss from the cancer specimen, which allows tumor-contaminated blood to remain within the peritoneal cavity
4. Lymph leak from transected lymphatic channels, which allows viable cancer cells to remain within the peritoneal cavity

4. OPTIMIZATION OF COLORECTAL CANCER RESECTION

An optimization of surgical technology in order to contain the malignant process can prevent iatrogenic recurrence in a majority of patients. First, adequate exposure is required so that the cancer specimen can be handled gently with minimal traction and thereby prevent disruption of the malignant tissue. Second, optimal containment requires complete hemostasis. No blood loss from the transection of blood vessels should be allowed. Electrosurgery should be used to transect tissue, which gives an additional margin of heat necrosis that will eliminate microscopic residual disease at the narrow margins of resection *(16,17)*. Third, conglomerate suture ligatures in continuity should be used to transect major vascular and lymphatic channels. This prevents the escape of cancer cells within leaking lymph channels. Fourth, adequate lateral margins of dissection are required to prevent the disruption of soft tissues that are in immediate contact with the primary malignancy. Generous utilization of peritonectomy procedures will provide the most adequate lateral margins *(18)*. These procedures allow surgeons to maintain a soft-tissue covering of the tumor as it is being resected. Finally, there must be adequate lymph node dissection. The en-bloc lymphadenectomy should go to the base of the major vessels so that persistence

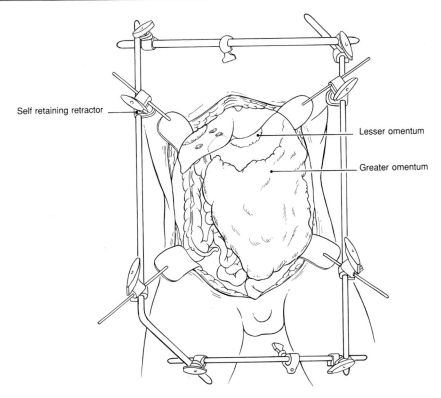

Fig. 2. Optimal exposure requires a midline incision, a self-retaining retractor to allow complete visualization of the operative field, and a second tier of retractors to remove viscera and other organs from the operative field.

or progression of disease within the abdominal or pelvic lymph node chains is prevented. For left colorectal cancer, a complete lymphadenectomy means resection of paracolic, intermediate, and inferior mesenteric nodes that are at the junction of the inferior mesenteric artery and aorta. In other parts of the colon, one must resect lymph nodes down to the origin of the middle colic, right colic, or ileocolic artery immediately adjacent to the superior mesenteric artery and vein.

The surgeon should not ligate any lymphatic or venous structures prior to the ligation of the relevant arterial structures. No venous hypertension should be elicited while the dissection is proceeding. Also, tissues surrounding large vascular structures should be ligated as a conglomerate of artery, vein, and lymphatic channels to prevent leakage of blood and lymph from the specimen side of the dissection. On the patient side of the dissection, large blood vessels should be ligated in continuity and then suture-ligated. Conglomerate ligation of blood vessels and lymphatic channels follows the principle of containment.

Optimal exposure is a necessary requirement of colorectal cancer surgery. Optimal exposure requires a complete midline incision, a self-retaining retractor to allow complete visualization of the operative field, and a second tier of retractors to remove viscera and other organs from the operative field (Fig. 2). Frequent irrigation of the operative field will remove blood from the tissues to be dissected so that they maintain a transparent quality. A bloodstained operative field promotes further blood loss because blood vessels cannot be seen prior to their transection. Finally, sometimes surgeons need better help than can be

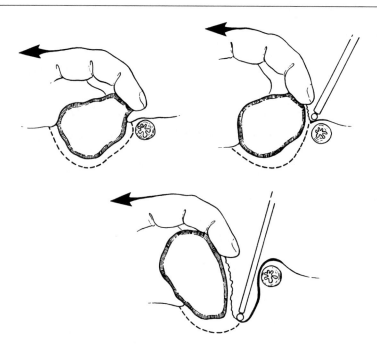

Fig. 3. Electrosurgery has replaced dissection with a scissors or knife in gastrointestinal cancer surgery. A lens-shaped (lenticular) defect is created by dissection with a ball tip if high-voltage electrosurgery on pure cut is used. Strong traction on the specimen will optimize the skeletonization of vital structures. A 0.5 to 1.0-mm layer of heat necrosis remains at the furthest extent of the dissection. This heat necrosis facilitates an adequate tumor-free margin of resection.

provided by resident assistance. Very difficult cases require expert assistance, such as that provided by a second experienced surgeon.

Optimal hemostasis is essential not only to preserve the translucent nature of the tissues and thereby facilitate exposure but also to prevent the dissemination of cancer cells contained within blood. The most dangerous bleeding, in terms of cancer dissemination, is that from transected veins and venules on the cancer specimen. Hemostasis is facilitated by using peritonectomy procedures, laser-mode electrosurgery, ligatures in continuity proximally and distally on all vessels, and a morsilization of fatty tissue surrounding small- and medium-sized blood vessels prior to ligation (Fig. 3).

A thorough knowledge of anatomy and the preservation of mesodermal planes is required within the abdomen and pelvis and within the retroperitoneal portion of the abdomen and pelvis. A prominent mesodermal layer exists posterior to the right colon. This layer must be respected when performing a right colectomy. A prominent mesodermal layer exists between the left colon and lower border of the pancreas, perirenal fat, the left paracolic gutter and left side of the pelvis. In addition, as the rectum becomes a retroperitoneal structure, the mesorectum persists and can guide the surgeon to dissect along the proper tissue plane so that there will be optimal clearance and containment of the cancerous process.

To summarize, optimal clearance and containment of primary colon and rectal cancer involves optimal exposure, complete hemostasis, adequate lymph node dissection, and adequate margins of resection. The technical requirements include but may not be limited to gentle handling of the cancer specimen, peritonectomy procedures to provide a biological dressing that will shroud the malignant process, preservation of the intact mesodermal envelope that will contain tumors in the portions of bowel that are associated with the retroperitoneum or pelvis, refusal to lyse potentially cancer-containing adhesions, electro-surgery to eliminate bleeding and provide a more adequate margin through heat necrosis, and conglomerate ligation of arterial, venous, and lymphatic channels on the specimen side of the dissection.

5. PREVENTION OF PERITONEAL CARCINOMATOSIS IN HIGH-RISK GROUPS

In some patients, there will be a high likelihood of subsequent peritoneal carcinomatosis determined at the time of the colorectal cancer exploration. Positive peritoneal cytology, cancerous involvement of the ovaries, visible evidence of peritoneal seeding on the surface of the specimen, bleeding from the surface of a necrotic tumor mass, adjacent organ involvement, intraoperative cancer spill from disruption of the specimen, and perforation of the malignancy through the primary cancer can be assumed to cause cancerous seeding of peritoneal surfaces.

Even though a complete lymphadenectomy has been performed, involved lymph nodes at the most distal margin of resection may be involved. Positive distal lymph nodes result in a high likelihood of cancerous lymph leak. It is unreasonable to expect cancer cells to be progressing within regional lymph nodes and for cancer cells to be absent from within the adjacent lymphatic channels. These lymphatic channels are inevitably transected as a result of the removal of the primary tumor. All of these conditions place the patient at high risk for subsequent progression of peritoneal carcinomatosis.

Whenever there is a high likelihood of peritoneal dissemination, the fact should be documented. In this instance, surgeons should use an intraoperative intraperitoneal chemotherapy wash as an essential part of the cancer surgery. The concept of eradicating the last cancer cell demands not only maximal surgical clearance and containment of the primary tumor but also the selective treatment with perioperative intraperitoneal chemotherapy of patients who are at high risk for microscopic residual disease.

6. TREATMENT OF PERITONEAL CARCINOMATOSIS FROM COLORECTAL CANCER

In patients who have carcinomatosis at the time of colon or rectal cancer resection, surgeons must accept a loss of containment of the primary tumor. However, in a selected group of patients, loco-regional containment can still be achieved. The successful treatment of peritoneal surface spread of large bowel cancer requires a combined approach that utilizes peritonectomy procedures and perioperative intraperitoneal chemotherapy. In addition, knowledgeable patient selection is mandatory. Both visceral and parietal peritonectomy procedures must be utilized in an attempt to resect all visible evidence of disease (18). Complete cytoreduction is essential for the treatment of peritoneal surface malignancy to result in long-term survival. However, peritonectomy procedures are utilized only in areas of visible implants. Small tumor nodules on the peritoneal surface are removed using electroevaporation. Involvement of visceral peritoneum requires resection of that portion of the bowel. A complete stripping of all the peritoneum including normal tissue is unnecessary and can result in a high incidence of postoperative complications. If all visible cancer can be removed, then the microscopic residual disease can be eradicated in a majority of patients by adequate perioperative intraperitoneal chemotherapy.

High-voltage electrosurgery is necessary for adequate peritonectomy (16). Removal of peritoneal surface disease using the traditional scissor or knife dissection will unnecessarily disseminate tumor emboli further. Surgery by electroevaporation leaves a margin of heat necrosis devoid of viable malignant cells. Also, in the absence of electrosurgery, profuse bleeding from stripped peritoneal surfaces may occur during the intraperitoneal wash with chemotherapy.

6.1. Conceptual Changes with the Use of Chemotherapy for Peritoneal Carcinomatosis

Changes in the use of chemotherapy in patients with peritoneal carcinomatosis have shown favorable results (19) (see Chapter 33). A change in route of drug administration has occurred: Chemotherapy is given intraperitoneally or combined intravenously and intraperitoneally. In this new strategy, intravenous chemotherapy alone is rarely indicated. Also, a change in timing has occurred because chemotherapy begins in the operating room and will continue for the first five postoperative days. There has been a change in selection criteria for treatment of patients with peritoneal carcinomatosis. The lesion size of the peritoneal implant is of crucial importance. Small lesions indicate treatment has been instituted at an early phase of the intraperitoneal dissemination process. The initiation of these treatments for peritoneal surface malignancy must occur as early as possible in the natural history of the disease in order to achieve the greatest benefits. A major change now needs to occur in the attitude of oncologists toward this manifestation of large bowel cancer. Peritoneal carcinomatosis may be cured with early application of combined treatments.

Recent reports by Pestieau and Sugarbaker suggest that early aggressive treatment of carcinomatosis may offer great benefits to these patients. Of 104 patients with peritoneal carcinomatosis from colon or rectal cancer, five patients (4.8%) had definitive treatment of the peritoneal surface spread of the cancer concomitant with resection of the primary lesion (20). Median survival for these patients has not been reached and their 5-yr survival rate is 100%. The remainder of the patients ($n = 99$) were referred for local and regional recurrence after their primary cancer had been removed and there was progression of carcinomatosis. Forty-four patients (42.3%) had a complete cytoreduction resulting in a 24-mo median survival and a 30% 5-yr survival ($p < 0.0001$). The other 55 patients (52.9%) had an incomplete cytoreduction resulting in a 12-mo median survival and a 0% 5-yr survival ($p < 0.0001$). In patients with peritoneal seeding occurring at the time of resection of the primary malignancy, peritonectomy procedures and perioperative intraperitoneal chemotherapy should be performed concomitantly (Fig. 4).

6.2. Peritoneal Space to Plasma Barrier

Intraperitoneal chemotherapy provides a high response at the peritoneal surface of the abdomen and pelvis as a result of the "peritoneal–plasma barrier." High-molecular-weight substances such as mitomycin C are confined to the abdominal cavity for long time periods and provide a dose-intensive therapy. The area-under-the-curve ratios of intraperitoneal to intravenous exposure are favorable. Table 1 presents the area under the curve (intraperitoneal/intravenous) for the drugs in routine clinical use in patients with peritoneal seeding. In our experience, these include 5-fluorouracil, mitomycin C, doxorubicin, cisplatin, paclitaxel, and gemcitabine.

6.3. Tumor Cell Entrapment

Sugarbaker presented the "tumor cell entrapment" hypothesis to explain the rapid progression of peritoneal surface malignancy in patients with microscopic or gross residual disease (21). This theory relates a high incidence and rapid progression of peritoneal implants

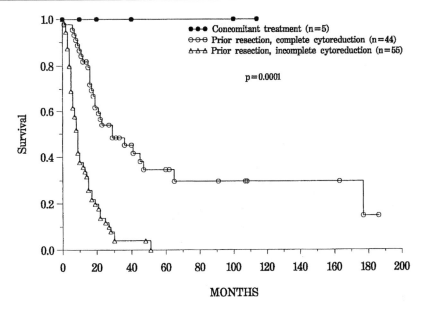

Fig. 4. In patients with peritoneal seeding occurring at the time of resection of the primary malignancy, peritonectomy procedures and perioperative intraperitoneal chemotherapy should be performed concomitantly. From ref. *20* with permission.

to entrapment of these tumor cells on traumatized peritoneal surfaces and a progression of the cells fixed at a particular anatomic site through growth factors that are involved in the wound-healing process. Reimplantation of malignant cells in patients with peritoneal carcinomatosis into peritonectomized surfaces must be expected unless intraperitoneal chemotherapy is used.

6.4. Patient Selection for Treatment of Peritoneal Carcinomatosis

The greatest impediment to lasting benefits from peritonectomy procedures and intraperitoneal chemotherapy is improper patient selection. In the past, numerous patients with advanced intra-abdominal disease have been treated with minimal benefit. Even with extensive cytoreduction and aggressive intraperitoneal chemotherapy, the patient with gross disease is not likely to show long-term survival. Patients who benefit must have minimal disease isolated to peritoneal surfaces, so that following peritonectomy, the chemotherapy is only required to eradicate microscopic residual disease. Partial responses are of little or no benefit in peritoneal surface malignancies. Complete and durable responses are the reasonable goals. The timing for the initiation of treatment has a great impact on the benefits achieved. Asymptomatic patients with small-volume peritoneal surface malignancy must be selected for treatment.

6.5. Quantitative Clinical Assessments of Peritoneal Carcinomatosis

The clinically most accurate quantitative assessment of peritoneal carcinomatosis is the peritoneal cancer index *(22)*. This assessment is a clinical integration of both peritoneal implant size and distribution of peritoneal surface malignancy (Fig. 5). It should be used in the decision-making process as the abdomen is explored *(23)*. Patients who have a low peritoneal cancer index should undergo cytoreductive surgery with curative intent. Those patients with a high peritoneal cancer index only receive debulking surgery with palliative

Table 1
Area-Under-the-Curve Ratios of Peritoneal Surface Exposure to Systemic
Exposure for Drugs Used to Treat Peritoneal Carcinomatosis

Drug	Molecular weight	Area-under-the-curve ratio
5-Fluorouracil	130	75
Gemcitabine	263	50
Cisplatin	300	20
Mitomycin C	334	75
Doxorubicin	544	500
Paclitaxel	808	1000

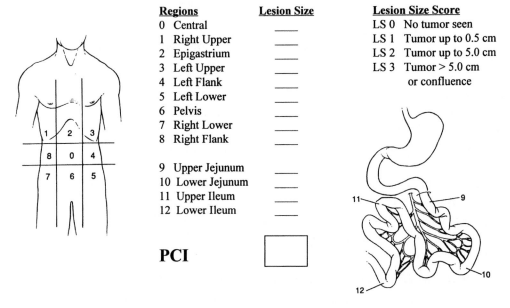

Fig. 5. Peritoneal cancer index is determined after the abdominal exploration is complete. It assists in making a surgical judgement to proceed or not with an attempt at complete cytoreduction.

intent. To arrive at a score, the size of intraperitoneal tumor nodules must be assessed in all of the 13 abdominal and pelvic regions. The lesion size (LS) score should be used. A LS-0 score means that no malignant deposits are visualized; a LS-1 score signifies the presence of tumor nodules less than 0.5 cm (the number of tumor nodules is not scored, only the size of the largest nodule); a LS-2 score signifies the presence of tumor nodules between 0.5 and 5.0 cm. A LS-3 score signifies tumor nodules > 5.0 cm in any dimension. In addition, confluence or layering of tumor within an abdominal or pelvic region indicates a LS-3 score. A LS score is determined for each of the 13 regions. The summation of the lesion size scores in each of the 13 abdomino-pelvic regions is the peritoneal cancer index for that patient. A maximum score is 39 or 13 × 3.

One caveat concerning scoring of the peritoneal cancer index should be mentioned. If cancer is found at a crucial anatomic site in which cytoreduction is impossible, then the patient will have a poor prognosis despite a low peritoneal cancer index. For example, deep invasion of the base of the bladder or disease deep into a pelvic side wall may, by itself, result in residual cancer even after maximal cytoreduction. Also, invasive cancer at numerous

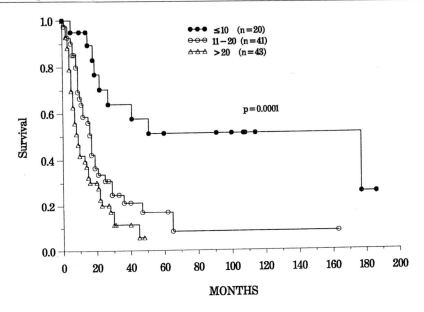

Fig. 6. Survival of patients with colorectal cancer and peritoneal carcinomatosis by the peritoneal cancer index. From ref. *20* with permission.

sites along the surface of the small bowel will confer a poor prognosis. Invasive cancer at a crucial anatomic site may function as a systemic disease equivalent in assessing the prognosis. Because long-term survival can only be achieved in patients in whom complete cytoreduction is carried out, residual disease at crucial anatomic sites may cause the surgeon to select palliative debulking rather than potentially curative cytoreduction despite a favorable score of the peritoneal cancer index *(23)*. The impact of the peritoneal cancer index on survival in patients with seeding from colorectal cancer is shown in Fig. 6.

6.6. Completeness of Cytoreduction Score

The second assessment used to measure prognosis with peritoneal carcinomatosis from large bowel cancer is the completeness of cytoreduction (CC) score. This information is of less value to the surgeon in planning treatment than the peritoneal cancer index. The CC score is not available until after the cytoreduction is complete rather than as the abdomen is being explored. However, if during exploration it becomes obvious that cytoreduction will not be complete, surgeons may decide that palliative debulking will provide symptomatic relief and less surgical risk. In other words, it would be inappropriate to continue with an aggressive cytoreduction. The CC score is the major prognostic indicator in treating large bowel cancer dissemination to peritoneal surfaces *(24)*.

In scoring the CC, the likelihood of effective chemotherapy must be considered. A CC-0 score indicates that no peritoneal seeding was exposed during the complete exploration. A CC-1 score indicates that the tumor nodules persisting after cytoreduction are < 2.5 mm. This is the nodule size thought to be penetrable by intraperitoneal chemotherapy. Therefore, a CC-0 or CC-1 cytoreduction is designated a complete cytoreduction. A CC-2 score indicates tumor nodules between 2.5 mm and 2.5 cm. A CC-3 score indicates tumor nodules > 2.5 cm or confluence of unresectable tumor nodules at any site within the abdomen or pelvis. CC-2 and CC-3 cytoreduction scores are considered incomplete cytoreduction (Fig. 7).

The impact of the CC score on the survival of patients with peritoneal carcinomatosis from colorectal cancer is shown in Fig. 8.

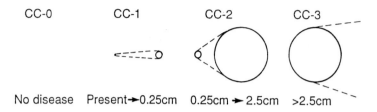

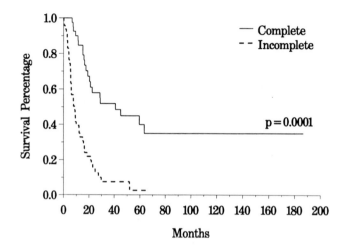

Fig. 7. Completeness of cytoreduction assessment is performed after the maximal surgical effort has been completed.

Fig. 8. Survival of patients with colorectal cancer and peritoneal carcinomatosis by the completeness of cytoreduction (CC) score. From ref. *24* with permission.

6.7. Current Methodology for Delivery of Heated Intraoperative Intraperitoneal Chemotherapy

In the operating room, heated intraoperative intraperitoneal mitomycin C chemotherapy can be used for patients with peritoneal carcinomatosis from colorectal cancer. Heat is part of the optimizing process and is used to bring as much dose intensity to the abdominal and pelvic surfaces as possible. Hyperthermia with intraperitoneal mitomycin C chemotherapy has several advantages. Hyperthermia increases the penetration of chemotherapy into tissues. As tissues soften in response to heat, the elevated interstitial pressure of a tumor mass decreases and allows improved drug penetration. Second, and probably most important, heat increases the cytotoxicity of mitomycin C chemotherapy. This synergism occurs only at the interface of heat and body tissue at the peritoneal surface. The thermal targeting is not produced at systemic sites around the body. The rationale for using heated intraperitoneal mitomycin C chemotherapy as a surgically directed modality in the operating room is presented in Table 2.

After the cancer resection is complete, the Tenckhoff catheter and closed-suction drains are placed through the abdominal wall and made watertight with a purse-string suture at the skin. Temperature probes are directed into the abdomen and pelvis and are secured to the skin edge. Using running no. 2 monofilament sutures, the skin edges are secured to the self-retaining retractor. A plastic sheet is incorporated into these sutures to create a covering for the abdominal cavity. A slit in the plastic cover is made to allow the surgeon's double-

Table 2
Rationale for the Use of Heated Intraoperative Intraperitoneal Chemotherapy

Heat increases drug penetration into tissue.
Heat increases the cytotoxicity of selected chemotherapy agents.
Heat has an antitumor effect by itself.
Intraoperative chemotherapy allows manual distribution of drug and heat uniformly to all surfaces of the abdomen and pelvis.
Renal toxicities of chemotherapy given in the operation room can be avoided by careful monitoring of urine output during chemotherapy perfusion.
The time that elapses during the heated perfusion allows a normalization of many parameters (temperature, blood clotting, hemodynamic, etc.).

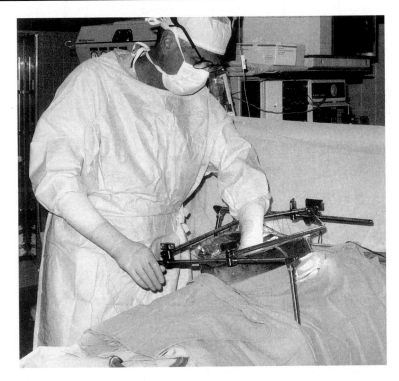

Fig. 9. Coliseum technique for the delivery of heated intraoperative intraperitoneal chemotherapy. The surgeon manually separates all surfaces to maintain uniformity of heat and chemotherapy throughout the abdomen and pelvis. He is required to "scrub" all surfaces to eliminate all adherent fibrin and blood clot.

gloved hand access to the abdomen and pelvis (Fig. 9). During the 90 min of perfusion, all the anatomic structures within the peritoneal cavity are uniformly exposed to heat and chemotherapy. The surgeon vigorously manipulates all the viscera to keep adherence of peritoneal surfaces to a minimum. Roller pumps force the chemotherapy solution into the abdomen through the Tenckhoff catheter and pull it out through the drains. The heat exchanger keeps the fluid infused at 44°C to 46°C so that the intraperitoneal fluid is maintained at 42°C to 43°C. The apparatus used for administering the heated intraoperative intraperitoneal chemotherapy is diagrammed in Fig. 10. The smoke evacuator is used to pull air from beneath the plastic cover through activated charcoal, preventing contamination of air in the operating room by chemotherapy aerosols.

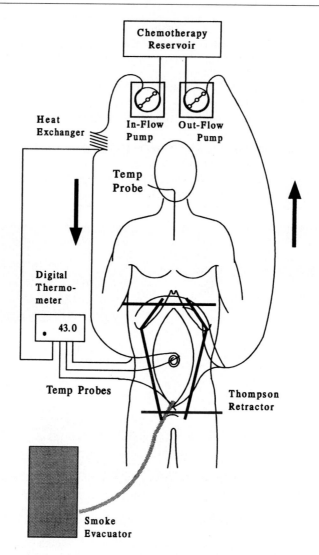

Fig. 10. Apparatus required for heated intraoperative intraperitoneal chemotherapy.

After the intra-abdominal heated chemotherapy with mitomycin C is complete, the abdomen is suctioned dry of fluid. The abdominal wall is then reopened and the retractors repositioned prior to performing anastomosis. It should be re-emphasized that no suture lines are constructed until after the chemotherapy perfusion is complete. The standardized orders for heated intraoperative intraperitoneal mitomycin C chemotherapy are given in Table 3.

6.8. Immediate Postoperative Abdominal Lavage

In patients with peritoneal carcinomatosis from large bowel cancer, we advocate early postoperative intraperitoneal 5-fluorouracil. The catheters that were positioned for intraoperative chemotherapy for drug instillation and abdominal drainage must be kept clear of blood clots and tissue debris. To accomplish this, an abdominal lavage is started in the operating room. This lavage utilizes the same tubes and drains that were positioned for heated intraoperative intraperitoneal chemotherapy. Large volumes of fluid are rapidly

Table 3
Standardized Orders for Heated Intraoperative Intraperitoneal Chemotherapy

Mitomycin Orders
1. For adenocarcinoma from appendiceal, colonic, rectal, gastric and pancreatic cancer; add mito-mycin _____ mg to 2 L of 1.5% dextrose peritoneal dialysis solution.
2. Dose of mitomycin C for men 12.5 mg/m^2, for women 10 mg/m^2.
3. Use a 33% dose reduction for heavy prior chemotherapy, marginal renal function, age >60 yr, extensive intraoperative trauma to small bowel surfaces, or prior radiotherapy.
4. Send 1 L of 1.5% dextrose peritoneal dialysis solution to test the perfusion circuit.
5. Send 1 L of 1.5% dextrose peritoneal dialysis solution for immediate postoperative lavage.
6. Send the above to operating room _____ at _____ AM/PM.

Table 4
Immediate Postoperative Abdominal Lavage

Day of Operation:
1. Run in 1000 mL 1.5% dextrose peritoneal dialysis solution as rapidly as possible. Warm to body temperature prior to instillation. Clamp all abdominal drains during infusion.
2. No dwell time.
3. Drain as rapidly as possible through the Tenckhoff catheter and abdominal drains.
4. Repeat irrigations every 1 h for 4 h, then every 4 h until returns are clear; then every 8 h until chemotherapy begins.
5. Change dressing at Tenckhoff catheter and abdominal drain skin sites using sterile technique once daily and as necessary.
6. Standardized precautions must be used for all body fluids from this patient.

infused and then drained from the abdomen after a short dwell time. The standardized orders for immediate postoperative abdominal lavage are given in Table 4. All intra-abdominal catheters are withdrawn before the patient is discharge from the hospital.

6.9. Early Postoperative Intraperitoneal 5-Fluorouracil

The standardized order for early postoperative intraperitoneal 5-fluorouracil are presented in Table 5. After the patient stabilizes postoperatively and after the drainage from the immediate postoperative abdominal lavage is no longer bloodstained, the 5-fluorouracil instillation begins. In some patients who have extensive small bowel trauma from lysis of adhesions, the early postoperative 5-fluorouracil is withheld for fear of fistula formation. During the first 6 h of intraperitoneal 5-fluorouracil administration, the patient turns every half-hour from the right side to the left side to maximize drug distribution through gravitational effects.

6.10. Second-Look Surgery

Patients are maintained on systemic chemotherapy after discharge from the hospital. The chemotherapy regimen of irinotecan, leucovorin, and 5-fluorouracil reported by Saltz and colleagues is recommended (25). After approx 6 mo on systemic treatment, the patient is recommended for a second-look procedure (22). At the time of second-look surgery, the abdomen is widely opened and all the peritoneal surfaces are visualized with a complete takedown of all adhesions. Additional cytoreduction is performed and additional visceral peritonectomies may be required. If a CC-0 or CC-1 cytoreduction can be achieved, then

Table 5
Early Postoperative Intraperitoneal Chemotherapy with 5-Fluorouracil

Postoperative days 1–5
1. Add to _____ mL 1.5% dextrose peritoneal dialysis solution:
   (a) _____ mg 5-fluorouracil (650 mg/m^2, maximal dose 1300 mg)
   (b) 50 meq sodium bicarbonate
2. Intraperitoneal fluid volume: 1 L for patients <2.0 m^2, 1.5 L for >2.0 m^2.
3. Drain all fluid from the abdominal cavity prior to instillation, then clamp abdominal drains.
4. Run the chemotherapy solution into the abdominal cavity through the Tenckhoff catheter as rapidly as possible. Dwell for 23 h and drain for 1 h prior to next instillation.
5. Use gravity to maximize intraperitoneal distribution of the 5-fluorouracil. Instill the chemotherapy with the patient in a full right lateral position. After 1/2 h, direct the patient to turn to the full left lateral position. Change position right to left every 1/2 h. If tolerated, use 10 degrees of Trendelenburg position. Continue turning for the first 6 h after instillation of chemotherapy solution.
6. Continue to drain abdominal cavity after final dwell until Tenckhoff catheter is removed.
7. Use 33% dose reduction for heavy prior chemotherapy, age >60 yr, or prior radiotherapy.

heated intraoperative intraperitoneal chemotherapy is used again. Early postoperative intraperitoneal 5-fluorouracil is also recommended after the reoperation. In some patients, the disease may suggest a "chemotherapy failure." In this situation, a change in the drugs used for intraperitoneal chemotherapy is recommended. Usually, a regimen of intraperitoneal cisplatin and doxorubicin is utilized.

7. PATIENT CARE CONSIDERATIONS

The major detrimental side effect of combined cytoreductive surgery and intraperitoneal chemotherapy is prolonged ileus. Patients may have a nasogastric tube in place, with large volumes of secretions being aspirated from the stomach for 2–4 wk postoperatively. For this reason, parenteral feeding is recommended for all of these patients. The length of time required for nasogastric suctioning is dependent on the extent of peritonectomy and the extent of prior abdominal adhesions that required lysis.

The most life threatening postoperative complication is small bowel fistula. Usually, these are side-wall perforations of the small bowel, but, occasionally, a colon or stomach perforation has occurred. Patients need to be aware of the possibility of fistula formation before cytoreductive surgery and intraperitoneal chemotherapy are contemplated. The incidence of anastomotic leak is very low.

The morbidity rate of cytoreductive surgery and intraperitoneal chemotherapy for colon cancer is approx 25% and the mortality rate is 1.5%. Mortality is usually related to neutropenia, which can occur from overly aggressive use of intraperitoneal 5-fluorouracil. In some patients who are age > 60 yr old, have received prior systemic chemotherapy, or prior radiation therapy, a dose reduction of the intraperitoneal 5-fluorouracil must be made *(26)*.

8. ETHICAL CONSIDERATIONS IN TREATING PERITONEAL CARCINOMATOSIS FROM COLON AND RECTAL CANCER

Currently, the phase II studies that show benefit in the prevention or treatment of peritoneal carcinomatosis demand that patients be treated. Patients recommended for treatment are

Table 6
Patients with Colorectal Cancer Recommended for Perioperative Intraperitoneal Chemotherapy

- Positive peritoneal cytology
- Ovarian involvement
- Peritoneal seeding on the serosal surface of the colon
- Rupture of a necrotic tumor mass
- Adjacent organ involvement
- Intraoperative tumor spill
- Perforation of the primary tumor
- Involved lymph nodes at the margin of excision
- Limited peritoneal seeding with a peritoneal cancer index of <20
- Limited peritoneal seeding so that a complete cytoreduction can be achieved

those identified in Table 6. Until clinical trials have been initiated, we also recommend that patients with bulky lymph node metastases or lymphatic dissemination that continues to the superior mesenteric vein or aorta be treated. The likelihood of tumor spill as a result of cancer cells leaking from lymphatic channels is so great that these low-morbidity/mortality treatments need to be initiated.

In patients with potentially curable large bowel cancer, intraperitoneal chemotherapy treatments should only be initiated as Institutional Review Board-approved randomized controlled studies. There is a strong rationale for treatment of patients with advanced malignancy, especially those patients in whom major surgical trauma is required for resection (i.e., have large tumors at the hepatic flexure, splenic flexure, or within the pelvis).

REFERENCES

1. Turnbull RB, Kyle K, Watson FR, and Spratt J. Cancer of the colon: the influence of the no-touch isolation technic on survival rates. *Ann. Surg.*, **166(3)** (1967) 420–427.
2. Phillips RKS, Hittinger R, Blesovsky L, Fry JS, and Fielding LP. Local recurrence following "curative" surgery for large bowel cancer: I. The overall picture. *Br. J. Surg.*, **71** (1984) 12–16.
3. McArdle CS and Hole D. Impact of variability among surgeons on postoperative morbidity and mortality and ultimate survival. *Br. J. Surg.*, **302** (1991) 1501–1505.
4. Hermanek P, Wieblet H, Staimmer D, Riedl S, and the German Study Group Colo-Rectal Carcinoma (SGCRC). Prognostic factors of rectum carcinoma—experience of the German multicentre study SGCRC. *Tumori*, **81(Suppl.)** (1995) 60–64.
5. Holm T, Johansson H, Cedermark B, Ekelund, G, and Rutqvist LE. Influence of hospital- and surgeon-related factors on outcome after treatment of rectal cancer with or without preoperative radiotherapy. *Br. J. Surg.*, **84** (1997) 657–663.
6. Porter GA, Soskolne CL, Yakimets WW, and Newman SC. Surgeon-related factors and outcome in rectal cancer. *Ann. Surg.*, **227(2)** (1998) 157–167.
7. Anthone G, Brophy M, Fals J, Vukasin P, Ortega A, Ross R, et al. Does designated surgical interest improve the surgical management of colorectal cancer? Work done at University of Southern California. Annual Meeting of the American Society of Colon and Rectal Surgeons, 1998.
8. Averbach AM, Jacquet P, and Sugarbaker PH. Surgical technique and colorectal cancer: impaction on local recurrence and survival. *Tumori*, **81(Suppl.)** (1995) 65–71.
9. Scott N, Jackson P, Al-Jaberi, Dixon MF, Quirke P, and Finan PJ. Total mesorectal excision and local recurrence: A study of tumour spread in the mesorectum distal to rectal cancer. *Br. J. Surg.*, **82** (1995) 1031–1033.
10. Heald RJ and Ryall RDH. Recurrence and survival after total mesorectal excision for rectal cancer. *Lancet*, **i** (1986) 1479–1482.
11. Gunderson LL and Sosin H. Areas of failure found at reoperation (second or symptomatic look) following "curative surgery" for adenocarcinoma of the rectum: clinicopathologic correlation and implications for adjuvant therapy. *Cancer*, **34** (1974) 1278–1292.

12. Pickren JW, Tsukada Y, and Lane WW. Liver metastasis: analysis of autopsy data. In *Liver Metastasis.* Weiss L and Gilbert HA (eds.), GK Hall, Boston, 1982, pp 2–18.

13. Lofgren EP, Waugh JM, and Dockerty MB. Local recurrence of carcinoma after anterior resection of the rectum and the sigmoid. *Arch. Surg.,* **74** (1957) 825–838.

14. Cole WH, Roberts SS, and Strehl FW. Modern concepts in cancer of the colon and rectum. *Cancer,* **19** (1966) 1347–1358.

15. Sugarbaker PH, Gianola FJ, Speyer JL, Wesley R, Barofsky I, and Meyers CE. Prospective randomized trial of intravenous versus intraperitoneal 5-fluorouracil in patients with advanced primary colon or rectal cancer. *Surgery,* **98** (1985) 414–421.

16. Sugarbaker PH. Laser-mode electrosurgery. In *Peritoneal Carcinomatosis: Principles of Management.* Sugarbaker PH (ed.), Kluwer, Boston, 1996, pp. 375–386.

17. Sugarbaker PH. Peritoneal carcinomatosis, sarcomatosis and mesothelioma. Surgical responsibilities. In *Surgical Oncology Multidisciplinary Approach to Difficult Problems.* Silverman H and Lieberman AW (eds.), Arnold, NY, 2002, pp. 175–205.

18. Sugarbaker PH. Peritonectomy procedures. *Ann. Surg.,* **221** (1995) 29–42.

19. Sugarbaker PH (ed.). *Intraperitoneal Chemotherapy and Cytoreductive Surgery: A Manual for Physicians and Nurses,* 3rd ed. Ludann Company, Grand Rapids, Michigan, 1998.

20. Pestieau SR and Sugarbaker PH. Treatment of primary colon cancer with peritoneal carcinomatosis: A comparison of concomitant versus delayed management. *Dis. Colon Rectum,* **43** (2000) 1341–1348.

21. Sugarbaker PH. Peritoneal carcinomatosis: natural history and rational therapeutic interventions using intraperitoneal chemotherapy. In *Peritoneal Carcinomatosis: Drugs and Diseases.* Sugarbaker PH (ed.), Kluwer, Boston, 1996, pp. 149–168.

22. Gomez Portilla A, Sugarbaker PH, and Chang D. Second-look surgery after cytoreductive and intraperitoneal chemotherapy for peritoneal carcinomatosis from colorectal cancer: analysis of prognostic features. *World J. Surg.,* **23(1)** (1999) 23–29.

23. Esquivel J and Sugarbaker PH. Elective surgery in recurrent colon cancer with peritoneal seeding: when to and when not to operate (editorial). *Cancer Therapeut.,* **1** (1998) 321–325.

24. Sugarbaker PH. Successful management of microscopic residual disease in large bowel cancer. *Cancer Chemother. Pharmacol.,* **43(Suppl.)** (1999) S15–S25.

25. Saltz LB, Cox JV, Blanke C, Rosen LS, Fehrenbacher L, Moore MJ, et al. Irinotecan plus fluorouracil and leucovorin for metastatic colorectal cancer. Irinotecan Study Group. *N. Engl. J. Med.,* **343** (2000) 905–914.

26. Stephens AD and Sugarbaker PH. Morbidity and mortality of cytoreductive surgery and hyperthermic intraoperative intraperitoneal chemotherapy with mitomycin C using the coliseum technique. *Ann. Surg. Oncol.,* **6(8)** (1999) 790–796.

23 Cryosurgical Ablation for the Management of Unresectable Hepatic Colorectal Metastases

Gregory D. Kennedy, Fred T. Lee, Jr.,
David Mahvi, and John E. Niederhuber

CONTENTS

1. INTRODUCTION

Nearly 15% of patients presenting with primary colorectal carcinoma will have synchronous metastases, and an additional 60% of patients with colorectal carcinoma will develop subsequent metastases to the liver. The natural history of hepatic metastases depends on several factors, including tumor histology, stage of primary tumor, the extent of liver metastases, the disease-free interval, and the presence or absence of extrahepatic disease. Patients with unresectable colorectal metastases to the liver have a very poor prognosis, with a median survival of 6–13 mo *(1)*. The preferred treatment for hepatic colorectal metastases is complete surgical resection, which can lead to a 5-yr survival of 25–40% (*see* Chapter 20) *(1–3)*. Unfortunately, only 10–30% of patients with isolated hepatic metastases have surgically resectable disease.

From: *Colorectal Cancer: Multimodality Management*
Edited by: L. Saltz © Humana Press Inc., Totowa, NJ

Driven by the low resectability rate and limited treatment options, recent therapeutic efforts have focused on more aggressive regional therapies for hepatic metastases from colorectal adenocarcinoma. Cryosurgery involves using a liquid-nitrogen-cooled probe to freeze a tumor, thereby rendering the cancer cells nonviable while sparing normal liver tissue. Accumulating evidence documents that cryosurgical ablation is a safe, efficacious treatment alternative for many patients with surgically unresectable tumors. In fact, cryoablation of selected patients with unresectable colorectal carcinoma isolated to the liver results in long-term survival similar to that achieved with surgically resected lesions. In this chapter, we review the available data supporting the use of cryosurgery for the treatment of liver metastases and outline some of the basic principles of patient selection and techniques for its use.

2. HISTORY

It is interesting to note that the application of cold for the treatment of cancer has its roots in the mid-1800s when the English physician James Arnott (1797–1883) used salt solutions containing crushed ice at a temperature in the range of $-18°C$ to $-24°C$ to freeze advanced cancers in accessible sites such as the breast and cervix (4). However, this therapeutic option was limited to surface tumors until the early 1960s when the automated cryosurgical unit cooled by liquid nitrogen was introduced by Cooper and Lee (5). The technology introduced by Cooper and Lee permitted the cooling process to be more rigorously controlled and monitored. As a result, many different specialties of medicine applied cryosurgery to a number of different disease processes. During this early period of investigation, a wide variety of solid tumors were treated with cryosurgery with considerable success (6).

Prior to 1985, using cryosurgery for liver tumors was limited because of difficulties in tumor localization, probe placement, and the complications that invariably arose because the freezing process could not be accurately monitored (7). Today, liver tumors can be accurately imaged with intraoperative ultrasound allowing highly specific probe placement and real-time imaging of the freezing process (8,9). Accordingly, cryosurgery has emerged as a viable therapeutic alternative for the treatment of patients with unresectable liver tumors and as an adjunct to be used in combination with resection.

3. BIOLOGY OF CRYOINJURY

Numerous animal studies have been performed to demonstrate the feasibility of cryosurgery of the liver. Despite all of these investigations, the exact mechanism of cellular death remains unknown. It is likely that cell death results from complex physiologic mechanisms involving ice crystal formation and cellular anoxia during the frozen state, followed by indirect microvascular thrombosis. Experimental evidence also suggests an adaptive immunologic tumor response in the postfrozen state (10,11). The overall results are cell membrane destruction, enzyme denaturation, osmotic dehydration, anoxia, and cellular necrosis (12). Using an animal model of hepatic metastases, Heise et al. at the University of Wisconsin have been able to demonstrate that tumor cells at the periphery of a cryoinduced lesion, which have escaped cold-induced necrosis, will undergo apoptosis. The specific apoptotic pathway activated by freezing remains to be identified (13).

Although the mechanism of cryodestruction is tissue-nonspecific, individual tissues have different sensitivities to cold-induced injury. For example, hepatocytes, bile duct epithelial cells, and connective tissue cells are resistant to temperatures as low as $-10°C$ but are completely destroyed at $-40°C$. In contrast, larger blood vessels seem to be unaffected by temperatures of these extremes (14,15). These observations have been attributed to the heat-sink effect of flowing blood preventing the vessel wall from freezing and have been exploited clinically. The heat-sink effect allows the treatment of tumors adjacent to essential blood vessels that cannot be resected, as resection of tumors in such locations would leave microscopically positive tumor margins.

4. REVIEW OF CLINICAL EXPERIENCE

In 1991, Ravikumar et al. reported the results of phase I/II clinical trials establishing the feasibility and accepted morbidity for cryosurgery (16). They reported on their initial experience with 24 patients with colorectal hepatic metastases treated with cryosurgery using intraoperative ultrasound (IOUS) guidance between 1985 and 1990. At a median follow-up of 24 mo, 29% of patients remained disease-free and an additional 34% were alive with disease, whereas 37% of patients had died. Tumor recurrence in the liver was seen in 35% of patients; however, only 8% of these were felt to be located at the previously treated site.

These data are supported by those published in 1991 by Onik at al. (17). In this retrospective review of their institution's experience, the authors were able to demonstrate a 22% disease-free survival rate at a median follow-up of 22 mo. Local recurrence was noted in 22% of all patients but was only seen in patients with metastatic tumors >4 cm. A study including 136 patients with colorectal metastases reported by Weaver et al. revealed a median survival for all patients of 23 mo with a range of 2–92 mo (18).

In 1997, Korpan published the results of a prospective, randomized trial comparing liver resection with cryosurgical ablation of liver metastases (19). One hundred twenty-three patients were entered into this trial, with 63 patients randomized to cryosurgery and 60 patients to conventional surgery. The majority of patients in each group had liver metastases arising from colorectal carcinoma (>60%) and all patients in the study received postoperative chemotherapy with 5-fluorouracil. The 3- and 5-yr survival rates for each group were reported as 60% and 44% for the cryosurgery group and 51% and 36% in the resection group. At 10-yr, 14% of patients in the cryosurgery group were alive vs 5% of patients in the resection group.

In 1997, Yeh et al. published their results from the Fox Chase Cancer Center on treatment of hepatic metastases with cryosurgical ablation (20). In this small retrospective analysis, the authors reviewed 24 patients who underwent cryosurgery for biopsy-confirmed metastases from adenocarcinoma of the colon and rectum. Twelve of their patients were treated with cryosurgery alone for unresectable disease, whereas the other 12 patients were treated with resection and cryosurgery of the resection margin. Median disease-free survival for both groups was reported to be 14 mo, with a 25% local recurrence rate. A summary of all available reported trials in which colorectal cancer is the predominantly treated tumor is found in Table 1.

Taken together, these data on the treatment of metastatic colorectal cancer involving the liver suggest that patients with unresectable disease should be treated aggressively using cryoablation, as their outcome may be no different than those patients who undergo resection alone. However, before this principle can be applied indiscriminately, an adequately powered prospective randomized trial comparing resection to state-of-the-art cryosurgery needs to be undertaken.

5. COMPETING ABLATIVE MODALITIES

In recent years, radiofrequency ablation (RFA) has been introduced as an alternative to cryosurgery for the treatment of hepatic colorectal metastases (see Chapter 24). RFA for

Table 1
Results for Cryosurgical Ablation of Colorectal Metastases to the Liver

Authors (ref.)	Type of Study	Year	No. of patients	No. of lesions treated	Recurrence rate (%)	Median follow-up (mo)	Survival rate disease-free (%)
Ravikumar et al. (16)	Prospective, nonrandomized	1991	32	NR[a]	8	24	29
Onik et al. (17)	Prospective, nonrandomized	1991	18	73	20	29	22
Weaver et al. (18)	Retrospective	1995	140	158	0	30	29
Yeh et al. (20)	Retrospective	1997	24	NR	25	NR	[b]
Korpan (19)	Prospective	1997	123	NR	NR	120	14
Adam (29)	Retrospective	1997	34	>55	44	16	20[c]
Cha (31)	Retrospective	2000	38	65	12	28	25

Note: The use of recurrence in this context refers to a recurrence within a previously treated lesion. Because of the retrospective nature of most investigations, the local recurrence rate should be used as the benchmark to compare results.

[a]NR = not reported.

[b]The authors state the median survival was not reached so it was not reported. However, they do report an overall disease-free survival of 23.5 mo.

[c]Median survival was not achieved at a follow-up of 16 mo. At the time of publication, the authors report a 20% disease-free survival. Potential bias is introduced by the author's self-admitted lack of IOUS experience and not involving a radiologist in their investigation. The authors have reported on their experience with cryoablation alone and cryoablation combined with resection of liver metastases. The majority of patients in this series underwent treatment of colorectal metastases. A 36% disease-free survival at 48 mo is demonstrated for patients undergoing cryoablation and resection vs 25% 48-mo disease-free survival for patients undergoing cryoablation alone ($p = 0.49$).

colorectal metastases is based on a similar concept to cryosurgery in that a small probe is placed into a metastatic lesion under ultrasound guidance. However, unlike cryosurgery, which depends on generation of cold temperatures, radio-frequency current delivered to a tumor is converted into heat, which results in tissue coagulation and tumor destruction (21) The clinical experience with RFA is not as extensive as that with cryosurgery, and the local recurrence rate, the only statistic that should be used to effectively compare the two competing modalities, has been shown to be from 50% to 100% (22–25). However, recent investigations from the M.D. Anderson Cancer Center studying the use of RFA for the treatment of both primary and metastatic liver tumors reported a local recurrence rate of only 1.8% when performed at the time of laparotomy with a Pringle maneuver (26).

Consistent with the observations made by Curley et al., investigations at the University of Wisconsin have demonstrated in a porcine model that decreasing blood flow to the liver through the use of a Pringle maneuver will increase the area and volume of a lesion generated by RFA (27). This phenomenon could account for the lower local recurrence rate demonstrated by Curley et al. Additional investigations at the University of Wisconsin have led to the development and testing of a bipolar RFA probe. This bipolar probe has been shown to generate larger and more reproducible lesions and, hopefully, will result in a lower local recurrence rate when used percutaneously (unpublished observations).

In summary, radio-frequency ablation is currently under investigation as an alternative to cryosurgery for the treatment of unresectable colorectal cancer metastases involving the liver. RFA has been shown in preliminary studies to have a lower complication rate than cryosurgery but a slightly higher local recurrence rate when used percutaneously. However, when used at the time of laparotomy, RFA has been shown to have a similar complication rate and local recurrence rate as cryosurgery (26). It is our contention that intraoperative use of RFA negates many of the advantages of the technology. It is also more difficult to use ultrasound to follow the generation of a lesion induced by RFA than it is to follow the distinct margins of an iceball generated during cryosurgery. For example, RFA performed percutaneously under transabdominal ultrasound guidance is an outpatient procedure because the heated probe cauterizes the probe tract, resulting in less postprocedure bleeding. For this reason, investigation into the development of newer, more effective probes as well as the optimal surgical procedure in which to perform the procedure will continue. In addition, if RFA is to be used at the time of laparotomy, it should be tested against cryosurgery, the current gold standard of ablative therapy, in a randomized controlled trial.

6. PRINCIPLES OF CRYOSURGERY

The primary objective of cryosurgical ablation is to destroy all malignant tissue while preserving normal tissue. Intraoperative ultrasound (IOUS) has made this objective a reality by not only allowing the surgeon to directly monitor the placement of the probe into the tumor but also allowing the surgeon to monitor progression of the freezing process. The newer technology of IOUS allows the detection and treatment of lesions as small as 0.4 cm, which historically would have been missed. Stone et al. demonstrated the importance of IOUS to liver surgery for the management of colorectal metastases (28). In this retrospective review of recurrent liver-only colorectal metastases, the authors were able to demonstrate that in 3 of 10 patients, 3 lesions were identified that would have otherwise been missed. Two of these lesions were resected without incident; therefore, the IOUS data changed the intraoperative management in 20% of cases.

Patient selection is the key component for the successful use of cryosurgery. General indications for cryosurgery can be found in Table 2. Lesion size and number has been an area of debate when utilizing cryosurgery for treatment of colorectal metastases. It is feasible to treat multiple lesions, as many as 10–15 lesions, during any 1 surgery; however the survival benefit when treating a high number of lesions has yet to be demonstrated (29). In an attempt to identify prognostic factors after cryotherapy for colorectal metastases, Seifert and Morris undertook a review of a prospectively collected database of 116 patients undergoing cryosurgery for colorectal metastases to the liver (30). The data indicated that lesion number did not portend a poor prognosis and, in fact, the patients in this study who had cryoablation of >3 lesions (58 total patients) had no difference in their outcome with a median follow-up of 20.5 mo. These limited data suggest that patients with multiple lesions should have all lesions treated if technically feasible, as those treated in this manner did as well as those patients with three or fewer lesions. However, a prospective randomized trial comparing cryoablation of multiple lesions to systemic chemotherapy or hepatic arterial chemotherapy ≥ cryotherapy of a subset of the lesions (as an attempt to decrease tumor burden) would be required to clarify this issue.

Like lesion number, lesion size and location have been areas of debate regarding patient selection for cryosurgery. Lesions larger than 5 cm have been shown to have a higher local recurrence rate (29) and to also be predictive of a poor prognosis (30). Treatment of patients with bilobar disease has also been controversial and it was initially thought that patients with extensive bilobar disease would have worse outcomes secondary to "silent" extrahepatic disease. In fact, Seifert and Morris looked at unilobar versus bilobar disease in their series and found no difference in 1, 2, or 3-yr survival between these two groups (30). This finding

Table 2
General Indications for Cryosurgery

- Documented metastatic liver disease
- Absence of extrahepatic disease
- Surgically unresectable disease
  - Limited hepatic reserve
  - Bilobar/multilobar disease
  - Tumor in close proximity to major vessels
- Tumor involving surgically resected margins

suggests that patients with bilobar disease are good candidates for cryotherapy and have no worse prognosis than patients with disease limited to one lobe of the liver.

Recently, the University of Wisconsin experience was reviewed, generating new information regarding the efficiency of resection with the addition of cryotherapy for patients with bilobar disease *(31)*. The majority of patients in this analysis had metastatic colorectal carcinoma that was treated with either cryoablation alone or a combination of cryoablation and resection of metastatic lesions. The authors were able to demonstrate no difference in survival between groups, regardless of lesion size or number and irrespective of the age of the patient. Furthermore, a comparison of patients undergoing resection alone vs cryoablation did not demonstrate a difference in survival. This suggests that although cryosurgery is not the new gold standard of treatment, it certainly provides a viable alternative for patients who would otherwise be considered unresectable.

When evaluating patients for cryosurgery, pulmonary metastases are often an issue, as many patients presenting with hepatic metastases will have synchronous metastases in their lungs. Special consideration must be given to this group of patients, especially if their liver disease is amenable to cryosurgery and their pulmonary disease amenable to resection (i.e., unilateral with few nodules that are easily resected). In 1992, McCormack et al. published their series of patients with pulmonary metastases of colorectal carcinoma who underwent pulmonary resection *(32)*. One hundred forty-four patients were included with 5- and 10-yr survival rates of 44% and 25%, respectively. In this trial, patients who were determined not to be resectable were treated with chemotherapy alone and had survival limited to 24 mo. A study from the National Cancer Center of Japan supported these findings, with 159 patients undergoing pulmonary resection for colorectal carcinoma metastases with 5- and 10-yr survival rates of 40.5% and 27%, respectively *(33)*. Furthermore, 33 patients in this series had hepatic metastases treated before their pulmonary metastases and had 5-yr survival rates of 33%. Taken together, these two series suggest that patients with resectable pulmonary metastases have excellent long-term survival and should be treated aggressively, including surgical treatment of hepatic metastases if indicated.

7. PREOPERATIVE EVALUATION

Patients who are candidates for cryosurgical ablation of colorectal hepatic metastases should undergo a routine preoperative evaluation to identify comorbidities. This includes a complete history and physical as well as routine laboratory evaluation, including tumor markers, with carcinoembryonic antigen (CEA) being the most important. In addition, it is imperative that the patient has no evidence of extrahepatic disease. A chest X-ray can be obtained to rule out pulmonary metastases; however, a chest computed tomogram (CT) is more sensitive and is appropriate to include in the initial investigations.

Extrahepatic abdominal disease should be ruled out and the extent of hepatic disease must be determined in the preoperative evaluation as well. A contrast-enhanced spiral CT of the abdomen is an examination that will allow both of these areas to be fully investigated and is the most commonly used modality in the preoperative assessment of patients with liver tumors. In addition, the sensitivity of spiral CT for the detection of liver tumors is ≥90%, with a specificity ≥80% *(34)*. Magnetic resonance imaging (MRI) has also been shown to be a promising tool for the evaluation of the hepatobiliary system. One randomized controlled trial comparing MRI to CT for the evaluation of liver tumors demonstrated CT to be more sensitive (78% vs 94%), however, this study used older MRI technology *(35)*. Future studies will hopefully clarify the most sensitive and specific test for detection of colorectal cancer metastases to the liver.

The role for positron-emission tomography (PET) in the initial workup of the patient with hepatic metastases of colon carcinoma is currently under investigation. In 1999, Fong et al. published the results of a prospective trial in which patients at high risk for unresectable disease (by clinical criteria) scheduled for elective hepatic resection for colorectal metastases were evaluated with PET preoperative workup *(36)*. In this trial, findings on 18F-fluorodeoxyglucose (FDG)–PET scanning influenced the clinical management in 16 patients (40%) and directly altered management in 9 cases (23%). These data suggest that PET is a useful study in patients at high risk for unresectable disease, which is likely to be the subset of patients considered for cryosurgery. However, prior to adding PET to the preoperative workup of all patients considered for cryosurgical ablation of hepatic metastases, a prospective, randomized trial should be performed to confirm its clinical utility in this patient population.

8. CRYOSURGICAL TECHNIQUE

Following the preoperative workup, the eligible patient is taken to the operating room for a laparotomy. A standard intra-abdominal exploration is performed, taking care to evaluate the primary resection site. A hilar lymph node dissection is performed if there is any indication of involved nodes and the liver is fully mobilized. At this time, an intraoperative ultrasound is crucial to allow further evaluation of the liver.

Experience with IOUS indicates that approx 7–35% more lesions are detected than with preoperative imaging modalities alone. Overall, the use of IOUS alters the planned operative procedure in 20–40% of cryosurgical patients *(37)*. A wide variety of equipment for performing IOUS is commercially available and each has its own advantages and disadvantages. For standard liver imaging 5.0- or 7.5-mHz I- or T-shaped, real-time, B-mode or linear-array transducers are commonly used. At the University of Wisconsin, we use state-of-the-art ultrasound equipment with dedicated operating room probes. We use one of three different ultrasound units: ATL 500 (Bothel, WA), Acuson Sequoia (Mountain View, CA), or GE Logiq 700 (Milwaukee, WI). The probes most frequently used in our institution are the T- or I-shaped high-frequency transducer *(9)*.

Placement of the cryoprobe is accomplished under ultrasound guidance and great care is taken to avoid major vascular structures (Fig. 1). IOUS is used to guide the 18-gauge Teflon-coated needle into position, approximately 1 cm beyond the distal margin. A guide wire is passed through the needle under ultrasound guidance. A peel-away sheath is inserted over the guidewire to allow for precise positioning of the probe, which is an especially useful technique for deep lesions. In order to get precise placement, we have borrowed a technique learned in prostate cryosurgery and place the needle and probe using a transverse approach. While the operator is scanning from the dome of the liver, the needle is placed into the lesion

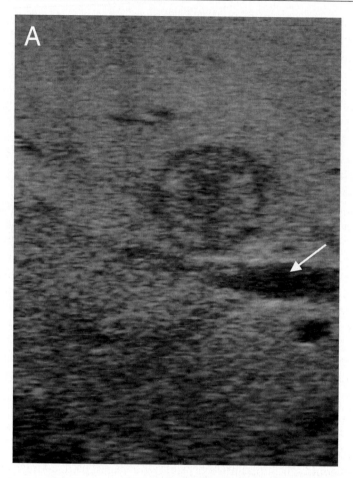

Fig. 1A. Panel **A** shows an IOUS of a metastatic lesion from a colorectal primary in a patient who also underwent resection of the opposite lobe. A major vascular structure can be seen in close proximity (solid arrow).

perpendicular to the ultrasound beam. Once the needle enters the beam, it can be followed into place. This allows one to visualize the needle placement in both the x- and y-axes while minimizing operator movement on the dome of the liver. The z-axis can then be checked, either by rotating the T-shaped transducer 90° or by using an I-shaped transducer, ensuring precise placement of the probe into the lesion. Using this technique has allowed one to achieve local recurrence rates in the low single digits *(31)*. Furthermore, if the lesion is too large to be encompassed by an iceball formed from one probe, as many as three separate probes can be placed to completely envelop the lesion using the above-described technique. At the University of Wisconsin, we favor a technique that involves introducing a 2.4-mm probe directly into a lesion using ultrasound guidance without passing a guidewire and sheath into the lesion. This "direct stick" technique saves time and allows for placement of up to eight separate probes into a single lesion. These additional probes can be placed in close proximity to the vessel to counteract the heat-sink effect seen when tumors are near large blood vessels. Placing the probes near the blood vessel increases the chance for obtaining tumoricidal temperatures along the tumor–vessel interface.

Once the probe is accurately placed under ultrasound guidance, the freezing process is started. The cryogen (usually liquid nitrogen or argon) is circulated through the insulated

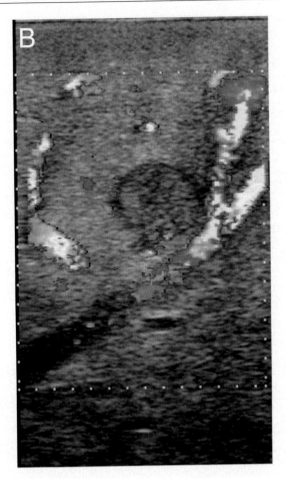

Fig. 1B. Panel **B** is a color-flow Doppler image of the same lesion prior to inserting the probe.

probe shaft to the uninsulated tip. This results in a tip temperature of –140°C to –196°C and adjacent tissue temperature of –100°C to –160°C. As the freezing begins, the iceball migrates outward from the tip of the probe and its progression is monitored by ultrasound. Characteristic changes include a rim of hyperechogenicity surrounding the iceball with posterior acoustic shadowing (Fig. 2).

Following four simple principles can maximize the actual tumoricidal effect. First, rapid freezing of the tumor must occur to temperatures ≤ –35°C. Second, the frozen state must be maintained for several minutes—we maintain the low temperature for at least 10 min. Third, the tumor should be slowly rethawed followed, by refreezing. Although the optimal number of freeze–thaw cycles is not entirely clear, it is accepted that one freeze–thaw cycle is suboptimal and most centers perform at least two freeze–thaw cycles *(16,38)*. Upon completion of the freezing process, the probe is removed, hemostasis is assured and the abdomen is closed.

9. POSTCRYOSURGICAL COMPLICATIONS

Complications following routine cryoablation of colorectal metastases are infrequent *(16,17)*. The most common complication seen is transient intraoperative hypothermia, which is easily prevented by using warming blankets and fluid warmers and increasing the operating room temperature.

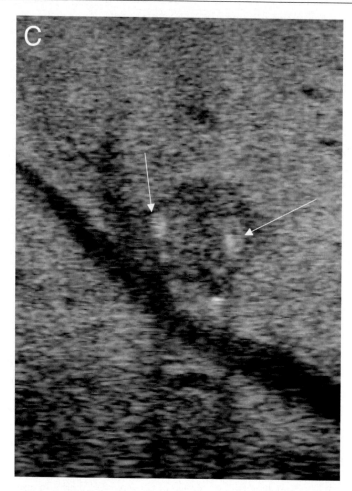

Fig. 1C. Panel **C** shows two probes (indicated by the arrows) precisely placed into the lesion to form an iceball that covers the entire lesion (panel **D**, *opposite page*).

If the cryolesion approaches the liver surface, cracking of the liver capsule and bleeding can occur. This is often easily managed by cautery, suture ligation, or packing the liver. The most common scenario in which this complication arises is in the cirrhotic patient with a rather noncompliant liver or in the patient with a large tumor. The placement of probes through normal liver prior to treating the tumor will usually prevent this complication.

Coagulapathy and myoglobinuria resulting in acute renal failure occur with an incidence of 1.4% and 3.7%, respectively *(39)*. These sequelae should be treated by full support of the patient with vigorous hydration, alkalinization of the urine, and osmotic diuresis. Prevention consists of good intraoperative hydration and liberal use of low-dose dopamine to improve renal perfusion in patients with limited cardiac or renal reserve.

Elevation of liver enzymes occurs in the immediate postoperative period but is transient in nature. Liver transaminases usually return to the normal range by 48 h. Bleeding, although rare, is a major complication that can occur from the cryoprobe tract. It can usually be controlled with simple intraoperative measures such as packing the cryoprobe tract with a procoagulant. An uncommon cause of bleeding may be from thrombocytopenia caused by the freezing process. Thrombocytopenia by itself need not be treated, but when it is associated with bleeding, it requires platelet transfusion.

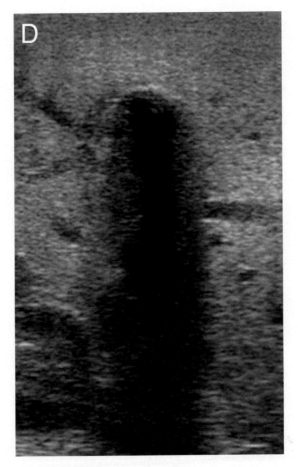

Fig. 1D.

Finally, cryoshock is a complex of multisystem organ failure, including renal failure and disseminated intravascular coagulapathy that occurs following cryosurgery. This syndrome is responsible for 18% of all deaths after hepatic cryotherapy. Fortunately, it is a relatively rare complication; in fact, a survey of all groups performing hepatic cryotherapy demonstrated cryoshock to have an incidence around 1% (21 of 2173 patients) *(40)*.

10. FOLLOW-UP AFTER CRYOSURGERY

Computed tomography scans should be obtained at 3-mo intervals for the first 1 yr and it is of utmost importance that the radiologist be familiar with the natural history of a cryo-induced lesion. If the patient shows no sign of recurrence, the interval can be increased to every 6 mo the second and third year. A patient that remains radiographically disease-free for 3 yr can then be followed every year with abdominal CT scans.

Radiographic changes of the cryo-induced lesion within 2 wk of surgery are quite distinct and well described by Kuszyk et al. *(41)*. The authors of this retrospective review evaluated the postoperative CT scans from 14 patients with 28 separate cryolesions. The mean number of hepatic cryolesions per patient was 2 with a range of 1–7. All 28 lesions identified were generally lower in attenuation than the surrounding hepatic parenchyma and extended to the liver surface. Identifiable foci of air were found in 36% of lesions. Additionally, 93% of the lesions generated in this series demonstrated high-attenuation areas consistent with

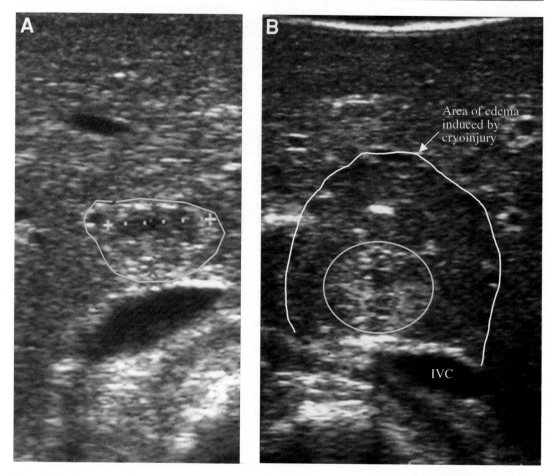

Fig. 2. Panel **A** shows an IOUS image of a metastatic lesion (outlined in yellow) prior to cryosurgery. Panel **B** shows the same lesion after cryosurgery. Note the changes that have occurred with the rim of hyperechogenicity around the lesion itself (indicated by a white and yellow outline, respectively).

hemorrhage. The shapes of the lesions on axial CT scans fell into one of three categories: wedge shaped, rounded, and teardrop. The most common appearance described by the authors was that of a wedge shape, seen in 15 of 28 lesions (54%).

After several weeks, the lesion undergoes liquefaction necrosis with eventual scarring. For several months postablation, the cryolesion demonstrates rim enhancement, which is the result of granulation tissue, inflammation, and regeneration of the liver immediately around the scar, giving it a vascular appearance. This rim should appear smooth, uniform, and concentric. Evidence of nodular tissue growth in the rim should be biopsied to rule out recurrence or persistence of tumor. Figure 3 shows a CT scan of a lesion precryosurgery and postcryosurgery.

Tumor markers (CEA) should be followed every 3 mo for the first year with the expectation that the levels will initially rise following the procedure. If the levels remain elevated, persistence of disease should be suspected and a thorough investigation should be undertaken.

The literature demonstrates that patients who undergo liver resection for recurrent colorectal metastases do quite well—with 5-yr survivals of 25–41% (*42–44*). Despite there being little data available for repeat cryosurgery for recurrent disease, most centers use the

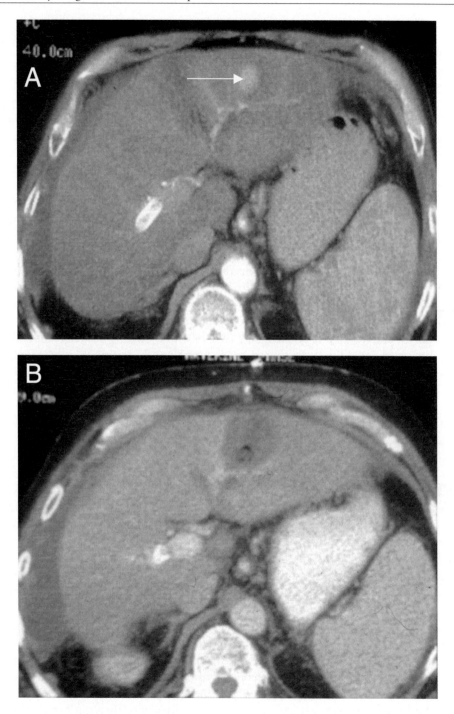

Fig. 3. Panel **A** shows a lesion precryosurgery (white arrow) and panel **B** is the same lesion approx 1 mo following cryosurgical ablation.

resectional data as proof of principle and perform the repeat cryosurgery. At the University of Wisconsin, we will perform repeat cryosurgery in highly selected patients. Furthermore, we have anecdotal evidence patients can enjoy long-term survival of 10 yr or better.

11. FUTURE DIRECTIONS

Recently, investigators have evaluated laparoscopic cryosurgery. Initial results with this technique have been favorable with good outcomes and low complication rates *(45,46)*. For this procedure to be successful, the surgeon must have a sensitive method for examining the liver. Because of this, laparoscopic ultrasound (LUS) probes have been developed. A recent publication from the University of Virginia investigated the sensitivity of LUS for detection of liver lesions *(47)*. In this study, the authors created lesions in the liver of a pig and compared the detection rate using LUS to the detection rate of IOUS and manual palpation. They found LUS to have a sensitivity of 94% in this animal model, with a specificity of 77%. In the second part of the study, the authors compared LUS to IOUS and manual palpation in 15 patients undergoing exploration for colorectal cancer. Similar to the pig model, the authors first examined the patients' livers using LUS, then performed laparotomies and examined the livers using IOUS and manual palpation. LUS found four of the five metastatic lesions for a sensitivity of 80% and a specificity of approx 91%. These results suggest that LUS is a sensitive modality for examining the liver and can be used to detect metastatic lesions. However, the sensitivity is less than that of IOUS with manual palpation, so the routine used of laparoscopic cryosurgery with LUS guidance cannot be recommended.

Investigations into minimally invasive techniques not involving laparoscopy are currently underway at the University of Wisconsin. In 1999, Lee et al. published their data on a minilaparotomy procedure performed in a porcine model *(48)*. In this study, the authors used prototype thin-shaft probes with sharp tips for direct puncture. IOUS was performed using an end-fire, convex-array 5.0-MHz transrectal transducer (Aloka SSD-2000; Aloka Ultrasound, Inc., Wallingford, CT). The ultrasound transducer and probe were passed into the animal's abdomen using a very small midline incision (approximately 2–4 cm on average). The authors were able to demonstrate adequate margins in more than 95% of all animals treated with either one or two probes. All animals treated survived the procedure and none suffered bleeding complications. This same group has also performed investigation on percutaneous cryosurgery under CT guidance in a similar porcine model *(49)*. Again, the authors were able to successfully treat all iatrogenically induced lesions with a mean margin of 1.7 cm. In this study, only one animal had a positive margin, which was secondary to equipment failure.

Tumor recurrence both in the liver and at the site of previously treated lesions is clearly a major obstacle in expanding the use of cryosurgery. Identification of antifreeze proteins (AFPs) and their utility in cryosurgery has provided a promising adjuvant therapy that may result in a clinical tool to decrease the local recurrence rate. The exact mechanism by which AFPs function to enhance the killing effect of cryotherapy is unknown, but the crystal structure of the relationship between the AFP and ice crystal may provide a potential mechanism *(50)*. AFPs cause the ice crystal to form in a needlelike structure, which hypothetically could be quite deleterious to the cell. These proteins have been shown to function in tissue culture but have never been demonstrated to be effective in humans. To date, only one trial has evaluated the activity of these proteins in an animal model *(51)*. In this study, rat livers were excised and perfused with either phosphate-buffered saline (PBS) or PBS supplemented with antifreeze proteins. The livers were then frozen using a flat-surfaced cryosurgical probe for either one or two freeze–thaw cycles. Upon completion of the freeze–thaw process, the livers were examined for viability using a two-color fluorescent dye assay that utilizes the plasma membrane integrity to differentiate between live and dead cells. After one freeze–thaw cycle, between 17% and 37% of cells were destroyed by freezing without AFP and this number did not change significantly with two freeze–thaw cycles. However, in the presence of AFP, one freeze–thaw cycle caused the cell death of 25–40% of cells, whereas two cycles increased this cell death to 40–70%. Obviously, conclusions are limited by the fact that this is an ex vivo model with normal livers that were chilled to 4°C prior to cryoablation. However, it does give some hope that AFPs may provide some benefit toward enhancement of cell death by the freezing process.

Regional therapy with chemotherapeutics delivered by a hepatic arterial infusion pump for colorectal cancer that has metastasized to the liver has been studied extensively *(52–58)*. Some centers have taken the hepatic arterial infusion (HAI) delivery system and applied it to the adjuvant setting in patients who have undergone hepatic resection with curative intent, in an attempt to decrease the recurrence rate.

One trial examining the role of adjuvant 5-FU delivered by HAI after cryosurgery is available and demonstrated that the therapy was feasible and well tolerated in this nonrandomized prospective analysis of 30 patients *(59)*. Experience at the University of Wisconsin indicates that chemotherapy can be safely delivered following cryosurgery or cryosurgery plus resection using continuous HAI (unpublished observations). Further investigation into this question is certainly warranted and the results are potentially quite exciting.

12. SUMMARY

Although resection remains the standard therapy for colorectal metastases to the liver, cryosurgery is a reasonable alternative for patients with unresectable disease. However, it is important to emphasize that cryosurgery is still very much a technology in development, which should not be applied indiscriminately. Patients should be carefully selected and the procedure undertaken by a skilled team with an intimate knowledge of hepatobiliary anatomy, physiology, and surgery. A skilled radiologist is an essential member of the cryosurgical team.

The immediate future for further development of cryosurgery includes the combination of surgical resection and cryoablation. Additionally, there is sufficient early clinical trial data to support enthusiasm for the use of hepatic arterial infusion chemotherapy as an "adjuvant" treatment for postresection and cryoablation patients. These multimodality approaches to patients with hepatic metastases appear to be significantly increasing the number of patients who gain long-term benefit and improved quality of life.

REFERENCES

1. Hughes KS, Simon R, Songhorabodi S, et al. Resection of the liver for colorectal carcinoma metastases: a multi-institutional study of patterns of recurrence. *Surgery*, **100(2)** (1986) 278–284.
2. Scheele J, Stangl R, and Altendorf-Hofmann A. Staging of resectable colorectal liver metastases [letter; comment]. *Surgery*, **119(1)** (1996) 118–120.
3. Rosen CB, Nagorney DM, Taswell HF, et al. Perioperative blood transfusion and determinants of survival after liver resection for metastatic colorectal carcinoma. *Ann. Surg.*, **216(4)** (1992) 493–504; discussion 504–505.
4. Arnott J. Practical illustrations of the remedial efficacy of a very low or anaesthetic temperature. *Lancet*, **2** (1850) 257–259.
5. Cooper I and Lee A. Cryostatic congelation: a system for producting a limited controlled region of cooling or freezing of biologic tissues. *J. Nerv. Ment. Dis.*, **133** (1961) 259–263.
6. Gage AA. History of cryosurgery. *Semin. Surg. Oncol.*, **14(2)** (1998) 99–109.
7. Onik G, Gilbert J, Hoddick W, et al. Sonographic monitoring of hepatic cryosurgery in an experimental animal model. *Am. J. Roentgenol.*, **144(5)** (1985) 1043–1047.
8. Ravikumar TS, Kane R, Cady B, et al. Hepatic cryosurgery with intraoperative ultrasound monitoring for metastatic colon carcinoma. *Arch. Surg.*, **122(4)** (1987) 403–409.
9. Lee FT Jr, Mahvi DM, Chosy SG, et al. Hepatic cryosurgery with intraoperative US guidance. *Radiology*, **202(3)** (1997) 624–632.

10. Jacob G, Li AK, and Hobbs KE. A comparison of cryodestruction with excision or infarction of an implanted tumor in rat liver. *Cryobiology*, **21(2)** (1984) 148–156.

11. Blackwood CE and Cooper IS. Response of experimental tumor systems to cryosurgery. *Cryobiology*, **9(6)** (1972) 508–515.

12. Rubinsky B, Lee CY, Bastacky J, and Onik G. The process of freezing and the mechanism of damage during hepatic cryosurgery. *Cryobiology*, **27(1)** (1990) 85–97.

13. Heise C, Warner T, Lee FJ, et al. Cryosurgical ablation induces tumor apoptosis, manuscript in preparation.

14. Weber SM, Lee FT Jr, Chinn DO, et al. Perivascular and intralesional tissue necrosis after hepatic cryoablation: results in a porcine model. *Surgery*, **122(4)** (1997) 742–747.

15. Gage AA, Fazekas G, Riley EE Jr. Freezing injury to large blood vessels in dogs. With comments on the effect of experimental freezing of bile ducts. *Surgery*, **61(5)** (1967) 748–754.

16. Ravikumar TS, Steele G Jr, Kane R, and King V. Experimental and clinical observations on hepatic cryosurgery for colorectal metastases. *Cancer Res.*, **51(23 Pt. 1)** (1991) 6323–6327.

17. Onik G, Rubinsky B, Zemel R, et al. Ultrasound-guided hepatic cryosurgery in the treatment of metastatic colon carcinoma. Preliminary results. *Cancer*, **67(4)** (1991) 901–907.

18. Weaver ML, Ashton JG, and Zemel R. Treatment of colorectal liver metastases by cryotherapy. *Semin. Surg. Oncol.*, **14(2)** (1998) 163–170.

19. Korpan NN. Hepatic cryosurgery for liver metastases. Long-term follow-up. *Ann. Surg.*, **225(2)** (1997) 193–201.

20. Yeh KA, Fortunato L, Hoffman JP, and Eisenberg BL. Cryosurgical ablation of hepatic metastases from colorectal carcinomas. *Am. Surg.*, **63(1)** (1997) 63–68.

21. Lorentzen T. A cooled needle electrode for radiofrequency tissue ablation: thermodynamic aspects of improved performance compared with conventional needls design. *Acad. Radiol.*, **3** (1996) 556–563.

22. Livraghi T, Goldberg SN, Monti F, et al. Saline-enhanced radio-frequency tissue ablation in the treatment of liver metastases. *Radiology*, **202(1)** (1997) 205–10.

23. Solbiati L, Ierace T, Goldberg SN, et al. Percutaneous US-guided radio-frequency tissue ablation of liver metastases: treatment and follow-up in 16 patients. *Radiology*, **202(1)** (1997) 195–203.

24. Nagata Y, Hiraoka M, Nishimura Y, et al. Clinical results of radiofrequency hyperthermia for malignant liver tumors. *Int. J. Radiat. Oncol. Biol. Phys.*, **38(2)** (1997) 359–365.

25. Mazziotti A, Grazi GL, Gardini A, et al. An appraisal of percutaneous treatment of liver metastases. *Liver Transplant Surg.*, **4(4)** (1998) 271–275.

26. Curley SA, Izzo F, Delrio P, et al. Radiofrequency ablation of unresectable primary and metastatic hepatic malignancies: results in 123 patients. *Ann. Surg.*, **230(1)** (1999) 1–8.

27. Chinn SB, Lee FT Jr, Kennedy GD, et al. Effect of vascular occlusion on radiofrequency ablation of the liver: results in a porcine model. *Am. J. Roentgenol.*, **176(3)** (2001) 789–795.

28. Stone MD, Cady B, Jenkins RL, et al. Surgical therapy for recurrent liver metastases from colorectal cancer. *Arch. Surg.*, **125(6)** (1990) 718–721; discussion 722.

29. Adam R, Akpinar E, Johann M, et al. Place of cryosurgery in the treatment of malignant liver tumors. *Ann. Surg.*, **225(1)** (1997) 39–48; discussion 48–50.

30. Seifert JK and Morris DL. Prognostic factors after cryotherapy for hepatic metastases from colorectal cancer. *Ann. Surg.*, **228(2)** (1998) 201–208.

31. Cha C, Lee FJ, Rikkers L, et al. Rationale for the combination of cryoablation with surgical resection of hepatic tumors: combined cryoablation with surgical resection. *J. Gastrointestinal Surg.* **5(2)** (2001) 206–213.

32. McCormack PM, Burt ME, Bains MS, et al. Lung resection for colorectal metastases. 10-year results. *Arch. Surg.*, **127(12)** (1992) 1403–1406.

33. Okumura S, Kondo H, Tsuboi M, et al. Pulmonary resection for metastatic colorectal cancer: experiences with 159 patients. *J. Thorac. Cardiovasc. Surg.*, **112(4)** (1996) 867–874.

34. Carter R, Hemingway D, Cooke TG, et al. A prospective study of six methods for detection of hepatic colorectal metastases. *Ann. R. Coll. Surg. Engl.*, **78(1)** (1996) 27–30.

35. Soyer P, Levesque M, Caudron C, et al. MRI of liver metastases from colorectal cancer vs. CT during arterial portography. *J. Comput. Assisted Tomogr.*, **17(1)** (1993) 67–74.

36. Fong Y, Saldinger PF, Akhurst T, et al. Utility of 18F-FDG positron emission tomography scanning on selection of patients for resection of hepatic colorectal metastases. *Am. J. Surg.*, **178(4)** (1999) 282–287.

37. McCarty TM and Kuhn JA. Cryotherapy for liver tumors. *Oncology (Huntingt.)*, **12(7)** (1998) 979–987.

38. Dutta P, Montes M, and Gage AA. Large volume freezing in experimental hepatic cryosurgery. Avoidance of bleeding in hepatic freezing by an improvement in the technique. *Cryobiology*, **16(1)** (1979) 50–55.

39. Ravikumar T, Kaleya R, and Kishinevsky A. Surgical ablative therapy of liver tumors. In *Cancer: Principles and Practice of Oncology*. Devita V, Hellman S, and Rosenberg S (eds.), Lipincott Williams & Wilkins, Cedar Knolls, NJ, 2000. Vol. 14, p. 12.

40. Seifert JK, Junginger T, and Morris DL. A collective review of the world literature on hepatic cryotherapy. *J. R. Coll. Surg. Edinb.*, **43(3)** (1998) 141–154.

41. Kuszyk B, Choti M, Urban B, et al. Hepatic tumors treated by cryosurgery: normal CT appearance. *Am. J. Radiol.*, **166** (1996) 363–367.

42. Yamamoto J, Kosuge T, Shimada K, et al. Repeat liver resection for recurrent colorectal liver metastases. *Am. J. Surg.*, **178(4)** (1999) 275–281.

43. Tuttle TM, Curley SA, and Roh MS. Repeat hepatic resection as effective treatment of recurrent colorectal liver metastases. *Ann. Surg. Oncol.*, **4(2)** (1997) 125–130.

44. Adam R, Bismuth H, Castaing D, et al. Repeat hepatectomy for colorectal liver metastases. *Ann. Surg.*, **225(1)** (1997) 51–60; discussion 60–62.

45. Heniford BT, Arca MJ, Iannitti DA, et al. Laparoscopic cryoablation of hepatic metastases. *Semin. Surg. Oncol.*, **15(3)** (1998) 194–201.

46. Tandan VR, Litwin D, Asch M, et al. Laparoscopic cryosurgery for hepatic tumors. Experimental observations and a case report. *Surg. Endoscopy*, **11(11)** (1997) 1115–1117.

47. Foley EF, Kolecki RV, and Schirmer BD. The accuracy of laparoscopic ultrasound in the detection of colorectal cancer liver metastases. *Am. J. Surg.*, **176(3)** (1998) 262–264.

48. Lee FT, Jr., Chosy SG, Weber SM, et al. Hepatic cryosurgery via minilaparotomy in a porcine model: an alternative to open cryosurgery [see comments]. *Surg. Endoscopy*, **13(3)** (1999) 253–259.

49. Lee FT Jr, Chosy SG, Littrup PJ, et al. CT-monitored percutaneous cryoablation in a pig liver model: pilot study. *Radiology*, **211(3)** (1999) 687–692.

50. Tatsutani K and Rubinsky B. A method to study intracellular ice nucleation. *J. Biomech. Eng.*, **120(1)** (1998) 27–31.

51. Pham L, Dahiya R, and Rubinsky B. An in vivo study of antifreeze protein adjuvant cryosurgery. *Cryobiology*, **38(2)** (1999) 169–175.

52. O'Connell MJ, Nagorney DM, Bernath AM, et al. Sequential intrahepatic fluorodeoxyuridine and systemic fluorouracil plus leucovorin for the treatment of metastatic colorectal cancer confined to the liver. *J. Clin. Oncol.*, **16(7)** (1998) 2528–2533.

53. Kemeny N, Conti JA, Sigurdson E, et al. A pilot study of hepatic artery floxuridine combined with systemic 5-fluorouracil and leucovorin. A potential adjuvant program after resection of colorectal hepatic metastases. *Cancer*, **71(6)** (1993) 1964–1971.

54. Lorenz M, Muller HH, Schramm H, et al. Randomized trial of surgery versus surgery followed by adjuvant hepatic arterial infusion with 5-fluorouracil and folinic acid for liver metastases of colorectal cancer. German Cooperative on Liver Metastases (Arbeitsgruppe Lebermetastasen) [see comments]. *Ann. Surg.*, **228(6)** (1998) 756–762.

55. Clavien P, Selzner M, and Morse M. Comment. *Ann. Surg.*, **230(4)** (1999) 607–608.

56. Ensminger WD, Rosowsky A, Raso V, et al. A clinical–pharmacological evaluation of hepatic arterial infusions of 5-fluoro-2'-deoxyuridine and 5-fluorouracil. *Cancer Res.*, **38(11 Pt.1)** (1978) 3784–3792.

57. van Laar JA, Rustum YM, Ackland SP, et al. Comparison of 5-fluoro-2'-deoxyuridine with 5-fluorouracil and their role in the treatment of colorectal cancer. *Eur. J. Cancer*, **34(3)** (1998) 296–306.

58. Kemeny N, Huang Y, Cohen AM, et al. Hepatic arterial infusion of chemotherapy after resection of hepatic metastases from colorectal cancer [see comments]. *N. Engl. J. Med.*, **341(27)** (1999) 2039–2048.

59. Stubbs RS, Alwan MH, and Booth MW. Hepatic cryotherapy and subsequent hepatic arterial chemotherapy for colorectal metastases to the liver. *HPB Surg.*, **11(2)** (1998) 97–104.

24

Radiofrequency Ablation of Colorectal Metastases to the Liver

Douglas L. Fraker

Contents

1. INTRODUCTION

The variety of techniques that have been developed and applied to treat metastatic colon cancer to the liver is a testament to the importance of this clinical problem and to the failure of any single technique to have provided a solution in this clinical situation. Radiofrequency thermal ablation (RFA) is one of the most recent techniques to be applied to the treatment of primary and metastatic disease in the liver. It can be categorized together with cryosurgical ablation and direction injection of alcohol, chemotherapeutics, or gene therapy vectors as a treatment that targets a specific area or region of the liver. These treatment strategies can be characterized as "subregional" regional therapy as opposed to vascular-based treatment that treat the entire liver. RFA is the opposite of cryoablation, as it uses heat generated by electrical current to directly destroy tissue, as opposed to cold temperatures to accomplish the same goal *(1)*.

In this chapter, the history and development of RFA technology, the current technology used for RFA, and the clinical results using this new treatment applied to colorectal metastases in the liver will be discussed. Although the focus of this chapter is on the treatment of colorectal metastases to the liver, much of the initial literature concerning treatment of liver tumors with RFA combine primary hepatoma *(2)* plus a variety of metastatic tumor types without discussing the results of each histology separately. In this regard, some of the data discussed will apply generally to a variety of metastases, including colorectal and primary hepatoma.

From: *Colorectal Cancer: Multimodality Management*
Edited by: L. Saltz © Humana Press Inc., Totowa, NJ

Table 1
Key Events in the Historical Development of RFA of Hepatic Tumors

1891	d'Arsonvol in Paris demonstrated that high-frequency alternating current creates heat
1892	and not painful muscle contraction.
1909	Doyon in Paris applies a biterminal electrode to a patient for the treatment of cancer.
1928	Bovie and Cushing design the prototype electrosurgical cautery unit in Boston.
1960–1980	Advances in solid-state transistor technology decrease size and increase reliability of electrosurgical devices.
1990	Retractable multiprong electrodes developed which create thermal lesions, up to 3 cm in size.
2000	New electrodes with high-energy generator increase size of thermal lesions up to 5 cm or more.

2. HISTORICAL DEVELOPMENT

Radiofrequency thermal ablation utilizes high-frequency alternating current to generate heat within tissues to the point where complete tissue destruction (cell death) occurs as coagulation necrosis. The use of heat in medicine dates back to antiquity, as direct application of heat was used to treat hemorrhage and tumors of the breast as early as 7000 BC. A major advance in the use of heat for treatment of a variety of diseases was made by d'Arsonval in Paris in the 1890s (Table 1). For the first time, d'Arsonval produced heat in tissues by applying a high-frequency alternating current instead of direct application of an externally heated object or substance *(3)*. Electrical currents from standard electrical outlets typically provide energy at 120 V with a 60-Hz alternating current. Application of such a current to human tissue causes pain resulting from nerve and muscle stimulation as experienced in an electrical shock. d'Arsonval demonstrated for the first time that increasing the frequency of the alternating current to 10,000 cycles/s (10 kHz) eliminates the pain of nerve and muscle stimulation and generates heat in the surrounding tissue. This heat is generated by rapid shifts in the direction of the ionized molecules in the tissue at such a high frequency that "molecular friction" is produced. This application of alternating current in a focused manner is the principal of RFA of tissues.

An important advance in this field occurred when Doyon, also working in Paris, developed a biterminal electrical system for the treatment of cancer in a human patient *(3)*. He constructed two opposing electrodes, one that was a smaller treatment electrode and a second that was a large dispersive electrode for the return current. This asymmetric electrode system produced tissue injury at the smaller electrode when energy is more focused while protecting the skin at the larger electrode where energy is dispersed over a large area. This approach eventually led to the development of an electricosurgical cautery unit by Bovie, who was working with Cushing in Boston in 1928 (Table 1). The same principles of monopolar electrocautery with a dispersive pad electrode and bipolar cautery developed by these pioneers are in use today as a standard surgical tool in operating rooms throughout the world. Technical advances in the 1960s and 1970s, such as development of solid-state transistors to replace bulky spark-gap condensers, led to a significant decrease in size of the electrocautery units as well as more reliable and reproducible energy production.

The final advance that led to the current interest in application of RFA to the treatment of hepatic tumors was the development of new electrode-designed technologies that can create reproducible three-dimensional thermal lesions as opposed to surface cautery *(4)*. Initial linear electrodes produce a cylinder of tissue destruction surrounding the device, which is relatively difficult to apply to more spherically shaped tumor metastases. The development of a technology with a retractable circular array of electrodes that can be advanced from a linear cylinder has allowed for production of a nearly spherical thermal lesion in hepatic and other tissues. Initial array electrode models created spherical lesions in the size range of 3 cm. Current technologies with second-generation electrode using more powerful generation create 5 cm or larger lesions *(5)*.

3. CURRENT TECHNOLOGY OF RFA DEVICES

The devices used currently for RFA of hepatic lesions utilize the principles delineated in the previous section describing the historical development of radiofrequency devices that resulted in this commonly available electrosurgical cautery units. Specifically, RFA requires a generator to produce a current, a monopolar treatment electrode, and a dispersive electrode for the return current *(6)*. Current generated between the two electrodes can be focused by the creation of a treatment electrode of a certain size and shape that allows significant impact on tissue in contact with this electrode. The frequency that is utilized with the current devices is in the range of 200–1200 kHz. The application of alternating current at these frequencies creates a back-and-forth motion of ions at the electrode–tissue interface that creates heat resulting from the friction caused by the rapid motion in the tissues. The electrode itself is not directly heated by the application of the electrical current, but, over time, with generation of heat in the surrounding tissue, it becomes hot. The rate of heat generated is proportional to the frequency of the alternating current applied between the two electrodes. The area of destruction or the so-called "thermal lesion" created is related to the size and shape of the electrode and to the output of energy from the generator.

Interstitial RFA differs from standard electrocautery units as the bovie cautery either touches or arcs current to the surface, whereas in interstitial RFA the electrode is inserted entirely within the tissue. Initial interstitial electrodes were linear and created a cylinder of tissue destruction or a sleeve of ablated tissue surrounding the electrode. Retractable multiprong electrodes allowed a more practical shaped thermal lesion to be created that is either spherical or elliptical *(7)*. These currently used electrodes are passed into tissues as a linear electrode but have retractable prongs stored within the hollow cavity of the tip of the electrode that can be deployed to create final orientation within the tissue (Fig. 1). Two prototype multiprong radiofrequency treatment electrodes have been developed that utilize a different approach in assessing the progress and completeness of the destruction of malignant tissue in the liver. Radiotherapeutics Corporation (Sunnyvale, CA) uses an algorithm with a stepwise increase in frequency of the alternating current that treats a given area until tissue impedance, which is resistant at current flow in the tissue, rises to a specific level (Fig. 2). As heat is created in the area of the active monopolar electrode, there is a progressive destruction as liquid substances within the tissue are vaporized. Initial tissue impedence is low, but as the treatment is applied and the tissue becomes more desiccated, impedence rises, as measured by monitoring devices on the opposing prongs of the electrode. When impedence reaches a specific point across opposing tips of the prongs of the electrode, it has been estimated that all viable tissue within that thermal lesion has been destroyed and this indicates completion of therapy, and the application of current is terminated.

A second corporation, RITA (Mountainview, CA) utilizes a similar multiprong electrode but has thermal coupling devices at the tips of the electrodes to measure tissue temperature at the site of radiofrequency ablation. The algorithm for creating a thermal lesion with

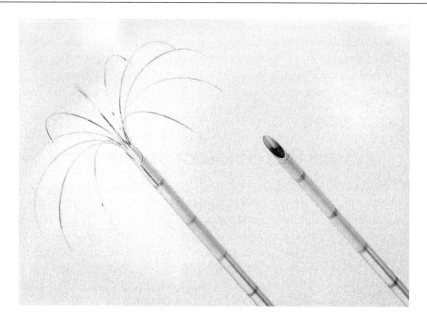

Fig. 1. This photograph shows the retractable prongs in a hollow electrode. A device in the handle of the electrode allows a prong to be advanced once the tip of the probe is inserted into the liver. The photograph shows the prongs retracted (right) and then fully advanced into a circular array (left).

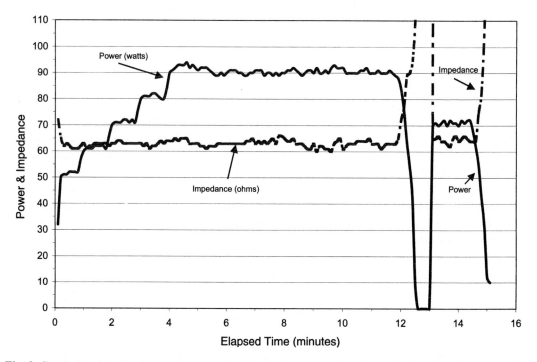

Fig. 2. Graph showing the changes in power from a generator as well as tissue impedence over time during RFA using a Radiotherapeutics device. It can be seen that as the impedence increases, the power dissipates. An initial treatment is performed, and after a 30-s interval, the power is restarted; when impedence increases a second time, the treatment is felt to be complete.

Table 2
Comparison of Types of Multiprong Electrodes Available for RFA of Hepatic Tumors

Company	Radiotherapeutics	RITA
End point when creating thermal lesion	Tissue impedence	Tissue temperature
Initial electrode characteristics		
No. of prongs	10	4
Diameter of thermal lesions	2 cm/3.5 cm	3.0 cm
Second-generation electrode characteristics		
No. of prongs	10	7
Size of lesion	4 cm	5 cm

the RITA device depends on reaching a certain temperature within the tissue and then continuing treatment for a defined period of time at that temperature. The differences and the specific details of the devices from these two major suppliers of RFA technology are given in Table 2.

Clearly, when applying RFA as the sole treatment for metastatic tumor within the liver, complete destruction of all viable tumor cells is mandatory for successful treatment. Any area of the tumor not completely destroyed by RFA will eventually regrow, causing a local failure at that site. The ability to judge which approach to creating RFA thermal lesion depends on accurate long-term follow-up of patients treated with these two or other devices, particularly monitoring the local relapse rate of lesions with similar characteristics.

4. TECHNIQUE OF RFA

Independent of the specific manufacturer of the RFA probes and generator, the general technique or the approach to the procedure is similar. One key component of RFA of a lesion in the liver is successful placement of the electrode within the tumor with the center point of the eventual array of electrodes located at the appropriate site. Radiofrequency ablation with placement of the electrode into the liver may occur in three types of clinical procedures: an open surgical procedure, a laparoscopic surgical procedure, and a percutaneous insertion typically performed in interventional radiology. For all of these situations, ultrasound is essential to verify that the tip of the electrode is placed into a precise point of the tumor, verified in three dimensions to create an appropriately placed thermal lesion relative to the tumor volume. Again, the application of RFA energy will destroy normal liver in an equivalent manner as tumor metastatic to the liver; therefore, appropriate destruction of tumor is completely dependent on the correct placement of the electrode. The advantages and disadvantages of these three approaches are listed in Table 3.

Percutaneous RFA has the advantage of minimal morbidity, as it avoids a general anesthetic and a surgical procedure (8). However, the percutaneous approach is limited in terms of the number of lesions and, in some ways, the location of lesions that can be treated. It is difficult to access a tumor metastasis that is deep or superior in the right lobe of the liver, as this area may be behind the inferior lung near the diaphragm, making it hard to see by ultrasound evaluation. Also, placement of a catheter and lesions in this location may transgress the lung, causing a pneumothorax or other potential pulmonary injury. Tumors that are located along the inferior surface of the liver may abut the hepatic flexure of the colon in the right lobe of the liver or the stomach and duodenum in the left lobe. Treatment of lesions located in this area may lead to injury to the adjacent bowel, and lesions in these locations cannot be treated percutaneously (Fig. 3).

Table 3
Advantages and Disadvantages of Approaches for Creation
of Radiofrequency Lesions in the Liver

	Advantages	*Disadvantages*
Percutaneous	• Low morbidity • No general anesthetic • Unable to treat surface lesions	• Incomplete staging • Unable to visualize and treat superior right lobe of liver
Open laparotomy	• Accurate staging • Ability to treat extensive disease • Access to place intra-arterial pump and do hepatic resection	• General anesthesia • Morbidity of laparotomy incision
Laparoscopic	• Accurate staging • Low morbidity	• General anesthesia • Specialized equipment and surgical skills

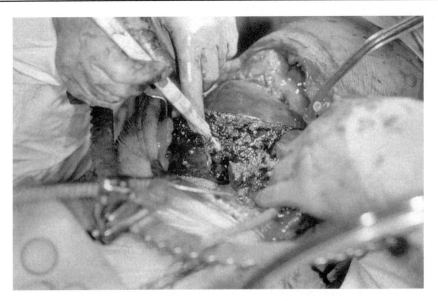

Fig. 3. An intraoperative photograph of a liver during an open ablation, showing the changes in the surface of the liver, with this lesion becoming somewhat charred by RFA treatment. A lesion such as this on the surface cannot undergo percutaneous treatment because of potential thermal injury to surrounding structures that can be dissected away during an open surgical procedure.

An open surgical technique, which is the most common way to administer RFA, obviously requires a general anesthetic and that the patient be healthy enough to tolerate a laparotomy. However, one major advantage of an open procedure is that it allows a more accurate staging, not only of the liver but also for extrahepatic disease. With an open technique, it is possible to mobilize the liver and retract structures so that essentially all areas of the liver, including the caudate lobe, would be accessible to RFA. Lesions that are on the surface of the liver, particularly along the inferior aspect where tumor may be in contact with the gall bladder or the right colon or stomach, may be treated with all adjacent areas dissected away and packed outside of the field so that no inadvertent thermal injury occurs. An open RFA technique can often be combined with a hepatic resection in which a single lesion located centrally that may be ablated within the contralateral lobe is resected. Finally, the open technique allows

Table 4

Calculated Volume of Sphere at Various Sizes Compared to Volume of a 3.5-cm Thermal Lesion

Diameter of lesion (cm)	Calculated volume (cm³)	Number of 3.5-cm thermal lesions needed to ablate the entire area
3.5	22.5	1.0
4	33.5	1.5
5	65.5	2.9
6	113.1	5.0
8	260.2	11.9
10	521.8	23.3

patients who have bilobar unresectable colorectal metastases to have an intra-arterial hepatic infusion pump placed at the same procedure *(9)* (Table 3).

Laparoscopic application of RFA combines some of the advantages of both the open surgical procedure as well as the percutaneous approach but requires significant expertise and training as well as adequate equipment for laparoscopic surgery and laparoscopic ultrasound *(10)*. A laparoscopic procedure is, by definition, a minimally invasive surgery and causes less morbidity than the open procedure and, in that way, is more similar to a percutaneous approach. However, laparoscopic approach allows better staging as well as better access with the use of laparoscopic ultrasound to all areas of the liver compared to the percutaneous technique. If one is using the laparoscopic approach, it is mandatory that laparoscopic ultrasound be available and that both the radiologist and the surgeon have to have skill in using this technique to appropriately place the electrode into the area of the tumor *(11)*.

One major criticism of RFA has been the maximal size of a thermal lesion that can be created, significantly limiting the ability to treat larger tumors that encompass the majority of the patients in need of such ablative techniques. The maximal size of a thermal lesion with complete destruction of the tumor with the initial versions of the multiprong retractable electrodes was in the range of 3–3.5 cm in diameter. Lesions larger than these could be treated only by overlapping multiple thermal spheres to encompass the entire tumor with a smaller rim of surrounding liver *(6)*. Because the volume of a sphere is directly related to the cube of the radius (volume of sphere = $[4/3]\pi r^3$), as the size of a tumor increases, the volume of the lesion rises quite rapidly. Table 4 describes the volume of a 3.5-cm thermal lesion and shows the number of these thermal lesions that would be necessary to treat lesions of a larger size. However, this calculation in Table 4 grossly underestimates the number of overlapping thermal lesions that are required to successfully ablate tumors of a given size. This underestimation occurs for two reasons. First, it is important to treat a rim of normal liver surrounding the tumor and not just the tumor itself. If one desires to treat a 0.5-cm rim of normal liver around the tumor to make certain that there is no viable tumor at the margins of the lesion, then the size of the diameter of the thermal lesion needed for a 5-cm tumor is 6 cm, and for a 6-cm tumor, it is 7 cm, and so on. The second problem is that these volume calculations assume that overlapping spheres can be created and combined such that each of the volumes treated is itself translated completely into the final thermal lesion. However, the geometry of overlapping spheres obviously would leave gaps in between the spheres such that to create a completely treated sphere 6 cm in diameter, it would take many more than the calculated five thermal lesions to completely encompass this size sphere with no untreated gaps.

The approach to a patient with metastatic colon cancer to the liver starts with the assessment of the number and size of the metastatic lesions. Although patients are often screened by computed tomography (CT) scans, the ability of CT scans to identify small tumor lesions is not as sensitive as a magnetic resonance imaging (MRI) scan with gadolinium enhancement. The CT scan or MRI scan would then need to be reviewed to determine the number and size of colon cancer metastases. The goal of RFA is to treat an area of normal liver surrounding the tumor; therefore, lesions must be smaller than 3 cm and preferably 2.5 cm to allow them to be treated completely with one thermal lesion *(12)*. For lesions >3 cm, the calculations given in Table 4 can be applied to estimate the number of thermal lesions that need to be created. For practical purposes, because each thermal lesion that is created takes between 15 and 30 min, including the heating time as well as placement of the electrode in the appropriate position, then creating 10 thermal lesions accounts for 2.5–5 h of RFA time. For most surgeons, ultrasound radiologists, and operating rooms, this would be near the maximal amount of time that could practically be allotted for such a technique. Therefore, patients who either because of the number of tumors or the size of their tumors have a need for greater than 10 thermal lesions to be created to treat all tumors, RFA may not be practical.

The majority of patients with colorectal cancer and metastases are treated with an open surgical technique, because almost by definition, they have multiple or bilobar lesions. If they do not have bilobar lesions and have reasonable performance status, they would, of course, be candidates for surgical resection. The operation is conducted by either a right subcostal or midline incision with exposure of the liver by dividing the falciform ligament and the triangular ligaments of the liver as required. Intraoperative ultrasound (IOUS) is then utilized both to confirm the number and presence of tumor metastases and to look for additional lesions missed by the preoperative imaging studies. One recent study reported that IOUS identified additional disease in 25/66 patients (38%) undergoing laparotomy for open RFA. Intraoperative ultrasound is also mandatory for placement of the electrodes as described earlier (Fig. 4). After correct positioning of the electrode in the center of a lesion with advancement of the final circumferential prongs, a treatment algorithm is then employed based on the design of the generator. For Radiotherapeutics RFA procedures, the algorithm depends on the creation of increased tissue impedence in the lesion; the design of the algorithm is shown in Fig. 5. For RITA, the algorithm is based on reaching a certain temperature and then treating for a certain period of time; the algorithm for RITA is shown in Fig. 6. For lesions that require overlapping thermal spheres because of their size, it is important to plan with the ultrasonographer how many thermal lesions are going to be required and what the orientation of these lesions are going to be relative to the size and shape of the metastatic tumor. After deciding the number and locations of the thermal lesions, the sequence of these lesions are created by starting with the deepest or farthest away point from the surface. This approach is used because the air released by the RFA obscures the ultrasound identification of the tissue inferior or deep into that area after the initial lesion is created *(13)* (Fig. 7). Therefore, if one started at the surface, it would be difficult to see in order to correctly place the electrode for the deeper locations. By starting at the deepest location, one can work backward toward the surface in an area that is still able to be well visualized by intraoperative ultrasound.

For lesions that did not reach the appropriate temperature or do not reach the tissue impedence that would signify the end of therapy, different techniques can be applied to facilitate complete RFA. For lesions near blood vessels in which the high flow through these intrahepatic vessels act to dissipate heat, one can apply a Pringle maneuver or occlusion

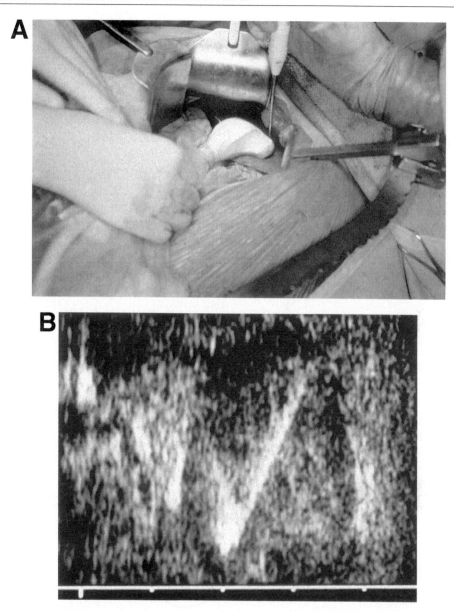

Fig. 4. Illustration of the use of an intraoperative ultrasound probe to guide the placement of radiofrequency electrode (**A**) with the tip placed into the center of the malignant lesion (**B**).

of the porta hepatis structures to limit blood flow into the liver *(14)*. By doing this, the dissipation of heat by vascular flow is diminished and successful treatment may proceed. It has been reported that vascular inflow occlusion has led to the creation of thermal lesions larger than would be predicted by the size of the electrode array. A second approach is to partially retract the prongs of the electrodes to a smaller size, and, as impedence or temperature increases with this smaller or more focused electrode, then to slowly readvance the prong into the surrounding tissue. By applying the energy of the generator through the treatment electrode at a smaller size, it allows a greater energy to be delivered for that surface volume and then the prongs can be fully deployed to complete the thermal lesion

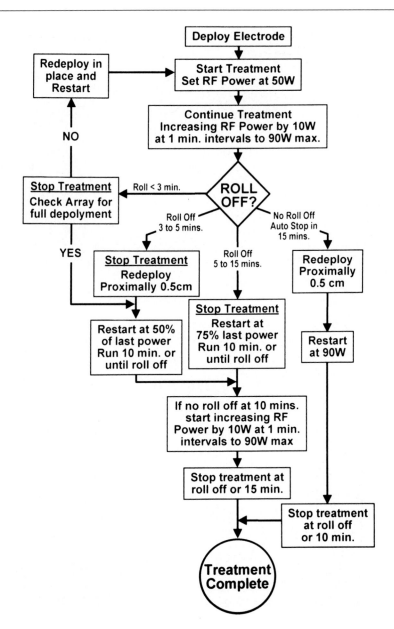

Fig. 5. Algorithm employed by the Radiotherapeutics Corp. to determine changes in power generated and times of treatment based on increases in tissue impedence.

of the appropriate size. Other investigators have injected saline into lesions at the time of RFA to augment the ablation *(15)*.

5. CLINICAL EXPERIENCE WITH RFA

Because RFA is a relatively new technique, clinical results reported in the literature are quite sparse with relatively minimal follow-up. Also, the initial application of RFA was primarily to treat hepatomas in cirrhotic patients who could not tolerate hepatic resection *(16,17)*. Therefore, there is a larger literature with more long-term follow-up for this histology than for patients with colorectal metastases *(18,19)*. The results of treatment of colorectal

For a 5 cm ablation:

Deploy to: (always 1st step)	Set Target Temp at:	Set Power at:	Set Timer at:	For a Duration of:
2 cm	80°	90 W	15.0	**Until Target Temp is reached** (you will hear a beep) then deploy to 3 cm
3 cm	105°	90 W	14.5	**Until Target Temp is reached** (you will hear a beep) then deploy to 4 cm
4 cm	110°	90 W	14.0*	**7 minutes at Target Temp** (after hearing the beep wait 7 min.) then deploy to to 5
5 cm	110°	110 W	7.0**	**7 minutes at Target Temp** (after hearing the beep wait 7 min.) then go to **Cool Down**

* Ensure that there is at least 14 minutes on the timer after deploying to 4 cm. If it is less than 14, increase to 14.)
** Ensure that there is at least 7 minutes on the timer after deploying to 5 cm. If it is less than 7, increase to 7.)

- Note: when deploying from 2 cm to 3 cm, 3 cm to 4 cm, and from 4 cm to 5 cm, there should be a drop in temperatures and a rise in power output. If this does not occur, Device may not be deployed properly. In this case, retract and redeploy to achieve these changes.

For a 4 cm ablation:

Deploy to:	Set Target Temp at:	Set Power at:	Set Timer at:	For a Duration of:
2 cm	80°	90 W	8.0	**Until Target Temp is reached** (you will hear a beep) then deploy to 3 cm
3 cm	105°	90 W	7.5	**Until Target Temp is reached** (you will hear a beep) then deploy to 4 cm
4 cm	110°	90 W	7.0**	**7 minutes at Target Temp**

** Ensure that there is at least 7 minutes on the timer after deploying to 4 cm. If it is less than 7, increase to 7.)

Fig. 6. Algorithm of the treatment employed by the RITA device in which temperature measured by thermal couples on the tips of the electrode determines the length of treatment.

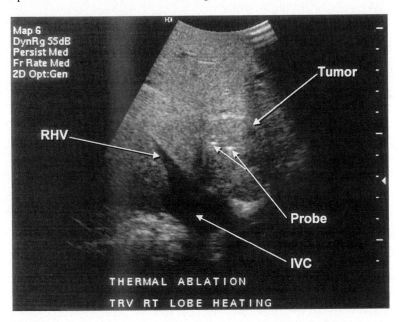

Fig. 7. Illustration of the prongs of the electrode in the tissue and the air that is generated during the destruction of a lesion near a major vein. The deep areas of the lesion need to be treated first, as the air generated by the initial thermal lesion obscures areas deep into that area visualized by ultrasound (IVC = inferior vena cava; RHV = right hepatic vein).

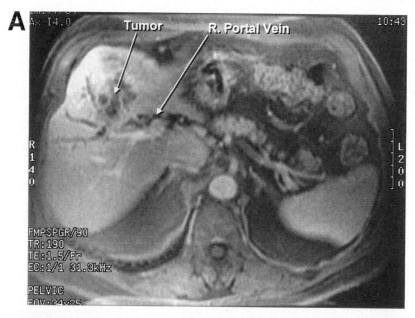

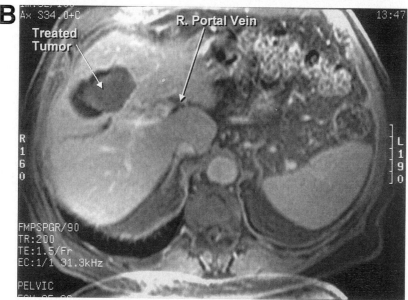

Fig. 8. Preoperative (**A**) and posttreatment (**B**) films of a lesion that has undergone RFA.

metastases are often included in institutional reports or series that combine treatment of colorectal metastases with RFA of other metastases to the liver as well as primary hepatomas. In many cases, it is difficult to extract the data specifically for colorectal carcinoma patients. Also, there is some difficulty in interpreting the response to RFA treatment using standard criteria. The most appropriate way to follow lesions treated by RFA is in terms of local progression or recurrence of treated lesions (20). It is not appropriate to report results of RFA in terms of the standard criteria for regression defining complete responses, partial responses, or minor responses. In fact, for inexperienced radiologists, the initial post-RFA CT or MRI scan is often read as progressive disease, as lesions appear larger than they were on the pretreatment scans (Fig. 8). If one successfully applies RFA to create a thermal lesion that includes the entire tumor and a surrounding rim of 0.5–1 cm of liver in all directions, the initial lesion will be increased by the size of this margin of normal liver. With complete destruction of the tumor and this surrounding rim of liver, the tissue becomes very hard and has a consistency of vulcanized rubber, with no blood flow within these areas. Therefore, resolution or disappearance of these RFA-treated areas appears to take quite some time and they appear as almost cystic lesions on follow-up imaging studies. The most appropriate way to follow these lesions in terms of imaging studies would need to account for metabolic activity or blood flow as a surrogate marker for viability *(21)*. Gadolinium-enhanced MRI scans or possibly positron-emission tomographic (PET) scans may provide such information and again size of the lesion is less important than areas of enhancement.

Because RFA obviously affects only on the areas where it is applied, progression of any tumors in other parts of the liver or in extrahepatic locations do not reflect the success of the radiofrequency treatment itself. Therefore, the most important data that are available in follow-up are lesion-per-lesion assessments of local recurrence evidenced by progressive enlargement of the areas on sequential scans, particularly in the setting of enhancement, which indicates viable tumor. The best and most mature series of RFA in the literature at this time comes from institutional reports from Curley et al. at M.D. Anderson Cancer Center in Houston *(22)*, Siperstein et al. initially at UCSF and most recently at the Cleveland Clinic *(23)*, Bilchik et al. at the John Wayne Cancer Institute in Santa Monica *(24)*, and deBaere et al. from France *(25)* (Table 5). All of these series combine patients with colorectal metastases, other metastases, and primary hepatomas. Curley et al. treated most patients with an open surgical approach and used percutaneous treatment for patients with small lesions or single lesions that were located in the periphery of the liver. These patients primarily had hepatomas in the setting of cirrhosis. Siperstein et al.'s patients were all treated by laparoscopic approach *(23)*. Bilchik et al. treated patients with combination approaches, including several patients who also had resection. deBaere et al. treated the majority of cases by percutaneous ablation, with one-third of the group having an open ablation.

In the series from M.D. Anderson, 2 out of 61 patients (3.2%) treated with colorectal metastases had regrowth of tumors treated by RFA or local recurrences *(22)*. One of these patients had a lesion that was >6 cm in size that required multiple overlapping treatment series. The second patient who recurred locally had a lesion that was located between the right and middle hepatic veins near the inferior vena cava at an area that may be difficult to treat or may have been protected by the high blood flow. In the series from Siperstein et al., there were 64 colorectal metastases treated in 18 patients *(23)*. Twelve of the 64 metastases regrew (17.6%) and the local recurrences happened in 7 of 18 patients (39%). In the series from Bilchik et al., 15 of 84 patients had recurrence *(24)* (17.5%). The distribution of the local recurrences among tumor histologies is not given nor are there any data in this series regarding tumor markers. However, it is noted that all of the local recurrences in Bilchik et al.'s series occurred in lesions >3 cm in size, in which overlapping thermal fields were applied. Roche had a similar overall recurrence rate of 17% with appropriate follow-up. In this series from Paris, the recurrence rate was almost twice as great for percutaneous RFA treatment (10%) than for open RFA (6%). Like Siperstein et al.'s and Bilchik et al.'s experience, almost all of the local recurrences occurred in larger lesions. The length of follow-up in the Siperstein series was 13.4 mo, which is similar to the follow-up of the M.D. Anderson and Paris series, with shorter follow-up in the Bilchik et al. series. Independent predictors of local failure in Siperstein et al.'s series included a lack of increased lesion size on a CT scan obtained 1 wk prior to following RFA. This early follow-up scan would be

Table 5

Clinical Series of RFA for Various Hepatic Tumors Including Colorectal Metastases

	Reference			
	22	23	24	25
Number of patients	123	44	84	68
Number of tumors	169	181	231	121
Tumor type	61 Colorectal (50%) 48 Hepatoma (39%) 14 Others (Distribution of patients)	64 Colorectal (35%) 11 Hepatoma (6%) 79 Neuroendocrine (44%) (proportion of tumor)	37 Colorectal (44%) 11 Hepatoma (13%) 10 Melanoma (12%) 26 Other (31%)	58 Colorectal 10 Other metastatic
Operative approach	92 Open (75%) 31 Percutaneous (25%)	100% Laparoscopy	39 Open (43%) 27 Laparoscopic (11%) 25 Percutaneous (27%)	21 Open 47 Percutaneous
Median size of tumors (range)	3.4 cm (0.5–12 cm)	<1–10 cm	2 cm (0.3–9 cm)	2.0 (0.5–4.2 cm)
Median follow-up	15 mo	12.9 mo	9 mo	13.7 mo
Local recurrence rate	3/109 (1.8%) (2 colorectal, 1 hepatoma)	28/181 Overall (15.4%) 10/64 Colorectal (28%) 0/11 Hepatoima (0%) 6/79 Neuroendocrine (7.5%) 4/27 Other (15%)	15/84 Patients (17.8%)	9/100 Lesions total (9%) 9/54 pts total (17%) 7/67 Percut. (10%)
Normalized tumor marker CEA/AFP	76/105 (72.4%)	7/18 Colorectal (39%) 3/11 Hepatoma (27%) 10/29 Overall (34%)	Not available	Not available
RFA device	Radiotherapeutics	RITA	RITA	Radionics
Complication	1 Hemorrhage into tissue	None	7 Complications (6%) 3 Hepatic abscesses, including 1 death 1 Hemorrhage 1 Myocardial infarct 1 Liver failure 1 Skin burn	3/68 Patients (4.4%) 2 Hepatic abscesses 1 Bile peritoneum

indicative of treatment of a rim of surrounding normal liver, and failure to make a larger lesion would be equivalent to failure to obtain an adequate margin in the thermal lesion. Additional variables that were associated with recurrence were histology of adenocarcinoma or sarcoma, as opposed to neuroendocrine tumors or hepatomas, which had better control *(23)*. Also, as would be expected, larger lesions and tumors with evidence of necrosis pretreatment had a greater tendency to recur.

In all series of RFA of hepatic lesions, including the four above-described large series, the toxicity of this technique is minimal, ranging from 0% to 8% of patients (Table 5). In comparing RFA to the more time-tested technique of cryosurgery, the overall safety with very minimal morbidity to the patient is one of the best reasons to promote this as an ablation technology. In the series from M.D. Anderson, there was one patient who required transfusions after an intrahepatic bleed into a hepatoma associated with major vessels *(22)*. There were no major complications seen in the Siperstein et al. series *(23)*. There was a higher rate of complications in the Bilchik et al. series, with a rate of 8% *(24)*. The most common complication was hepatic abscess formation that occurred in three patients. Two of these three were after percutaneous ablations. One hepatic abscess occurred in a patient who had a lesion near the dome of the liver and it caused not only necrosis of the tumor but led to diaphragm necrosis and an abscess in this area, resulting in the demise of the patient, with the death directly related to RFA, as stated by the authors. They felt that it would have been more appropriate to do an open RFA in this location and this would have avoided the diaphragm injury and, hopefully, the fatal sequence of events. A second abscess was related to a percutaneous ablation that caused disruption of an adjacent bile duct and required biliary stenting and percutaneous drainage. The final abscess was a delayed recurrence 5 mo after treatment of a large hepatoma with an open technique. Other complications included hemorrhage from the treatment site, a skin burn in a percutaneous ablation where they were ablating the treatment tract, and two complications not directly related to RFA of a perioperative myocardial infarction and liver failure in a patient who had a combined major hepatic lobar resection *(24)*. The complication rate was somewhat less in the series from deBaere at 4.4%, again having two patients with hepatic abscesses similar to the rate seen on a per lesion basis from Bilchik et al. *(24)*. These were treated with percutaneous drainage and antibiotics with no untoward effects. They also had a complication of a bile leak, causing bilo-peritoneum. In summary, the most common complications seen with RFA appears to be an infection in the ablated lesions and this appears to occur at the rate of 1.3% of lesions treated when all series are combined.

One recent study reported a nonrandomized direct comparison within a single institution of the efficacy and morbidity of RFA and cryosurgery. Cryosurgery treatment of 88 tumors in 54 patients resulted in a 40% complication rate, including one treatment-related death, 10 intrahepatic abscesses, 8 pleural effusions, 2 pneumothoraces, 2 perihepatic abscesses, 2 episodes of bleeding, and 2 episodes of renal failure *(26)*. The complications of RFA in this study were minimal, occurring in 3/92 patients (3.3%). These were two perihepatic abscesses and one episode of bleeding. When the complication rates of RFA, which ranged between 0% and 8% are compared to the 40% complication rate from cryosurgery *(27)*, this is clearly one of the major benefits of RFA. A direct comparison of the advantages and disadvantages of these two ablative techniques are listed in Table 6.

6. CONCLUSIONS

The field of RFA is currently a moving target in which the initial reports with adequate follow-up now appearing in the medical literature at the same time that current practice

Table 6
Comparison of the Advantages and Disadvantages of Cryosurgery
and RFA to Treat Metastatic and Primary Liver Tumors

	Cryosurgery	*RFA*
Cost	Very expensive (unit price $300,000)	Less expensive (unit price $20,000)
Toxicity	Moderate (postcryosyndrome)	Minimal
Probe size	Moderate–large	Small
Lesion Size	Large—up to or >10 cm	Limited—reliable at <3 cm, but new technology may increase this to 5 cm
Lesion location	Limited to more peripheral selected lesions	Able to treat more central lesions. Limited by tumor adjacent to bile ducts
Efficacy	Long-term follow-up available	Short follow-up time
	Local recurrence rate of 3–10% with 5-yr follow-up	3–28% Recurrence rate with 1-yr follow-up

is being modified with second- and third-generation electrodes and generators. The initial reports are quite favorable for this new technique in terms of a very acceptable complication rate ranging from 0% to 8% in the literature surveyed; only one death could be directly attributed to a complication from this procedure. The efficacy with the initial generators appears to be quite favorable in almost all series for lesions treated with a single thermal lesion; that is, for lesions that are <3 cm in size targeted with a 3 to 3.5-cm electrode, there is almost uniform control of the disease with follow-up now between 12 and 16 mo. However, there are variable results in trying to overlap treatment fields and for lesions larger than 3 cm. In general, the recurrence rates can be as high as 30–40% when this is attempted and this is clearly the most important limitation of RFA at this time. However, there is intense investigation among manufacturers and investigators utilizing RFA to make larger probes *(5)* as well as ensuring that the treatment algorithms lead to complete destruction of all tissue within the thermal lesion *(4)*. If the newer-generation probes and generators can achieve the same degree of local control in larger lesions, RFA will become an increasingly important technique in treating primary and metastatic liver tumors.

The eventual role for radiofrequency thermal ablation in the armamentarium of treatments directed against colorectal liver metastases remains to be determined and is dependent on technological advances as well as adequate clinical trials with appropriate follow-up *(1,28)*. Initial attempts are being made in North America to incorporate RFA and for prospective multi-institutional studies (Table 7). One study sponsored by the Arrow International Corporation utilizes RFA for bilobar liver metastases that are unresectable in combination with intra-arterial fluorodeoxyuridine (FUDR) delivered by an intrahepatic infusion pump. A second trial sponsored by the American College of Surgeons Oncology Group that is currently under review approaches a similar patient population with, again, maximal tumor ablation combining RFA and/or cryosurgery based on investigator preference combined with tumor resection as needed. In this phase II trial, patients will also receive intra-arterial FUDR delivered by a intrahepatic infusion pump, but this will also be combined with systemic irinotecan (CPT-11). These initial phase II efforts with appropriate data auditing and review will provide very good information about the efficacy of RFA combined with regional chemotherapy and systemic chemotherapy. These initial studies with the current technology will then hopefully define the randomized trials to clearly delineate which patient population is benefited in terms of survival by RFA of unresectable metastatic colorectal lesions to the liver.

Table 7
Ongoing or Proposed Multi-Institutional Trials Incorporating RFA for Colorectal Metastases

Principal investigator	Kelly McMasters	Ken Tanabe
Sponsor	Arrow Corporation	American College of Surgeons Oncology Group
Entry criteria	2–8 Hepatic metastases < 6 cm No extrahepatic disease	2–10 Hepatic metastases < 5 cm No extrahepatic disease
Treatment	Completion ablation/resection of gross disease by RFA Intra-arterial FUDR	Complete ablation/resection of gross disease by RFA or cryosurgery Intra-arterial FUDR Systemic CPT-11
Open in June 2001	Yes	No

REFERENCES

1. McGahan JP and Dodd GD. Radiofrequency ablation of the liver: current status. *Am. J. Roentgenol.*, **176** (2001) 3–16.
2. Giorgio A, Francica G, Tarantino L, and de Stefano G. Radiofrequency ablation of hepatocellular carcinomas lesions. *Radiology*, **218** (2001) 918–919.
3. Siperstein AE and Gitominski A. History and technological aspects of radiofrequency thermoablation. *Cancer J.*, **6** (2000) S293–S303.
4. Goldberg SN, Solbiati L, Hahn PF, Cosman E, Conrad JE, Fogle R, et al. Large volume tissue ablation with radiofrequency by using a clustered, internally cooled electrode technique: laboratory and clinical experience in liver metastases. *Radiology*, **209** (1998) 371–379.
5. Berber E, Flesher NL, and Siperstein AE. Initial clinical evaluation of the RITA 5-centimeter radiofrequency thermal ablation catheter in the treatment of liver tumors. *Cancer J.*, **6** (2000) S319–S329.
6. Scudamore C. Volumetric radiofrequency ablation: technical considerations. *Cancer J.*, **6** (2000) S316–S318.
7. Rossi S, Buscarini E, Garbagnati F, DiStasi M, Quaretti P, Rago M, et al. Percutaneous treatment of small hepatic tumors by an expandable RF needle electrode. *Am. J. Roentgenol.*, **170** (1998) 1015–1022.
8. Caturelli E. Percutaneous ablative therapies for small hepatocellular carcinoma: radiofrequency or percutaneous ethanol injection. *Radiology*, **216** (2000) 304–306.
9. Heslin MJ, Medina-Franco H, Parker M, Vickers S, Aldrete J, and Urist MM. Colorectal hepatic metastases: resection, local ablation, and hepatic artery infusion pump are associated with prolonged survival. *Arch. Surg.*, **136** (2001) 318–323.
10. Curley SA, Davidson BS, Fleming RY, Izzo F, Stephens LC, Tinkey P, et al. Laparoscopically guided bipolar radiofrequency ablation of areas of porcine liver. *Surg. Endoscopy*, **11** (1997) 729–733.
11. Siperstein A, Garland A, Engle K, Rogers S, Berber E, String A, et al. Laparoscopic radiofrequency ablation of primary and metastatic liver tumors. *Surg. Endosc.*, **14** (2000) 400–405.
12. Ravikumar TS, Kaleye R, and Kishinevsky A. Surgical ablative therapy of liver tumors. In *Cancer: Principles & Practice of Oncology.* 5th ed. Devita VT, Hellman S, and Rosenberg SA (eds.), Lippincott-Raven, New York, 2000, Vol. 14.
13. Rhim H and Dodd GD. Radiofrequency thermal ablation of liver tumors. *J. Clin. Ultrasound*, **27** (1999) 221–229.
14. Patterson EJ, Scudamore CH, Owen DA, Nagy AG, and Buczkowski AK. Radiofrequency ablation of porcine liver *in vivo:* effects of blood flow and treatment time on lesion size. *Ann. Surg.*, **237** (1998) 559–565.
15. Livraghi T, Goldberg SN, Monti F, Bizzini A, Lazzaroni S, Meloni F, et al. Saline-enhanced radiofrequency tissue ablation in the treatment of liver metastases. *Radiology*, **202** (1997) 205–210.
16. Curley SA, Izzo F, Ellis LM, Vauthey JN, and Vallone P. Radiofrequency ablation of hepatocellular cancer in 110 patients with cirrhosis. *Ann. Surg.*, **232** (2000) 381–391.
17. Rossi S, DiStasi M, Buscarini E, Quaretti P, Garbagnati F, Squassante L, et al. Percutaneous RF interstitial thermal ablation in the treatment of hepatic cancer. *Am. J. Roentgenol.*, **167** (1996) 759–768.
18. Solbiati L, Goldberg SN, Ierace T, Livraghi T, Meloni F, Dellanoce M, et al. Hepatic metastases: percutaneous radiofrequency ablation with cooled tip electrodes. *Radiology*, **205** (1997) 367–373.

19. Solbiati L, Ierace T, Goldberg SN, Sironi S, Livraghi T, Fiocca R, et al. Percutaneous US-guided radiofrequency tissue ablation of liver metastases: treatment and follow-up in 16 patients. *Radiology*, **202** (1997) 195–203.

20. Jiao LR, Hansen PD, Havlik R, Mitry RR, Pignatelli M, and Habib N. Clinical short-term results of radiofrequency ablation in primary and secondary liver tumors. *Am. J. Surg.*, **177** (1999) 303–306.

21. Berber E, Foroutani A, Garland AM, Rogers SJ, Engle KL, Ryan TL, et al. Use of CT Hounsfield unit density to identify ablated tumor after lapoaroscopic radiofrequency ablation of hepatic tumors. *Surg. Endoscopy*, **14** (2000) 799–803.

22. Curley SA, Izzo F, Deirio P, Ellis LM, Granchi J, Vallone P, et al. Radiofrequency ablation of unresectable primary and metastatic hepatic malignancies. *Ann. Surg.*, **230** (1999) 1–8.

23. Siperstein A, Garland A, Engle K, Rogers S, Berber E, Foroutani A, et al. Local recurrence after laparoscopic radiofrequency thermal ablation of hepatic tumors. *Ann. Surg. Oncol.*, **7** (2000) 106–113.

24. Wood TF, Rose DM, Chung M, Allegra DP, Foshag LJ, and Bilchik AJ. Radiofrequency ablation of 231 unresectable hepatic tumors: indications, limitations, and complications. *Ann. Surg. Oncol.*, **7** (2000) 593–600.

25. deBaere T, Elias D, Dromain C, El Din MG, Kuoch V, Ducreux M, et al. Radiofrequency ablation of 100 hepatic metastases with a mean follow-up of more than 1 year. *Am. J. Roentgenol.*, **175** (2000) 1619–1625.

26. Pearson AS, Izzo F, Fleming D, Ellis LM, Delrio P, Roh MS, et al. Intraoperative radiofrequency ablation or cryoablation for hepatic malignancies. *Am. J. Surg.*, **178** (1999) 592–599.

27. Sarantou T, Bilchik A, and Ramming KP. Complications of hepatic cryosurgery. *Semin. Surg. Oncol.*, **14** (1998) 156–162.

28. Bilchik AJ, Wood TF, Allegra D, Tsioulias GJ, Chung M, Rose DM, et al. Cryosurgical ablation and radiofrequency ablation for unresectable hepatic malignant neoplasms: a proposed algorithm. *Arch. Surg.*, **135** (2000) 657–662.

IV MEDICAL ONCOLOGY

25

5-Fluorouracil and Its Biomodulation in the Management of Colorectal Cancer

Jean L. Grem

CONTENTS

Until the availability of irinotecan (*see* Chapter 28), 5-fluorouracil (5-FU) and 5-fluoro-2′-deoxyuridine (FdUrd) were the only commercially available treatment options that represented standard therapy for advanced colorectal cancer. 5-FU has generally been given by the intravenous (iv) route because of poor oral bioavailability, whereas FdUrd has been used mostly for regional therapy to the liver or peritoneal cavity. Greater understanding of the metabolic activation of 5-FU, its mechanism(s) of action, and clinical pharmacology has generated rational strategies that involve its combination with other drugs capable of either enhancing its metabolism or cytotoxic effects.

1. CELLULAR AND CLINICAL PHARMACOLOGY OF 5-FU

1.1. Intracellular Metabolism

5-Fluorouracil requires cellular uptake and metabolic activation to form its cytotoxic metabolites. 5-FU enters cells by either nonfacilitated diffusion or a facilitated transport system for both purine and pyrimidine bases. The nucleoside metabolites, 5-fluoro-2′-deoxyuridine (FdUrd) and 5-fluorouridine (FUrd), require the facilitated nucleoside transport systems for cellular entry. 5-FU is metabolized using the same enzymes involved in the anabolism and catabolism of uracil (Fig. 1) *(1)*. Thymidine phosphorylase, which is homologous to platelet-derived endothelial cell growth factor, catalyzes the reversible conversion of 5-FU to FdUrd *(2)*. Thymidine kinase adds a phosphate group to the 5′-carbon of the deoxyribose ring to form 5-fluoro-2′-deoxyuridine monophosphate (FdUMP). Thymidylate kinase converts FdUMP to the diphosphate form, and nucleoside diphosphate kinase then forms FdUTP. 5-FU is converted to the ribonucleotide level by one of two pathways.

From: *Colorectal Cancer: Multimodality Management*
Edited by: L. Saltz © Humana Press Inc., Totowa, NJ

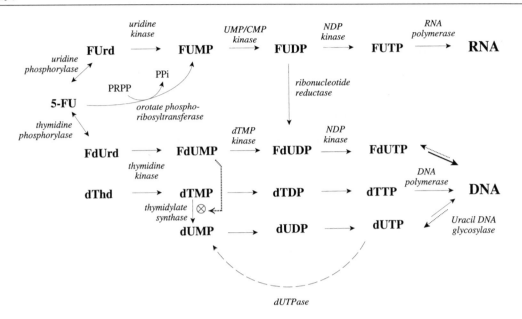

Fig. 1. Intracellular metabolism of 5-FU.

Uridine phosphorylase transforms 5-FU into FUrd; uridine kinase then catalyzes the formation of 5-fluorouridine monophosphate (FUMP). Orotate phosphoribosyltransferase directly forms FUMP by transferring a ribose 5′-monophosphate group from 5′-phosphoribosyl-1-pyrophosphate (PRPP) to 5-FU. Further metabolism to the diphosphate (FUDP) and triphosphate (FUTP) forms is mediated by UMP/CMP kinase and nucleoside diphosphate kinase, respectively. FUTP is readily incorporated into RNA. Ribonucleotide reductase converts FUDP to FdUDP, which represents another pathway for the formation of FdUMP. 5-FU nucleotide sugars, including FUDP-glucose, FUDP-hexose, FUDP-acetylglucosamine and FdUDP-*n*-acetylglucosamine, can also be formed, but the extent of their incorporation into proteins and lipids is not well understood.

Acid phosphatases, alkaline phosphatases, and 5′-nucleotidases convert the nucleotide derivatives of 5-FU back to the nucleoside level. Pyrimidine phosphorylases catalyze the reversible conversion of pyrimidine bases to nucleosides: Uridine phosphorylase converts uridine and fluorouridine (FUrd) to uracil and 5-FU, with release of ribose-1-phosphate, whereas thymidine phosphorylase converts thymidine, deoxyuridine, and FdUrd to thymine, uracil, and 5-FU, respectively, with release of 2′-deoxyribose-1-phosphate. FdUrd can also serve as a substrate for uridine phosphorylase. Dihydropyrimidine dehydrogenase (DPD) catalyzes the catabolism of 5-FU to dihydrofluororacil, and its importance is discussed in Chapter 26.

1.2. Mechanisms of Action

5-Fluorouracil is incorporated into both nuclear and cytoplasmic RNA species; the extent of this RNA incorporation correlates with cytotoxicity in some cell culture and in vivo models *(1,3)*. 5-FU-RNA incorporation results in a variety of effects, including interference with the conversion of high-molecular-weight nuclear RNA species to lower-molecular-weight rRNA, inhibition of mRNA polyadenylation (which decreases the stability of mRNA), and alteration of the secondary structure of RNA *(4–11)*. Covalent complexes that form between 5-FU-containing tRNA molecules and enzymes involved in posttranslational modification

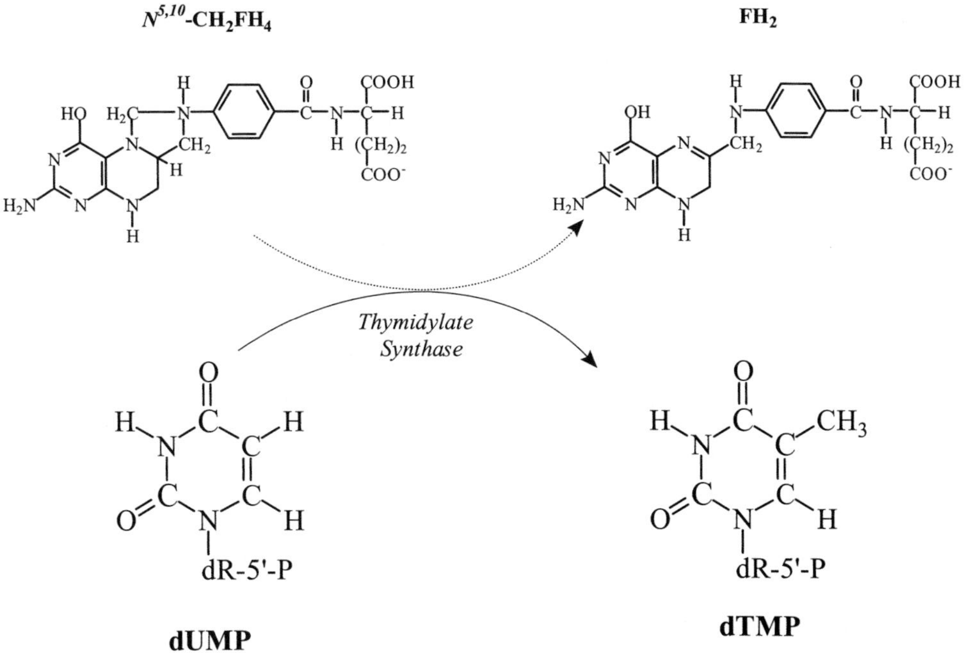

Fig. 2. *De novo* synthesis of thymidylate.

of uracil residues inhibit these enzymes *(12,13)*. RNA synthesis may be inhibited with 5-FU in a concentration- and time-dependent fashion *(14,15)*. The decrease in mRNA expression is often accompanied by a decrease in the corresponding protein level, but 5-FU-mediated alterations in protein expression can also occur rapidly in the absence of a clear effect on mRNA expression, presumably as a result of posttranscriptional effects *(16)*. Both qualitative and quantitative changes in protein synthesis have been demonstrated *(5,15,17)*. Incorporation into uracil-rich small nuclear RNA species interferes with normal splicing *(17–20)*. Induction of programmed cell death is usually the result of DNA-directed events of 5-FU, but induction of apoptosis in some tissues may be related to RNA-directed effects *(21)*.

Thymidylate synthase (TS) is responsible for the *de novo* production of thymidine 5′-monophosphate from 2′-deoxyuridine 5′-monophosphate (dUMP) through the transfer of a methyl group from 5,10-methylene tetrahydrofolate (Fig. 2) *(22)*. Inhibition of TS by FdUMP is an important mechanism of 5-FU action. In contrast to the interaction of TS with the natural substrate, dUMP, the ternary complex formed between the enzyme, FdUMP, and the reduced folate cofactor is only slowly reversible *(22,23)*. The intracellular levels of 5,10-methylene tetrahydrofolate and the extent of its polyglutamation affect the stability of the ternary complex. Expansion of the reduced folate pools with pharmacologic doses of 5-formyl-tetrahydrofolate (leucovorin, folinic acid) represents a clinically useful strategy to enhance the cytotoxicity of 5- FU *(23–25)*. TS inhibition depletes the pools of both thymidine 5′-monophosphate (dTMP, thymidylate) and thymidine 5′-triphosphate (dTTP), which interferes with DNA synthesis and repair. Thymidine can be directly converted to dTMP by thymidine kinase, thus bypassing inhibition of the *de novo* pathway, and pharmacologic concentrations of thymidine (10–30 μ*M*) are frequently used in preclinical models to provide protection against TS inhibition. Whereas salvage of extracellular thymidine represents a potential mechanism of circumventing TS inhibition, the circulating levels of thymidine in humans are much lower and are thought to be insufficient to afford protection *(26)*.

Inhibition TS is accompanied by accumulation of dUMP, which can also be metabolized to the 5′-triphosphate level (dUTP) *(27–30)*. Incorporation of 2′-deoxyuridine 5′-triphosphate (dUTP) and FdUTP into DNA results in damage to nascent DNA *(1)*. The extent of uracil misincorporation into DNA is limited by dUTP pyrophosphatase (dUTPase), which catalyzes the hydrolysis of (F)dUTP to (F)dUMP and inorganic pyrophosphate (PPi) *(31,32)*. Uracil-DNA-glycosylase hydrolyzes the (F)uracil–deoxyribose glycosyl bond of the (F)dUMP residues in DNA, resulting in an apyrimidinemic site *(33)*. Endonucleolytic cleavage of the base-free deoxyribose site leads to a single-strand break. In the face of thymidine triphosphate depletion, the efficiency of the repair of such strand breaks is reduced. Misincorporated 5-FU is removed more slowly from DNA than uracil *(33)*. FdUTP also inhibits the activity of uracil–DNA–glycosylase *(34)*. Accumulation of deoxyadenosine triphosphate accompanies TS inhibition *(35–38)*. The combined effects of deoxyribonucleotide imbalance (high dATP, low dTTP, high dUTP) and misincorporation of (F)dUTP into DNA result in a number of deleterious effects on both DNA synthesis and the integrity of nascent DNA *(28,35–39)*.

Genotoxic stress resulting from TS inhibition can activate programmed cell death pathways *(38,40–43)*. Different patterns of parental DNA damage are seen in various cell lines, including internucleosomal DNA laddering and high-molecular-weight DNA fragmentation (fragments ranging from about 50 kb to 1–3 Mb). Differences in the activities of endonucleases and DNA-degradative enzymes in a given cell line are thought to account for these distinct patterns of parental DNA fragmentation. Some cancer cells are readily disposed to undergo apoptosis, and genotoxic stress results in rapid and uniform induction of programmed cell death, with classic DNA laddering. Many cancer cell lines derived from common solid tumors including colon cancer, in contrast, appear to undergo delayed programmed cell death that requires several days. The duration of the genotoxic insult influences whether induction of cytostatis or programmed cell death occurs. A possible explanation for delayed apoptosis is that originally sublethal damage to genes that are necessary for cell survival may eventually result in cell death with additional rounds of DNA replication *(44,45)*.

Factors operating downstream from TS, such as overexpression of the cellular oncoproteins bcl-2 and mutant p53, influence the cellular response to TS inhibition *(46,47)*. Disruption of the signal pathways that sense genotoxic stress and/or trigger the induction of programmed cell death may render cancer cells inherently resistant to 5-FU. In some cancer cell lines, "thymineless" death is mediated by Fas–Fas ligand interactions *(48,49)*.

Because TS is needed for DNA replication, its activity is typically higher in proliferating than in noncycling cells. In continuously proliferating cancer cells, TS activity varies by about four- to eightfold from resting phase to synthetic phase *(50)*. When nonproliferating cells are synchronized and stimulated to enter the DNA synthetic phase of the cell cycle, TS content increases by up to 20-fold *(51,52)*. 5-FU exposure in preclinical models is accompanied by an acute increase in TS content, which may permit recovery of enzymatic activity *(53–56)*. The increase in total TS content is a function of 5-FU concentration and time of exposure. Serial tumor biopsies obtained from patients before and during treatment with 5-FU/LV (leucovorin) have also shown an increase in TS protein 24 h after dosing *(57,58)*. This phenomenon is thought to be the result of translational autoregulation, although increased stability of TS protein has been noted in some models *(55,56,59,60)*. TS protein binds to specific regions in its corresponding mRNA, which suppresses translation. TS protein bound in the ternary complex cannot interact with its mRNA, thus allowing translation of new TS protein to proceed.

Table 1
Clinical Schedules of Intravenous 5-FU

Schedule	Infusion type	Daily dose (mg/m²)
Daily for 5 d q 4–5 wk	Bolus	500
		425 (+ LV 20)
		370–400 (+ LV 200)
Weekly for 6 of 8 wk	Bolus	750
		600 (+ LV 500/2 h)
		500 (+ LV 500/2 h)
24 h q wk	Infusion	2600
		2300–2600 (+ LV 50–500/24 h)
48 h q wk	Infusion	1750
72 h q 3 wk	Infusion	2300
		2000 (+ LV 500/24 h)
96 h q 3 wk	Infusion	1000
120 h q 3 wk		750
Daily × 28 d q 5 wk	Infusion	300
		200 (+ LV 20 q wk)
Bolus → 22 h d 1, 2 q 2 wk	Mixed	400 → 600 (+LV 200/2 h)
Bolus → 48 h d 1 q 2 wk	Mixed	400 → 2400–3000 (+ LV 400/2 h)

The contribution of DNA- and/or RNA-directed mechanisms to 5-FU cytotoxicity is influenced by the patterns of intracellular metabolism, which can differ among various host and tumor tissues. 5-FU concentration and duration of exposure both influence the mechanism of cytotoxicity. Short-term, high-concentration exposures are thought to favor RNA-directed 5-FU toxicity, whereas DNA-directed effects are felt to be more prominent with longer exposures to lower drug concentrations *(61–63)*. However, these pathways are not mutually exclusive, and more than one mechanism of action may contribute to cytotoxicity *(64,65)*. Some patients who experience tumor progression during bolus 5-FU may respond to infusional schedules, suggesting that clinical resistance to bolus 5-FU does not necessarily confer resistance to other schedules *(66,67)*. The combination of bolus and infusional 5-FU represents another strategy to improve outcome by potentially allowing more than one cytotoxic mechanism to occur *(63,68)*.

The principal mechanism of action of 5-FU with various clinical schedules has not been clearly defined. However, the improved response rates observed with LV modulation of bolus 5-FU therapy, the correlation between high TS expression in tumor tissue and insensitivity to 5-FU-based therapy *(69–71)*, and the clinical activity of antifolate-based TS inhibitors provide clear evidence that TS is an important therapeutic target.

1.3. Clinical Pharmacology

5-Fluorouracil has been given by a variety of clinical schedules (Table 1) *(3)*. The clearance of 5-FU is mediated by the cytosolic enzyme dihydropyrimidine dehydrogenase (DPD), which converts 5-FU to dihydrofluorouracil (DHFU). The activity of DPD thus influences the amount of 5-FU available for anabolism. Clinical pharmacology studies indicate wide interpatient variation in both 5-FU clearance and DPD activity and pharmacogenetic and diurnal variations in DPD activity be contributing factors.

The pharmacokinetics of 5-FU are influenced by the dose and schedule of administration. After iv bolus injection of 370–720 mg/m^2 5-FU, peak plasma concentrations reach several hundred micromolar *(72–76)*. Thereafter, clearance occurs rapidly, and the primary half-life is 8–14 min. Whether given by bolus or continuous infusion, 5-FU readily penetrates the extracellular space, cerebrospinal fluid, and third-space accumulations such as ascites or pleural effusions. The volume of distribution ranges between 13 and 18 L. The vast majority of the parent drug is cleared through catabolism, and only a small portion is excreted unchanged in the urine.

Because 5-FU catabolism by DPD is saturable, the clearance is faster with infusion compared to bolus injection. Clearance increases as the dose rate decreases and it ranges from 2000 to 3000 mL/min/m^2 with various schedules of infusional 5-FU. The tolerated daily dose of 5-FU decreases as the duration of infusion increases. With protracted infusion of 300 mg/m^2/d, the achieved steady-state plasma levels range from 0.1 to 0.4 μ*M (77–79)*. Daily doses of 1000 mg/m^2/d for 96 h or 750 mg/m^2/d for 120 h are commonly used, and an intermittent schedule is necessary; steady-state plasma levels range from about 1 to 3.4 μ*M (80–83)*. Continuous infusion of 1750–2300 mg/m^2/d result in plasma levels ranging from about 5 to 9 μ*M (84–86)*.

The nonlinear elimination kinetics leads to the following with increasing 5-FU dose: a decrease in total-body clearance, a longer plasma half-life, and an increase in the area under the plasma concentration time curve *(74,86–91)*. The implication is that as the dose increases, the decrease in clearance and the increase in area under the curve (AUC) will change disproportionately.

The incidence of serious clinical toxicity tends to increase with higher systemic exposure *(74–76,78–79,92–96)*. However, some patients have toxicity despite relatively low 5-FU systemic exposure, whereas other patients with relatively high 5-FU systemic exposures do not experience untoward toxicity; clearly, other factors must contribute to the clinical toxicity.

Differences in 5-FU metabolism in host and tumor tissues are likely to be important determinants of both clinical toxicity and antitumor activity. FdUMP and FUTP have a more prolonged intracellular retention than the parent drug. 5-FU that has been incorporated into RNA appears to be retained in a stable fashion, whereas the duration of TS inhibition is much more variable. There is currently limited information that correlates the intracellular pharmacodynamics of 5-FU with either clinical toxicity or antitumor effect. Certain noninvasive methods such as nuclear magnetic resonance imaging (MRI) and positron-emission tomography (PET) should facilitate the conduct of such pharmacodynamic studies.

Hepatic arterial infusion, portal venous infusion, and intraperitoneal administration of 5-FU and FdUrd offer more a selective exposure to specific tumor-bearing sites to high local concentrations of drug *(97–99)*. Regional therapy to the liver is discussed in Chapter 32.

2. BIOCHEMICAL OR PHARMACOLOGIC STRATEGIES TO MODULATE 5-FU

2.1. Leucovorin Modulation of 5-FU

As mentioned earlier, inhibition of TS by FdUMP is a crucial mechanism of 5-FU action. Under normal circumstances, TS transfers a methyl group from 5,10-methylene tetrahydrofolate to the carbon-5 position of dUMP, followed by dissociation of the ternary complex and the release of free enzyme and the products of the reaction (Fig. 2). In

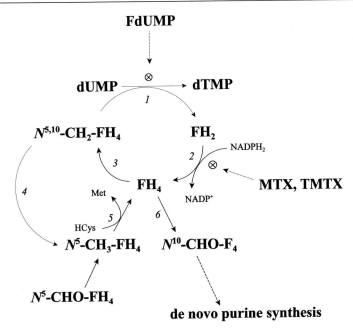

Fig. 3. Reduced folate metabolism. Abbreviations: (F)dUMP, (fluoro)deoxyuridine monophosphate; dTMP, thymidine monophosphate; MTX, methotrexate; FH_2, dihydrofolate; FH_4, tetrahydrofolate; $-CH_2$, methylene; -CHO, formyl; $-CH_3$, methyl, HCys, homocysteine; Met, methionine. The enzymes are (1) thymidylate synthase, (2) dihydrofolate reductase, (3) serine hydroxymethyltransferase, (4) N^5,N^{10}-methylene tetrahydrofolate reductase, (5) methionine synthase, (6) N^{10}-formyl-tetrahydrofolate synthetase.

contrast, the TS–FdUMP–folate ternary complex is only slowly reversible, and its stability is influenced by the intracellular level of 5,10-methylene tetrahydrofolate and the extent of its polyglutamation *(100)*. Pharmacologic concentrations of LV expand the intracellular pools of 5,10–methylene tetrahydrofolate (monoglutamates and polyglutamates) and thereby enhance the degree and duration of FdUMP-mediated TS inhibition (Fig. 3) *(101–105)*. A LV concentration of 10 μM is often cited as the optimal target concentration with short exposures to 5-FU, but the concentration of LV required for modulation of 5-FU cytotoxicity decreases as the exposure to 5-FU increases.

Two of the most commonly employed 5-FU/LV regimens involve either weekly administration of an iv bolus 5-FU given at the midpoint of a 2-h iv infusion of high-dose LV or a monthly (daily for 5 d every 4–5 wk) schedule of iv bolus LV and 5-FU. With the monthly schedule, the recommended doses of 5-FU are 370–400 mg/m^2 with 200 mg/m^2 LV and 425 mg/m^2 with 20 mg/m^2 LV. Pharmacokinetic data for several schedules of iv LV are shown in Table 2 *(106–108)*.

A meta-analysis of the value of bolus 5-FU/LV in patients with advanced colorectal cancer employed individual data provided by the principal investigators from nine randomized trials *(109)*. All 1381 patients entered in these trials were included on a strictly intent-to-treat basis. A highly statistically significant advantage in response rate was observed with LV-modulated 5-FU (22.5% vs 11.1%), but this did not translate into a significant difference in median survival (11.5 vs 11.0 mo).

The results of 14 randomized trials comparing 5-FU administered by iv bolus either as a single agent or modulated by LV have been published *(110–123)*. Two trials included patients

Table 2
Pharmacokinetic Data with IV or Oral Administration of Leucovorin

Ref.	Leucovorin dose	d-5-formyl-FH$_4$	l-5-formyl-FH$_4$	l-5-methyl-FH$_4$
107	50 mg iv push			
	C_p at 1 h (μM)	6.2	2.1 μM	0.8–1.0
	half-life (min)	451 ± 24	31.6 ± 1.1	227 ± 20
	AUC^a(min•mg/L)	2303	78.3 ± 7.4	310 ± 35
108	500 mg/m^2 iv over 2 h			
	C_{max} (μM)	97.7 ± 34.3	28.8 ± 12.7	20.8 ± 6.8
	half-life (min)	534	96	
109	200 mg/m^2 iv push			
	C_{max} (μM)	97.7 ± 34.3	43	1–2
	half-life (min)	659 ± 59	alpha: 20 ± 2	beta: 362 ± 59
			beta: 122 ± 20	

^{a}AUC = area under the curve.

with nonmeasurable disease *(118,121)*. Based on the number of eligible and assessable patients reported in each trial, the combined data for all 14 trials indicate a response rate of 13.8% in patients treated with 5-FU alone (Table 3) and 25.3% in patients treated with 5-FU/LV (Table 4). For time to progression, the median of the reported values was 6.0 mo for 5-FU/LV and 4.2 mo for 5-FU alone, whereas the median of the reported survival times was 12.4 mo for 5-FU/LV and 11.0 mo for 5-FU alone.

The next generation of trials sought to define the optimal 5-FU/LV schedule. A randomized trial conducted by the North Central Cancer Treatment Group (NCCTG) compared the monthly schedule of low-dose LV/5-FU with the weekly schedule of high-dose LV/5-FU *(124)*. In this trial, the overall response rate was 34% and 31% in patients treated with the monthly and weekly schedules, respectively. Both the median time to tumor progression (about 4.4 mo and about 6.3 mo) and median survival (9.3 and 10.7 mo) were somewhat longer with the weekly schedule, but they did not reach statistical significance. The response rates for the monthly and weekly schedules of 5-FU + LV from the 14 randomized studies shown in Table 4 are similar: 25.0% ± 1.6% and 25.7% ± 1.9%. Therefore, the data suggest that these two schedules of 5-FU/LV are therapeutically equivalent in advanced colorectal cancer, although the spectrum of toxicity differs. Dose-limiting diarrhea is more frequent with the weekly schedule and severe mucositis is uncommon. In contrast, mucositis tends to be dose limiting with the monthly schedule, although diarrhea also occurs. Until recently, the monthly schedule has been regarded as the "gold standard" for pivotal trials in colorectal cancer in the United States based on one randomized study that demonstrated a survival advantage with LV-modulated 5-FU *(125)*. In addition, the low-dose monthly regimen is less costly. The weekly schedule remains popular, however, and is more convenient for some patients. Increased awareness of the potential for life-threatening diarrhea with the weekly schedule has led to greater vigilance during therapy, with interruption of treatment if early signs of toxicity occur. A disadvantage of the monthly schedule is that clinical toxicity usually occurs after all 5 d of treatment have been given. Consequently, many oncologists believe the weekly regimen is easier to manage.

High-dose vs low-dose LV on a particular schedule has been addressed in several trials. Three randomized trials have directly compared 20 mg/m^2 of racemic (*d,l*–) LV or

Table 3
Fourteen Randomized Trials Comparing Intravenous Bolus 5-FU ± Leucovorin: 5-FU Alone Arm

Trial	Patients entered	CR + PR vs no. assessable	Median TTP (mo)	Median survival (mo)
Weekly				
Martoni *(110)*	30	1 of 30	5.0	7.0
Nobile *(109,111)*	73	6 of 73	—	—
Valone *(112)*	55	10 of 52	4.5	11.3
Laufman *(113)*	112	23 of 109	3.7	12.4
Monthly				
Petrelli *(114)*	23	2 of 19	—	12
Petrelli *(115)*	113	13 of 107	—	10.6
Erlichman *(116)*	64	4 of 61	2.9	9.6
Doroshow *(117)*	40	5 of 40	3.9	12.7
Poon *(118)*	70	4 of 39[†]	4.0	7.7
Labianca *(119)*	90	9 of 90	6.0	11.5
Di Costanzo *(109,120)*	90	14 of 90	4.9	—
Leichman *(121)*	93	17 of 60[†]	6.0	14.0
Petrioli *(122)*	91	16 of 86		7.5
Borner *(123)*	157	13 of 139	3.9	10.0
Total no. or	1101	137 of 995	4.0	10.6
median (range)		13.8 ± 2.2%	(2.9–6.0)	(7.0–14.0)

Note: In the trial reported by Valone, an initial 5-d loading course of 5-FU was given followed at d 28 by weekly injections of 5-FU. The term "assessable" reflects eligible patients with measurable disease in whom response to therapy could be determined. [†] designates those trials that included patients with both measurable and nonmeasurable disease. The mean and 95% confidence interval for the response rate are shown.

10 mg/m^2 of pure *l*-LV with a 10-fold higher dose given with 370–425 mg/m^2 5-FU on the monthly schedule *(126–129)*. No advantage with high-dose LV was seen in any of these trials with respect to response rate, time to progression, or survival. Two randomized trials compared 20 or 25 mg/m^2 LV with 500 mg/m^2 LV given over 2 h with bolus 5-FU 500 or 600 mg/m^2 iv given at the midpoint of the infusion *(116,129)*. Although the response rate was somewhat higher with the higher LV dose in both trials, the difference was not significant, and there was no difference in survival.

In contrast to the advanced-disease setting, bolus 5-FU/LV has improved survival when used as adjuvant therapy for high-risk colon cancer. Because the North American randomized trials using the weekly schedule have employed high-dose LV (500 mg/m^2/2 h) *(130,131)*, it may be unwise to extrapolate that low-dose LV given on the weekly schedule would result in a disease-free and overall survival benefit as adjuvant therapy in patients with colorectal cancer A benefit with both high-dose (200 mg/m^2) and low-dose (20 mg/m^2) LV modulation of 5-FU has been seen in adjuvant colon cancer trials evaluating the monthly schedule.

In order to test the value of different adjuvant chemotherapy regimens, a multicenter trial termed QUASAR (quick and simple and reliable) was conducted in the United Kingdom using a 2 × 2 factorial design: Patients received a fixed dose of 375 mg/m^2 5-FU in combination with either 175 or 25 mg *l*-LV with or without levamisole. Participating physicians selected either a daily 5-d schedule repeated every 4 wk for six cycles, or a weekly schedule for 30 wk. Over 4900 patients with stage II or II colorectal cancer were entered in this trial between 1994 and 1997. Although this was a nonrandomized comparison with respect

Table 4
Fourteen Randomized Trials Comparing Intravenous Bolus 5-FU ± Leucovorin: 5-FU/LV Arm

Trial	Patients entered	No. CR/PR vs no. assessable	Median TTP (mo)	Median survival (mo)
Weekly				
Petrelli (115)	30	12 of 30	—	12.0
Petrelli: LD LV (116)	115	21 of 112	—	10.4
Petrelli: HD LV (116)	115	33 of 109	—	12.7
Martoni (110)	34	9 of 34	6.0	10.0
Nobile (100,111)	75	16 of 75	—	—
Laufman (113)	106	31 of 101	5.1	12.4
Leichman (121)	89	12 of 60[†]	6.0	14.0
Monthly				
Erlichman (116)	66	21 of 64	5.1	12.6
Valone (112)	107	19 of 107	5.5	10.7
Doroshow (117)	39	16 of 39	5.4	14.2
Poon: LD LV (118)	73	16 of 37[†]	7.0	12.0
Poon: HD LV (118)	69	9 of 35[†]	7.0	12.2
Labianca (119)	92	19 of 92	6.0	11.0
Di Costanzo (109,120)	91	12 of 91	5.8	—
Leichman (121)	89	16 of 61[†]	6.0	14.0
Petrioli (122)	94	27 of 81		13.5
Borner (123)	152	30 of 134	6.2	12.4
Total no. or median (range)	1436	319 of 1262 (25.3 ± 2.4%)	6.0 (5.1–7.0)	12.3 (10.4–14.0)

Note: Although the doses of 5-FU and LV varied among the trials, they are organized into weekly or monthly schedules (daily for 5 d every 28–35 d). The term "assessable" reflects eligible patients with measurable disease in whom response to therapy could be determined. Trials that included patients with both measurable and nonmeasurable disease are shown by †. The response rate and 95% confidence interval are shown.

to the schedule of 5-FU/LV, a similar proportion of patients were treated on each arm (weekly, 2370; monthly, 2559) and the two groups were well balanced for stage (B or C), site (colon or rectum), dose of LV, use of levamisole or placebo, gender and age. There were no differences in either 3-yr recurrence rates (35.6% weekly vs 35.5% monthly, odds ratio = 0.99) or overall survival (70.6% weekly vs 71.0% monthly, odds ratio = 0.97) (132). The incidence of serious diarrhea, stomatitis, myelosuppression, and dermatologic toxicities was significantly higher with the monthly schedule of 5-FU/LV. In this trial, higher doses of LV produced no extra benefit, and dose reductions for toxicity were required more frequently in patients receiving high-dose LV (42% vs 17%) (133).

Another issue concerns the formulation of LV. In the United States, the commercial formulation is a racemic mixture of the nonphysiologic stereoisomer, *d*-LV, and the active stereoisomer, *l*-LV. Both stereoisomers enter cells via the reduced folate carrier and are substrates for folylpolyglutamate synthase, raising the potential for competition. However, preclinical studies have demonstrated that a 20- to 200-fold excess of *d*-LV did not affect the uptake, metabolism, or polyglutamation of *l*-LV (133–135). Several randomized trials have directly compared *d,l*-LV and *l*-LV as modulators of 5-FU. The NCCTG conducted a three-arm study that compared iv administration of 200 mg/m^2 *d,l*-LV, 100 mg/m^2 *l*-LV, or 500 mg/m^2 *d,l*-LV given orally (136). Another trial compared 100 mg/m^2 of either racemic or *l*-LV with weekly 5-FU of 400 mg/m^2/2 h (137). No advantage was seen with *l*-LV in

Table 5
Randomized Trials of Biochemical Modulation of 5-FU
Showing No Advantage for the Experimental Arm

Ref.	Regimen 5-FU given IV; doses in mg/m²	No. patients (measurable)	Response rate (%)	TTP (mo)	Survival (mo)
137	5-FU 400/2 h + 100 *d,l*-LV iv q wk	125	25	6.2	14.5
	5-FU 400/2 h + 100 *l*-LV iv q wk	123	32	8.0	15.0
136	5-FU 370 + 200 *d,l*-LV iv d 1-5 q 4-5 wk	309 (170)	34	6	12
	5-FU 370 + 500 *d,l*-LV po d 1–5 q 4–5 wk	310 (174)	34	6	12
	5-FU 370 + 100 *l*-LV iv d 1–5 q 4–5 wk	308 (140)	28	6	12
121	5-FU 2600/24 h q wk	88 (63)	24	6	15
	Same + PALA 250 24 h prior	87 (63)	14	4	11
138	5-FU 2600/24 h q wk	224 (123)	13		14.8
	Same + PALA 250 24 h prior	229 (133)	10		12.9
139	5-FU 600 + LV 300 iv d 2–4 q 3 wk	93	15		11.6
	Same + dipyridamole 75 mg po tid d 1–5	85	13		9.3
140	5-FU 600 + LV 500 iv q wk × 6 of 8 wk	81	22	4.8	10.4
	Same + hydroxyurea 35 mg/kg po in 3 doses q 8 h starting 6 h post	81	30	5.1	11.7

either of these trials (Table 5). Thus, data from both preclinical and clinical studies suggest that there is no benefit of using pure *l*-LV, although *l*-LV is the available formulation in some countries.

More recent randomized trials in colorectal cancer have compared various agents such as raltitrexed, UFT, capecitabine, high-dose intermittent infusional 5-FU schedules, or irinotecan/5-FU/LV with the monthly schedule of bolus 5-FU/LV. Figure 4 shows the response rates, median time to disease progression, and median survival for the control arm of monthly bolus 5-FU/LV in 10 randomized trials, and data from the first-generation trials that compared bolus 5-FU with or without LV on the monthly schedule *(141–151)*. Although the response rates and time to disease progression appears to be worse in the more recent trials compared to that reported in the first-generation trials, the survival is similar. A possible explanation may be differences in response criteria and imaging modalities. Another factor may be the recent availability of effective second-line therapy for patients who have failed 5-FU/LV; perhaps patients are removed from therapy sooner than they would have been in the past. Nevertheless, these findings support survival as a reliable end point in assessing the worth of therapies as first-line treatment of advanced colorectal cancer.

2.2. Methotrexate/5-FU

Sequence-dependent synergy has been noted in preclinical studies with methotrexate (MTX) preceding 5-FU; the opposite sequence was antagonistic *(1,152)*. Inhibition of TS reduces consumption of reduced folate cofactors that would otherwise be used in the conversion of dUMP to dTMP (Fig. 3). Availability of reduced folates permits continued purine biosynthesis despite MTX-mediated inhibition of dihydrofolate reductase. In contrast, administration of MTX prior to 5-FU inhibits purine biosynthesis. Consequently, an increase in the intracellular levels of PRPP occurs, which is normally used in the first committed step of *de novo* purine synthesis. Increased availability of PRPP favors the conversion of 5-FU to FUMP.

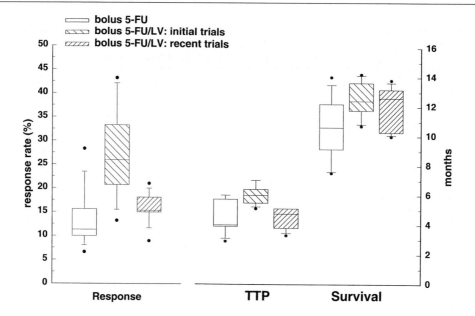

Fig. 4. Clinical results with monthly schedules of bolus 5-FU alone or with leucovorin modulation: Comparison of first-generation and recent phase III trials. In the first-generation phase III trials, the experimental regimen of 5-FU modulated by LV was compared to the standard arm of bolus 5-FU alone. In recently reported clinical trials, the monthly schedule of bolus 5-FU/LV served as the control arm to which other experimental arms were compared. The data for the first-generation trials are from refs. *110–123* and the data for the recent trials are from refs. *141–151*. The data are presented in boxplot format; the median value is displayed; the top and bottom of the rectangles are the 75th and 25th percentiles; the top and bottom whiskers are the 90th and 10th percentiles; the outliers are shown by the solid circle.

A number of phase III trials in advanced colorectal cancer have compared methotrexate given at various intervals prior to 5-FU, with mixed results. One study suggested that a 24-h interval between MTX and 5-FU was optimal for expansion of PRPP pools *(153)*. Another trial in advanced colorectal cancer demonstrated that a 24-h interval between MTX and 5-FU was superior to a 1-h interval *(154)*. In general, when higher than standard doses of MTX are used, LV rescue has been employed for protection against MTX-associated toxicity. A meta-analysis of 8 randomized trials involving 1178 patients comparing 5-FU alone with MTX-modulated 5-FU (± LV rescue) revealed a significantly higher response rate (19% vs 10%) and a survival advantage (median, 10.7 vs 9.1 mo) in favor of MTX/5-FU *(155)*. Because many of the MTX-containing arms involved LV rescue, it is unclear whether the benefit might have been the result of the use of LV rather than MTX, *per se.*

The rationale for using LV rescue is the notion that delayed administration of LV may selectively rescue normal tissues from MTX toxicity. However, the potential for LV rescue of tumor tissue remains a concern. Substitution of the lipophilic antifolate trimetrexate for MTX in regimens involving sequential antifolate followed by 5-FU with LV rescue may be advantageous, because trimetrexate and LV do not compete for transport or polyglutamation. Sequence-dependent synergism has been reported with trimetrexate given prior to 5-FU in several preclinical models *(156,157)* A phase I trial of sequential trimetrexate, LV and bolus 5-FU recommended 110 mg/m² trimetrexate over 30 min followed 24 h later by 500 mg/m² LV iv, 600 mg/m² 5-FU iv, and 10 mg/m² oral LV every 6 h for 7 doses weekly for 6 of 8 wk *(158)*. Phase II studies in patients with patients with previously untreated colorectal cancer using trimetrexate with slightly lower doses of 5-FU/LV were associated with response rates of 36% and 42%, respectively *(159,160)*. The benefit of this three-drug combination versus 5-FU/LV alone is being tested in randomized clinical trials in previously untreated colorectal cancer *(161)*.

2.3. Administration of 5-FU by Continuous Infusion

Concentration and duration of exposure are important determinants of 5-FU-associated cytotoxicity *(1,162,163)*. Because the half-life of 5-FU in plasma is very short, potentially cytotoxic concentrations are maintained for only about 2 h after bolus administration, whereas continuous infusion allows sustained plasma exposure. Several randomized trials have shown improved activity with infusional over bolus 5-FU in terms of response rate without a survival advantage *(164–166)*. A meta-analysis of 6 randomized trials involving 1219 patients with colorectal cancer compared bolus and infusional 5-FU. The response rate was significantly higher with infusional 5-FU (22% vs 14%) and there was a small but statistically significant advantage in median survival (12.1 vs 11.3 mo) *(167)*. Hand–foot syndrome occurred significantly more often with infusional 5-FU (34% vs 13%), whereas grade 3–4 myelosuppression complicated bolus 5-FU therapy more frequently (4% vs 31%) *(168)*.

Several intermittent, high-dose infusional regimens have also been evaluated, including weekly high-dose 5-FU given over 24 or 48 h, and an every 2 wk schedule involving bolus and infusional 5-FU *(138,141,142,169,170)*. A randomized phase II trial from the Southwest Oncology Group (SWOG) indicated that two arms featuring either 300 mg/m^2 5-FU given as a protracted infusion or 2600 mg/m^2 given as a weekly 24-h infusion were at least as effective as iv bolus 5-FU ± LV and were better tolerated *(121)*. Preliminary results from a five-armed phase III trial conducted jointly by the Eastern Cooperative Oncology Group (ECOG) and the Cancer and Leukemia Group B (CALGB) demonstrated that 2600 mg/m^2 5-FU given on a weekly 24-h infusion schedule was associated with median survival comparable to LV-modulated bolus 5-FU but was much better tolerated than the two bolus 5-FU/LV arms *(138)*.

Aranda et al. reported that a high-dose weekly 5-FU infusion (3500 mg/m^2/48 h) was superior to the monthly bolus 5-FU/LV regimen in terms of response rate and time to progression *(141)*. De Gramont and colleagues developed a regimen that contained a 400 mg/m^2 5-FU bolus, 200 mg/m^2/2 h LV followed by 600 mg/m^2 5-FU over 22 h on d 1 and 2 every 2 wk. A randomized trial demonstrated that this regimen was associated with significantly higher response rates and a longer time to progression compared to monthly bolus 5-FU/LV *(142)*.

The question of whether LV modulation is beneficial in the setting of infusional 5-FU regimens has been addressed in two trials. Two of the seven arms tested by the SWOG in advanced colorectal cancer patients involved protracted infusion of 5-FU given alone (300 mg/m^2/d) or at a reduced dose (200 mg/m^2/d) with weekly 20 mg/m^2 LV *(121)*. There were no differences in response rate (30% and 28%), median time to progression (6 and 6 mo) or survival (15 and 14 mo) (Fig. 5). A German Cooperative Oncology Group (AIO) added high-dose 500 mg/m^2 LV as a 2-h infusion to the weekly high-dose 24-h 5-FU infusional regimen developed by Ardalan, which served as the control arm in a series of randomized phase III trials *(170)*. An intergroup phase III trial conducted in Europe compared 2600 mg/m^2 5-FU given as a weekly 24-h infusion alone or with 2-h infusion of high-dose LV. Preliminary results suggest that the LV-modulated 24-h infusion arm had a significantly higher response rate (20% vs 10%) and a longer time to progression (6.4 vs 4.4 mo) at the

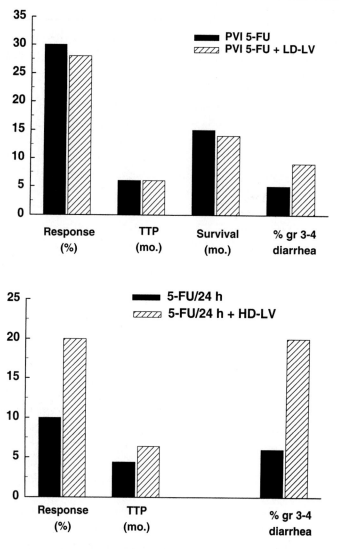

Fig. 5. The impact of leucovorin on the therapeutic activity of infusional 5-FU. The data for protracted infusional 5-FU is from ref. *121*, and the data for the 24-h weekly 5-FU schedule is from ref. *171*.

cost of a higher incidence of grade 3–4 diarrhea *(171)*. These findings suggest no benefit when weekly low-dose LV is added to a protracted infusion of 5-FU, but response rates appear to be improved when LV is added to a weekly 24-h infusion.

In summary, a number of infusional 5-FU regimens have been developed that are useful in the therapy of patients with colorectal cancer. In general, these regimens have a more favorable toxicity profile compared to bolus 5-FU/LV. A disadvantage of this approach is catheter-related complications. About 15–20% of patients will require catheter removal for thrombosis, sepsis, malposition, or breakage, and an additional 10–15% of patients will have infections requiring antibiotic treatment without the need for catheter removal. Prophylaxis with low-dose warfarin (1 mg po daily) has been shown to significantly reduce the incidence of venogram-proven catheter-associated thrombosis *(172)*. Nevertheless, the inconvenience and potential morbidity associated with indwelling venous catheters and the need for a pump has fueled the interest in developing oral 5-FU regimens that can simulate the iv infusional schedules (*see* Chapter 27).

2.4. Unsuccessful Modulation Strategies

Despite a logical rationale, a number of strategies to modulate 5-FU have failed to demonstrate a benefit in preclinical studies (Table 5). For example, preclinical studies suggested that interferon increased the cytotoxicity of 5-FU, associated with enhanced DNA damage *(173)*. High response rates in phase II studies *(174)* led to numerous randomized trials that compared interferon-α-modulated 5-FU with or without LV on a variety of schedules. Preliminary results have been presented from a meta-analyses using primary data from 3254 patients entered in randomized trials evaluating the worth of interferon-α as a modulator of 5-FU *(175)*. Three trial designs were identified. The first 2 compared the same schedule of 5-FU ± interferon-α or 5-FU/LV ± interferon-α, with 5-FU alone given either by bolus or continuous infusion, and included 12 trials involving 1766 patients. No difference in either response rate (25% vs 24%) or median survival (11.4 mo vs 11.5 mo) was noted in the absence or presence of interferon, respectively *(175)*. The third trial design featured a comparison between 5-FU/LV and 5-FU/interferon-α; 7 trials involving 1488 patients were analyzed. An advantage in favor of 5-FU plus LV over 5-FU plus interferon was seen in terms of tumor response (23% vs 18%, $p = 0.042$), and the survival benefit was of borderline significance *(175)*. Thus, interferon-α does not increase the efficacy of either 5-FU or 5-FU/LV in patients with metastatic colorectal cancer. Further, a randomized trial comparing the worth of interferon-α in combination with 5-FU/LV as adjuvant therapy of colon cancer involving over 2100 patients showed no significant benefit to the interferon-containing arm in terms of either 4-yr disease-free (70% vs 69%) or survival (81% vs 80%) *(176)*. Patients receiving 5-FU/LV/interferon were also more likely to stop therapy early for toxicity (22% vs 6%). Enhanced clinical toxicity was commonly seen in the arms containing interferon-α in nearly all phase III trials, suggesting non-selective enhancement of 5-FU toxicity.

N-Phosphonacetyl-L-aspartic acid (PALA) is an inhibitor of aspartate carbamoyltransferase. Although PALA had negligible activity as a single agent, it remained of interest as a potential modulator of 5-FU *(177)*. Initial studies using higher doses of PALA with lower doses of 5-FU showed no advantage for the combination. Renewed interest centered on using the lowest biochemically active dose of PALA in combination with near-maximum doses of 5-FU *(169,178)*. Two randomized trials have compared a high-dose 24-h weekly infusion of 2600 mg/m^2 5-FU alone or combined with 250 mg/m^2 PALA given 24 h prior to 5-FU; neither showed an advantage with PALA *(121,138)*.

Inhibition of nucleoside transport has been evaluated as a strategy to augment 5-FU toxicity by preventing influx of potential rescue nucleosides, such as thymidine, and by trapping 5-fluorodeoxyuridine and deoxyuridine within the cell *(1,179)*. A phase III trial that compared 600 mg/m^2 5-FU with 300 mg/m^2 LV iv d 2–4 every 3 wk alone or with 75 mg dipyridamole po three times daily on d 1–5 showed no advantage with the addition of dipyridamole *(139)*. These negative results are most likely the result of differences in free drug availability in cell culture models versus in vivo. The concentration of free dipyridamole required for optimal modulation of 5-FU cytotoxicity in vitro is several orders of magnitude higher than that which can be achieved in vivo. The apparent explanation is that dipyridamole is extensively protein bound by acid-1-α glycoprotein; the latter is abundant in human plasma but is not present in fetal bovine serum. Additional studies are being pursued by some investigators, but the information to date suggests that this strategy is unlikely to be successful using currently available nucleoside transport inhibitors.

Hydroxyurea, an inhibitor of ribonucleotide reductase, has been proposed as a modulator of 5-FU based on its ability to decrease deoxyribonucleotide triphosphate pools and to prevent conversion of fluorodeoxyuridine diphosphate to its corresponding deoxyribonucleotide

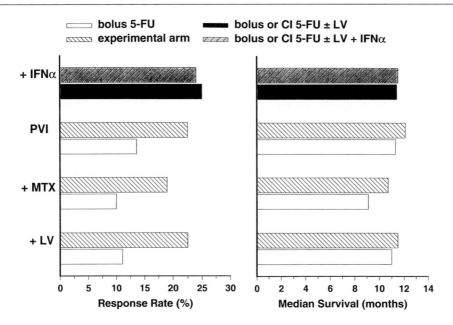

Fig. 6. Response rates and median survival from four meta-analyses in colorectal cancer. The response rate and median survival are shown from meta-analyses comparing either bolus 5-FU alone with either leucovorin (LV) modulation *(109)*, methotrexate modulation (MTX) *(155)* or administration by protracted continuous iv infusion (PCI) *(167)*, or comparing the worth of interferon combined with 5-FU given by either bolus or CI ± leucovorin modulation *(175)*.

derivative *(140)*. A recent phase III trial that evaluated 5-FU/LV (600/500 mg/m^2) given weekly for 6 of 8 wk alone or with hydroxyurea (35 mg/kg given in three divided oral doses every 8 h starting 6 h after 5-FU) showed no significant improvements in response rate, time to progression, or survival *(180)*.

In summary, a variety of approaches have been used in an effort to improve the therapeutic activity of 5-FU by either adding agents that were intended to enhance the cytotoxicity of 5-FU or by altering the schedule of administration. Figure 6 summarizes the results of four meta-analyses that focused on systemic approaches to increase the therapeutic effect of 5-FU. Three meta-analyses included bolus 5-FU alone as the control arm, and the response rates and median survival ranged from 10% to 13.6% and 9.1 to 11.3 mo, respectively. In contrast, in the experimental arm, the response rates and median survival ranged from 19% to 22.5% and 10.7 to 12.1 mo, respectively. The meta-analysis of interferon-α as a modulator was somewhat more complex because the control arm represented either bolus or infusional 5-FU alone or modulated by LV, whereas the experimental arm included interferon-α. Nonetheless, the response rates and median survival with the best systemic regimen in each meta-analysis did not exceed 25% and 12.1 mo, respectively, suggesting that a plateau has been reached with strategies that focus on modulating 5-FU.

3. COMBINATION OF 5-FU WITH OTHER ACTIVE AGENTS

In contrast to the use of biochemical modulators, which are intended to enhance the metabolism of 5-FU, 5-FU has been also been combined with other active cytotoxic agents or modalities. A number of interactions have been reported to result in more than additive cytotoxicity in preclinical models, and, in general, the biochemical and molecular effects of 5-FU complement the cytotoxic effects of the second agent.

3.1. Interaction with Cisplatin

Synergistic cytotoxicity has been seen with the combination of cisplatin and 5-FU in several preclinical models *(181–188)*. The apparent basis of the interaction has varied in different models, but enhancement of DNA-directed toxicity has been a common finding *(182,187,188)*. In ovarian cancer cells, a 1-h incubation with cisplatin (10 μ*M*) was accompanied by about 2.5-fold increases in intracellular levels of tetrahydrofolate and 5,10-methylene tetrahydrofolate and greater TS ternary-complex formation *(182)*. The basis for this phenomenon was thought to result from the inhibition of methionine uptake by cisplatin. In turn, *de novo* synthesis of methionine from homocysteine is stimulated, resulting in metabolism of 5-methyltetrahydrofolate to tetrahydrofolate, which is then converted to 5,10-methylene tetrahydrofolate (Fig. 3). In other models, the combination of 5-FU and cisplatin is associated with enhanced DNA damage as a result of the inhibition of the repair of cisplatin-induced DNA crosslinks *(185,188)*.

In some models, pre-exposure to 5-FU before cisplatin was superior to the opposite sequence *(183–186,188)*. In a murine colon cancer model, administration of 5-FU (35 mg/kg) followed 24 h later by cisplatin (3 mg/kg) given weekly for 5 doses significantly reduced the tumor burden compared to either drug alone, whereas initial administration of cisplatin led to inferior antitumor effects but greater host toxicity *(183)*. In NCI H548 colon cancer cells, pre-exposure to 5-FU for 24 h followed by cisplatin for 2 h produced more than additive cytotoxicity and a greater degree of DNA fragmentation compared to the opposite sequence *(188)*. A 24-h pre-exposure of human squamous cancer cells to 5-FU followed by cisplatin after a 24- to 48-h drug-free interval led to optimal cytotoxicity and significantly reduced repair of cisplatin–DNA crosslinks compared to cisplatin alone or 5-FU followed immediately by cisplatin *(185)*. The observation that thymidine did not antagonize the interaction in concert with the requirement for a 48-h interval suggested that RNA-directed effects might be involved. 5-FU has been shown to inhibit the mRNA expression of ERCC1, an enzyme involved in nucleotide excision repair, and γ-glutamylcysteine synthetase in cisplatin-resistant cancer cells. Thus, 5-FU-mediated interference with the expression of DNA repair enzymes might represent another mechanism of enhancing cisplatin-associated DNA damage *(189)*. Other models indicate that concurrent exposure to both drugs was useful *(182–187)*.

Promising results seen with 5-FU plus cisplatin in phase II studies in patients with advanced colorectal cancer led to a number of randomized studies. In general, cisplatin has been given on d 1, whereas several schedules of 5-FU have been employed: bolus injection, infusion for 120 h, or protracted infusion. No significant improvement in response rate or survival was seen in the phase III setting in colorectal cancer, although toxicity was generally greater *(190–194)*. IF 5-FU is functioning to primarily enhance the DNA-damage associated with cisplatin, perhaps these negative results are not surprising, as cisplatin is not active against colorectal cancer. 5-FU/cisplatin combinations are clearly beneficial in diseases in which both agents have single-agent activity, including squamous cell cancers arising in the anus, head and neck, esophagus, and cervix.

Oxaliplatin is a new platinum analog that has shown additive or synergistic cytotoxic properties with 5-FU in both in vitro and in vivo studies *(195,196)*. More importantly, there is evidence of clinical synergy between oxaliplatin and 5-FU in metastatic colorectal cancer. Objective responses have been seen when oxaliplatin is added to a 5-FU-based regimen on which patients have had documented tumor progression *(197–200)*. Results from several European randomized trials in advanced colorectal cancer showed a significant improvement in the response rate and time to progression when oxaliplatin is added to 5-FU/LV as first-line therapy, although this did not result in a significant survival advantage *(201–203)*. Ongoing phase III trials are testing the contribution of oxaliplatin to 5-FU/LV as adjuvant therapy. In advanced disease, several combinations of oxaliplatin/5-FU/LV are being evaluated. The basis for the differential activity of oxaliplatin in colorectal cancer compared to the inactivity of cisplatin and carboplatin is not entirely clear, but oxaliplatin's diaminocyclohexane moiety is thought to form bulkier DNA adducts that are more difficult to repair. In addition, oxaliplatin retains activity against some cancer cell lines that are resistant to cisplatin and against tumor cells with defective nucleotide mismatch repair.

3.2. Interaction of 5-FU with Ionizing Radiation

Heidelberger et al. initially reported that growth-inhibitory doses of radiotherapy in rodent tumors can be rendered curative by the addition of 5-FU *(204)*. The synergistic interaction between 5-FU and irradiation has been confirmed by other investigators in a variety of model systems *(205–215)*. In general, combined treatment with 5-FU and radiotherapy leads to dose- and time-dependent enhancement of cell killing, and radiosensitization requires exposure to 5-FU for a period exceeding the cell-doubling time *(205,206)*. However, the optimal schedule for 5-FU radiosensitization in preclinical models varies depending on the model system employed *(207)*. Most often, however, more prolonged exposure to fluoropyrimidines is associated with optimal effects *(214,215)*. FdUMP-mediated inhibition of TS with resulting dTTP pool depletion and deoxyribonucleotide imbalance, increased DNA damage, inhibition of DNA repair, and accumulation of cells in the S phase appear to be important features of radiosensitization. As mentioned earlier, the RNA-directed effects of 5-FU might also play a role by altering the expression of proteins required for DNA repair.

5-Fluorouracil given alone or in combination with other agents (including cisplatin or mitomycin C) during radiotherapy has demonstrated efficacy in patients with either squamous cell cancers arising in the anal canal, cervix, head and neck, and esophagus or adenocarcinomas arising in the rectum *(216–221)*. Diverse schedules of 5-FU have been employed: bolus administration of 5-FU on the first and final 3 d of radiation, 96- to 120-h continuous infusion for the first and last week of radiation, and prolonged infusion throughout the period of radiation therapy. A randomized trial in high-risk rectal cancer patients comparing 5-FU given by intermittent bolus injections with protracted infusion during postoperative radiation therapy to the pelvis demonstrated significant improvements in time to relapse and survival in favor of the infusional arm *(221)*.

3.3. Gemcitabine and 5-FU

Gemcitabine is a deoxycytidine analog that contains two fluorine atoms at the 2'-position of the deoxyribose moiety *(222)*. It is metabolized to two active metabolites: gemcitabine diphosphate, which inhibits ribonucleotide reductase, and gemcitabine triphosphate, which incorporates into DNA and functions as a masked chain terminator. DNA incorporation appears to be required for induction of programmed cell death. A prior study demonstrated antagonism when colon cancer cells were pre-exposed to 5-FU followed by exposure to either cytarabine or fazarabine; like gemcitabine, these two agents are deoxycytidine analogs that exert cytotoxicity after incorporation into DNA *(223)*. In contrast, administration of the deoxycytidine analogs first followed by 5-FU was synergistic. The basis for the sequence-dependent antagonism was 5-FU-associated inhibition of cytarabine incorporation into DNA. In HT29 colon cancer cells, sequential exposure to gemcitabine for 4 h followed by FdUrd for 24 h led to more than additive cytotoxicity and marked S-phase accumulation *(43)*. The

Table 6
Clinical Schedules of Gemcitabine/5-FU

Ref.	Gemcitabine (mg/m²/30 min) (unless otherwise stated)	LV (mg/m²)	5-FU (mg/m²)	Schedule
224	1000	No	600 Bolus	Weekly × 3 of 4 wk
225	1500 at 10 mg/m²/min	No	600 Bolus	Weekly × 2 of 3 wk
226	1000	25	600 Bolus	Weekly × 3 of 4 wk
227	800 (30 min after 5-FU)	20	340 Bolus	Weekly
228	900/90 min (after LV)	100/h	450 Bolus at 30 min of LV	Weekly × 6 of 8 wk
229	1000 d 1, 8, 15	No	200/24 h d 1–15	Repeat q 4 wk
230	600 d 1, 8, 15	No	150/24 h d 1–21	Repeat q 4 wk
231	1000 d 1, 8, 15	No	200/24 h d 1–21	Repeat q 4 wk
232	900 d 1, 8, 15	No	200/24 h daily	Repeat q 4 wk
233	1000	200	750/24 h	Weekly × 4 of 6 wk
234	1000 d 1, 8, 15	No	500/24 h d 1–5	Repeat q 4 wk

cells subsequently progressed through the cell cycle after a 22-h drug-free interval. FdUrd-mediated TS, dTTP depletion, and imbalance in the ratio of dATP to dTTP were greater when gemcitabine preceded FdUrd. Nascent DNA damage was greater with gemcitabine followed by FdUrd compared to either drug alone. Delayed induction of high-molecular-mass DNA damage was observed 72 and 96 h after sequential exposure to gemcitabine and FdUrd, consistent with postmitotic apoptosis.

Several clinical schedules of gemcitabine combined with 5-FU have been evaluated (Table 6) (224–234). These trials were not designed to test the possible contribution of sequence of drug administration on either pharmacodynamic or clinical toxicity end points. Gemcitabine was administered first in all but two trials, although the timing of drug administration was very close regardless of sequence. Gemcitabine does not appear to be active as a single agent in the treatment of colorectal cancer; therefore, its potential role when combined with 5-FU with or without LV in this disease setting remains to be determined.

3.4. 5-FU and Taxanes

Several preclinical studies have described sequence-dependent antagonism between pacli-taxel and 5-FU (235–237). Sequential 24-h exposures to paclitaxel followed by FUra led to additive effects in four different human cancer cell lines using the 3-(4,5-dimethylthiazol-2-yl)-2,5 diphenyl tetrazolium bromide (MTT) assay, whereas the opposite sequence was antagonistic in three of the four cell lines (235). Concurrent continuous exposure of both BCap37 breast cancer cells and KB human epidermoid cancer cells to 100 nM paclitaxel and 10 μM 5-FU inhibited the oligonucleosomal DNA fragmentation typically seen with paclitaxel alone at 48 and 72 h (236). Although 5-FU alone did not produce noticeable changes in the cell-cycle profile, it diminished the ability of paclitaxel to produce G2/M blockade and prevented apoptosis. In MCF-7 human breast cancer cells, sequential 24-h exposures to paclitaxel followed by 5-FU led to synergistic cytotoxicity; the opposite sequence was antagonistic (237). A 24-h 5-FU exposure produced S-phase accumulation and pre-exposure to 5-FU diminished the paclitaxel-associated G2/M phase block and prevented the induction of parental DNA fragmentation. In contrast, double-stranded DNA fragmentation was seen at 48 h when cells were exposed to paclitaxel for an initial 24-h period, and the DNA damage was not prevented by subsequent exposure to 5-FU.

Table 7
Clinical Schedules of Taxanes Combined with 5-FU

Ref.	Taxane (mg/m²)	LV (mg/m²)	5-FU (mg/m²)	Schedule
238	Docetaxel 85 d 1	No	750/24 h d 1–5	Repeat q 3 wk
239	Docetaxel 85 d 1	No	750/24 h d 1–5	Repeat q 3 wk
240	Docetaxel 70 d 1	No	800/24 h d 1–5	Repeat q 3 wk
241	Docetaxel 50 d 1	No	500/24 h d 1–5	Repeat q 3–4 wk
242	Docetaxel 60 d 1	No	300 Bolus d 1–3 or 1–5	Repeat q 4 wk
243	Paclitaxel 175 d 1, 22	500/2 h	2000/24 h q wk × 6	Repeat q 50 d
244	Paclitaxel 175 d 1, 22	500/2 h	2000/24 h q wk × 6	Repeat q 50 d
245	Paclitaxel 175 d 1	No	1500/3 h d 2	Repeat q 3 wk
246	Paclitaxel 225 d 1	No	500 wk 1–3	Repeat q 3 wk
247	Paclitaxel 175 d 1	300/1 h d 1–3	350 d 1–3	Repeat q 3 wk
248	175 d 1	500/30 min d 2–5	370 d 2–5	Repeat q 3 wk

Note: In each of these trials, docetaxel was given by 1-h infusion, whereas paclitaxel was given by 3-h infusion.

Taken together, the preclinical data suggest the importance of administering paclitaxel first to establish G2/M arrest prior to giving 5-FU. Several schedules of either docetaxel or paclitaxel in combination with 5-FU have been developed (Table 7) *(238–248)*. Docetaxel has most commonly been given as a 1-h infusion on d 1 followed by a 120-h infusion of 5-FU every 3 wk. Paclitaxel has generally been administered over 3-h once every 3 wk, and has been combined with either a weekly schedule of 5-FU given as a 24-h infusion or by bolus injection. As an alternative, paclitaxel has been given d 1 with bolus 5-FU alone or modulated by LV for 3 or 4 d every 3 wk. Two trials have delayed the administration of 5-FU until the day after taxane therapy *(245,248)*. Each of these regimens has been associated with clinical activity. The taxanes have limited single-agent activity in adenocarcinomas arising in the large intestine; therefore, the clinical potential of this combination in this disease is not clear.

3.5. Irinotecan and 5-FU

Irinotecan belongs to the camptothecin class of anticancer drugs, which interact with the nuclear enzyme topoisomerase I. Irinotecan has single-agent activity in colorectal cancer when used as both initial therapy and in patients whose disease has progressed on 5-FU therapy; this drug was initially approved by the Food and Drug Administration based on its activity in patients with 5-FU-refractory colorectal cancer *(249–251)*. The rationale for the combination of irinotecan and 5-FU alone or with LV modulation is that each has single-agent activity, the mechanisms of action differ, and irinotecan has activity against some 5-FU/LV-resistant tumors. Irinotecan has recently received approved as a component of first-line therapy for advanced colorectal cancer based on two pivotal trials that compared combined therapy with irinotecan and LV-modulated 5-FU against 5-FU/LV alone; each trial showed an advantage of the combined regimen in terms of response rate, time to progression, and survival *(148,252)*.

In North America, there is greater experience with the weekly schedule of irinotecan; therefore, it was combined with a weekly schedule of bolus 5-FU modulated by low-dose LV (to reduce potential 5-FU/LV-associated diarrhea) *(148)*. In France, the de Gramont schedule of mixed bolus and infusional 5-FU modulated by high-dose LV is the standard, whereas in Germany, the weekly schedule of 5-FU given by 24-h infusion is popular. Therefore, the combination arm in the European phase III trial employed either a weekly or every-other-week schedule of irinotecan, 5-FU, and LV *(252)*. Further details concerning the role of irinotecan in the clinical therapy of colorectal cancer can be found in Chapter 28.

A number of preclinical studies have been performed to investigate the interaction of 5-FU or other TS inhibitors with irinotecan (in vivo) or SN-38 (the active metabolite of irinotecan required for in vitro studies). These studies suggest that optimal cytotoxicity is observed when irinotecan or SN-38 exposure precedes exposure to the TS inhibitor *(253–257)*. For example, sequential 4-h exposures of HCT-8 ileocecal cancer cells to SN-38 followed by raltitrexed was more effective than concurrent exposure or the opposite sequence *(253)*. The sequence-dependent synergism was more prominent when raltitrexed exposure was delayed for 24 h after SN-38 exposure. The cytotoxicity of 24-h exposures to irinotecan and 5-FU in various sequences was studied in three human colorectal cancer cell lines *(254)*. Sequential irinotecan followed by 5-FU produced the greatest cytotoxicity and DNA damage, whereas administration of 5-FU first led to antagonism. In a rat colon tumor model, irinotecan and 5-FU were given by iv push weekly for 4 wk according to three different sequences: simultaneous administration, 5-FU given 24 h prior to irinotecan, and irinotecan given 24 h prior to 5-FU. When the two drugs were combined at half of their individual maximally tolerated doses, the complete regression rate was 95% when irinotecan preceded 5-FU, but it was only 38% with the opposite sequence; intermediate results were observed with simultaneous administration (62% tumor regression) *(256)*. The apparent explanation for the sequence-dependent cytotoxicity is the requirement for active DNA synthesis to convert topoisomerase I inhibitor-mediated stabilization of cleavable complexes into a lethal event. Whereas the current clinical schedules of irinotecan/5-FU/LV clearly represent a therapeutic advance in colorectal cancer, the preclinical data suggest that simultaneous administration of topoisomerase 1 and TS inhibitors may not be optimal. It is therefore possibile that improvements in the therapeutic results may be realized with alternate schedules of irinotecan/5-FU.

REFERENCES

1. Grem JL. 5-Fluorinated pyrimidines. In *Cancer Chemotherapy and Biotherapy. Principles and Practice.* Chabner BA and Longo DL (eds.), Lippincott–Raven, Philadelphia, 1996, pp. 149–210.
2. Miyadera K, Sumizawa T, Haraguchi M, Yoshida H, Konstanty W, Yamada Y, et al. Role of thymidine phosphorylase activity in the angiogenic effect of platelet derived endothelial cell growth factor/thymidine phosphorylase. *Cancer Res.,* **55** (1995) 1687–1690.
3. Glazer RI and Lloyd LS. Association of cell lethality with incorporation of 5-fluorouracil and 5-fluorouridine into nuclear RNA in human colon carcinoma cells in culture. *Mol. Pharmacol.,* **21** (1982) 468–473.
4. Kanamaru R, Kakuta H, Sato T, Ishioka C, and Wakui A. The inhibitory effects of 5-fluorouracil on the metabolism of preribosomal and ribosomal RNA in L-1210 cells in vitro. *Cancer Chemother. Pharmacol.,* **17** (1986) 43–46.
5. Will CL and Dolnick BJ. 5-Fluorouracil inhibits dihydrofolate reductase precursor mRNA processing and/or nuclear mRNA stability in methotrexate-resistant KB cells. *J. Biol. Chem.,* **264** (1989) 21,413–21,421.
6. Armstrong RD, Lewis M, Stern SG, and Cadman EC. Acute effect of 5-fluorouracil on cytoplasmic and nuclear dihydrofolate reductase messenger RNA metabolism. *J. Biol. Chem.,* **261** (1986) 7366–7371.
7. Ghoshal K and Jacob ST. Specific inhibition of pre-ribosomal RNA processing in extracts from the lymphosarcoma cells treated with 5-fluorouracil. *Cancer Res.,* **54** (1994) 632–636.
8. Ghoshal K and Jacob ST. An alternative molecular mechanism of action of 5-fluorouracil, a potent anticancer drug. *Biochem. Pharmacol.,* **53** (1997) 1569–1575.
9. Danenberg PV, Shea LCC, and Danenberg K. Effect of 5-fluorouracil substitution on the self-splicing activity of Tetrahymena ribosomal RNA. *Cancer Res.,* **50** (1990) 1757–1763.

10. Takimoto CH, Voeller DB, Strong JM, Anderson L, Chu E, and Allegra CJ. Effects of 5-fluorouracil substitution on the RNA conformation and in vitro translation of thymidylate synthase messenger RNA. *J. Biol. Chem.*, **28** (1993) 21,438–21,422.

11. Schmittgen TD, Danenberg KD, Horikoshi T, Lenz H-J, and Danenberg PV. Effect of 5-fluoro- and 5-bromouracil substitution on the translation of human thymidylate synthase mRNA. *J. Biol. Chem.*, **269** (1994) 16,269–16,275.

12. Santi DV and Hardy LW. Catalytic mechanism and inhibition of tRNA uracil-5-methyltransferase: evidence for covalent catalysis. *Biochemistry*, **26** (1987) 8599–8606.

13. Samuelsson T. Interactions of transfer RNA pseudouridine synthases with RNAs substituted with fluorouracil. *Nucleic Acids Res.*, **19** (1991) 6139–6144.

14. Geoffroy FJ, Allegra CJ, Singha B, and Grem JL. Enhanced cytotoxicity with interleukin-1α and 5-fluorouracil in HCT116 colon cancer cells. *Oncol. Res.*, **6** (1994) 581–591.

15. Fujishima H, Niho Y, Kondo T, Tatsumoto T, Esaki T, Masumoto N, et al. Inhibition by 5-fluorouracil of ERCC1 and gamma-glutamylcysteine synthetase messenger RNA expression in a cisplatin-resistant HST-1 human squamous carcinoma cell line. *Oncol. Res.*, **9** (1997) 167–172.

16. Jin Y, Heck DE, DeGeorge G, Tian Y, and Laskin JD. 5-Fluorouracil suppresses nitric oxide biosynthesis in colon carcinoma cells. *Cancer Res.*, **56** (1996) 1978–1982.

17. Doong SL and Dolnick BJ. 5-Fluorouracil substitution alters pre-mRNA splicing in vitro. *J. Biol. Chem.*, **263** (1988) 4467–4473.

18. Patton JR. Ribonucleoprotein particle assembly and modification of U2 small nuclear RNA containing 5-fluorouridine. *Biochemistry*, **32** (1993) 8939–8944.

19. Wu XP and Dolnick BJ. 5-Fluorouracil alters dihydrofolate reductase pre-mRNA splicing as determined by quantitative polymerase chain reaction. *Mol. Pharmacol.*, **44** (1993) 22–29.

20. Lenz H-J, Manno DJ, Danenberg KD, and Danenberg PV. Incorporation of 5-fluorouracil into U2 and U6 snRNA inhibits mRNA precursor splicing. *J. Biol. Chem.*, **269** (1994) 31,962–31,968.

21. Pritchard DM, Watson AJM, Potten CS, Jackman AL, and Hickman JA: Inhibition of uridine but not thymidine of p53-dependent intestinal apoptosis initiated by 5-fluorouracil: evidence for the involvement of RNA perturbation. *Proc. Natl. Acad. Sci. USA*, **94** (1997) 1795–1799.

22. Carreras CW and Santi DV. The catalytic mechanism and structure of thymidylate synthase. *Annu. Rev. Biochem.*, **64** (1995) 721–762.

23. Santi DV, McHenry CS, Raines RT, and Ivanetich KM: Kinetics and thermodynamics of the interaction of 5-fluouro-2'-deoxyuridylate and thymidylate synthase. *Biochemistry*, **26** (1987) 8606–8613.

24. Ullman B, Lee M, Martin DW Jr, and Santi DV. Cytotoxicity of 5-fluoro-2'-deoxyuridine: requirement for reduced folate cofactors and antagonism by methotrexate. *Proc. Natl. Acad. Sci. USA*, **75** (1978) 980–983.

25. Radparvar S, Houghton PJ, and Houghton JA. Effect of polyglutamylation of 5,10-methylenetetrahydrofolate on the binding of 5-fluoro-2-deoxyuridylate to thymidylate synthase purified from a human colon adenocarcinoma xenograft. *Biochem. Pharmacol.*, **38** (1989) 335–342.

26. Grem JL, Hoth D, Hamilton MJ, King SA, and Leyland-Jones B. An overview of the current status and future directions of clinical trials of 5-fluorouracil and folinic acid. *Cancer Treat. Rep.*, **71** (1987) 1249–1264.

27. Howell SB, Mansfield SJ, and Taetle R. Significance of variation in serum thymidine concentration for the marrow toxicity of methotrexate. *Cancer Chemother. Pharmacol.*, **5** (1981) 221–226.

28. Grem JL, Mulcahy RT, Miller EM, Allegra CJ, and Fischer PH. Interaction of deoxyuridine with fluorouracil and dipyridamole in a human colon cancer cell line. *Biochem. Pharmacol.*, **38** (1989) 51–59.

29. Curtin NJ, Harris AL, and Aherne GW. Mechanism of cell death following thymidylate synthase inhibition: 2'-deoxy-5'-triphosphate accumulation, DNA damage, and growth inhibition following exposure to CB3717 and dipyridamole. *Cancer Res.*, **51** (1991) 2346–2352.

30. Aherne G W, Hardcastle A, Raynaud F, and Jackman AL. Immunoreactive dUMP and TTP pools as an index of thymidylate synthase inhibition; effect of tomudex (ZD1694) and a nonpolyglutamated quinazoline antifolate (CB30900) in L1210 mouse leukaemia cells. *Biochem. Pharmacol.*, **51** (1996) 1293–1301.

31. Harris JM, McIntosh EM, and Muscat GE. Structure/function analysis of a dUTPase: catalytic mechanism of a potential chemotherapeutic target. *J. Mol. Biol.*, **2** (1999) 275–287.

32. Canman CE, Lawrence TS, Shewach DS, Tang HY, and Maybaum J. Resistance to fluorodeoxyuridine-induced DNA damage and cytotoxicity correlates with an elevation of deoxyuridine triphosphatase activity and failure to accumulate deoxyuridine triphosphate. *Cancer Res.*, **53** (1993) 5219–5224.

33. Mauro DJ, De Riel JK, Tallarida RJ, and Sirover MA. Mechanisms of excision of 5-fluorouracil by uracil DNA glycosylase in normal human cells. *Mol. Pharmacol.*, **43** (1993) 854–857.

34. Wurzer JC, Tallarida RJ, and Sirover MA: New mechanism of action of the cancer chemotherapeutic agent 5-fluorouracil in human cells. *J. Pharmacol. Exp. Ther.*, **269** (1994) 39–43.

35. Yoshioka A, Tanaka S, Hiraoka O, et al: Deoxyribonucleoside triphosphate imbalance—fluorodeoxyuridine-induced DNA double strand breaks in mouse FM3A cells and the mechanism of cell death. *J. Biol. Chem.*, **262** (1987) 8235–8241.

36. Houghton JA, Tillman DM, and Harwood FG. Ratio of 2′-deoxyadenosine-5′-triphosphate/thymidine-5′-triphosphate influences the commitment of human colon carcinoma cells to thymineless death. *Clin. Cancer Res.*, **1** (1995) 723–730.

37. Wadler S, Horowitz R, Mao X, and Schwartz EL. Effect of interferon of 5-fluorouracil-induced perturbations in pools of deoxynucleotide triphosphates and DNA strand breaks. *Cancer Chemother. Pharmacol.*, **38** (1996) 529–535.

38. Ismail A-SA, Van Groeningen CJ, Hardcastle A. Modulation of fluorouracil cytotoxicity by interferons alpha and γ. *Mol. Pharmacol.*, **53** (1998) 252–261.

39. Jones S, Willmore E, and Durkacz BW. The effects of 5-fluoropyrimidines on nascent DNA synthesis in Chinese hamster ovary cells monitored by pH-step alkaline and neutral elution. *Carcinogenesis*, **15** (1994) 2435–2438.

40. Ayusawa D, Arai H, Wataya Y, and Sento T. A specialized form of chromosomal DNA degradation induced by thymidylate stress in mouse FM3A cells. *Mutat. Res.*, **200** (1988) 221–230.

41. Canman CE, Tang HY, Normolle DP, Lawrence TS, and Maybaum J. Variations in patterns of DNA damage induced in human colorectal tumor cells by 5-fluorodeoxyuridine: implications for mechanisms of resistance and cytotoxicity. *Proc. Natl. Acad. Sci. USA*, **89** (1992) 10,474–10,478.

42. Li Z-R, Yin M-B, Arredendo MA, Schöber C, and Rustum YM. Down-regulation of c-myc gene expression with induction of high molecular weight DNA fragments by fluorodeoxyuridine. *Biochem. Pharmacol.*, **48** (1994) 327–334.

43. Ren Q-F, Kao V, and Grem J. Cytotoxicity and DNA fragmentation associated with sequential gemcitabine and 5-fluoro-2'-deoxyuridine in HT29 colon cancer cells. *Clin. Cancer Res.*, **4** (1998) 2811–2818.

44. Catchpoole DR and Stewart BW. Etoposide-induced cytotoxicity in two human T-cell leukemic lines: delayed loss of membrane permeability rather than DNA fragmentation as an indicator of programmed cell death. *Cancer Res.*, **53** (1993) 4287–4296.

45. Darzynkiewicz Z. Methods in analysis of apoptosis and cell necrosis. In *The Purdue Cytometry CD-ROM Vol. 3*. Parker J and Stewart C (eds.), Purdue University Press, West Lafayette, IN, 1997.

46. Lowe SW, Ruley HE, Jacks T, and Housman DE. p53-Dependent apoptosis modulates the cytotoxicity of anticancer agents. *Cell*, **74** (1993) 957–967.

47. Fisher TC, Milner AE, Gregory CD, et al. Bcl-2 modulation of apoptosis induced by anticancer drugs: resistance to thymidylate stress is independent of classical resistance pathways. *Cancer Res.*, **53** (1993) 3321–3326.

48. Houghton JA, Harwood FG, and Tillman DM. Thymineless death in colon carcinoma cells is mediated via Fas signaling. *Proc. Natl. Acad. Sci. USA*, **94** (1997) 8144–8149.

49. Tillman DM, Petak I, and Houghton JA. A Fas-dependent component in 5-fluorouracil/leucovorin-induced cytotoxicity in colon carcinoma cells. *Clin. Cancer Res.*, **5** (1999) 425–430.

50. Cadman E and Heimer R. Levels of thymidylate synthetase during normal culture growth of L1210 cells. *Cancer Res.*, **46** (1986) 1195–1198.

51. Rode W, Scanlon KJ, Moroson BA, and Bertino JR. Regulation of thymidylate synthetase in mouse leukemia cells (L1210). *J. Biol. Chem.*, **255** (1980) 1305–1311.

52. Jenh C-H, Rao LG, and Johnson LF: Regulation of thymidylate synthase enzyme synthesis in 5-fluorodeoxyuridine-resistant mouse fibroblasts during the transition from the resting to growing state. *J. Cell Physiol.*, **122** (1985) 149–154.

53. Chu E, Zinn S, Boarman D, and Allegra CJ. Interaction of interferon and 5-fluorouracil in the H630 human colon carcinoma cell line. *Cancer Res.*, **50** (1990) 5834–5840.

54. Van der Wilt CL, Pinedo HM, Smid K, and Peters GJ: Elevation of thymidylate synthase following 5-fluorouracil treatment is prevented by the addition of leucovorin in murine colon tumors. *Cancer Res.*, **52** (1992) 4922–4928.

55. Chu E, Koeller DM, Casey JL, et al. Autoregulation of human thymidylate synthase messenger RNA translation by thymidylate synthase. *Proc. Natl. Acad. Sci. USA*, **88** (1991) 8977–8981.

56. Chu E, Koeller DM, Johnston PG, Zinn S, and Allegra CJ. Regulation of thymidylate synthase in human colon cancer cells treated with 5-fluorouracil and interferon-gamma. *Mol. Pharmacol.*, **43** (1993) 527–533.

57. Swain SM, Lippman ME, Chabner BA, Drake JC, Steinberg SM, and Allegra CJ. Fluorouracil and high-dose leucovorin in previously treated patients with metastatic breast cancer. *J. Clin. Oncol.*, **7** (1989) 890–899.

58. Alexander HR, Grem JL, Hamilton JM, et al. Thymidylate synthase protein expression association with response to neoadjuvant chemotherapy and resection for locally advanced gastric and gastroesophageal adenocarcinoma. *Cancer J.*, **1** (1995) 49–54.

59. Kitchens ME, Forsthoefel AM, Rafique Z, Spencer HT, and Berger FG. Ligand-mediated induction of thymidylate synthase occurs by enzyme stabilization. Implications for autoregulation of translation. *J. Biol. Chem.*, **274** (1999) 12,544–12,547.

60. Kitchens ME, Forsthoefel AM, Barbour KW, Spencer HT, and Berger FG. Mechanisms of acquired resistance to thymidylate synthase inhibitors: the role of enzyme stability. *Mol. Pharmacol.*, **56** (1999) 1063–1070.

61. Aschele C, Sobrero A, Faderan MA, and Bertino JR. Novel mechanisms of resistance to 5-fluorouracil in human colon cancer (HCT-8) sublines following exposure to two different clinically relevant dose schedules. *Cancer Res.*, **52** (1992) 1855–1864.

62. Sobrero AF, Aschele C, Guglielmi AP, Mori AM, Melioli GG, Rosso R, et al. Synergism and lack of cross-resistance between short-term and continuous exposure to fluorouracil in human colon adenocarcinoma cells. *J. Natl. Cancer Inst.*, **85**, 1937–1944.

63. Sobrero AF, Aschele C, and Bertino JR. Fluorouracil in colorectal cancer—a tale of two drugs: implications for biochemical modulation. *J. Clin. Oncol.*, **15** (1997) 368–381.

64. Evans RM, Laskin JD, and Hakala MT. Assessment of growth-limiting events caused by 5-fluorouracil in mouse cells and in human cells. *Cancer Res.*, **40** (1980) 4113–4122.

65. Ren Q-F, Van Groeningen CJ, Geoffroy F, Allegra CJ, Johnston PG, and Grem JL. Determinants of cytotoxicity with prolonged exposure to fluorouracil in human colon cancer cells. *Oncol. Res.*, **9** (1997) 77–88.

66. Thirion P, Cunningham D, Findlay M, et al. Pooled analysis of phase II trials with low-dose 5-fluorouracil continuous infusion as a second line chemotherapy in advanced colorectal cancer. *Proc. Am. Soc. Clin. Oncol.*, **17** (1998) 272a (abstract).

67. Nobile MT, Barzacch MC, Sanguineti O, et al. Activity of high dose 24 hour 5-fluorouracil infusion plus l-leucovorin in advanced colorectal cancer. *Anticancer Res.*, **18** (1998) 517–521.

68. de Gramont A, Bosset JF, Milan C, et al. Randomized trial comparing monthly low-dose leucovorin and fluorouracil bolus with bimonthly high-dose leucovorin and fluorouracil bolus plus continuous infusion for advanced colorectal cancer: a French intergroup study. *J. Clin. Oncol.*, **15** (1997) 808–815.

69. Johnston PG, Lenz H-J, Leichman CG, Danenberg KD, Allegra CJ, Danenberg PV, et al. Thymidylate synthase gene and protein expression correlate and are associated with response to 5-fluorouracil in human colorectal and gastric tumors. *Cancer Res.*, **55** (1995) 1407–1412.

70. Lenz H-J, Leichman CG, Danenberg KD, et al. Thymidylate synthase mRNA level in adenocarcinoma of the stomach: a predictor for primary tumor response and overall survival. *J. Clin. Oncol.*, **14** (1995) 176–182.

71. Leichman CG, Lenz H-J, Leichman L, et al. Quantitation of intratumoral thymidylate synthase expression predicts for disseminated colorectal cancer response and resistance to protracted-infusion fluorouracil and weekly leucovorin. *J. Clin. Oncol.*, **15** (1997) 3223–3229.

72. MacMillan WE, Wolberg WH, and Welling PG. Pharmacokinetics of fluorouracil in humans. *Cancer Res.*, **38** (1978) 3479–3482.

73. Heggie GD, Sommadossi J-P, Cross DS, Huster WJ, and Diasio RB. Clinical pharmacokinetics of 5-fluorouracil and its metabolites in plasma, urine, and bile. *Cancer Res.*, **47** (1987) 2203–2206.

74. van Groeningen CJ, Pinedo HM, Heddes J, et al. Pharmacokinetics of 5-fluorouracil assessed with a sensitive mass spectrometric method in patients on a dose escalation schedule. *Cancer Res.*, **48** (1988) 6956–6961.

75. Grem JL, McAtee N, Balis FM, et al: A pilot study of interferon alfa-2a in combination with fluorouracil plus high-dose leucovorin in metastatic gastrointestinal carcinoma. *J. Clin. Oncol.*, **9** (1991) 1811–1820.

76. Grem JL, McAtee N, Murphy RF, et al. Dose-intensification of 5-fluorouracil/high-dose leucovorin with granulocyte-macrophage colony stimulating factor in metastatic gastrointestinal cancer. *J. Clin. Oncol.*, **12** (1994) 560–568.

77. Harris BE, Song R, Soong SJ, and Diasio RB. Relationship between dihydropyrimidine dehydrogenase activity and plasma 5-fluorouracil levels with evidence for circadian variation of enzyme activity and plasma drug levels in cancer patients receiving 5-fluorouracil by protracted continuous infusion. *Cancer Res.*, **50** (1990) 197–201.

78. Yoshida T, Araki E, Iigo M, et al. Clinical significance of monitoring serum levels of 5-fluorouracil by continuous infusion in patients with advanced colonic cancer. *Cancer Chemother. Pharmacol.*, **26** (1990) 352–354.

79. Grem JL, McAtee N, Balis F, et al. A phase II study of continuous infusion 5-fluorouracil and leucovorin with weekly cisplatin in metastatic colorectal carcinoma. *Cancer*, **72** (1993) 663–668.

80. Fraile RJ, Baker LH, Buroker TR, Horwitz J, and Vaitkevicius VK. Pharmacokinetics of 5-fluorouracil administered orally by rapid intravenous and by slow infusion. *Cancer Res.*, **40** (1980) 2223–2228.

81. Petit E, Milano G, Levi F, Thyss A, Bailleul F, and Schneider M. Circadian rhythm-varying plasma concentration of 5-fluorouracil during a five-day continuous venous infusion at a constant rate in cancer patients. *Cancer Res.*, **48** (1988) 1976–1980.

82. Fleming RF, Milano G, Thyss A, Etienne MC, Renee N, Schneider M, et al. Correlation between dihydropyrimidine dehydrogenase activity in peripheral mononuclear cells and systemic clearance of fluorouracil in cancer patients. *Cancer Res.*, **52** (1992) 2899–2902.

83. Erlichman C, Fine S, and Elhakim T. Plasma pharmacokinetics of 5-FU given by continuous infusion with allopurinol. *Cancer Treat. Rep.*, **70** (1986) 903–904.

84. Remick SC, Grem JL, Fischer PH, et al. Phase I trial of 5-fluorouracil and dipyridamole administered by 72-hour concurrent continuous infusion. *Cancer Res.*, **50** (1990) 2667–2672.

85. Grem JL, McAtee N, Steinberg SM, et al. A phase I study of continuous infusion 5-fluorouracil plus calcium leucovorin in combination with *n*-(phosphonacetyl)-L-aspartate in metastatic gastrointestinal adenocarcinoma. *Cancer Res.*, **53** (1993) 4828–4836.

86. Collins JM, Dedrick RL, King FG, Speyer JL, and Myers CE. Nonlinear pharmacokinetic models for 5-fluorouracil in man: intravenous and intraperitoneal routes. *Clin. Pharmacol. Ther.*, **28** (1980) 235–246.

87. McDermott BJ, van der Berg HW, and Murphy RF. Nonlinear pharmacokinetics for the elimination of 5-fluorouracil after intravenous administration in cancer patients. *Cancer Chemother. Pharmacol.*, **9** (1982) 173–178.

88. Schwartz PM, Turek PJ, Hyde CM, Cadman EC, and Handschumacher RE. Altered plasma kinetics of 5-FU at high dosage in rat and man. *Cancer Treat. Rep.*, **69** (1985) 133–136.

89. Cohen JL, Irwin LW, Marshall OJ, Darvey H, and Bateman JR. Clinical pharmacology of oral and intravenous 5-fluorouracil (NSC-19893). *Cancer Chemother. Rep.*, **58** (1974) 723–731.

90. Finch RE, Bending MR, and Lant AF. Plasma levels of 5-fluorouracil after oral and intravenous administration in cancer patients. *Br. J. Clin. Pharmacol.*, **7** (1979) 613–617.

91. Fraile RJ, Baker LH, Buroker TR, Horwitz J, and Vaitkevicius VK. Pharmacokinetics of 5-fluorouracil administered orally by rapid intravenous and by slow infusion. *Cancer Res.*, **40** (1980) 2223–2228.

92. Almersjo OE, Gustavsson BG, Regardh CG, and Wahlen P. Pharmacokinetic studies of 5-fluorouracil after oral and intravenous administration in man. *Acta Pharmacol. Toxicol.*, **46** (1980) 329–336.

93. Thyss A, Milano G, Renee N, Vallicioni J, Schneider M, and Demard F. Clinical pharmacokinetic study of 5-FU in continuous 5-day infusions for head and neck cancer. *Cancer Chemother. Pharmacol.*, **16** (1986) 64–66.

94. Trump DL, Egorin MJ, Forrest A, Willson JK, Remick S, and Tutsch KD. Pharmacokinetic and pharmacodynamic analysis of fluorouracil during 72-hour continuous infusion with and without dipyridamole. *J. Clin. Oncol.*, **9** (1991) 2027–2035.

95. Santini J, Milano G, Thyss A, et al. 5-FU therapeutic monitoring with dose adjustment leads to an improved therapeutic index in head and neck cancer. *Br. J. Cancer*, **59** (1989) 287–290.

96. Fety R, Rolland F, Barberi-Heyob M, et al. Clinical impact of pharmacokinetically-guided dose adaptation of 5-fluorouracil: results from a multicentric randomized trial in patients with locally advanced head and neck carcinomas. *Clin. Cancer Res.*, **4** (1998) 2039–2045.

97. Wagner JG, Gyves JW, Stetson PL, Walker-Andrews SC, Wollner IS, Cochran MK, et al. Steady-state nonlinear pharmacokinetics of 5-fluorouracil during hepatic arterial and intravenous infusions in cancer patients. *Cancer Res.*, **46** (1986) 1499–1506.

98. Ensminger WD, Rosowsky A, Raso VO, et al. A clinical pharmacological evaluation of hepatic arterial infusion of 5-fluoro-2'-deoxyuridine and 5-fluorouracil. *Cancer Res.*, **38** (1978) 3784–3792.

99. Goldberg JA, Kerr DJ, Watson DG, Willmott N, Bates CD, McKillop JH, et al. The pharmacokinetics of 5-fluorouracil administered by arterial infusion in advanced colorectal hepatic metastases. *Br. J. Cancer*, **61** (1990) 913–915.

100. Danenberg PV and Danenberg KD. Effect of 5,10-methylenetetrahydrofolate and the dissociation of 5-fluorodeoxyuridylate binding of human thymidylate synthetase. Evidence for an ordered mechanism. *Biochemistry*, **17** (1978) 4018–4024.

101. Houghton JA, Schmidt C, and Houghton PF. The effect of derivatives of folic acid on the fluorodeoxyuridylate–thymidylate synthetase covalent complex in human colon xenografts. *Eur. J. Cancer Clin. Oncol.*, **18** (1982) 347–354.

102. Yin M-B, Zakrzewski SF, and Hakala MT. Relationship of cellular folate cofactor pools to the activity of 5-fluorouracil. *Mol. Pharmacol.*, **23** (1983) 190–197.

103. Cao S, Frank C, and Rustum YM. Role of fluoropyrimidine schedule and (6R,S)leucovorin dose in a preclinical animal model of colorectal carcinoma. *J. Natl. Cancer Inst.*, **88** (1996) 430–436.

104. Drake JC, Voeller DM, Allegra CJ, et al. The effect of dose and interval between 5-fluorouracil and leucovorin on the formation of thymidylate synthase ternary complex in human cancer cells. *Br. J. Cancer*, **71** (1995) 1145–1150.

105. Keyomarsi K and Moran R. Folinic acid augmentation of the effects of fluoropyrimidines on murine and human leukemic cells. *Cancer Res.*, **46** (1986) 5229–5235.

106. Straw JA, Szapary D, and Wynn WT. Pharmacokinetics of the diastereoisomers of leucovorin after intravenous and oral administration to normal subjects. *Cancer Res.*, **44** (1984) 3114–3119.

107. Trave F, Rustum YM, Petrelli NJ, et al. Plasma and tumor tissue pharmacology of high dose intravenous leucovorin calcium in combination with fluorouracil in patients with advanced colorectal carcinoma. *J. Clin. Oncol.*, **6** (1988) 1181–1188.

108. Machover D, Goldschmidt E, Chollet P, et al. Treatment of advanced colorectal and gastric adenocarcinomas with 5-fluorouracil and high-dose folinic acid. *J. Clin. Oncol.*, **4** (1986) 685–696.

109. Piedbois P, Buyse M, Rustum Y, et al., for The Advanced Colorectal Cancer Meta-Analysis Project: Modulation of fluorouracil by leucovorin in patients with advanced colorectal cancer: evidence in terms of response rate. *J. Clin. Oncol.*, **10** (1992) 896–903.

110. Martoni A, Cricca A, Guaraldi M, et al. Randomized clinical trial with a weekly regimen of 5-FU vs 5-FU plus intermediate-dose folinic acid in the treatment of advanced colorectal cancer. *Ann Oncol.*, **3** (1992) 87–88.

111. Nobile MT, Vidili MG, Sobrero A, et al. 5-Fluorouracil alone or combined with high dose folinic acid in advanced colorectal cancer patients. A randomized trial. *Proc. Am. Soc. Clin. Oncol.*, **7** (1988) 97 (abstract).

112. Valone FH, Friedman MA, Wittlinger PS, et al. Treatment of patients with advanced colorectal carcinomas with fluorouracil alone, high-dose leucovorin plus fluorouracil, or sequential methotrexate, fluorouracil, and leucovorin: a randomized trial of the Northern California Oncology Group. *J. Clin. Oncol.*, **7** (1989) 1427–1436.

113. Laufman LR, Bukowski R, Collier MA, et al. A randomized, double-blind trial of fluorouracil plus placebo versus fluorouracil plus oral leucovorin in patients with metastatic colorectal cancer. *J. Clin. Oncol.*, **11** (1993) 1888–1892.

114. Petrelli N, Herrera L, Rustum Y, et al. A prospective randomized trial of 5-fluorouracil versus 5-fluorouracil and high-dose leucovorin versus 5-fluorouracil and methotrexate in previously untreated patients with advanced colorectal carcinoma. *J. Clin. Oncol.*, **5** (1987) 1559–1565.

115. Petrelli N, Douglass HD, Herrera L, et al. The modulation of fluorouracil with leucovorin in metastatic colorectal carcinoma. A prospective randomized Phase III trial. *J. Clin. Oncol.*, **7** (1991) 1419–1426.

116. Erlichman C, Fine S, Wong A, et al. A randomized trial of fluorouracil and folinic acid in patients with metastatic colorectal carcinoma. *J. Clin. Oncol.*, **6** (1988) 469–475.

117. Doroshow JH, Multhauf P, Leong L, et al. Prospective randomized comparison of fluorouracil versus fluorouracil and high-dose continuous infusion leucovorin calcium for the treatment of advanced measurable colorectal cancer in patients previously unexposed to chemotherapy. *J. Clin. Oncol.*, **8** (1990) 491–501.

118. Poon MA, O'Connell MJ, Moertel CG, et al. Biochemical modulation of fluorouracil: evidence of significant improvement of survival and quality of life in patients with advanced colorectal carcinoma. *J. Clin. Oncol.*, **7** (1989) 1407–1418.

119. Labianca R, Pancera E, Aitini E, et al. Folinic acid + 5-fluorouracil (5-FU) versus equidose 5-FU in advanced colorectal cancer. Phase III study of "GISCAD" (Italian Group for the Study of Digestive Tract Cancer). *Ann. Oncol.*, **2** (1991) 673–679.

120. Di Costanzo F, Bartolucci R, Sofra M, et al. 5-Fluorouracil alone vs high dose folinic acid and 5-FU in advanced colorectal cancer: a randomized trial of the Italian Oncology Group for Clinical Research. *Proc. Am. Soc. Clin. Oncol.*, **8** (1989) 106 (abstract).

121. Leichman CG, Fleming TR, Muggia FM, et al. Phase II study of fluorouracil and its modulation in advanced colorectal cancer: a Southwest Oncology Group Study. *J. Clin. Oncol.*, **131** (1995) 1303–1311.

122. Petrioli R, Lorenzi M, Aquino A, et al. Treatment of advanced colorectal cancer with high-dose intensity folinic acid and 5-fluorouracil plus supportive care. *Eur. J. Cancer*, **31A** (1995) 2105–2108.

123. Borner MM, Castiglione M, Bacchi M, et al. The impact of adding low-dose leucovorin to monthly 5-fluorouracil in advanced colorectal carcinoma: results of a phase III trial. Swiss Group for Clinical Cancer Research (SAKK). *Ann. Oncol.*, **9** (1998) 535–541.

124. Buroker TR, O'Connell MJ, Wieand HS, et al. Randomized comparison of two schedules of fluorouracil and leucovorin in the treatment of advanced colorectal cancer. *J. Clin. Oncol.*, **12** (1994) 14–20.

125. Poon MA, O'Connell MJ, Wieand HS, et al. Biochemical modulation of fluorouracil with leucovorin: confirmatory evidence of improved therapeutic efficacy in advanced colorectal cancer. *J. Clin. Oncol.*, **9** (1991) 1967–1972.

126. Labianca R, Cascinu S, Frontini L, et al. High- versus low-dose levo-leucovorin as a modulator of 5-fluorouracil in advanced colorectal cancer: a "GISCAD" phase III study. *Ann. Oncol.*, **8** (1997) 169–174.

127. Ychou M, Fabro-Peray P, Perney P, et al: A prospective randomized study comparing high- and low-dose leucovorin combined with same-dose 5-fluorouracil in advanced colorectal cancer. *Am. J. Clin. Oncol.*, **21** (1998) 233–236.

128. Jäger E, Heike M, Bernhard H, et al. Weekly high-dose leucovorin versus low-dose leucovorin combined with fluorouracil in advanced colorectal cancer: results of a randomized multicenter trial. *J. Clin. Oncol.*, **14** (1996) 2274–2279.

129. Wolmark N, Rockette H, Fisher B, et al. The benefit of leucovorin-modulated fluorouracil as postoperative adjuvant therapy for primary colon cancer: results from National Surgical Adjuvant Breast and Bowel Project Protocol C-03. *J. Clin. Oncol.*, **10** (1993) 1879–1887.

130. Haller DG, Catalano PJ, Macdonald JS, and Mayer RJ. Fluorouracil, leucovorin and levamisole adjuvant therapy for colon cancer: final results of INT-0089. *Proc. Am. Soc. Clin. Oncol.*, **17** (1998) 256a (abstract).

131. Kerr DJ, Gray R, McConkey C, and Barnwell J. Adjuvant chemotherapy with 5-fluorouracil,L-folinic acid and levamisole for patients with colorectal cancer: non-randomised comparison of weekly versus four-weekly schedules—less pain, same gain. *Ann. Oncol.*, **11** (2000) 947–955.

132. Quasar Collaborative Group: Comparison of fluorouracil with additional levamisole, higher-dose folinic acid, or both, as adjuvant chemotherapy for colorectal cancer: a randomised trial. *Lancet*, **355** (2000) 1588–1596.

133. Bertrand J and Jolivet J. Lack of interference by the unnatural isomer of 5-formyltetrahydrofolate with the effects of the natural isomer in leucovorin preparations. *J. Natl. Cancer Inst.*, **81** (1989) 1175–1178.

134. Zhang Z-G and Rustum YM. Effects of diastereoisomers of 5-formyl-tetrahydrofolate on cellular growth, sensitivity to 5-fluoro-2′-deoxyuridine, and methylenetetrahydrofolate polyglutamate levels in HCT-8 cells. *Cancer Res.*, **51** (1991) 3476–3481.

135. Boarman DM and Allegra CJ. Intracellular metabolism of 5-formyltetrahydrofolate in human breast and colon cell lines. *Cancer Res.*, **52** (1992) 36–44.

136. Goldberg RM, Hatfield AK, Kahn M, et al. Prospectively randomized North Central Cancer Treatment Group trial of intensive-course fluorouracil combined with the l-isomer of intravenous leucovorin, oral leucovorin, or intravenous leucovorin for the treatment of advanced colorectal cancer. *J. Clin. Oncol.*, **15** (1997) 3320–3329.

137. Scheithauer W, Kornek G, Marczell A, et al. Fluorouracil plus racemic leucovorin versus fluorouracil combined with the pure l-isomer of leucovorin for the treatment of advanced colorectal cancer: a randomized phase III study. *J. Clin. Oncol.*, **15** (1997) 908–914.

138. O'Dwyer PJ, Manola J, Valone FH, et al. Fluorouoracil modulation in colorectal cancer: lack of improvement with *N*-phosphonacetyl-*l*-aspartic acid or oral leucovorin or interferon, but enhanced therapeutic index with weekly 24-hour infusion schedule—An Eastern Cooperative Oncology Group/Cancer and Leukemia Group B Study. *J. Clin. Oncol.*, **19** (2001) 2413–2421.

139. Köhne CH, Hiddemann W, Schöller J, et al. Failure of orally administered dipyridamole to enhance the antineoplastic activity of 5-fluorouracil in combination with folinic acid in patients with advanced colorectal cancer. A prospective randomized trial. *J. Clin. Oncol.*, **13** (1995) 1201–1208.

140. Moran RG, Danenberg PV, and Heidelberger C. Therapeutic response of leukemic mice treated with fluorinated pyrimidines and inhibitors of deoxyuridylate synthesis. *Biochem. Pharmacol.*, **31** (1982) 2929–2935.

141. Aranda E, Diaz-Rubio E, Cervantes A, et al. Randomized trial comparing monthly low-dose leucovorin and fluorouracil bolus with weekly high-dose 48-hour continuous-infusion fluorouracil for advanced colorectal cancer: a Spanish Cooperative Group for Gastrointestinal Tumor Therapy (TTD) study. *Ann. Oncol.*, **9** (1998) 727–731.

142. de Gramont A, Bosset JF, Milan C, et al. Randomized trial comparing monthly low-dose leucovorin and fluorouracil bolus with bimonthly high-dose leucovorin and fluorouracil bolus plus continuous infusion for advanced colorectal cancer: a French intergroup study. *J. Clin. Oncol.*, **15** (1997) 808–815.

143. Cocconi G, Cunningham D, van Cutsem E, et al. Open, randomized multicenter trial of raltitrexed versus fluorouracil plus high-dose leucovorin in patients with advanced colorectal cancer. *J. Clin. Oncol.*, **16** (1998) 2943–2952.

144. Cunningham D, Zalcberg JR, Rath U, et al: Final results of a randomised trial comparing "Tomudex"® (raltitrexed) with 5-fluorouracil plus leucovorin in advanced colorectal cancer. *Ann. Oncol.*, **7** (1996) 961–965.

145. Pazdur R and Vincent M. Raltitrexed versus 5-fluorouracil and leucovorin in patients with advanced colorectal cancer: results of a randomized, multicenter, North American Trial. *Proc. Am. Soc. Clin. Oncol.*, **16** (1997) 228a (abstract).

146. Hoff PM, Ansari R, Batist G, et al. Comparison of oral capecitabine versus intravenous fluorouracil plus leucovorin as first-line treatment in 605 patients with metastatic colorectal cancer: results of a randomized phase III study. *J. Clin. Oncol.*, **19** (2001) 2282–2292.

147. Twelves C, Boyer M, Findlay M, et al. Capecitabine (Xeloda™) improves medical resource use with 5-fluorouracil plus leucovorin in a phase III trial conducted in patients with advanced colorectal cancer. *Eur. J. Cancer*, **37** (2001) 597–604.

148. Twelves C, Harper P, Van Cutsem E, et al. A phase III trial of Xeloda™ (capecitabine) in previously untreated advanced/metastatic colorectal cancer. *Proc. Am. Soc. Clin. Oncol.*, **18** (1999) 263a (abstract).

149. Pazdur R, Douillard J-Y, Skillings JR, et al. Multicenter phase III study of 5-fluorouracil or UFT™ in combination with leucovorin in patients with metastatic colorectal cancer. *Proc. Am. Soc. Clin. Oncol.*, **18** (1999) 263a (abstract).

150. Carmichael J, Popiela T, Radstone D, et al. Randomized comparative study of Orzel® (oral uracil/tegafur (UFT™) plus leucovorin (LV)) versus parenteral 5-fluorouracil plus LV in patients with metastatic colorectal cancer. *Proc. Am. Soc. Clin. Oncol.*, **18** (1999) 264a (abstract).

151. Saltz LB, Cox JV, Blanke C, et al. Irinotecan plus fluorouracil and leucovorin for metastatic colorectal cancer. *N. Engl. J. Med.*, **343** (2000) 905–914.

152. Bertino JR. Biomodulation of 5-fluorouracil with anitfolates. *Semin. Oncol.*, **24(Suppl. 18)** (1997) S18-52–S18-56.

153. Kemeny N, Ahmed T, Michaelson R, et al. Activity of sequential low-dose methotrexate and fluorouracil in advanced colorectal carcinoma. attempt at correlation with tissue and blood levels of phosphoribosylpyrophosphate. *J. Clin. Oncol.*, **2** (1984) 311–315.

154. Marsh JC, Bertino JR, Katz KH, et al. The influence of drug interval on the effect of methotrexate and fluorouracil in the treatment of advanced colorectal cancer. *J. Clin. Oncol.*, **9** (1991) 371–380.

155. Advanced Colorectal Cancer Meta-analysis Project. Meta-analysis of randomized trials testing the biochemical modulation of fluorouracil by methotrexate in metastatic colorectal cancer. *J. Clin. Oncol.*, **12** (1994) 960–969.

156. Elliot WL, Howard CT, Kykes DJ, and Leopold WR. Sequence and schedule-dependent synergy of trimetrexate in combination with 5-fluorouracil in vitro and in mice. *Cancer Res.*, **15** (1989) 5586–5590.

157. Romanini A, Li WW, Colofiore JR, et al. Leucovorin enhances cytotoxicity of trimetrexate/fluorouracil, but not methotrextae/fluorouracil, in CCRF-CEM cells. *J. Natl. Cancer Inst.*, **84** (1992) 1033–1038.

158. Conti JA, Kemeny N, Seiter K, et al. Trial of sequential trimetrexate, fluorouracil, and high-dose leucovorin in previously treated patients with gastrointestinal carcinoma. *J. Clin. Oncol.*, **12** (1994) 695–700.

159. Blanke CD, Kasimis B, Schein P, et al. Phase II study of trimetrexate, fluorouracil, and leucovorin for advanced colorectal cancer. *J. Clin. Oncol.*, **15** (1997) 915–920.

160. Szelenyi H, Hohenberger P, Lochs H, et al. Sequential trimetrexate, 5-fluorouracila and folinic acid are effective and well-tolerated in metastatic colorectal carcinoma. The phase II study group of the AIO. *Oncology*, **58** (2000) 273–279.

161. Punt CJA , Keizer HJ, Douma J, et al. Multicenter randomized trial of 5-fluorouracil and leucovorin with or without trimetrexate as first line treatment in patients with advanced colorectal cancer. *Proc. Am. Soc. Clin. Oncol.*, **18** (1999) 262a (abstract).

162. Santelli G and Valeriote F. Schedule-dependent cytotoxicity of 5-fluorouracil in mice. *J. Natl. Cancer Inst.*, **76** (1986) 159–164.

163. Moran RG and Scanlon KL. Schedule-dependent enhancement of the cytotoxicity of fluoropyrimidines to human carcinoma cells in the presence of folinic acid. *Cancer Res.*, **51** (1991) 4618–4623.

164. Lokich JJ, Ahlgren JD, Gullo JJ, et al. A prospective randomized comparison of continuous infusion fluorouracil with a conventional bolus schedule in metastatic colorectal carcinoma: a Mid-Atlantic Oncology Program Study. *J. Clin. Oncol.*, **7** (1989) 425–432.

165. Hansen RM, Ryan L, Anderson T, et al. Phase III study of bolus versus infusion fluorouracil with or without cisplatin in advanced colorectal cancer. *J. Natl. Cancer Inst.*, **88** (1996) 668–674.

166. Rougier P, Paillot B, LaPlanche A, et al. 5-Fluorouracil (5-FU) continuous intravenous infusion compared with bolus administration. Final results of a randomised trial in metastatic colorectal cancer. *Eur. J. Cancer*, **33** (1997) 1789–1793.

167. Meta-Analysis Group In Cancer. Efficacy of intravenous continuous infusion of fluorouracil compared with bolus administration in advanced colorectal cancer. *J. Clin. Oncol.*, **16** (1998) 301–308.

168. Meta-Analysis Group In Cancer. Toxicity of fluorouracil in patients with advanced colorectal cancer. Effect of administration schedule and prognostic factors. *J. Clin. Oncol.*, **16** (1998) 3537–3541.

169. Ardalan B, Singh G, Silberman HA. Randomized phase I and phase II study of short-term infusion of high-dose fluorouracil with or without n-(phosphonacetyl)-L-aspartic acid in patients with advanced pancreatic and colorectal cancer. *J. Clin. Oncol.*, **6** (1988) 1053–1058.

170. Kohne CH, Schoffski P, Wilke H, et al. Effective biomodulation by leucovorin of high-dose infusion fluorouracil given as a weekly 24-hour infusion: results of a randomized trial in patients with advanced colorectal cancer. *J. Clin. Oncol.*, **16** (1998) 418–426.

171. Schmöll HJ, Köhne CH, Lorenz M, et al. Weekly 24h infusion of high-dose 5-fluorouracil with or without folinic acid vs. bolus 5-FU/FA (NCCTG/Mayo) in advanced colorectal cancer: a randomized Phase III trial of the EORTC, GITCCG and the AIO. *Proc. Am. Soc. Clin. Oncol.*, **19** (2000) 241A (Abstract).

172. Bern MM, Lokich JJ, Wallach SR, et al. Very low doses of warfarin can prevent thrombosis in central venous catheters. A randomized prospective trial. *Ann. Intern. Med.*, **112** (1990) 423–428.

173. Grem JL, van Groeningen CJ, Ismail AA, et al. The role of interferon-alpha as a modulator of fluorouracil and leucovorin. *Eur. J. Cancer*, **31A(7/8)** (1995) 1316–1320.

174. Wadler S, Lembersky B, Atkins M, et al. Phase II trial of fluorouracil and recombinant interferon alfa-2a in patients with advanced colorectal carcinoma: an Eastern Cooperative Oncology Group study. *J. Clin. Oncol.*, **9** (1991) 1806–1810.

175. Meta-Analysis Group in Cancer. Alpha-interferon does not increase the efficacy of 5-fluorouracil in advanced colorectal cancer. *Br. J. Cancer*, **84** (2001) 611–620.

176. Wolmark N, Bryant J, Smith R, et al. Adjuvant 5-fluorouracil and leucovorin with or without interferon alfa- 2a in colon carcinoma: National Surgical Adjuvant Breast and Bowel Project protocol C-05, *J. Natl. Cancer Inst.*, **90** (1998) 1810–1816.

177. Grem JL, King SA., O'Dwyer PJ, et al. *N*-(Phosphonoacetyl)-ʟ-aspartate (PALA): a review of its biochemistry and clinical activity. *Cancer Res.*, **48** (1988) 4441–4454.

178. Casper ES, Vale K, Williams LJ, et al: Phase I and clinical pharmacological evaluation of biochemical modulation of 5-fluorouracil with *n*-(phosphonacetyl)-ʟ-aspartic acid. *Cancer Res.*, **43** (1983) 2324–2329.

179. Grem JL. Biochemical modulation of 5-fluorouracil by dipyridamole: preclinical and clinical experience. *Semin. Oncol.*, **19(Suppl. 3)** (1992) 56–65.

180. Di Costanzo F, Gasperoni S, Malacarne P, et al. High-dose folinic acid and 5-fluorouracil alone or combined with hydroxyurea in advanced colorectal cancer. A randomized trial of the Italian Oncology Group for Clinical Research. *Am. J. Clin. Oncol.*, **21** (1998) 369–375.

181. Schabel FM, Trader MW, Laster WR Jr, et al. *cis*-Dichlorodiammineplatinum(II) combination chemotherapy and cross-resistance studies with tumors of mice. *Cancer Treat. Rep.*, **63** (1979) 1459–1473.

182. Scanlon KJ, Newman EM, Lu Y, and Priest DG. Biochemical basis for cisplatin and 5-fluorouracil synergism in human ovarian carcinoma cells. *Proc. Natl. Acad. Sci. USA*, **83** (1986) 8923–8925.

183. Pratesi G, Gianni L, Manzotti C, and Zunino F. Sequence dependence of the antitumor and toxic effects of 5-fluorouracil and *cis*-diamminedichloroplatinum combination on primary colon tumors in mice. *Cancer Chemother. Pharmacol.*, **20** (1988) 237–241.

184. Palmeri S, Trave F, Russello O, et al. The role of drug sequence in therapeutic selectivity of the combination of 5-fluorouracil and cisplatin. *Sel. Cancer Ther.*, **5** (1989) 169–177.

185. Esaki T, Nakano S, Tatsumoto T, et al. Inhibition by 5-fluorouracil of *cis*-diamminedichloroplatinum(II)-induced DNA interstrand cross-link removal in a HST-1 human squamous carcinoma cell line. *Cancer Res.*, **52** (1992) 6501–6506.

186. Kuroki M, Nakano S, Mitsugi K, et al. In vivo comparative therapeutic study of optimal administration of 5-fluorouracil and cisplatin using a newly established HST-1 human squamous-carcinoma cell line. *Cancer Chemother. Pharmacol.*, **29** (1992) 273–276.

187. Tsai C-M, Hsiao S-H, Frey CM, et al. Combination cytotoxic effects of *cis*-diamminedichloroplatinum(II) and 5-fluorouracil with and without leucovorin against human non-small cell lung cancer cell lines. *Cancer Res.*, **53** (1993) 1079–1084.

188. Johnston PG, Geoffroy F, Drake J, Voeller D, Grem JL, and Allegra CJ. The cellular interaction of 5-fluorouracil and cisplatin in a human colon carcinoma cell line. *Eur. J. Cancer*, **32A** (1996) 2148–2154.

189. Fujishima H, Niho Y, Kondo T, Tatsumoto T, Esaki T, Masumoto N, et al. Inhibition by 5-fluorouracil of ERCC1 and gamma-glutamylcysteine synthetase messenger RNA expression in a cisplatin-resistant HST-1 human squamous carcinoma cell line. *Oncol. Res.*, **9** (1997) 167–172.

190. Loehrer PJS, Turner S, Kubilis P, et al. A prospective randomized trial of fluorouracil versus fluorouracil plus cisplatin in the treatment of metastatic colorectal cancer. A Hoosier Oncology Group trial. *J. Clin. Oncol.*, **6** (1988) 642–648.

191. Lokich JJ, Ahlgren HD, Cantrell J, et al. A prospective randomized comparison of protracted infusional 5-fluorouracil with or without weekly bolus cisplatin in metastatic colorectal carcinoma. *Cancer*, **67** (1991) 14–19.

192. Kemeny N, Israel K, Niedzwiecki D, et al. Randomized study of continuous infusion fluorouracil versus fluorouracil plus cisplatin in patients with metastatic colorectal cancer. *J. Clin. Oncol.*, **8** (1990) 313–318.

193. Diaz-Rubio E, Jimeno J, Anton A, et al. A prospective randomized trial of continuous infusion 5-fluorouracil (5- FU) versus 5-FU plus cisplatin in patients with advanced colorectal cancer. A trial of the Spanish Cooperative Group for Digestive Tract Tumor Therapy (T.T.D.). *Am. J. Clin. Oncol.*, **15** (1992) 56–60.

194. Hansen RM, Ryan L, Anderson T, et al. Phase III study of bolus versus infusion fluorouracil with or without cisplatin in advanced colorectal cancer. *J. Natl. Cancer Inst.*, **88** (1996) 668–674.

195. Raymond E, Buquet-Fagot F, Djelloul C, et al. Antitumor activity of oxaliplatin in combination with 5-fluorouracil and the thymidylate synthase inhibitor AG337 in human colon, breast and ovarian cancers. *Anticancer Drugs*, **8** (1997) 876–885.

196. Fischel JL, Etienne MC, Formento P, et al. Search for the optimal schedule for the oxaliplatin/5-fluorouracil association modulated or not by folinic acid. Preclinical data. *Clin. Cancer Res.*, **4** (1998) 2529–2535.

197. de Gramont A, Vignoud J, Tournigand C, et al. Oxaliplatin with high-dose leucovorin and 5-fluorouracil 48-hour continuous infusion in pretreated metastatic colorectal cancer. *Eur. J. Cancer*, **33** (1997) 214–219.

198. deBraud F, Munzone E, Nole F, et al. Synergistic activity of oxaliplatin and 5-fluorouracil in patients with metastatic colorectal cancer with progressive disease while on or after 5-fluorouracil. *Am. J. Clin. Oncol.*, **21** (1998) 279–283.

199. Andre T, Louvet C, Raymond E, et al. Bimonthly high-dose leucovorin, 5-fluorouracil infusion and oxaliplatin (FOLFOX3) for metastatic colorectal cancer resistant to the same leucovorin and 5-fluorouracil regimen. *Ann. Oncol.*, **9** (1998) 1251–1253.

200. Andre T, Bensmaine MA, Louvet C, et al. Multicenter phase II study of bimonthly high-dose leucovorin, fluorouracil infusion, and oxaliplatin for metastatic colorectal cancer resistant to the same leucovorin and fluorouracil regimen. *J. Clin. Oncol.*, **17** (1999) 3560–3568.

201. de Gramont A, Figer A, Seymour M, et al. Leucovorin and fluorouracil with or without oxaliplatin as first-line treatment in advanced colorectal cancer. *J. Clin. Oncol.*, **18** (2000) 2938–2947.

202. Levi F, Zidani R, and Misset JL. Randomised multicentre trial of chronotherapy with oxaliplatin, fluorouracil, and folinic acid in metastatic colorectal cancer. International Organization for Cancer Chronotherapy. *Lancet*, **350** (1997) 681–686.

203. Giacchetti S, Perpoint B, Zidani R, et al. Phase III multicenter randomized trial of oxaliplatin added to chronomodulated fluorouracil–leucovorin as first-line treatment of metastatic colorectal cancer. *J. Clin. Oncol.*, **18** (2000) 136–144.

204. Heidelberger C, Griesvach L, Montag BJ, et al. Studies on fluorinated pyrimidines. II. Effects on transplanted tumors. *Cancer Res.*, **18** (1958) 305–317.

205. Byfield JE, Calabro-Jones P, Klisak I, and Kulhanian F. Pharmacologic requirements for obtaining sensitization of human tumor cells in vitro to combined 5-fluorouracil or ftorafur and x-rays. *Int. J. Radiat. Oncol. Biol. Phys.*, **8** (1982) 1923–1933.

206. Ishikawa T, Tanaka Y, Ishitsuka H, and Ohkawa T. Comparative antitumor activity of 5-fluorouracil and 5′-deoxyfluorouridine in combination with radiation therapy in mice bearing colon 26 adenocarcinoma. *Cancer Res.*, **80** (1989) 583–591.

207. Smalley SR, Kimler BF, and Evans RG. 5-Fluorouracil modulation of radiosensitivity in cultured human carcinoma cells. *Int. J. Radiat. Oncol. Biol. Phys.,* **20** (1991) 207–211.

208. Bruso CE, Shewach DS, and Lawrence TS. Fluorodeoxyurine-induced radiosensitization and inhibition of DNA double-strand break repair in human colon cancer cells. *Int. J. Radiat. Oncol. Biol. Phys.*, **19** (1990) 1411–1417.

209. Lawrence T, Heimburger D, and Shewach DL. The effects of leucovorin and dipyridamole on fluoropyrimidine-induced radiosensitization. *Int. J. Radiat. Oncol. Biol. Phys.*, **20** (1991) 377–381.

210. Miller EM and Kinsella TJ. Radiosensitization by fluorodeoxyuridine. effects of thymidylate synthase inhibition and cell synchronization. *Cancer Res.*, **52** (1992) 1687–1694.

211. Davis MA, Tang HY, Maybaum J, and Lawrence TS. Dependence of fluorodeoxyuridine-mediated radiosensitization on S phase progression. *Int. J. Radiat. Biol.*, **67** (1995) 509–517.

212. Lawrence TS, Davis MA, and Loney TL. Fluoropyrimidine-mediated radiosensitization depends on cyclin E-dependent kinase activation. *Cancer Res.*, **56** (1996) 3203–3206.

213. Hwang HS, Davis TW, Houghton JA, and Kinsella TJ. Radiosensitivity of thymidylate synthase-deficient human tumor cells is affected by progression through the G1 restriction point into *S*-phase: implications for fluoropyrimidine radiosensitization. *Cancer Res.*, **60** (2000) 92–100.

214. Lawrence TS, Tepper JE, and Blackstock AW. Fluoropyrimidine-radiation interactions in cells and tumors. *Semin. Radiat. Oncol.*, **7** (1997) 260–266.

215. Rich TA. Irradiation plus 5-fluorouracil. Cellular mechanisms of action and treatment schedules. *Sem. Radiat. Oncol.*, **7** (1997) 267–273.

216. UKCCCR Anal Cancer Trial Working Party. Epidermoid anal cancer: results from the UKCCCR randomized trial of radiotherapy alone versus radiotherapy, 5-fluorouracil and mitomycin C. *Lancet*, **348** (1996) 1049–1054.

217. Bartelink H, Roelofsen F, Eschwege F, et al. Concomitant radiotherapy and chemotherapy is superior to radiotherapy alone in the treatment of locally advanced anal cancer: results of a phase III randomized trial of the European Organization for Research and Treatment of Cancer Radiotherapy and Gastrointestinal Cooperative Groups. *J. Clin. Oncol.*, **15** (1997) 2040–2049.

218. Flam M, John M, Pajack TF, et al. Role of mitomycin in combination with fluorouracil and radiotherapy, and of salvage chemoradiation in the definitive nonsurgical treatment of epidermoid carcinoma of the anal canal: results of a phase III randomized intergroup study. *J. Clin. Oncol.*, **14** (1996) 2527–2539.

219. Morris M, Eifel PJ, Lu J, Grigsby PW, et al. Pelvic radiation with concurrent chemotherapy compared with pelvic and para-aortic radiation for high-risk cervical cancer. *N. Engl. J. Med.*, **340** (1999) 1137–1143.

220. Cooper JS, Guo MD, Herskovic A, et al. Chemoradiotherapy of locally advanced esophageal cancer. Long-term follow-up of a prospective randomized trial (RTOG 85-01). Radiation Therapy Oncology Group. *J. Am. Med. Assoc.*, **281** (1999) 1623–1627.

221. O'Connell MJ, Martenson JA, Wieand HS, et al. Improving adjuvant therapy for rectal cancer by combining protracted infusion fluorouracil with radiation therapy after curative surgery. *N. Engl. J. Med.*, **33** (1994) 502–507.

222. Plunkett W, Huang P, Searcy CE, and Gandhi V. Gemcitabine: preclinical pharmacology and mechanisms of action. *Semin. Oncol.*, **23(5Suppl. 10)** (1996) 3–15.

223. Grem JL and Allegra CJ. Sequence-dependent interaction of 5-fluorouracil and arabinosyl-5- azacytosine or 1-beta-D-arabinofuranosylcytosine. *Biochem. Pharmacol.*, **42** (1991) 409–418.

224. Cascinu S, Silva RR, Barni S, et al. A combination of gemcitabine and 5-fluorouracil in advanced pancreatic cancer, a report from the Italian Group for the Study of Digestive Tract Cancer (GISCAD). *Br. J. Cancer*, **80** (1999) 1595–1598.

225. Cascinu S, Frontini L, Labianca R, et al. A combination of a fixed dose rate infusion of gemcitabine associated to a bolus 5-fluorouracil in advanced pancreatic cancer, a report from the Italian Group for the Study of Digestive Tract Cancer (GISCAD). *Ann. Oncol.*, **11** (2000) 1309–1311.

226. Berlin JD, Adak S, Vaughn DJ, et al. A phase II study of gemcitabine and 5-fluorouracil in metastatic pancreatic cancer: an Eastern Cooperative Oncology Group Study (E3296). *Oncology*, **58** (2000) 215–218.

227. Poplin E, Roberts J, Tombs M, et al. Leucovorin, 5-fluorouracil, and gemcitabine: a phase I study. *Invest. New Drugs*, **17** (1999) 57–62.

228. Madajewicz S, Hentschel P, Burns P, et al. Phase I chemotherapy study of biochemical modulation of folinic acid and fluorouracil by gemcitabine in patients with solid tumor malignancies. *J. Clin. Oncol.*, **18** (2000) 3553–3557.

229. Rinaldi DA, Lormand NA, Brierre JE, et al. A phase I trial of gemcitabine and infusional 5-fluorouracil (5-FU) in patients with refractory solid tumors: Louisiana Oncology Associates protocol no. 1 (LOA-1). *Am. J. Clin. Oncol.*, **23** (2000) 78–82.

230. Rini BI, Vogelzang NJ, Dumas MC, et al. Phase II trial of weekly intravenous gemcitabine with continuous infusion fluorouracil in patients with metastatic renal cell cancer. *J. Clin. Oncol.*, **18** (2000) 2419–2426.

231. Kurtz JE, Kohser F, Negrier S, et al. Gemcitabine and protracted 5-FU for advanced pancreatic cancer. A phase II study. *Hepatogastroenterology*, **47** (2000) 1450–1453.

232. Oettle H, Arning M, Pelzer U, et al. A phase II trial of gemcitabine in combination with 5-fluorouracil (24-hour) and folinic acid in patients with chemonaive advanced pancreatic cancer. *Ann. Oncol.*, **11** (2000) 1267–1272.

233. Hidalgo M, Castellano D, Paz-Ares L, et al. Phase I–II study of gemcitabine and fluorouracil as a continuous infusion in patients with pancreatic cancer. *J. Clin. Oncol.*, **17** (1999) 585–592.

234. Matano E, Tagliaferri P, Libroia A, et al. Gemcitabine combined with continuous infusion 5-fluorouracil in advanced and symptomatic pancreatic cancer: a clinical benefit-oriented phase II study. *Br. J. Cancer*, **82** (2000) 1772–1775.

235. Kano Y, Akutsu M, Tsunoda S, et al. Schedule-dependent interaction between paclitaxel and 5-fluorouracil in human carcinoma cell lines in vitro. *Br. J. Cancer*, **74** (1996) 704–710.

236. Johnson KR, Wang L, Miller MC III, Willingham MC, and Fan W. 5-fluorouracil interferes with paclitaxel cytotoxicity against human solid tumor cells. *Clin. Cancer Res.*, **3** (1997) 1739–1745.

237. Grem JL, Nguyen D, Monahan BP, Kao V, and Geoffroy FJ. Sequence-dependant antagonism between fluorouracil and paclitaxel in human breast cancer cells. *Biochem. Pharmacol.*, **58** (1999) 477–486.

238. Van Den Neste E, de Valeriola D, Kerger J, et al. A phase I and pharmacokinetic study of docetaxel administered in combination with continuous intravenous infusion of 5-fluorouracil in patients with advanced solid tumors. *Clin. Cancer Res.*, **6** (2000) 64–71.

239. Lortholary A, Maillard P, Delva R, et al. Docetaxel in combination with 5-fluorouracil in patients with metastatic breast cancer previously treated with anthracycline-based chemotherapy. A phase I, dose-finding study. *Eur. J. Cancer*, **36** (2000) 1773–1780.

240. Colevas AD, Adak S, Amrein PC, et al. A phase II trial of palliative docetaxel plus 5-fluorouracil for squamous-cell cancer of the head and neck. *Ann. Oncol.*, **11** (2000) 535–539.

241. Ando M, Watanabe T, Sasaki Y, et al. A phase I trial of docetaxel and 5-day continuous infusion of 5-fluorouracil in patients with advanced or recurrent breast cancer. *Br. J. Cancer*, **77** (1998) 1937–1943.

242. Petit T, Aylesworth C, Burris H, et al. A phase I study of docetaxel and 5-fluorouracil in patients with advanced solid malignancies. *Ann. Oncol.*, **10** (1999) 223–229.

243. Klaassen U, Wilke H, Harstrick A, et al. Paclitaxel in combination with weekly 24-hour infusional 5-fluorouracil plus leucovorin in the second-line treatment of metastatic breast cancer: results of a phase II study. *Ann. Oncol.*, **9** (1998) 45–50.

244. Bokemeyer C, Lampe CS, Clemens MR, et al. A phase II trial of paclitaxel and weekly 24 h infusion of 5-fluorouracil/folinic acid in patients with advanced gastric cancer. *Anticancer Drugs*, **8** (1997) 396–399.

245. Murad AM, Petroianu A, Guimaraes RC, et al. Phase II trial of the combination of paclitaxel and 5-fluorouracil in the treatment of advanced gastric cancer: a novel, safe, and effective regimen. *Am. J. Clin. Oncol.*, **22** (1999) 580–586.

246. Cascinu S, Ficarelli R, Safi MA, et al. A phase I study of paclitaxel and 5-fluorouracil in advanced gastric cancer. *Eur. J. Cancer*, **33** (1997) 1699–1702.

247. Johnson DH, Paul D, and Hande KR. Paclitaxel, 5-fluorouracil, and folinic acid in metastatic breast cancer: BRE-26, a phase II trial. *Semin. Oncol.*, **24** (1997) S22–S25.

248. Takimoto CH, Morrison GB, Frame JN, et al. A phase I and pharmacokinetic trial of paclitaxel and 5-fluorouracil plus leucovorin in patients with solid tumors. *Proc. Am. Soc. Clin. Oncol.*, **14** (1995) 471 (abstract).

249. Pitot HC. US pivotal studies of irinotecan in colorectal carcinoma. *Oncology (Huntington)*, **12** (1998) 48–53.

250. Cunningham D, Pyrhonen S, James RD, et al. Randomised trial of irinotecan plus supportive care versus supportive care alone after fluorouracil failure for patients with metastatic colorectal cancer. *Lancet*, **352** (1998) 1413–1418.

251. Rougier P, Van Cutsem E, Bajetta E, et al. Randomised trial of irinotecan versus fluorouracil by continuous infusion after fluorouracil failure in patients with metastatic colorectal cancer. *Lancet*, **352** (1998) 1407–1412 [published erratum appears in *Lancet*, **352** (1998) 1634].

252. Douillard JY, Cunningham D, Roth AD, et al. Irinotecan combined with fluorouracil compared with fluorouracil alone as first-line treatment for metastatic colorectal cancer: a multicentre randomised trial. *Lancet*, **355** (2000) 1041–1047.

253. Aschele C, Baldo C, Sobrero AF, Debernardis D, Bornmann WG, and Bertino JR. Schedule-dependent synergism between raltitrexed and irinotecan in human colon cancer cells in vitro. *Clin. Cancer Res.*, **4** (1998) 1323–1330.

254. Mans DR, Grivicich I, Peters GJ, and Schwartsmann G. Sequence-dependent growth inhibition and DNA damage formation by the irinotecan-5-fluorouracil combination in human colon carcinoma cell lines. *Eur. J. Cancer*, **35** (1999) 1851–1861.

255. Pavillard V, Formento P, Rostagno P, et al. Combination of irinotecan (CPT11) and 5-fluorouracil with an analysis of cellular determinants of drug activity. *Biochem. Pharmacol.*, **56** (1998) 1315–1322.

256. Cao S and Rustum YM. Synergistic antitumor activity of irinotecan in combination with 5-fluorouracil in rats bearing advanced colorectal cancer: role of drug sequence and dose. *Cancer Res.*, **60** (2000) 3717–3721.

257. Houghton JA, Cheshire PJ, Hallman JD, 2nd, et al. Evaluation of irinotecan in combination with 5-fluorouracil or etoposide in xenograft models of colon adenocarcinoma and rhabdomyosarcoma. *Clin. Cancer Res.*, **2** (1996) 107–118.

26 Clinical Implications of Dihydropyrimidine Dehydrogenase on 5-Fluorouracil Pharmacology

Robert B. Diasio

Contents

1. INTRODUCTION

Over the past decade, there has been increasing evidence of the importance of the pyrimidine catabolic pathway in regulating the metabolism of 5-fluorouracil (5-FU) and thus critically influencing the pharmacology of 5-FU and other fluoropyrimidine drugs *(1)*. Dihydropyrimidine dehydrogenase or DPD (also known as, dihydrouracil dehydrogenase, dihydrothymine dehydrogenase, uracil reductase, E.C. 1.3.1.2) is the initial rate-limiting enzymatic step in the catabolism of not only the widely used antimetabolite cancer chemotherapy drug 5-FU but also the naturally occurring pyrimidines uracil and thymine *(2–3)*. As shown in Fig. 1, DPD occupies an important position in the regulation of the metabolism of 5-FU, converting over 85% of a standard intravenous dose of administered 5-FU to dihydrofluorouracil (5-FUH$_2$), an inactive metabolite, in an enzymatic step that physiologically is essentially irreversible *(4,5)*. Although DPD is critical in regulating 5-FU metabolism, 5-FU cytotoxic action is dependent on the anabolism of 5-FU to the "active" nucleotides 5-fluorodeoxyuridine monophosphate (FdUMP), 5-fluorouridine triphosphate (FUTP), and 5-fluorodeoxyuridine triphosphate (FdUTP). These important "active" metabolites are, in turn, responsible for inhibition of cell replication through primarily inhibition of thymidylate synthase and secondarily through incorporation into RNA or DNA.

From: *Colorectal Cancer: Multimodality Management*
Edited by: L. Saltz © Humana Press Inc., Totowa, NJ

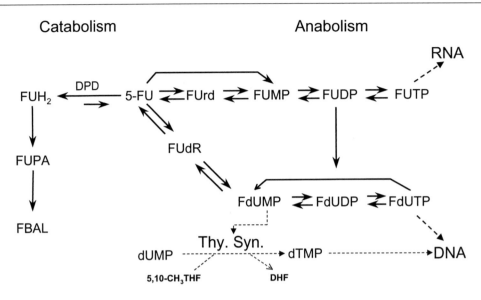

Fig. 1. Metabolic overview illustrating the critical position of DPD in the metabolism of 5-FU as well as the natural pyrimidines uracil and thymine. More than 85% of administered 5-FU is catabolized via DPD.

2. CLINICAL EVIDENCE OF IMPORTANCE OF DPD TO 5-FU PHARMACOLOGY

Although preclinical studies *(1,2,4,5)* of 5-FU metabolism demonstrated that DPD was the rate-limiting step in the catabolism of 5-FU, thus suggesting a potentially important role in 5-FU pharmacology, it is the more recent clinical studies of 5-FU that have demonstrated that DPD has an important role in the clinical pharmacology of 5-FU (Table 1). In particular, it is clear that DPD accounts for much of the variability that has been noted in clinical studies with 5-FU. This includes both intrapatient variability as well as interpatient variability.

With the increased use of ambulatory pumps for protracted infusions of 5-FU over the past two decades, pharmacokinetic studies had demonstrated that 5-FU levels often varied during an infusion despite 5-FU being delivered at a constant rate *(6)*. The basis for this was initially not clear, but variation in DPD was considered because of its important role in the regulation of 5-FU metabolism. DPD activity has been shown to follow a circadian pattern in both animals and humans *(7–9)*. Preclinical studies in rats on a 12-h light/12-h dark schedule had demonstrated that hepatic levels of DPD follow a pattern that can be plotted on a cosine wave *(7)*. This pattern was completely reversed in another group of rats on an inverted 12-h light/12-h dark schedule. In patients receiving continuous infusion of 5-FU by automated pumps, sampling of serum 5-FU over a 24-h period has been shown to also exhibit circadian patterns when plotted on a cosine wave *(9)*. DPD activity in peripheral blood mononuclear cells obtained at the same time-points from the same patients have been shown also to follow a circadian pattern that was essentially inverse to the 5-FU circadian pattern (Fig. 2). The data from this study suggested that perhaps DPD was responsible for the circadian variation in 5-FU. This has led some chemotherapists to propose time-modified 5-FU infusions to optimize drug delivery during a 24-h period. Such regimens have been popularized by oncologists in Europe who have suggested a potential benefit in the treatment of certain human cancers *(10)*.

For the past four decades that 5-FU has been used clinically, it is notable that there has been wide variation in the published reports of the clinical pharmacokinetics of 5-FU. The

Table 1
Importance of DPD in 5-FU Metabolism

- Variability in 5-FU blood levels during the day while receiving continuous (protracted) infusion of 5-FU. Circadian variation of 5-FU related to circadian variation of DPD; implication for time-modified therapy.
- Variability of 5-FU clinical pharmacokinetics ($t_{1/2}$ and clearance) related to variability in DPD.
- Variability in 5-FU bioavailability related to variability in DPD.
- Variability of 5-FU catabolism due to variability in gene expression of DPD secondary to sequence changes in the DPD gene; genetic deficiency of DPD (pharmacogenetic syndrome).
- Variability in 5-FU antitumor activity (i.e., resistance) may be related to variability in DPD expression in the tumor.
- DPD is a potential therapeutic target for improving 5-FU therapy.

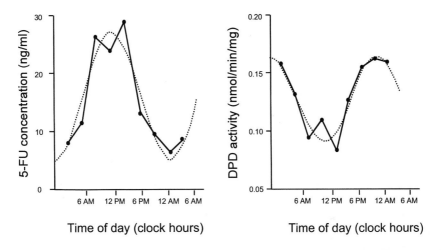

Fig. 2. Circadian pattern of DPD with inverse circadian pattern of serum 5-FU from a patient receiving a protracted infusion of 5-FU 300 mg/m² by ambulatory pump. (Adapted from ref. *9.*)

basis for this variability has been confusing. Carefully executed studies in our own clinical research center setting have demonstrated similar variability in 5-FU pharmacokinetics with half-lives ($t_{1/2}$) ranging from around 4 min to 25 min after an intravenous bolus (Table 2) *(11)*. Because DPD occupies a critical position in the 5-FU metabolic pathway (*see* Fig. 1), it was hypothesized that the variation in pharmacokinetic characteristics might be secondary to variability of DPD enzyme activity among different individuals. Population studies were initially undertaken to assess DPD enzyme activity in easily accessible tissues (e.g., peripheral blood mononuclear [PBM] cells) from healthy individuals, with subsequent studies examining DPD activity in human cadaver liver specimens. DPD was shown to vary from individual to individual, with a normal distribution pattern ("bell-shaped curve") that was approx a sixfold variation from the lowest to the highest values (Fig. 3) *(12,13)*. Essentially the same pattern of DPD activity has also been observed in the PBM cells of both breast and colorectal cancer patients who have been tested, although, interestingly, the normal distribution is shifted to the left with a lower median DPD activity in the breast cancer patient population *(14)*. The mechanism for this latter observation is currently unknown, but it does not appear to be related to age, menopausal status, concurrent hormonal therapy, or chemotherapy. The wide variation in DPD activity observed in the above-described

Table 2
Clinical Pharmacokinetics of 5-FU

Patients	$t_{1/2}$ (min)	Clearance (mL/min/m²)
1	16.5	376
2	8.9	707
3	7.6	596
4	11.4	431
5	26.7	335
6	7.9	633
7	7.9	558
8	5.3	1014
9	23.9	567
10	12.6	726
Mean ± SD	12.9 ± 7.3	594 ± 198

Note: Data adapted from ref. *11*.

populations is thought to account for the wide variation in the $t_{1/2}$ (and pharmacokinetics) that has been observed in patients treated with 5-FU *(11)*.

One of the most unexpected observations in clinical pharmacologic studies of 5-FU had been the apparent variability in absorption of 5-FU after oral administration. Over the years this has led to the recommendation that 5-FU not be administered by the oral route *(3)*. Because 5-FU is a relatively small (molecular weight) molecule with a pK_a that should favor excellent absorption and bioavailability, one would predict that the absorption of 5-FU should be efficient and the bioavailability excellent, with little variability. Recent studies examining the potential use of oral fluoropyrimidine drugs have demonstrated that variation in DPD activity is likely responsible for the apparent variable bioavailability of 5-FU, with the use of DPD inhibitors permitting a pharmacokinetic pattern produced by oral administration of 5-FU that was essentially the same as that produced by intravenous administration, resulting in essentially 100% bioavailability when potent irreversible DPD inhibitors were used *(15)*.

Although most patients tolerate 5-FU reasonably well, over the past four decades there have been an increasing number of patients noted who developed severe, at times life-threatening, toxicity after standard doses of 5-FU *(16–19)*. Because these patients demonstrated exaggerated normal toxic side effects as if they had received an overdose of drug, it was hypothesized that these patients were deficient in a catabolic enzyme that resulted in more 5-FU being present over time. Initial studies in these affected patients demonstrated elevated uracil and thymine levels suggesting deficiency of the first step in pyrimidine catabolism, DPD *(16–18)*. Subsequent studies demonstrated that many of these patients were indeed deficient in DPD. It is clear now that an additional small percentage (<3%) of the population has DPD activity significantly below the normal distribution that characterizes most of the population *(19)*. These individuals are at significant risk if they develop cancer and are given 5-FU. This is a true pharmacogenetic syndrome, with symptoms not being recognized until exposure to the drug *(19)*.

Although it has long been well known that variability in the activity of pyrimidine anabolic enzymes is important in determining the antitumor effectiveness of 5-FU, much less attention has been focused on the variability in the activity of the pyrimidine catabolic enzymes. Of interest was the hypothesis that increasing levels of DPD expression in tumors

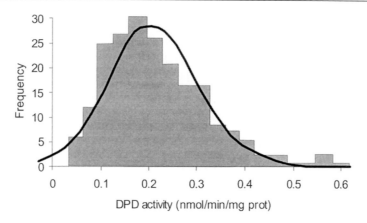

Fig. 3. Pattern of DPD activity in population of 104 healthy individuals demonstrating wide sixfold variation in DPD activity. (Adapted from ref. *12*.)

should increase resistance to 5-FU. In fact, tumors that are resistant to 5-FU have been shown to express increased levels of DPD activity *(20)*. With the development of more sensitive methods for assessing DPD in small-needle-biopsy-sized tumor specimens through the use of quantitative polymerase chain reaction (PCR) to measure DPD mRNA, increased expression of DPD mRNA has been demonstrated in tumors from patients who were resistant to 5-FU *(21)*.

3. UTILIZING UNDERSTANDING OF DPD TO DEVELOP A PHARMACOLOGIC STRATEGY

The observed variable DPD levels in both normal and tumor tissues provide a rationale for the oncologist to either alter the dose of the fluoropyrimidine drug or inhibit DPD in order to minimize the variability in 5-FU pharmacology. The presence of increased tumor DPD suggests the need to increase the dose of 5-FU (or a prodrug of 5-FU) to overcome the increased catabolism of 5-FU within the tumor by enabling enough 5-FU to be available within the tumor to be converted to active anabolites (*see* Fig. 1). An alternative approach is to use known inhibitors of DPD, usually with a lower dose of 5-FU, to directly inhibit 5-FU degradation within the tumor, permitting the 5-FU that is present, even if present in low concentrations, to be converted to active 5-FU anabolites. Inhibiting DPD in 5-FU-susceptible host tissue such as gastrointestinal (GI) mucosa and bone marrow should also make dosing from patient to patient less variable, the latter being accomplished through lessening the variability in pharmacokinetics, bioavailability and the resultant host toxicity.

Over the years, there have been many attempts to synthesize effective inhibitors of DPD *(22)*. Unfortunately, many of these compounds have proven to be very toxic. In the past several years, there have been several fluoropyrimidine drugs using DPD inhibition introduced into the clinic. These drugs, referred to as DPD inhibitory fluoropyrimidines (DIF), include UFT, Eniluracil, S-1, and BOF-A2 *(23)*. These drugs differ both in the mechanism of DPD "inhibition" as well as in the degree of inhibition produced. The rationale for using DIF drugs is that there is a source of 5-FU, either from 5-FU itself or from a "prodrug" that is converted to 5-FU together with another drug that interferes with (or inhibits) the otherwise rapid catabolism of 5-FU. This permits oral delivery of 5-FU (potentially oral bioavailability >70%) and results in less variability in the pharmacokinetics of the fluoropyrimidines. In addition, by inhibiting the catabolic pathway, more 5-FU can enter the anabolic pathway, potentially increasing the antitumor effect. This is theoretically important for tumors that are resistant secondary to an increase of intratumoral DPD (*see* earlier discussion).

UFT was the first of the DIF drugs to be synthesized and is the one most studied *(24,25)*. This oral fluoropyrimidine is a combination of the naturally occurring pyrimidine uracil with the fluoropyrimidine Tegafur (Ftorafur) in a 4:1 molar ratio. The presence of uracil in excess of 5-FU results in competition at the level of DPD such that 5-FU, which is formed from Tegafur, theoretically should not be rapidly degraded and therefore should remain present for a more prolonged period. Although not true inhibition of DPD, the competition between 5-FU and uracil for DPD produces an effect similar to what one achieves with a true DPD inhibitor. In contrast to the true DPD inhibitors and inactivators, the effect on DPD is more rapidly reversible. This rapidly reversible inhibition may avoid some of the problems that were seen with the earlier DPD inhibitors and may account for a more favorable toxicity profile compared to some of the earlier DPD inhibitors *(22)* as well as some of the newer DIF drugs. There is now extensive data from Japan as well as Europe, South America, and the United States demonstrating that orally administered UFT has antitumor activity in several tumor types (particularly breast and colon cancer), either as a single agent or combined with leucovorin *(26)*. Studies thus far have shown that it is at least as effective as intravenously infused 5-FU. Furthermore the toxicity profile has proven quite tolerable with the typical fluoropyrimidine toxicities (e.g., diarrhea and nausea) seen at the maximum tolerated dose (MTD). Of note is the paucity of other toxicities, in particular hand–foot syndrome, neurologic, and cardiotoxicity *(27)*. Although not well understood, some of these toxicities may be secondary to 5-FU catabolites. 5-FU catabolites are less likely to form from UFT and, therefore, these toxicities are not typically observed.

Although DPD is clearly an important factor *(28)*, it is probably a more rational approach to monitor multiple factors (including not only DPD but also the target thymidylate synthase [TS] and possibly enzymatic steps leading to anabolism of 5-FU to active nucleotide anabolites) that are known to predict 5-FU effectiveness and base the decision on these taken together. In particular, the use of immunohistochemical assessment or quantitative PCR of multiple targets may provide a valuable method by which to approach this. A recent study in which patients on a clinical trial for advanced colorectal cancer were assessed clinically for response to 5-FU + leucovorin and independently assessed for DPD, TS, and the enzyme thymidine phosphorylase demonstrated a very high degree of prediction of response based on these markers *(21)*. Patients with had relatively "low" expression of all of these markers responded to the regimen, whereas those patients who had elevation of any one marker were essentially unresponsive and progressed earlier (*see* Fig. 4). It is likely that this assessment of multiple markers will become the approach used in the future.

4. POTENTIAL BENEFIT FROM DECREASING FORMATION OF 5-FU CATABOLITES

The use of DPD inhibitors together with 5-FU has other potential theoretical clinical benefits by lessening toxicities thought to be caused by downstream catabolites of 5-FU (*see* Fig. 1). Many of the common fluoropyrimidine toxicities are thought to be the result of anabolism of 5-FU nucleotides (*see* Fig. 5), with the inhibition of thymidylate synthase by FdUMP resulting in S-phase inhibition. Because rapidly growing cells (e.g., oral and gastrointestinal mucosa, certain hematopoietic cells) have a relatively large fraction of cells in the S phase, these cells are particularly sensitive to the effects of 5-FU with toxicities, such as mucositis, stomatitis, gastrointestinal side effects (such as nausea, vomiting, and

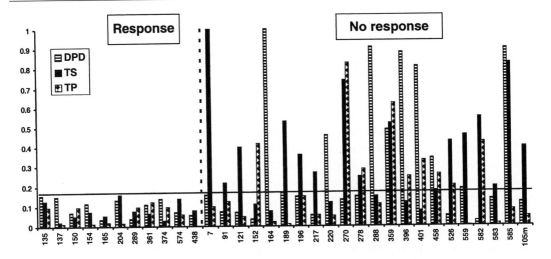

Fig. 4. Quantitative PCR mRNA pattern of DPD, TS, and thymidine phosphorylase (TP) from tumor specimens of patients treated with a Mayo Clinic regimen of 5-FU + leucovorin. Patients who responded had relatively low mRNA expression of the three markers (below horizontal line), whereas patients who were unresponsive had elevation of one or more of these markers. (Adapted from ref. *21.*)

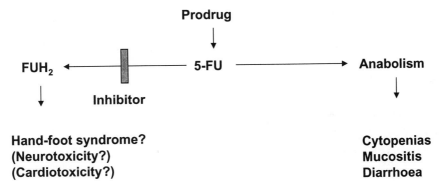

Fig. 5. Toxicities associated with 5-FU secondary to anabolism and possibly secondary to catabolism. Potential effect of inhibiting DPD is shown.

diarrhea), leukopenia and sometimes thrombocytopenia, typically being seen. In contrast to these toxicities, there are other toxicities that have been suggested to be possibly related to catabolites of 5-FU. These have included neurotoxicity manifested as cerebellar ataxia and at times decreased consciousness, which has been suggested to be caused by further metabolism of the 5-FU-catabolite α-fluoro-β-alanine (FBAL) (*see* Fig. 1) to fluorocitrate and subsequently fluoroacetate by metabolism within the Krebs cycle *(29)*. Although this appears to be biochemically possible, the evidence that this does occur and is responsible for the neurotoxicity of 5-FU remains indirect at best. 5-FU-related cardiotoxicity has also been suggested to be secondary to 5-FU catabolites. As with neurotoxicity, the evidence in support of this is somewhat inconclusive. Thus if neurotoxicity and cardiotoxicity are indeed caused by 5-FU catabolites, then the addition of a DPD inhibitor might lessen these toxicities while preserving 5-FU activity. One other toxicity that may be related to the effect of a 5-FU catabolite is hand–foot syndrome. Of interest is the decreased evidence of hand–foot syndrome observed when DPD inhibitors are used with 5-FU, in contrast to what is observed with oral 5-FU administration without DPD inhibition (e.g., Capecitabine [Xeloda]) or protracted intravenous infusion of 5-FU where hand–foot syndrome is more common, Whether this is caused by a 5-FU catabolite is unclear at the present time, but it will need to be further evaluated in the future.

5. CONCLUSION

Dihydropyrimidine dehydrogenase is the initial rate-limiting enzyme in the catabolism of 5-FU, accounting for catabolism of over 85% of an administered dose of 5-FU. DPD has an important role in regulating the availability of 5-FU for anabolism. It is now clear that DPD also accounts for much of the variability observed with the therapeutic use of 5-FU. This includes variable 5-FU levels over 24 h during a continuous infusion, the widely reported variability in 5-FU pharmacokinetics, the observed variable bioavailability that has led to the recommendation that 5-FU not be administered as an oral agent, variability at the level of the gene that is associated with pharmacogenetic syndrome, and, finally, the observed variability in both toxicity and drug response (resistance) after the same 5-FU dose. Knowledge of the DPD level as well as the levels of other potentially important molecular markers (e.g., thymidylate synthase) may permit adjustments in the 5-FU dose or modulation of the 5-FU dose that can result in an increase in the therapeutic efficacy of the 5-FU drug. DPD has also been a potentially attractive target for modulating 5-FU metabolism and, hence, potentially its efficacy and toxicity. Although some of the DIF drugs are approved in various locations worldwide (e.g., UFT, S-1), no DIF drugs are approved in the United States at present. Finally, it should be noted that several fluoropyrimidine toxicities may be caused by 5-FU catabolites, leading to the suggestion that potential use of DPD inhibition may lessen the chance of these toxicities.

REFERENCES

1. Diasio RB, Lu Z, Zhang R, and Shahinian HS. Fluoropyrimidine catabolism. In *Concepts and Mechanisms, and New Targets for Chemotherapy.* Muggia FM (ed.), Kluwer Academic, Norwell, MA, 1995.
2. Daher GC, Harris BE, and Diasio RB. Metabolism of pyrimidine analogues and their nucleosides. In *Metabolism and Reactions of Anticancer Drugs.* Vol. 1. *The International Encyclopedia of Pharmacology and Therapeutics.* Powis G (ed.), Pergamon, Oxford, 1994, Chap. 2.
3. Diasio RB and Harris BE. Clinical pharmacology of 5-flurouracil. *Clini. Pharmacokin.*, **16** (1989) 215–237.
4. Lu Z-H, Zhang R, and Diasio RB. Purification and characterization of dihydropyrimidine dehydrogenase from human liver. *J. Biol. Chem.*, **267** (1992) 17,102–17,109.
5. Sommadossi JP, Gewirtz DA, Diasio RB, Aubert C, Cano JP, and Goldman ID. Rapid catabolism of 5-fluorouracil in freshly isolated rat hepatocytes as analyzed by high performance liquid chromatography. *J. Biol. Chem.*, **257** (1982) 8171–8176.
6. Kawai M, Rosenfeld J, McCulloch P, and Hillcoat BL. Blood levels of 5-fluorouracil during intravenous infusion. *Br. J. Cancer*, **36** (1976) 346–347.
7. Harris BE, Song R, He Y, Soong S-J, and Diasio, RB. Circadian rhythm of rat liver dihydropyrimidine dehydrogenase: possible relevance to fluoropyrimidine chemotherapy. *Biochem. Pharm.*, **37** (1988) 4759–4763.
8. Harris BE, Song R, Soong S-J, and Diasio RB. Circadian variation of 5-fluorouracil catabolism in isolated perfused rat liver. *Cancer Res.*, **49** (1989) 6610–6614.
9. Harris BE, Song R, Soong SJ, and Diasio RB. Relationship of dihydropyrimidine dehydrogenase activity and plasma 5-fluorouracil levels: evidence for circadian variation of 5-fluorouracil levels in cancer patients receiving protracted continuous infusion. *Cancer Res.*, **50** (1990) 197–201.
10. Giacchetti S, Perpoint B, Zidani R, Le Bail N, Faggiuolo R, Focan C, et al. Phase III multicenter randomized trial of oxaliplatin added to chronomodulated fluorouracil–leucovorin as first-line treatment of metastatic colorectal cancer. *J. Clin. Oncol.*, **18** (2000) 136–147.
11. Heggie GD, Sommadossi JP, Cross DS, Huster WJ, and Diasio RB. Clinical pharmacokinetics of 5-fluorouracil and its metabolites in plasma, urine, and bile. *Cancer Res.*, **47** (1987) 2203–2206.

12. Lu Z, Zhang R, and Diasio RB. Dihydropyrimidine dehydrogenase activity in human peripheral blood mononuclear cells and liver: population characteristics, newly identified patients, and clinical implication in 5-fluorouracil chemotherapy. *Cancer Res.*, **53** (1993) 5433–5438.

13. Lu Z, Zhang R, and Diasio RB. Dihydropyrimidine dehydrogenase activity in human liver: population characteristics and clinical implication in 5-FU chemotherapy. *Clin. Pharmacol. Ther.*, **58** (1995) 512–522.

14. Lu Z, Zhang R, Carpenter JT, and Diasio RB. Decreased dihydropyrimidine dehydrogenase activity in population of patients with breast cancer: implications for 5-FU-based chemotherapy. *Clin. Cancer Res.*, **4** (1998) 325–329.

15. Baccanari DP, Davis ST, Knick VC, and Spector T. 5-Ethynyluracil: effects on the pharmacokinetics and antitumor activity of 5-fluorouracil. *Proc. Natl. Acad. Sci. USA*, **90** (1993) 11,064–11,068.

16. Diasio RB, Beavers TL, and Carpenter JT. Familial deficiency of dihydropyrimidine dehydrogenase: biochemical basis for familial pyrimidinemia and severe 5-fluorouracil-induced toxicity. *J. Clin. Invest.*, **81** (1988) 47–51.

17. Harris BE, Carpenter JT, and Diasio RB. Severe 5-fluorouracil toxicity secondary to dihydropyrimidine dehydrogenase deficiency: a potentially more common pharmacogenetic syndrome. *Cancer*, **68** (1991) 499–501.

18. Takimoto CH, Lu Z-H, Zhang R, Liang MD, Larson LV, Cantilena LR Jr, et al. Severe neurotoxicity following 5-fluorouracil-based chemotherapy in a patient with dihydropyrimidine dehydrogenase deficiency. *Clin. Cancer Res.*, **2** (1996) 477–481.

19. Lu Z and Diasio RB. Polymorphic drug metabolizing enzymes. In *Principles of Antineoplastic Drug Development and Pharmacology.* Schilsky RL, Milano GA, and Ratain MJ (eds.), Marcel Dekker, New York, 1996.

20. Jiang W, Lu Z, He Y, and Diasio RB. Dihydropyrimidine dehydrogenase activity in hepatocellular carcinoma; implication for 5-fluorouracil-based chemotherapy. *Clin. Cancer Res.*, **3** (1997) 395–399.

21. Salonga D, Danenberg KD, Johnson M, Metzger R, Groshen S, Tsao-Wei DD, et al. Gene expression levels of dihydropyrimidine dehydrogenase and thymidylate synthase together identify a high percentage of colorectal tumors responding to 5-fluorouracil. *Clin. Cancer Res.*, **6** (2000) 1322–1327.

22. Naguib FNM, el Kouni MH, and Cha S. Enzymes of uracil catabolism in normal and neoplastic human tissues. *Cancer Res.*, **45** (1985) 5405–5412.

23. Diasio RB. Oral administration of fluorouracil: a new approach utilizing modulators of dihydropyrimidine dehydrogenase activity. *Cancer Therap.*, **2** (1999) 97–106.

24. Majima H. Phase I and preliminary phase II study of coadministration of uracil and FT-207 (UFT therapy). *Gan To Kagaku Ryoho.*, **7** (1980) 1383–1387.

25. Takino T. Clinical studies on the chemotherapy of advanced cancer with UFT (uracil plus futraful preparation). *Gan To Kagaku Ryoho.*, **7** (1980) 1804–1812.

26. Gonzalez Baron M, Colmenarejo A, Feliu J, et al. Preliminary results of phase I clinical trial. UFT modulated by folinic acid (PO) in the treatment of advanced colorectal cancer. *Therap. Res.*, **13** (1992) 451–458.

27. Pazdur R, Lassere Y, Diaz-Canton E, et al. Phase I trials of uracil–tegafur (UFT) using 5- and 28-day administration schedules: Demonstration of schedule-dependent toxicities. *Anti-Cancer Drugs*, **7** (1996) 728–733.

28. Pazdur R, Lassere Y, Diaz-Canton E, et al. Phase I trial of uracil–tegafur (UFT) plus oral leucovorin: 14-day schedule. *Invest. New Drugs*, **15** (1997) 123–128.

29. Koenig H and Patel A. Biochemical Basis for fluorouracil neurotoxicity. *Arch. Neurol.*, **23** (1970) 155–160.

27 Oral Fluoropyrimidines in Colorectal Cancer

John L. Marshall

CONTENTS

1. INTRODUCTION

5-Fluorouracil (5-FU) has been the most significant drug in the management of colorectal cancer for the previous 40 yr. Its mechanism of action, toxicity profile, mechanisms of resistance, and clinical utility have been clearly defined through many clinical trials and basic science research efforts (*see* Chapters 25 and 26). It is established in the key role of systemic therapy in both the metastatic setting as well as the adjuvant setting for colorectal cancer. Likewise, it is used for many other cancers of the gastrointestinal (GI) tract, head and neck region, and breast cancer. For the past 10–15 yr, the focus of research has been on improving the clinical efficacy of 5-FU through biochemical modulation. The addition of such agents as leucovorin have demonstrated improvement in response rates but have only minimally advanced survival outcomes (*1–3*). Alterations in dose and schedule of 5-FU have likewise resulted in improvement in response rates without large changes in survival outcomes. Most significantly, prolonged infusions of low-dose 5-FU have been found to generate a lower-toxicity profile as well as equal or improved clinical outcomes, including a survival advantage (Table 1) (*4*). Unfortunately, the administration of intravenous 5-FU chronically is somewhat tedious and burdensome for patients and physicians alike. Logically, the development of an oral 5-FU equivalent would have dramatic implications for the therapy of colon cancer as well as for patient quality of life (*5*).

From: *Colorectal Cancer: Multimodality Management*
Edited by: L. Saltz © Humana Press Inc., Totowa, NJ

Table 1
5-FU Bolus vs 5-FU CI in Colorectal Cancer: Meta-Analysis

Six trials (n = 1219)	5-FU bolus	5-FU CI	p-value
Response rate[a] (%)	14	22	<0.002
Survival[a] (months)	11.3	12.1	<0.04
Toxicity: grade 3–4 neutropenia[b] (%)	31	4	<0.0001
Hand–foot syndrome[b] (%)	13	34	<0.0001

[a]Data from Meta-analysis Group in Cancer. *J. Clin. Oncol.*, **16** (1998) 1301–1308.
[b]Data from Meta-analysis Group in Cancer. *J. Clin. Oncol.*, **16** (1998) 3537–3541.

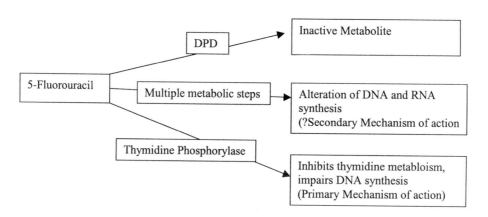

Fig. 1. Metabolism of 5-fluorouracil.

This chapter will focus on the development of drugs that allow for the oral delivery of 5-FU. The compounds that have been developed approach the problem of oral delivery from different angles, resulting in compounds with potential clinical differences as well. One of the agents is already approved for use in much of the world and others have sought approval or are soon to seek approval for use in cancer patients. Therefore, it is critical to understand the different agents, the advantages and disadvantages of each, and to review the current clinical experience with the compounds.

2. DIHYDROPYRIDINE DEHYDROGENASE

Dihydropyridine dehydrogenase (DPD) is an enzyme found predominantly in the liver but widely present in other human tissues, particularly the GI tract (*see* Chapter 26). This enzyme is responsible for the catabolism of 5-FU to its inactive metabolite *(6)*.

Approximately 80% of all 5-FU administered is catabolized by DPD. The remaining 20% of 5-FU is anabolized to active species which are responsible for its antitumor activity (Fig. 1) *(7)*. In principle, 5-FU is orally bioavailable, but because of the large first-pass effect through the liver and metabolism by DPD, it is difficult to predict how much 5-FU would reach the systemic circulation. A second issue surrounding DPD is the fact that it is variably expressed in patients. In other words, some patients have high levels of DPD expression and activity, whereas others have very low levels. There are rare patients who express no DPD. This latter

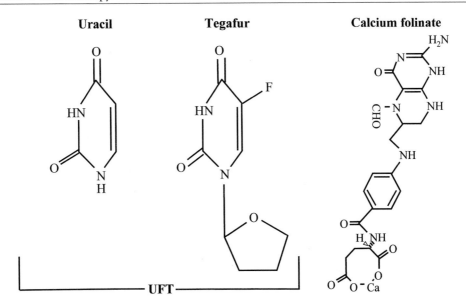

Fig. 2. Chemical structures of uracil, Tegafur, and calcium folinate.

group is obviously extremely sensitive to 5-FU and occasionally suffer fatal or near-fatal complications when given standard doses of intravenous (IV) 5-FU *(8–10)*.

In order to successfully deliver an oral fluoropyrimidine, one must design agents that either bypass or, in some way, inhibit DPD. Two compounds (UFT and S-1) utilize agents that are competitive inhibitors of DPD. A third compounds (which has now been withdrawn from clinical development) (eniluracil) reversibly inhibits DPD. The fourth compound (capecitabine) is, in fact, DPD "resistant" is the result of modifications in the structures of molecule. The specifics of the mechanisms of action, pharmacology, and structure will be described in detail in the following sections. It is important to note that these agents will have different side-effect profiles and different risks in patients because of these differences on DPD.

3. DPD INHIBITORS

3.1. Tegafur and UFT

Tegafur is a furanyl nucleoside analog of 5-FU initially introduced many years ago (Fig. 2). It is absorbed intact from the GI tract and is then converted to 5-FU in vivo by hepatic microsomal cytochrome P-450 enzymes. The initial clinical trials with this compound revealed unacceptable toxicity, namely severe gastrointestinal and central nervous system toxicities *(11)*. It also failed to result in significant persistent levels of 5-FU. Clinical activity has been observed with his compound in 5-FU-sensitive malignancies and a more protracted administration schedule has helped with toxicity.

In order to improve the toxicity profile and efficacy of this compound, a combination agent utilizing Tegafur and uracil, a competitive inhibitor of DPD, in a fixed combination of 1:4 molar ratio has been developed *(12)* (Fig. 2). Preclinical studies demonstrated that this combination, called UFT, resulted in significant improvements in the tumor to normal tissue and tissue to serum ratios of 5-FU *(13,14)*. This compound was explored in a series of clinical trials showing it to have similar single-agent activity to that of iv 5-FU. One trial has been performed using this compound in the adjuvant setting in patients with stage 2 and stage 3

Table 2
Phase III Results of Orzel vs 5-FU/Leucovorin

	Orzel	*5-FU/Leucovorin*
No. of patients	598	598
Dose	300 mg/m UFT/90 LV tid 28 d on, 7 d off	425 mg/m 5-FU + 20 mg/m LV d 1–5 q 28 d
Response rates	12% US study 11% European study	15% US study 9% European study
Survival	No difference	
Toxicity	Significantly less neutropenia and mucositis	

colon cancer compared to surgery alone with significant improvements in disease-free survival rates *(15)*. UFT (uracil, 5-FU, tegafur) has been commercially available in Japan for many years.

As stated earlier, significant evidence exists supporting the positive impact of leucovorin in combination with 5-FU *(16)*, resulting in improved response rates. The mechanism of action for this improvement is thought to be through enhanced binding of the active metabolite of 5-FU to its target enzyme, thymidine synthase. Leucovorin, a reduced folate, enhances this binding through the formation of a ternary complex. Therefore, it is logical to pursue combinations of the oral fluoropyrimidines such as UFT with leucovorin. In summary, UFT demonstrates a clinical impact similar to that of iv 5-FU but with a significantly lower-toxicity profile. Most notable is that this compound does not cause hand–foot syndrome commonly seen with capecitabine.

3.2. Clinical Trials of UFT

Phase I trials of single-agent UFT examined both a 5-d schedule repeated every 21 d and a 28-d schedule repeated every 35 d *(17)*. In each trial, the dose was divided by 3 and administered three times daily at 8-h intervals. Granulocytopenia was the dose-limiting toxicity for the 5-d regimen and diarrhea was dose limiting for the 28-d regimen. This parallels the toxicity seen with iv 5-FU. The recommended phase II dose for UFT administered without leucovorin was 800 mg/m/d for the 5-d schedule and 360 mg/m/d for the 28-d schedule. In subsequent studies, UFT was combined with oral leucovorin using the 28-d schedule repeated every 35 d *(18)*. Again, diarrhea was dose limiting and the recommended phase II dose was UFT 300 mg/m/d plus leucovorin 90 mg/d. In phase II studies of UFT plus oral leucovorin in advanced colorectal cancer, response rates ranged from 25% to 42% *(19,20)*. Toxicity was low, with manageable diarrhea being dose limiting. There was no significant myelosuppression, mucositis, or hand–foot syndrome seen. The compound was found to be safe in the elderly *(21)*. Two phase III trials have been performed in patients with previously untreated metastatic colorectal cancer *(22,23)* (Table 2). To summarize the results, UFT plus oral leucovorin closely simulates the response rate to iv 5-FU and leucovorin given on the daily times five regimen. Importantly however, the toxicity of the oral regimen is significantly less than the intravenous regimen, and the overall patient quality of life was superior. An important fact in reviewing these results is that the response rate seen with iv 5-FU and leucovorin was lower than has been seen in many other randomized trials.

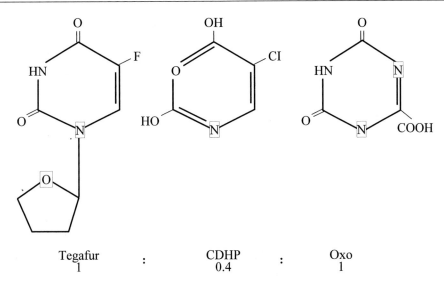

Tegafur   :   CDHP   :   Oxo
1   0.4   1

Fig. 3. Chemical structure of S-1.

4. S-1

S-1 is a another oral antitumor agent composed of Tegafur as in UFT but contains two other compounds, CDHP (5-chloro-2,4-dohydroxypyrimidine) and potassium oxonate (Oxo) in a molar ratio of 1:0.4:1 (Fig. 3). CDHP is a reversible inhibitor of DPD and Oxo inhibits the conversion of UFT to 5-FU in the GI tract, reducing the local GI toxicity *(24)*. The latter two compounds do not have any antitumor activity themselves and act as modulators. Preclinical studies performed showed a higher response rate observed in mice than had been seen previously with other 5-FU-like compounds. S-1 has been shown to exert a potent antitumor effect with low gastrointestinal toxicity in experimental tumor models *(25)*.

On the basis of phase I and early phase II clinical trials, a dose of 80 mg/m/d given in two divided doses after breakfast and supper using a 28-d consecutive oral regimen was recommended *(26,27)*. The dose-limiting toxicities were diarrhea and neutropenia. Pharmacokinetic analysis showed no fluctuations in pharmacokinetics or any drug accumulation *(28)*. Further clinical studies have not been published in manuscript form, but several abstracts have been produced. In one study, a 16% response rate was observed in patients with colorectal cancer treated with 50–75 mg of S-1 twice daily for 28 d followed by a 14-d rest. Many of these patients had received prior therapy *(29)*. A 35% response rate was reported in a second study using a lower dose of 40–60 mg in previously untreated metastatic colorectal cancer *(30)*. Continued development of this compound is underway in Japan, Europe, and the United States.

5. ENILURACIL

Eniluracil is a compound that offers an alternative approach to the inhibition of DPD. This compound is a small molecule that has been shown to be an irreversible inhibitor of DPD *(31)* (Fig. 4). The effects of eniluracil on DPD were demonstrated in an early clinical trial of patients who were scheduled to undergo primary colorectal tumor resection *(32)*. These patients received oral eniluracil 10 mg/m^2 twice daily for 3 d before surgery. Both

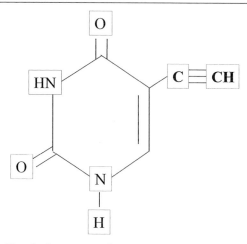

Fig. 4. Chemical structure of eniluracil (5-ethynyluracil, 5-EU).

mononuclear cells and tumor tissue were obtained. Measurements of DPD activity and plasma uracil were obtained as a primary end point. In all patients who received eniluracil, there was no detectable tumor DPD activity recorded when compared to the untreated patients. The same was seen in mononuclear cells. Plasma uracil changed, dramatically increasing over 200 times. This study provided definitive evidence of complete inhibition of DPD in human tumors. In a different approach, to monitor the intratumoral effects of eniluracil, another study was performed utilizing positron-emission tomography (PET) scanning to determine the pharmacokinetics of F-18-labeled fluorouracil *(33)*. In comparison to patients untreated with eniluracil, the treated patients had marked retention of 5-FU in tumors compared to normal liver and other tissues. However, another significant finding of this study was the reduction in uptake in normal liver and kidneys compared with the tumors. This would suggest a selective effect on tumor tissue.

5.1. Clinical Trials of Eniluracil

In an initial phase I study using a 28-d schedule of oral 5-FU administered twice daily in combination with oral eniluracil followed by a 7-d break, the recommended phase II dose of 5-FU was 1 mg/m^2 twice daily with eniluracil 20 mg twice daily *(34)*. Extensive pharmacokinetics were performed as a part of this trial, showing that 5-FU given by this route achieves steady-state levels similar to that with protracted intravenous administration of 5-FU. The phase II study was then performed in patients with metastatic colorectal cancer that were previously untreated or refractory to 5-FU leucovorin *(35)*. They were enrolled in two separate cohorts. Twenty-four patients had not previously received chemotherapy or had received adjuvant chemotherapy > 6 mo prior to enrollment. Fifty-one patients had disease refractory to iv 5-FU leucovorin. The treatment schedule was seven consecutive daily doses of eniluracil 20 mg/d with once daily oral 5-FU given on d 2–6 repeated every 4 wk. One-half of the patients in each cohort also received 50 mg/d of oral leucovorin on d 2–6. The 5-FU dose was 25 mg/m^2 without leucovorin and 20 mg/m^2 when given with leucovorin. Five of the 24 previously untreated patients responded, but no responses were seen in the previously treated group. Fifteen patients did demonstrate stable disease. Only 7% of patients experienced grade 3 diarrhea. Myelosuppression was frequent and dose limiting. Neutropenic sepsis was seen in 13.5% of patients. This study showed the parallel

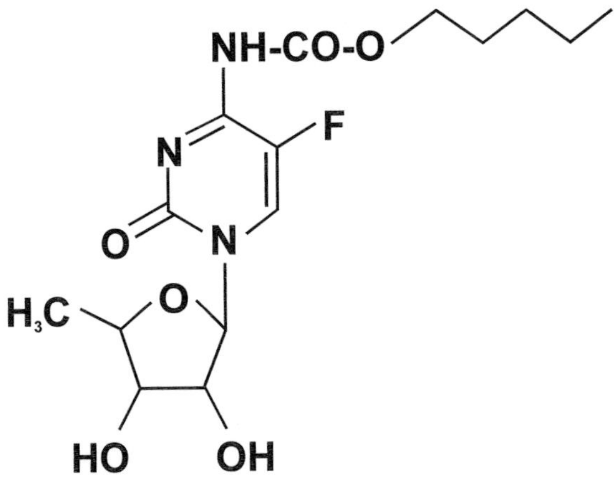

Fig. 5. Chemical structure of capecitabine.

in toxicity and efficacy between this oral regimen given for 5 d and the daily times five iv 5-FU and leucovorin (Mayo Clinic).

In a second phase II trial performed exclusively in untreated, metastatic colon cancer patients and using the 28-d treatment schedule (1.0 or 1.15 mg/m 5-FU) repeated every 5 wk, a 25% partial response rate was achieved with an additional 36% of the patients maintaining stable disease *(36)*. The median duration of progression-free (22.6 wk) and overall survival (59 wk) were comparable to results with iv 5-FU. No difference was observed between the two doses in terms of response, with the 1.15-mg/m dose resulting in slightly higher frequency of hematologic toxicity.

Recently, a phase III trial comparing iv 5-FU and leucovorin to eniluracil and oral 5-FU using the 28-d schedule has completed accrual. The results of this study are critical in the determination of whether this compound gets approval within the United States for use in colon cancer. By not only inhibiting the DPD within the systemic circulation and liver but also within the tumors themselves, it was hoped that this compound would result in improved response rates or other measures of improved clinical outcome. Unfortunately, although incomplete and not published, the preliminary results of this study were negative; namely there was no advantage seen with eniluracil and oral 5-FU as compared to iv 5-FU. Therefore further development of this compound has been stopped.

6. CAPECITABINE

Capecitabine (N^4-pentyloxycarbonyl-5'-deoxy-5-fluorocytidine) is a novel fluoropyrimidine carbamate that is converted to 5-FU selectively in tumors through a cascade of three enzymes *(37)* (Fig. 5). Using rational design and unique tissue localization patterns of key enzymes, capecitabine was developed to be selectively activated within tumor tissues. Capecitabine is absorbed unchanged through the gastrointestinal tract and is metabolized in the liver to 5'-deoxy-5-fluorocytidine (5'-DFCR) by a carboxylesterase. It is then converted to doxifluridine (5'-DFUR) by a cytidine deaminase found in high concentrations in the liver and various types of solid tumors. Finally, it is converted from 5'-DFUR to 5-FU by thymidine phosphorylase, which was known to be markedly elevated in tumor tissues as compared to normal tissues (Fig. 6). The intermediate metabolites do not have significant cytotoxicity and, therefore, 5-FU is the dominant cytotoxic species. This design was

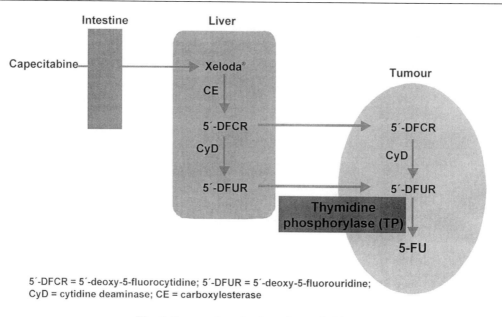

5´-DFCR = 5´-deoxy-5-fluorocytidine; 5´-DFUR = 5´-deoxy-5-fluorouridine;
CyD = cytidine deaminase; CE = carboxylesterase

Fig. 6. Enzymatic activation of capecitabine.

undertaken to improve the safety profile of 5-FU, to allow for oral bioavailability of the drug and possibly allow for an increased tumor efficacy based on selective delivery of the drug *(38)*.

Preclinical studies have demonstrated significant activity of capecitabine in both 5-FU-sensitive and 5-FU-resistant tumors *(39)*. A study was performed that investigated tissue localization of the three enzymes in humans as well as the selective activation of the compound to 5-FU *(40)*. In this study, 19 patients requiring surgical resection of either their primary colon tumor or colon cancer metastases to the liver received 1255 mg/m^2 of capecitabine twice daily orally for 5–7 d prior to surgery. On the day of surgery, samples of tumor tissue, adjacent healthy tissue, and blood samples were collected from each patient 2–12 h after the last dose of capecitabine had been administered. These tissues were then analyzed using high-performance liquid chromatography (HPLC) for the concentration of 5-FU. In addition, the activities of key enzymes, including thymidine phosphorylase and DPD, were measured. The results showed consistent upregulation of thymidine phosphorylase in colorectal tumor tissue as compared to adjacent normal tissue. The one exception to this was within the liver where thymidine phosphorylase levels were roughly equivalent to metastatic tumor. On average, the level of 5-FU in the tumor was 3.2 times higher than in the adjacent healthy tissue in primary colorectal tumors but only 1.4 times higher in metastases. The mean tissue to plasma 5-FU concentration ratios exceeded 20 for colorectal tumors and ranged from 8 to 10 for other tissues (Fig. 7). This study, performed in humans, documents the selective activation of capecitabine in patients with colorectal cancer.

6.1. Clinical Trials of Capecitabine

A series of phase I studies were performed using this compound in patients with advanced metastatic cancer. In one study, capecitabine was administered twice daily as an outpatient for 2 wk in a row followed by 1 wk of rest *(41)*. Thirty-four patients with solid tumors were enrolled. The result showed that at a dose of 2510 mg/m^2 daily toxicity was acceptable. Dose-

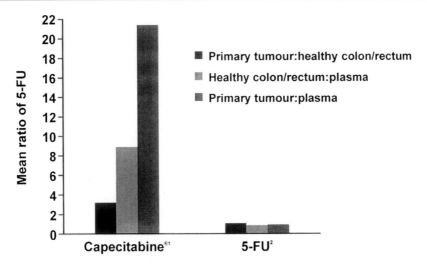

'Schüller J et al. Cancer Chemother Pharmacol 2000 (in press)
'Kovach JS, Beart RW Jr. Invest New Drugs 1989;7:13–25

Fig. 7. Mean ratios of 5-FU concentrations following administration of capecitabine and 5-FU in humans. Data for capecitabine from Schüller J, et al. *Cancer Chemother. Pharmacol.* (2000), in press. Data for 5-FU from Kovach JS and Beart RW Jr. *Invest. New Drugs,* **7** (1999) 13–25.

limiting toxicities of diarrhea abdominal pain and leukopenia were observed. Palmar–plantar erythrodyesthesia (hand–foot syndrome) was observed at the higher dose levels in patients after prolonged treatment. Objective tumor responses were observed. The recommended phase II dose for the schedule was 2510 mg/m divided into two doses administered daily for 14 d with 1 wk off. A second phase I trial sought to define the toxicity profile of capecitabine in combination with leucovorin *(42)*. The same basic treatment schedule was used with a 2-wk period of treatment followed by 1 wk of rest. The dose-limiting toxicities of diarrhea, nausea, vomiting, and hand–foot syndrome were observed at doses above 2000 mg/m/d, making the recommended phase II dose 1650 mg/m/d of capecitabine plus 60 mg/d of leucovorin. Pharmacokinetics showed rapid GI absorption and conversion to the active drug. Leucovorin had no effect on the pharmacokinetics of capecitabine. Clinical responses were likewise seen. In a third trial, the impact of food on the absorption and metabolism of capecitabine was investigated and found to play a significant role. The recommendation is to take the medicine with food, as was done in the trials, but the absence of food may, in fact, increase the absorption of capecitabine, altering its clinical profile *(43)*.

In order to determine the optimum dose and schedule to take on to more definitive testing a phase II randomized trial was performed comparing three different schedules of capecitabine in patients with previously untreated advanced colorectal cancer *(44)*. The three schedules were (1) 1331 mg/m^2/d continuously, (2) 2510 mg/m/d, 2 wk on and 1 wk off, and (3) 1675 mg/m^2/d plus oral leucovorin 60 mg/d two wk on and 1 wk off. One hundred nine patients were randomized on this study, with equal distribution among the three arms. The greatest toxicity was observed in the arm with capecitabine plus leucovorin, with an increase in diarrhea and hand–foot syndrome. Tumor responses were seen in all three arms. The intermittent single-agent schedule was proposed for phase III evaluation (arm 2) based on the higher-dose intensity, the slightly superior response rate and time to progression, and overall acceptable toxicity.

Two phase III studies have been performed in patients with previously untreated metastatic colorectal cancer comparing capecitabine 2500 mg/m/d, 2 wk on and 1 wk off, to the 5-FU

Table 3
Phase III Results of Capecitabine vs 5-FU/Leucovorin

	Capecitabine	*5-FU/Leucovorin*
No. of patients	602	602
Dose	2500 mg/m bid 14 d on 7 d off	425 mg/m 5-FU + 20 mg/m LV d 1–5 q 28 d
Response rates	24.8%[b] (25.5%)[b] "North	15.5% (111.6%) "North
Investigator (IRR[a])	American" study 26.6%[b] (18.9%) "Europe/Australia" study	American" study 17.9% (15%) "Europe/Australia" study
Survival	No difference	
Toxicity	Significantly less neutropenia, diarrhea, mucositis	Significantly less hand–foot syndrome

[a]IRR = independent radiology review.
[b]Statistically significant.

iv 425 mg/m and 20 mg/m leucovorin daily × 5 (Mayo Clinic regimen). One study was performed primarily in North America (United States, Canada, Mexico, and Brazil) *(45)* and the other study was performed in Europe, Israel, Australia, and Taiwan *(46)*. Both studies were designed in an identical fashion, with 602 patients accrued to each study. Patients were randomized to receive either capecitabine or iv 5-FU with leucovorin. All patients were diagnosed with previously untreated metastatic colorectal cancer or had received adjuvant chemotherapy at least 12 mo previously (Table 3). Two different responses were reported: those of the investigators who were treating the patients and those of an independent review committee who reviewed the scans in a blinded fashion. It is important to note that although there was a significant improvement in response rates with capecitabine, there was no difference in time to progression or overall survival between the two arms. The toxicity that was observed was an increase in hand–foot syndrome in patients treated with capecitabine, but a significant reduction in fever/neutropenia, diarrhea, and mucositis when compared to iv 5-FU. The time to onset of grade 3 and 4 toxicities was later with capecitabine compared to iv 5-FU leucovorin. Based on the data from these two trials, this compound is likely to become approved for front-line usage in metastatic colorectal cancer.

Currently, several clinical trials are ongoing to define the role of capecitabine in combination with other chemotherapeutic agents such as CPT-11 and oxaliplatin. Combination trials of capecitabine in radiation therapy are ongoing. Trials utilizing capecitabine in the adjuvant setting are planned.

7. COMPARING ORAL TO INTRAVENOUS 5-FU

The clinical studies that have been performed so far suggests that oral fluoropyrimidines are equally active in patients with metastatic colorectal cancer when compared to iv 5-FU and leucovorin. The trials with UFT and leucovorin suggest equivalance to iv 5-FU and leucovorin, whereas capecitabine appears to result in a higher response rate. No trial of an oral agent has yet shown an improvement in survival compared to iv 5-FU. Therefore, the primary motivation for changing to an oral agent would be patient convenience and lower toxicity profile. The clinical trials that have been performed to date confirm the improvement in toxicity profile as well as patient acceptance. A more widespread usage of oral fluoropyrimidines is inevitable.

Although outside the scope of this chapter, reimbursement for oral chemotherapeutic agents has become a significant hurdle for their wider application. It is clear that physicians and their staff will play a central role in patient education and follow-up when patients are on home-based oral therapies *(47)*. Currently, there is no mechanism for physicians to be reimbursed for this service, creating in some areas a disincentive for the use of these more "patient-friendly" therapies. Significant effort is required to ensure an improved mechanism of reimbursement for these compounds as they become more widely available.

8. ORAL FLUOROPYRIMIDINES IN COMBINATION THERAPY

Several clinical trials have now been performed that support the role of infusional 5-FU in combination with radiation therapy as being superior to bolus dosing *(48)*. This is logical, as the 5-FU half-life is extremely short and the opportunity for synergy with radiation is greater when protracted infusion is used. It also may allow for less toxicity. Therefore, it is likely that the use of oral fluoropyrimidines would further simplify and improve this process.

To date, there have only been a limited number of published studies combining oral fluoropyrimidines with radiation therapy. The two compounds that have been in clinical trial included UFT with leucovorin *(49)* and capecitabine. A study has been published of UFT combined with radiation in pancreatic cancer *(50)* and there are several ongoing studies combining this drug with radiation in preoperative and postoperative rectal cancer. The results of these latter studies are not available. The pancreatic cancer study showed this combination to be safe and well-tolerated without significant toxicity. The recommended dose of 300 mg/m three times daily combined with leucovorin was associated with very limited toxicity. Given the fact that UFT is a direct precursor of 5-FU and requires very little activation, it is not surprising that these results appear similar to what one could achieve with intravenous protracted infusion 5-FU. On the other hand, capecitabine requires more significant metabolic activation and relies on thymidine phosphorylase to convert it to 5-FU. In fact, a preclinical study demonstrated that radiation enhanced the activity of thymidine phosphorylase in tumor tissues as compared to normal surrounding tissues, suggesting that this may further improve the therapeutic index of capecitabine when given in combination with radiation *(51)*. Clinical trials are ongoing in a variety of settings combining capecitabine with radiation but have not yet been published. The results from these trials are eagerly awaited.

As with radiation, multiple trials are currently ongoing combining oral fluoropyrimidines with other cytotoxic chemotherapeutic agents such as CPT-11, oxaliplatin, gemcitabine, docetaxel, and others. Trials have only been published in abstract form but suggest a high level of tolerability with these combinations without significant impact on pharmacokinetics.

9. ADJUVANT THERAPY

The use of oral fluoropyrimidines has been limited primarily to patients with metastatic disease where they have shown at least equivalence to iv 5-FU in efficacy with significantly less toxicity. The logical next step would be to consider these compounds in the adjuvant setting. Clinical trials comparing iv 5-FU and leucovorin to capecitabine and UFT plus leucovorin are under way. In order to gain approval for adjuvant therapy, these trials must confirm at least equivalent survival outcomes compared to iv 5-FU. As capecitabine requires metabolic activation, it is possible that certain clones of metastatic disease will not overexpress thymidine phosphorylase, creating a selective survival advantage for these cells that would not be seen with intravenous 5-FU or UFT. Although this scenario is unlikely, the trial results will be critical to confirm the equivalency of these compounds. If proven effective, this would be a clear advantage with regard to patient toxicity and overall quality of life in the adjuvant setting. Trials of CPT-11 and oxaliplatin in the adjuvant setting are further complicating the development of the oral fluoropyrimidines in the adjuvant setting. With so many new agents proving useful in colorectal cancer, it is difficult to know what the standard of care for adjuvant therapy will become. However, one would predict that it would include a combination of an oral fluoropyrimidine with CPT-11 and/or oxaliplatin. Participation in clinical trials is essential to move this field forward as quickly as possible.

10. CONCLUSIONS

Oral fluoropyrimidines represent an extremely exciting advance in the management of colorectal cancer as well as other malignancies. There are at least two new agents with great potential for use, each having a slightly different mechanism of action and, therefore, possibly different clinical efficacy and toxicity profile. Understanding the distinctions between the compounds is important when deciding on which to use in various clinical scenarios. It is important to recognize that these compounds have not yet resulted in a survival advantage for patients with metastatic colorectal cancer but may be superior in the adjuvant setting or in other combination settings. They do have a significantly lower toxicity profile. A significant amount of clinical work still needs to be performed in order to more clearly establish the specific roles of these compounds in the standard practice and management of cancer patients. However, it appears certain that these compounds will replace iv 5-FU in most clinical scenarios. Insurers, patients, and oncology practices must adapt to the changing therapies with the interest of patients and patient comfort coming first.

REFERENCES

1. Leichman CG, Fleming TR, Muggia FM, et al. Phase II study of fluorouracil and its modulation in advanced colorectal cancer: a Southwest Oncology Group study [see comments]. *J. Clin. Oncol.*, **13** (1995) 1303–1311.
2. Mayer RJ. Chemotherapy for metastatic colorectal cancer. *Cancer*, **70** (1992) 1414–1424.
3. Buyse M, Carlson RW, and Piedbois P. Meta-analyses of published results are unreliable [letter; comment]. *J. Clin. Oncol.*, **17** (1999) 1646–1647.
4. Cancer Meta-analysis group. Toxicity of fluorouracil in patients with advanced colorectal cancer: effect of administration schedule and prognostic factors. *J. Clin. Oncol.*, **16** (1998) 3537–3541.
5. Liu G, Franssen E, Fitch MI, et al. Patient preferences for oral versus intravenous palliative chemotherapy. *J. Clin. Oncol.*, **15** (1997) 110–115.
6. Beck A, Etienne MC, Cheradame S, et al. A role for dihydropyrimidine dehydrogenase and thymidylate synthase in tumour sensitivity to fluorouracil [see comments]. *Eur. J. Cancer*, **10** (1994) 1517–1522.
7. Heggie GD, Sommadossi JP, Cross DS, et al. Clinical pharmacokinetics of 5-fluorouracil and its metabolites in plasma, urine, and bile. *Cancer Res.*, **47** (1987) 2203–2206.
8. Diasio RB and Lu Z. Dihydropyrimidine dehydrogenase activity and fluorouracil chemotherapy [editorial; comment]. *J. Clin. Oncol.*, **12** (1994) 2239–2242.
9. Diasio RB, Van Kuilenburg AB, Lu Z, et al. Determination of dihydropyrimidine dehydrogenase (DPD) in fibroblasts of a DPD deficient pediatric patient and family members using a polyclonal antibody to human DPD. *Adv. Exp. Med. Biol.*, **370** (1994) 7–10.
10. Takimoto CH, Lu ZH, Zhang R, et al. Severe neurotoxicity following 5-fluorouracil-based chemotherapy in a patient with dihydropyrimidine dehydrogenase deficiency. *Clin. Cancer Res.*, **2** (1996) 477–481.
11. Friedman MA and Ignoffo RJ. A review of the United States clinical experience of the fluoropyrimidine, ftorafur (NSC-148958). *Cancer Treat. Rev.*, **7** (1980) 205–213.
12. Damjanov N and Meropol NJ. Oral therapy for colorectal cancer: how to choose [in process citation]. *Oncology (Huntingt.)*, **14** (2000) 799–807; discussion 807–820.

13. Taguchi T. UFT: biochemical modulation for 5-fluorouracil (5-FU). *Chin. Med. J. (Engl.)*, **110** (1997) 294–296.
14. Taguchi T. Clinical application of biochemical modulation in cancer chemotherapy: biochemical modulation for 5-FU. *Oncology*, **54** (1997) 12–18.
15. Nakazato H, Koike A, and Suzuki H. Efficacy of oral UFT as adjuvant chemotherapy to curative resection of colorectal cancer: a prospective randomized clinical trial. *Proc. Am. Assoc. Clin. Oncol.*, **16** (1997) 279a.
16. Anonymous. Modulation of fluorouracil by leucovorin in patients with advanced colorectal cancer: evidence in terms of response rate. Advanced Colorectal Cancer Meta-Analysis Project [see comments]. *J. Clin. Oncol.*, **10** (1992) 896–903.
17. Pazdur R, Lassere Y, Diaz-Canton E, et al. Phase I trials of uracil–tegafur (UFT) using 5 and 28 day administration schedules: demonstration of schedule-dependent toxicities. *Anticancer Drugs*, 7 (1996) 728–733.
18. Meropol NJ, Rustum YM, Petrelli NJ, et al. A phase I and pharmacokinetic study of oral uracil, ftorafur, and leucovorin in patients with advanced cancer. *Cancer Chemother. Pharmacol.*, **37** (1996) 581–586.
19. Pazdur R. Phase II study of UFT plus leucovorin in colorectal cancer. *Oncology*, **54** (1997) 19–23.
20. Pazdur R, Lassere Y, Rhodes V, et al. Phase II trial of uracil and tegafur plus oral leucovorin: an effective oral regimen in the treatment of metastatic colorectal carcinoma. *J. Clin. Oncol.*, **12** (1994) 2296–2300.
21. Diaz-Rubio E, Sastre J, Abad A, et al. UFT plus or minus calcium folinate for metastatic colorectal cancer in older patients. *Oncology (Huntingt.)*, **13** (1999) 35–40.
22. Carmichael J, Popiela T, Radstone D, et al. Randomized comparative study of ORZEL® (oral uracil/tegafur (UFTTM) plus leucovorin (LV)) versus parenteral 5-fluorouracil (5-FU) plus LV in patients with metastatic colorectal cancer. *Proc. Am. Assoc. Clin. Oncol.*, **18** (1999) 1015.
23. Pazdur R, Douillard J, Skillings J, et al. Multicenter phase III study of 5-fluorouracil (5-FU) or UFTTM in combination with leucovorin (LV) in patients with metastatic colorectal cancer. *Proc. Am. Assoc. Clin. Oncol.*, **18** (1999) 1009.
24. Shirasaka T, Shimamoto Y, and Fukushima M. Inhibition by oxonic acid of gastrointestinal toxicity of 5-fluorouracil without loss of its antitumor activity in rats. *Cancer Res.*, **53** (1993) 4004–4009.
25. Takechi T, Nakano K, Uchida J, et al. Antitumor activity and low intestinal toxicity of S-1, a new formulation of oral tegafur, in experimental tumor models in rats. *Cancer Chemother. Pharmacol.*, **39** (1997) 205–211.
26. Hirata K, Horikoshi N, Aiba K, et al. Pharmacokinetic study of S-1, a novel oral fluorouracil antitumor drug. *Clin. Cancer Res.*, **5** (1999) 2000–2005.
27. Hoff P, Wenske C, Medgyesy D, et al. Phase I and pharmacokinetic (PK) study of the novel oral fluoropyrimidine, S-1. *Proc. Am. Assoc. Clin. Oncol.*, **18** (1999) 665.
28. Peters G, Van Groeningen C, and Schomage J. Phase I clinical and pharmacokinetic study of S-1, an oral 5-fluorouracil-based antineoplastic agent. *Proc. Am. Assoc. Clin. Oncol.*, **16** (1997) 227.
29. Horikoshi N, Mitachi Y, and Sakata Y. S-1, new oral fluoropyrimidine is very active in patients with advanced gastric cancer (early phase II study). *Proc. Am. Assoc. Clin. Oncol.*, **15** (1996) 466.
30. Baba H, Ohtsu A, and Sakata Y. Late phase II study of S-1 in patients with advanced colorectal cancer in Japan. *Proc. Am. Assoc. Clin. Oncol.*, **17** (1998) 206.
31. Saleem A, Abaogye E, and Yap J. In vivo modulation of 5-fluorouracil pharmacokinetics by eniluracil: an inactivator of dihydopyrimidine dehydrogenase. *Br. J. Cancer*, **80** (1999) 94.
32. Ahmed FY, Johnston SJ, Cassidy J, et al: Eniluracil treatment completely inactivates dihydropyrimidine dehydrogenase in colorectal tumors. *J. Clin. Oncol.*, **17** (1999) 2439–2245.
33. Saleem A, Yap J, Osman S, et al. Modulation of fluorouracil tissue pharmacokinetics by eniluracil: in-vivo imaging of drug action. *Lancet*, **355** (2000) 2125–2131.
34. Baker SD, Diasio RB, O'Reilly S, et al. Phase I and pharmacologic study of oral fluorouracil on a chronic daily schedule in combination with the dihydropyrimidine dehydrogenase inactivator eniluracil. *J. Clin. Oncol.*, **18** (2000) 915–926.
35. Schilsky RL, Bukowski R, Burris H III, et al. A multicenter phase II study of a five-day regimen of oral 5- fluorouracil plus eniluracil with or without leucovorin in patients with metastatic colorectal cancer [in process citation]. *Ann. Oncol.*, **11** (2000) 415–420.
36. Mani S, Hochster H, Beck T, et al: Multicenter phase II study to evaluate a 28-day regimen of oral fluorouracil plus eniluracil in the treatment of patients with previously untreated metastatic colorectal cancer. *J. Clin. Oncol.*, **18** (2000) 2894–2901.
37. Miwa M, Ura M, Nishida M, et al. Design of a novel oral fluoropyrimidine carbamate, capecitabine, which generates 5-fluorouracil selectively in tumours by enzymes concentrated in human liver and cancer tissue. *Eur. J. Cancer*, **34** (1998) 1274–1281.
38. Verweij J. Rational design of new tumoractivated cytotoxic agents. *Oncology*, **57(Suppl. 1)** (1999) 9–15.
39. Ishikawa T, Utoh M, Sawada N, et al. Tumor selective delivery of 5-fluorouracil by capecitabine, a new oral fluoropyrimidine carbamate, in human cancer xenografts. *Biochem. Pharmacol.*, **55** (1998) 1091–1097.

40. Schuller J, Cassidy J, Dumont E, et al. Preferential activation of capecitabine in tumor following oral administration to colorectal cancer patients. *Cancer Chemother. Pharmacol.*, **45** (2000) 291–297.
41. Mackean M, Planting A, Twelves C, et al. Phase I and pharmacologic study of intermittent twice-daily oral therapy with capecitabine in patients with advanced and/or metastatic cancer. *J. Clin. Oncol.*, **16** (1998) 2977–2985.
42. Cassidy J, Dirix L, Bissett D, et al. A Phase I study of capecitabine in combination with oral leucovorin in patients with intractable solid tumors. *Clin. Cancer Res.*, **4** (1998) 2755–2761.
43. Reigner B, Verweij J, Dirix L, et al. Effect of food on the pharmacokinetics of capecitabine and its metabolites following oral administration in cancer patients. *Clin. Cancer Res.*, **4** (1998) 941–948.
44. Van Cutsem E, Findlay M, Osterwalder B, et al. Capecitabine, an oral fluoropyrimidine carbamate with substantial activity in advanced colorectal cancer: results of a randomized phase II study. *J. Clin. Oncol.*, **18** (2000) 1337–1345.
45. Cox J, Pazdur R, Thibault A, et al. A phase III trial of XELODA™ (capecitabine) in previously untreated advanced/metastatic colorectal cancer. *Proc. Am. Assoc. Clin. Oncol.*, **18** (1999) 1016.
46. Twelves C, Harper P, Van Cutsem E, et al. A phase III trial (SO14796) of Xeloda™ (capecitabine) in previously untreated advanced/metastatic colorectal cancer. *Proc. Am. Assoc. Clin. Oncol.*, **18** (1999) 1010.
47. Mrozek-Orlowski ME, Frye DK, and Sanborn HM. Capecitabine: nursing implications of a new oral chemotherapeutic agent. *Oncol. Nurs. Forum*, **26** (1999) 753–762.
48. O'Connell MJ, Martenson JA, Wieand HS, et al. Improving adjuvant therapy for rectal cancer by combining protracted- infusion fluorouracil with radiation therapy after curative surgery. *N. Engl. J. Med.*, **331** (1994) 502–507.
49. Hoffmann W, Schiebe M, Dethling J, et al. UFT plus calcium folinate plus radiotherapy for recurrent rectal cancer. *Oncology (Huntingt.)*, **13** (1999) 125–126.
50. Childs HA III, Spencer SA, Raben D, et al. A phase I study of combined UFT plus leucovorin and radiotherapy for pancreatic cancer. *Int. J. Radiat. Oncol. Biol. Phys.*, **47** (2000) 939–944.
51. Sawada N, Ishikawa T, Sekiguchi F, et al. X-ray irradiation induces thymidine phosphorylase and enhances the efficacy of capecitabine (Xeloda) in human cancer xenografts. *Clin. Cancer Res.*, **5** (1999) 2948–2953.

28 Irinotecan in the Treatment of Colorectal Cancer

Leonard B. Saltz

Contents

1. INTRODUCTION

Irinotecan, also known as CPT-11, is a semisynthetic derivative of the plant alkaloid camptothecin. The antitumor activity of the camptothecin derivatives is accomplished via inhibition of the nuclear enzyme topoisomerase I (topo I). Topo I facilitates DNA uncoiling for replication and transcription by binding to DNA and causing reversible single-stranded DNA breaks (1). Under normal circumstances, these single-stranded breaks are transient and readily reversible. However, in the presence of irinotecan or its active metabolite, SN-38 (2), these single-stranded breaks are stabilized and potentiated. This stabilization is also reversible and nonlethal. However, if a replication fork collides with one of these stabilized single-stranded breaks, double-stranded breaks and DNA fragmentation occurs, leading to cell death (3).

Phase I clinical trials were first begun in Japan, where the compound was initially synthesized (4,5). Subsequently, phase I development was also initiated in the United States (6,7) and France (8). Because antitumor activity was demonstrated in these early phase I trials in advanced, treatment-refractory colorectal cancer, an extensive worldwide development program of irinotecan in this disease was launched.

From: *Colorectal Cancer: Multimodality Management*
Edited by: L. Saltz © Humana Press Inc., Totowa, NJ

2. IRINOTECAN AS A SINGLE AGENT IN COLORECTAL CANCER

The first phase II study of irinotecan in patients with metastatic colorectal cancer was reported by Shimada et al. *(9)*. In this trial, 81% of the patients had fluorouracil-refractory disease. A major objective response rate of 22% was seen in these treatment-refractory patients. Of the relatively small number of chemotherapy-naive patients treated, 27% responded. A confirmatory trial in patients with fluorouracil-refractory disease was conducted in the United States. In this trial involving 43 patients with fluorouracil-refractory colorectal cancer, a major objective response rate of 23% was observed *(10)*. An additional 31% of patients on this therapy achieved either a minor clinical regression or stable disease, bringing the population of patients who experienced some antitumor activity on this trial to 54%. At about the same time, a trial in colorectal cancer patients conducted in France utilizing a 350-mg/m^2 starting dose once every 3 wk reported results for 165 fluorouracil-refractory patients and 48 chemotherapy-naive patients *(11)*. The response rate on this trial was 18% for both chemotherapy-naive and fluorouracil-refractory patients.

The results of three trials of nearly identical design, all conducted within the United States and inclusive of the above-described American trial *(10)*, were subsequently combined for analysis, resulting in a dataset of 304 fluorouracil-refractory colorectal cancer patients *(12)*. The major objective response rate in this pooled analysis was 13%, with an additional 49% of patients achieving either a minor response or stabile disease. These pooled phase II data led to the initial provisional registration of irinotecan in the United States for the treatment of fluorouracil-refractory colorectal cancer.

The confirmatory evidence of the usefulness of irinotecan in fluorouracil-refractory disease was provided by two randomized trials conducted primarily in Europe. In a trial conducted largely in those countries where best supportive care (BSC) was the routine standard practice for fluorouracil-refractory colorectal cancer, patients were randomized to receive either BSC alone or BSC plus irinotecan *(13)*. Overall survival was the primary end point of this study. The median overall survival for the irinotecan group was modestly superior by approx 3 mo. This difference was statistically significant. The chance of a patient being alive 1 yr after randomization was 36% for those patients receiving irinotecan, and this was 2.5 times greater in the irinotecan-treated group. Furthermore, formal quality-of-life measurements, as assessed using the EORTC QLQ-C30 questionnaire, showed superior quality-of-life measurements for the irinotecan-treated patients vs those receiving BSC.

In a parallel trial conducted in areas of Europe where an infusional fluorouracil regimen was the routine standard second-line therapy for colorectal cancer, 5-fluorouracil (5-FU)-refractory colorectal cancer patients were randomized to receive an infusional fluorouracil regimen vs irinotecan *(14)*. Again, there was a modest survival advantage for the irinotecan group and this difference was statistically significant. One-year survival for the irinotecan-treated patients was 1.4 times that of the infusion 5-FU group. Quality-of-life data were similar for both groups.

3. FIRST-LINE IRINOTECAN AS A SINGLE AGENT

Most of the early development of irinotecan focused on single-agent use as a salvage therapy for fluorouracil-refractory disease. However, phase II studies of single-agent irinotecan in chemotherapy-naive patients with metastatic colorectal cancer were also performed in the United States. At Memorial Sloan-Kettering Cancer Center, 41 patients received a starting dose of 125 mg/m^2 of irinotecan weekly for 4 wk, followed by a 2-wk break *(15)*. Major objective responses were observed in 13 patients (32%, 95% confidence interval [CI] = 18–46%), and an additional 44% of patients demonstrated some lesser degree of antitumor activity (minor response or stable disease). Median duration of response was 8 mo and the median survival was 12 mo. Diarrhea and neutropenia were found to be the major dose-limiting toxicities. In this trial, diarrhea was largely controlled when strict use of aggressive loperamide support was instituted, based on work reported from France that demonstrated the utility of an intensive loperamide-based antidiarrheal regimen for the management of irinotecan-induced late-onset diarrhea *(16,17)*.

Concurrent with the Memorial Sloan-Kettering study, a trial was also conducted at the Mayo Clinic, using the same entry criteria and treatment regimen. Very similar results were reported, with major objective responses seen in 8 of 31 patients (26%, 95% CI = 12–45%). In this trial as well, a median duration of response of 8 mo and a median survival of 12 mo was reported *(18)*.

Thus, by the mid-1990s, three independent trials had been able to demonstrate that irinotecan was active as a single agent in the first-line treatment of metastatic colorectal cancer *(11,15,18)*. Response rates, however, did not appear to be substantially different from those achievable with then-standard fluorouracil-based treatments, and survival appeared to be similar to historical controls as well. For this reason, there was little enthusiasm for use of irinotecan as a single agent in first-line treatment *(19)*. Efforts were therefore turned to the development of irinotecan plus fluorouracil combinations for the first-line treatment of metastatic colorectal cancer.

4. TOXICITY OF IRINOTECAN

Diarrhea and neutropenia are the most common dose-limiting toxicities of irinotecan. To put the incidence and severity of these toxicities in proper perspective, it is best to evaluate them in comparison with the toxicities of other chemotherapy regimens used in the treatment of colorectal cancer. Diarrhea, neutropenia, and mucositis are the most common dose-limiting toxicities with 5-FU, and the toxicities of 5-FU-based regimens have been widely reported *(20)*. Recognizing that these are nonrandomized comparisons of toxicity data for both irinotecan and fluorouracil/leucovorin, the comparison can still provide a useful barometer.

The overall incidence of dose-limiting diarrhea in the initial trial of chemotherapy-naive patients from Memorial Sloan–Kettering was 29% *(15)*. Of 193 fluorouracil-refractory patients who received the 125-mg/m^2 starting dose of irinotecan, 34% developed grade 3–4 diarrhea *(12)*. By comparison, the incidence of severe diarrhea in fluorouracil-based treatments in similar patient populations does not appear to be substantially different. The North Central Cancer Treatment Group (NCCTG) reported a large, multicenter phase III trial of the two most widely used schedules (in the United States) of fluorouracil plus leucovorin in chemotherapy-naive colorectal cancer patients *(20)*. In this trial, dose-limiting diarrhea occurred in 32% of patients receiving weekly fluorouracil plus high-dose leucovorin (LV) and in 20% of patients receiving daily × 5 low-dose leucovorin. Similar toxicity rates were reported for these 5-FU/LV regimens in another large multicenter study *(21)*.

Much of the early data regarding irinotecan toxicity was generated during the initial development phase of the drug. There have been two major changes in clinical practice that have occurred since the earlier clinical trials of irinotecan that can be expected to reduced the incidence of severe diarrhea. One change is that clinicians have by now developed extensive experience with irinotecan. This presumably will lead to greater familiarity with the toxicity profile of the drug. Clinicians are now better at picking up early signs of gastrointestinal toxicity and adjusting doses accordingly, and this would be expected to improve the safety profile of the drug. Another important change is the widespread use of intensive loperamide at the first signs of diarrhea. Use of loperamide early in the development of diarrhea and for extended periods of time is now widely recognized as a necessary supportive measure with irinotecan administration *(16)*. Given these changes, it is likely that the above-referenced studies indicate a higher rate of diarrhea than might be anticipated today.

Neutropenia is the other major dose-limiting toxicity of irinotecan; however, this was rarely a major clinical problem in the single-agent trials. In the Memorial Sloan–Kettering single-agent, first-line trial, three patients (7%) experienced grade 4 neutropenia *(15)*. Only one patient (2%) developed neutropenic fever. In the Mayo Clinic study of 31 chemotherapy-naive patients, 9% developed grade 4 neutropenia and 3% experienced neutropenic fevers *(18)*. In the pooled analysis of 304 phase II fluorouracil-refractory colorectal cancer patients, grade 4 neutropenia was seen in 12% of patients, and 3% developed neutropenic fever. One treatment-related death (0.3%), which was the result of neutropenic sepsis, occurred in the 304 5-FU-refractory patients. This death rate compares favorably with the treatment-related mortality of 7 deaths out of 372 patients (1.9%) *(21)* and 8 deaths out of 620 patients (1.3%) *(22)* reported in two large multicenter trials of fluorouracil-based chemotherapy in first-line colorectal cancer patients.

In a three-arm randomized North American trial discussed in more detail below, the primary objective was to evaluate the combination of irinotecan/fluorouracil/leucovorin *(22)*. However, this study contained a standard fluorouracil/leucovorin arm and an irinotecan-alone arm. It therefore provides the first direct randomized comparison between single-agent irinotecan and a standard 5-FU/LV regimen. Although grade 3 and 4 diarrhea were more frequent with irinotecan, grade 4 neutropenia, neutropenic fevers, and grade 3 mucositis were all more severe with the standard (Mayo Clinic schedule) 5-FU/LV regimen. The overall incidence of dose-limiting toxicity was similar between fluorouracil/leucovorin and irinotecan, and treatment-related deaths occurred in 1% of patients on each of these treatments. Thus, although the patterns of toxicity were somewhat different, the overall degree of toxicity experienced by patients with either fluorouracil/leucovorin or with irinotecan was similar.

5. SINGLE-AGENT SCHEDULES

Irinotecan has been developed on a number of different schedules. One hundred twenty-five milligrams per square meter weekly for 4 wk followed by a 2-wk rest and 350 mg/m^2 once every 3 wk have been the most widely studied. Although many different schedules have been studied, a remarkable consistency of results has been seen between these, both in terms of efficacy and toxicity, although it must be remembered that comparison of different phase II trials is necessarily inaccurate. Thus far, there have been no adequately powered studies that provide a randomized direct comparison of different irinotecan administration schedules, and no data are available to suggest superiority of any one irinotecan administration schedule over another. At this time, it would appear that irinotecan is not a particularly schedule-dependent drug.

6. IRINOTECAN/FLUOROURACIL COMBINATIONS

The activity of irinotecan in fluorouracil-refractory disease suggested that the concurrent first-line administration of irinotecan and fluorouracil might provide a regimen with superior antitumor activity, if such a regimen were tolerable. Several groups of investigators therefore designed and conducted phase I studies of the combination of irinotecan and fluorouracil.

Irinotecan	125 mg/m^2	90 min iv infusion
Leucovorin	20 mg/m^2	iv bolus
Fluorouracil	500 mg/m^2	iv bolus

Fig. 1. Weekly bolus administration schedule of irinotecan, leucovorin, and fluorouracil. All drugs given weekly × 4, repeated every 6 wk. (Adapted from ref. *23*.)

At the time that these combinations were being developed, far less was known about the toxicities and schedule dependence (or lack thereof) of irinotecan than of fluorouracil. For this reason, our group at Memorial Sloan–Kettering Cancer Center chose to use the schedule of irinotecan that had been selected for initial development in North America, which was a weekly bolus regimen on a 4-wk on, 2-wk off schedule, and to add fluorouracil and leucovorin to this 6-wk schedule. Because of concerns about possible overlapping gastrointestinal toxicity (especially diarrhea), a low dose of leucovorin was selected, as low-dose leucovorin regimens had been shown to have a lower incidence of diarrhea than high-dose leucovorin regimens.

A phase I trial was conducted in which escalating doses of fluorouracil were added to fixed doses of irinotecan and leucovorin. The end result was a regimen that utilized full-dose (125 mg/m^2) weekly irinotecan with 500 mg/m^2 fluorouracil and 20 mg/m^2 leucovorin, with all drugs given weekly for 4 consecutive weeks followed by a 2-wk break (Fig. 1) *(23)*. Pharmacokinetic studies were performed in this trial to look at levels of irinotecan and SN-38, as well as the glucuronidated (inactivated) SN-38 levels, when patients were given either irinotecan alone (d 1 of cycle 1 only) or irinotecan plus fluorouracil and leucovorin. Thus, each patient served as his/her own internal control for these pharmacokinetic studies. The results indicated conclusively that there was no substantial pharmacokinetic effect of fluorouracil on the metabolism of irinotecan to SN-38 or on the glucuronidation of SN-38.

This weekly combination schedule of irinotecan, leucovorin, and fluorouracil has now been evaluated in a three-arm, multicenter, multinational phase III trial in comparison with fluorouracil plus leucovorin (daily × 5 low-dose leucovorin "Mayo Clinic" schedule) and against irinotecan alone *(22)*. As expected from earlier phase II data, the response rate of single-agent irinotecan was similar to that seen with a standard 5-FU-based regimen. Progression-free survival and overall survival were also essentially the same for those treated with first-line irinotecan versus those treated with fluorouracil plus leucovorin. The antitumor activity seen with the irinotecan, fluorouracil, and leucovorin combination was, however, superior. Data are shown in Table 1. The major objective response rate was nearly doubled as compared to fluorouracil plus leucovorin alone (50% vs 28%, $p < 0.0001$), and both progression-free survival and overall survival were significantly improved (for survival, $p < 0.04$, difference favoring the irinotecan combination). At any given time on study, patients treated with irinotecan/5-FU/LV had a 19% reduction in the risk of death relative to those treated with 5-FU/LV alone (hazard ratio 0.81, 95% CI = 0.65–0.99).

Examination of confirmed response rates by subgroup analyses showed that for every subgroup evaluated, including patients with poor performance status, extensive metastatic disease, prior adjuvant therapy, or abnormal baseline laboratory values, the response rate with irinotecan/5-FU/LV was approximately double that with 5-FU/LV alone *(24)*. Progression-free survival was also found to be improved with combination irinotecan/5-FU/LV in all patient subgroups *(24)*.

Table 1
Results of Phase III North American Trial of Irinotecan/LV/5-FU

	Irinotecan/LV/5-FU (N = 222)	LV/5-FU (N = 221)	CPT-11 (N = 223)
Overall response rate	50%	28%	29% ($p < 0.0001$)
Confirmed response rate	39%	21%	18% ($p < 0.0001$)
PFS (median)	7.0 mo	4.3 mo	4.2 mo ($p < 0.005$)
Overall survival	14.8 mo	12.6 mo	12.0 mo ($p < 0.05$)
Gr4 neutropenia	24%	43%	12%
Neutropenic fever	7%	15%	6%
Gr3 diarrhea	15%	6%	18%
Gr4 diarrhea	8%	7%	13%
Gr3/4 mucositis	2%	17%	2%
Gr3/4 vomiting	10%	4%	12%

Note: PFS, progression-free survival; mo, months; Gr, grade.
Source: ref. 22.

Toxicity data, also shown in Table 1, were of particular interest in that the combination of irinotecan/5-FU/LV was not found to be significantly different in overall toxicity from the standard 5-FU/LV regimen. More grade 3 and 4 diarrhea as well as grade 3 vomiting were seen with the irinotecan/5-FU/LV combination; however, more grade 4 neutropenia, neutropenic fever, and grade 3 mucositis were seen with the standard 5-FU/LV regimen. Similar patterns were seen in comparison of the irinotecan-only arm to 5FU/LV. Treatment-related deaths occurred at a rate of less than 1% in all treatment arms.

A parallel trial of first-line combination treatment with irinotecan plus fluorouracil and leucovorin was conducted in Europe *(25)*. In this study, each study site chose one of two infusional regimens for administration of 5-FU/LV according to local clinical practice or preference. These included either the 24-h infusion once-weekly regimen of the Arbeitsgemeinschaft Internische Onkologie (AIO) cooperative German group for oncology *(26)*, or the 48-h infusion every-2-wk regimen of de Gramont *(27)*. Each of these 5-FU/LV regimens had been previously studied in a phase I manner in combination with irinotecan *(28,29)*. Once a site selected its preferred regimen (either AIO or de Gramont), patients at the site were randomized to receive that schedule of 5-FU/LV, plus or minus irinotecan. After initial treatment, doses in all treatment arms of both studies could be adjusted according to specified guidelines to accommodate individual patient tolerance to the study drugs.

The overall response rate again showed a near-doubling with combination irinotecan/ 5-FU/LV versus 5-FU/LV alone (*see* Table 2) (49% vs 31%, $p < 0.001$). The median duration of confirmed objective tumor response from time of randomization was about 9 mo across all treatment arms. Progression-free survival was significantly longer for patients who received irinotecan/5-FU/LV compared with those who received 5-FU/LV (median 6.7 mo vs 4.4 mo, $p < 0.001$). Comparison of survival with irinotecan/5-FU/LV vs 5-FU/LV showed that survival was significantly ($p < 0.03$) longer with irinotecan/5-FU/LV therapy than with 5-FU/LV, with the risk of death at any time of the study being decreased by 23% for the irinotecan/5-FU/LV patients relative to those treated with 5-FU/LV alone (hazard ratio = 0.77, 95% CI = 0.60–0.98).

In order to more fully explore the potential benefits of first-line combination irinotecan/ 5-FU/LV vs 5-FU/LV, a meta-analysis of the North American and European phase III

Table 2
Results of European Phase III Trial of Irinotecan/5-FU/LV in Colorectal Cancer

	Irinotecan/5-FU/LV	*5-FU/LV*
Overall response rate	49%	31% ($p < 0.001$)
Confirmed response rate	35%	22% ($p < 0.001$)
Progression-free survival	6.7 mo	4.4 mo ($p < 0.001$)
Overall survival	17.4 mo	14.1 mo ($p < 0.05$)
Neutropenia grade 4	9%	1%
Neutropenic fever	5%	1%
Grade 3 diarrhea	17%	6%
Grade 4 diarrhea	6%	5%
Grade 3/4 mucositis	3%	3%
Vomiting grade 3–4	6%	3%

Source: ref. 25.

studies was performed *(30)*. In this analysis, the combined analysis of the survival data showed a median survival of 15.9 mo for irinotecan/5-FU/LV vs 13.3 mo for 5-FU/LV alone ($p = 0.003$, stratified log-rank test).

It was noted in comparing these two studies that the irinotecan/5-FU/LV curve separates from the 5-FU/LV curve later in the North American trial than in the European trial. The explanation for this finding is not immediately clear but may possibly be accounted for by the greater proportion of patients with ECOG Performance Status 2 in the North American trial. These poorer performance status patients generally had survival times <6 mo with either therapy. If only patients with ECOG Performance Status 0-1 are considered, survival results for the irinotecan/5-FU/LV arms are quite similar (medians of 17.2 mo and 17.4 mo in the North American and European trials, respectively) *(31)*.

7. CONCURRENT VS SEQUENTIAL FLUOROURACIL/IRINOTECAN TREATMENT

Although poststudy treatment was not a formal component of the first-line combination trials, data on poststudy chemotherapy on the North American trial were obtained. Of the patients receiving single-agent fluorouracil plus leucovorin up front on this trial, 55% received either irinotecan or an irinotecan-based regimen as part of their second-line poststudy chemotherapy. This number is very consistent with marketing surveys performed during the last year of the study accrual, which indicated that 56% of patients who received fluorouracil for colorectal cancer went on to receive second-line irinotecan. Of the patients receiving first-line irinotecan, approx 70% received second-line fluorouracil. Thus, the survival benefits seen for concurrent fluorouracil plus irinotecan administration are seen despite this large crossover. The study, therefore, can be seen as accurately reflecting the benefits of concurrent versus sequential administration of fluorouracil and irinotecan.

It is important to remember that not all patients who progress through a first-line treatment will then be physically or emotionally well enough to receive second-line therapy. Many patients will have a significant deterioration in performance status that will preclude second-line therapy. A patient progressing with a bowel obstruction, decreased nutritional intake, or increased serum bilirubin level will not be able to receive second-line irinotecan. Because the majority of available data do not support a clinically meaningful synergy between irinotecan and fluorouracil (the effects appear to be additive), it is possible that much of the benefit seen in terms of survival may be the result of the larger number of patients exposed to both irinotecan and fluorouracil when concurrent first-line administration is used.

Other schedules of irinotecan/fluorouracil combinations have now been reported (28,29, 32,33), and some of these have now entered phase III trials. One schedule that had been developed at the Mayo Clinic employed a dose of irinotecan on day 1, followed by bolus doses of fluorouracil and leucovorin on d 2–5 repeated every 21 d. This schedule was based on cell culture data suggesting a possible benefit to sequencing of the agents, with irinotecan followed by fluorouracil. Although this schedule was initially included in the six-arm NCI intergroup trial N9741, early toxicity data led to closure of that arm and further investigations of this daily × 5 irinotecan/fluorouracil schedule are not planned. At present, no randomized comparisons of different irinotecan/fluorouracil combination schedules with each other have been completed. Therefore, there are no compelling data available establishing a preference of the weekly bolus schedule vs the biweekly infusion schedule.

8. IRINOTECAN/FLUOROURACIL COMBINATIONS IN THE ADJUVANT SETTING

With the establishment of irinotecan/fluorouracil/leucovorin combinations as effective therapy for metastatic disease, there is considerable enthusiasm for the evaluation of these regimens in the postsurgical treatment of high-risk resected patients. It is reasonable to anticipate that the higher response rates and modest survival advantages demonstrated in stage 4 disease could translate into higher postsurgical cure rates, as a higher degree of eradication of minimal residual disease could expected. The National Cancer Institute intergroup is currently conducting a phase III trial of the weekly bolus irinotecan/fluorouracil/leucovorin schedule versus standard weekly 5-FU/LV for resected stage III patients. European investigators have also launched a phase III trial of the biweekly 48 h infusion schedule of irinotecan/fluorouracil/leucovorin in the adjuvant setting.

Irinotecan appears to have potent radiation sensitization properties and has been explored in a number of combined modality regimens with radiation therapy as a potential adjuvant treatment for rectal cancer. At Memorial Sloan–Kettering Cancer Center, a low-dose daily schedule of irinotecan, piloted in a phase I study (34), has been explored in conjunction with preoperative pelvic radiotherapy (35). A phase I study of infusional 5-FU with weekly bolus irinotecan and concurrent pelvic radiation therapy has also been reported (36,37), and other doses and schedules of irinotecan plus concurrent radiation therapy are being explored (38).

It is important to point out, however, that the long-term consequences of irinotecan therapy remain unknown at this time. The use of irinotecan in the adjuvant setting for colon or rectal cancer therefore remains a promising investigational approach, but it seems premature at this time to adopt this approach as standard for locally advanced disease and its use in this setting should remain largely confined to clinical trials.

9. TOLERANCE OF IRINOTECAN: SPECIAL CASES

The metabolism of irinotecan and its active metabolite, SN-38 is almost exclusively hepatically mediated. SN-38 is inactivated by glucuronidation to SN-38G and this inactive metabolite is secreted into the bile (39). Several factors can have a profound effect on the metabolism of irinotecan, with resultant effects on either toxicity or efficacy.

Biliary obstruction or hepatic dysfunction can substantially impair excretion of irinotecan and its metabolites. As such, elevated bilirubin is a strong relative contraindication to irinotecan therapy. Studies designed to establish appropriate parameters for dose modifications in hepatic dysfunction are in progress, however, in the absence of published data to provide guidance, use of irinotecan in patients with abnormal bilirubin should be undertaken with extreme caution, if at all.

One particularly vulnerable population of patients is those with Gilbert's disease, an inborn error of metabolism that prevents glucuronidation and results in an abnormal indirect bilirubin level. These patients are extremely limited in their ability to conjugate and thereby inactivate SN-38 and may develop profound or even life-threatening toxicity from even a single dose of irinotecan. On rare occasions, mild Gilbert's disease may produce intermittent elevations in total bilirubin levels, such that the serum bilirubin is normal when evaluated pretreatment, but a relative deficiency in glucuronidation may still be present. This should be suspected in patients with unusually severe toxicity to their first treatment of irinotecan, and bilirubin fractionation should be performed to look for this *(40)*.

Once excreted into the bile, SN-38 and SN-38G undergo some degree of enterohepatic circulation. Slowed gastrointestinal transit time may therefore have the effect of increasing enterohepatic reabsorption and so may yield increased toxicity. Patients with intestinal obstruction are therefore poor candidates for irinotecan or irinotecan-based combinations.

Under normal circumstances, irinotecan is processed by the 3A/4 component of the cytochrome P-450 enzymes in the liver to a minor metabolite known as APC *(41)*. This can take on clinically significant proportions, however, if overactivity of the 3A/4 P450 enzymes is induced. Strong inducers of this enzyme system, such as phenobarbitol, can cause irinotecan to be substantially inactivated, leading to subtherapeutic blood levels of SN-38.

10. FUTURE DIRECTIONS

Much current research in the use of irinotecan centers around its combination with newer agents. Combinations with oxaliplatin (*see* Chapter 29) are being actively explored. At the time of this writing, the current intergroup trial for advanced disease is comparing first-line irinotecan/5-FU/LV (weekly bolus regimen) to an infusional schedule of oxaliplatin 5-FU/LV (de Gramont schedule) and a regimen of irinotecan plus oxaliplatin. Combinations with other active agents such as raltitrexed have also been reported *(42)*.

Antiangiogenesis agents such as anti-vascular endothelial growth factor (VEGF) monoclonal antibody or the tyrosine kinase inhibitor SU5416 are currently in phase III trials in colon cancer, given in conjunction with irinotecan/fluorouracil/leucovorin (*see* Chapter 39).

Among the more interesting and encouraging findings is the report that combinations of irinotecan plus the antiepidermal growth factor receptor (EGFR) monoclonal antibody IMC-C225 is able to produce response in some patients in whom irinotecan alone has failed. In a phase II trial of 121 patients with documented irinotecan-refractory colorectal cancer, a preliminary report indicated a response rate of 17% when patients were given the identical dose and schedule of irinotecan that had failed, plus weekly infusions of IMC-C225 *(43)*. First-line trials of IMC-C225 plus irinotecan/5-FU/leucovorin have now been initiated.

11. CONCLUSION

As more data become available, the role of irinotecan in colorectal cancer is evolving and changing. Current data strongly support the use of irinotecan/fluorouracil/leucovorin combinations in the first-line treatment of metastatic colorectal cancer. Irinotecan/5-FU/LV combinations have now been shown in two large randomized trials to be superior to 5-FU/LV alone in terms of response rate, progression-free survival, and overall survival. These combinations may well prove to be useful in the adjuvant setting and in other gastrointestinal malignancies as well, and investigations to explore these possibilities are in progress. Given the superiority of first-line combination therapy, use of irinotecan as a second-line agent is likely to become far less frequent, and the challenge ahead will be to identify new agents for salvage therapy after first-line failure, as well as new and better agents for the initial therapy of colorectal cancer.

In addition, the role of molecular profiling of tumors in order to anticipate sensitivity or resistance to fluorouracil, irinotecan, and other agents is likely to increase (*see* Chapter 34) *(44–46)*. At present, the identification of molecular markers for CPT-11 sensitivity or resistance has not been successful, but efforts are continuing in this field. These molecular evaluations will undoubtedly play an important roll in the selection or exclusion of irinotecan and other agents as a component of first-line therapy in colorectal cancer.

REFERENCES

1. Pommier Y, Tanizawa A, and Kohn KW. Mechanisms of topoisomerase I inhibition by anticancer drugs. In *Advances in Pharmacology.* Liu LF (ed.), Academic, New York, 1994, Vol. 29B, pp. 73–92.
2. Khana R, Morton CL, Danks MK, and Potter PM. Proficient metabolism of irinotecan by a human intestinal carboxylesterase. *Cancer Res.*, **60(17)** (2000) 4725–4728.
3. Takimoto CH, Kieffer LV, Kieffer ME, Arbuck SG, and Wright J. DNA topoisomerase I poisons. *Cancer Chemother. Biol. Response Modif.*, **18** (1999) 81–124.
4. Negoro S, Fukuoka M, Masuda N, Takada M, Kusunoki Y, Matsui K, et al. Phase I study of weekly intravenous infusions of CPT-11, a new derivative of camptothecin, in the treatment of advanced non-small-cell lung cancer. *J. Natl. Cancer Inst.*, **83** (1991) 1164–1168.
5. Ohe Y, Sasaki Y, Shinkai T, et al. Phase I study and pharmacokinetics of CPT-11 with 5-day continuous infusion. *J. Natl. Cancer Inst.*, **84** (1992) 972–974.
6. Rothenberg ML, Kuhn JG, Burris HA III, Nelson J, Eckardt JR, Tristan-Morales M, et al. Phase I and Pharmacokinetic trial of weekly irinotecan. *J. Clin. Oncol.*, **11** (1993) 2194–2204.
7. Rowinsky EK, Grochow LB, Ettinger DS, Sartorius SE, Lubejko BG, Chen TL, et al. Phase I and pharmacological study of the novel topoisomerase inhibitor 7-ethyl-10-[4-(1-piperidino)-1-piperidino]carbonyloxycamptothecin (CPT-11) administered as a ninety minute infusion every three weeks. *Cancer Res.*, **54** (1994) 427–436.
8. Abigerges D, Carbot GG, Armand JP, Mathieu-Boue A, Re M, Gouyette A, et al. Phase I and pharmacologic studies of the camptothecin analogue irinotecan administered every three weeks in cancer patients. *J. Clin. Oncol.*, **13** (1995) 210–221.
9. Shimada Y, Yoshino M, Wakui A, et al. Phase II study of irinotecan, a new camptothecin derivative, in metastatic colorectal cancer. *J. Clin. Oncol.*, **11** (1993) 909–913.
10. Rothenberg ML, Eckert JR, Kuhn JG, et al. Phase II trial of Irinotecan in patients with progressive or rapidly recurrent colorectal cancer. *J. Clin. Oncol.*, **14** (1996) 1128–1135.
11. Rougier Ph, Bugat R, Douillard JY, et al. A phase II study of CPT-11 (irinotecan) in the treatment of advanced colorectal cancer in chemotherapy-naive patients and patients pretreated with 5-FU-based chemotherapy. *J. Clin. Oncol.*, **15** (1997) 333–340.
12. Von Hoff DD, Rothenberg ML, Pitot HC, et al. Irinotecan therapy for patients with previously treated metastatic colorectal cancer. Overall results of FDA-reviewed pivotal U.S. clinical trials. *Proc. Am. Soc. Clin. Oncol.*, **16** (1997) a803.
13. Cunningham D, et al. Randomized trial of irinotecan plus supportive care versus supportive care alone after fluorouracil failure for patients with metastatic colorectal cancer. *Lancet*, **352** (1998) 1413.
14. Rougier P, et al. Randomised trial of irinotecan versus fluorouracil by continuous infusion after fluorouracil failure in patients with metastatic colorectal cancer. *Lancet*, **352** (1998) 1407.
15. Conti JA, Kemeny NE, Saltz LB, et al. Irinotecan is an active agent in untreated patients with metastatic colorectal cancer. *J. Clin. Oncol.*, **14** (1996) 709–715.
16. Abigerges D, Armand JP, Chabot GG, et al. High dose intensity irinotecan administered as a single dose every 3 weeks: the Institute Gustave Roussy experience. *Proc. Am. Soc. Clin. Oncol.*, **12** (1993) 133.

17. Gandia D, Abigerges D, Armand JP, et al. Irinotecan induced cholinergic effects in cancer patients. *J. Clin. Oncol.*, **11** (1993) 196–197.

18. Pitot HC, Wender MJ, O'Connel, et al. A phase II trial of CPT-11 (irinotecan) in patients with metastatic colorectal carcinoma: a North Central Cancer Treatment Group (NCCTG) study. *Proc. Am. Soc. Clin. Oncol.*, **13** (1994) a573.

19. Saltz LB. Irinotecan in the first-line treatment of colorectal cancer. *Oncology*, **12(8 Suppl. 6)** (1998) 54–58.

20. Buroker TR, O'Connell MJ, Wieand HS, et al. Randomized comparison of two schedules of fluorouracil and leucovorin in the treatment of advanced colorectal cancer. *J. Clin. Oncol.*, **12** (1994) 14–20.

21. Leischman CG, Fleming TR, Muggia FM, et al. Phase II study of fluorouracil and its modulation in advanced colorectal cancer: a Southwest Oncology Group Study. *J. Clin. Oncol.*, **13** (1995) 1303–1311.

22. Saltz LB, Cox J, Blanke CB, et al. Irinotecan plus fluorouracil and leucovorin in metastatic colorectal cancer. *N. Engl. J. Med.*, **353** (2000) 905–914.

23. Saltz L, Kanowitz J, Kemeny N, Spriggs D, Schaaf L, Eng M, et al. A phase I clinical and pharmacologic trial of irinotecan, 5-fluorouracil, and leucovorin in patients with advanced solid tumors. *J. Clin. Oncol.*, **14** (1996) 2959–2967.

24. Knight RD, Miller LL, Pirotta N, et al. First-line irinotecan (C), fluorouracil (F), leucovorin (L) especially improves survival (OS) in metastatic colorectal cancer (MCRC) patients (PT) with favorable prognostic indicators. *Proc. Am. Soc. Clin. Oncol.*, **19** (2000) 991a.

25. Douillard JY, Cunningham D, Roth AD, et al. Irinotecan combined with fluorouracil compared with fluorouracil alone as first-line treatment for metastatic colorectal cancer: a multicentre randomised trial. [erratum appears in *Lancet*, **355** (2000) 1372]. *Lancet*, **355** (2000) 1041–1047.

26. Köhne CH, Schöffski P, Wilke H, et al. Effective biomodulation by leucovorin of high-dose infusion fluorouracil given as a weekly 24-hour infusion: results of a randomized trial in patients with advanced colorectal cancer. *J. Clin. Oncol.*, **16** (1998) 418–426.

27. de Gramont A, Bosset JF, Milan C, et al. Randomized trial comparing monthly low-dose leucovorin and fluorouracil bolus with bimonthly high-dose leucovorin and fluorouracil bolus plus continuous infusion for advanced colorectal cancer: a French intergroup study. *J. Clin. Oncol.*, **15** (1997) 808–815.

28. Vanhoefer U, Harstrick A, Kohne K, et al. Phase I study of a weekly schedule of irinotecan, highdose leucovorin, and infusional fluorouracil as first-line chemotherapy in patients with advanced colorectal cancer. *J. Clin. Oncol.*, **17** (1999) 907–913.

29. Ducreaux M, Ychou M, Seitz J-F, et al. Irinotecan combined with bolus fluorouracil, continuous infusion fluorouracil, and high dose leucovorin every two weeks (LV5FU2 regimen): a clinical dose-finding and pharmacokinetic study in patients with pretreated metastatic colorectal cancer. *J. Clin. Oncol.*, **17** (1999) 2901–2908.

30. Saltz LB, Douillard J, Pirotta N, et al. Combined analysis of two phase III randomized trials comparing irinotecan (C), fluorouracil (F), leucovorin (L) vs F alone as first-line therapy of previously untreated metastatic colorectal cancer (MCRC). *Proc. Am. Soc. Clin. Oncol.*, **19** (2000) 242a.

31. Saltz LB, Douillard J-Y, Pirotta N, et al. Irinotecan plus fluorouracil/leucovorin for metastatic colorectal cancer: a new survival standard. *Oncologist*, **6** (2001) 81–91.

32. Paz-Ares L, Sastre J, Diaz-Rubio E, et al. Phase I dose-finding study of irinotecan over a short iv infusion combined with fixed dose of 5-fluorouracil protracted continuous iv infusion in patients with advanced solid tumors. *Proc. Am. Soc. Clin. Oncol.*, **16** (1997) a874.

33. Rothenberg M, Pazdur R, Rowinsky EK, et al. A phase II multicenter trial of alternating cycles of irinotecan and 5-FU/LV in patients with previously untreated metastatic colorectal cancer. *Proc. Am. Soc. Clin. Oncol.*, **16** (1997) a944.

34. Saltz L, Early E, Kelsen D, et al. Phase I study of chronic daily low dose irinotecan. *Proc. Am. Soc. Clin. Oncol.*, **16** (1997) 200a (abstract).

35. Minsky BD, O'Reilly E, Wong D, et al. Daily low-dose irinotecan plus pelvic irradiation as preoperative treatment of locally advanced rectal cancer. *Proc. Am. Soc. Clin. Oncol.*, **18** (1999) 266a (abstract).

36. Mitchell E, Ahmad N, Fry R, et al. Combined modality therapy of locally advanced or recurrent adenocarcinoma of the rectum: preliminary report of a phase I trial of chemotherapy with CPT-11, 5FU, and concomitant irradiation. *Proc. Am. Soc. Clin. Oncol.*, **18** (1999) 247a (abstract).

37. Mitchel EP. Irinotecan in preoperative combined modality therapy for locally advanced rectal cancer. *Oncology*, **14(Suppl. 14)** (2000) 56–61.

38. Rich TA and Kirichenko AV. Camptothecin schedule and timing of administration with irradiation. *Ocology*, **15 (Suppl. 5)** (2001) 37–41.

39. Ratain M. Insights into the pharmacokinetics and pharmacodynamics of irinotecan. *Clin. Cancer Res.*, **6(9)**(2000) 3393–3394.

40. Iyer L, King C, Tephley T, and Ratain MJ. UGT isoform 1.1 glucuronidates SN-38, the active metabolite of irinotecan. *Proc. Am. Soc. Clin. Oncol.*, **16** (1997) a707.

41. Rivory LP, Riou JF, Haaz MC, Sable S, Vuihorgue M, Comercu A, et al. Identification and properties of a major plasma metabolite (CPT-11) isolated from plasma of patients. *Cancer Res.*, **56** (1995) 3689–3694.

42. Ford HE, Cunningham D, Ross PJ, et al. Phase I study of irinotecan and raltitrexed in patients with advanced gastrointestinal tract adenocarcinoma. *Br. J. Cancer*, **83(2)** (2000) 146–152.

43. Saltz L, Rubin M, Hochster H, et al. Cetuximab (IMC-C225) plus irinotecan is active in CPT-11-refractory colorectal cancer that expresses the epidermal growth factor receptor. *Proc. Am. Soc. Clin. Oncol.*, **20** (2001) (abstract).

44. Leichman G, Lenz H-J, Leichman L, Danenberg K, Baranda J, Groshen S, et al. Quantitation of intratumoral thymidylate synthase expression predicts for disseminated colorectal cancer response and resistance to protracted-infusion fluorouracil and weekly leucovorin. *J. Clin. Oncol.*, **15** (1997) 3223–3229.

45. Danenberg K Metzger R, Salonga D, Lenz H-J, Leichman L, Leichman G, et al. Thymidine phosphorylase expression in colorectal tumors together with that of thymidylate synthase predict tumor response to 5-fluorouracil. *Proc. Am. Assoc. Cancer Res.*, **38** (1997) 614.

46. Saltz L, Danenberg K, Paty P, Kelsen D, Kemeny N, Salonga D, et al. High thymidylate synthase expression does not preclude activity of CPT-11 in colorectal cancer. *Proc. ASCO*, **17** (1998) 281a.

29   Oxaliplatin in the Treatment of Colorectal Cancer

Stacy D. Jacobson, Steven R. Alberts, and Richard M. Goldberg

CONTENTS

1. INTRODUCTION

Oxaliplatin is one member of a class of antineoplastic agents distinguished by the presence of a platinum complex containing a 1,2-diaminocyclohexane (DACH) carrier ligand (Fig. 1). In the 1970s, these drugs were found to be active in cisplatin-resistant cell lines *(1)*. In part, because one of the first agents in this class to be tested, tetraplatin, had an unfavorable toxicity profile in phase I studies, little further study of the DACH–platinum compounds occurred in the 1970s *(2)*. During the 1980s, George Mathe at the Hopital Paul Brousse performed in vitro experiments that led him to initiate human trials with oxaliplatin. These trials provided the first indications of the drug's potential clinical utility *(3)*.

Since then, oxaliplatin has been subjected to intensive study in patients with a wide range of primary tumor types, and is available by prescription in 17 countries worldwide for the treatment of advanced colorectal adenocarcinoma. Oxaliplatin combined with 5-fluorouracil (5-FU) and leucovorin is now being compared to standard therapy with 5-FU and leucovorin

From: *Colorectal Cancer: Multimodality Management*
Edited by: L. Saltz © Humana Press Inc., Totowa, NJ

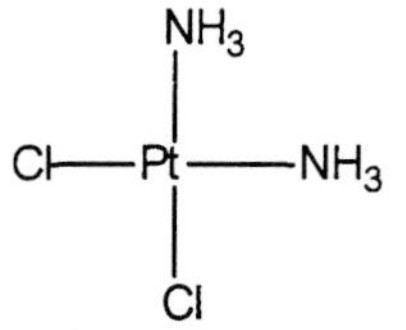

CISPLATIN
(cis-dichloro-diammine platinum: CDDP)

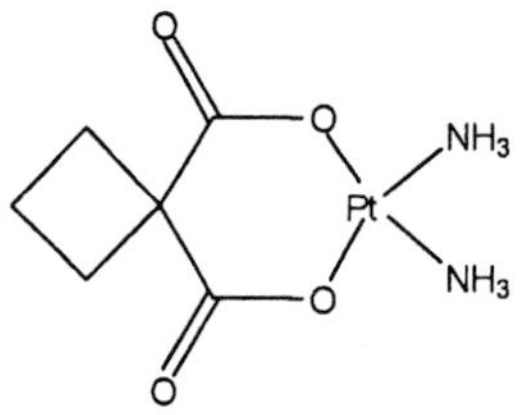

CARBOPLATIN
(Cisdiammine 1-1 cyclobutane dicarboxylatoplatine II: CBDCA)

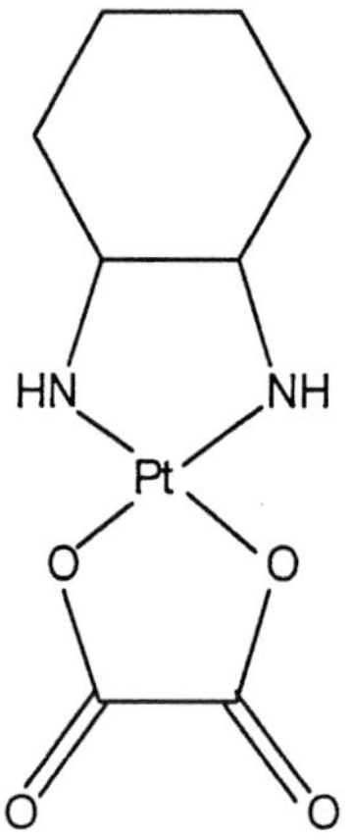

OXALIPLATIN
(1,2-diammino cyclohexane oxalotoplatine II: I-OHP)

Fig. 1. Chemical structures of cisplatin, carboplatin, and oxaliplatin.

in the adjuvant setting in patients with resected stage II or III colon cancer in phase III trials ongoing in both the United States and in Europe. In the United States, this agent has not been approved by the Federal Drug Administration (FDA) for any indication. Despite this, there is strong demand for the drug through clinical trials, via a company-sponsored compassionate-use treatment program or as administered under the supervision of a physician from a country where the agent is legally available.

This chapter reviews the pharmacology and pharmacokinetic data available on oxaliplatin. The preclinical studies in human tumor xenografts and cell cultures that indicate oxaliplatin has a broad activity spectrum (including activity against gastrointestinal cancers originating from sites other than the colon) are also detailed. The clinical development of oxaliplatin is traced sequentially through phase I, II, and III trials in which the drug was administered both as a single agent and in combination with other antineoplastic agents. The associated drug toxicity both when administered alone and in combination with other chemotherapy agents is reviewed. Areas for future research are also delineated.

2. PRECLINICAL STUDIES OF OXALIPLATIN

Many platinum-based compounds were synthesized in the 1970s in an attempt to overcome both innate and acquired resistance to cisplatin and to moderate the spectrum of toxicity, especially nephrotoxicity and hematologic toxicity associated with cisplatin administration. One family of compounds, the "DACH" family, was synthesized by substituting the amine groups of cisplatin with a 1,2-diaminocyclohexane group, also termed a DACH ligand. Conners et al. reported on the activity of a large number of platinum compounds, including those of the DACH family against PC-6 plasma cell lines in 1972 and showed that many of these compounds had a therapeutic index comparable to that of cisplatin *(4)*. Since then, many studies have been performed to construct DACH–platinum compounds as well as to ascertain which compounds are active and which of the active compound's isomers has the best toxicity profile and antitumor effect.

In 1977, Burchenal authored the initial report of activity of the two agents 1,2-diaminocyclohexylplatinum malonate and 1,2-cyclohexyldiaaminoplatinum sulfate in leukemia cell lines that were resistant to cisplatin *(5)*. Multiple subsequent studies reported activity of the DACH–platinum compound. However, these studies used isomeric mixtures of the compounds, and, therefore, the experiments demonstrated relatively low therapeutic indices *(6–8)*. Kidani et al. separated these DACH–platinum compounds into trans and cis isomers, with further separation of the trans isomer into its two optical isomers, trans-*d* and trans-*l (9,10)*. This work was important because subsequent studies reported differential antitumor activity for these isomers. A number of 1,2-DACH–platinum complexes (dichloro, dibromo, oxalato, malanato, sulfato, dinitrato, glucuronato) were synthesized and tested on L-1210 leukemia cells in mice. The trans-*l* compounds proved to be more potent than the cis or trans-*d* isomers in the L-1210 cell lines *(11)*. Conversely, when tested against sarcoma-180 tumors in mice, the cis isomer was the most active. In this study, different complexes were synthesized (dichloro, oxalato, malanato), and platinum (oxalato) (*cis*-DACH) was identified as having a very high therapeutic index and good solubility *(12)*. Vollano et al. corroborated the finding that the trans-*l* form of DACH–platinum compounds had a higher therapeutic index against L-1210 cells *(13)*. Additional investigations confirmed that both the isomeric configuration and the leaving group are important determinants of the activity and toxicity of the DACH compounds *(14)*.

It is also apparent that the activity and toxicity of the various isomers may be tumor dependent. This finding was corroborated and extended by Pendyala et al., who studied the effectiveness of the three isomers on a variety of human cell lines, including L-1210, HT 29 colon cancer, and A-2780 ovarian cancer *(15)*. In all but one cell line, the trans-*l* isomer had the greatest relative molar potency. In A-2780 lines with some resistance to oxaliplatin, the trans-*l* and trans-*d* isomers had the same potency, and both were more active than the cis isomer. Interestingly, in the A-2780 cell line that was made "resistant" to oxaliplatin by chronic exposure to the drug in culture, resistance was seen with the trans-*d* and cis isomers but not the trans-*l* isomer. However, the oxaliplatin resistant L-1210 cells exhibited resistance to all isomers, in the order of *l*-oxaliplatin>*d*-oxaliplatin>*cis*-oxaliplatin. In cell lines made resistant to cisplatin, the L-1210 murine cells were sensitive to all oxaliplatin isomers, whereas the human A-2780 cells showed low-level resistance to the cis isomer only. The authors also found that platinum accumulation and DNA binding in the A-2780 cells was greatest for the *l*-isomer. These studies suggest that conformational changes along with the structure of the leaving group (chloro, oxalato, malonato, etc.) resulted in different activity, toxicity, and resistance patterns in human tumor xenografts.

A number of studies were performed to determine the activity of oxalato (*trans*-l-1, 2-diaminocyclohexane) platinum (II) (oxaliplatin) in other cell lines and animal tumor models. These studies have consistently demonstrated the drug's activity in many tumor types and its lack of cross-resistance with cisplatin. The studies using tumor cell lines inoculated into mice are summarized in Table 1.

Table 1
Studies Using Tumor Cell Lines Inoculated into Mice

Cell line	Oxaliplatin	Cisplatin	Ref.
L-1210 (iv/ip)	++	+	16
P-388 (leukemia)	+	+	
Lewis lung Ca	+	+	
Colon 26	+	++	
Colon 36	+	+	
Fibrosarc M5076	++	+	
L-1210 (resistant to CDDP)[a]	++	–	
Melanoma B-16	+	++	
L-1210 (ip)	++	+	3
L-1210 (iv)	+	+	
L-1210 (intracerebral)	++	–	
L-1210 (resistant to CDDP)	–	–	
L40 AkR leukemia	+	+	
LGC lymphoma	+	–	
Glioma-26	–	–	
B16 melanoma	–	–	
MA 16-C mammary	–	–	
3LL Lewis lung	–	–	
HT-29 human colon	++	+	17
FLC erythroleukemia	++	+	
Hu K562 leukemia	++	+	
Hu MCF-7 breast Ca	++	+	
MA 16-C mammary	+	–	18
Neuroblastoma	+	++	19
Germ cell 1777NRp	++	+	20
Germ cell H12DDP (intermediate resistance to CDDP)	++	+	
1411HP (high resistance to CDDP)	+	+	
H12.1 (CDDP sensitive)	+	+	

Note: ++: more active based on survival times or tumor weight; +: active; –: inactive.
[a]CDDP, cisplatin.

In order to broaden the knowledge base of the comparative activity of a variety of platinum compounds across primary tumor types, Rixe et al. conducted a large study using the cell lines of the NCI's Anticancer Drug Screen (21). Cisplatin-resistant cell lines (KB3-1 cervical cancer and A-2780 ovarian cancer) were less than one-tenth as resistant to DACH compounds (tetraplatin and oxaliplatin) than they were to cisplatin or carboplatin. In the cisplatin-resistant cell lines, there was reduced accumulation of all platinated compounds, even at higher extracellular concentrations. The authors postulated that the differential accumulation of platinum agents could account for the low levels of cross-resistance observed with members of the DACH family. Using cell lines with unknown platinum sensitivity, they found increased sensitivity of many colon cancer cell lines to oxaliplatin as compared to cisplatin. Conversely, cells originating in the central nervous system were less sensitive to oxaliplatin. These results suggest that the mechanisms of action of oxaliplatin and mechanisms of resistance to oxaliplatin may differ in cells originating from different tissues.

Raymond et al. employed an in vitro human tumor cloning assay to determine the activity of oxaliplatin at concentrations of 0.5–50 µg/mL on a variety of human tumors in vitro. The specimens were exposed to oxaliplatin for either 1 h or continuously for 14 d. Oxaliplatin activity was concentration dependent and the agent was twofold more active when cells were exposed to the agent continuously for 14 d. How this can be applied clinically requires further study, but this suggests the potential utility of continuous infusion regimens using this agent. Among the tumors that responded to oxaliplatin were colon, non-small-cell lung cancer, breast, and gastric primaries, as well as tumors typically refractory to other platinum-based agents, such as melanomas, renal cell, and sarcomas. Oxaliplatin also showed activity in tumors resistant to 5-FU, irinotecan, paclitaxel, doxorubicin, and cyclophosphamide. It is known that loss of mismatch repair activity leads to resistance to cisplatin; however, this was not observed in vitro with oxaliplatin. The authors suggest that this may be one factor contributing to the different spectrum of activity between these two agents (22).

The promising activity led to initial animal studies of the agent's toxicity patterns. Mathe et al. also demonstrated that the marked nephrotoxicity in animals treated with cisplatin was not observed in mice or in baboons treated with oxaliplatin (3). No hematologic, cardiac, or hepatic toxicity was seen in mice or baboons (18).

3. MECHANISM OF ACTION

Based on the results of the in vitro and xenograft screens reported earlier and the preliminary indications of the reasonable nature of the agent's toxicity, particularly in comparison to cisplatin, additional mechanistic research was begun to understand how and why it differed from other platinum compounds. Like cisplatin and carboplatin, oxaliplatin forms intrastrand platinum–DNA adducts that inhibit DNA synthesis (23). The intrastrand links occur between two adjacent guanine residues or two adjacent guanine–adenine base pairs. In cell culture experiments, the DACH carrier ligand is associated with enhanced intracellular accumulation of platinum, increased DNA–platinum binding, increased tolerance of DNA adducts, and decreased repair of DNA adducts when compared to platinum-based drugs, which lack the DACH carrier ligand (24,25). Oxaliplatin adducts may also be more cytotoxic than cisplatin- or carboplatin-induced adducts, as indicated by the finding that there are 2-fold to 10-fold fewer adducts observed at equimolar and equitoxic concentrations of cisplatin (21,25,26).

Initially, oxaliplatin forms monoadducts with the guanine bases in DNA. These are then converted to stable diadducts. These diadducts block both DNA replication and transcription. The agent's activity is felt to result because these diadducts, like the DNA–platinum complexes formed with other platinum-based agents, protrude into the major groove in the DNA (21,23–28). However, the DACH carrier ligand confers a different activity and toxicity profile than is observed with other platinum-based agents that lack the ligand. These differences are felt to result principally because of the DACH ligand's greater bulkiness that results in steric hindrance of repair mechanisms as well as its enhanced hydrophobic properties (24,25).

Oxaliplatin–DNA adducts appear to efficiently prevent the binding of mismatch repair (MMR) protein complexes and, subsequently, the repair of platinum-induced lesions in DNA. This appears to activate apoptotic pathways instead of permitting error correction via the MMR pathway (29). The elucidation of the cell-signaling pathways that lead to apoptosis is under investigation and is beyond the scope of this review (30).

3.1. Mechanisms of Oxaliplatin Resistance

Described mechanisms of resistance to platinum compounds include decreased drug diffusion across cells, increased efflux of drug, increased drug inactivation, increased quenching of DNA monoadducts, increased excision repair, and increased postreplication repair (also termed "postreplication bypass"). Cisplatin and oxaliplatin are largely noncross-resistant, a phenomenon that may be explained by the large DACH ligand on oxaliplatin. Although the same type of adducts are formed by CDDP and oxaliplatin, there are some important differences. In many cases of cisplatin resistance, DNA elongation occurs despite the presence of cisplatin–DNA adducts, a phenomenon termed "replicative bypass" (24,26,31). Bulkier oxaliplatin–DNA adducts appear to defeat the mechanism of replicative bypass. The DACH ligand decreases the rate of conversion of monoadducts to diadducts and impairs the cell's ability to tolerate the damage induced by unrepaired platinum–DNA adducts (27,29).

Deficiency of genes that encode mismatch repair enzymes has been shown to confer resistance to cisplatin, but not oxaliplatin (24,26). When the mismatch repair complex attaches to a cisplatin–DNA adduct in order to correct or permit bypass of the drug-induced DNA damage in a cisplatin-sensitive cell, it is thought that futile cycling occurs. This is a process of repeated ineffectual excision and resynthesis of the strand of DNA opposite the damaged strand. The gaps in the DNA that the cisplatin–DNA adducts cause ultimately result in cell death (32). In cisplatin-resistant cells and in mismatch-repair-deficient cells, the excision and resynthesis process does not occur effectively. DNA elongation proceeds despite the existence of DNA base-pair mismatches and cells do not enter an apoptotic pathway. When a bulkier oxaliplatin–DNA adduct forms in the DNA of a cell with competent mismatch repair, the mismatch repair enzymes cannot gain access to the area of damage, preventing repair or replicative bypass and this ineffectual repair process leads to apoptosis (32–34). Defective mismatch repair resulting from germline mutations in the hMLH1 or hMSH2 genes such as is observed in patients with the syndrome hereditary nonpolyposis colon cancer (HNPCC or Lynch syndrome) leads to cisplatin resistance because such cells are tolerant of DNA damage and do not enter an apoptotic pathway. Such cells are not intrinsically oxaliplatin resistant (35). In summary, the mismatch repair system does not appear to detect oxaliplatin–DNA adduct formation and, therefore, alteration in the competence of this repair mechanism does not affect sensitivity of cell lines to oxaliplatin in the same way as the alteration can lead to cisplatin resistance.

3.2. Biotransformation

Platinum-based antineoplastic drugs must undergo intracellular activation before they can bind to DNA. When injected into the bloodstream of an organism, oxaliplatin undergoes spontaneous nonenzymatic conversion. The oxalate group is displaced by weak nucleophiles (bicarbonate, dihydrogen phosphate) to form reactive unstable intermediates (36). Two species of DACH–platinum can then be formed, depending on the local chloride concentration: monoaqua 1,2-DACH monochloroplatinum and 1,2-DACH–platinum dichloride. The diaquated species predominates intracellularly because of relatively lower intracellular chloride concentrations, whereas the monoaqua form predominates in the higher chloride environment of the blood. The aquated compounds form the complexes that appear to result in the antineoplastic activity with intracellular molecules, including guanine bases on DNA, or bind irreversibly with blood cells and plasma proteins. The unbound, or ultrafilterable, platinum is responsible for the cytotoxic effect of oxaliplatin. The platinum that is bound to red blood cells or plasma proteins is inactive and is taken up in tissues or excreted in the urine

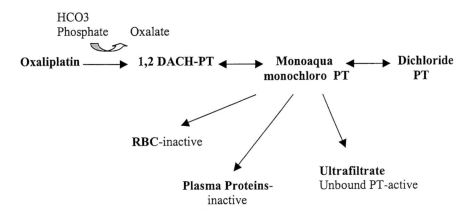

Fig. 2. Biotransformation of oxaliplatin.

(37,38). Biotransformation is depicted in Fig. 2. After infusion, approx 85% of oxaliplatin is bound to plasma proteins, mostly to albumin and γ-globulins. The amount of protein binding increases over time. Seventy percent of injected platinum is protein bound 2 h after infusion. This percentage of bound platinum increases to 95% after 5 d *(38–40)*.

3.3. Circadian Variation and Oxaliplatin Administration

Circadian rhythms in biologic systems have been used as a basis for varying drug infusion rates to maximize drug activity and minimize normal tissue toxicity. The concept of chronomodulation assumes two things. The first assumption is that normal tissues have daily rhythms of activity and rest. The second assumption is that neoplastic cells do not share the same biorhythms as normal tissue. In clinical oncology, chronomodulation has been felt mainly to apply to differential changes that occur during the day in enzymes that degrade 5-fluorouracil in normal tissues. This difference can be exploited to the patient's advantage by maximizing infusion of a drug when the potential toxicity to normal tissues is likely to be at a minimum, thus permitting maximal drug doses to be administered.

The investigators at the Hopital Paul Brousse had long been intrigued with circadian variation in organisms and have designed regimens whereby they hoped to exploit these rhythms to optimize the therapeutic effect of various agents. They established in both mouse and humans that cisplatin and other antineoplastic drug tolerance was dependent on the time of day when the agent is administered *(41,42)*. An example of their work is a study of 404 rats living under controlled conditions with 12-h alternating, fixed cycles of light and darkness daily. Oxaliplatin was injected into these rats at various times from the hour of light onset and toxicity was monitored by assessment of leukocyte and erythrocyte counts, renal function, histopathologic study of organs, mortality, and pharmacokinetics. The optimal time for oxaliplatin administration was determined to be 16 h after light onset based on reduced toxicity. Pharmacokinetics were not dependent on when in the circadian cycle the drug was administered *(43)*. This group has also looked at 5-FU injection according to circadian rhythm and found that the optimal time to maximize infusion of this agent is during the interval from midnight to 4:00 AM.

3.4. Pharmacokinetics

The pharmacokinetics (PK) of oxaliplatin has been extensively studied, and for details, readers are referred to an excellent review by Graham et al. *(44)*. After biotransformation of oxaliplatin, the drug's metabolites are cleared mainly by renal excretion. Renal clearance accounts for about half of the total plasma clearance. The remaining oxaliplatin is distributed into tissues. There is minimal excretion of oxaliplatin or its metabolites into the feces *(38)*. Oxaliplatin is not a substrate for cytochrome P-450 enzymes (CYP450), and therefore drugs that induce or inhibit this system should have no effect on the metabolism of oxaliplatin.

The volume of distribution of platinum is high. This is mainly because the metabolites of oxaliplatin are lipophilic and, consequently, bind irreversibly to proteins, DNA, and other cellular molecules. As described earlier, much of the platinum in an injected dose becomes sequestered inside the red blood cells (RBCs). This proportion of platinum that is sequestered inside RBCs is irreversibly bound and does not interact with malignant cells. Because of the binding to tissues and RBCs, the terminal half-life for oxaliplatin is quite long, on the order of 27 h. Table 2 provides a summary of various PK parameters of oxaliplatin after both infusion of 130 mg/m^2 every 3 wk and 85 mg/m^2 every 2 wk *(44)*.

3.5. Oxaliplatin in Special Patient Populations

Graham et al. studied the influence of age, gender, renal, and hepatic function (ALT) on the pharmacokinetics of oxaliplatin. Twenty-six patients received oxaliplatin 130 mg/m^2 over 2 h. The glomerular filtration rate (GFR) of these patients ranged from 42.8 to 113.8 mL/min. GFR was found to be a major determinant of both renal platinum clearance and total-body clearance. Oxaliplatin clearance was not affected by the patient's age, gender, or hepatic function *(45)*. Massari et al. studied the influence of renal dysfunction on platinum clearance. These investigators noted that patients with moderate renal dysfunction had a significant increase in area under the curve (AUC) and decreased clearance compared to those with normal renal function. However, there was no excess toxicity reported in the patients with renal impairment *(46)*.

4. OXALIPLATIN COMBINED WITH OTHER AGENTS

4.1. Preclinical Studies

A number of studies have suggested a synergistic or additive effect when oxaliplatin is combined with other chemotherapy agents in cell culture or mouse models. Oxaliplatin is additive or synergistic with many drugs used to treat colon cancer, including 5-FU, CPT-11, and other experimental thymidylate synthase inhibitors. These studies are summarized in Table 3.

Raymond et al. noted that the combination of oxaliplatin with thymidylate synthesis (TS) inhibitors (AG337 and ZD1694) led to less cytotoxic potentiation than was observed with 5-FU. They also identified the fact that the reversion of cisplatin- and oxaliplatin-induced DNA interstrand crosslinks was retarded by the active metabolite of irinotecan, SN-38. They concluded that development of 5-FU/oxaliplatin and topoisomerase-I inhibitor/oxaliplatin combinations was warranted *(47)*.

An intriguing report by Taron et al. showed that colon cancer cells made resistant to 5-FU in vitro can be made just as sensitive as the parental cell line when oxaliplatin is added to 5-FU. This phenomenon is sequence dependent and is more pronounced when the oxaliplatin is given before 5-FU. This group also reported that the synergism seen with oxaliplatin and 5-FU and oxaliplatin plus topotecan was independent of the 5-FU-resistant phenotype, p53 status, and whether or not the cells were DNA–mismatch repair proficient (HT29) or deficient (LoVo) *(51,52)*.

Table 2
Pharmacokinetics of Oxaliplatin

	130 mg/m² q wk	*85 mg/m² q 2wk*
C_{max} [a] (plasma) mean	2.59–3.22 µg/mL	
AUC[b] 0–48	50.4–71.5 µg/mL • h	
C_{max} ultrafiltrate	1.21 ± 0.10 µg/mL (cycle 5)	0.681 ± 0.077 µg/mL (cycle 3)
C_{max} plasma	3.61 ± 0.43 µg/mL	1.92 ± 0.338 µg/mL
C_{max} RBC	3.25 ± 0.49 µg/mL	2.67 ± 0.798 µg/mL
AUC ultrafiltrate	11.9 ± 4.60 µg/mL • h (cycle 1)	4.25 ± 1.18 µg/mL • h
AUC plasma	207 ± 60.9 µg/mL • h	118 ± 8.97 µg/mL • h
AUC RBC	1326 ± 570 µg/mL • h	252 ± 34.6 µg/mL • h
$T_{1/2}$[c] a	0.28 h	
$T_{1/2}$ b	16.3 h	
$T_{1/2}$ γ(terminal)	273 h	
Clearance	9.34 ± 2.85 to 13.3 ± 3.9 L/h	18.5 ± 4.71 L/h
Vd[d]	349–812 L	295 L

[a] C_{max}, maximum clearance.
[b] AUC, area under the curve.
[c] $T_{1/2}$, half-life.
[d] V_d, volume of distribution.

4.2. Pharmacokinetics/Drug Interactions

Oxaliplatin does not appear to influence the clearance of 5-FU. 5-FU and oxaliplatin pharmacokinetics (PK) were reported in a study using the style of 5-FU infusion popularized by de Gramont, in which 5-FU is initially administered as a loading dose followed by a short-term 5-FU infusion plus or minus oxaliplatin. In this case, drug administration was as follows: 350 mg of leucovorin (LV), 400 mg/m² 5-FU bolus, 2400 mg/m² 5-FU infusion over 46 h. Oxaliplatin was administered at a dose of 85 mg/m² over 2 h with LV. There was no difference in any PK parameter for 5-FU with or without oxaliplatin *(59)*. Papamichael et al. also studied PK in 16 patients receiving 5-FU/LV with or without oxaliplatin (200 mg/m² LV, 400 mg/m² 5-FU, then 600 mg/m² 5-FU over 22 h; oxaliplatin dose not specified). In this study, the presence of oxaliplatin did significantly decrease 5-FU AUC, but it did not affect nonlinear clearance *(60)*. Metzger et al. noted that chronomodulation can affect the PK of oxaliplatin, with lower C_{max} and lower AUC and longer $T_{1/2}$ of platinum seen with peak delivery at 0100 compared to 0700 or 1600 h. Chronomodulation takes into account diurnal rhythms of differential drug metabolism. The authors suggested that high extraplasmic diffusion of oxaliplatin during early night hours may account for the increased toxicity that was seen in their trial *(61)*.

Lokliec et al. studied the PK of both agents in patients receiving both CPT-11 and oxaliplatin in a phase I trial *(62)*. These investigators found no significant differences in clearance for either drug when administered alone or in combination. This was expected based on the knowledge that these drugs are metabolized and excreted in different ways.

5. CLINICAL TRIALS

5.1. Phase I Trials

The above-reviewed preclinical data suggested that oxaliplatin satisfied the criteria for clinical testing; it was active in tumors that were cisplatin resistant and did not cause

Table 3
Preclinical Studies of Oxaliplatin in Combination with Other Agents

Cell line	Drug added	Effect	Ref.
In vitro			
MDA-MB-231 breast	5-FU	Synergistic	47,48
HT29 colon	5-FU	Synergistic	
	AG337	Synergistic	
	(TS inhibitor)		
HT29 (5-FU resistant), CaCO₂	5-FU	Synergistic	
	AG337	Synergistic	
A-2780 ovarian	5-FU	Synergistic	
(parental and CDDP resistant)			
MCF-7 breast	5-FU	Additive	
MCF-mdr (doxo resistant)	5-FU	Additive	
2008 ovarian	5-FU	Synergistic	
2008-C13 (CDDP resistant)	5-FU	None	
HCT116 colon	Gemcitabine	Synergistic	49
Colo 320	Gemcitabine	Synergistic (gem-oxal sequence)	
		Additive (oxal-gem sequence)	
CEM leuk	Gemcitabine	Synergistic (oxal-gem sequence)	
		Antagonism (gem-oxal sequence)	
HT29 colon	CPT-11 (SN-38)	Synergistic	50
	SN-38	Synergistic	47
HT29/LoVo colon	Topotecan	Synergistic	51,52
HT295FUR (5-FU resistant)	Topotecan	Synergistic	
LoVo5FUR (5-FU resistant)	Topotecan	Synergistic	
HT29/LoVo colon	5-FU	Synergistic	
HT295FUR	5-FU	Synergistic	
LoVo5FUR (5-FU resistant)	5-FU	Additive (when 5-FU given first)	
KB/A-2780 human	Cisplatin	Additive/synergistic	21
Various tumors, Evassay	5-FU	Synergistic	53
(human lung, ovarian, breast, GI, melanoma)			
	DFDC	Synergistic	
	Topotecan	Synergistic	
hu colon ca	Raltitrexed	Antagonistic	54
IGROV-1 hu ovarian	Topotecan	Supraadditive	55
In vivo			
HT29 xenograft	5-FU	Additive	47
GR mouse mammary model	5-FU	Additive	
DHD/K12-TRb colon, rat model	5-FU	Synergistic	56
DHD/K12-TRb colon, rat model	MitoC	Synergistic	
HD/K12-TRb colon, rat model	Cyclophos	Synergistic	
L-1210 leukemia mouse model	Cyclophos	Synergistic	57
	5-FU	None	
MV-522 hu lung xenograft	Taxol	Additive	58
	Tirapazamine/ taxol	Additive	
GR mouse mammary	SN38	Low additive	47
GR mouse mammary	AG337	Additive	
	ZD1694		
	(TS inhibitors)		

nephrotoxicity. These findings led to the first phase I study, reported in 1986 by Mathe et al. *(63)*. Twenty-three patients with a variety of tumor types were treated using a somewhat unconventional design since intrapatient dose-escalation was permitted. The objective of this trial was to confirm tolerance of the highest dose of the maximally efficient dose range (MEDR) seen in mice. Most of these patients were heavily pretreated with prior chemotherapy. Patients started at 0.45 mg/m^2 (one-tenth the MEDR in mice) and were escalated to 15 mg/m^2 by d 11. Oxaliplatin was then given every 3 wk, with dose escalations from 22.5 to 67 mg/m^2 (subtoxic dose in mice). Eleven patients reached the highest dose level. Patients who did not continue treatment had progressive disease. The median total dose given was 500 mg/m^2.

This regimen was well tolerated, with no treatment-related deaths, anaphylaxis, nephrotoxicity, or neutropenia. Other toxicities were mild. Hematologic toxicity was only seen at doses exceeding 45 mg/m^2 and included one patient with grade 1 thrombocytopenia and three patients with grade 1–2 anemia. Nausea and vomiting were seen in all patients treated with more than 45 mg/m^2. No maximum tolerated dose (MTD) was identified, but the recommended starting dose for phase II trials was 67 mg/m^2. One patient with melanoma had a complete response to therapy, and one patient with metastatic breast cancer had a partial response. Four of the 23 patients had a minor response or stable disease. This study identified the agent as one that merited further clinical study.

Extra et al. conducted a phase I trial in 44 patients with a variety of malignancies *(64)*. Most patients were chemotherapy veterans, having been heavily pretreated. The starting dose of 45 mg/m^2 was escalated to 200 mg/m^2. Oxaliplatin was given every 4 wk, over 1–6 h. The longer infusions were used for doses over 60 mg/m^2 to reduce gastrointestinal side effects. Again, no treatment-related deaths or nephrotoxicity were observed. Nausea and vomiting occurred at all doses, with 23/43 patients experiencing grade 3 or 4 toxicity. Gastrointestinal toxicity was not influenced by the duration of infusion. Hematologic toxicity was mild with no grade 3 or 4 leukopenia observed, and only one patient had grade 4 thrombocytopenia. Thrombocytopenia was dose related and was noted to occur in 13% of patients treated at dose level 135–150 mg/m^2 and in 28% treated at 175–200 mg/m^2. Only transient grade 1–2 renal toxicity was observed in five patients. Other toxicities reported included transient mild increases in liver enzymes (6/43), fever (3/43), and phlebitis (1/43).

In this study, a novel pattern of sensory neurotoxicity became apparent and was the dose-limiting side effect. Patients described paresthesias and dysesthesias in the extremities and perioral area, initiated or exacerbated by exposure to cold. A sensation of choking or inability to swallow, now termed "pharyngolaryngeal-dysesthesia," was identified. These neurologic findings were observed at doses exceeding 135 mg/m^2 and could occur during or after the infusion. The incidence of neurotoxicity for different dose levels of oxaliplatin is shown in Table 4.

After the first course at which neurologic symptoms were noted, the paresthesias were generally short-lived. However, symptoms lasted longer with subsequent cycles. Grade 3 neurotoxicity was seen in 1/21 patients with cumulative dose <270mg/m^2, 0/11 at 270–540 mg/m^2, and 5/9 at doses >540 mg/m^2. The authors noted the dysesthesias involved the extremities, forearms, legs, mouth, and throat. One patient had transient laryngeal symptoms after two cycles and five patients experienced this after four cycles. Of these five patients, four developed marked ataxia. Electromyograms (EMG) were conducted in six patients, revealing an axonal sensory neuropathy. In this study, there was no relationship between prior cisplatin exposure and the development of neurotoxicity.

This neuropathy differs from cisplatin-associated neuropathy in that symptoms occurring after oxaliplatin infusion are acute in onset. Symptoms are exacerbated by cold and are

Table 4
Incidence of Neurotoxicity for Different Dose Levels of Oxaliplatin

Dose (mg/m^2)	Incidence (first course)	Courses (N)	Courses with neurotoxicity (grade)			
			0	1	2	3
135	50%	39	15	19	4	1
150	64%	28	6	14	5	3
175	71%	22	3	12	5	2
200	100%	10	1	6	2	1

Source: ref. 64.

reversible. The above-described neurotoxicity improved after 6 mo; however, the authors stated that some long-term deficits persisted. Because of neurotoxicity, the authors defined the recommended dose at 130 mg/m^2. They also recommended careful evaluation of neurologic symptoms, especially above the cumulative dose of 500 mg/m^2, as more constant and potentially disabling symptoms were seen at these doses. In this study, four patients had a partial response to therapy (urothelial, esophageal, lung) and four patients had stable disease. Two of these patients had experienced disease progression on cisplatin-based therapy in the past.

A third phase I study was conducted in France by Caussanel et al. using continuous infusion of oxaliplatin given in a circadian rhythm as well as at a constant rate (65). Preclinical data in rats suggested that giving oxaliplatin in a circadian rhythm decreased toxicity, as discussed later in this subsection (43). Twenty-five patients were enrolled, with 23 evaluated for response. Patients were randomized to a 5-d infusion of oxaliplatin, given either by constant rate or administration via circadian rhythm, with peak delivery of drug at 1600 h. The starting dose was 125 mg/m^2, and doses were escalated by 25 mg/m^2 per cycle as tolerated, with a maximum dose of 200 mg/m^2. Four of 11 patients on the circadian arm reached the maximum dose (median MTD-175 mg/m^2) and none of those on constant rate infusion reached the maximum dose (median MTD-150 mg/m^2).

Toxicities were similar to those observed in prior trials, with most patients experiencing nausea, vomiting, and neuropathy. There were no toxic deaths, nor was alopecia, auditory, or renal toxicity observed. Sixty-seven percent of all courses were associated with nausea and/or vomiting. The authors reported <10% hematologic toxicity. In 42% of courses, patients experienced cold-induced paresthesias, and in 30% of courses, there was grade II or higher neuropathy observed. In 14% of courses, patients noted some functional impairment as a result of distal sensory loss. The authors described a grading scale for peripheral paresthesias designed to take the duration of symptoms into account:

  Grade I: moderate intensity, lasting less than 2 wk
  Grade II: moderate intensity, with incomplete recovery 2 wk after course onset
  Grade III: beginning of functional impairment

In 13 courses, the dose was decreased 25 mg/m^2 because of persistent symptoms, and paresthesias resolved within 2 mo. When comparing the two schedules, the circadian schedule resulted in a lower incidence of paresthesias (2% vs 28% of courses) and less neutropenia (2% vs 19% of courses). Of note, there were no severe neuropathies (ataxia) or laryngopharyngeal-dysesthesias observed even at the highest dose level, as had been seen with conventional dosing. Other toxicities were not significantly different between the two arms.

Preliminary pharmacokinetic data was obtained in one patient given 20 mg/m^2/d for 5 d first by continuous infusion, then by circadian rhythm 3 wk later. The AUC was 30% greater with the circadian delivery. However, the mean level of residual platinum 2 wk postinfusion was higher after the constant-rate infusion. The authors concluded that plasma pharmacokinetics do not explain why doses can be safely escalated in the circadian delivery. In this study, there were two partial responses observed in patients with breast cancer, and one minor response seen in a patient with hepatocellular cancer. All responders were treated with circadian rhythm schedule.

The authors concluded that circadian rhythm delivery of continuous venous infusion oxaliplatin is well tolerated, and higher doses of oxaliplatin can be administered with less neuropathy, gastrointestinal, and hematologic toxicity than with constant-rate infusion or conventional bolus administration. The recommended dose for phase II trials using circadian rhythm delivery was 175 mg/m^2.

Three other phase I trials have been conducted, as reported by Raymond et al. in a review of preclinical and clinical studies using oxaliplatin *(66)*. Taguchi treated 20 patients with 20–180 mg/m^2 over 2 h every 3–4 wk. The MTD was 180 mg/m^2 and the recommended therapeutic dose was 175 mg/m^2. Again, neurotoxicity was dose limiting. Two other unpublished trials using high-dose oxaliplatin were also conducted. Chevalier and Armand treated a total of 10 patients with ≥175 mg/m^2. Acute transient or laryngopharyngo-dysesthesia was seen during the infusion. Severe nausea and vomiting were seen in 33% of patients, and severe neurotoxicity in 20%. Hematologic toxicity was mild.

These phase I trials established the safety and described the toxicities seen with oxaliplatin given as a single agent. As found in preclinical studies, there was no renal toxicity observed, and routine pretreatment hydration was felt to be unnecessary. There was no ototoxicity or alopecia, and hematologic toxicity was mild. Nausea and vomiting were very common and not influenced by the rate of infusion. However, these studies did not use 5HT3 receptor antagonists, and in more recent studies, the incidence of nausea and vomiting has decreased with the widespread use of these newer antiemetics. The dose-limiting toxicity with bolus delivery is the unique neuropathy of two distinct clinical types. There is an immediate syndrome of digital and oral paresthesias that occurs during or soon after oxaliplatin infusion, is exacerbated by exposure to cold, and is reversible. It is dose dependent and cumulative. With longer drug exposure, more typical stocking-glove sensory neuropathy can occur and become persistent. The recommended dose given by bolus for phase II studies was 130 mg/m^2. With circadian delivery, the MTD was higher (175 mg/m^2), nausea and vomiting were dose limiting, and the recommended dose for future circadian modulated trials was 175 mg/m^2. A summary of the three early phase I trials is shown in Table 5.

5.2. Single-Agent Phase II Trials

Diaz-Rubio et al. conducted a multicenter phase II trial in 25 patients with metastatic colorectal cancer who were of good functional status and had not been treated previously for advanced disease *(67)*. Patients were given 130 mg/m^2 oxaliplatin over 2 h every 3 wk. Dose reductions of 25% were applied for grade 3 neutropenia, thrombocytopenia, neuropathy, or grade 2 renal toxicity. Dose reductions of 50% were applied for grade 4 hematologic toxicity or grade 3 renal toxicity. Treatment was discontinued for grade 4 nonhematologic toxicity. Responses to therapy were assessed using computed tomography (CT) scans every 3 wk, and these scans were reviewed by independent radiologists. The response rate was 20% when assessed by investigators and 12% when assessed by independent reviewers. Results are shown in Table 6.

Table 5
Summary of Phase I Studies of Single-Agent Oxaliplatin

Author (ref.)	No. evaluated	Dose (mg/m^2)	MTD	RD	DLT	Responses
Mathe et al. (63)	23	0.45–67	NR	>67	None	Melanoma (CR)^c, breast (PR)^d
Extra et al. (64)	43	45–200	200	130	Neuropathy	Urothelial (PR), esophageal (PR), lung (PR), head/neck (PR),
Caussanel et al. (65)	13^a	125–200	150		Nausea/vomiting/	Breast (2) (PR),
	12^b	125–200	175	175	Neutropenia	HCC^e (minor)

^{a}Continuous venous infusion (CVI), constant rate × 5 d.
^{b}CVI × 5 d, circadian rhythm.
^{c}Complete response.
^{d}Partial response.
^{e}Hepatocellular cancer.

Table 6
Summary of Results from the Diaz-Rubio et al. (67) Phase II Trial

Patients receiving full dose	96.7%
Median number cycles	5 (range 1–9)
Median cumulative dose per patient	650 mg/m^2 (130–1170)
Overall RR investigators (independent reviewers)	20% (12%)
CR	1/25 (0/25)
PR	4/25 (3/25)
Stable	8/25 (12/25)
Median TTP in responders	6 mo (range 4–9)
Median PFS	4 mo (range 2–7)
Median OS	14.5 mo

Toxicities were similar to those reported in phase I trials, with laryngopharyngeal-dysesthesias (92%) and grade 1–2 peripheral neuropathy (75%) occurring very commonly. One patient experienced hypersensitivity (generalized erythema) during the sixth cycle, which occurred again when the patient was retreated with oxaliplatin. One patient experienced severe laryngeal-dysesthesia and shortness of breath requiring hospitalization. This patient was retreated without incident when oxaliplatin was administered via a prolonged infusion. Three patients experienced grade 3–4 vomiting, and one patient had grade 3 diarrhea. All other toxicities were grade 1–2. Again, mild neutropenia occurred in only 20% and thrombocytopenia in 24% of treated patients. Neuropathic symptoms resolved within a median of 9 wk from the discontinuation of therapy. Other neurologic symptoms reported included cramps, Lhermitte's sign, and loss of reflexes. There was no alopecia, ototoxicity, or nephrotoxicity reported.

Becouarn et al. conducted a multicenter phase II trial in 38 previously untreated patients with metastatic colorectal cancer (68). Patients were treated with 130 mg/m^2 over 2 h every 3 wk. Responses were evaluated over three cycles and confirmed by independent review. Doses were adjusted according to hematologic, neurologic, and any other grade 3–4 toxicities. Most patients had good performance status and had not been treated with prior adjuvant chemotherapy. The response rate was 24%. Other results are shown in Table 7.

Table 7
Results from Becouarn et al. *(68)* Phase II Trial

Overall RR	24.3%
CR	0/37
PR	13/37
Stable	15/37
Median time to achieve response	3 cycles
Median duration of response	7 mo (84–447 + d)
Median PFS	4 mo (22–447 + d)
Overall survival (OS)	395 d (28–573 + d)
1 yr OS	73.7%

Toxicity was similar to that seen in previous trials. There were no treatment-related deaths, but three patients had therapy terminated as a result of therapy-related side effects, including anaphylactoid reaction, thrombocytopenia, and neurotoxicity. Given the known unique patterns of neurotoxicity observed in prior treatment trials with oxaliplatin, the authors devised a specific toxicity scale to evaluate these symptoms.

Grade 1: dysesthesias or paresthesias that completely regressed before the next cycle, or cramps/pseudospasms graded as mild

Grade 2: dysesthesias or paresthesias that persisted between courses, or cramps/ pseudospasms graded as moderate

Grade 3: dysesthesias or paresthesias that were associated with functional impairment, or cramps/pseudospasms graded as severe

Neurosensory toxicity was the most common toxicity, with 37/38 patients experiencing symptoms. Grade 3 neurotoxicity was observed in 13% of patients. Both cold-induced and cold-unrelated paresthesias were observed. Neurotoxicity was noted to be cumulative and led to dose reductions in 10% of patients. Pharyngolaryngeal-dysesthesia and cramping was common (21/38, 19/38 respectively) but only 2.6% of patients had grade 3 toxicity. Four months after completion of therapy, severe neurotoxicity regressed completely in two patients, diminished to grade 1–2 in two patients, and remained stable in one patient.

Thrombocytopenia was the most common hematologic toxicity, with 19/38 patients experiencing some degree of abnormality and 3/38 with grade 3–4 toxicity. No bleeding episodes were noted, nor were transfusions required. Grade 3 neutropenia occurred in only 5% of patients (1% of cycles) and was associated with severe infection in two patients. Grade 3–4 vomiting occurred in 8%, grade 3 stomatitis in 3%, and grade 3 diarrhea in 3% of patients. Other toxicities noted included mild alopecia in two patients, three grade 1–2 skin toxicities, and four transient grade 1 increases in creatinine.

Machover et al. reported two consecutive phase II trials of patients with metastatic colorectal cancer who had progressed on prior 5-FU-based regimens *(69)*. A total of 109 patients were treated with 130 mg/m^2 over 2 h every 3 wk. Some patients had been treated with two or more chemotherapy regimens for metastatic disease. Dose reductions were made for grade 3 hematologic toxicity or neurotoxicity. Any grade 4 toxicity led to discontinuation of the drug. Responses were assessed by CT scan of all measurable lesions by the investigators and confirmed by independent radiologist review. The response rate was 10–11%. Other results are shown in Table 8.

Again, the most common toxicity seen in both trials was neuropathy. The authors used a grading scale similar to the Becouarn et al. trial, with grade 1—dysesthesia/paresthesia,

Table 8
Results from Machover et al. (69) Phase II Trials

	Study 1	Study 2
Number of patients	58	51
Median cumulative dose	650 mg/m^2	390 mg/m^2
Response rate	11%	10%
CR	0/58	0/51
PR	6/58	5/51
Stable	23/58	16/51
Time to achieve response	6 wk	6–12 wk
Time to progression	5–13 mo	4–9 mo
Median OS	8.2 mo	NR

transient (less than 7 d), grade 2—symptoms transient (less than 14 d), grade 3—symptoms persisting during the drug-free interval between courses, and grade 4—severe dysesthesia/hypoesthesia with functional impairment. Sensory neuropathy was seen in 96–98% of all patients; grade 3 toxicity was seen in 31% of patients in study 1 and 18% in study 2. This consisted predominantly of dysesthesia of the limbs and oropharynx, again exacerbated by exposure to cold. Neurotoxicity was cumulative in incidence and severity. Of those available for follow-up, all patients with severe neurotoxicity had either resolution or improvement in symptoms within 6 mo of finishing the study. The authors recommended discontinuation of therapy if grade 3 neurotoxicity developed.

In all patients, hematologic toxicity was mild, with only 10/109 having grade 3–4 neutropenia, and no patient experienced grade 3–4 thrombocytopenia. Nausea, vomiting, and diarrhea were also common, but mild. A total of 10 patients had grade 3 diarrhea and 25/109 had grade 3–4 nausea/vomiting. Other toxicities included five patients with grade 1 transient increase in creatinine and one patient with shortness of breath during the infusion and mild anemia.

In preclinical studies, it was shown that oxaliplatin administered by infusion according to circadian rhythms had less toxicity than did conventional dosing. As described earlier, this was confirmed clinically in a phase I trial, where patients treated with circadian-rhythm-modulated oxaliplatin had less neurotoxicity and hematologic toxicity and with the circadian administration, which also allowed for higher drug delivery doses than did constant infusion. Levi et al. conducted a multicenter phase II trial using this regimen in 29 patients with metastatic disease, most of whom had failed prior regimens (70). Patients were treated with 5-d infusions of 30 mg/m^2/d every 3 wk. Doses were escalated as tolerated up to 35 mg/m^2/d at the second course and 40 mg/m^2/d at the third course. The peak amount of drug was infused by a programmable pump at 1600 h each day. The primary end point of this trial was the response rate, as determined by CT or ultrasound evaluation performed after every third course. The scans that were used to assess response to therapy were reviewed by a panel of independent radiologists.

Eight patients were taken off of therapy because of progressive disease prior to the third cycle. Twelve of 21 patients were able to tolerate dose escalation to 35 mg/m^2/d and 8 of 21 patients had dose escalations to 40 mg/m^2/d. All responses occurred in pretreated patients and at doses of 35 mg/m^2/d or higher. The response rate in this study was 10%. Other results are shown in Table 9.

Table 9
Results from Levi et al. *(70)* Phase II Study

Median no. of Courses	3 (2–9)
Median total dose	500 mg/m^2 (275–1550)
Response rate	3/29 (10%)
CR	0
PR	3/29
Stable	7/29
TTP	20–29 wk
Median PFS	20 wk
Median OS (est.)	40 wk

Hematologic toxicity was mild, with 97–98% of courses having no toxicity. Only one course was associated with grade 3 neutropenia and thrombocytopenia. Grade 1–2 nausea and vomiting were seen in 59% of courses, and grade 3–4 in only two courses. Grade 3–4 diarrhea was seen in six courses, and one patient withdrew because of this toxicity. There was no nephrotoxicity. Peripheral sensory neuropathy was the most common side effect, seen in 79% of courses. This was graded in the same manner as described by Machover et al. *(69)*. In most patients, these dysesthesias resolved within 1–2 wk (grade 1–2). However, in 12% of courses, the dysesthesias did not resolve prior to the next cycle (grade 3). Three courses were associated with functional impairment (grade 4). Thirteen patients did not reach the highest dose level in this study because of grade II or higher neuropathy. Again, this toxicity was found to be cumulative; the authors noted a doubling of incidence with a cumulative dose of 700–1550 mg/m^2. Two patients experienced muscle cramps of the jaw and/or shoulders during the infusion, which recurred upon rechallenge in one patient despite retreatment at a lower dose.

Schmilovich et al. reported results of the experience using single-agent oxaliplatin in patients with 5-FU-resistant metastatic colorectal cancer treated in Argentina under an extended access program *(71)*. Thirty-nine patients were treated with 130 mg/m^2 oxaliplatin every 3 wk, with 38 patients evaluable. There were no treatment-related deaths and toxicity was mild. The overall response rate was 8.4%, with median survival of 7.4 mo.

In summary, in phase II trials of oxaliplatin as a single agent, the drug was well tolerated and active. This was true whether oxaliplatin was administered every three weeks or every 2 wk and by chronomodulated infusion over 5 d or as a constant short term infusion. Response rates ranged from 8 to 24%. The lower rates were in pretreated patients and the highest rate in those previously untreated for advanced colorectal cancer. Preclinical data provided compelling evidence that oxaliplatin had synergistic interactions with a number of other agents including 5-fluorouracil and irinotecan leading to the next generation of studies with multiple agents.

5.3. Phase II Trials of Combinations with 5-FU

The phase II trials of oxaliplatin administered with 5-FU/LV (leucovorin) can be divided into those that pursued one of two treatment strategies; chronomodulated infusion over multiple days or flat (unchronomodulated) short-infusion therapy. The principal proponents of the chronomodulated approach have been Levi and his colleagues. De Gramont and his collaborators have experimented with a series of regimens of flat short-term oxaliplatin infusion administered with varying infusion 5-FU/LV regimens that they have termed

FOLFOX 1 to 7. There have also been several studies in which oxaliplatin had been administered with bolus 5-FU/LV in a manner designed to correspond to the standard bolus approaches of 5-FU ± LV favored in the United States. Oxaliplatin with 5-FU/LV has been tested in legions of small phase II trials that enrolled 10–50 patients mainly conducted in Europe. In contrast to the plethora of phase II studies that have been reported in abstract form or as full reports in the literature, results from only a few phase III trials are available. For the purposes of this discussion, selected phase II trials will be discussed and divided into those that treated patients with a chronomodulated infusion and those that used a flat short-term infusion.

5.3.1. Oxaliplatin Chronomodulated Infusion Regimens

One of the initial reports on clinical experience with a chronomodulated regimen of 5-FU and oxaliplatin came from Levi and colleagues published in 1992 *(72)*. In this study, 93 patients were treated with 700 mg/m^2/d 5-FU, 300 mg/m^2/d LV, and 25 mg/m^2/d oxaliplatin for 5 consecutive days every 21 d. Toxicity included grade 3 diarrhea in 18% of courses and emesis in 34% of courses. Paresthesias occurred in 58% of courses and were noted to be mild in most cases. However, 14 patients discontinued treatment because of neurologic toxicity. Two patients died of toxicity, both related to diarrhea and dehydration. The response rate was 54% and 18 patients subsequently underwent resection for cure.

Levi and his group have developed an aggressive surgical approach in the management of their patients with potentially resectable metastases (described later in this chapter). In some cases, operating several times during the course of treatment for metastatic colorectal cancer in an attempt to render individuals free of disease. If patients who are felt to be sufficiently fit to withstand surgery have sufficient tumor shrinkage on chemotherapy to permit resection of metastatic disease, this aggressive surgical strategy is recommended. This combined chemotherapeutic and surgical approach could potentially influence median survival favorably, even if patients eventually relapse after treatment. The median survival in this trial was 15 mo.

A randomized phase II trial of flat versus chronomodulated infusion, both administered over 5 consecutive days, was then performed *(73)*. In this study, 92 patients were treated with a 5-d continuous infusion of 5-FU at a lower starting dose of 600 mg/m^2/d, 300 mg/m^2/d LV, 20 mg/m^2/d oxaliplatin every 21 d. If no WHO grade ≥ 2 toxicity was encountered, the 5-FU was increased to 700 mg/m^2/d and oxaliplatin to 25 mg/m^2/d. Forty-seven patients were randomized to a flat rate and 45 to a chronomodulated infusion schedule. In the chronomodulated, therapy the oxaliplatin was administered between 1015 and 2145 h and peak levels of the 5-FU + LV were given from 2215 to 0945 hours using a variable-rate programmable infusion device known as the IntelliJect pump. Response was assessed after every third treatment course.

Dose-limiting toxicity of stomatitis occurred 8.7 times more frequently on the flat compared to the chronomodulated schedule. No differences between the incidence and severity of nausea and vomiting, diarrhea, or skin toxicity were noted. Grade 3 or 4 toxicity was seen in less than 5% of patients. The reported incidence of severe paresthesias was 53% vs 22.8%. The response rate was 32% for the flat infusion and 53% for the chronomodulated infusion. In this trial, resection for cure was done in 23% of patients on the flat infusion and in 38% on the chronomodulated schedule. The median survival for all patients was 14.9 vs 19 mo. This trial provided clinical data to corroborate the potential of chronomodulation with these agents and led to additional trials. However, this trial was a phase II study and was not adequately powered to permit definitive comparisons between flat and chronomodulated infusion strategies.

Levi et al. pooled and updated data from this trial and a second study *(74,75)*. In the combined analysis, 140 patients were treated with the flat infusion and 138 with the chronomodulated infusion schedule. The objective response rates were 30% vs 51% and the resection rate was 13% vs 23%. Median survival was 16.5 vs 18.6 mo and 13% vs 15% of patient were alive at 5 yr after study entry.

This group then tried to intensify treatment into a 4-d treatment course and compress the cycle length to 14 d *(76)*. The initial dose for each of the 90 patients enrolled in this trial was 700 mg/m^2/d 5-FU, 300 mg/m^2/d LV, and 25 mg/m^2/d oxaliplatin for 4 d every 14 d. Responses were assessed after every fourth treatment cycle. Toxicity with the higher dose intensity administered in this program was more troublesome. Two patients died of gastrointestinal toxicity and dehydration. Nineteen percent of patients ceased treatment because of neuropathy. Grade 3–4 toxicities in the form of diarrhea were observed in 41% and mucositis was noted in 30% of patients. Grade 3–4 neutropenia occurred in 13% of patients. However, the confirmed objective response rate was 66%, among the highest rates that have ever been reported in advanced colorectal cancer, and 42% of patients underwent surgery for attempted resection of all known disease. There was a complete resection documented in 34% of the total patient group. The median survival was 18.5 mo, with 4% of patients in sustained complete remission at a median follow-up time of 3.5 yr.

Another French group has published work using chronomodulated drug delivery schedules *(77)*. In this trial, 50 patients with metastatic colorectal cancer, 37 of whom were pretreated, were given a regimen consisting of 300 mg/m^2 /d LV, 700 mg/m^2/d 5-FU, and 25 mg/m^2/d oxaliplatin for 4 d every 2 wk. The drugs were delivered via a pump programmed to maximize peak flow rates of oxaliplatin at 4:00 PM and 5-FU at 4:00 AM. The median 5-FU drug dose was 3200 mg/m^2 per course, indicating that dose escalation was possible in many patients. The response rate was 48%, including a 40% response rate in 5-FU-pretreated patients. Toxicity was moderate with grade 3 hand–foot syndrome in 14%, peripheral neuropathy in 28%, grade 3–4 nausea and vomiting in 36%, and diarrhea in 7%.

Despite the high response rates observed with the chronomodulated approach, it has not been widely accepted outside of France. This is in part the result of the complexity of the approach that requires long-term intravenous access with multiple ports and the use of a programmable pump. Such devices have not yet been FDA approved in the United States. There has also been some degree of skepticism that the potential to exploit circadian variation is important enough to warrant the complexities of administration associated with its use.

5.3.2. Oxaliplatin Regimens with a Flat Infusion Strategy

Aimery de Gramont and his colleagues at the Hopital Saint-Antoine in Paris have performed a series of clinical trials with a variety of 5-FU, LV, and oxaliplatin regimens, which they have termed FOLFOX 1–7. These studies are based on the administration of folinic acid (LV), followed by a loading dose and 1–2 d infusion of 5-FU with a short infusion of oxaliplatin on the first day of each cycle. These investigators have favored the infusion of 5-FU based on the theoretical consideration that a drug such as 5-FU, with a half-life of 14 min, will more effectively interfere with tumor cell replication when drug exposure is prolonged via administration by continuous infusion. Additionally, one of the infusion regimens tested by this group had a favorable toxicity and activity profile when compared in a phase III study of 200 patients to bolus 5-FU therapy. The infusion program modestly improved both time to progression and the response rate, although no significant survival advantage was apparent in this study (78).

The initial regimen tested was termed FOLFOX 1 (79). It prescribed 130 mg/m^2 oxaliplatin and 500 mg/m^2 LV followed by 1500–2000 mg/m^2 5-FU over 22 h. The LV and 5-FU were repeated on the second day of a 2-wk cycle. Oxaliplatin was administered every other cycle. Initially, the lower dose of 5-FU was used and this dose was escalated if no grade 3 toxicity was observed. This pilot trial included only 13 patients and identified a 31% response rate.

The investigators then decreased the oxaliplatin dose but gave the drug with every cycle in their next trial with the regimen termed FOLFOX 2 (80). In this study, 46 patients were treated after progression on 5-FU and leucovorin. In 24 patients, several prior 5-FU exposures had occurred prior to enrollment. In 22 patients, oxaliplatin was added to the same 5-FU regimen on which they had manifest progressive disease. The protocol prescribed treatment with 100 mg/m^2 oxaliplatin on d 1, 500 mg/m^2 LV followed by 1.5-2.0 g/m^2 5-FU for 2 consecutive days every 2 wk. The response rate was 46%, including 10 of the 22 (43%) patients in whom the only difference between first- and second-line therapy was the addition of oxaliplatin. The median progression-free survival was 7 mo, and the median overall survival was 17 mo. Using the WHO scale, grade 3 or 4 toxicity was peripheral neuropathy in 9%, nausea in 4%, diarrhea in 9%, mucositis in 13%, neutropenia in 39%, febrile neutropenia in 9%, thrombocytopenia in 11%, and alopecia in 9%. The high response rate in the cohort of patients who had oxaliplatin added to their prior 5-FU regimen suggested that the synergy between 5-FU and oxaliplatin observed in vitro was also relevant in patients.

The next two regimens tested were designed to reduce the dose of leucovorin and to reduce the dose of oxaliplatin administered in hopes of moderating toxicity. The experience with these two regimens was reported in a single article (81). One hundred patients were initially treated with one of two first-line regimens of LV/5-FU. Among those 40 patients treated with the FOLFOX 3 treatment program, the initial first-line therapy was 500 mg/m^2 LV and 1.5–2.0 g/m^2 5-FU over 22 h on d 1 and 2 of every 2 wk. At progression, 85 mg/m^2 oxaliplatin every 2 wk was added. Fifty-seven patients were treated with FOLFOX 4, after initial progression on a regimen consisting of 200 mg/m^2 LV and 400 mg/m^2 5-FU as a loading dose over 2 h, followed by 600 mg/m^2 over 22 h on d 1 and 2 of every 2 wk. Similarly, after progression on the second regimen, patients were retreated with the same LV/5-FU program, with the addition of 85 mg/m^2 oxaliplatin on d 1. The response rate was 18% for the first regimen and 23% for the second. The median response duration was 7 mo and the median survival approached 11 mo. Toxicity included peripheral neuropathy of grade 3 in 21% and neutropenia in 15% on the first regimen and 37% on the second regimen. Grade 3 nausea and vomiting affected 5% and 7%, respectively, of patients and diarrhea was rarely troublesome. These regimens did not seem to represent a major advance over FOLFOX 2.

The FOLFOX 4 regimen was also tested by Souglakos and colleagues, with similar results (82). In this study of 33 patients, the response rate was 30% and median survival was not yet reached at the time of the report. Toxicity included grade 3–4 neutropenia in 48%, febrile neutropenia in 3%, and peripheral neuropathy in 9% of patients.

FOLFOX 5 was an identical regimen to FOLFOX 4 with the exception that the oxaliplatin dose was increased to 100 mg/m^2 every 2 wk. This regimen was never actually tested. Instead, FOLFOX 6 was created in an attempt to simplify the program. FOLFOX 4 required visits to the clinic for treatment on 2 subsequent days. Some patients returned to the clinic on the third day to have their pumps disconnected. With FOLFOX 6, the program called for administration of 100 mg/m^2 oxaliplatin and 400 mg/m^2 LV, followed by bolus

400 mg/m^2 5-FU as a loading dose followed by a 46-h infusion of 2.4–3.0 g/m^2 5-FU with every 2 wk cycles *(83)*. Sixty patients with progressive disease on or soon after treatment with LV/5-FU were treated. The response rate was 27%, with a median progression-free interval of 5 mo and median survival of 11 mo. The NCI-CTC grade 3 and 4 toxicities observed were peripheral neuropathy 16%, nausea 7%, diarrhea 7%, mucositis 5%, neutropenia 24%, and thrombocytopenia 2%. The lower response rate observed with FOLFOX 6 as compared to FOLFOX 2 was thought to be related in part to patient selection and, in part, to the lower dose intensity of oxaliplatin in the later regimen.

In an attempt to increase the dose intensity of oxaliplatin and limit hematologic toxicity, de Gramont and his group are now testing FOLFOX 7 in which the oxaliplatin dose is increased and the 5-FU dose is reduced. The FOLFOX 7 regimen is 100 mg/m^2 oxaliplatin and 400 mg/m^2 LV, followed by bolus 400 mg/m^2 5-FU as a loading dose followed by a 46-h infusion of 2.4 g/m^2 5-FU with every 2 wk cycles *(84)*. A 44% response rate in previously treated patients was observed in this study, which was ongoing at the time of the reported abstract.

The FOLFOX series of trials have all enrolled patients who had prior therapy for advanced colorectal cancer. Therefore, the high reported response rates are provocative. Additional testing is in progress using this approach both in the United States and in Europe. FOLFOX 4 is being tested in the adjuvant setting in Europe against 5-FU and leucovorin alone. In the United States, FOLFOX 4 is being compared to a 5-FU, leucovorin, and irinotecan regimen, as well as to irinotecan and oxaliplatin in first-line treatment of advanced disease. In Europe, de Gramont and colleagues are testing a strategy of treatment in which oxaliplatin is given in an intermittent fashion rather than continuously in an attempt to ameliorate the cumulative neurotoxicity in a trial known as the OPTIMOX study.

5.3.3. Oxaliplatin, Leucovorin, and Bolus 5-Fluorouracil Regimens

A number of small trials have been done that combine a 5-FU bolus regimen with LV and oxaliplatin in an attempt to build a regimen more like those commonly employed in the United States, where 5-FU infusion is less often chosen than it is in Europe. One advantage to this type of administration schedule is the elimination of the need for central venous access in many patients. These studies can be divided into those based on the Mayo Clinic regimen (425 mg/m^2/d 5-FU administered following 20 mg/m^2/d LV for 5 consecutive days) vs those based upon the Roswell Park Memorial Institute (RPMI) regimen (600 mg/m^2/d 5-FU administered following 500 mg/m^2/d LV given weekly).

One study using the Mayo Clinic-type program called for administration of 130 mg/m^2 oxaliplatin on d 1 followed by 100 mg/m^2/d LV and 400–500 mg/m^2/d 5-FU on d 1–5 repeated every 3 wk. A 20% response rate was noted in 29 heavily pretreated patients with modest toxicity noted. This study was still in progress at the time that the abstract was reported *(85)*. Another trial treated patients who had progressed on the Mayo Clinic 5-FU/LV treatment with 130 mg/m^2 oxaliplatin on d 1 followed by 20 mg/m^2/d LV and 320 mg/m^2/d 5-FU, both administered on d 1–5 every 3 wk. Of 115 patients, 13% responded to therapy and the median survival was 10 mo. Toxicity was noted as similar to that seen with 5-FU/LV alone, with the exception of the incidence of grade 3 neuropathy in 8% of patients *(86)*. A third study treated 73 patients with 25 mg/m^2/d LV and 425 mg/m^2/d 5-FU on d 1–4 with 130 mg/m^2 oxaliplatin on d 1 every 3 wk. In these patients, only 40% of whom had prior exposure to 5-FU in the adjuvant setting, the response rate was 32%. The median time to progression was 8 mo and median survival was 12 mo. The major grade 3–4 toxicities included neurosensory (3%), diarrhea (12%), nausea/vomiting (8%), and sepsis (3%) *(87)*.

Three trials have been reported in abstract form that used a weekly treatment schedule based on the RPMI approach. In one study, patients previously untreated for metastatic colorectal cancer received weekly LV at 20 mg/m^2/d and 5-FU at 500 mg/m^2/d, with 85 mg/m^2/d oxaliplatin every other week for 3 of every 4 wk. This ongoing study was reported after 11 patients had been enrolled, only 5 of whom could be evaluated for response. However, all five patients responded to the treatment. Toxicity was modest, but the accuracy was hampered by the fact that the trial was ongoing (88). Another study with the same regimen enrolled 31 patients, of which 22 were chemotherapy naive, and found a 14% response rate. Toxicity exceeding grade 2 was diarrhea (6%), neuropathy (9%), and thrombocytopenia (6%) (89). The studies that have employed bolus-type regimens of 5-FU/LV with oxaliplatin are largely immature, and it is difficult to draw definitive activity or toxicity conclusions from these interim reports. However, the National Surgical Adjuvant Breast and Bowel Program (NSABP) is currently enrolling patients with stage II and stage III colon cancer on an adjuvant study comparing the RPMI 5-FU/LV program to a weekly bolus regimen of 5-FU/LV and bimonthly oxaliplatin.

5.3.4. OTHER OXALIPLATIN, 5-FLUOROURACIL, AND LEUCOVORIN REGIMENS

A group of Greek investigators developed a regimen based on a 24-h high-dose infusion of 5-FU program that is used commonly in Germany and other countries in Europe (90). This trial treated 32 patients with metastatic colorectal cancer who had relapsed after or during chemotherapy with 5-FU and/or irinotecan using 500 mg/m^2 LV and 2.5 g/m^2 5-FU by 24-h infusion with 50 mg/m^2 oxaliplatin on d 1, 8, 15, 22, 29, and 36 repeated every 50 d. The objective response rate was 13%. Median time to progression was 3 mo and median survival was 9 mo. Grade 3–4 toxicity included diarrhea in 52%, nausea and vomiting in 28%, thrombocytopenia in 11%, and neutropenia in 10%. No grade 3–4 neurotoxicity was recorded, but 50% of patients experienced some sensory neuropathy. Three patients refused further treatment because of toxicity.

A number of programs have been designed around the world to permit access to oxaliplatin for compassionate use, particularly in countries where the agent has not been approved for prescription use. In these programs, patients are permitted to receive the drug in combination or alone without enrollment in a formal protocol, with entry criteria and the exact treatment regimen determined by the treating physician. An example of this experience is the compassionate-use program in Germany (91). In this experience, there were 34 patients who received oxaliplatin after progression either on or shortly after treatment with irinotecan at 8 German oncologic centers. Patients were treated at physician discretion with oxaliplatin alone or in combination with a 5-FU and leucovorin program. The response rate was 12% and the median time to progression was 3 mo. Despite the small number of patients treated by diverse regimens, the authors concluded that the outcomes appeared to favor the use of oxaliplatin combined with 5-FU and LV over oxaliplatin alone.

6. PHASE III TRIALS

6.1. Chronomodulated Infusion

Two phase III trials comparing 5-FU/LV alone vs 5-FU/LV with oxaliplatin have been completed. These trials used different schedules and doses of 5-FU/LV. These two trials were recently presented by the Oncologic Drugs Advisory Committee (ODAC) to the United States Federal Drug Admininstration (FDA) in hopes of obtaining recommendation for FDA approval for oxaliplatin + 5-FU in the treatment of advanced colorectal cancer. Neither trial showed an overall benefit in patient survival over 5-FU and LV alone, and ODAC did not recommend the combination for FDA approval. However, these trials did meet their statistical goals, which were to show superior response rates and/or progression-free survival to those observed with the same 5-FU/LV regimen without oxaliplatin.

The first trial was from France and was reported by Giachetti et al. on behalf of the group associated with Levi *(92)*. Two hundred patients with previously untreated metastatic colorectal cancer were enrolled in this multicenter trial. Eligibility included bidimensionally measurable disease, performance score ≤2, and adequate marrow, renal, and hepatic function. Patients who had received adjuvant therapy more than 6 mo from entry were eligible. Ineligibility criteria included age over 76, prior treatment for metastatic disease, second malignancies, or history of peripheral sensory neuropathy.
Patients were randomized to one of two arms:

Arm A: 5-FU (700 mg/m^2/d) and LV (300 mg/m^2/d) infused from 2215 to 0945 h, peak delivery by programmable pump at 0400 h, d 1–5, q 21 d

Arm B: oxaliplatin (125 mg/m^2/d) infused from 1000 to 1600 h, d 1, q 21 d and 5-FU (700 mg/m^2/d) and CF (300 mg/m^2/d) delivered as in arm A, d 1–5, q 21 d

The primary endpoint of the trial was response rate, which was assessed every three cycles by standard WHO criteria. Secondary endpoints included overall survival, progression-free survival, and toxicity. The data were analyzed with intent-to-treat method.

Neuropathy was graded so as to take into account both the intensity and duration of symptoms by a third scale devised for this trial:

Grade 1a: peripheral paresthesias of moderate intensity lasting less than 7 d
Grade 1b: paresthesias of moderate intensity lasting 8–14 d
Grade 1c: incomplete recovery between courses or mild hypoesthesias of the extremities
Grade 2: early functional impairment

Doses were modified for grade 3–4 toxicity (except for alopecia/neuropathy) as follows: 5-FU was reduced by 100 mg/m^2 and oxaliplatin by 25 mg/m^2; oxaliplatin was reduced by 25 mg/m^2 for grade 1c sensory neuropathy and, if persistent, was reduced again by 25 mg/m^2. Treatment was discontinued if neurotoxicity persisted beyond this or for any grade 2 neurotoxicity. Treatment was also discontinued for other persistent hematologic and nonhematologic toxicity within 6 wk after the last course. Patients with progressive disease or who were rendered surgically resectable were taken off study and resected when possible and were then followed for progression and survival. Discontinuation of treatment for any reason was considered treatment failure.

Three patients were ineligible and one patient on arm B did not receive oxaliplatin. Patient characteristics were similar between groups. Notable exceptions included more patients with elevated carcinoembryonic antigen (CEA) exceeding 10 ng/mL in the oxaliplatin group (B) and more patients who had been treated with adjuvant chemotherapy in group A. The median age of patients was 61yr (range 29–75), and most had PS 0–1. The median duration of follow-up was 47 mo (35–67 mo). Toxicity was generally mild in arm A, with less than a 5% incidence of grade 3–4 toxicity. Diarrhea was the most common toxicity in arm B, with 43% experiencing grade 3–4 toxicity. Nausea and vomiting were also common in arm B, despite treatment with standard antiemetics; 25% experienced grade 3–4 toxicity. Hematologic toxicity was mild in both treatment arms, with neutropenia and thrombocytopenia only occurring in 1–2% overall. Mild increases in serum transaminase levels were observed in 60% of patients in arm B and 24% in arm A. Only two patients in both arms experienced grade 3–4 hepatotoxicity. As had been observed in prior trials, there was no clinically meaningful renal toxicity. Grade 1–2 alopecia was seen in five patients—one on arm A and

Table 10
Results of Phase III Study of Giachetti et al. *(92)*

	Arm 1: 5-FU/LV	*Arm 2: 5-FU/LV/OXAL*
No. of patients	100	100
No. evaluable	92	88
Median no. of courses	6	8
Overall response rate	16%	53% (*p* <0.001)
CR	0/100	3/100
PR	16/100	50/100
Stable	45/100	24/100
Percentage with confirmed response at 9 wk	12%	34% (*p* <0.001)
Median time to best response	6 mo (4.3–7.4)	5 mo (4.3–5.5)
Median PFS	6.1 mo (4–7.4)	8.7 mo (7.4–9.2)
Median OS	19.9 mo (14–25.7 mo)	19.4 mo (15.4–23.4 mo)

four patients on arm B. There was one treatment-related death on each arm. However, there were 12 treatment-related withdrawals from the study on arm B.

There were 45 patients in arm B who had grade 1c or grade 2 sensory neurotoxicity. Onset of grade 1c neuropathy was seen from 250 mg/m^2 to 1625 mg/m^2 (median 716 mg/m^2). Ten of these patients withdrew from the trial (four with grade 1c and six with grade 2). The median cumulative dose in these patients was 1075 mg/m^2 (range 675–1650 mg/m^2). Other reported neurotoxicity included one patient with masseter contractions during the second course of therapy, for 4 d, and one patient with acute "spasms." An independent radiology review of patients scans was performed in 91% of cases and was used to determine response rates as shown in Table 10.

An important point to note in this trial is that crossover was allowed for patients with progression on 5-FU/LV. Fifty-seven patients who progressed on arm 1 were subsequently treated with 5-FU/CF and oxaliplatin. Also, more surgeries for cure were attempted in patients on the oxaliplatin-containing arm (32 vs 21). The authors noted that complete resection of metastatic disease was performed in 17 patients on arm A and in 21 patients on arm B. As determined by multivariate analysis, age and treatment arm were significant prognostic factors for response to therapy. Prognostic factors for survival were performance status and extent of liver metastasis.

In summary, this randomized multicenter phase III trial using chronomodulated 5-FU/LV confirmed the high response rates seen in phase II trials combining 5-FU/LV with oxaliplatin. Response rates were increased threefold in the combination arm compared to 5-FU/LV alone. The trial was not designed to detect differences in overall survival, and the fact that over half of the patients crossed over to receive oxaliplatin at progression on arm 1 makes overall survival data difficult to interpret. Also, the overall median survival of nearly 20 mo is longer than that seen in other trials using 5-FU-based therapy. However, progression-free survival was significantly longer in the combination arm. Overall, the oxaliplatin-containing arm did have more toxicity. The most common side effect was diarrhea, and the cumulative dose-limiting toxicity was sensory peripheral neuropathy. This neuropathy did not affect dose intensity until late in treatment, as it occurred at a mean dose of 1100 mg/m^2, or about 6 mo worth of treatment. The authors did not report whether the 13 patients who developed functional impairments (grade 2 neurotoxicity) had improvement or resolution of symptoms with time.

6.2. Flat Infusion

De Gramont et al. recently reported the results of a phase III study, in which first-line 5-FU/LV given bimonthly was compared to 5-FU/LV/oxaliplatin *(93)*. The bimonthly regimen consisted of a loading dose plus infusion of 5-FU given with LV and was employed here as the control arm of the trial. In a previous trial, known as the French Intergroup Trial, this regimen has been reported to result in higher response rates and longer progression-free survival than the Mayo Clinic regimen, but it did not lead to a significant difference in overall survival. The Mayo Clinic regimen prescribed bolus 5-FU/ LV for 5 consecutive days monthly. In this next-generation trial, the experimental regimen from the French Intergroup Trial was compared to the same program to which biweekly oxaliplatin was added. The schedule was that prescribed by the FOLFOX 4 program described earlier. At 35 institutions in Europe, 420 patients with metastatic colon or rectal cancer were enrolled. Eligible patients had PS 0–2, age 18–75, with measurable disease. Prior adjuvant chemotherapy was permitted but must have been completed at least 6 mo prior to enrollment. The regimens consisted of either arm A (200 mg/m^2 LV over 2 h, followed by bolus 400 mg/m^2/d 5-FU and an infusion of 600 mg/m^2/d 5-FU over 22 h) or arm B (FOLFOX 4, which used the same 5-FU regimen, with oxaliplatin given at 85 mg/m^2 over 2 h concurrent with LV). Either regimen was repeated every 2 wk.

Chemotherapy doses were reduced for NCI Common Toxicity Criteria grade >3 diarrhea, stomatitis, dermatitis, neutropenia, or for persistent paresthesia, temporary painful paresthesia, or functional impairment. If neurologic symptoms persisted, oxaliplatin was omitted until recovery. Each patient was assessed for response after every four cycles or every 8 wk using World Health Organization criteria. Magnetic resonance imaging (MRI)/CT scans were reviewed through a program of independent blinded review by at least two radiologists.

Four patients on arm A and three patients on arm B were unable to be assessed for response. These patients were included for an intent-to-treat analysis. The median age of enrolled patients was 63 yr (range 20–76). Most patients had PS 0–1 and had a primary tumor of the colon (rather than rectum) with liver metastasis. Other characteristics were well balanced between the two arms. The results are displayed in Table 11.

Approximately 60% of patients in each arm in this study received other chemotherapy at the time that they manifested progression with regimens containing either oxaliplatin or irinotecan. The median overall survival for those who did not receive further chemotherapy at progression in arm A (*n* = 132 patients) was 12.2 mo, and in arm B (*n* = 148 patients), it was 14.8 mo (*p* = 0.04). Independent prognostic factors for improved overall survival were low LDH level, good PS, low alkaline phosphatase, and a limited number of involved metastatic sites.

Patients in arm B experienced more grade 3–4 neutropenia, diarrhea, mucositis, and neuropathy than those in arm A. The authors reported one death resulting from gastrointestinal/ hematologic toxicity from treatment in arm B. Neurotoxicity was very common in patients receiving oxaliplatin, with 68% experiencing some degree of toxicity. Patients experienced cumulative neurosensory or cold-related dysesthesias, pharyngolaryngeal dysesthesia, laryngospasms, cramps, and Lhermitte's sign. Grade 3 neurotoxicity was reversible in 74% of patients, with a median time to recovery of 13 wk. Elderly patients (>65 yr old) did not

Table 11
Results of Phase III Study from de Gramont et al. *(93)*

	Arm A: 5-FU/LV	Arm B: 5-FU/LV/OXAL
No. of patients	210	210
No. evaluable	206	207
Overall response rate		
Assessable	22.3%	50.7%
Intent to treat	21.9%	50.0% ($p = 0.0001$)
CR	1/210 (.5%)	3/210 (1.4%)
PR	45/210 (21.4%)	102/210 (48.6%)
Stable	107/210 (51%)	67/210 (31.9%)
Median time to best response	12 wk	9 wk
Duration of response	46.1 wk	45.1 wk
Median PFS	6.2 mo	9 mo ($p = 0.0001$)
External review	6.0 mo	8.2 mo ($p = 0.0003$)
Median OS	14.7 mo	16.2 mo ($p = 0.12$)
1-yr survival	61%	69%

experience greater toxicity compared to younger patients, except for the observation of more grade 3–4 diarrhea in older patients.

Patient quality of life (QOL) was also examined using EORTC QLQ-C30 every fourth treatment cycle. This instrument assesses the frequency and severity of common symptoms related to colon cancer, as well as estimating the patient's ability to accomplish activities necessary for independent daily living. Median QOL scores were not different between the two arms. However, time to deterioration of global health status was significantly prolonged in arm B.

The Levi and de Gramont trials both establish the improved relative activity of two methods of combining 5-FU/LV with oxaliplatin with respect to response rates and time to tumor progression. In both of these trials, the end points set out at the time of the trials' design to measure the success of the experimental regimens were achieved. Neither trial indicated a statistically significant improvement in survival but neither was adequately powered to achieve that goal. In addition, the end point of survival was obscured by second-line therapies, usually with drugs proven to be active in the secondary therapy of colorectal cancer such as irinotecan or oxaliplatin. Many patients were taken to the operating room for removal of metastatic lesions in the liver or lung or in both locations. This surgical intervention potentially also influenced the survival of many patients in a manner that is difficult to predict from current experience.

7. OXALIPLATIN TRIALS IN LIVER LIMITED METASTATIC COLORECTAL CANCER

In an autopsy series of 1541 patients dying of colorectal carcinoma, 44% of the cases had metastases involving the liver. In 46% of these cases (20% overall), liver metastases was the only site of metastatic disease *(94)*. Without chemotherapy treatment, patients with liver metastases have a median survival of less than 1 yr *(95–97)*. Patients with limited involvement of the liver generally have a better survival, perhaps reflecting lead-time bias or tumor heterogeneity. Untreated, 77% of limited disease patients are alive at 1 yr, 14–23% at 3 yr, and 2–8% at 5 yr *(98,99)*.

7.1. Treatment of Unresectable Liver Disease

Patients with unresectable metastatic colorectal cancer confined to the liver may be candidates for regional infusion therapy. Studies of individuals with colon cancer confined to the liver treated with chemotherapy infusion through the hepatic artery have demonstrated higher tumor response rates than treatment with systemic chemotherapy, although the demonstration of an overall survival advantage remains controversial *(100)*. Potential toxicities associated with this form of therapy include chemical hepatitis as well as biliary sclerosis. Drug infusion via the hepatic artery can also expose the duodenum and stomach to chemotherapy, resulting in gastritis or ulcer formation. In spite of a reduction in the toxic complications in current trials, previous prospective randomized studies have failed to consistently demonstrate a survival advantage when hepatic artery infusion is compared to intravenous 5-FU *(100)*. The lack of improvement in survival can be explained by patient crossover, inclusion of patients with extrahepatic disease, and extensive floxuridine (FUDR) toxicity secondary to higher doses involved in these earlier studies. Additional trials are underway, including the use of oxaliplatin as an agent for hepatic artery infusion *(101)*, to better define the role of regional therapy and its impact on overall survival. Given the potential side effects from the regional therapy with hepatic artery infusion, as well as the need for exploratory laparotomy for catheter placement and idiosyncratic hepatic vascular anatomy that precludes satisfactory liver perfusion, continued improvement in systemic therapy in this patient population is appropriate.

Systemic therapy with oxaliplatin has become an important component of therapy for patients with hepatic metastases, particularly in Europe, as noted earlier. Bismuth, a surgeon working with Levi et al., has reported on a series of patients undergoing surgical resection of initially unresectable hepatic metastases from colorectal carcinoma after neoadjuvant chemotherapy with a combination of infusional oxaliplatin, 5-FU, and LV *(102,103)*. In the most recent update of this study, the outcome of 151 patients with unresectable liver-only metastases was reported *(102)*. Oxaliplatin, 5-FU, and LV produced an objective response in 89 (59%) of these patients. Surgery with curative intent was performed on 77 (50%) of these patients. At the time of surgery, an objective response was confirmed in 61 patients, including 2 patients with a complete response. Forty-eight patients (32%) were able to undergo a complete resection of their liver metastases. Gross total resection of liver metastases, but with microscopically positive margins, was possible in an additional 10 patients. Tumor resection was technically impossible in the remaining 19 patients.

Tumor recurred in 72% of the 58 patients undergoing resection, including 1 patient with a complete response. The median time to relapse was 12 mo. For the 77 patients undergoing surgery, the median overall survival was 48 mo, with a 5-yr survival of 50%. The median overall survival for the 58 patients undergoing resection had not been reached at the time of this report. The estimated 5-yr survival for this group was 58%.

7.2. Role of Hepatic Artery Infusion in Resectable Disease

In patients with potentially resectable liver-only disease at initial presentation, surgery alone can result in long-term survival, but will likely cure no more than a small portion of patients with stage IV disease *(104,105)*. A 5-yr survival rate of 25–37% has been reported in a number of studies, with a median survival of 24–42 mo *(106)*. For patients who do recur after undergoing liver resection, 41% of recurrences involve only the liver *(107)*. This suggests that more intensive regional therapy may be of benefit in reducing the risk of hepatic recurrence *(106,108–110)*. Recent studies of patients receiving hepatic artery infusion (HAI) therapy after resection have reported an improved survival as well as a decrease in hepatic

Table 12
Sites of Recurrent Colorectal Carcinoma in a Randomized Trial of Combined HAI
and Systemic Therapy vs Systemic Therapy Alone After Resection of Hepatic Metastases *(29)*

Site of recurrence	Combined group	Systemic group
Lung	15 (20%)	17 (21%)
Liver	7 (9%)	30 (37%)
Ovaries	4 (5%)	1 (1%)
Bone	3 (4%)	3 (4%)
Pelvis	4 (5%)	7 (9%)
Lymph nodes	3 (4%)	10 (12%)
Other	6 (8%)	6 (7%)

recurrence compared to patients receiving systemic therapy. The rationale for these studies comes from the observation of benefit from regional therapy for patients with unresectable liver metastases from colorectal cancer.

Two randomized trials of HAI following surgical resection of hepatic metastases from colorectal cancer have recently been reported. IN a study from Memorial Sloan-Kettering Cancer Center, patients were randomized to systemic chemotherapy alone (5-FU with or without LV) vs systemic chemotherapy combined with HAI FUDR *(111)*. Seventy-four patients were randomized to combined therapy and 82 to systemic therapy. A significant benefit was seen in patients receiving combined therapy. The median survival in the group receiving combined therapy was 72.2 mo compared to 59.3 mo for those receiving systemic therapy alone. At 2 yr, the rate of survival free of hepatic recurrence was 90% in the combined therapy group compared to 60% in the systemic therapy only group ($p < 0.001$). However, recurrence rates outside the liver appeared similar in both groups (Table 12). In a separate study published only in abstract, patients with 2–4 resected hepatic metastases were randomized to resection alone vs HAI with FUDR combined with systemic infusion of 5-FU *(112)*. This study also showed a marked decrease in the incidence of hepatic recurrence with HAI as well as a significant improvement in recurrence-free survival.

The recent experience with HAI combined with systemic chemotherapy suggests that, despite improved disease-free survival, both intrahepatic and extrahepatic recurrence of colorectal carcinoma continues to be a problem for patients under going resection of hepatic metastases. As such, better systemic regimens are needed. The combination of oxaliplatin, 5-FU, and LV, as reviewed earlier, has shown promising activity for both intrahepatic and extrahepatic metastases. Clinical trials of HAI oxaliplatin are underway. In one of these trials the tolerability of a 5-FU and LV given via a hepatic artery catheter over 2 h on d 1, followed by oxaliplatin given through the same catheter over 4 h on d 2 of the treatment cycle, is being assessed *(101)*. The efficacy of this approach is yet to be determined. Taking a slightly different approach, the NCCTG is currently assessing the activity of systemic oxaliplatin, 5-FU, and LV alternating with HAI FUDR. With the demonstrated activity of oxaliplatin these approaches hold the potential of further decreasing the rate of recurrent metastatic colorectal cancer.

8. ADJUVANT THERAPY

To date, there are no trials that have been reported examining the role of oxaliplatin in the adjuvant setting. A number of studies are in progress. The de Gramont group is conducting a two-arm study that they have named the MOSAIC trial. Patients are randomized to get 200 mg/m^2 LV on d 1, then a 5-FU loading dose of 400 mg/m^2, followed by two consecutive 22-h infusions of 600 mg/m^2 5-FU with or without 85 mg/m^2 oxaliplatin given every other week (FOLFOX 4). This trial will complete accrual of 2000 patients in 2000 or early 2001. Analysis will likely not occur until 2003 or 2004.

The NSABP is conducting an adjuvant study using a weekly bolus schedule of 5-FU modeled on the RPMI high-dose-leucovorin program. The randomization is between 500 mg/m^2/d LV and 500 mg/m^2/d 5-FU weekly for 6 of 8 wk and that regimen plus oxaliplatin 85 mg/m^2/d. This trial opened in March 2000 and will likely complete accrual by 2002.

9. OXALIPLATIN COMBINATION WITH OTHER AGENTS

9.1. Oxaliplatin/CPT-11

A number of trials combining oxaliplatin with other chemotherapy agents are currently underway or have recently been reported. Most of the reports are from meeting abstracts and are outlined in Table 13. The combination of oxaliplatin and CPT-11 has been developed based on preclinical observations. When evaluated in vitro, this combination has shown greater additive inhibition in a human colon cancer HT29 cell line (115). Pre-exposure of the cells to oxaliplatin enhanced the toxic effect of SN-38. In this study, DNA damage induced by oxaliplatin resulted in the finding of a higher likelihood of prolonged DNA elongation and a higher percentage of S-phase arrest when SN-38 was added.

Building on this observation, several phase I trials have been reported (114,115). Wasserman et al. have reported on two independent but identical phase I trials in which oxaliplatin and CPT-11 were given on 1 d every 3 wk (114). Two different maximum tolerated doses (MTD) were determined (Table 1). However, based on further patient accrual, the investigators recommended 110 mg/m2 oxaliplatin and 200 mg/m^2 CPT-11 for phase II trials. At this MTD, no patient experienced grade 4 neutropenia persisting for more than 7 d. However, 23% of patients had febrile neutropenia and 46% of patients experienced grade 3–4 diarrhea. It should be noted that the recommended dose of oxaliplatin is higher in the published article than that reported in the meeting abstract (114,116). The every-3-wk schedule is currently included as one arm of a phase III study of first-line therapy for metastatic colorectal cancer.

This same group of investigators performed two separate phase I trials using the same combination given on an every-2-wk schedule in order to try and increase the dose intensity (116,117). In the abstracts from these two trials, the recommended phase II dose for the every-2-wk schedule was determined to be 85 mg/m^2 oxaliplatin and 175 mg/m^2 CPT-11. In the trial conducted by Wasserman et al., 1 complete response (CR) and 6 partial responses (PR) were seen in 11 patients (9 refractory to 5-FU) at the recommended dose level (116).

Similar response rates were seen in the trial reported by Goldwasser et al. (117). A weekly schedule of oxaliplatin and CPT-11 has been evaluated by Kemeny et al. and recently reported in a meeting abstract (115). A more dose-intense schedule has been reported by Scheithauer et al. in which weekly oxaliplatin and CPT-11 are given together with granulocyte-colony stimulating factor (G-CSF) support (Table 1). In a group of 36 patients refractory to 5-FU and LV, 42% achieved an objective clinical response. With the use of G-CSF, per the study guidelines, only 6% of patients developed grade 4 neutropenia. Grade 3 diarrhea occurred in 19% of patients. Additional patient enrollment with the weekly and biweekly schedules has been undertaken to better determine the toxicities associated with these schedules.

Table 13
Table 13
Summary of Studies Combining Oxaliplatin with Other Agents

Reference	Combination	Response	Comments
	Oxaliplatin/CPT-11		
(114)	Two identical phase I studies maximum tolerated dose (MTD) (q 3 wk): (1) OXAL 110 mg/m^2, CPT-11 200 mg/m^2 d 1 (2) OXAL 110 mg/m^2, CPT-11 250 mg/m^2 d 1	Colorectal cancer: PR 29%	Authors recommend MTD 1

(116)	Three phase I studies MTD:
	(1) q 3 wk (2 studies) OXAL 85 mg/m^2, CPT-11 200 mg/m^2 day 1
	(2) q 2 wk OXAL 85 mg/m^2, CPT-11 175 mg/m^2 d 1
		Q 3 wk
		  PR 35%
		Q 2 wk
		  CR 9%
		  PR 55%	

(145)	Phase II study (q 4 wk) • OXAL 85 mg/m^2 d 1, 15 • CPT-11 80 mg/m^2 d 1, 8, 15 • G-CSF (5 µg/kg/d × 5 d)	36 5-FU refractory patients CR 6% PR 36%	Grade 4 neutropenia 6%; 36% of patients had delays in treatment
(115)	Phase I study, MTD (q 6 weeks): • OXAL 60 mg/m^2 d 1, 8, 15, 22 • CPT-11 65 mg/m^2 d 1, 8, 15, 22	PR 26%; study ongoing	Diarrhea and neutropenic fever dose limiting
(117)	Phase I study, MTD (q 2 wk): • OXAL 85 mg/m^2 d 1 • CPT-11 175 mg/m^2 d 1	CR 9% PR 45%	
	Oxaliplatin/CPT-11/5-FU		
(118)	Phase I study, MTD (q 2 wk): • OXAL 85 mg/m^2 d 1 • CPT-11 180 mg/m^2 d 1 • CF 200 mg/m^2 1, 2 • 5-FU 400 mg/m^2 d 1, 2 bolus 600 mg/m^2 d 1, 2 PVI	9 objective responses (5 colorectal cancer)	
(119)	Phase I study (q 3 wk): • OXAL 85 mg/m^2 d 1 • CPT-11 200 mg/m^2 d 1 • CF 200 mg/m^2 d 1 • 5-FU 2000 mg/m^2 96 h PVI		On-going study
(120)	Phase II study (q 4 wk) • OXAL 120 mg/m^2 d 1 • CPT-11 250 or 300 mg/m^2 d 1 • 5-FU different schedules (IA or IV)	CR 9% PR 49%	64% Previously treated; significant toxicity with 3 deaths in IA group
	Oxaliplatin/UFT and Oxaliplatin/Capecitabine		
(128)	Phase II study (q 4 wk) • OXAL 85 mg/m^2 d 1, 14 • CF 250 mg/m^2 IV 1 • CF 7.5 mg PO q12 h d 1–14 • UFT 300–390 mg/m^{2}d, d 1–14	Unavailable	
(134)	Phase I, MTD (q 3 wk): • OXAL 130 mg/m^2 d 1 • Capecitabine 2000 mg/m^2/d, d 1–14	PR in 5 of 9 patients	

Table 13 *(continued)*

Reference	Combination	Response	Comments
	Oxaliplatin/Raltitrexed		
(139)	Phase II study (q 3 wk) • Raltitrexed 3 mg/m^2 d 1 • OXAL 130 mg/m^2 d 1	CR 2% PR 60%	2 Treatment-related deaths 2 possibly related deaths
(137)	Phase I/II study (q 3 wk): • Raltitrexed 3 mg/m^2 d 1 • OXAL 130 mg/m^2 d 1	At MTD Overall response 46%	
(136)	Phase I study (q 2 wk), MTD: • Raltitrexed 3 mg/m^2 d 1 • OXAL 130 mg/m^2 d 1	No responses in patients	
(138)	Phase I study (q 2 wk), MTD: • OXAL 130 mg/m^2 d 1 • Raltitrexed 3 mg/m^2 d 1 • CF 250 mg/m^2 d 2 • 5-FU 1200 mg/m^2 d 2	1 CR and 8 PR in 41 patients	4 of 8 patients developed grade 3–4 neutropenia
	Oxaliplatin/Topotecan		
(144)	Phase I study, MTD: • OXAL 85 mg/m^2 d 1 • Topotecan 0.9 mg/m^2/d CIV × 3 d	No responses	

9.2. Oxaliplatin/CPT-11/5-FU

Trials assessing a more drug-intensive regimen of oxaliplatin, CPT-11, and 5-FU, with or without LV, are currently underway or have recently been reported (Table 1). In the studies that have been reported, all as meeting abstracts, an every-2-, every-3-, or every-4-wk schedule has been used *(118–120)*. With the 2-wk schedule, the toxicity appeared tolerable, with grade 4 neutropenia of 7 or more days duration and grade 4 diarrhea occurring in two out of nine patients *(118)*. The every-3-wk schedule used oxaliplatin and CPT-11 combined with a 4-d continuous infusion of 5-FU *(119)*. Neutropenia and diarrhea were the dose-limiting toxicities. No objective responses were seen in a group of patients with heavily pretreated gastrointestinal malignancies, including seven patients with colorectal cancer.

The every-4-wk schedule appeared to be the most toxic *(120)*. In this study, oxaliplatin and CPT-11 were combined with either 2500 mg/d 5-FU given as a hepatic artery infusion or 2600 mg/m^2 5-FU and 500 mg/m^2 CF given intravenously on d 1 and 15. For patients receiving the hepatic artery infusion, 64.7% experienced grade 3–4 neutropenia/thrombocytopenia and 52.9% experienced grade 3–4 diarrhea. Three out of 17 patients in this group died as a result of toxicity. In patients who received intravenous 5-FU and LV, grade 3–4 neutropenia/thrombocytopenia occurred in 41.2% and 43.7% of patients at CPT-11 doses of 300 mg/m^2 and 250 mg/m^2, respectively.

9.3 Oxaliplatin and UFT or Capecitabine

UFT is a fixed combination (4 : 1 molar ratio) of tegafur and uracil (*see* Chapter 27) Tegafur (ftorafur) is a furanyl nucleoside analog of 5-FU. It is absorbed through the gastrointestinal tract and then converted to 5-FU by hepatic microsomal cytochrome P-450 enzymes and by soluble enzyme hydrolysis in the cytosol *(121)*. Uracil is a competitive inhibitor of dihydropyrimidine dehydrogenase. In preclinical studies, UFT produced significantly higher levels of 5-FU in tumors compared to healthy tissues and serum *(122)*. Phase II and III trials of UFT and LV have shown evidence of clinical activity in patients with advanced or metastatic colorectal cancer *(123–127)*.

A trial of UFT and LV combined with oxaliplatin (Table 1) was recently completed *(128)* and the plan for a separate trial was recently reported *(129)*. When used as first-line therapy for advance colorectal cancer, significant diarrhea and nausea/vomiting occurred at the higher dose level of 390 mg/m^2/d UFT d 1–14, but became more tolerable when a dose of 300 mg/m^2/d was used. At this dose level, grade 3–4 diarrhea and nausea/vomiting occurred in 18% and 9% of patients, respectively. The response rate to this treatment was not reported in the abstract.

Capecitabine (N_4-pentoxycarbonyl-5′-deoxy-5-fluorocytidine) is an oral fluoropyrimidine that is absorbed intact and sequentially converted to 5-FU in a 3-step process as reviewed elsewhere *(130)*. Colorectal tumors appear to express a high level of thymidine phosphorylase, one of the enzymes involved in the conversion of capecitabine to 5-FU, resulting in a higher level of 5-FU in the tumor compared to healthy tissue. In preclinical studies, this difference in enzyme levels resulted in tumor concentration of 5-FU that were greater with capecitabine than with equivalent doses of 5-FU. Similar results have been shown in clinical studies. In a group of 19 patients given capecitabine for 1 wk prior to surgical resection of their primary tumor and/or liver metastases, 5-FU concentrations were 3.2 and 1.4 times higher in the primary tumor and liver metastases, respectively, compared to healthy tissue *(131)*. A recent international phase III trial compared capecitabine to 5-FU 450 mg/m^2 modulated with LV 20 mg/m^2 given intravenously d 1–5 every 4 wk in patients with previously untreated advanced or metastatic colorectal cancer *(132)*. A response rate of 23% was seen with capecitabine compared to 16 percent for modulated 5-FU ($p = 0.02$). Survival data were not available at the time of this report. Grade 3–4 toxicity for capecitabine consisted mainly of hand-foot syndrome and diarrhea, while that for modulated 5-FU consisted of neutropenia, stomatitis, and diarrhea.

Building upon the activity of capecitabine in colorectal cancer, a phase I study was recently completed evaluating the MTD of capecitabine and oxaliplatin *(133)*. In this study, with oxaliplatin given once every 3 wk and capecitabine given as a twice-a-day dose for 2 wk, the MTD was determined to be 130 mg/m^2 oxaliplatin and 2000 mg/m^2 capecitabine. The dose-limiting toxicity was diarrhea. Five of nine patients with colorectal cancer obtained a partial response.

9.4. Oxaliplatin and Raltitrexed

Raltitrexed is a novel, direct, and specific quinazoline antifolate inhibitor of thymidylate synthase (TS). The potent cytotoxic activity of raltitrexed is dependent upon active uptake in the cells via a reduced folate carrier and subsequent metabolism to polyglutamates (tri-, tetra- and pentaglutamates). These polyglutamates are approx 60-fold more active than the parent compound and are not effluxed readily from cells *(134)*. This property of the drug makes it possible to give a brief infusion of the drug once every 3 wk. A series of phase III trials of raltitrexed have recently been reported *(135)*. These studies have shown clinical activity equivalent to 5-FU and LV.

Several phase I studies have evaluated the combination of raltitrexed and oxaliplatin *(136–138)*. In a phase I study of patients with advanced cancer and a separate phase I/II study of patients with advanced colorectal cancer, the MTD of raltitrexed and oxaliplatin was determined (Table 1). Forty-six percent of the 48 patients in the phase I/II study treated at the MTD had a partial response *(137)*. Grade 3–4 neutropenia occurred in 19% of patients at the MTD. Other less common toxicities included peripheral neuropathy, increase in transaminases, diarrhea, stomatitis, and vomiting. In a separate phase II trial of raltitrexed and oxaliplatin in 63 evaluable, previously untreated patients with metastatic colorectal cancer, an overall response rate of 61.9% was observed *(139)*. Grade 3–4 neutropenia occurred in 16.5% of patients, nausea in 10.5%, and diarrhea in 9%. The median duration of response was 8.1 mo.

A phase I trial of oxaliplatin and raltitrexed on d 1 and 5-FU and LV on d 2 every 2 wk was recently reported as a meeting abstract (Table 1) *(138)*. At the high doses used, four of eight patients developed dose-limiting toxicity. Objective responses were seen in 9 out of 41 patients. Further evaluation of this regimen is indicated.

9.5. Oxaliplatin and Topotecan

Topotecan is a semisynthetic water-soluble analog of camptothecin. The camptothecin family of drugs inhibit topoisomerase I. Topisomerase I-targeting drugs stabilize a covalent DNA-topoisomerase I complex leading to DNA single-strand breaks and cell death *(140)*. Several phase II trials have been performed to assess the activity of topotecan as a single agent in patients with colorectal cancer. In a Southwest Oncology Group trial (SWOG 9241), 48 patients with untreated advanced colorectal cancer received topotecan as first line therapy *(141)*. Given at a standard dose of 1.5 mg/m^2/d for 5 d every 3 wk only two partial responses were seen (4%). In a separate study of high dose topotecan (3.5 mg/m^2/d for 5 d every 3 wk) and G-CSF, no major responses were seen in 16 evaluable patients with colorectal cancer refractory to 5-FU-based therapy *(142)*.

In a preclinical study, the combination of oxaliplatin and topotecan showed highly synergistic activity in both 5-FU-sensitive and 5-FU-resistant human colon cancer cell lines *(143)*. A phase I study of oxaliplatin combined with a 3-d continuous infusion of topotecan (Table 1) in patients with 5-FU refractory colorectal cancer showed significant toxicity and no apparent activity *(144)*.

9.6. Oxaliplatin Combined with Novel Agents

Oxaliplatin, combined with novel agents, has been evaluated in several preclinical studies. When combined with ZD-1839, an epidermal growth factor receptor-selective tyrosine kinase inhibitor, in a human colon cancer cell line culture (GEO), a supra-additive growth-inhibitory effect was noted *(146)*. The addition of ZD-1839 produced an approx 3.5-fold increase in oxaliplatin-induced apoptosis. A similar supra-additive effected was noted when LY231514 (MTA) was combined with oxaliplatin *(147)*. MTA is a multitargeted antifolate that has shown promising activity when combined with other agents in phase I and II trials *(148)*. A Cancer and Leukemia Group B (CALGB) phase II study of oxaliplatin, 5-FU, leucovorin and trastuzumab is currently accruing patients with refractory colorectal cancer.

10. OXALIPLATIN COMBINED WITH RADIATION

There is preliminary information reported in abstract form that oxaliplatin may have activity as a radiation sensitizer. In the single study on this subject, radiation survival data were generated for HT-29 colon cancer cells treated with single graded doses of radiation in the presence or absence of various doses of oxaliplatin in vitro. Clonogenic assays were examined at 14 d and were normalized for drug cytotoxicity. In vivo experiments followed in which mice bearing human tumor xenografts were then treated with 5 Gy alone or in combination with intraperitoneal oxaliplatin. The radiation-sensitizing effect was measured using a tumor-growth-delay assay. In both circumstances, there was enhanced radiation lethality when cells or animals were exposed to oxaliplatin compared to radiation alone *(149)*.

Three dose-finding studies are underway in which oxaliplatin is employed as a radiation sensitizer. In one trial, the drug is combined with raltitrexed, LV, and 5-FU. The other two studies combine oxaliplatin with 5-FU/LV and radiation. Small numbers of patients have been entered on these trials to date and the results remain preliminary. Indications of activity have been observed *(150–152)*.

11. TOXICITY

Phase I and II studies of oxaliplatin administered as a single agent are reviewed above. These studies have established the safety and toxicity profile of oxaliplatin and the findings from these trials have been extended in phase III trials. Early studies showed that this platinum analog has very different toxicities from cisplatin. Specifically, oxaliplatin does not cause renal toxicity or alopecia, and the neurotoxicity observed with oxaliplatin is generally reversible. In most early studies, nausea and vomiting were common; however, this side effect has decreased with the widespread use of 5HT3 receptor antagonists. Hematologic toxicities are also very mild. In most studies, grade 1–2 neutropenia and/or thrombocytopenia has been observed in <25% of patients, with infectious or bleeding complications very rare.

The dose-limiting toxicity of oxaliplatin is an unusual neurotoxicity. Patients experience paresthesias and dysesthesias in the extremities and perioral area, initiated or exacerbated by exposure to cold. This was observed at doses ≥ 135 mg/m^2 and could occur during or after the infusion. It is dose dependent, reversible, and cumulative. These symptoms can occur in up to 78% of patients. Patients can develop a more persistent sensory neuropathy that typically causes difficulty in fine finger movements and usually occurs after a cumulative dose of 850 mg/m^2. This clinically significant neuropathy was seen in <20% of patients in the pivotal trial by de Gramont et al. *(93)*. Grade 3 neurotoxicity was reversible in 74% of patients, with a median time to recovery of 13 wk. Some patients have also experienced acute laryngopharyngeal symptoms during infusion of oxaliplatin. These dysesthesias cause a feeling of dysphagia or dyspnea and are quite uncommon. Seldom patients will have laryngospasm that is usually associated with an anaphylactic reaction to the agent. Patients should be instructed to avoid cold liquids and food, and to wear gloves in cold weather to minimize these events. Additionally, the duration of oxaliplatin infusion can be prolonged from 2 to 6 h, a strategy that will ameliorate acute neurologic toxic effects in many patients.

The neuropathy observed with oxaliplatin differs from CDDP-associated neuropathy in that symptoms occurring after oxaliplatin infusion are acute at onset, are exacerbated by cold, and are generally reversible. For most patients, neurotoxicity improves or resolves in weeks to months, but a minority will have some persistent symptoms. The mechanism of this neuropathy is unknown, but oxaliplatin does cause axonal sensory changes seen on EMG. The mechanism of this toxicity was studied in 22 patients receiving oxaliplatin by performing EMGs before and during treatment. Patients were also receiving 5-FU. Sensory damage was seen at a cumulative total dose of 410 mg/m^2 and confirmed at 862 mg/m^2. Total dose, but not dose intensity, was correlated with the development of sensory changes on EMG studies *(153)*.

Gabapentin is a drug commonly used to treat neuropathic pain. A group from Italy reported some initial success in treating patients with oxaliplatin-induced neuropathy *(154)*. Fifteen patients with metastatic colorectal cancer with no history of neuropathy were treated

Table 14
Other Uncommon Toxicities of Oxaliplatin seen in Phase I and II Trials

Mild transient increase in liver enzymes	Lhermitte's sign
Mild transient increase in creatinine	Loss of deep tendon reflexes (DTR)
Diarrhea	Laryngospasm
Muscle cramps	Phlebitis
Fever	Anaphylactoid reaction
Shortness of breath during infusion	Stomatitis
Erythema/skin toxicity	Mild alopecia

with a bimonthly oxaliplatin and 5-FU regimen. Seven patients have experienced grade 1–2 neuropathy after the third cycle and were treated with gabapentin 100 mg twice daily, which could be increased another 100 mg/d if symptoms did not improve. All patients had resolution of symptoms and have continued on with treatment without recurrence of symptoms. This may represent an approach to treat this dose-limiting toxicity seen with oxaliplatin and certainly deserves further study.

Although the vast majority of neurotoxicity seen with oxaliplatin is peripheral or oral, there have been reports of central nervous system (CNS) toxicity. Four patients receiving the FOLFOX 4 regimen were reported to have CNS toxicity (Lhermitte's sign, genitosphincteral deficiency, and proprioception deficits). This was only seen at cumulative doses >1000 mg/m^2, and symptoms resolved in all patients within weeks after discontinuing treatment *(155)*. Other uncommon toxicities were reported in phase I and phase II trials and are listed in Table 14.

There have been seven reports of oxaliplatin-induced anaphylaxis. Five were reported by Tournigard et al. in 1998. Patients were aged 59–77, both males and females, receiving oxaliplatin in doses of 85–100 mg/m^2. Symptoms including hypotension, flushing, sweating, and tachycardia were observed after cycles 5–12 of the drug. Two patients had return of symptoms with reintroduction of oxaliplatin. The authors estimated that the incidence of this toxicity was 2% of those receiving oxaliplatin *(156)*. An additional case was reported from France, in a 55-yr-old man receiving bimonthly oxaliplatin plus 5-FU. During the sixth cycle, the patient developed an anaphylactic reaction, which responded to supportive treatment and discontinuation of the drug *(157)*. Finally, Medioni et al. from France reported an anaphylactic reaction in a 63-yr-old man receiving his sixth cycle of oxaliplatin/5-FU/LV. He also quickly responded to supportive treatment *(158)*.

Hemolytic anemia was reported in two patients receiving oxaliplatin. The first patient was on a bimonthly regimen that included 100 mg/m^2 oxaliplatin, 400 mg/m^2 5-FU bolus followed by 22-h infusion of 600 mg/m^2, and FA 200 mg/m^2. The patient developed hemolysis after 45 courses of this regimen, with back pain, fever, and drop in hemoglobin after oxaliplatin infusion. Coomb's test was positive and a blood smear showed no schistocytes. Positive agglutination between allogenic red blood cells and the patient's serum seen only with oxaliplatin points to an immune-complex-mediated hemolysis. The patient died despite transfusions, steroids, dialysis, and hemofiltration *(159)*. The second patient had received chronomodulated 5-FU/CF/oxaliplatin for a number a courses when she presented with hemolytic crisis 5 d after infusion. The patient was treated with steroids and gradually recovered *(160)*. This rare toxicity has been reported with other platinum agents and is probably the result of an immunoglobulin (IGG)-drug-dependent antibody.

12. SUMMARY AND FUTURE DIRECTIONS

Oxaliplatin is currently approved for the treatment of colorectal cancer in numerous countries around the world. There are clear signs of its activity in vitro, in human tumor xenograft models, and in many of the over 50,000 patients who have been exposed to the drug worldwide. Additional research needs to be done to determine the preferred schedule of administration and the best ways to combine oxaliplatin with other agents. Studies to address these issues are in progress and many were detailed in this chapter. One example of a strategy in progress is a trial by de Gramont and colleagues (the OPTIMOX study). In it, patients are treated with a 5-FU/LV and oxaliplatin regimen and then the oxaliplatin is temporarily held to permit neurologic toxicity to resolve before the patient is exposed to that agent again. Among the most important tasks for the future include the presentation of convincing data to the US FDA that meets the regulatory requirements that would permit the drug to be licensed.

REFERENCES

1. Burchenal JH, Kalaher K, O'Toole T, and Chisholm J. Lack of cross-resistance between certain platinum coordination compounds in mouse leukemia. *Cancer Res.*, **37** (1977) 3455–3457.
2. O'Rourke TJ, Weiss GR, New P, et al. Phase I clinical trial of ormaplatin (tetraplatin, NSC 363812). *Anticancer Drugs*, **5** (1994) 520–526.
3. Mathe G, Kidani Y, Noji M, et al. Antitumor activity of l-OHP in mice. *Cancer Lett.*, **27** (1985) 135–143.
4. Connors TA, Jones M, Ross WCJ, et al. New platinum complexes with anti-tumor activity. *Chem. Biol. Interact.*, **5** (1972) 415–424.
5. Burchenal, JH, Kalaher K, O'Toole T, et al. Lack of cross-resistance between certain platinum coordination compounds in mouse leukemia. *Cancer Res.*, **37** (1977) 3455–3457.
6. Gale GR, Walker EM, Atkins L, et al. Antileukemic properties of dichloro (1,2) diaminocyclohexane platinum(II). *Res. Commun. Chem. Pathol. Pharmacol.*, **7(3)** (1974) 529–538.
7. Cleare MJ and Hoeschele JD. Studies on the antitumor activity of group VIII transition metal complexes. *Bioinorg. Chem.*, **2** (1973) 187–210.
8. Speer RJ, Ridgway H, Stewart DP, et al. Sulfato 1,2-diaminocyclohexane platinum (II): A potential new antitumor agent. *J. Clin. Hematol. Oncol.*, **7** (1976) 210–219.
9. Kidani Y, Noji M, and Tashiro T. Antitumor activity of platinum (II) complexes of 1,2-diaminocyclohexane isomers. *Gann*, **71** (1980) 637–643.
10. Kidani Y, Inagaki Y, and Tsukagoshi, S. Examination of anti-tumor activities of platinum complexes of the 1,2-diaminocyclohexane isomers and their related compounds. *Gann*, **67** (1976) 921–922.
11. Kidani Y, Inagaki K, and Saito R. Synthesis and antitumor activities of platinum (II) compounds of 1,2-diaminocyclohexane isomers and their related derivatives. *J. Clin. Hematol. Oncol.*, **7** (1977) 197–209.
12. Kidani Y, Inagaki K, Iigo M, et al. Antitumor activity of 1,2-diaminocyclohexane-platinum complexes against sarcoma-180 ascites form. *J. Med. Chem.*, **21(12)** (1978) 1315–1318.
13. Vollano JF, Al-Baker S, Dabrowiak JC, and Schurig JE. Comparative anti-tumor studies on platinum (II) and platinum (IV) complexes containing 1,2-diaminocyclohexane. *J. Med. Chem.*, **30** (1987) 716–719.
14. Siddik ZH, al-Baker S, Burditt TL, and Khokhar AR. Differential antitumor activity and toxicity of isomeric 1,2-diaminocyclohexane platinum (II) complexes. *J. Cancer Res. Clin. Oncol.*, **120** (1993) 12–16.
15. Pendyala L, Kidani Y, Perez R, et al. Cytotoxicity, cellular accumulation and DNA binding of oxaliplatin isomers. *Cancer Lett.*, **97** (1995) 177–184.
16. Tashiro T, Kawada Y, Sakurai Y, Kidani Y. Antitumor activity of a new platinum complex, oxalato (trans-l-1, 2-diaminocyclohexane)platinum (II): new experimental data. *Biomed. Pharmacother.*, **43** (1989) 251–260.
17. Silvestro L, Anal H, Sommer F, et al. Comparative effects of a new platinum analog, l-OHP with CDDP on various cells: correlation with intracellular accumulation. Abstracts of the Third International Conference of Anticancer Research, 1990, p. 1376.
18. Mathe G, Kidani Y, Segiguchi M, et al. Oxalato-platinum or l-OHP, a third generation platinum complex: an experimental and clinical appraisal and preliminary comparison with cis-platinum and carboplatinum. *Biomed. Pharmacother.*, **43** (1989) 237–250.
19. Riccardi A, Ferlini D, Meco D, et al. Antitumor activity of oxaliplatin in neuroblastoma cell lines. *Eur. J. Cancer*, **35(1)** (1999) 86–90.

20. Dunn TA, Schmoll HJ, Grunwald V, et al. Comparative cytotoxicity of oxaliplatin and cisplatin in non-seminomatous germ cell cancer cell lines. *Invest. New Drugs*, **15** (1997) 109–114.

21. Rixe O, Ortuzar W, Alvarez M, et al. Oxaliplatin, tetraplatin, cisplatin, and carboplatin: spectrum of activity in drug-resistant cell lines and in the cell lines of the NCI's anticancer drug screen panel. *Biochem. Pharm.*, **52** (1996) 1855–1865.

22. Raymond E, Lawrence R, Izbicka E, et al. Activity of oxaliplatin against human tumor colony-forming units. *Clin. Cancer Res.*, **4** (1998) 1021–1029.

23. Woynarowski JM, Chapman WG, Napier C, et al. Sequence- and region-specificity of oxaliplatin adducts in naked and cellular DNA. *Mol. Pharm.*, **54** (1998) 770–777.

24. Gibbons GR, Page JD, Mauldin SK, et al. Role of carrier ligand in platinum resistance in L1210 cells. *Cancer Res.*, **50** (1990) 6497–6501.

25. Schmidt W and Chaney SG. Role of carrier ligand in platinum resistance of human carcinoma cell lines. *Cancer Res.*, **53** (1993) 799–805.

26. Mamenta EL, Poma EE, Kaufmann WK, et al. Enhanced replicative bypass of platinum-DNA adducts in cisplatin-resistant human ovarian carcinoma cell lines. *Cancer Res.*, **54** (1994) 3500–3505.

27. Page JD, Husain I, Sancar A, et al. Effect of the diaminocyclohexane carrier ligand on platinum adduct formation, repair, and lethality. *Biochemistry*, **29** (1990) 1016–1024.

28. Saris CP, van de Vaart PJ, Rietbrook RC, et al. In vitro formation of DNA adducts by cisplatin, lobaplatin, and oxaliplatin in calf thymus DNA in solution and in cultured human cells. *Carcinogenesis*, **17** (1996) 2763–2769.

29. Scheeff ED, Briggs JM, and Howell SB. Molecular modeling of the intrastrand guanine–guanine DNA adducts produced by cisplatin and oxaliplatin. *Mol. Pharm.*, **56(3)** (1999) 633–643.

30. Nehme A, Baskaran R, Nebel S, et al. Induction of JNK and c-Abl signalling by cisplatin and oxaliplatin in mismatch repair-proficient and -deficient cells. *Br. J. Cancer*, **79** (1999) 1104–1110.

31. Vaisman A, Varchenko M, Chaney SG, et al. Correlation between mismatch repair defects and increased replicative bypass in cisplatin resistant cell lines. *Proc. AACR*, **38** (1997) A2091.

32. Drummond JT, Anthoney A, Brown R, and Modrich P. Cisplatin and adriamycin resistance are associated with MutLa and mismatch repair deficiency in an ovarian tumor cell line. *J. Biol. Chem.*, **271** (1996) 19,645–19,648.

33. Raymond E, Faivre S, Woynarowski JM, and Chaney S. Oxaliplatin: mechanism of action and antineoplastic resistance. *Semin. Oncol.*, **25(2, Suppl. 5)** (1998) 4–12.

34. Anthoney DA, McIlwrath AJ, Gallagher WM, et al. Microsatellite instability, apoptosis, and loss of p53 function in drug-resistant tumor cells. *Cancer Res.*, **56** (1996) 1374–1381.

35. Brassett C, Joyce JA, Froggatt NJ, et al. Microsatellite instability in early onset and familial colorectal cancer. *J. Med. Genet.*, **33** (1996) 981–985.

36. Mauldin SK, Plescia M, Richard F, et al. Displacement of the bidentate malonate ligand from (*d,l*-trans-1,2-diaminocyclohexane) malonatoplatinum (II) by physiologically important compounds in vitro. *Biochem. Pharm.*, **37(17)** (1988) 3321–3333.

37. Calvert H. Platinum complexes in cancer medicine: pharmacokinetics and pharmacodynamics in relation to toxicity and therapeutic activity. *Cancer Surveys*, **17** (1993) 189–217.

38. Misset JL, Brienza S, Taamma A, et al. Pharmacokinetics, urinary and fecal excretion of oxaliplatin in cancer patients. *Proc. AACR*, **37** (1996) 183 (abstract).

39. Gamelin E, Le Bouil A, Boisdron-Celle M, et al. Cumulative pharmacokinetic study of oxaliplatin, administered every three weeks, combined with 5-fluorouracil in colorectal cancer patients. *Clin. Cancer Res.*, **3** (1997) 891–899.

40. Pendyala L and Creaven PJ. In vitro cytotoxicity, protein binding, red blood cell partitioning, and biotransformation of oxaliplatin. *Cancer Res.*, **53** (1993) 5970–5976.

41. Levi F, Boughattas NA, and Blazsek I. Comparative murine chronotoxicity of anticancer agents and related mechanism. *Annu. Rev. Chronopharmacol.*, **4** (1987) 283–331.

42. Hrushesky W, Levi F, and Halberg F. Circadian-stage dependence of cis-diamminedichloroplatinum lethal toxicity in rats. *Cancer Res.*, **42** (1982) 945–949.

43. Boughattas NA, Levi F, Fournier C, et al. Circadian rhythm in toxicities and tissue uptake of 1,2-diamminocyclohexane (trans-1)oxalatoplatinum(II) in mice. *Cancer Res.*, **49** (1989) 3362–3368.

44. Graham MA, Lockwood GF, Greenslade D, et al. Clinical pharmacokinetics of oxaliplatin: a critical review. *Clin. Cancer Res.*, **6** (2000) 1205–1218.

45. Graham MA, Lockwood F, Cunningham D, et al. Pharmacokinetics of oxaliplatin in special patient populations. *Proc. ASCO*, **18** (1999) 189a (abstract).

46. Massari C, Brienza S, Rotarski M, et al. Pharmacokinetics of oxaliplatin in patients with normal versus impaired renal function. *Cancer Chemother. Pharmacol.*, **45** (2000) 157–164.

47. Raymond E, Djelloul S, Buquet-Fagot C, et al. Oxaliplatin and cisplatin in combination with 5FU, specific thymidylate synthase inhibitors (AG337, ZD1694) and topoisomerase I inhibitors (SN38, CPT-11), in human colonic, ovarian and breast cancers. *Proc. AACR*, **37** (1996) 291 (abstract).

48. Raymond E, Buquet-Fagot C, Djelloul S, et al. Antitumor activity of oxaliplatin in combination with 5FU and the thymidylate synthase inhibitor AG337 in human colon, breast, and ovarian cancers. *Anticancer Drugs*, (1997) **8** 867–885.

49. Faivre S, Raymond E, Woynarowski JM, and Cvitkovic E. Supraadditive effect of gemcitabine in combination with oxaliplatin in human cancer cell lines. *Cancer Chemother. Pharmacol.*, (1999) **44** 117–123.

50. Zeghari-Squalli N, Raymond E, Cvitkovic E, and Goldwasser F. Cellular pharmacology of the combination of the DNA topoisomerase inhibitor SN-38 and the diaminocyclohexane platinum derivative oxaliplatin. *Clin. Cancer Res.*, 5 (1999) 1189–1196.

51. Plasencia C, Taron M, Abad A, et al. Synergism of oxaliplatin with either 5FU or topoisomerase I inhibitor in sensitive and 5FU-resistant colorectal cell lines is independent of DNA-mismatch repair and p53 status. *Proc. ASCO*, **19** (2000) 204a (abstract).

52. Taron M, Plasencia C, Abad A, et al. Preclinical synergy of oxaliplatin, topotecan, and 5-fluorouracil in sensitive and 5-FU resistant HT29 cell line. *Proc. ASCO*, **18** (1999) 170a (abstract).

53. Evans SS, Chow Y, Su Z, et al. Oxaliplatin vs. cisplatin activity in human tumors. *Proc. ASCO*, **19** (2000) 228a (abstract).

54. Jackman AL, Kimbell R, and Ford HER. Combination of raltitrexed with other cytotoxic agents: rationale and preclinical observations. *Eur. J. Cancer*, **35(Suppl. 1)** (1999) S3–S8.

55. Goldwasser F, Bozec L, Zeghari-Squalli N, and Misset J. Cellular pharmacology of the combination of oxaliplatin with topotecan in the IGROV-1 human ovarian cancer cell line. *Anticancer Drugs*, **10** (1999) 195–201.

56. Genne P, Duchamp O, Brienza S, et al. Oxaliplatin in combination with 5FU, mitomycin C or cyclophosphamide in a model of peritoneal carcinomatosis induced by colon cancer cells in BD IX rats. *Proc. AACR*, **38** (1997) 319 (abstract).

57. Gale GR, Walker EM, Atkins L, et al. Antileukemic properties of dichloro(1,2) diaminocyclohexane) platinum(II). *Res. Commun. Chem. Pathol. Pharmacol.*, **7(3)** (1974) 529–538.

58. Debner J, Dexter D, Mangold G, et al. Evaluation of oxaliplatin–tirapazamine–taxol combinations in the MV-522 human lung carcinoma xenograft model. *Proc. AACR*, **37** (1997) 312 (abstract).

59. Joel SP, Richards F, and Seymour M. Oxaliplatin (l-OHP) does not influence the pharmacokinetics of 5-fluorouracil. *Proc. ASCO*, **19** (2000) 192a (abstract).

60. Papamichael D, Joel SP, Seymour MT, et al. Pharmacokinetic interaction between 5-fluorouracil and oxaliplatin. *Proc. ASCO*, **17** (1998) 202 (abstract).

61. Metzger G, Massari C, Renee N, et al. Variations in platinum plasma levels depending on chronomodulated oxaliplatin peak time. *Proc. ASCO*, **16** (1997) 244a (abstract).

62. Lokiec F, Wasserman E, Cvitkovic E, et al. Final results of the pharmacokinetic study of both CPT-11 and LOHP in combination during a phase I trial in gastrointestinal cancer patients. *Proc. ASCO*, **17** (1998) 202a (abstract).

63. Mathe G, Kidani Y, Triana K, et al. A phase I trial of trans-1-diaminocyclohexane oxalato-platinum (l-OHP). *Biomed. Pharmacother.*, **40** (1986) 372–376.

64. Extra JM, Espie M, Calvo F, et al. Phase I study of oxaliplatin in patients with advanced cancer. *Cancer Chemotherapy Pharmacol.*, **25** (1990) 299–303.

65. Caussanel JP, Levi F, Brienza S, et al. Phase I trial of 5-day continuous venous infusion of oxaliplatin at circadian rhythm-modulated rate compared with constant rate. *J. NCI*, **82(12)** (1990) 1046–1050.

66. Raymond E, Chaney, SG, Taamma A, and Cvitkovic E. Oxaliplatin: a review of preclinical and clinical studies. *Ann. Oncol.*, **9** (1998) 1053–1071.

67. Diaz-Rubio E, Sastre J, Zaniboni A, et al. Oxaliplatin as single agent in previously untreated colorectal carcinoma patients: a phase II multicentric study. *Ann. Oncol.*, (1998) **9** 105–108.

68. Becouarn Y, Ychou M, Ducreux M, et al. Phase II trial of oxaliplatin as first line chemotherapy in metastatic colorectal cancer patients. *J. Clin. Oncol.*, **16** (1998) 2739–2744.

69. Machover D, Diaz-Rubio E, de Gramont A, et al. Two consecutive phase II studies of oxaliplatin for treatment of patients with advanced colorectal carcinoma who were resistant to previous treatment with flouropyrimidines. *Ann. Oncol.*, **7** (1996) 95–98.

70. Levi F, Perpoint B, Garufi C, et al. Oxaliplatin activity against metastatic colorectal cancer. A phase II study of 5-day continuous venous infusion at circadian rhythm modulated rate. *Eur. J. Ca.*, **29A(9)** (1993) 1280–1284.

71. Schmilovich A, Chacon R, Coppola F, et al. Expanded access program single agent oxaliplatin in 5FU resistant advanced colorectal cancer patients. *Proc. ASCO*, **17** (1998) 272a (abstract).

72. Levi F, Misset J-L, Brienza S, et al. A chronopharmacologic phase II clinical trial with 5-flourouracil, folinic acid, and oxaliplatin using an ambulatory multichannel programmable pump. *Cancer*, **69** (1992) 893–900.

73. Levi FA, Zidani R, Vannetzel J-M, et al. Chronomodulated versus fixed infusion-rate delivery of ambulatory chemotherapy with oxaliplatin, fluorouracil, and folinic acid (leucovorin) in patients with colorectal cancer metastases: a randomized multi-institutional trial. *J. Natl. Cancer Inst.*, **86** (1994) 1608–1617.

74. Levi FA, Zidani R, Misset J, et al. Randomised multicentre trial of chronotherapy with oxaliplatin, fluoruracil, and folinic acid in metastatic colorectal cancer: for the International Organization for Cancer Chronotherapy. *Lancet*, **350** (1997) 681–686.

75. Levi FA, Zidani R, Llory J, et al. Final efficacy update at 7 years of flat vs chronomodulated infusion (chrono) of oxaliplatin, 5-fluorouracil and leucovorin as first line treatment of metastatic colorectal cancer. *Proc. Am. Soc. Clin. Oncol.*, (2000) **19**, 242a (abstract).

76. Levi F, Zidani R, Brienza S, et al. A multicenter evaluation of intensified, ambulatory, chronomodulated chemotherapy with oxaliplatin, 5-fluorouracil, and leucovorin as initial treatment of patients with metastatic colorectal carcinoma. *Cancer*, **85** (1999) 2532–2540.

77. Bertheault-Cvitkovic F, Jami A, Ithzaki M, et al. Biweekly intensified ambulatory chronomodulated chemotherapy with oxaliplatin, fluorouracil, and leucovorin in patients with metastatic colorectal cancer. *J. Clin. Oncol.*, **14** (1996) 2950–2958.

78. de Gramont A, Bosset JF, Milan C, et al. Randomized trial comparing monthly low-dose leucovorin and fluorouracil bolus with bimonthly fluorouracil bolus plus continuous infusion for advanced colorectal cancer: a French intergroup study. *J. Clin. Oncol.*, **15** (1997) 808–815.

79. de Gramont A, Gastiaburu J, Tournigand C, et al. Oxaliplatin with high-dose folinic acid and 5-fluorouracil 48 h infusion in pretreated metastatic colorectal cancer. *Proc. Am. Soc. Clin. Oncol.*, **13** (1994) 220 (abstract).

80. de Gramont A, Vignoud J, Tournigand C, et al. Oxaliplatin with high-dose leucovorin and 5-fluorouracil 48-hour continuous infusion in pretreated metastatic colorectal cancer. *Eur. J. Cancer*, **33** (1997) 214–219.

81. Andre T, Bensmaine MA, Louvet C, et al. Multicenter phase II study of bimonthly high-dose leucovorin, fluorouracil infusion, and oxaliplatin for metastatic colorectal cancer resistant to the same leucovorin and fluoruracil regimen. *J. Clin. Oncol.*, **17** (1999) 3560–3568.

82. Souglakos J, Kouroussis C, Ziras N, et al. First-line treatment with 5-fluorouracil (5-FU), leucovorin (LV), and oxaliplatin (L-OHP) in advanced colorectal cancer (ACC): a multicenter phase II study. *Proc. Am. Soc. Clin. Oncol.*, **19** (2000) 302a (abstract).

83. Maindrault-Goebel F, Louvet C, Andre T, et al. Oxaliplatin added to the simplified bimonthly leucovorin and 5-fluorouracil regimen as second-line therapy for metastatic colorectal cancer (FOLFOX6). *Eur. J. Cancer*, **35** (1999) 1338–1342.

84. Maindrault-Goebel F, de Gramont A, Louvet C, et al. High-dose oxaliplatin with the simplified 48 h bimonthly leucovorin (LV) and 5-fluorouracil (5FU) regimens (FOLFOX) in pretreated metastatic colorectal cancer. *Proc. Am. Soc. Clin. Oncol.*, **18** (1999) 265a (abstract).

85. Zaniboni A, Meriggi F, Aitini E, et al. Oxaliplatin (OX) and 5-day 5-fluorouracil (5-FU) + leucovorin (LV) as salvage treatment for advanced colorectal cancer (ACC), preliminary results. *Proc. Am. Soc. Clin. Oncol.*, **19** (2000) 304a (abstract).

86. Van Cutsem E, Szanto J, Roth A, et al. Evaluation of the addition of oxaliplatin (OXA) to the same Mayo or German 5FU regimen in advanced refractory colorectal cancer (ARCRC). *Proc. Am. Soc. Clin. Oncol.*, **18** (1999) 234a (abstract).

87. Marantz A, Lopez J, Ivulich C, et al. First-line chemotherapy with 5-fluorouracil (5FU), leucovorin (LV), and oxaliplatin (l-OHP) in metastatic colorectal cancer (MCC) patients (pts). *Proc. Am. Soc. Clin. Oncol.*, **19** (2000) 271a (abstract).

88. Hochster H, Chachoua A, Wernz J, et al. Oxaliplatin with weekly bolus 5 FU and low-dose leucovorin (LV): early report of high activity in first line therapy of advanced colorectal cancer (ACRC). *Proc. Am. Soc. Clin. Oncol.*, **19** (2000) 289a (abstract).

89. Giornelli G, Roca E, Chacon M, et al. Bimonthly oxaliplatin (L-OHP) and weekly bolus 5-fluorouracil (5-FU) and folinic acid (FA) in patients (Pts) with metastatic colorectal cancer (CRC): a feasible and active regimen. *Proc. Am. Soc. Clin. Oncol.*, **19** (2000) 295a (abstract).

90. Janinis J, Papakostas P, Samelis G, et al. Second-line chemotherapy with weekly oxaliplatin and high-dose 5-flourouracil with folinic acid in metastatic colorectal carcinoma: a Hellenic Cooperative Oncology Group (HeCOG) phase II feasibility study. *Ann. Oncol.*, **11** (2000) 163–167.

91. Kretzschmar A, Mezger J, Thuss-Patience PC, et al. Oxaliplatin (OX) after irinotecan (Iri): antitumor activity and clinical benefit of 3rd and higher-line chemotherapy with Ox for patients (pts) with metastatic colorectal cancer (MCC) after failure of iri. *Proc. Am. Soc. Clin. Oncol.*, **18** (1999) 259a (abstract).

92. Giacchetti S, Perpoint B, Zidani R, et al. Phase III multicenter randomized trial of oxaliplatin added to chronomodulated fluourouracil-leucovorin as first-line treatment of metastatic colorectal cancer. *J. Clin. Oncol.*, **18(1)** (2000) 117–147.

93. de Gramont A, Figer A, Seymour M, et al. Leucovorin and fluorouracil with or without oxaliplatin as first-line treatment in advanced colorectal cancer. *JCO*, **18(16)** (2000) 2938–2947.

94. Weiss L, Grundmann E, Torhorst J, et al. Haematogenous metastatic patterns in colonic carcinoma: an analysis of 1541 necropsies. *J. Pathol.*, **150** (1986) 195–203.

95. Finan PJ, Marshall RJ, Cooper EH, and Giles GR. Factors affecting survival in patients presenting with synchronous hepatic metastases from colorectal cancer: a clinical and computer analysis. *Brit. J. Surg.*, **72** (1985) 373–377.

96. Goslin R, Steele G, Zamcheck N, et al. Factors influencing survival in patients with hepatic metastases from adenocarcinoma of the colon or rectum. *Dis. Colon Rectum*, **25** (1982) 749–754.

97. Bengtsson G, Carlsson G, Hafstrom L, and Jonsson PE. Natural history of patients with untreated liver metastases from colorectal cancer. *Am. J. Surg.*, **141** (1981) 586–589.

98. Wagner JS, Adson MA, Van Heerden JA, et al. The natural history of hepatic metastases from colorectal cancer. A comparison with resective treatment. *Ann. Surg.*, **199** (1984) 502–508.

99. Wood CB, Gillis CR, and Blumgart LH. A retrospective study of the natural history of patients with liver metastases from colorectal cancer. *Clin. Oncol.*, **2** (1976) 285–288.

100. Anonymous. Reappraisal of hepatic arterial infusion in the treatment of nonresectable liver metastases from colorectal cancer. Meta-analysis group in Cancer. *J. Natl. Cancer Inst.*, **88** (1996) 252–258.

101. Kern W, Beckert B, Lang N, et al. Phase I and pharmacokinetic study of hepatic arterial infusion with oxaliplatin, folinic acid, and 5-fluorouracil in patients with hepatic metastases from colorectal cancer. *Proc. Am. Soc. Clin. Oncol.*, **19** (2000) 289a (abstract).

102. Giacchetti S, Itzhaki M, Gruia G, et al. Long-term survival of patients with unresectable colorectal cancer liver metastases following infusional chemotherapy with 5-fluorouracil, leucovorin, oxaliplatin and surgery. *Ann. Oncol.*, **10** (1999) 663–669.

103. Bismuth H, Adam R, Levi F, et al. Resection of nonresectable liver metastases from colorectal cancer after neoadjuvant chemotherapy. *Ann. Surg.*, **224** (1996) 509–520.

104. Rosen CB, Nagorney DM, Taswell HF, et al. Perioperative blood transfusion and determinants of survival after liver resection for metastatic colorectal carcinoma. *Ann. Surg.*, **216** (1992) 493–504.

105. Anonymous. Resection of the liver for colorectal carcinoma metastases: a multi-institutional study of indications for resection. Registry of Hepatic Metastases. *Surgery*, **103** (1988) 278–288.

106. Fong Y. Surgical therapy of hepatic colorectal metastasis. *CA Cancer J. Clin.*, **49** (1999) 231–255.

107. Hughes KS, Simon R, Songhorabodi S, et al. Resection of the liver for colorectal carcinoma metastases: a multi-institutional study of patterns of recurrence. *Surgery*, **100** (1986) 278–284.

108. Hughes K, Scheele J, and Sugarbaker PH. Surgery for colorectal cancer metastatic to the liver. Optimizing the results of treatment. *Surg. Clin. N. Am.*, **69** (1989) 339–359.

109. Leslie KA, Rossi R, Hughes K, Tsao J. Survival expectancy of patients alive 5 years after hepatic resection for metastatic colon carcinoma: report from the registry of hepatic metastases. *Proc. ASCO*, **14** (1995) A477 (abstract).

110. Fong Y, Cohen AM, Fortner JG, et al. Liver resection for colorectal metastases. *J. Clin. Oncol.*, **15** (1997) 938–946.

111. Kemeny N, Huang Y, Cohen AM, et al. Hepatic arterial infusion of chemotherapy after resection of hepatic metastases from colorectal cancer. *N. Engl. J. Med.*, **341** (1999) 2039–2048.

112. Kemeny MM, Adak S, Lipsitz S, et al. Results of the intergroup [Eastern Cooperative Oncology Group (ECOG) and Southwestern Oncology Group (SWOG)] prospective randomized study of surgery alone versus continuous heaptic artery infusion of FUDR and continuous systemic infusion of 5FU after hepatic resection for colorectal liver metastases. *Proc. ASCO*, **18** (1999) 264a (abstract).

113. Zeghari-Squalli N, Raymond E, Cvitkovic E, Goldwasser F. Cellular pharmacology of the combination of the DNA topoisomerase I inhibitor SN-38 and the diaminocyclohexane platinum derivative oxaliplatin. *Clin. Cancer Res.*, **5** (1999) 1189–1196.

114. Wasserman E, Cuvier C, Lokiec F, et al. Combination of oxaliplatin plus irinotecan in patients with gastrointestinal tumors: results of two independent phase I studies with pharmacokinetics. *J. Clin. Oncol.*, **17** (1999) 1751–1759.

115. Kemeny N, Tong W, Stockman J, et al. Phase I trial of weekly oxaliplatin and irinotecan in previously untreated colorectal cancer. *Proc. ASCO*, **19** (2000) 245a (abstract).

116. Wasserman E, Kalla SL, Misset J, et al. Oxaliplatin (L-OHP) and irinotecan (CPT-11) phase I/II studies: results in 5 FU refractory (FR) colorectal cancer (CRC) patients (pts). *Proc. ASCO*, **18** (1999) 238a (abstract).

117. Goldwasser F, Gross M, Tigaud JM, et al. CPT-11/oxaliplatin (L-OHP) combination every two weeks: final results of a phase I study in advanced digestive malignancies. *Proc. ASCO*, **18** (1999) 176a (abstract).

118. Conroy T, Seitz JF, Capodano G, et al. Phase I study of triplet combination of oxaliplatin + irinotecan + LV5FU2 in patients with metastatic solid tumors. *Proc. ASCO*, **19** (2000) 921G (abstract).

119. Lerebours F, Cottu P, Hocini H, et al. Oxaliplatin (OXA), irinotecan (CPT11), and 4-day continuous infusion of 5-fluorouracil (CIVFU) every three weeks (Q3W): a phase I study in advanced gastrointestinal tumors. *Proc. ASCO*, **19** (2000) 313a (abstract).

120. Calvo E, Gonzalez-Cao M, Cortes J, et al. Combined irinotecan, oxaliplatin, 5-FU in patients (PTS) with metastatic colorectal cancer (MCC). *Proc. ASCO*, **19** (2000) 259a (abstract).

121. Sayed YM and Sadee W. Metabolic activation of *R,S*-1-(tetrahydro-2-furanyl)-5-fluorouracil (ftorafur) to 5-fluorouracil by soluable enzymes. *Cancer Res.*, **43** (1983) 4039–4044.

122. Taguchi T. Clinical application of biochemical modulation in cancer chemotherapy: biochemical modulation for 5-FU. *Oncology*, **54** (1997) 12–18.

123. Gonzalez-Baron M, Feliu J, de la Gandara I, et al. Efficacy of oral tegafur modulation by uracil and leucovorin in advanced colorectal cancer. A phase II study. *Eur. J. Cancer*, **31A** (1995) 2215–2219.

124. Saltz LB, Leichman CG, Young CW, et al. A fixed-ratio combination of uracil and Ftorafur (UFT) with low dose leucovorin. An active oral regimen for advanced colorectal cancer. *Cancer*, **75** (1995) 782–785.

125. Pazdur R, Lassere Y, Rhodes V, et al. Phase II trial of uracil and tegafur plus oral leucovorin: an effective oral regimen in the treatment of metastatic colorectal carcinoma. *J. Clin. Oncol.*, **12** (1994) 2296–2300.

126. Pazdur R, Douillard JY, Skillings JR, et al. Multicenter phase III study or 5-fluorouracil (5-FU) or UFT in combination with leucovorin (LV) in patients with metastatic colorectal cancer. *Proc. ASCO*, **18** (1999) 263a (abstract).

127. Carmichael J, Popiela T, Radstone D, et al. Randomized comparative study of Orzel (oral uracil/tegafur (UFT) plus leucovorin (LV)) versus parenteral 5-fluorouracil (5-FU) plus LV in patients with metastatic colorectal neoplasms. *Proc. ASCO*, **18** (1999) 527 (abstract).

128. Garcia-Giron C, Feliu J, Vincent JM, et al. Phase II trial of oxaliplatin-UFT-leucovorin (OXA-UFT-LV) combination in first line treatment of advanced colorectal cancer (ACC). *Proc. Am. Soc. Clin. Oncol.*, **19** (2000) 293a (abstract).

129. Hoff PM and Pazdur R. Oxaliplatin and UFT/oral calcium folinate for advanced colorectal carcinoma. *Oncology*, **13** (1999) 48–50.

130. Miwa M, Ura M, Nishida M, et al. Design of a novel oral fluoropyrimidine carbamate, capecitabine, which generates 5-fluorouracil selectively in tumours by enzymes concentrated in human liver and cancer tissue. *Eur. J. Cancer*, **34** (1998) 1274–1281.

131. Schuller J, Cassidy J, Dumont E, et al. Preferential activation of capceitabine in tumor following oral administration to colorectal cancer patients. *Cancer Chemother. Pharmacol.*, **45** (2000) 291–297.

132. Cox JV, Pazdur R, Thibault A, et al. A phase III trial of xeloda (capecitabine) in previously untreated advanced/metastatic colorectal cancer. *Proc. Am. Soc. Clin. Oncol.*, **18** (1999) 265a (abstract).

133. Diaz-Rubio E, Evans J, Tabernero J, et al. Phase I study of capecitabine in combination with oxaliplatin in patients with advanced or metastatic solid tumors. *Proc. Am. Soc. Clin. Oncol.*, **19** (2000) 198a (abstract).

134. Jackman AL, Farrugia DC, Gibson W, et al. ZD1694 (tomudex): a new thymidilate synthase inhibitor with activity in colorectal cancer. *Eur. J. Cancer*, **31** (1995) 1277–1282.

135. Cunningham D. Mature results from three large controlled studies with raltitrexed ('Tomudex). *Brit. J. Cancer*, **77** (1998) 15–21.

136. Fizazi K, Ducreux M, Ruffie P, et al. Phase I, dose-finding, and pharmacokinetic study of raltitrexed combined with oxaliplatin in patients with advanced cancer. *J. Clin. Oncol.*, **18** (2000) 2293–2300.

137. Scheithauer W, Kornek GV, Ulrich-Pur H, et al. Promising therapeutic potential of oxaliplatin + raltitrexed in patients with advanced colorectal cancer (ACC): results of a phase I/II trial. *Proc. Am. Soc. Clin. Oncol.*, **19** (2000) 257a (abstract).

138. Catalano G, Casaretti R, De Lucia L, et al. Oxaliplatin (L-OHP) and tomudex (TOM) followed by levo-leucovorin (LLV)-modulated 5-fluorouracil (5FU) I.V. bolus every 2 weeks. A dose finding study in advanced colorectal carcinoma (ACC). *Proc. Am. Soc. Clin. Oncol.*, **19** (2000) 272a (abstract).

139. Douillard JY, Michel P, Gamelin E, et al. Raltitrexed ('Tomudex') plus oxaliplatin: an active combination for first-line chemotherapy in patients with metastatic colorectal cancer. *Proc. Am. Soc. Clin. Oncol.*, **19** (2000) 250a (abstract).

140. Hsiang YH, Lihou MG, and Liu LF. Arrest of replication forks by drug-stabilized topoisomerase I-DNA cleavable complexes as a mechanism of cell killing by camptothecin. *Cancer Res.*, **49** (1989) 5077–5082.

141. Macdonald JS, Benedetti JK, Modiano M, and Alberts DS. Phase II evaluation of topotecan in patients with advanced colorectal cancer. A Southwest Oncology Group trial (SWOG 9241). *Invest. New Drugs*, **15** (1997) 357–359.

142. Rowinsky EK, Baker SD, Burks K, et al. High-dose topotecan with granulocyte-colony stimulating factor in fluoropyrimidine-refractory colorectal cancer: a phase II and pharmacodynamic study. *Ann. Oncol.*, **9** (1998) 173–180.

143. Taron M, Plasencia C, Abad A, et al. Preclinical synergy of oxaliplatin (OXA), topoisomerase I-inhibitor (topotecan) and 5-fluorouracil in sensitive and 5-fluorouracil resistant HT29 cell line. *Proc. Am. Soc. Clin. Oncol.*, **18** (1999) 170a (abstract).

144. Szelenyi H, Huetter G, Staab HJ, et al. Oxaliplatin in combination with continuous infusion of topotecan in patients with 5-FU refractory metastatic colorectal carcinoma: a phase IB study. *Proc. Am. Soc. Clin. Oncol.*, **19** (2000) 229a (abstract).

145. Scheithauer W, Kornek GV, Raderer M, et al. Combined irinotecan and oxaliplatin plus granulocyte colony-stimulating factor in patients with advanced fluoropyrimidine/leucovorin-pretreated colorectal cancer. *J. Clin. Oncol.*, **17** (1999) 902–906.

146. Ciardiello F, Caputo R, Bianco R, et al. Antitumor effect and potentiation of cytotoxic drugs activity in human cancer cells by ZD-1839 (Iressa), an epidermal growth factor receptor-selective tyrosine kinase inhibitor. *Clin. Cancer Res.*, **6** (2000) 2053–2063.

147. Teicher BA, Chen V, Shih C, et al. Treatment regimens including the multitargeted antifolate LY231514 in human tumor xenografts. *Clin. Cancer Res.*, **6** (2000) 1016–1023.

148. O'Dwyer PJ, Nelson K, and Thornton DE. Overview of phase II trials of MTA in solid tumors. *Sem. Oncol.*, **26** (1999) 99–104.

149. Hess S and Blackstock W. Oxaliplatin: in vitro and in vivo evidence of its radiation sensitizing activity—preclinical observations relevant to ongoing clinical trials. *Proc. Amer. Assoc. Cancer Res.*, **41** (2000) 53.

150. Catalano G, Cari R, Lucia P, et al. Oxaliplatin (L-OHP) and tomudex (TOM) followed by levo-leucovorin modulated 5-fluorouracil (5-FU I.V. bolus every 2 weeks. A dose finding study in advanced colorectal carcinoma (ACC). *Proc. Am. Soc. Clin. Oncol.*, **19** (2000) 272a (abstract).

151. Carraro S, Roca E, Cartelli C, et al. Oxaliplatin (OXA), 5-fluorouracil (5-FU) and leucovorin (LV) plus radiotherapy in unresectable rectal cancer (URC): preliminary results. *Proc. Am. Soc. Clin. Oncol.*, **19** (2000) 291a (abstract).

152. Glynne-Jones R, Falk S, Maughan T, et al. Results of preoperative radiation and oxaliplatin in combination with 5-fluorouracil (5-FU) and leucovorin (LV) in locally advanced rectal cancer: a phase I study. *Proc. Am. Soc. Clin. Oncol.*, **19** (2000) 310a (abstract).

153. Garufi C, Pietrangeli A, Brienza S, et al. Electrophysiological evaluation of oxaliplatin neurotoxicity. *Proc. ASCO*, **18** (1999) (abstract).

154. Mariani G, Garrone C, Granetto C, et al. Oxaliplatin induced neuropathy: could gabapentin be the answer? *Proc. ASCO*, **19** (2000) 609a (abstract).

155. Taieb S, Freyer G, Rambaud,L, et al. Central neurotoxicity induced by oxaliplatin: report on 4 cases. *Proc. ASCO*, **19** (2000) 312a (abstract).

156. Tournigand C, Maindrault-Goebel F, Louvet C, et al. Severe anaphylactic reactions to oxaliplatin. *Eur. J. Cancer*, **34(8)** (1998) 1297–1298.

157. Larzilliere I, Brandissou S, Breton P, et al. Anaphylactic reaction to oxaliplatin: A case report. *Am. Jo. Gastroent.*, **94(11)** (1999) 3387–3388.

158. Medioni J, Coulon MA, Morere, JF, et al. Anaphylaxis after oxaliplatin. *Ann. Oncol.*, **10** (1999) 610.

159. Desrame J, Brouset H, Darodes de Tally P, et al. Oxaliplatin-induced haemolytic anaemia. *Lancet*, **354** (1999) 1179–1180.

160. Garufi C, Vaglio S, Brienza S, et al. Immunohemolytic anemia following oxaliplatin administration. *Ann. Onc.*, **11(4)** (2000) 497.

30 TS Inhibitors and Antifolates

Hugo E. R. Ford and David Cunningham

Contents

1. INTRODUCTION

For many years, the chemotherapy of colorectal cancer has depended almost exclusively on the use of antimetabolite drugs. These drugs interfere with the normal metabolic processes within cells and are principally divided into two classes: the nucleoside analogs, such as 5-fluorouracil (5-FU) and gemcitabine, and the antifolates, which are discussed in this chapter.

A large number of pathways involved in the synthesis of purines and pyrimidines for incorporation into nucleic acids are dependent on the transfer of one-carbon units between molecules. This is accomplished enzymatically, with the use of reduced folates as cofactors (Fig. 1). Therefore, these pathways are highly attractive targets for anticancer chemotherapy. Structural analogs of folic acid can bind to the folate-binding sites of these enzymes with an inhibitory effect and some of the earliest cytotoxic drugs to be developed were antifolate antimetabolites such as aminopterin and methotrexate. Recent advances in the understanding of underlying biochemical mechanisms as well as improvements in drug synthesis have allowed the development of a number of novel antifolate compounds targeting specific enzymes in these pathways.

Among the most studied of these enzymes is thymidylate synthase (TS), which catalyzes the reductive methylation of 2'-deoxyuridine-5'-monophosphate (dUMP) to 2'-deoxythymidine-5'-monophosphate (thymidylate, dTMP), with 5,10-methylene tetrahydrofolate acting as the methyl donor. This enzyme is known to be one of the principle targets for 5-FU, which, via its metabolite 5-fluoro-2'-deoxyuridine-5'-monophosphate (FdUMP),

From: *Colorectal Cancer: Multimodality Management*
Edited by: L. Saltz © Humana Press Inc., Totowa, NJ

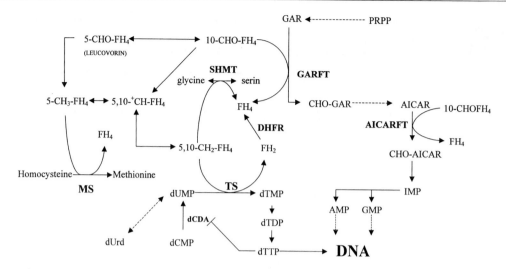

Fig. 1. Role of reduced folates in purine and pyrimidine biosynthesis. Abbreviations: FH_4, tetrahydrofolate; FH_2, dihydrofolate; TS, thymidylate synthase; DHFR, dihydrofolate reductase; SHMT, serine hydroxy-methyltransferase; GARFT, glycinamide ribonucleotide formyltransferase; AICARFT, aminoimidazole carboxamide ribonucleotide formyltransferase; MS, methionine synthetase; DCDA, deoxycytidylate deaminase; PRPP, phosphoribosyl pyrophosphate; IMP, inositol monophosphate; AMP, adenosine monophosphate; GMP, guanidine monophosphate; LV, leucovorin; DUrd, 2'-deoxyuridine.

forms a stable ternary complex with the enzyme and the folate cofactor. Infused 5-FU, which is thought to act predominantly through the inhibition of TS, has antitumor activity at least as great as more toxic bolus regimens *(1)* which appear to be associated with a greater degree of incorporation of 5-FU metabolites into RNA *(2)*. This suggests that non-TS-mediated mechanisms may play a significant part in the toxicity of 5-FU and has led to considerable interest in the development of those mechanisms, which have greater specificity for TS. By comparison with most folate-dependent enzyme inhibitors, pure inhibitors of TS are potentially DNA-specific, as thymidylate is the only nucleotide specifically required for DNA synthesis. Other enzymes have also been targeted, including dihydrofolate reductase (DHFR) and two of the principle enzymes in the purine synthetic pathway, glycinamide ribonucleotide formyltransferase (GARFT) and aminoimidazole carboxamide ribonucleotide formyltransferase (AICARFT).

2. FOLATE TRANSPORT

Natural folates are taken up into the cell by the reduced folate carrier (RFC) and rapidly polyglutamated by the enzyme folylpolyglutamate synthetase (FPGS). These polyglutamates may be hydrolyzed by γ-glutamyl hydrolase (GGH) to lower chain-length forms *(3)* (Fig. 2). The longer-chain-length polyglutamates are retained intracellularly, as they are not transported out of the cell by the RFC. Transport and polyglutamation may affect sensitivity to individual antifolates, and as such, the enzymes affecting these processes are important factors to consider in the design of anticancer drugs. For example, under-expression of FPGS or overexpression of GGH are potential mechanisms of resistance to polyglutamated antifolates, especially where the polyglutamated drug has a higher affinity for the target enzyme than the parent molecule. Rational drug design has been a feature of the development of antifolates and allows the clinician to exploit these factors and thus overcome potential mechanisms of resistance.

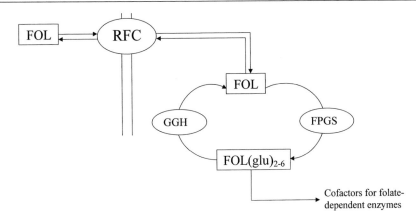

Fig. 2. Uptake and polyglutamation of natural folates. Abbreviations: FOL, reduced folates; FOL(glu)$_n$, polyglutamated folates; RFC, reduced folate carrier; FPGS, folylpolyglutamate synthetase; GGH, γ-glutamyl hydrolase.

3. DIHYDROFOLATE REDUCTASE INHIBITORS

In general, DHFR inhibitors have poor single-agent response rates in colorectal cancer, but a number of researchers have observed that these drugs have the ability to biomodulate the action of 5-FU. Administration of a DHFR inhibitor prior to 5-FU causes an increase in intracellular levels of 5-phosphoribosyl-1-pyrophosphate (PRPP). This allows for an increased production of active metabolites of 5-FU, potentially leading to increased cytotoxicity *(4)*. As an added effect, levels of the TS cofactor 5,10-methylene tetrahydrofolate are increased, which may augment TS inhibition by facilitating the binding of FdUMP to the enzyme *(5)*.

3.1. Methotrexate

Methotrexate (Fig. 3) was developed as an inhibitor of DHFR. Polyglutamated forms of the drug have been found to inhibit TS and AICARFT, however, and it is likely that DHFR inhibition is not the sole cytotoxic mechanism *(6)*. Methotrexate has limited single-agent activity in colorectal cancer, and trials have mostly centered on its use as a biomodulator for 5-FU *(see* above). A number of studies have compared the results obtained from treatment with 5-FU-based chemotherapy with or without the addition of methotrexate *(7–11)*. Results have conflicted somewhat, but only one large study has shown a statistically significant survival benefit for the addition of methotrexate *(7)*. This study compared methotrexate plus 5-FU to 5-FU alone, and studies using leucovorin (LV) modulated 5-FU as a control arm have not suggested any advantage to the addition of methotrexate. A meta-analysis of 1178 patients treated in randomized trials of 5-FU vs 5-FU plus methotrexate confirmed a modest survival advantage for methotrexate plus 5-FU over 5-FU alone, but not LV-modulated 5-FU *(12)*. In view of the increased toxicity and inconvenience seen with the methotrexate-modulated regimens and the possibility of competitive inhibition between methotrexate and LV for uptake and polyglutamation, methotrexate modulation of 5-FU is not widely practiced.

3.2. Trimetrexate

Unlike methotrexate, which utilizes the same transport and polyglutamation pathways as natural folates, trimetrexate (Fig. 3) is a lipophilic compound transported into the cell

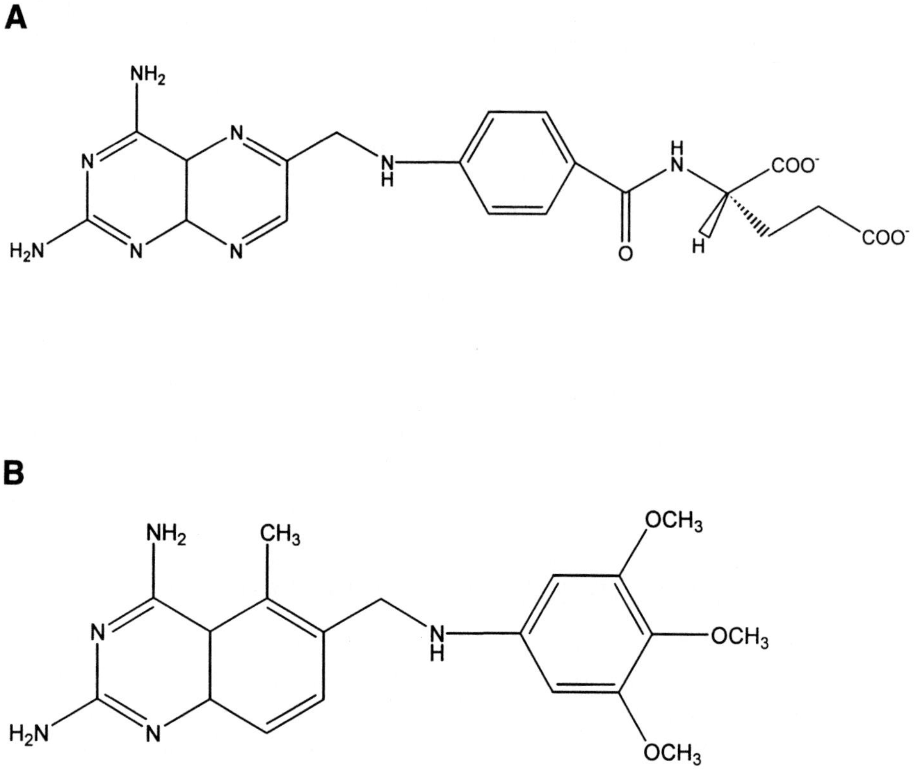

A

B

Fig. 3. Structure of DHFR inhibitors methotrexate (**A**) and trimetrexate (**B**).

by diffusion and is not polyglutamated *(13)*. This overcomes the known mechanisms of resistance to methotrexate arising from reduced carrier-mediated transport or polyglutamate formation and also circumvents any potential competitive inhibitory interaction between methotrexate and leucovorin when the two agents are coadministered. Although single-agent phase II evaluation again showed limited single-agent activity in colorectal cancer *(14)*, trimetrexate has also been used as a biological modifier with 5-FU. Phase II evaluation has been carried out using the combination of 110 mg/m^2 trimetrexate followed after 24 h by 200 mg/m^2 leucovorin, 500 mg/m^2 5-FU, and 7 oral doses of 15 mg leucovorin at 6-hourly intervals beginning 6 h after the 5-FU. This cycle is repeated weekly for 6 wk followed by a 2-wk rest. Two studies have reported response rates of 50% *(15)* and 36% *(16)*, respectively. This led to the initiation of a randomized study comparing this schedule to 200 mg/m^2 leucovorin and 600 mg/m^2 5-FU iv bolus again given for 6 wk of an 8-wk cycle. Initial reports have suggested that there may be a modest improvement in progression-free survival in the trimetrexate arm of the study *(17)*.

3.3. Edatrexate and Piritrexim

Edatrexate and Piritrexim are analogs of methotrexate developed as DHFR inhibitors. Although active in other tumor types, neither of them has significant single-agent activity in colorectal cancer.

4. THYMIDYLATE SYNTHASE INHIBITORS

4.1. CB3717

CB3717 (N^{10}-propargyl-5,8-dideazafolic acid) was the first quinazoline-based inhibitor of TS to enter clinical study. Although a very potent inhibitor of the enzyme and with very encouraging signs of clinical activity in early clinical study, a few patients developed unpredictable and life-threatening nephrotoxicity, which was thought to be the result of precipitation of the drug in the renal tubules *(18)*. Development of CB3717 was therefore discontinued and research effort focused on developing analogs that would retain high levels of potency with increased solubility.

4.2. Raltitrexed

Raltitrexed (Fig. 4) was the result of the ensuing development program aimed at producing a TS inhibitor that would retain the inhibitory potency and FPGS substrate activity of CB3717, but with increased solubility. Raltitrexed as a monoglutamate has a k_i for isolated TS of 60–90 nM *(19)*; however, it is an excellent substrate for FPGS, and the higher chain-length polyglutamated forms are up to 70-fold more potent than the parent compound. In vitro studies have also demonstrated that TS inhibitory activity is maintained after short exposures to the drug followed by extracellular drug removal, providing evidence for intracellular drug retention through polyglutamation *(20)*. This property was confirmed by subsequent in vivo studies *(21)*, and in view of this an infrequent (3-weekly) dosing schedule was chosen for clinical trials. Further preclinical data have shown that raltitrexed can act as a radiosensitizing agent, and clinical studies combining raltitrexed with fractionated radiotherapy have been instituted *(22)*.

Two large phase I studies with raltitrexed were conducted. Both trials showed the dose-limiting toxicities of raltitrexed to be lethargy, diarrhea, and myelosuppression. In the European study *(23)*, the maximum tolerated dose (MTD) was 3.5 mg/m^2, with a recommended dose for further evaluation of 3.0 mg/m^2 3-weekly. In the other study, carried out in the United States *(24)*, although the dose-limiting toxicity (DLTs) were identical, the MTD was higher at 4.5 mg/m^2. Thus, the recommended dose for further evaluation from this study was 4.0 mg/m^2 3-weekly. This dose level was abandoned after excess toxicity in phase III trials and the current recommended dose is 3.0 mg/m^2 3-weekly.

Pharmacokinetic analysis from the initial phase I studies was limited in value, as a lack of data from late time-points made measurement of the very long terminal half-life ($t_{1/2}$) of raltitrexed impossible. Further studies were subsequently carried out using ^{14}C-labeled raltitrexed *(25)*, which revealed a terminal $t_{1/2}$ of 257 h. In addition, a study of the pharmacokinetics of raltitrexed in patients with renal impairment revealed that in patients with creatinine clearance less than 65 mL/min, the area under the curve (AUC) and $t_{1/2}$ were approximately doubled. Furthermore, there were more adverse events in the group with impaired renal function *(26)*. This study has led to the current recommendation that patients with creatinine clearance less than 25 mL/min should not receive raltitrexed and that patients with creatinine clearance between 25 and 64 mL/min should receive a modified dose of 1.5 mg/m^2 4-weekly.

Phase II studies with 3.0 mg/m^2 raltitrexed 3-weekly showed a broad spectrum of clinical activity, with particularly encouraging response rates in breast (23%) *(27)* and colorectal

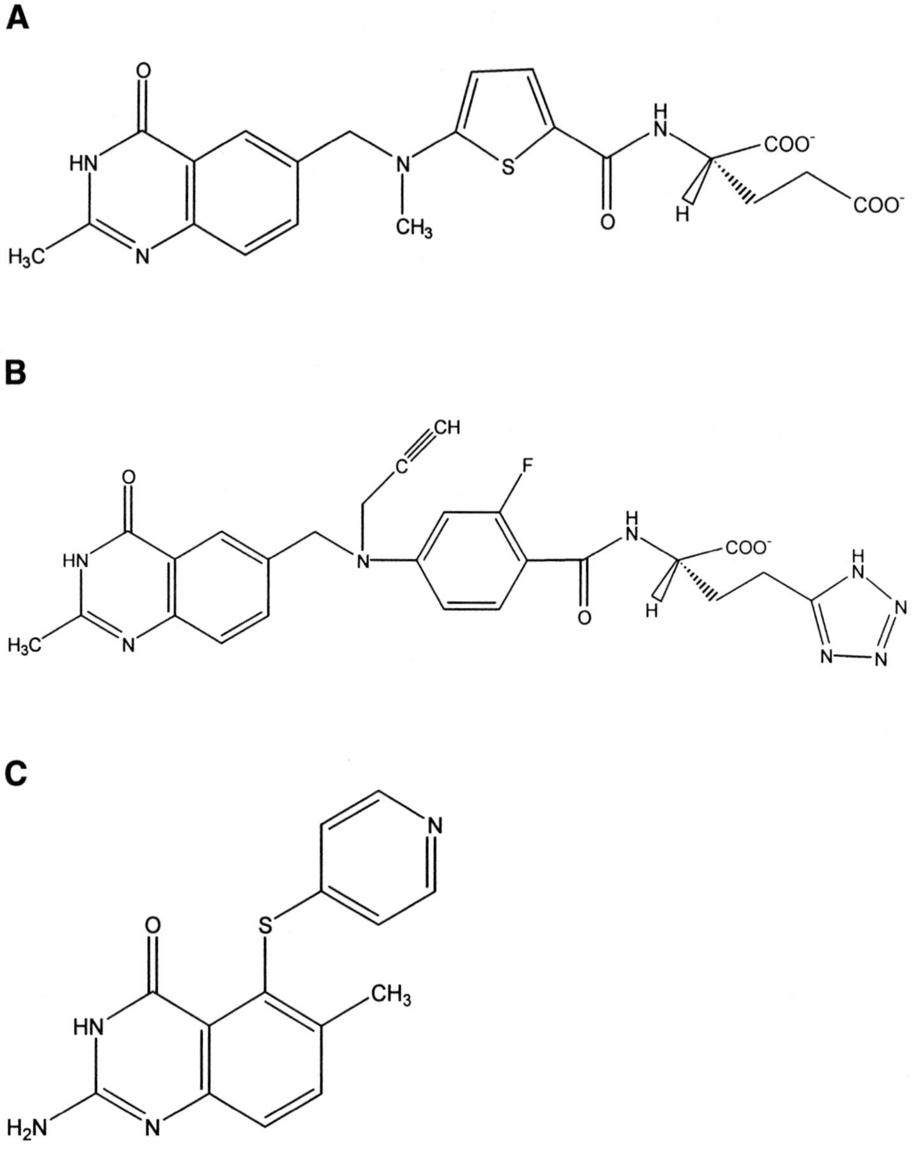

A

B

C

Fig. 4. Structure of TS inhibitors raltitrexed (**A**), ZD9331 (**B**), and nolatrexed (**C**).

(26%) cancer *(28)*, leading to a series of phase III studies comparing raltitrexed to standard 5-FU-based regimens.

Initially, three multicenter phase III studies were conducted. One of these studies was initially designed as a three-arm study, comparing the standard Mayo Clinic schedule of 5-FU and leucovorin with raltitrexed 3.0 mg/m^2 or 4.0 mg/m^2. Toxicity in the 4.0-mg/m^2 group necessitated the early closure of this arm of the trial, however. Only data from the 3.0-mg/m^2 arm were included in the data analyzed from this study, which nevertheless showed inferior overall and progression-free survival in the raltitrexed arm. There is some evidence that the initial toxicity seen in the high-dose arm affected subsequent clinical decision-making, and the results of this study should therefore be interpreted with caution *(29)*.

Two further phase III studies were carried out as part of the initial development process: In the European study (30), patients were randomized to receive either 3.0 mg/m^2 raltitrexed 3-weekly or 425 mg/m^2 5-FU and 20 mg/m^2 leucovorin daily × 5 repeated every 28 d. The results from this study showed similar response rates and survival times between the two arms, with a significant reduction in the rates of leukopenia and stomatitis in the raltitrexed arm. In an international trial (31), patients were randomized to receive either 3.0 mg/m^2 raltitrexed 3-weekly or 400 mg/m^2 5-FU and 200 mg/m^2 leucovorin given daily for the first 5 d of a 28-d cycle. In this trial, response rates and overall survival were again similar, but there was a modest but statistically significant difference in progression-free survival in favor of the 5-FU arm. Toxicity was again substantially reduced in the patients treated with raltitrexed. Subsequently, the UK MRC group carried out a large randomized study comparing 3.0 mg/m^2 raltitrexed to two different infused 5-FU regimens (32). Nine hundred five patients were randomized in this trial, and a preliminary analysis has shown no significant differences in overall survival between the arms. The comparative data from all four studies is shown in Table 1.

4.2.1. Toxicity of Raltitrexed

The striking finding from all studies with raltitrexed has been that although the incidence of severe toxicity is very low (and has been significantly less than for 5-FU in all the studies for which data are available), the morbidity in those patients who experience toxicity is very high. All studies have reported the most significant toxicities of raltitrexed to be myelosuppression, diarrhea, and asthenia. Asymptomatic elevation in hepatic transaminases is common following treated with raltitrexed, but it is usually self-limiting and does not normally require dose modification. Less commonly, cutaneous toxicity may occur. This usually takes the form of an apparent bilateral lower-limb cellulitis and may be so severe as to prevent further treatment with raltitrexed, although systemic steroid therapy may be beneficial. The combination of grade 4 diarrhea and neutropenia is rare, occurring in approx 3% of patients treated with raltitrexed (33). Mortality from this condition is, however, extremely high, unless intensive supportive therapy is promptly administered. It has been shown that an increase in adverse events may follow failure to adhere to recommended dose modifications in the case of impaired renal function or in subsequent cycles following an initial episode of toxicity (34). In addition, a small proportion of patients without any apparent predisposition will experience life-threatening toxicity from raltitrexed. Therefore, it is vital that patients be adequately assessed and monitored both pretreatment and while on therapy in order to minimize the incidence of severe toxicity. Should significant toxicity occur, there should be a low threshold for admission to hospital. In the event of grade 3–4 diarrhea combined with neutropenia, it is recommended that 25 mg/m^2 leucovorin should be administered every 6 h in addition to other supportive measures. This has been shown to reduce the severity and duration of raltitrexed toxicity in rodents, presumably by its competitive effect on polyglutamate homeostasis and transport (35).

4.3. ZD9331

In vitro studies have shown that cell lines expressing low levels of FPGS are relatively resistant to raltitrexed (36). To overcome this potential resistance mechanism, ZD9331 was developed with the aim of achieving a similar degree of potency to raltitrexed without the need for polyglutamation. ZD9331 is not a substrate for FPGS and has a k_i for isolated TS of approx 1 nM (37). It has been shown to retain activity in cell lines deficient in FPGS and

Table 1
Phase III Clinical Trials with Raltitrexed in Advanced Colorectal Cancer

Authors and study regimen	No. of patients	Response rate (%)	OS (mo)	PFS (mo)	Leukopenia (%)	Stomatitis (%)	Diarrhea (%)
Cunningham et al, 1996	439						
425 mg/m² 5-FU +20 mg/m² LV daily ×5 q 28 d	216	16.7	10.2	3.6	30[a]	22[a]	14
3.0 mg/m² raltitrexed q 21 d	223	19.3	10.1	4.8	14[a]	2[a]	14
Reported in Cunningham, 1998	427						
425 mg/m² 5-FU +20 mg2 LV daily ×5 q 28 d	210	15.2	12.7[a]	5.3[a]	41[a]	10	12
4.0 mg/m² raltitrexed or 3.0 mg/m² q 21 d	217	14.3	9.7[a]	3.1[a]	16[a]	3	9
Cocconi et al., 1998	495						
400 mg/m² 5-FU + 200 mg/m² LV daily ×5 q d	248	18.0	12.3	5.1[a]	13	16[a]	19
3.0 mg/m² raltitrexed q 21 d	247	19.0	10.9	3.9[a]	6	2[a]	10
Maughan et al., 1999	905						
5-FU + LV (de Gramont schedule) q 14 d	303	24	10	6[a,b]	NK[c]	NK	NK
300 mg/m²/d 5-FU continuous infusion (Lokich)	301	26	10	6[a,b]	NK	NK	NK
3.0 mg/m² raltitrexed q 21 d	301	20	10	5[a,b]	NK	NK	NK

[a]Statistically significant.
[b]Progression-free survival (PFS) was not a study end point.
[c]NK, not known.

showed activity against colorectal, breast, and ovarian cancer in phase I trials *(38,39)*. Like raltitrexed, ZD9331 has a long $t_{1/2}$ of up to 75 h in man, although, in contrast with raltitrexed, this occurs as a result of slow plasma clearance rather than through tissue retention. DLTs are myelosuppression and diarrhea. The recommended dose for phase II evaluation of ZD9331 is 130 mg/m^2 given on d 1 and 8 of a 3-wk schedule. The response data from phase II studies with ZD9331 are not available at the time of writing.

4.4. Nolatrexed (AG337, Thymitaq™)

Nolatrexed was the product of a research program aimed at the development of a lipophilic TS inhibitor that would not require active transport into the cell. The compound was developed by computer modeling using X-ray crystallographic analysis of the structure of bacterial TS and has no substrate activity for either the RFC or FPGS. It is a potent inhibitor of isolated TS, with a k_i of approx 11 nM *(40)*. It is rapidly eliminated from the plasma, requiring prolonged iv administration *(41)*. The intravenous schedule used in the phase II studies quoted was 800 mg/m^2 d as a 5-d continuous infusion repeated every 3 wk. Oral administration was also explored and found to be feasible *(42)*. In phase II studies, nolatrexed demonstrated some activity against colorectal cancer and other tumor types *(43)*. Despite this, the drug is not planned for further development.

5. FUTURE DIRECTIONS WITH TS INHIBITORS

5.1. Scheduling

Preclinical work has shown that prolonged TS inhibition appears to result in improved efficacy. Studies of elevation of plasma 2′-deoxyuridine, a surrogate marker of TS inhibition, suggests that TS is inhibited for between 5 and 8 d following a single dose of either raltitrexed or ZD9331 *(44)*. The schedule chosen for further development of ZD9331 incorporates dosing on d 1 and 8, following which, recovery generally occurs between d 15 and 21. This schedule should provide near continuous TS inhibition (Fig. 5). In addition, studies of raltitrexed have been carried out with administration on a 14-d schedule *(45)*, providing TS inhibition for at least 10/14 d. Further trials will be required to show whether modifying drug schedules in this way will result in improved efficacy; however, it is likely that alternative regimens will become available that may have particular benefits in combination therapy.

5.2. Drug Combinations

The relatively low incidence of toxicity and convenient administration profile of raltitrexed makes it an ideal candidate for use in combination with other agents. A number of drug combinations with raltitrexed have shown promising results, and some of these are now discussed.

5.2.1. RALTITREXED/IRINOTECAN

In vitro studies showed pronounced synergy between raltitrexed and SN-38, the active metabolite of irinotecan. This synergy was only seen when SN-38 preceded raltitrexed *(46)*. Phase I evaluation, with both drugs given in this sequence as short infusions on a 3-weekly schedule, in patients with gastrointestinal (GI) tract cancer (predominantly colorectal) showed remarkably little toxicity. Diarrhea and neutropenia were uncommon and the DLT was asthenia. A response rate of 20% was seen in heavily pretreated patients, across all dose levels *(47)*. Phase II evaluation of this combination at the recommended doses of 350 mg/m^2 irinotecan and 3.0 mg/m^2 raltitrexed 3-weekly is ongoing.

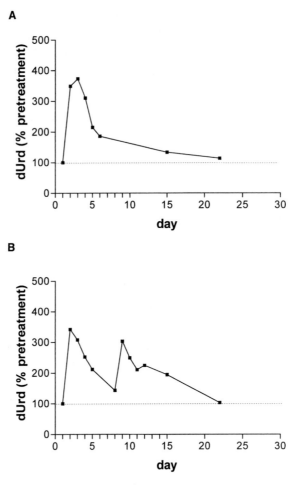

Fig. 5. Mean plasma 2′-deoxyuridine elevation after 3.0 mg/m^2 raltitrexed (**A**) and 130 mg/m^2 ZD9331 d 1 and 8 (**B**).

5.2.2. RALTITREXED/OXALIPLATIN

A phase I study of the combination of raltitrexed and oxaliplatin showed that the two drugs could be given together without modification of the single-agent doses, and significant activity was seen in mesothelioma as well as pancreatic and renal carcinoma (48). Phase II evaluation of the combination of 130 mg/m^2 oxaliplatin and 3.0 mg/m^2 raltitrexed 3-weekly has been carried out in advanced colorectal cancer and showed the impressive objective response rate of 57.3%. Overall toxicity from this combination appeared relatively mild, although NCI-CTC grade 3–4 diarrhea and neutropenia were seen in 9% and 16.5% of patients, respectively (49).

5.2.3. RALTITREXED/5-FU

As with methotrexate, there is evidence that the ternary complex formed by FdUMP, raltitrexed, and TS is more stable than that formed with the folate cofactor (50), which could cause potentiation of TS inhibition by 5-FU. In addition, there is some evidence for non-cross-resistance between 5-FU and raltitrexed. In vitro studies suggested a sequence-specific interaction between the drugs, and optimum cytotoxic effects were achieved when 5-FU was given after raltitrexed *(51)*. Studies have been performed to evaluate the combination of 5-FU and raltitrexed in advanced colorectal cancer. In one phase I study *(52)*, which evaluated the combination of raltitrexed followed by bolus 5-FU given 3-weekly. In the first part of the study, the raltitrexed dose was fixed at 3.0 mg/m², and the 5-FU was dose-escalated, and, subsequently, the 5-FU dose was fixed at 1200 mg/m², and the raltitrexed was dose-escalated. The DLT was neutropenia in both arms of the study, and the MTD was 3.0 mg/m² raltitrexed/1350 mg/m² 5-FU in the first arm and 6.0 mg/m² raltitrexed/1200 mg/m² 5-FU in the second arm. Significant activity was seen in the study, with 1 complete response and 4 partial responses out of a total of 54 patients treated. The recommended dose for further evaluation from this study was 5.5 mg/m² raltitrexed/1200 mg/m² 5-FU 3-weekly. A second study *(53)* evaluating 5-FU on a weekly times 5 schedule followed by a 1-wk rest and raltitrexed prior to the 5-FU on wk 2 and 5 gave a recommended dose of 2600 mg/m² 5-FU and 2.6 mg/m² raltitrexed, with neutropenia again the DLT. The objective response rate in this study of chemotherapy-naive patients was 46%, with very little toxicity seen in the group treated at the recommended dose. Interestingly, both these studies showed that the AUC and peak plasma concentration (C_{max}) of 5-FU are significantly increased when raltitrexed is coadministered.

5.3. Targeted Therapy

Clinical studies with 5-FU have demonstrated that the pattern of gene expression in tumors is highly relevant to tumor response rates (*see* Chapter 34). The TS mRNA levels, as measured by real-time reverse transcription–polymerase chain reaction (RT-PCR) have been shown to predict response to 5-FU/LV with a response rate of 52% in patients with a TS/β-actin ratio $< 4.1 \times 10^3$, compared with 0% in patients with higher levels of TS expression *(54)*. In the same group of patients, high levels of TP and DPD gene expression were found independently to predict lack of response to 5-FU/LV *(55,56)*. A similar study of response to raltitrexed showed a response rate of 5/7 (71%) in low-TS-expressing patients, compared to 1/13 (8%) in the higher-TS expressing group *(57)*. This difference was statistically significant ($p = 0.009$). No relationship was seen between DPD or TP gene expression and response in this study, suggesting that a proportion of patients with disease likely to be 5-FU resistant may respond to raltitrexed. Although one retrospective study showed only 1 response to 5-FU and mitomycin C out of 50 patients pretreated with raltitrexed *(58)*, preliminary data from a prospective study of raltitrexed following 5-FU failure showed objective responses in 7/45 (16%) of patients *(59)*, although the previous treatment regimens in this study were not standardized and no firm conclusions can be drawn from these data at this stage. Taken together, however, there is increasing evidence that patients' treatments could be optimized by pretreatment tumor gene expression analysis. Further studies are required to know whether this approach will prove superior to first-line combination therapy.

6. GARFT/AICARFT INHIBITORS

6.1. Lometrexol

Lometrexol (5,10-dideazatetrahydrofolate, DDATHF) (Fig. 6) is a potent inhibitor of purine biosynthesis, acting through GARFT inhibition. It showed evidence of activity against colorectal cancer in a phase I study *(60)*. Thrombocytopenia is the DLT, and a pattern of cumulative toxicity was seen, which was reversible with leucovorin administration. This toxicity limited initial development, but subsequent investigators have shown that coadministration of oral folic acid reduces toxicity and allows therapeutic dosing *(61)*. A

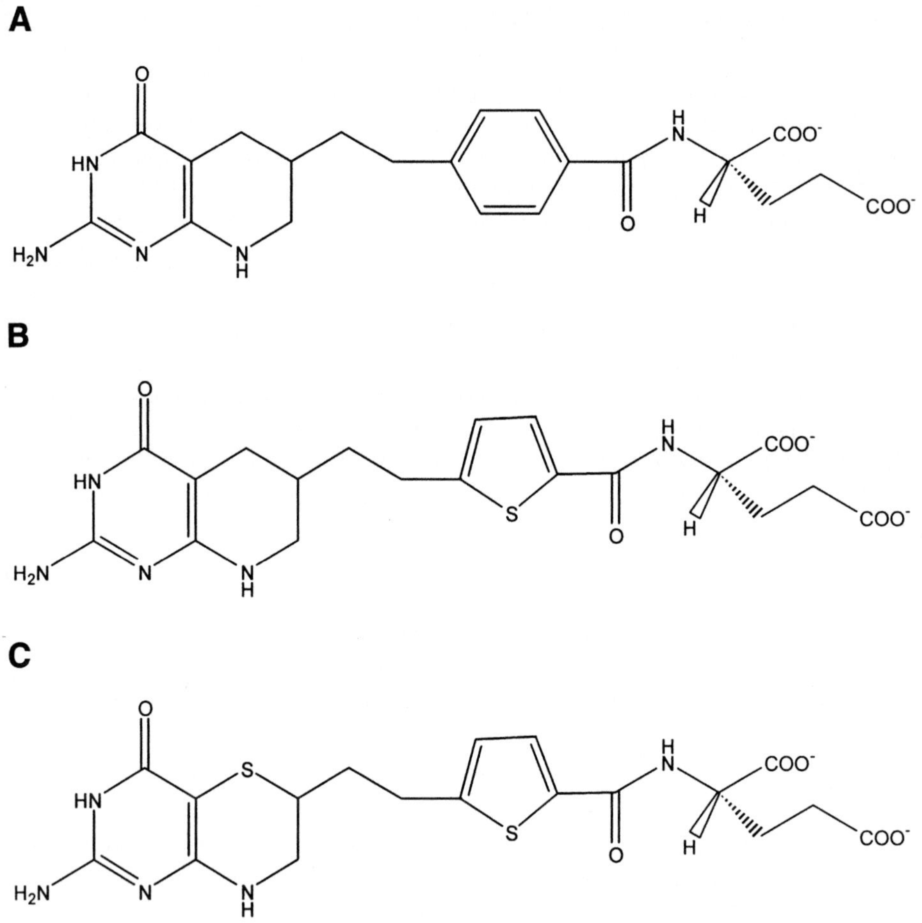

A

B

C

Fig. 6. Structure of GARFT inhibitors lometrexol (**A**), LY309887 (**B**), and AG2034 (**C**).

dose of 10.4 mg/m^2 weekly with 3 mg/m^2/d folic acid has been recommended for phase II evaluation *(62)*, although the development of the drug has been discontinued in favor of the more potent and potentially less toxic inhibitor LY309887.

6.2. LY309887

LY309887 (2′,5′-thienyl-5,10-dideazatetrahydrofolate) was developed as a less toxic GARFT inhibitor than lometrexol. It demonstrates a ninefold increase in GARFT inhibitory activity over lometrexol (k_i 6.5 n*M*) and has an increased affinity for the α-folate receptor (α-FR), another membrane-bound folate-binding protein that may be overexpressed in some tumor types *(63)*. Although it retains FPGS substrate activity, the first-order rate constant is lower, and preclinical studies have shown less hepatic drug accumulation. The drug is highly active against colon cancer cell lines and has the potential to display less toxicity than lometrexol. A phase I study has shown DLTs of myelosuppression and neuropathy, and the MTD is 8 mg/m^2, with a recommended phase II dose of 6 mg/m^2 LY309887 3-weekly with 5 mg folic acid daily for 14 d starting 7 d prior to LY309887. Increasing the dose of folic acid to 25 mg/d × 14 d did not allow further dose-escalation. Efficacy data on this compound is currently limited *(64)*.

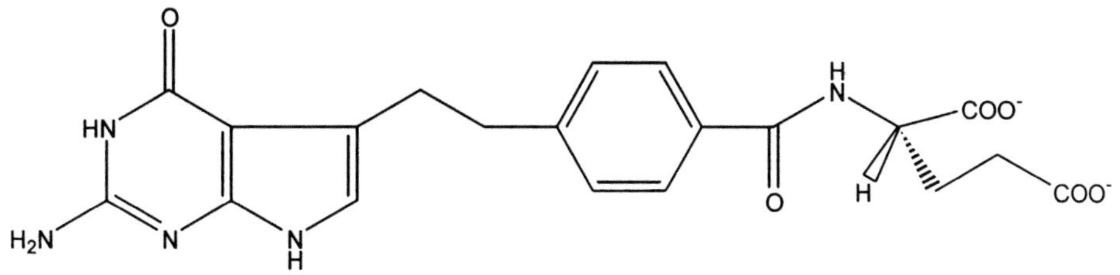

Fig. 7. Structure of pemetrexed.

6.3. AG2034

AG2034 is a second-generation inhibitor of GARFT developed using crystallographic analysis of the enzyme structure. It enters the cell via the RFC and has good substrate activity for FPGS *(65)*. A phase I study has so far demonstrated less severe toxicity than with lometrexol, although data on activity are limited. DLTs are myelosuppression, gastrointestinal, and lethargy. AG2034 is planned for phase II evaluation at a dose of 5.0 mg/m^2 3-weekly *(66)*.

6.4. AG2009

AG2009 is a specific inhibitor of AICARFT designed through computer modeling, using X-ray crystallography of the enzyme structure. No clinical data are yet available.

7. MULTITARGETED ANTIFOLATE

7.1. Pemetrexed (LY231514 and MTA)

The pyrrolo-[2,3-*d*]-pyrimidine pemetrexed (Fig. 7) was developed as an analog of lometrexol, but preclinical studies showed it to be a potent inhibitor of TS *(67)*. It is a good substrate for FPGS, and as with raltitrexed, the polyglutamated drug shows increased potency compared to the parent compound. However, the effect of pemetrexed is only partially reversed by the addition of thymidine, suggesting that cytotoxicity is not entirely the result of TS inhibition. In addition, clinical studies demonstrated responses in patients with disease resistant to 5-FU and raltitrexed *(68)*. Pemetrexed has been shown to have inhibitory activity against GARFT and DHFR and, to a lesser extent, against AICARFT and C-1 synthetase *(69)*. Two phase II studies were carried out in colorectal cancer using pemetrexed doses of 500–600 mg/m^2 3-weekly, and response rates of 15.4% *(70)* and 17% *(71)*, respectively, were seen. The DLTs are fatigue and neutropenia, with skin rash and gastrointestinal mucosal toxicity also significant. Interestingly, the incidence of antiproliferative toxicity with MTA appears to be strongly associated with high pretreatment levels of homocysteine (indicative of low levels of reduced folates), suggesting that relative folate deficiency may be a significant predisposing factor for toxicity *(72)*.

8. SUMMARY

There are a wide variety of folate-based antimetabolites available, several of which are active in colorectal cancer (Table 2). The most advanced in the development of these drugs are the TS inhibitors, of which raltitrexed is the lead compound. Initial enthusiasm has been somewhat tempered by the relatively high incidence of treatment-related mortality seen with raltitrexed, and the suggestion of inferior progression-free survival compared with 5-FU in

Table 2
Properties of Antifolates with Potential Utility in Colorectal Cancer Chemotherapy

Drug	Major target	Other targets	Uptake	Polyglutamation	Phase II response rate (single agent)	Current status in colorectal cancer
Methotrexate	DHFR	TS AICARFT	Active	Yes	<10%	Not widely used
Trimetrexate	DHFR		Passive	No	<10%	Phase III as biological modulator with 5-FU
Raltitrexed	TS		Active	Yes	26%	Licensed in many countries
ZD9331	TS		Active	No	N/K	Phase II
Nolatrexed	TS		Passive	No	<10%	Discontinued after phase II
Lometrexol	GARFT		Active	Yes	N/K	Discontinued after phase I
LY309887	GARFT		Active	Yes	N/K	Phase I completed
AG2034	GARFT		Active	Yes	N/K	Phase II
AG2009	AICARFT				N/K	Phase I
Pemetrexed	TS	GARFT DHFR AICARFT C-1 synthetase	Active	Yes	15–17%	Phase II completed

580

some studies. Nevertheless, it appears likely that by dose modification based on pretreatment renal function and with appropriate monitoring of toxicity, the morbidity associated with raltitrexed may be minimized. Therefore, raltitrexed as a single agent provides a genuine alternative to 5-FU, especially where the latter is contraindicated, and there are increasing signs that the activity and convenience of delivery of raltitrexed in combination therapy will make it a useful part of clinicians' armamentarium for the treatment of advanced disease in the future. Results obtained from trials of the combinations of raltitrexed and oxaliplatin or irinotecan bear comparison with the equivalent 5-FU-based regimens. In addition, the rational processes involved in the design of TS inhibitors have produced a range of unique compounds with known properties that lend themselves to a targeting approach to chemotherapy. Although the mass applications of this therapeutic advance are, at present, limited, improvements in diagnostic technology allowing automation of gene-expression profiling has the potential to make these assays more widely available. Utilizing this is likely to become ever more practical as the role the various folate-binding enzymes play in drug resistance becomes clearer. Newer schedules and second-generation compounds are likely to provide improved activity, and a greater understanding of the mechanisms involved in the toxicity seen with this class of compounds should add further benefits. The role of non-TS-targeted drugs, especially those targeted at purine biosynthesis, is less clear at present; however, in vitro and early clinical data suggest great potential for future development in the clinic. The advent of combination chemotherapy as a standard of care in colorectal cancer increases the opportunity to use a variety of antimetabolites and drugs directed at other targets in conjunction to achieve improved patient benefit. Arriving at the optimum combination or treatment strategy is one of the great challenges currently facing clinicians and researchers.

REFERENCES

1. Anonymous. Efficacy of intravenous continuous infusion of fluorouracil compared with bolus administration in advanced colorectal cancer. Meta-analysis Group In Cancer. *J. Clin. Oncol.*, **16(1)** (1998) 301–308.
2. Aschele C, Sobrero A, Faderan MA, and Bertino JR. Novel mechanism(s) of resistance to 5-fluorouracil in human colon cancer (HCT-8) sublines following exposure to two clinically relevant dose schedules. *Cancer Res.*, **52** (1992) 1855–1864.
3. McGuire JJ and Coward JK. Pteroylpolyglutamates: biosynthesis, degradation and function. *Folates Pterins*, **1** (1984) 135–190.
4. Cadman E, Heimer R, and Davis L. Enhanced 5-fluorouracil nucleotide formation after methotrexate administration: explanation for drug synergism. *Science*, **205** (1979) 1135–1137.
5. Fernandes DJ and Bertino JR. 5-Fluorouracil-methotrexate synergy: enhancement of 5-fluorodeoxyuridylate binding to thymidylate synthase by dihydropteroylglutamates. *Proc. Natl. Acad. Sci. USA*, **77(10)** (1980) 5663–5667.
6. Allegra CJ, Hoang K, Yeh GC, Drake JC, and Baram J. Evidence for direct inhibition of purine biosynthesis in human MCF-7 breast cancer cells as a principal mode of metabolic inhibition by methotrexate. *J. Biol. Chem.*, **262(28)** (1987) 13,520–13,526.
7. Anonymous. Superiority of sequential methotrexate, fluorouracil, and leucovorin to fluorouracil alone in advanced symptomatic colorectal carcinoma: a randomized trial. The Nordic Gastrointestinal Tumor Adjuvant Therapy Group. *J. Clin. Oncol.*, **7(10)** (1989) 1437–1446.
8. Glimelius B. Biochemical modulation of 5-fluorouracil: a randomized comparison of sequential methotrexate, 5-fluorouracil and leucovorin versus sequential 5-fluorouracil and leucovorin in patients with advanced symptomatic colorectal cancer. The Nordic Gastrointestinal Tumor Adjuvant Therapy Group. *Ann. Oncol.*, **4(3)** (1993) 235–240.
9. Machiavelli, M., Leone BA, Romero A, et al. Advanced colorectal carcinoma. A prospective randomized trial of sequential methotrexate, 5-fluorouracil and leucovorin versus 5-fluorouracil alone. *Am. J. Clin. Oncol.*, **14(3)** (1991) 211–217.
10. Poon MA, O'Connell MJ, Moertel CG, et al. Biochemical modulation of fluorouracil: evidence of improved survival and quality of life in patients with advanced colorectal carcinoma. *J. Clin. Oncol.*, **7** (1989) 1407–1418.

11. Petrelli N, Herrera L, Rustum Y, et al. A prospective randomized trial of 5-fluorouracil versus 5-fluorouracil and methotrexate in patients with advanced colorectal carcinoma. *J. Clin. Oncol.*, **5** (1987) 1559–1565.

12. Anonymous. Meta-analysis of randomized trials testing the biochemical modulation of fluorouracil by methotrexate in metastatic colorectal cancer. Advanced Colorectal Cancer Meta-Analysis Project. *J. Clin. Oncol.*, **12(5)** (1994) 960–969.

13. Jackson RC, Fry DW, Boritzki TJ, et al. Biochemical pharmacology of the lipophilic antifolate, trimetrexate. *Adv. Enzyme Regul.*, (1984) **22** 187–206.

14. Ajani JA, Abbruzzese JL, Faintuch JS, et al. A phase II study of trimetrexate therapy for metastatic colorectal carcinoma. *Cancer Invest.*, **8(6)** (1990) 619–621.

15. Blanke CD, Kasimis B, Schein P, Capizzi R, and Kurman M. Phase II study of trimetrexate, fluorouracil, and leucovorin for advanced colorectal cancer. *J. Clin. Oncol.*, **15(3)** (1997) 915–920.

16. Szelenyi H, Hohenberger P, Lochs H, et al. Sequential trimetrexate, 5-fluorouracil and folinic acid are effective and well tolerated in metastatic colorectal carcinoma. The phase II study group of the AIO. *Oncology*, **58(4)** (2000) 273–279.

17. Punt CJ, Keizer HJ, Douma J, et al. Multicenter randomized trial of 5-fluorouracil (5FU) and leucovorin (LV) with or without trimetrexate (TMTX) as first line treatment in patients (pts) with advanced colorectal cancer (ACC). *Proc. Am. Soc. Clin. Oncol.*, **18** (1999) A1006 (abstract).

18. Calvert AH, Alison DL, Harland SJ, et al. A phase I evaluation of the quinazoline antifolate thymidylate synthase inhibitor, N^{10}-propargyl-5,8-dideazafolic acid, CB3717. *J. Clin. Oncol.*, **4(8)** (1986) 1245–1252.

19. Jackman AL, Taylor GA, Gibson W, et al. ICI D1694, a quinazoline antifolate thymidylate synthase inhibitor that is a potent inhibitor of L1210 tumor cell growth in vitro and in vivo: a new agent for clinical study. *Cancer Res.*, **51(20)** (1991) 5579–5586.

20. Jackman AL, Kimbell R, Brown M, Brunton L, and Boyle FT. Quinazoline thymidylate synthase inhibitors: methods for assessing the contribution of polyglutamation to their in vitro activity. *Anticancer Drug Des.*, **10(7)** (1995) 555–572.

21. Aherne GW, Ward E, Lawrence N, et al. Comparison of plasma and tissue levels of ZD1694 (Tomudex), a highly polyglutamatable quinazoline thymidylate synthase inhibitor, in preclinical models. *Br. J. Cancer*, **77(2)** (1998) 221–226.

22. Teicher BA, Ara G, Chen YN, Recht A, and Coleman CN. Interaction of tomudex with radiation in vitro and in vivo. *Int. J. Oncol.*, **13(3)** (1998) 437–442.

23. Clarke SJ, Hanwell J, de Boer M, et al. Phase I trial of ZD1694, a new folate-based thymidylate synthase inhibitor, in patients with solid tumors. *J. Clin. Oncol.*, **14(5)** (1996) 1495–1503.

24. Grem JL, Sorensen JM, Cullen E, et al. A Phase I study of raltitrexed, an antifolate thymidylate synthase inhibitor, in adult patients with advanced solid tumors. *Clin. Cancer Res.*, **5(9)** (1999) 2381–2391.

25. Beale P, Judson I, Hanwell J, et al. Metabolism, excretion and pharmacokinetics of a single dose of [^{14}C]-raltitrexed in cancer patients. *Cancer Chemother. Pharmacol.*, **42(1)** (1998) 71–76.

26. Judson I, Maughan T, Beale P, et al. Effects of impaired renal function on the pharmacokinetics of raltitrexed (Tomudex ZD1694). *Br. J. Cancer*, **78(9)** (1998) 1188–1193.

27. Smith I, Jones A, Spielmann M, et al. A phase II study in advanced breast cancer: ZD1694 ("Tomudex") a novel direct and specific thymidylate synthase inhibitor. *Br. J. Cancer*, **74(3)** (1996) 479–481.

28. Zalcberg JR, Cunningham D, Van Cutsem E, et al. ZD1694: a novel thymidylate synthase inhibitor with substantial activity in the treatment of patients with advanced colorectal cancer. Tomudex Colorectal Study Group. *J. Clin. Oncol.*, **14(3)** (1996) 716–721.

29. Cunningham D. Mature results from three large controlled studies with raltitrexed ("Tomudex"). *Br. J. Cancer*, **77(Suppl. 2)** (1998) 15–21.

30. Cunningham D, Zalcberg JR, Rath U, et al. Final results of a randomised trial comparing "Tomudex" (raltitrexed) with 5-fluorouracil plus leucovorin in advanced colorectal cancer. "Tomudex" Colorectal Cancer Study Group [published erratum appears in *Ann. Oncol.*, **8(4)** (1997) 407], *Ann. Oncol.*, **7(9)** (1996) 961–965.

31. Cocconi G, Cunningham D, Van Cutsem E, et al. Open, randomized, multicenter trial of raltitrexed versus fluorouracil plus high-dose leucovorin in patients with advanced colorectal cancer. Tomudex Colorectal Cancer Study Group. *J. Clin. Oncol.*, **16(9)** (1998) 2943–2952.

32. Maughan TS, James RD, Kerr D, et al. Preliminary results of a multicentre randomised trial comparing 3 chemotherapy regimens (de gramont, lokich and raltitrexed) in metastatic colorectal cancer. *Proc. Am. Soc. Clin. Oncol.*, **18** (1999) 262a (abstract).

33. Ford HE and Cunningham D. Safety of raltitrexed [letter; comment]. *Lancet*, **354(9192)** (1999) 1824–1825.

34. Garcia-Vargas JE, Sahmoud T, Smith MP, and Green S. Qualitative and chronological assessment of toxicities during treatment with raltitrexed (Tomudex) in 861 patients: implications for patient management. *Eur. J. Cancer*, **35(Suppl. 4)** (1999) S72 (Abstract).

35. Farrugia DC, Aherne GW, Brunton L, Clarke SJ, and Jackman AL. Leucovorin rescue from raltitrexed (tomudex)-induced antiproliferative effects: in vitro cell line and in vivo mouse studies [in process citation]. *Clin. Cancer Res.*, **6(9)** (2000) 3646–3656.

36. Jackman AL, Kelland LR, Kimbell R, et al. Mechanisms of acquired resistance to the quinazoline thymidylate synthase inhibitor ZD1694 (Tomudex) in one mouse and three human cell lines. *Br. J. Cancer*, **71(5)** (1995) 914–924.

37. Jackman AL, Kimbell R, Aherne GW, et al. Cellular pharmacology and in vivo activity of a new anticancer agent, ZD9331: a water-soluble, nonpolyglutamatable, quinazoline-based inhibitor of thymidylate synthase. *Clin. Cancer Res.*, **3(6)** (1997) 911–921.

38. Goh BC, Ratain MJ, Bertucci D, et al. Phase I study of ZD9331 on a 5-day short infusion schedule given every 3 weeks. *Proc. Am. Soc. Clin. Oncol.*, (1999) **19** A653 (abstract).

39. Rees C, Beale P, Trigo J, et al. Phase I Trial of ZD9331, a non-polyglutamatable thymidylate synthase (TS) inhibitor given as a five day continuous infusion every 3 weeks. *Proc. Am. Soc. Clin. Oncol.*, **18** (1999) A657 (abstract).

40. Webber SE, Bleckman TM, Attard J, et al. Design of thymidylate synthase inhibitors using protein crystal structures: the synthesis and biological evaluation of a novel class of 5-substituted quinazolinones. *J. Med. Chem.*, **36(6)** (1993) 733–746.

41. Rafi I, Taylor GA, Calvete JA, et al. Clinical pharmacokinetic and pharmacodynamic studies with the nonclassical antifolate thymidylate synthase inhibitor 3, 4-dihydro-2-amino-6-methyl-4-oxo-5-(4-pyridylthio)-quinazolone dihydrochloride (AG337) given by 24-hour continuous intravenous infusion. *Clin. Cancer Res.*, **1(11)** (1995) 1275–1284.

42. Rafi I, Boddy AV, Calvete JA, et al. Preclinical and phase I clinical studies with the nonclassical antifolate thymidylate synthase inhibitor nolatrexed dihydrochloride given by prolonged administration in patients with solid tumors. *J. Clin. Oncol.*, **16(3)** (1998) 1131–1141.

43. Belani CP, Lembersky B, Ramanathan R, et al. A phase II trial of Thymitaq (AG337) in patients with adenocarcinoma of the colon. *Proceedings of the Annual Meeting of the American Society of Clinical Oncology*, (1997) p. A965 (abstract).

44. Jackman AL, Ford HER, Farrugia DC, et al. The effects of raltitrexed (Tomudex), ZD9331(Vamidex) and 5-FU on plasma dUrd, a surrogate marker of thymidylate synthase inhibition. *Proc. Am. Soc. Clin. Oncol.*, **19** (2000) A712.

45. Farrugia DC, Tischkowitz M, Ford HER, et al. Phase I study of raltitrexed (Tomudex) given every 14 days (q14)—a schedule for combination. *Br. J. Cancer*, **80(Suppl. 2)** (1999) 35 (abstract).

46. Aschele C, Baldo C, Sobrero AF, Debernardis D, Bornmann WG, and Bertino JR. Schedule-dependent synergism between raltitrexed and irinotecan in human colon cancer cells in vitro. *Clin. Cancer Res.*, **4(5)** (1998) 1323–1330.

47. Ford HE, Cunningham D, Ross PJ, et al. Phase I study of irinotecan and raltitrexed in patients with advanced gastrointestinal tract adenocarcinoma. *Br. J. Cancer*, **83(2)** (2000) 146–152.

48. Fizazi K, Ducreux M, Ruffie P, et al. Phase I, dose-finding, and pharmacokinetic study of raltitrexed combined with oxaliplatin in patients with advanced cancer. *J. Clin. Oncol.*, **18(11)** (2000) 2293–2300.

49. Douillard JY, Michel P, Gamelin E, et al. Raltitrexed ("Tomudex") plus oxaliplatin: an active combination for first line chemotherapy in patients with metastatic colorectal cancer. *Proc. Am. Soc. Clin. Oncol.*, **19** (2000) 250a (abstract).

50. van der Wilt CL, Pinedo HM, Kuiper CM, Smid K, and Peters GJ. Biochemical basis for the combined antiproliferative effects of AG337 or raltitrexed and 5-fluorouracil. *Proc. Am. Assoc. Cancer Res.*, (1995) 379 (abstract).

51. Jackman AL, Kimbell R, and Ford HE. Combination of raltitrexed with other cytotoxic agents: rationale and preclinical observations. *Eur. J. Cancer*, **35(Suppl. 1)** (1999) S3–S8.

52. Schwartz GK, Bertino J, Kemeny N, et al. Phase I trial of sequential raltitrexed ("Tomudex") followed by 5-FU in patients with advanced colorectal cancer. *Proc. Am. Soc. Clin. Oncol.*, **19** (2000) 252a (abstract).

53. Mayer S, Vanhoefer U, Hilger R, et al. Extended phase I study of raltitrexed and infusional 5-FU in patients with metastatic colorectal cancer. *Proc. Am. Soc. Clin. Oncol.*, **19** (2000) 299a (abstract).

54. Leichman CG, Lenz HJ, Leichman L, et al. Quantitation of intratumoral thymidylate synthase expression predicts for disseminated colorectal cancer response and resistance to protracted-infusion fluorouracil and weekly leucovorin. *J. Clin. Oncol.*, **15(10)** (1997) 3223–3229.

55. Metzger R, Danenberg K, Leichman CG, et al. High basal level gene expression of thymidine phosphorylase (platelet-derived endothelial cell growth factor) in colorectal tumors is associated with nonresponse to 5-fluorouracil. *Clin. Cancer Res.*, **4(10)** (1998) 2371–2376.

56. Salonga D, Danenberg KD, Johnson M, et al. Colorectal tumors responding to 5-fluorouracil have low gene expression levels of dihydropyrimidine dehydrogenase, thymidylate synthase, and thymidine phosphorylase. *Clin. Cancer Res.*, **6(4)** (2000) 1322–1327.

57. Jackman AL, Ford HER, Cunningham D, et al. Individualizing treatment approaches with antifolate antimetabolites. *Br. J. Cancer*, **83(Suppl. 1)** (2000) 19 (abstract).

58. Farrugia DC, Norman AR, and Cunningham D. Single agent infusional 5-fluorouracil is not effective second-line therapy after raltitrexed (Tomudex) in advanced colorectal cancer [see comments]. *Eur. J. Cancer*, **34(7)** (1998) 987–991.

59. Horikoshi N, Aiba K, Kurihaba M, et al. Phase II study of Tomudex in chemotherapy pretreated patients with advanced colorectal cancer. *Proc. Am. Soc. Clin. Oncol.*, **18** (1999) 257a (abstract).

60. Ray MS, Muggia FM, Leichman CG, et al. Phase I study of (6R)-5,10-dideazatetrahydrofolate: a folate antimetabolite inhibitory to de novo purine synthesis. *J. Natl. Cancer Inst.*, **85(14)** (1993) 1154–1159.

61. Laohavinij S, Wedge SR, Lind MJ, et al. A phase I clinical study of the antipurine antifolate lometrexol (DDATHF) given with oral folic acid. *Invest. New Drugs*, **14(3)** (1996) 325–335.

62. Roberts JD, Poplin EA, Tombes MB, et al. Weekly lometrexol with daily oral folic acid is appropriate for phase II evaluation. *Cancer Chemother. Pharmacol.*, **45(2)** (2000) 103–110.

63. Mendelsohn LG, Shih C, Schultz RM, and Worzalla JF. Biochemistry and pharmacology of glycinamide ribonucleotide formyltransferase inhibitors: LY309887 and lometrexol. *Invest. New Drugs*, **14(3)** (1996) 287–294.

64. Halford S, Harper P, Highley M, et al. A phase I and pharmacokinetic study of LY309887 given every 3 weeks with folic acid. *Proc. Am. Soc. Clin. Oncol.*, **18** (1999) 170a (abstract).

65. Boritzki TJ, Barlett CA, Zhang C, and Howland EF. AG2034: a novel inhibitor of glycinamide ribonucleotide formyltransferase. *Invest. New Drugs*, **14(3)** (1996) 295–303.

66. Roberts JD, Shibata S, Spicer DV, et al. Phase I study of AG2034, a targeted GARFT inhibitor, administered once every 3 weeks. *Cancer Chemother. Pharmacol.*, **45(5)** (2000) 423–427.

67. Taylor EC, Kuhnt D, Shih C, et al. A dideazatetrahydrofolate analogue lacking a chiral center at C-6, *N*-[4-[2-(2-amino-3,4-dihydro-4-oxo-7H-pyrrolo[2,3-d]pyrimidin-5-yl)ethyl]benzoyl]-L-glutamic acid, is an inhibitor of thymidylate synthase. *J. Med. Chem.*, **35(23)** (1992) 4450–4454.

68. Rinaldi DA, Burris HA, Dorr FA, et al. Initial phase I evaluation of the novel thymidylate synthase inhibitor, LY231514, using the modified continual reassessment method for dose escalation. *J. Clin. Oncol.*, **13(11)** (1995) 2842–2850.

69. Shih C, Chen VJ, Gossett LS, et al. LY231514, a pyrrolo[2,3-d]pyrimidine-based antifolate that inhibits multiple folate-requiring enzymes. *Cancer Res.*, **57(6)** (1997) 1116–1123.

70. John W, Picus J, Blanke CD, et al. Activity of multitargeted antifolate (pemetrexed disodium, LY231514) in patients with advanced colorectal carcinoma: results from a phase II study. *Cancer*, **88(8)** (2000) 1807–1813.

71. Cripps C, Burnell M, Jolivet J, et al. Phase II study of first-line LY231514 (multi-targeted antifolate) in patients with locally advanced or metastatic colorectal cancer: an NCIC Clinical Trials Group study. *Ann. Oncol.*, **10(10)** (1999) 1175–1179.

72. Niyikiza C, Walling J, Thornton D, Seitz D, and Allen R. LY231514 (MTA): relationship of vitamin metabolite profile to toxicity. *Proc. Am. Soc. Clin. Oncol.*, **17** (1998) 558a (abstract).

Adjuvant Therapy for Colon Cancer

Kyle Holen and Leonard B. Saltz

CONTENTS

1. INTRODUCTION

The risk of clinical failure following a potentially curative resection of colon cancer is not the result of an actual reoccurrence of a *de novo* colon cancer but rather of the clinical progression of previously undetected metastatic disease. At the time of resection, small, undetectable areas of disease may be present that will grow and be identifiable only at a later date. Patients who do not have residual microscopic metastases are cured by their operation alone, yet those who have untreated residual microscopic metastases would be expected to eventually be diagnosed with stage IV colon cancer. Key components of effective adjuvant therapies are the identification of those patients with residual micrometastases and the discovery of better ways to eliminate residual disease.

The most important prognostic factor in anticipating the likelihood of future gross metastatic disease is currently the stage of the tumor at the time of resection *(1)*. Stage I tumors (Dukes' A and B1) have not penetrated the full thickness of the bowel wall and have not spread to regional lymph nodes. These tumors have up to a 90% or greater cure rate with surgery alone. Higher-risk tumors that have either penetrated the full thickness of the bowel wall (stage II, Dukes' B2) or spread to regional lymph nodes (stage III, Dukes' C) have a much greater risk of recurrence after surgical resection. In these patients, the possible role of adjuvant therapy requires careful consideration. Other less validated and, at this time, less predictive prognostic indicators of the rate of recurrence include the use of carcinoembryonic antigen (CEA) levels preoperatively, the extent of vascular invasion on microscopic evaluation, thymidylate synthase levels, Ki-67, p53, expression and others *(2–4)*.

From: *Colorectal Cancer: Multimodality Management*
Edited by: L. Saltz © Humana Press Inc., Totowa, NJ

Historically, adjuvant treatments have developed from effective chemotherapy used in the metastatic setting. As a new therapy shows efficacy in the metastatic setting, it is reasonable that it might be able to clear minimal residual disease after a complete surgical resection. In the chapter that follows, we will review the evidence regarding the relative merits of the available adjuvant treatment strategies in the different stages of colon cancer. The adjuvant treatment of rectal cancer is discussed in Chapter 11 by Janjan.

2. EARLY TRIALS

Cooperative groups started forming in the late 1950s to investigate a "promising therapeutic concept"—adjuvant treatment. These early trials were published in the 1960s and 1970s and used a wide array of schedules and chemotherapies. One of the earliest trials by Holden et al. used triethylenethiophosphoramide (Thiotepa) and showed no benefit in 5-yr survival (5). Another negative trial described the use of nitrogen mustard and other alkylating agents administered either during or shortly after surgery (6). Floxuridine (FUDR) given only at the time of operation and in the immediate postoperative period produced no improvement in 5-yr survival (7). It is not surprising that these trials were negative; clinical data on the efficacy of these agents in advanced disease were often not available at that time and many of the agents investigated then are now known to have little or no antitumor activity in colorectal cancer. Also, many agents were used at suboptimal doses or for only brief periods of time. Finally, many of these early trials were insufficiently powered to detect small differences in outcome.

3. FLUOROURACIL

Fluorouracil (see Chapter 25) was first used in the adjuvant setting in a trial by the Veterans Administration Surgical Adjuvant Group (8). In this study, the fluorouracil was administered to patients for two cycles at 2 and 8 wk postoperatively. Each cycle consisted of a 12-mg/kg bolus given on 5 successive days. All stages of disease were included in this trial, including those with gross residual disease after resection. Although differences were seen between the groups that received chemotherapy and those that were observed, these did not reach statistical significance. The heterogeneous patient population and the short duration of treatment make interpretation of this trial difficult.

Soon after the completed enrollment of the above trial, another trial in a more select group of patients used a longer duration of fluorouracil. In this trial, by Higgins et al., fluorouracil was given as soon after surgical resection as possible, to those with "high-risk" tumors, defined as those with Dukes' B or C colon carcinoma (9). The dose was 12 mg/kg given daily for 5 d repeated every 6–8 wk. Similar to the prior study, a small survival benefit was shown, but it did not reach statistical significance. Given the results of these two trials, Moertel suggested in 1975 that there was little reason to continue adjuvant studies using fluorouracil as a single agent (10).

Two large trials were later published by the Gastrointestinal Tumor Study Group (GTSG) and the National Surgical Adjuvant Breast and Bowel Project (NSABP) using combinations of agents with fluorouracil (11,12). These combinations included fluorouracil, semustine, and bacillus Calmette-Guerin (BCG) in the former trial and fluorouracil, semustine, and vincristine (MOF) in the latter trial. The GTSG trial treated all Dukes' B2 and C colon cancers under four different arms: close observation, BCG alone, chemotherapy with fluorouracil and semustine, or chemotherapy and BCG. After over 5 yr of follow-up, no differences were seen in any of the treatment arms. In the NSABP trial, protocol C-01,

Dukes' B and C colon cancers were included and randomization occurred to one of the following three arms: close observation alone, chemotherapy with MOF, or BCG. In this trial, those who received postoperative BCG did no better than those in the observation alone arm. Those in the chemotherapy arm, however, had a better survival than those in the observation arm. The 5-yr survival for chemotherapy was 67%, and for observation, it was 59% ($p = 0.05$). The toxicities of chemotherapy were not trivial, as could be expected with vincristine, semustine and fluorouracil. Forty-four percent of those in the chemotherapy arm had a white blood count (WBC) less than 2500 cells/mm^3, 54% had platelet counts less than 100,000, 65% had controllable nausea and vomiting, 6% had intractable nausea and vomiting, three patients died of leukemia, and three others were diagnosed with myelo dyplastic syndrome (MDS). Yet, this trial was significant because it was the first trial to show a modest benefit in support of adjuvant chemotherapy.

A major problem with many of these trials is that they often did not have adequate power to detect small differences in survival. Hence, a large meta-analysis was performed to try to detect such a difference *(13)*. This meta-analysis was done in 1988 and included all randomized trials of adjuvant therapy in colorectal cancer. Seventeen trials with treatments encompassing a wide array of therapies, doses, and schedules were included, many of these would be considered less than ideal treatments compared to today's 5-fluorouracil (5-FU) schedules. Analysis showed a small, nonsignificant benefit of therapy in terms of overall survival, with a mortality odds ratio of 0.83 in favor of therapy (95% confidence interval [CI] = 0.70–0.98). This meta-analysis suggested that adjuvant chemotherapy may play an important role in improving survival in the adjuvant setting, but much larger trials would be needed to prove such benefit.

4. FLUOROURACIL BIOMODULATION

4.1. Fluorouracil with Levamisole

Levamisole is an anthelmintic that is used in both animals and humans. It attracted the interest of investigators because of its putative immunomodulatory effects *(14)*. Preliminary studies showed some promising results using combination levamisole and fluorouracil in the adjuvant setting *(15)*. Therefore a large, multicenter, confirmatory trial was initiated. This trial, known as intergroup 0035, randomized patients to fluorouracil plus levamisole or to no additional therapy after resection of Dukes' B2 or C colon cancer *(16)*. Those with Dukes' C colon cancer could also be randomized to levamisole as a single agent; 1296 patients were randomized, 325 with B2 disease and 971 with C disease. The treatment consisted of observation alone, 50 mg levamisole every 8 hr for 3 d repeated every 2 wk for the levamisole-alone arm, or levamisole on the same schedule combined with 5-FU given 450 mg/m^2 daily for 5 d followed 28 d later by 48-weekly 5-FU injections at 450 mg/m^2 in the 5-FU and levamisole arm. Early results published in 1990 showed no statistically significant difference between the groups with B2 disease, but those with Dukes' C disease treated with levamisole and fluorouracil had a 41% reduction in disease recurrence over observation, which was highly statistically significant ($p = 0.0001$). Furthermore, there was a 33% reduction in mortality ($p = 0.0064$). These striking results lead the NIH to release a consensus statement declaring adjuvant therapy as standard of care for all patients with node-positive colon cancer in the absence of medical or psychiatric contraindications to such treatment *(17)*. Follow-up analysis published in 1995 confirmed the early results with similar figures after 7 yr of follow-up: a 40% reduction in disease recurrence rate ($p = 0.0001$) and a 33% reduction in mortality for stage III patients ($p = 0.0007$) *(18)*.

4.2. Fluorouracil with Leucovorin

Several clinical trials performed between 1987 and 1991 showed a response advantage when fluorouracil was used in combination with leucovorin in the treatment of patients with advanced colorectal cancer *(19–22)*. On the basis of these results, this combination was chosen as an experimental treatment in adjuvant trials. The National Surgical Adjuvant Breast and Bowel Project (NSABP) initiated a randomized clinical trial (protocol C-03) to evaluate the efficacy of 1 yr of fluorouracil and leucovorin as compared to MeCCNU, vincristine, and fluorouracil (MOF) as adjuvant therapy for patients with Dukes' B and C carcinoma of the colon *(23)*. The results of this trial, published in 1993, demonstrated a clear advantage in the fluorouracil and leucovorin arm, with an 84% 3-yr survival in the fluorouracil and leucovorin arm and a 77% survival in the MOF arm ($p = 0.003$). The North Central Cancer Treatment Group (NCCTG) published a randomized trial comparing fluorouracil with low-dose leucovorin to observation in 1997 *(24)*. There was a clear benefit in favor of adjuvant fluorouracil and leucovorin in time to relapse ($p = 0.01$) and survival ($p = 0.02$) with no treatment-related deaths.

Further demonstrating the benefit of adjuvant fluorouracil and leucovorin was a publication by the International Multicentre Pooled Analysis of Colon Cancer Trials (IMPACT) investigators *(25)*. This publication combined the data from three independently randomized trials by the Gruppo Interdisciplinare Valutazione Interventi Oncologia (GIVIO), the National Cancer Institute Canada Clinical Trials Group (NCIC-CTG), and the Fondation Francaise de Cancerologie Digestive (FFCD). Dukes' B and C patients were randomized to Mayo Clinic regimen fluorouracil and leucovorin or observation. There were significant advantages favoring the group who received chemotherapy over observation in both disease-free survival and overall survival, with a mortality reduction for the entire study population (both Dukes' B and C patients) of 22% (95% CI-3–38%; $p = 0.029$). As expected, most of the benefit was seen in Dukes' C patients, with a mortality reduction of 29% (95% CI = 6–46%).

Further studies carried out through the NSABP attempted to illicit the difference, if any, between the fluorouracil with levamisole regimen and the fluorouracil with leucovorin schedule. NSABP trial C-04 was a direct comparison between the two schedules and also included a third arm with the three drugs fluorouracil, levamisole, and leucovorin *(26)*. This trial, published in 1999, disclosed only a slight difference in disease-free survival favoring fluorouracil and leucovorin over fluorouracil and levamisole with no significant difference in overall survival. The three-drug regimen did not provide any additional benefit over fluorouracil and leucovorin.

Another trial that compared the three-drug regimen fluorouracil, leucovorin, and levamisole to fluorouracil and levamisole was conducted by the NCCTG *(27)*. This trial randomized patients with stage II and stage III colon cancer to either the three- or two-drug schedule and to either 6 or 12 mo of therapy in a 2×2 design. There were no differences overall between those treated for 6 mo vs 12 mo.

Arguably, the trial with the most significant impact in setting the current standard of care is the intergroup INT-0089 study, which evaluated four different treatment arms and has thus far been published in abstract form only *(28)*. This trial randomized high-risk stage II and stage III colon cancer patients to receive one of the following schedules: fluorouracil plus levamisole for 52 wk, weekly fluorouracil plus high-dose leucovorin for 32 wk (500 mg/m^2 fluorouracil and 500 mg/m^2 leucovorin weekly for 6 wk, repeated every 8 wk for four cycles), daily $\times$ 5 fluorouracil plus low-dose leucovorin for 24 wk (425 mg/m^2 fluorouracil and 20 mg/m^2 leucovorin for 5 consecutive days (Mayo Clinic Schedule), repeated every 28 d for six cycles), and a daily × 5 schedule of fluorouracil plus low-dose leucovorin as above but with the addition of levamisole. The only significant difference among the four arms was the 5-yr overall survival comparison of fluorouracil/leucovorin/levamisole and fluorouracil/levamisole, favoring the three-drug regimen (65% vs 60%; $p = 0.0054$). The results highlight that the 52 wk fluorouracil plus levamisole regimen is not superior to the shorter fluorouracil and leucovorin regimens and that the addition of levamisole to fluorouracil plus leucovorin does not provide a benefit over fluorouracil plus leucovorin alone.

Given the scores of trials evaluating chemotherapy in the adjuvant setting, which schedule is most effective? Both levamisole and leucovorin used in conjunction with fluorouracil have proven efficacy in multiple randomized intergroup studies. At the present time, leucovorin-biomodulated fluorouracil is generally accepted as the current standard of care for adjuvant stage III colon cancer, given as six cycles of fluorouracil and leucovorin daily for 5 d every 28 wk or four cycles of fluorouracil and leucovorin weekly for 6 wk every 8 wk.

5. STAGE II PATIENTS

The controversy surrounding the treatment of those with stage II colon cancer continues to inspire heated debate. The reason for this controversy is many-fold. First, the benefit, if any, is small. Most patients with stage II colon cancer are cured with surgery alone. Second, there are relatively large numbers of noncancer deaths in this population. Finally, the two pivotal reviews large enough to show such a small difference in survival published differing conclusions.

The first, a pooled analysis of four different trials initiated by the National Surgical Adjuvant Breast and Bowel Project (NSABP), analyzed 1565 Dukes' B patients from four widely different treatment groups. As discussed in an editorial that accompanied the article, the authors used highly unorthodox statistical methods, methods which "might set to red all the statistical stop lights in sight" *(29)*. The Dukes' B patients were divided into two groups: the *superior* group, those in the superior arms of each trial, and the *inferior* group, those in the inferior arms of each trial. The cumulative odds of death in the Dukes' B patients was 0.70, favoring the *superior* treatment group, with a 95% confidence interval that did not cross 1. Despite this finding, it is difficult to say with certainty that treatment in this cumulative analysis provided a real benefit over observation. The trials were not designed to evaluate treatment effect in the B2 subset prospectively. As well, the treatments administered were very different and more than half of the patients were not randomized to an observation arm. It may be possible that the Dukes' B patients treated in the *inferior* group had a higher mortality from the inferior chemotherapy than they would have if they were in an observation arm. For these reasons, it is difficult to draw any definitive conclusions from this analysis.

The second article, by the IMPACT B2 investigators *(30)*, was an analysis of the stage B2 patients from the initial three pooled trials published in the IMPACT study *(25)*, as well as the B2 patients from two additional studies—the NCCTG *(24)* study outlined earlier and a trial published from the University of Sienna *(31)*. One thousand sixteen patients with B2 colon cancer were randomized to either fluorouracil and leucovorin or observation. The treatment arms were all similar, ranging from 370 to 425 mg/m^2 of fluorouracil plus 20–200 mg/m^2 leucovorin daily for 5 d every 28–35 d. Chemotherapy was given for 6 cycles, except in the Sienna trial, in which 12 cycles were given. The results show a 3%

improvement in 5-yr event-free survival (EFS) and a 2% improvement in overall survival (OS) for the treated group; however, these differences did not reach statistical significance. The conclusion, therefore, was that further studies evaluating the efficacy of adjuvant therapy in B2 patients should appropriately contain a no-treatment control arm.

It is possible that the IMPACT study did not reach significance because it was underpowered to show such a small difference between the two arms. The clinical relevance of such a small difference, even if statistically significant, is debatable. Thousands more patients would be necessary to show a 2% survival difference, and prospective, randomized studies with such large numbers of patients are cumbersome and costly. Retrospective analyses, although potentially limited, can nonetheless provide useful information about a large number of patients when randomized data are not feasible. A recent report using a SEER–Medicare cohort analyzed 3725 resected stage II colon cancer patients *(32)*. Similar to the results noted by the IMPACT B2 investigators, the 5-yr overall survival difference was 2% but did not reach statistical significance with a hazard ratio of 0.93 (95% CI = 0.81–1.07). These results, taken together with the IMPACT B2 study, demonstrate a continued need for observation as a control arm in stage II patients.

At present, we lack the necessary information to make a definitive statement regarding adjuvant treatment of stage II patients. Certain prognostic factors, however, have been correlated with higher risk for recurrence in patients with stage II tumors. These factors have included bowel perforation or obstruction by the tumor at presentation *(33)*, vascular invasion noted on histology *(34)*, an elevated CEA preoperatively, poorly differentiated histology *(30)*, a high S-phase fraction, the presence of an 18q deletion *(35)*, thymidylate synthase levels, Ki-67, p53 expression, and others *(36)*. The presence of one or more of these risk factors is likely to correlate with a higher risk of recurrence. It is not clear, however, that adjuvant therapy in these higher-risk Dukes' B2 patients can reduce that risk. In the absence of definitive data, clinical judgment and thorough patient education regarding the risks and benefits of such treatment must be employed. In appropriately informed and selected patients, it may be reasonable to offer adjuvant chemotherapy to Dukes' B2 patients with established high-risk prognostic factors, recognizing that this would necessarily be happening in the absence of definitive supportive data.

6. INVESTIGATIONAL AGENTS

6.1. Portal Vein Infusion

Cancer cells originating in the colon are able to access the liver via the portal venous system, along the same channels used by nutrients traveling from the bowel to the liver. Up to half of all relapsing patients present with hepatic metastases as the first site of failure. Because tumors less than 5 mm obtain their blood supply from both the hepatic artery and portal vein *(37,38)*, the delivery of chemotherapy directly into the portal vein would, therefore, be a reasonable approach to explore for the administration of adjuvant treatment.

Phase I trials proved that fluorouracil can be given safely to patients via the portal circulation and follow-up studies not only confirmed this fact but also showed that a substantially larger amounts of fluorouracil can be administered this way than can be given intravenously because of "first pass clearance" by the liver *(39)*. Initial small trials were promising, but they did not convincingly prove survival advantages for Dukes' C patients *(40,41)*.

A larger trial, designed and run by the NSABP *(42)*, enrolled 1158 Dukes' A, B, and C patients and randomized them to receive either a 7-d portal infusion of fluorouracil

(600 mg/m^2/d) or to surgery alone. A small but statistically significant survival advantage in the group receiving intraportal chemotherapy was noted; yet, interestingly, the incidence of hepatic metastases was not different between the two groups.

In another trial by the Swiss Group for Clinical Cancer Research (SAKK), similar results were demonstrated *(43)*. Five hundred thirty-three patients were assigned to receive intraportal mitomycin and fluorouracil or surgery alone. No difference in the incidence of hepatic metastases was found, and there was a modest improvement in overall survival (66% vs 55%; $p = 0.026$). The conclusion drawn from these studies was that part of the benefit obtained with a single course of adjuvant chemotherapy via the portal vein for patients with operable colorectal carcinoma was most likely the result of the systemic effects of the portal chemotherapy.

To better elucidate small advantages, if any, from intraportal chemotherapy, a meta-analysis was done combining 10 studies and including over 4000 patients. There was only a modest (4%) improvement in 5-yr overall survival for the patients receiving portal infusion and, again, this was attributed to the decreased rate of all recurrences (local relapses, liver metastases, and other distant metastases), suggesting that the benefit seen is the result of the systemic effects of portal chemotherapy. At present, the use of intraportal adjuvant chemotherapy should be regarded as of unproven benefit and its use should be limited to investigational settings.

6.2. Intraperitoneal Treatment

The rationale behind using adjuvant intraperitoneal chemotherapy for colon cancer is two fold. First, those with tumor involving the peritoneal surfaces are at high risk for recurrence *(44)* and this approach delivers higher concentrations to these tumors. Second, the peritoneal cavity is drained by portal lymphatics into the portal vein, thereby administering higher concentrations directly into the liver. Because floxuridine (FUDR) and, to a lesser extent, fluorouracil have a high first-pass metabolism, these drugs are good potential candidates for intraperitoneal therapy. Because of hepatic clearance, pharmacologic investigations have shown concentrations in the peritoneal cavity 200- to 400-fold greater than those found systemically.

One of the first trials evaluating intraperitoneal therapy by Sugarbaker et al. showed a decreased incidence of peritoneal metastases following peritoneal therapy; however, this did not result in a survival advantage *(45)*. This study was limited by its small size and because initiation of chemotherapy up to 2 full months following surgery was permitted. Such delays in treatment could increase the chance of spread of tumor outside the peritoneal cavity and permit the establishment of hepatic micrometastases with a hepatic arterial blood supply.

To circumvent such delays, a pilot study was initiated using a combination of immediate postoperative intraperitoneal floxuridine and leucovorin plus systemic fluorouracil and levamisole *(46)*. The treatment given included intraperitoneal floxuridine and leucovorin therapy twice daily for 3 consecutive days repeated every other week for three cycles. The levamisole was given orally and initiated with the second intraperitoneal cycle and fluorouracil was given as a bolus injection daily for 5 consecutive days beginning with the third ip cycle. The doses of systemic fluorouracil were escalated in a stepwise fashion, and after d 29 from the start of fluorouracil, weekly fluorouracil and every-other-week levamisole were started and continued to complete 1 yr of therapy.

The treatment was well tolerated, with no apparent increase in perioperative morbidity. At a median follow-up of 24 mo, 24 of 28 patients were alive and free of disease.

A somewhat larger randomized trial similar to the trial by Sugarbaker et al. has been published *(47)*. This trial enrolled 241 patients with resected stage III or high-risk stage II colon cancer. The two treatment arms were a standard arm of fluorouracil and levamisole given for 6 mo and an investigational arm of intravenous bolus fluorouracil and leucovorin given on d 1–4 and intraperitoneal fluorouracil and leucovorin on d 1 and 3, all repeated every 4 wk. No significant difference was noted in the 45 stage II patients. The 196 stage III patients, however, had a significant improvement in both disease-free survival ($p = 0.0014$) and overall survival ($p = 0.0005$) in favor of the investigational arm. The results of this small trial suggest that ip strategies may be useful in the adjuvant therapy of colon cancer. Further investigations are needed to better evaluate its utility and safety.

6.3. Edrecolomab

Current theory holds that immune therapy is more effective on small-volume disease and, therefore, should be perfectly suited for adjuvant treatment. The reduction in colon cancer recurrence with vaccines and antibodies has remained elusive *(48)*.

Edrecolomab is a murine IgG2a monoclonal antibody directed against the 17-1A antigen. Studies have shown it to be well tolerated in patients with terminal malignancies and have shown that it induces antibody-dependent cellular cytotoxicity with human effector cells and prevents outgrowth of human tumor xenografts in mice. In *Lancet* in 1994, Riethmüller et al. reported a randomized trial of edrecolomab versus no treatment in Dukes' C colon cancer patients. After 5 yr, the recurrence rate in the observation arm was 66.5% and 48.7% in the edrecolomab group, a statistically significant difference ($p = .03$). It also had a significant effect on survival, with 64% alive in the edrecolomab group at 5 yr and 49% alive in the observation arm. The treatment was very well tolerated, with infrequent toxicities. The question, however, was whether this effect seen with edrecolomab was equivalent to what had been previously shown with fluorouracil and leucovorin.

Therefore, a randomized phase III trial with three arms was developed to compare the following adjuvant therapies: the combination of the two regimens (fluorouracil, leucovorin, and edrecolomab) vs the single agents (fluorouracil and leucovorin or edrecolomab). The results after 3 yr of follow-up were reported at the 2001 annual meeting of the American Society of Clinical Oncology *(49)*. The combination treatment had a slightly less, but nonsignificant overall and disease-free survival (DFS) compared to fluorouracil and leucovorin alone (OS 74.7% vs 76.1%, $p = 0.528$; DFS 63.8% vs 65.5%, $p = 0.220$) and that edrecolomab as a single agent was inferior to fluorouracil and leucovorin (OS 70.1% vs 76.1%, $p = 0.05$, DFS 53.0% vs 65.5% $p < 0.001$).

Vaccine treatments also have a theoretical advantage in the role of adjuvant treatments, working best on small-volume disease. However, there currently are no large randomized trials underway to assess efficacy in the adjuvant setting. For a complete discussion on vaccine and other immune therapies in colon cancer, *see* Chapter 41.

6.4. Newer Chemotherapies

Both oxaliplatin and irinotecan in combination with fluorouracil and leucovorin have improved the response rates in metastatic colon cancer. The irinotecan combination has also afforded stage IV patients a survival benefit when compared to fluorouracil and leucovorin in two randomized trials *(50,51)*. Both drugs, therefore, have excellent potential as treatments in the adjuvant setting. Trials are currently underway to test these hypotheses. A multicenter, intergroup, phase III trial randomizes patients to receive either standard fluorouracil and leucovorin as 6-weekly bolus injections every 8 wk for four cycles versus the combination of irinotecan, fluorouracil and leucovorin as 4-weekly injections every 6 wk for five cycles (CALGB 89803). This trial has completed accrual and final results are awaiting maturation of the data. Early-warning systems built into the trial detected higher than expected early-death rates in the irinotecan-containing arm, at 2.2% *(52)*. The combination of irinotecan and fluorouracil/leucovorin remains investigational for adjuvant treatment and, at this time, is not recommended for adjuvant treatment outside of a clinical trial.

Capecitabine, an oral fluoropyrimidine, has recently been shown to be equivalent to fluorouracil and leucovorin in the metastatic setting with a considerable benefit in toxicity and is currently being evaluated in the adjuvant setting *(53)*.

7. DIRECTED THERAPIES

Exciting developments in the metastatic setting are therapies that are tailored to specific characteristics of an individual tumor. Directed therapies have the potential to substantially reduce the toxicities of treatment and at the same time not compromise, or even improve upon, efficacy. As an example, those colon cancers that have a high thymidine synthase gene expression more rapidly clear fluorouracil and are less likely to respond to fluorouracil treatment *(54)*. Irinotecan or oxaliplatin may be a preferred therapy in this setting. Furthermore, more than 70% of colon cancers overexpress the endothelial growth factor receptor (EGFR). For those tumors with EGFR overexpression, targeted therapy with an agent such as cetuximab, a monoclonal antibody that binds to the EGFR, may be able to clear any residual disease after a surgical resection. ZD1839 (Iressa) also works on the EGF pathway. It is a small molecule with excellent oral bioavailability and acts as an EGFR-selective tyrosine kinase inhibitor. As a tyrosine kinase inhibitor, it is a potent and selective inhibitor of tumor cell growth in culture. In preclinical in vivo studies, ZD1839 has remarkable antitumor activity in human tumor xenografts. These targeted therapies are currently being evaluated in the metastatic setting and may eventually be tried postsurgically.

8. CONCLUSION

It is clear that therapy with fluorouracil-based regimens provides the best chance at cure for those diagnosed with colon cancer that has spread to regional lymph nodes. The standard of care remains fluorouracil and leucovorin, given either daily for 5 d every 4 wk or weekly for 6 wk every 8 wk. Patients with stage II disease have a better prognosis overall than those with stage III; yet, adjuvant therapy cannot be universally recommended. Investigational therapies, including portal vein infusion, intraperitoneal treatment, and novel agents such as irinotecan, oxaliplatin, capecitabine, edrecolomab, and others, remain unproven at this time in terms of safety and efficacy as adjuvant treatment.

Despite our progress, the data remain sobering. Greater than a third of patients with resected stage III colon cancer will die from their disease despite adequate chemotherapy. Thus, further advances in the field are imperative. With more active anticolorectal cancer agents appearing ever increasingly, we can expect developments at a more rapid pace. Once these therapies are deemed effective in the metastatic setting, we will need to carefully evaluate them in the adjuvant setting, to see if they will provide improved efficacy with adequate safety.

REFERENCES

1. Willet CG, Tepper JE, and Cohen AM. Failure pattern following curative resection of colonic carcinoma. *Ann. Surg.*, **200** (1984) 685–690.
2. Minsky B, Mies C, Rich T, et al. Potentially curative surgery of colon cancer: the influence of blood vessel invasion. *J. Clin. Oncol.*, **6(1)** (1988) 119–127.
3. Allegra CJ, Paik S, Parr A, et al. Prognostic value of thymidylate synthase (TS), Ki-67, and p53 in patients with Dukes B & C colon cancer. *Proc. Amer. Soc. Clin. Oncol.*, **491** (2001) (abstract).
4. Allegra CA, Paik S, and Parr A. Prognostic value of thymidylate synthase (TS), Ki-67, and p53 in patients (Pts) with Dukes' B & C colon cancer. American Society of Clinical Oncology Annual Meeting, 2001, abstract 491.
5. Holden WD, Dixon WJ, and Kuzma JW. The use of triethylenethiophosphoramide as an adjuvant to the surgical treatment of colorectal carcinoma. *Ann. Surg.*, **165** (1967) 481–503.
6. Mrazek R, Economou S, McDonald GO, Slaughter DP, and Cole WH. Prophylactic and adjuvant use of nitrogen mustard in the surgical treatment of cancer. *Ann. Surg.*, **150** (1959) 745–755.
7. Dwight R, Humphrey E, Higgins G, et al. FUDR as an adjuvant to surgery in cancer of the large bowel. *J. Surg. Oncol.*, **5** (1973) 243–249.
8. Higgins GA, Dwight RW, Smith JV, et al. Fluorouracil as an adjuvant to surgery in carcinoma of the colon. *Arch. Surg.*, **102** (1971) 339–343.
9. Higgins G, Humphrey E, Juler G, et al. Adjuvant chemotherapy in the surgical treatment of large bowel cancer. *Cancer*, (1976) 1461–1476.
10. Moertel C, Schutt A, Hahn R, et al. Brief communication—therapy of advanced colorectal cancer with a combination of 5-fluorouracil, methyl-1,3-cis(2-chlorethyl)-1-nitrosurea, and vincristine. *J. Natl. Cancer Inst.*, **54** (1975) 69–71.
11. Gastrointestinal Tumor Study Group. Adjuvant therapy of colon cancer—results of a prospecdtively randomized trial. *N. Engl. J. Med.*, **310** (1984) 737–743.
12. Wolmark N, Fisher B, Rockette H, et al. Postoperative adjuvant chemotherapy or BCG for colon cancer: Results from NSABP protocol C-01. *J. Natl. Cancer Inst.*, **80** (1988) 30–36.
13. Buyse M, Zeleniuch-Jacquotte A, and Chalmers TC. Adjuvant therapy of colorectal cancer. Why we still don't know. *JAMA*, **259** (1988) 3571–3578.
14. Renoux G. The general immunopharmacology of levamisole. *Drugs*, **19** (1980) 89–99.
15. Laurie JA, Moertel CG, Fleming TR, et al. Surgical adjuvant therapy of large-bowel carcinoma: an evaluation of levamisole and the combination of levamisole and fluorouracil: the North Central Cancer Treatment Group and the Mayo Clinic. *J. Clin. Oncol.*, **7** (1989) 1447–1456.
16. Moertel CG, Fleming TR, Macdonald JS, et al. Levamisole and fluorouracil for adjuvant therapy of resected colon carcinoma. *N. Engl. J. Med.*, **322** (1990) 352–358.
17. NIH Consensus Conference. Adjuvant therapy for patients with colon and rectal cancer. *JAMA*, **264** (1990) 1444–1450.
18. Moertel CG, Fleming TR, Macdonald JS, et al. Fluorouracil plus levamisole as effective adjuvant therapy after resection of stage III colon carcinoma: a final report. *Ann. Intern. Med.*, **122** (1995) 321–326.
19. Petrelli N, Herrera L, Rustum Y, et al. Prospective randomized trial of 5-fluorouracil vversus 5-fluorouracil and high-dose leucovorin versus 5-fluorouracil and methotrexate in previously untreated patients with advanced colorectal carcinoma. *J. Clin. Oncol.*, **5** (1987) 1559–1656.
20. Erlichman C, Fine S, Wong A, et al. A randomized trial of flourouracil and folinic acid in patients with metastatic colorectal carcinoma. *J. Clin. Oncol.*, **6** (1988) 469–475.
21. Poon MA, O'Connell MJ, Moertel CG, et al. Biochemical modulation of fluorouracil: evidence of significant improvement of survival and quality of life in patients with advanced colorectal carcinoma. *J. Clin. Oncol.*, **7** (1989) 1407–1418.
22. Doroshow JF, Molthauf P, Leong L, et al. Prospective randomized comparison of fluorouracil versus fluorouracil and high-dose continuous infusion leucovorin calcium for the treatment of advanced measurable colorectal cancer in patients previously unexposed to chemotherapy. *J. Clin. Oncol.*, **8** (1990) 491–501.
23. Wolmark N, Rockette H, Fisher B, et al. The benefit of leucovorin-modulated fluorouracil as postoperative adjuvant therapy for primary colon cancer: results from National Surgical Adjuvant Breast and Bowel Project Protocol C-03. *J. Clin. Oncol.*, **11(10)** (1993) 1879–1887.
24. O'Connell MJ, Mailliard JA, Kahn MJ, et al. Controlled trial of fluorouracil and low-dose leucovorin given for 6 months as postoperative adjuvant therapy for colon cancer. *J. Clin. Oncol.*, **15** (1997) 246–250.
25. International Multicentre Pooled Analysis of Colon Cancer (IMPACT) investigators. Efficacy of adjuvant fluorouracil and folinic acid in colon cancer. *Lancet*, **345** (1995) 939–944.

26. Wolmark N, Rockette H, Mamounas E, et al. Clinical trial to assess the relative efficacy of fluorouracil and leucovorin, fluorouracil and levamisole, and fluorouracil, leucovorin, and levamisole in patients with Dukes' B and C carcinoma of the colon: results from National Surgical Adjuvant Breast and Bowel Project C-04. *J. Clin. Oncol.*, **17(11)** (1999) 3553–3559.

27. O'Connell M, Laurie J, Kahn M, et al. Prospectively randomized trial of postoperative adjuvant chemotherapy in patients with high-risk colon cancer. *J. Clin. Oncol.*, **16(1)** (1998) 295–300.

28. Haller DG, Catalano PJ, MacDonald JS, et al. Fluorouracil (FU), leucovorin (LV), and levamisole (LEV) adjuvant therapy for colon cancer: five-year final repost of INT-0089. *Proc. Am. Soc. Clin. Oncol.*, **17** (1998) 256a.

29. Harrington DP. The tea leaves of small trials. *J. Clin. Oncol.*, **17** (1999) 1336–1338.

30. International Multicentre Pooled Analysis of B2 Colon Cancer Trials (IMPACT B2) Investigators. Efficacy of adjuvant fluorouracil and folinic acid in B2 colon cancer. *J. Clin. Oncol.*, **17** (1999) 1356–1363.

31. Francini G, Petrioli R, Lorenzini L, et al. Folinic acid and 5-fluorouracil as adjuvant therapy in colon cancer. *Gastroenterology*, **106** (1994) 899–906.

32. Schrag D, Gelfand S, Bach P, et al. Adjuvant chemotherapy for stage II colon cancer: insight from a SEER-Medicare cohort. *Proc. Am. Soc. Clin. Oncol.*, **20** (2001) 488.

33. Willet CG, Tepper JE, and Cohen AM. Obstructive and perforative colonic carcinoma: patterns of failure. *J. Clin. Oncol.*, **3** (1985) 379–384.

34. Minsky B, Mies C, Rich T, et al. Potentially curative surgery of colon cancer: the influence of blood vessel invasion. *J. Clin. Oncol.*, **6** (1988) 119–127.

35. Jen J, Kim H, Piantadosi S, et al. Allelic loss of chromosome 18q and prognosis in colorectal cancer. *N. Engl. J. Med.*, **331** (1994) 213–221.

36. Allegra CJ, Paik S, Parr A, et al. Prognostic value of thymidylate synthase (TS), Ki-67, and p53 in patients with Dukes B & C Colon Cancer. *Proc Amer. Soc. Clin. Oncol.*, (2001) (abstract).

37. Ackerman NB. The blood supply of experimental liver metastases. Changes in vascularity with increasing tumor growth. *Surgery*, **75** (1974) 589–597.

38. Basserman R. Changes of vascular pattern of tumors and surrounding tissue during different phases of metastatic growth. *Cancer Res.*, **100** (1986) 256–264.

39. Almersjo O, Brandberg A, and Gustavsson B. Concentration of biologically active 5-fluorouracil in the general circulation during continuous portal infusion in man. *Cancer Lett.* **1** (1975) 113.

40. Taylor I, Rowling JT, and West C. Adjuvant cytotoxic liver perfusion for colorectal cancer. *Br. J. Surg.*, **66** (1979) 833–837.

41. Taylor I, Machin D, Mullee M, Trotter G, Cooke T, and West C. A randomized controlled trial of adjuvant portal vein cytotoxic perfusion in colorectal cancer. *Br. J. Surg.*, **72** (1985) 359–363.

42. Wolmark N, Rockette H, Wickerman DL, et al. Adjuvant therapy of Dukes' A, B, and C adenocarcinoma of the colon with portal vein fluorouracil hepatic infusion: preliminary results of the National Surgical Adjuvant Breast and Bowel Project Protocol C-02. *J. Clin. Oncol.*, **8** (1990) 1466–1475.

43. Swiss Group for Clinical Cancer Research. Long term results of a single course of adjuvant intraportal chemotherapy for colorectal cancer. *Lancet*, **345** (1995) 349–352.

44. Tong D, Russel AH, Dawson LE, et al. Second laparatomy for proximal colon cancer: sites of recurrence and implications for adjuvant therapy. *Am. J. Surg.*, **145** (1983) 382–386.

45. Sugarbaker P, Gianola F, Speyer J, et al. Prospective randomized trial of intravenous versus intraperitoneal fluorouracil in patients with advanced primary colon or rectal cancer. *Surgery*, **98** (1985) 414–421.

46. Kelsen D, Saltz L, Cohen A, et al. A phase I trial of immediate postoperative intraperitoneal floxuridine and leucovorin plus systemic 5-fluorouracil and levamisole after resection of high risk colon cancer. *Cancer*, **74** (1994) 2224–2233.

47. Scheithauer W, Kornek G, Marczell A, et al. Combined intravenous and intraperitoneal chemotherapy with fluorouracil + leucovorin vs. fluorouracil + levamisole for adjuvant therapy of resected colon carcinoma.

48. Moertel, CG. Vaccine adjuvant therapy for colorectal cancer: "very dramatic" or ho-hum. *J. Clin. Oncol.*, **11(3)** (1993) 385–386.

49. Punt, CJA, Nagy A, Douillard JY, et al. Edrecolomab (17-1A Antibody) alone or in combination with 5-fluorouracil base chemotherapy in the adjuvant treatment of stage III colon cancer: results of a phase III study. *Proc. Am. Soc. Clin. Oncol.*, **20** (2001) 487.

50. Saltz L, Cox J, Blanke C, et al. Irinotecan plus fluorouracil and leucovorin for metastatic colorectal cancer. *N. Engl. J. Med.*, **343** (2000) 905–914.

51. Doulliard J, Cunningham D, Roth A, et al. Irinotecan combined with fluorouracil compared with fluorouracil alone as first-line treatment for metastatic colorectal cancer: a multicentre randomised trial. *Lancet*, **355** (2000) 1041–1047.

52. Sargent D, Niedzwiecki D, O'Connell M, and Schilsky RL. Recommendation for caution with irinotecan, fluorouracil, and leucovorin for colorectal cancer. *N. Engl. J. Med.*, **345** (2001) 144–145.
53. Hoff PM, Ansari R, Batist G, Cox J, et al. Comparison of oral capecitabine versus intravenous fluorouracil plus leucovorin as first-line treatment in 605 patients with metastatic colorectal cancer: results of a randomized phase III study. *J. Clin. Oncol.*, **19(8)** (2001) 2282–2292.
54. Leichman L, Lenz H-J, Leichman CG, Groshen S, Danenberg KD, Baranda J, et al. Quantitation of intratumoral thymidylate synthase expression predicts for resistance to protracted infusion of 5-fluorouracil and weekly leucovorin in disseminated colorectal cancers. *Eur. J. Cancer*, **31** (1995) 1306–1310.

32 Hepatic Artery Infusion

M. Margaret Kemeny and Nancy E. Kemeny

CONTENTS

INTRODUCTION
IMPLANTABLE HEPATIC ARTERY INFUSION PUMP
HAI FOR UNRESECTABLE METASTASES
HEPATIC RESECTION AND HEPATIC ARTERY INFUSION
REFERENCES

1. INTRODUCTION

It is known that when patients die of metastatic colorectal cancer, most patients have liver metastases. In general, the treatment of liver metastases with systemic chemotherapy is identical to the treatment of disseminated colorectal cancer. However, there exists a group of patients who have liver-only metastases, and for those patients, regional approaches of treatment have been successfully pursued in many cases.

At least 20% of patients with colorectal cancer will develop liver metastases only (1). This means that each year in the United States, over 20,000 patients will have colorectal cancer with metastases only to the liver. To put this number in perspective, this represents more patients than all of the patients with esophageal cancer each year in the United States. It is almost the same number as all patients who get stomach cancer each year in the United States. Thus, liver metastases from colorectal cancer can be looked at as a disease entity by itself.

Treatment of metastatic disease, especially to the liver, has interested scientists for many years, because it does seem that even though the liver is the site of blood-borne metastases, it still can be the only site of metastatic disease. Therefore, treatment of the regional disease that eradicates the tumor can result in a cure. This is a very important concept because radical local therapies generally are reserved for primary tumor situations in which they can result in a cure, and metastases are usually considered proof of tumor dissemination that are not amenable to local therapies.

Historically, the first surgical attempts at regional therapy were resection of solitary liver metastases. This became more common in the 1960s because of advances in surgical and anesthetic techniques. The results from early studies indicated that at least 25% of patients would remain disease-free after hepatic resection (2,3). With new surgical tools to facilitate hepatic resection, the guidelines for resection became broadened and surgeons began to look at removing more than a solitary metastasis. Several large studies were completed in

From: *Colorectal Cancer: Multimodality Management*
Edited by: L. Saltz © Humana Press Inc., Totowa, NJ

the 1990s that showed that certainly patients with two to three lesions could do as well as patients with solitary lesions and that a 30% 5-yr survival could be expected for those patients *(4–6)*. More recent work has included patients with even more than four lesions *(4,5)*. Surgical techniques are not just limited to resection, but are beginning to include various ablative measures to destroy the tumors, including cryosurgery and, more recently, radio-frequency ablation *(7,8)*.

While the work was proceeding with hepatic resection, other groups of oncologists were beginning to look carefully at regional infusion of chemotherapy for liver metastases. The development in 1969 of the non-battery-powered mechanism for a totally implantable hepatic artery infusion pump spurred the possibilities of easily using hepatic artery infusion as a long-term therapy. After this pump went into production in the 1970s, hepatic artery infusion began to be much more common. Thousands of patients have been treated with hepatic artery infusion using various chemotherapy agents and several studies have looked at its place in the treatment of colon cancer.

2. IMPLANTABLE HEPATIC ARTERY INFUSION PUMP

2.1. Pump Characteristics

The basic design of the original pump was a two-chambered unit made out of titanium. One chamber was the drug fluid chamber, which could be accessed from the outside of the pump. The other chamber was the charging fluid chamber, which was filled with Freon and totally sealed off. The mechanism driving the pump was one of mechanical energy that was supplied on each refill of the pump. The fluid to fill the pump would be put into the drug chamber by means of a percutaneously placed needle. This would fill up the drug chamber and push out the bellows that compressed the charging chamber. The compressed Freon would then exert its energy by pushing up on the diaphragm in the device, which would slowly push out fluid through the catheter of the pump (*see* Fig. 1). The activity of the Freon at body temperature was well regulated and would be constant every day until the pump went dry. The first pumps used were made by the Infusaid Corporation and they had a 50-cm^3 reservoir. They also had a side port by which one could inject directly into the catheter.

In recent years, other designs of these pumps have appeared, generally with different placements of the side port. In the pump made by Arrow, the port is part of the pump mechanism and it can only be accessed from the central needle inlet, but one needs to use a special catheter needle (*see* Fig. 2).

2.2. Operative Pump Placement

All patients needed a hepatic arteriogram prior to placement of the pump including an arteriogram of the celiac axis and the superior mesenteric artery. In the normal anatomy the common hepatic artery is a branch of the celiac axis and the gastroduodenal artery is the first branch off the common hepatic, followed by the bifurcation of the hepatic into the right and left hepatic arteries. The superior mesenteric arteriogram is needed to be sure that there are no accessory right hepatic arteries coming off the superior mesenteric artery.

A study of arteriograms done in 100 consecutive patients who were going for pump placement showed that only 50% of patients had the normal hepatic arteriovasculature *(9)*. The most common deviation was that of a right hepatic artery branching off of the superior mesenteric artery, which was either an accessory (i.e., in addition to the right hepatic artery, which bifurcates off the common hepatic) or a replaced right hepatic (there is no right hepatic artery off the common hepatic). An accessory or replaced left hepatic artery was the next

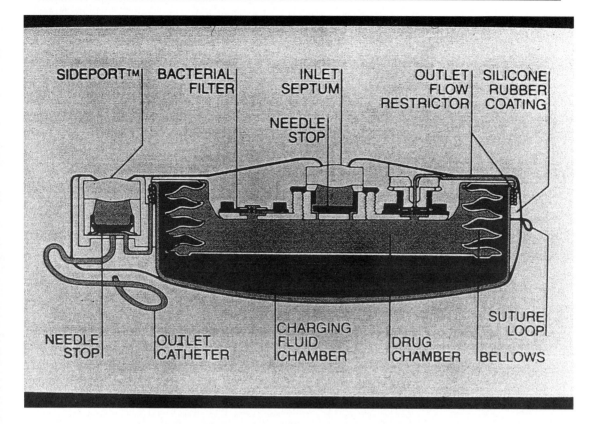

Fig. 1. Cross-section diagram of the Infusaid pump.

most frequent anomaly, usually as a branch off the left gastric artery. A final arterial anomaly, which could cause difficulty placing the pump, was a trifurcation, where the gastroduodenal artery and the bifurcation of the right and left hepatic arteries came off at exactly the same place. This was troublesome for pump placement because the flow from the catheter that was lying in the gastroduodenal artery could go entirely into one or the other of the hepatic branches instead of equally into both branches.

When the arterial anatomy is normal, the catheter is placed into the gastroduodenal artery. If there is an accessory or replaced artery, then, usually, the accessory artery is tied off and the catheter is still placed into the gastroduodenal artery. If both arteries are replaced and there is no gastroduodenal artery then a catheter is placed directly into the largest of the replaced vessels and the other is tied off.

The procedure for pump placement includes a cholecystectomy, because 30% of patients who did not have their gallbladder removed experienced acalculous cholecystitis during hepatic artery infusion (HAI) in the early experience with the pumps. The lymph nodes in the porta hepatic should be biopsied. If they are positive for tumor, the pump will probably not be beneficial for that patient because this signifies extrahepatic disease.

The pump pocket will be placed superficial to the fascia, generally in the left upper quadrant of the abdomen. This area is optimal for the pump because it does not get in the way of subsequent computed tomography (CT) or magnetic resonance imaging (MRI) scans of the liver used to evaluate whether the liver metastases are responding to pump therapy.

Pump Refill
Correct Needle Placement

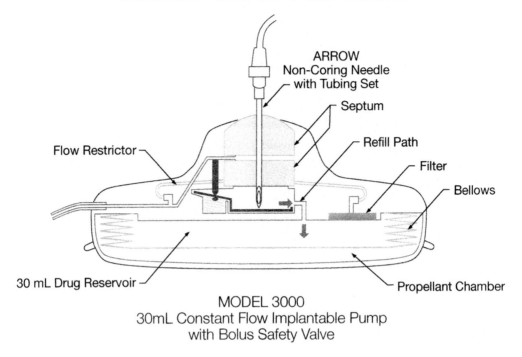

MODEL 3000
30mL Constant Flow Implantable Pump
with Bolus Safety Valve

Fig. 2. Cross-section diagram of the Arrow pump, showing the bolus needle design.

The pump should be kept in a warmer throughout the first part of the operation because if the pump is not warm (i.e., at least body temperature), then there will be no positive pressure in the catheter and there may be retrograde flow from the artery into the pump catheter. This may cause clotting of the catheter. When the pocket is ready for implantation, the pump should be primed with a Heparin solution of 30 cm^3 of 1000 U/cm^3 of heparin (30,000 U of heparin).

The catheter is put into the gastroduodenal artery. To check for correct placement of the catheter, 5–10 cm^3 of 50% fluroscein is injected into the side port of the pump, followed with 10 cm^3 of a heparin solution of 100 U/cm^3, and an ultraviolet lamp (Wood's lamp) should be used to visualize the liver. Both lobes of the liver must light up; also, the stomach should not light up.

If the whole liver does not light up with the fluroscein, then an unrecognized accessory artery is probably present. It must be found and ligated. If the defect is in the left lobe, then the artery can be found in the gastroheptic ligament between the esophagus and the hepatic artery. If the defect is in the right lobe, then the artery will be found behind the portal vein, in the posterior aspect of the porta hepatis.

To check pump placement postoperatively, a nuclear medicine scan using macroaggregate albumin labeled with technetium is injected into the side port and a scan is taken. The liver should light up with this method.

Patients can start on pump treatments as soon as the medical oncologist wishes. Usually, treatment commences 1 wk after the implantation day. The pump should be refilled every 2 wk.

2.3. Long-Term Surgical Complications

The pump can flip inside the pocket making it impossible to access. If this happens early in the course, it can be flipped mechanically without entering the pocket. Later on, this is harder to do and the pocket might have to be entered surgically to flip the pump over and sew it in place. This is an extremely rare occurrence but should be kept in mind as a reason for access problems.

There have been rare cases when the pump has been in place for over a year that the catheter has eroded through the wall of the duodenum. These patients usually complain of abdominal pain, leading to endoscopy. At endoscopy, the catheter can be seen in the duodenum through the scope. Surgery is required to remove the catheter and repair the duodenum.

If the catheter is placed too low in the gastroduodenal artery, the chemotherapy from the pump pools in the gastroduodenal artery instead of going directly into the hepatic artery. Because the concentration of chemotherapy is so high and because of the pooling, the wall of the artery can be eroded. This not only can cause bleeding, but also chemotherapy can extravasate into the abdomen and cause pain and, occasionally, pancreatitis *(10)*. This is usually diagnosed by a CT scan that shows a hematoma in the area of the gastroduodenal artery. If this complication occurs, the pump must be emptied and no further fluid should be placed in it. This will allow the catheter to clot and it may also stop the bleeding. The patient should be followed to be sure that there is no further bleeding. The pump can be removed at any time after this event. If the bleeding continues, then an abdominal exploration may be necessary to remove the catheter and tie off the gastroduodenal artery.

Pump pocket infections occur rarely during the course of treatment. At the first sign of infection (erythema over the pump pocket), systemic antibiotics need to be started. If the infection does not resolve, then the pump needs to be moved to a new location, in a newly created pocket. The old pocket should be opened and drained.

3. HAI FOR UNRESECTABLE METASTASES

3.1. Rationale

The rationale of hepatic arterial therapy is based on the information that once hepatic metastases grow beyond 3 mm, they are fed predominantly by the hepatic artery, whereas normal hepatocytes are fed predominantly by the portal vein *(11)*. The liver may be the initial stop for metastatic spread through the portal vein. Agents that are taken up by the liver and have a high first-pass extraction as well as high total-body clearance are the most useful agents. When evaluating drugs, taking into account the above-mentioned factors, the most active drug is 5-fluoro-2-deoxyuridine (FUDR), which has a 60–90% first-pass liver extraction rate and an estimated 100- to 400-fold increase in hepatic exposure when used for hepatic arterial infusion *(12)* (Table 1).

3.2. Trials

Eight randomized trials have been performed looking at the use of HAI of chemotherapy in the treatment of unresectable hepatic metastases from colorectal cancer (Table 2). In the trial at Memorial Sloan-Kettering, 162 patients were randomized to HAI of FUDR or

Table 1
Drugs Used for Hepatic Arterial Infusion

Drug	Estimated increased exposure by hepatic arterial infusion (-fold)
Fluorouracil	5–10
5-Fluoro-2-deoxyuridine	100–400
Bischloroethylnitrosurea	6–7
Mitomycin C	6–8
Cisplatin	4–7
Doxorubicin	2

Table 2
Randomized Trials of HAI vs Systemic Chemotherapy
for Hepatic Metastases from Colorectal Cancer

Authors (ref.)	N	Agents	Response rate (%)	Survival (mo.)
Kemeny et al.	162	HAI FUDR vs	52	17
(13)		iv FUDR	20	12
Chang et al.	64	HAI FUDR vs	62	—
(15)		iv FUDR	17	—
Hohn et al.	143	HAI FUDR vs	42	16
(14)		iv FUDR	10	15
Martin et al.	69	HAI FUDR vs	48	12.6
(16)		iv 5-FU/LV	21	10.5
Kemeny et al.	41	HAI FUDR vs	55	13.8
(17)		iv 5-FU	20	11.6
Rougier et al.	163	HAI 5-FU vs	49	14
(19)		iv 5-FU	14	10
Allen-Mersch et al.	100	HAI 5-FU vs	50	13
(20)		iv 5-FU/palliation	0	7.3
Lorenz et al.	168	HAI 5-FU/LV vs	45	18.7
(21)		HAI FUDR vs	43	12.7
		iv 5-FU	19.7	17.6

systemic FUDR infusion (13). All patients underwent surgical exploration to confirm the absence of extrahepatic disease and to have a hepatic arterial catheter placed for HAI therapy, either initially or after systemic chemotherapy failure. A partial response was seen in 52% of patient's treated with HAI and in 20% treated with systemic chemotherapy. Of note, 60% of patients on the systemic arm crossed over to receive HAI. The survival based on the initial randomization was 17 mo for the HAI group and 12 mo for the systemic arm. In patients who crossed over to HAI after progressing on systemic therapy, the median survival was 18 mo vs 8 mo in patients who were not able to be crossed over because of technical problems with the hepatic arterial catheter.

The Northern California Oncology group (NCOG) performed a similar study using FUDR via HAI or systemic infusion (14). A partial response of 42% was seen with HAI therapy and 10% with systemic therapy with no difference in survival, but, again, most of the patients were crossed over to pump therapy after they failed systemic therapy. Those patients who were crossed over to HAI had a doubling of survival compared to those who did not cross over.

At the National Cancer Institute, 64 patients, including some patients with positive portal lymph nodes, were randomized to HAI of FUDR vs systemic FUDR *(15)*. Response rates were 62% and 17% in the HAI and systemic arms, respectively. Actuarial 2-yr survival was 22% and 15% respectively. However, in a subset analysis excluding patients with portal lymph node involvement, the 2-year survival was significantly better in patients treated with HAI (47% vs 13%, respectively).

The Mayo Clinic also reported a small study that enrolled only 69 patients. Response rates were 48% and 21% with the HAI and systemic groups, respectively. In addition, a significant increase in time to hepatic progression was noted with HAI therapy, 15.7 mo vs 6 mo for patients on systemic therapy. There was no difference in survival, but survival results were difficult to interpret because 50% of patients randomized to the HAI did not receive treatment for reasons including pump failure and extrahepatic disease *(16)*.

At the City of Hope, 41 patients with nonresectable liver metastases received HAI versus systemic chemotherapy *(17,18)* In the group receiving HAI of FUDR, the response rate was 55%, with a median survival of 13.8 mo. Patients treated with systemic chemotherapy had a 20% response rate and a median survival of 11.6 mo. As in the other studies, patients were allowed to cross over to pump therapy if they failed systemic infusion.

A French trial randomized 163 patients to HAI of FUDR vs systemic bolus 5-fluorouracil (5-FU) with response rates of 49% and 14%, respectively. The median time to hepatic progression was 15 and 6 mo, and 2-yr survival was 22% and 10% ($p < 0.02$) in the HAI and systemic groups, respectively. Median survival was 14 and 10 mo in the HAI and systemic groups, respectively; however, patients in the systemic group were sometimes treated only when they became symptomatic *(19)*.

In an English trial that randomized patients to HAI of FUDR vs conventional therapy, quality of life as well as overall survival were measured *(20)* A significant improvement in survival was seen in the HAI group, 405 d, vs 226 d in the systemic group. In addition, a good quality of life in patients receiving HAI of FUDR was significantly prolonged measured by physical symptoms, anxiety, and depression. However, only 22% in the conventional-treatment arm received systemic chemotherapy. The authors concluded that in addition to the survival benefit seen with HAI, it was well tolerated, leading to a better and longer sustained performance status.

The German Cooperative Group randomized 168 patients to HAI of FUDR vs 5-FU and leucovorin (LV) administered by either HAI or systemic infusion *(21)*. An intention to treat analysis was used, although only 70% patients randomized to 5-FU/LV and 68.5% randomized to HAI of FUDR were treated as assigned. Median survival was 12.7, 18.7, and 17.6 mo for HAI of FUDR, HAI of FU+LV and systemic FU+ LV, respectively. Tumor response was 43.2%, 45%, and 19.7% for the three groups respectively. The development of extrahepatic disease was 40.5%, 12.5%, and 18.3%, respectively. Toxicity data indicated that 5-FU/LV therapy was much more toxic than FUDR. It is difficult to interpret the results of the HAI FUDR group because there is no information on details of their treatment, such as number of cycles and pump complications and the dose modification scheduled was very primitive.

A meta-analysis combining the results of seven trials supports the use of HAI of FUDR in the treatment of nonresectable liver metastases from colorectal cancer *(22)* A significantly better response rate of 41% was achieved with HAI of FUDR compared with a 14% response rate with systemic 5-FU. Median survival was significantly increased to 16 mo with HAI vs 13 mo with systemic therapy.

3.3. Hepatic Toxicity

Hepatic artery infusion therapy is associated with hepatic toxicity evidenced by the necrosis and cholestasis seen on biopsies or a pericholangitic process and fibrosis of biliary radicals. These changes may resolve if the drug is withdrawn and the patient is given a treatment rest. However, in later stages, the patient can develop changes similar to idiopathic sclerosing cholangitis *(23)*. If the patient develops jaundice that does not resolve and ERCP reveals fibrosis of the main biliary radical, stenting of the biliary tree should be performed.

Liver function tests (LFT) must be monitored very carefully. A method for decreasing the dosing of chemotherapy or for ceasing treatment is included in Table 3.

In order to decrease hepatic toxicity, the use of dexamethasone was evaluated in a randomized study. Using dexamethasone with FUDR *(24)*, decreased frequency of bilirubin elevations to 9% from 30% ($p = 0.07$) with FUDR alone in a randomized study. The response rate was increased from 40–71% ($p = 0.03$) and survival rate was increased from 15–23 mo.

Alternating-drug regimens is another method to decrease hepatotoxicity from HAI of FUDR. By utilizing HAI of FUDR on d 1–8 followed by hepatic arterial bolus of 5-FU on d 14, 21, and 28 via the side port, every 35 d, Stagg et al. improved toxicity *(25)*. There were no treatment terminations with this regimen and 50% of patients responded with a median survival of 22 mo. Metzgar et al., using an infusion of 5-FU and mitomycin C, found that median survival was 18 mo with a partial response rate of 57% in his patients. Sclerosing cholangitis did not occur, but mucositis and leukopenia did *(26)*.

3.4. Addressing Extrahepatic Recurrence

One of the main criticisms of HAI therapy is the occurrence of extrahepatic disease. Combination systemic chemotherapy and HAI has been attempted to reduce the rate of extrahepatic recurrence. In one trial, HAI of FUDR alone was compared with concurrent HAI and systemic FUDR. Although both groups achieved a response rate of 60%, the rate of extrahepatic disease was significantly less in the group treated with intravenous and HAI therapy, 56% vs 79%, with HAI alone *(27)*. In another study, patients with unresectable hepatic metastases were treated with HAI of FUDR and systemic 5-FU/LV delivered 1 wk after the start of HAI of FUDR *(28)*. The response rate was 62%. The incidence of extrahepatic progression was 45%. Another study, at Memorial Sloan–Kettering Cancer Center, combined systemic irinotecan (CPT-11) with HAI of FUDR + dexamethasone in 38 patients with unresectable hepatic metastases from colorectal cancer *(29)*. All of them had been treated with iv 5-FU/LV and 16 had prior CPT-11. Partial responses were seen in 74% of patients analyzed, but extrahepatic disease still developed. However, this was a group of heavily pretreated patients.

3.5. Cost

Total treatment of intramuscular FUDR costs, including the cost of the pump, procedure, hospitalization, chemotherapy, follow-up, and toxic effect came to about $30,000 for 1 yr. This is in line with the costs of newer chemotherapeutic regimens, including CPT-11, which, on average, costs $54,000 for 1 yr of treatment, including the cost of drug and drug administration, in the United States *(30)*. Therefore, when compared to the costs of treatment for other severe medical illnesses and other regimens for colorectal cancer, HAI falls within

Table 3
FUDR Dose Modification Schedule

SGOT (Reference values)	</= 50 U/L	> 50 U/L	Check at pump emptying or day of planned treatment (take higher value)
FUDR dose: 100%	0–<3X ref.	0–<2X ref.	
80%	3–<4X ref.	2–<3X ref.	
50%	4–<5X ref.	3–<4X ref.	
Hold	>/= 5X ref.	>/= 4X ref.	
Alkaline Phosphatase:	</= 90 U/L	> 90 U/L	
FUDR dose: 100%	0–<1.5X ref.	0–<1.2X ref.	
50%	1.5–<2.0X ref.	1.2–<1.5X ref.	
Hold	>/= 2.0X ref.	>/= 1.5X ref.	
Total Bilirubin:	</= 1.2 mg/dL	>1.2 mg/dL	
FUDR dose: 100%	0–<1.5X ref.	0–<1.2X ref.	
50%	1.5–<2.0X ref.	1.2–<1.5X ref.	
Hold	>/= 2.0X ref.	>/= 1.5X ref.	

Note: Reference values defined as the values obtained the day of the last dose of FUDR. To determine if dose modification is necessary, compare the value obtained the day the pump is emptied or the day it is to be filled, whichever is higher.

Recommendations on restarting treatment: If resulting from an abnormal SGOT, only restart when level has fallen to 4X reference value (if reference ≤ 50 U/L) or within 3X reference value (if reference > 50). If started, we recommend reinitiation at 50% of the last FUDR dose given.

If resulting from an abnormal alkaline phosphatase, restart once level has fallen to 1.5X reference value (if reference ≤ 90 U/L) or 1.2X reference value (if reference > 90 U/L). If started, recommence at 25% of last FUDR dose given.

If resulting from an abnormal bilirubin, restart once level has fallen to 1.5X reference value (if reference ≤ 1.2 mg/dL) or within 1.2X reference value (if > 1.2 mg/dL). Restart chemotherapy at 25% of last FUDR dose. However, if a marked abnormality of the bilirubin compared to reference exceeding 2X reference value (in patients with reference value ≤ 1.2) or 1.5X reference value (in patients with reference value > 1.2) occurs, then the next cycle should not be administered. Instead, levels should be rechecked at 14 d. If the bilirubin continues to be normal, FUDR can be restarted at 25% of the usual dose.

the range of accepted therapies. A regimen that combines HAI of fluoropyrimidine with newer agents, such as irinotecan and/or oxaliplatin, will be expected to have higher total costs.

3.6. Conclusions

Metastatic colorectal cancer continues to be a difficult problem to manage. Newer chemotherapeutic agents like irinotecan and oxaliplatin have improved outcomes over fluorouracil-based treatment, but a majority of patients still succumb to their disease within 2 yr. The work summarized here outlines options that can be used in the loco-regional management of metastatic colorectal cancer.

Hepatic arterial infusion of FUDR and dexamethasone has been shown to be a viable treatment option for patients with metastatic colorectal cancer to the liver. Multiple studies have demonstrated an increased response rate with HAI that is up to three times higher than the responses attainable with systemic 5-FU-based chemotherapy. The toxicity can be managed effectively by ensuring proper technique with pump placement and the use of dexamethasone in order to decrease portal inflammation. In addition, it is an economically viable option, especially when compared to other therapies for severe conditions.

The impact of HAI on survival has been difficult to ascertain. Many trials allowed crossover in those patients who progressed. An ongoing trial conducted by the Cancer and Leukemia Group B (CALGB) will attempt to address whether or not this therapy influences survival by not allowing crossover in its design. Quality-of-life measures, molecular markers, including thymidylate synthetase, and a cost-effectiveness analysis will also be examined. Systemic failure has been an ongoing dilemma in patients treated with hepatic arterial infusion. Further clinical trials will need to be done incorporating systemic chemotherapy and HAI in the treatment of advanced colorectal cancer.

4. HEPATIC RESECTION AND HEPATIC ARTERY INFUSION

4.1. Clinical Trials

With advancing surgical technique, large liver resections can be done with a very respectable operative mortality and approximately one-third or more of patients who undergo these operations will survive for 5 yr and, perhaps, even be cured of their disease (see Chapter 20). However, because the majority of patients were not cured, new approaches needed to be explored to try to increase the cure rate after resection. Several reports have looked into the location of recurrence after liver resection. It is clear that over half of the patients who have recurrent disease have the recurrence in the liver after liver resections. Decreasing the numbers of patients who fail in the liver would seem like a good strategy for increasing survival after liver resection.

Because the multitude of trials done on hepatic artery infusion had shown better response rates of liver metastases to hepatic artery infusion than with any other chemotherapy route, it was a logical step to try to use hepatic artery infusion after hepatic resection to see if the number of liver recurrences could be reduced. In an early single-institution, prospective, randomized trial, patients with solitary resectable liver metastases were randomized to resection alone or resection followed by HAI of FUDR. In the same study, patients with multiple hepatic metastases that were resectable were randomized to resection followed by HAI or to HAI without resection. There were only 11 patients with solitary metastases in this study and 25 patients with multiple resectable lesions, clearly too small a number to reach any definitive conclusions about this treatment. However, this study did show that for patients who got hepatic resection followed with HAI, not one of those patients recurred in the liver, whereas over 50% of the patients recurred in the liver in the small group that had resection alone (17,18). This study raised the possibility that HAI after hepatic resection may decrease the incidence of liver recurrence.

Because of these findings, a larger intergroup study with participation of ECOG (Eastern Cooperative Oncology Group) and SWOG (Southwestern Oncology Group) was performed from 1991 to 1997. In this study patients, with one to three resectable hepatic metastases were randomized between hepatic resection alone or hepatic resection followed by HAI of FUDR and systemic chemotherapy utilizing 5-FU. Because of the international scope of this study (Australia was part of ECOG), it was decided that an intraoperative randomization would be impossible and that patients could only be randomized preoperatively. The problem with this approach was that many patients who were randomized preoperatively could not be included in the study because, at operation, they did not fulfill the criteria for resection. These patients did not get the therapy to which they were assigned and were placed off protocol. Thus, of the 109 patients who were randomized, 53 patients were placed in the surgery-alone arm, and of those 53, 45 actually had a hepatic resection. The rest were placed off protocol because of having more than three metastases, having extrahepatic disease or unresectable disease. For the 56 patients in the hepatic resection plus chemotherapy arm, 18 patients had to be placed off protocol because of the same reasons. Patients in the chemotherapy arm received four courses of FUDR given by HAI. The starting dose was 0.1 mg/kg/d for 14 d, followed by 14 d of heparin infusion, and then the second cycle was 0.2 mg/kg/d for 14 d. The next two cycles remained at the 0.2-mg level. Patients were also treated with systemic therapy starting with a continuous 2-wk infusion of 5-FU given intravenously at a dose of 200 mg/m^2. This was infused during the 2-wk break when the heparin infusion was being given intraarterially. After the four courses of HAI, the systemic infusion was then escalated to 300 mg/m^2 for eight additional courses. The overall 4-yr survival, 4-yr recurrence-free survival, and 4-yr liver-recurrence-free survival were 61.3%, 47.5%, and 66.9%, respectively, for the chemotherapy arm vs 52.7%, 25.2%, and 43%, respectively, for the control arm (significant for the latter two). Thus the patients with hepatic artery infusion and systemic therapy after hepatic resection had a significantly better recurrence-free survival rate and hepatic-disease-free survival rate than the patients who had resection only *(31)*.

Almost simultaneous with this intergroup trial, a similar single-institution study was done at Memorial Sloan–Kettering. In this randomized trial, HAI of FUDR and dexamethasone and systemic administration of 5-FU with or without LV was compared to similar systemic chemotherapy alone after the resection of hepatic metastases. The end points of the study were overall survival, survival free of hepatic progression, and overall progression-free survival at 2 yr. Because this was a single-institution study, patients were able to be randomized intraoperatively and only the patients who fit the criteria were randomized and treated. One hundred fifty-six patients were enrolled into this study. Over a quarter of the patients had greater than four hepatic lesions. Treatment in the combined-modality arm consisted of 320 mg/m^2 5-FU and 200 mg/m^2 LV, followed by HAI of FUDR and dexamethasone, initiated 2 wk after systemic therapy. Patients received pump infusion for 14 d. After the 2 wk of therapy, the pump was emptied and the patients were given 1 wk of rest before reinitiating the systemic therapy. In the systemic-treatment group, 5-FU was administered at 375 mg/m^2 with the same dose of LV for 5 d every 4 wk. A total of six cycles were scheduled for each group. In patients previously treated with 5-FU and LV, 5-FU was administered as a 5-d continuous infusion at a dose of 850 mg/m^2 in the HAI group and 1000 mg/m^2 in the systemic group.

Patients were stratified according to the number of liver metastases (1, 2, 4, > 4) and type of previous chemotherapy (none, 5-FU ± Levamisole, or 5-FU ± LV).

Actuarial survival at 2 yr was significantly increased with combined-modality therapy (86% vs 72%, $p = 0.03$). Univariate analysis showed an unadjusted risk ratio of 2.13 for death in the systemic group compared with the HAI and systemic therapy group. Additionally, increased survival was seen with the HAI and systemic therapy group of 72.2 mo as opposed to 59.3 mo in the systemic therapy group. After adjustment for location of the primary tumor and lesions greater or equal to 5 cm, the risk ratio for death in the systemic therapy group compared to the HAI and systemic therapy group was statistically significant at 2.34 ($p = 0.027$). Hepatic recurrence was also greatly decreased in the patients treated with HAI and systemic therapy. Comparing the HAI and systemic-therapy-arm with the systemic therapy only arm, the actuarial rate of survival free from hepatic recurrence at 2 yr was 90% and 60%, respectively. Median time free from hepatic recurrence has not been reached in the HAI and systemic therapy arm, but was reported at 42.7 mo in patients treated with systemic therapy alone. Overall progression-free survival at 2 yr was 57% in the HAI and systemic therapy group and 42% in the systemic therapy group. Although equivalent numbers of patients in each group progressed in the lungs (15 patients in the HAI and systemic group vs 17 patents in the systemic group), 7 patients and 30 patients progressed in the liver in the HAI and systemic group versus the systemic-alone group, respectively.

More patients in the HAI plus systemic therapy group compared to the systemic alone therapy group experienced diarrhea (29% vs 14%) and nausea (10% vs 5%). Twenty-nine patients required hospitalization in the HAI plus systemic treatment arm compared to 18 patients receiving systemic treatment alone.

Hepatic enzyme elevations in the HAI plus systemic group occurred in the following: 29% had a doubling of the serum alkaline phosphatase, 65% had a tripling of the aspartate aminotransferase levels, and 18% had increases in their serum bilirubin to > 3.0 mg/dL. Biliary abnormalities returned to normal in all but four patients who required biliary stents. Two patients in the systemic therapy group required biliary stents.

This study again demonstrated there was a benefit for hepatic artery infusion after hepatic resection with a decrease in the amount of recurrence in the liver and an increase in 2-yr overall survival *(32)*.

A study from the German Cooperative Group on Liver Metastases randomized patients to hepatic resection alone versus hepatic resection plus HAI infusion of 5-FU and LV. All patients were stratified according to number of liver metastases (1–2, 3–6) and the site of the primary tumor (colon or upper rectum, mid or lower rectum). One hundred thirteen patients were assigned to each group. Despite the initial randomization, 24 (21%) in the HAI arm and 18 (16%) patients in the control group did not receive the assigned treatment. In the group randomized to adjuvant treatment, it was not performed for the following reasons: anatomic variants, documentation of extrahepatic disease at the time of surgery, technical complications with port placement, and patient refusal after randomization. In the group randomized to resection alone, reasons for not following the randomized assignment were unresectable disease, microscopic residual disease, and extrahepatic disease. In the control group, 3 patients received HAI FU/LV and 10 received palliative systemic chemotherapy.

If the entire group of patients is considered there is no difference in median survival. However, in the group receiving HAI of 5-FU/LV the median time to liver progression doubled compared to the control group: 44.8 mo vs 23.3 mo. Additionally, median time to progression of disease or death was increased in the group receiving adjuvant HAI of 5-FU/LV: 20 mo vs 12.6 mo.

The results of this randomized trial must be interpreted with caution. Of the 113 patients randomized, 73 (64%) had chemotherapy data available, and only 34 (30%) patients completed the assigned protocol. This suggests that the power to detect a difference, even with an intention-to-treat analysis, was not adequate, given that the majority of patients did not receive their assigned treatment *(33)*.

Also, HAI therapy was given in a different way than in the Memorial study and the Intergroup study. The German patients received a continuous infusion of 5-FU for 5 d, combined with a 15-min infusion of LV at 200 mg/m^2/d every 28 d. This was quite different than the 14-d infusion of FUDR used in both of the American studies and may also account for the difference in results of these three studies.

4.2. Conclusions

The two prospective randomized studies from the United States showed a significant benefit for HAI of FUDR after liver resection both to reduce hepatic recurrence and to prolong recurrence-free survival. New investigations on different systemic drugs and combinations need to be completed to try to build on these improvements, so that further systemic control can be achieved as well as hepatic control. This may lead to more patients who achieve a cure in the setting of hepatic metastases from the combined therapies of surgical removal, HAI, and intravenous chemotherapies.

REFERENCES

1. Kemeny NE, Kemeny MM, and Lawrence TS. Liver metastases. In *Clinical Oncology*. Abeloff MD, Armitage JO, Lichter AS, and Niederhuber JE (eds.), Churchill Livingstone, New York, 2000, pp. 886–921.
2. Adson MA, van Heerden JA, Adson JH, et al. Resection of hepatic metastases from colorectal cancer. *Arch. Surg.*, **119** (1984) 647–651.
3. Hughes KS, Scheele J. and Sugarbaker PH. Surgery for colorectal cancer metastatic to the liver: Optimizing the result of treatment. *Surg. Clin. North Am.*, **69** (1989) 339–359.
4. Nordlinger B, Guiguet, M., Valliant JC, Balladur P, Boudjema KE, Bachellier P, et al. Surgical resection of colorectal carcinoma metastases to the liver. A prognostic scoring system to improve case selection, based on 1568 patients. *Assoc. Fr. Chir. Cancer*, **77** (1996) 1254–1262.
5. Fong Y, Fortner J, Sun RL, Brennan MF, and Blumgart LH. Clinical score for predicting recurrence after hepatic resection for metastatic colorectal cancer: Analysis of 1001 consecutive cases. *Ann. Surg.*, **230** (1999) 309–318.
6. Scheele J. Stang R, Altendorf-Hofmann A, and Paul M. Resection of colorectal liver metastases. *World J. Surg.*, **19** (1995) 59–71.
7. Curley SA, Izzo F, Delrio P, Ellis L, Granch J, Vallone P, et al. Radiofrequency ablation of unresectable primary and metastatic hepatic malignancies: results of 123 patients. *Ann. Surg.*, **230(1)** (1999) 1–8.
8. Pearson AS, Izzo F, Fleming RY, Ellis LM, Delrio P, Roh MS, et al. Intraoperative radiofrequency ablation or cryoablation for hepatic malignancies. *Am. J. Surg.*, **178(6)** (1999) 592–599.
9. Kemeny MM, Hogan JM, Goldberg DA, Lieu C, Beatty JD, Kokal WA, et al. Continuous hepatic artery infusion with an implantable pump: problems with hepatic artery anomalies. *Surgery*, **99(4)** (1986) 501–504.
10. Kemeny MM and Brennan MF. The surgical complications of chemotherapy in the cancer patient. *Curr. Prob. Surg.*, **24(10)** (1987) 607–675.
11. Breedis C and Young C. Blood supply of neoplasms in the liver. *Am. J. Pathol.*, **30** (1954) 969–985.
12. Ensminger WD, Rosowsky A, and Raso V. Clinical pharmacological evaluation of hepatic arterial infusions of 5-fluoro-2-deoxyuridine in patients with liver metastases from colorectal carcinoma. *Ann. Int. Med.*, **107** (1987) 459–465.
13. Kemeny N, Daly J. Oderman P, et al. Randomized study of intrahepatic versus systemic infusion of fluorodeoxyuridine in patients with liver metastases from colorectal carcinoma. *Ann. Int. Med.*, **107** (1987) 459–465.
14. Hohn D, Stagg R, Friedman M, et al. A randomized trial of continuous versus hepatic intraarterial floxuridine in patients with colorectal cancer metastases to the liver: the Northern California Oncology Group trial. *J. Clin. Oncol.*, **7** (1989) 1646–1654.
15. Chang AE, Schneider PD, and Sugarbaker PH. A prospective randomized trial of regional versus systemic continuous 5-flurorxyuridine chemotherapy in the treatment of colorectal liver metastases. *Ann. Surg.*, **206** (1987) 685–693.
16. Martin JK Jr, O'Connell MJ, Wieand HS, et al. Intra-arterial floxuridine vs systemic fluorouracil for hepatic metastases from colorectal cancer. A randomized trial. *Arch. Surg.*, **125** (1990) 1022.
17. Wagman L, Kemeny M, Leong L, et al. A prospective randomized evaluation of the treatment of colorectal cancer metastatic to the liver. *J. Clin. Oncol.*, **8** (1990) 1885–1893.
18. Kemeny M, Goldberg D, Beatty JD, et al. Results of a prospective randomized trials of continuous regional chemotherapy and hepatic resection as treatment of hepatic metastases from colorectal primaries. *Cancer*, **57** (1986) 492–498.
19. Rougier P, Laplanche A, Huguier M, et al. Hepatic arterial infusion of floxuridine in patients with liver metastases from colorectal carcinoma: long-term results of a prospective randomized trial. *J. Clin. Oncol.*, **10** (1992) 1112–1118.
20. Allen-Mersh TG, Earlam S, Fordy C, et al. Quality of life and survival with continuous hepatic artery floxuridine infusion for colorectal liver metastases. *Lancet*, **344** (1994) 1255–1260.
21. Lorenz M, Muller H, et al. Randomized, multicenter trial of fluorouracil plus leucovorin administered either via hepatic arterial or intravenous infusion versus fluorordeoxyuridine administered via hepatic

arterial infusion in patients with nonresectable liver metastases from colorectal cancer. *J. Clin. Oncol.*, **18** (2000) 243–254.

22. Meta-Analysis Group in Cancer. Reappraisal of hepatic arterial infusion in the treatment of nonresectable liver metastases from colorectal cancer. *J. Natl. Cancer Inst.*, **88** (1996) 252–258.

23. Kemeny M Battifora H, Flayney D, et al. Sclerosing cholangitis after continuous hepatic artery infusion of FUDR. *Ann. Surg.*, **202** (1985) 176–181.

24. Kemeny N, Seiter K, Diedzweikei D, et al. A randomized trial of intrahepatic infusion of floxuridine (FUDR) with dexamethasone vs. FUDR alone in the treatment of metastatic colorectal cancer. *Cancer*, **69** (1992) 327–334.

25. Stagg RJ, Venook AP, Chase JL, et al. Alternative hepatic intra-arterial floxuridine and fluorouracil: a less toxic regimen for treatment of liver metastases from colorectal cancer. *J. Natl. Cancer Inst.*, **83** (1991) 423–428.

26. Metzgar U, Weder W, Rothlin M, and Largiader F. Phase II study of intra-arterial fluorouracil and mitomycin-C for liver metastases of colorectal cancer. *Recent Results Cancer Res.*, **121** (1991) 198–204.

27. Safi F, Bittner R, Roscher R, et al. Regional chemotherapy for hepatic metastases from colorectal carcinoma (continuous intra-arterial versus continuous intra-arterial/intravenous therapy. *Cancer*, **64** (1989) 379–387.

28. O'Connell M, Nagorney D, Barmath A, et al. Sequential intrahepatic fluorodeoxyuridine and systemic fluorouracil plus leucovorin for the treatment of metastatic colorectal cancer confined to the liver. *J. Clin. Oncol.*, **16** (1998) 2528–2533.

29. Ron IG, Kemeny N, Tong B, et al. Phase I/II study of the escalating doses of systemic irinotecan (CPT-11) with hepatic arterial infusion of floxuridine (FUDR) and dexamethasone (D), with or without cryosurgery for patients with unresectable hepatic metastases from colorectal cancer. *Proc. ASCO*, **18** (1999) 236a.

30. Kemeny N and Ron IG. Hepatic arterial chemotherapy in metastatic colorectal patients. *Semin. Oncol.*, **26** (1999) 524–535.

31. Kemeny MM, Adak S, Lipsitz S, Gray B, MacDonald J, and Benson AB III. Results of the intergroup (Eastern Cooperative Oncology Group (ECOG) and Southwest Oncology Group (SWOG) prospective randomized study of surgery alone versus continuous hepatic artery infusion of FUDR and continuous systemic infusion of 5FU after hepatic resection for colorectal liver metastases. *Proc. ASCO*, **18** (1999) 1012.

32. Kemeny N, Huang Y, Cohen A, et al. Hepatic arterial infusion of chemotherapy after resection of hepatic metastases from colorectal cancer. *N. Engl. J. Med.*, **341** (1999) 2039–2048.

33. Lorenz, M, Staib-Sebler E, Koch B, Gog, C, Waldeyer M, and Encke A. The value of postoperative hepatic arterial infusion following curative liver resection. *Anticancer Res.*, **17** (1997) 3825–3834.

33

Intraportal and Intraperitoneal Chemotherapy for Colon Cancer

Werner Scheithauer

CONTENTS

1. INTRAPORTAL CHEMOTHERAPY

1.1. Rationale of Intraportal Chemotherapy

Metachronous liver metastases are present at the time of initial diagnosis of colorectal cancer in approx 25–30% of patients (1). Similarly, the liver is the most common and sometimes the only site of distant failure after potential curative surgical resection (2). Colorectal cancer metastases reach the liver via the portal vein and such dissemination may occur preoperatively and intraoperatively. Operative stress and immediate postoperative decrease in immune defense, in fact, have been shown in some experimental models to improve the survival of malignant cells and to facilitate their growth in the liver (3). Fisher and Turnbull discovered tumor cells in the mesenteric venous blood of 32% of patients at the time of colorectal cancer resection (4), and in 1957, Dukes found evidence of venous spread in 17% of operative rectal cancer specimens (5). Despite continuing controversies, established metastases seem to be fed primarily by the hepatic artery, whereas micrometastases are likely to depend on the portal venous blood (6,7). Thus, early postoperative regional administration of chemotherapeutic agents into the portal vein (resulting in high anticancer drug concentrations) might be particularly beneficial, destroying suspected tumor cells in the liver before established tumor growth can take place. Ideally, treatment should be commenced shortly after resection of the primary tumor, because micrometastases are more sensitive to a given drug due to a shorter cell-cycle time, better accessibility to drugs, and a smaller chance of harboring resistance (8,9).

The above-mentioned theoretical advantages of early postoperative intraportal chemotherapy have been investigated in animal studies. Intraportal administration of carcinosarcoma cells in Walker rats immediately followed by a single injection of meclorethamine via the same route resulted in a 50% reduction in liver tumor takes (10). The safety and the

From: *Colorectal Cancer: Multimodality Management*
Edited by: L. Saltz © Humana Press Inc., Totowa, NJ

pharmacological basis of portal vein infusion (PVI) was subsequently established in 1975 by Almersjö and co-workers *(11)*.

1.2. Clinical Trials of Intraportal Chemotherapy in Colorectal Cancer

Nonrandomized studies of PVI, using either mechlorethamine *(12)* or thiotepa *(13)*, were undertaken in the 1950s but were abandoned because of concerns about toxicity. The first randomized trial to test cytotoxic PVI of fluorouracil (FU) was initiated in 1975 *(7)*. Two hundred forty-four eligible patients with primary stage I to III colon or rectal carcinoma were randomly assigned to either surgery alone or to surgery plus a 1-wk continuous infusion of FU (1 g/d) administered via a catheter that had been inserted into the portal vein; in addition, intravenous heparin (5000 U/d) was given in order to prevent portal vein thrombosis. After a median follow-up of 4 yr, 53 patients had died with recurrent disease in the control group and 25 in the infusion group. The liver was the predominant site of recurrence and its incidence was significantly lower in the treatment group (5 vs 22 patients). Similarly, overall survival seemed improved in the infusion group, although a subset analysis suggested that this advantage was accrued mainly for patients with stage II colon carcinoma.

The Australian and New Zealand Trial evaluated 372 patients with colon cancer randomly allocated to observation alone or to immediate postoperative chemotherapy with 600 mg/m^2/d FU × 7 given intravenously or intraportally *(14)*. Exclusion totaled as many as 175 patients (47%) for various reasons, including nonmalignant disease, stage I or IV tumors, or inadequate follow-up. The incidence of liver metastases was not reported. The overall test for survival differences among the three arms was of borderline significance ($p = 0.67$), but the pairwise comparisons between the PVI arm and the other two were significant ($p = 0.04$ vs control and $p = 0.03$ vs systemic therapy). Four-year survival was about 35% for controls and 80% for PVI, with the difference being most apparent for patients with stage III disease. Mature results of this study to determine the magnitude and duration of benefits more precisely have not yet been published.

Another study investigating adjuvant intraportal chemotherapy was conducted by the Swiss Group for Clinical Cancer Research (SAKK) *(15,16)*. From 1981 to 1987, 505 eligible patients with histologically proven adenocarcinoma of the colorectum who were candidates for a curative en-bloc resection were randomly allocated to a control or to a chemotherapy group, receiving immediate postoperative intraportal continuous infusional 500 mg/m^2/d FU × 7 with 5000 IU of heparin. On the first day of therapy, a 10-mg/m^2 bolus of mitomycin C was also administered. After a median follow-up duration of 96 mo *(17)*, the 5-yr disease-free survival rate was 57% for treated patients compared with 48% for untreated controls ($p = 0.05$); the respective values for overall survival were 66% and 55% ($p = 0.026$). Adjuvant therapy reduced the risk of recurrence by 21% and the risk of death by 26%. The beneficial effect was greatest in colon cancer patients with regional lymph node metastases. In a subsequent trial of the Swiss group, conducted between 1987 and 1993, surgery alone, PVI of FU + mitomycin C, and systemic intravenous FU + mitomycin C were compared: 769 patients were randomized. Preliminary results of this trial were disappointing, because after a median follow-up of 5 yr the significant advantage of PVI observed in the first trial could not be confirmed/reproduced. The 5-yr overall survival for PVI, systemic infusion, and control was 68%, 74%, and 72%, respectively *(18)*. The authors believed that the reduced effect of chemotherapy in their second trial might be explained by improved surgical treatment results. Disease-free and overall survival in the control arm, in fact, were 1.3-fold higher compared with the first trial, despite similar inclusion criteria.

In 1990, Wereldsma and colleagues published the results of a Dutch multi-institutional trial. Three hundred seventeen patients were randomized intraoperatively after curative en-bloc resection into one of three arms: surgery alone, intraportal FU plus heparin at the same dose, route and schedule as was used by Taylor et al., or urokinase 10,000 U given over 24 h *(19)*. After a median follow-up duration of 44 mo, the FU/heparin group had a lower rate of liver metastases than the other groups. In a multivariate Cox regression analysis correcting for stage, tumor site, age, and gender, the chance of developing liver metastases after PVI with FU/heparin was one-third of the chance in the control group ($p = 0.001$). However, the decrease in hepatic recurrences did not translate into a survival advantage.

The North Central Cancer Treatment Group (NCCTG) and Mayo Clinic have also reported a randomized trial of 224 patients with stage II and III colorectal cancer in which the PVI of FU plus heparin (allowing a delay until the fifth postoperative day) was compared with a surgery-alone control group *(20)*. After a median follow-up of 5.5 yr, the frequency of liver metastases and the overall survival rate were similar for the two groups.

One of the largest randomized studies investigating the therapeutic concept of perioperative PVI of FU and heparin has been conducted by the NSABP *(21)*. Between 1984 and 1988, a total of 1158 patients with colon cancer without evidence of metastatic disease have been included; they were randomized preoperatively to receive PVI of 600 mg/m^2/d FU plus heparin 5000 U for 7 consecutive days beginning within 6 h of completion of surgery or no treatment. Two hundred seventeen patients were excluded after randomization for stage IV or benign disease, and 43 were ineligible for other reasons. After an average time on study of 89.7 mo, the 5-yr disease-free survival for patients randomized to surgery alone was 60%, compared to 68% for those randomized to FU ($p = 0.01$). The 5-yr overall survival time in the two arms were 71% and 76%, respectively ($p = 0.03$). Rather, in contradiction to the rationale of loco-regional treatment, the beneficial effects in survival could not be attributed to a decrease in the rate of hepatic recurrence. The investigators thought that the advantage of treatment was probably related to a systemic effect of FU.

Fielding and co-workers performed a randomized three-group comparison (control, PVI of 1 g/d FU plus heparin 10,000 U/d, and PVI of heparin alone) *(22)*. There was no reduction in liver metastases or increased overall survival in either active treatment arm of the study. In agreement with the first published analysis of the NSABP trial *(21)*, however, after the third year of follow-up, a beneficial effect was noted for the combined treatment in the subgroup of patients with stage III tumors. The survival advantage was 16% compared with surgery-only controls ($p > 0.03$). Unfortunately, these encouraging data could not be confirmed in a more recent update of the NSABP results *(23)* and also seem to contrast with the outcome of the recently published studies of the European Organization for Research and Treatment of Cancer (EORTC).

After demonstrating the feasibility and safety of PVI of heparin plus FU in a three-group randomized pilot trial involving 235 curatively resected colon cancer patients *(24)*, the Gastro-Intestinal Tract Cancer Cooperative Group (GITCGG) of the EORTC started another randomized controlled multicenter trial: 1235 eligible patients with colon and rectal cancer were randomly assigned surgery plus PVI (500 mg/m^2 FU plus 5000 IU heparin daily for 7 d) or surgery alone. As in their pilot project, no difference in terms of disease-free survival at 5 yr (67% vs 65%), overall survival (73% vs 72%), and the number of patients with liver metastases (79 vs 76) were detectable between the control and the PVI groups *(25)*.

A meta-analysis involving about 4000 patients who were enrolled in randomized trials initiated before 1987, in which short-term continuous postoperative PVI was compared with

Table 1
Prospective Trials of Portal Vein Infusion Chemotherapy

Studies (ref.)	Treatment	Stage type	Eligible patients	Hepatic recurrence (%)	5-yr survival (%)
Taylor et al. (1985)	Control	I–III	127	17.3	42
(7)	FU/heparin		117	4.3, $p = 0.001$	72, $p = 0.002$
Wereldsma (1990)	Control	I–III	102	23	64
(19)	FU/heparin		99	7, $p = 0.01$	72, n.s.
	Urokinase		103		
SAKK (1995)	Control	I–III	253	14.6	55
(17)	FU/MMC/heparin		252	12.3, n.s.	66, $p = 0.02$
Beart et al. (1990)	Control	II, III	109	13	68
(20)	FU/heparin		110	15, n.s.	68, n.s.
Wolmark (1990)	Control	I–III	459	5.9	71
(21)	FU/heparin		442	7, n.s.	76, $p = 0.03$
Nitti et al. (1997)	Control	I–III	72	15.3	69
(24)	Heparin		57	22.8	61
	FU/heparin		70	11.4, n.s.	71, n.s.
Fielding et al. (1992)	Control	I–III	145		77
(22)	Heparin		123		72.7
	FU/heparin		130	n.s.	81.7, n.s.
Rougier et al. (1998)	Control	I–III	619	12.8	73
(25)	FU/heparin		616	12.5, n.s.	72, n.s.
Laffer et al. (1998)	Control	I–III ⎫			72
(18)	PVI FU/MMC/heparin	⎬	769		68
	iv FU/MMC	⎭		n.s.	74, n.s.

Note: FU = 5-fluorouracil; MMC = mitomycin C, n.s. = not statistically significant.

no further treatment, has shown that only the first trial found a significant increase in survival (23). The remaining nine hypothesis-testing trials yielded an absolute survival difference of only 3.6% ($p = 0.04$). Similarly, in contrast to the highly significant reduction in liver metastases seen in the initial study (79% reduction; $p = 0.00000007$), the reduction found in the nine hypothesis testing trials was not significant (14% reduction; $p = 0.2$). At that time, it was concluded that results are encouraging but not definitive.

Meanwhile, the available information has been substantially increased by several additional above-mentioned trials (Table 1), as well as by preliminary results of the Adjuvant X-ray and Infusion Study (AXIS) of the UK Coordinating Committee on Cancer Research (UKCCCR). Between November 1989 and December 1997, 3583 patients were randomized to PVI of FU plus heparin versus control (26). Additionally, rectal cancer patients could be randomized to preoperative or postoperative radiotherapy or no adjuvant radiotherapy. As it concerns PVI, the estimated survival benefit at 5 yr was 2.5%, and the hazard ratio was 0.91 ($p = 0.2$) with the benefit appearing greatest for colon cancer (4.0%). Long-term follow-up of this trial and an update of the meta-analysis should provide a definitive answer (i.e., be able to define reliably the size of any survival benefit achievable with PVI).

To determine whether the combination of PVI plus systemic iv therapy is superior to either modality given alone in patients with colon cancer, a randomized trial was started in 1992 (27). Patients were randomized intraoperatively to PVI of 500 mg/m^2/d FU

× 7 + heparin, 100 mg/m^2 l-leucovorin + 370 mg/m^2 FU both given iv on 5 consecutive days every 4 wk × 6, or PVI + iv chemotherapy. One thousand ninety-four cases were confirmed as eligible. A preliminary analysis performed at a median follow-up time of 35 mo failed to show a significant difference in event-free ($p = 0.26$) and overall survival ($p = 0.18$) and, thus, any synergism between regional and systemic treatment.

2. INTRAPERITONEAL CHEMOTHERAPY

2.1. Rationale of Intraperitoneal Chemotherapy

Intraperitoneal (ip) delivery of chemotherapeutic agents seems to be a reasonable therapeutic strategy in the management of colon cancer for various reasons: First, in addition to disease progression through lymphatics and the vascular compartment, the pattern of disease spread includes direct involvement of the peritoneal cavity: second-look and autopsy assessments, in fact, have demonstrated unsuspected intraperitoneal ± hepatic metastases in as many as 45% of patients *(28–30)*. Second, phase I and pharmacokinetic studies with various anticancer agents, including the fluorinated pyrimidines, have demonstrated presence of tumoricidal drug doses in the abdominal cavity for a prolonged time after instillation *(30)*; using FU or, to a greater extent, floxouridine, 200- to 400-fold greater ip areas under the curve (AUCs) could be achieved compared with those after intravenous therapy *(31,32)*. Additionally, FU is a soluble compound of relatively low molecular weight with an ideal "tumor penetration profile" compared to many other cytotoxic agents *(33)*. Third, cytotoxic agents delivered into the peritoneal cavity principally exit that compartment through the portal circulation. Intraperitoneal drug delivery may thus not only protect peritoneal surfaces but also counteract occult metachronous liver metastases by achieving high intraportal/intrahepatic drug concentrations: After ip administration of fluorinated pyrimidines, up to 10 times the level of drugs is seen in the portal vein than is noted in the peripheral blood *(34,35)*; Archer and co-workers have reported that ip delivery of FU produces comparable portal vein pharmacokinetics as direct intraportal vein administration *(36)*. Fourth, because of the (desired) high portal and liver extraction rate, drug concentrations in the plasma are low, thus reducing the risk of systemic toxicity. Accordingly, the ip route permits the use of FU doses as high as 1.5 times those administered intravenously without toxicity *(34)*; alternatively, systemic IV chemotherapy can be coadministered in order to counteract loco-regional plus systemic micrometastases.

2.2. Clinical Trials of Intraperitoneal Chemotherapy in Colon Cancer

In a small randomized controlled trial involving 66 patients with a high risk of recurrence following resection of colon cancer, Sugarbaker et al. investigated the efficacy of adjuvant intraperitoneal FU compared with intravenous administration of the agent *(34)*. In patients receiving ip chemotherapy, the tolerable dose of drug was markedly increased without an increase in adverse side effects. No difference in disease-free or overall survival was noted between the two treatment groups, although there was a significant decrease in the incidence of recurrence within the peritoneal cavity in patients treated by the intraperitoneal route as documented by second-look surgery. Biopsy-proven recurrent peritoneal carcinomatosis occurred in 2/10 vs 10/11 patients in the ip and iv arm, respectively ($p < 0.003$). This favorable local effect did not translate into an important clinical benefit because of recurrence/progression in the liver, lymph nodes, and outside the cavity, where there was no pharmacokinetic advantage associated with regional drug delivery.

Intraperitoneal FU has also been examined in a nonrandomized trial as adjuvant therapy following resection of hepatic metastases from colorectal cancer, with no evidence of benefit compared with a carefully selected historical control population *(37)*. Similarly, in a trial examining ip FU in patients with unresectable liver metastases from colon cancer, there was no evidence of a benefit from treatment *(38)*. In an effort to enhance the therapeutic potential of regional treatment, ip FU has been administered in combination with leucovorin *(39)* as well as with adjuvant external beam radiation *(40)*. Furthermore, 5-fluoro-2′deoxyuridine (FUDR) has been examined for ip administration, both as single agent *(41)* and in combination with leucovorin, with a marked pharmakokinetic advantage for cavity exposure being observed *(42)*.

2.3. Clinical Trials of Combined Intraperitoneal and Systemic Intravenous Chemotherapy

A number of clinical investigational efforts have been undertaken to determine the therapeutic potential of combined ip and systemic intravenous (iv) chemotherapy. Regional FU has been given simultaneously with continuous iv infusion of the drug, taking maximal advantage of both routes of delivery *(43)*. In another pilot phase I study, Kelsen et al. examined the use of immediate postoperative intraperitoneal floxuridine and leucovorin in 26 patients with colon cancer and a high risk for developing recurrent disease *(44)*. Regional therapy was initiated 2–5 d following surgery and was administered twice daily for 3 d. Therapy was repeated at 2-wk intervals for a total of three courses. Approximately 1 mo following the initiation of the ip regimen, patients also received systemic iv FU plus levamisole. The regional drug delivery program appeared to be well tolerated, with only minor local toxicities. There was no increase in postoperative morbidity and no operative mortality. It seems noteworthy that after a median duration of 18 mo, only four patients had recurrent disease and there was no documented recurrence within the peritoneal cavity.

The first randomized study of adjuvant combined regional and systemic iv chemotherapy in colon cancer was undertaken in Austria *(45)*. Between 1988 and 1990, 121 patients with stage III or high-risk stage II (T4N0M0) were randomly assigned for observation (which was considered standard care until the NIH consensus conference in 1990) or postoperative treatment with 200 mg/m^2 leucovorin plus 350 mg/m^2 FU both given iv (d 1–4) and ip (d 1 and 3) every 4 wk for a total of six courses. After a median follow-up time of almost 5 yr, results suggested an improved disease-free (75% vs 58%; $p = 0.06$) and overall survival (78% vs 63%; $p = 0.05$) in favor of adjuvant treatment. A reduced rate of locoregional and intrahepatic tumor recurrences was noted in the experimental arm, with the benefit appearing greatest in patients with stage III disease. Treatment-associated toxicity was infrequent and generally mild, with only 5% experiencing severe (WHO grade III) adverse reactions.

Based on the encouraging results, a second confirmatory trial of this particular combined ip/iv treatment regimen was initiated *(46)*: The surgery-alone control arm of the former study was replaced by "standard chemotherapy" with FU/levamisole given for a duration of 6 mo. A total of 241 patients, again with resected stage III or high-risk stage II colon cancer, were enrolled. After a median follow-up duration of 4 yr, both an improvement in disease-free survival ($p = 0.0014$) and a survival advantage ($p = 0.0005$), with an estimated 43% reduction in mortality rate in favor of the investigational arm was noted among the 196 patients with stage III tumors. The sample size of patients with stage II disease was considered much too small to elucidate such effect. In agreement with its theoretical concept and the results of the previous trial, ip/iv FU/LV was particularly effective in reducing locoregional (9 vs 25) tumor recurrences and, to a lesser degree, also intrahepatic

(14 vs 23 patients) recurrences. The superior treatment effect when compared to most PVI studies was thought to be related to use of a more effective cytotoxic drug regimen using biochemical modulation of FU, the additive effects of ip plus iv drug administration, as well as the much longer duration of cytotoxic treatment (i.e., 180 rather than 5–7 d, as generally used in trials of adjuvant PVI).

The therapeutic potential of a short-term perioperative ip and iv FU regimen was investigated in a very recently published multicenter randomized trial *(47)*. Two hundred sixty-seven patients with stages II and III colon cancer either received iv 1 g FU intraoperatively, followed by ip 600 mg/m^2/d FU × 6 on d 4–10, or just underwent resection alone. Survival curves were superimposed during the first 3 yr and began diverging thereafter. Five-yr overall survival rates, however, were not significantly different (74% vs 69%). A beneficial effect was only noted in terms of disease-free survival in patients with stage II cancers (89% vs 73%; $p = 0.05$). The authors concluded that perioperative ip/iv short-term chemotherapy should be combined with prolonged systemic treatment to reduce both local and distant recurrences.

This treatment strategy is currently being investigated in the EORTC trial 40911, in which 1850 patients with resected Astler–Coller Stage B2/C colorectal cancer have been entered until thus far. In this double randomized study, patients are randomly assigned to receive or not receive early adjuvant regional chemotherapy (either PVI or ip FU, which is left to the investigators' discretion) plus long-term adjuvant systemic chemotherapy (with FU/levamisole or FU/L-leucovorin). The major study objective is to compare overall and disease-free survival and recurrence rates in patients receiving early postoperative regional therapy prior to systemic treatment vs those who receive only systemic therapy.

2.4. Other Clinical Experiences with Intraperitoneal Therapy

Sugarbaker and co-workers have reported extensive experience with multiagent hyperthermic intraoperative intraperitoneal chemotherapy (HIIC) following aggressive surgical resection of pseudomyxoma peritonei *(see* Chapter 22) *(48)*. A similar intensive combined-modality approach has also been used by this study group for the treatment of peritoneal carcinomatosis from colon cancer with excellent long-term disease-free and overall survival results in a subset of these patients. It remains uncertain, however, what role ip treatment played in the therapeutic outcome. Patients selected for this aggressive local–regional therapeutic approach may not be comparable to other individuals affected by this disease because of potentially more favorable biologic features and differences in performance status and other prognostically important factors. Furthermore, survival might have been improved by debulking/cytoreductive surgery itself rather than subsequent hyperthermic ip chemotherapy *(49)*. Because HIIC can be associated with substantial morbidity even in experienced hands *(50)*, this intensive therapeutic strategy remains clearly investigational and warrants further investigation in well-designed controlled clinical trials.

3. CONCLUSIONS

Adjuvant regional chemotherapy in colorectal cancer, either in the form of perioperative portal vein infusion or of intraperitoneal drug administration, has a profound rational. With approx 10,000 patients having been involved in various randomized studies, the former approach has already undergone extensive clinical evaluation. Although an updated meta-analysis is not yet available, accumulating data including the results of several recently reported large multicenter studies suggest that the size of any survival benefit associated with PVI must be very small, apparently even if combined with conventional postoperative iv chemotherapy *(27)*. One possible explanation for the lack of a more successful realization of this theoretically appealing therapeutic concept may be that PVI regimens should have been optimized first, before attempting to reproduce encouraging pilot data obtained with an empirical regimen. For example, prolonging the duration of treatment, increasing the dose, and/or use of combined administration of FU with biomodulators or other drugs might have resulted in an improved therapeutic outcome. This and other questions remain unanswered unless readdressed and reanalyzed reliably in additional randomized trials, which, however, again would require several thousands of patients.

As it concerns intraperitoneal ± systemic intravenous chemotherapy, only a few studies have been reported until today. Therapeutic results in resected high-risk colon cancer are encouraging, although the study population seems too small to draw any firm conclusions. Thus, clearly, further large multicenter trials will be necessary to determine the true benefits of ip treatment with or without systemic chemotherapy. To avoid the above-mentioned potential problem associated with PVI, additional preclinical and clinical studies in order to define the best suited ip ± iv regimen should be encouraged. Important questions are related to the most effective and best tolerated drug or combination to be used for ip administration [FU/leucovorin, floxouridine with its higher first-pass extraction by the liver, or irinotecan, which has recently been shown to be highly effective in mouse models for counteracting peritoneal seeding and liver metastases *(51)*], improved drug delivery systems [such as the novel polymeric carrier solution icodextrin that seems to allow safe and prolonged ip infusion of chemotherapeutic drugs *(52)*], prevention of potential acute and long-term complications (e.g., risk of infection, adhesion formation), as well as definition of the optimal infusion volume and duration of treatment.

REFERENCES

1. Bengmark S and Hafenström L. The natural history of primary and secondary malignant tumors of the liver. The prognosis for patients with hepatic metastases from colonic and rectal carcinoma by laparotomy. *Cancer*, **23** (1969) 198–204.
2. Cedarmark BJ, Schultz SS, Bakshi S, et al. Value of liver scan in the follow-up of patients with adenocarcinoma of the colon and rectum. *Surg. Gynecol. Obstet.*, **144** (1977) 745–748.
3. Taylor I, Rowling J, and West C. Adjuvant cytotoxic liver perfusion for colorectal cancer. *Br. J. Surg.*, **66** (1979) 833–837.
4. Fisher ER and Turnbull RB. The cytological demonstration and significance of tumor cells in the mesenteric venous blood in patients with colorectal cancer. *Surg. Gynecol, Obstet.*, **100** (1955) 102–106.
5. Dukes CE. Discussion on major surgery in carcinoma of the rectum, with or without colostomy, excluding the anal canal and including the rectosigmoid. *Proc. R. Soc. Med.*, **50** (1957) 1031.
6. Storer EH and Akin TJ. Chemotherapy of hepatic neoplasm on the umbilical portal vein. *Am. J. Surg.*, **111** (1966) 56–58.
7. Taylor I, Machin D, Mullee M, et al. A randomized controlled trial of adjuvant portal vein cytotoxic perfusion in colorectal cancer. *Br. J. Surg.*, **72** (1985) 359–363.
8. Norton L and Simon R. Tumor size, sensitivity to therapy, and design of treatment schedules. *Cancer Treat. Rep.*, **61** (1977) 1307–1317.
9. Salmon SE. Kinetics of minimal residual disease. *Recent Results Cancer Res.*, **67** (1979) 5–15.
10. Cruz EP, McDonald GO, and Cole WH. Prophylactic treatment of cancer: the use of chemotherapeutic agents to prevent tumor metastases. *Surgery*, **40** (1956) 291–296.
11. Almersjö O, Brandenberg A, and Gustavsson B. Concentration of biologically active 5-fluorouracil in general circulation during continuous portal infusion in men. *Cancer Lett.*, **1** (1975) 113–118.
12. Morales F, Bell M, McDonald GO, and Cole WH. The prophylactic treatment of cancer at the time of operation. *Ann. Surg.*, **146** (1957) 588–595.
13. Holden WD and Dixon WJ. A study on the use of triethylenethiophosporamide as an adjuvant to surgery in the treatment of colorectal cancer. *Cancer Chemother. Rep.*, **16** (1962) 129–134.

14. Gray BN, deZwart J, Fisher R, et al. The Australia and New Zealand trial of adjuvant chemotherapy in colon cancer. In *Adjuvant Therapy of Cancer*. 5th ed. Grune & Stratton, New York, 1987, p. 537.

15. Metzger U, Mermillod B, Aeberhard P, et al. Intraportal chemotherapy in colorectal carcinoma as an adjuvant modality. *World J. Surg.*, **11** (1987) 452–458.

16. Metzger U, Laffer U, Castiglione M, and Senn HJ. Adjuvant intraportal chemotherapy for colorectal cancer: 4-year results of the randomized Swiss study. *Proc. Am. Soc. Clin. Oncol.*, **8** (1989) 105 (abstract).

17. Swiss Group for Clinical Cancer Research (SAKK). Long term results of single course of adjuvant intraportal chemotherapy for colorectal cancer. *Lancet* **345** (1995) 349–353.

18. Laffer U, Maibach R, Metzger U, et al. Randomized trial of adjuvant perioperative chemotherapy in radically resected colorectal cancer (SAKK 40/87). *Proc. Am. Soc. Clin. Oncol.*, **17** (1998) 256a (abstract).

19. Wereldsma JCJ, Bruggink EDM, Meijer WS, et al. Adjuvant portal liver infusion in colorectal cancer with 5-fluorouracil/heparin versus urokinase versus control. *Cancer*, **65** (1990) 425–432.

20. Beart RW, Moertel CG, Wieand HS, et al. Adjuvant therapy for resectable colorectal carcinoma with fluorouracil administered by portal vein infusion. *Arch. Surg.*, **125** (1990) 897–901.

21. Wolmark N, Rockette H, Wickerman DL, et al. Adjuvant therapy of Dukes A, B, and C adenocarcinoma of the colon with portal vein fluorouracil hepatic infusion: preliminary results of NSABP protocol C-02. *J. Clin. Oncol.*, **8** (1990) 1466–1475.

22. Fielding LP, Hittinger R, Grace RH, and Fry JS. Randomized controlled trial of adjuvant chemotherapy by portal-vein infusion after curative resection for colorectal adenocarcinoma. *Lancet*, **340** (1992) 502–506.

23. Liver Infusion Meta-analysis Group. Portal chemotherapy for colorectal cancer: a meta-analysis of 4000 patients in 10 studies. *J. Natl. Cancer Inst.*, **89** (1997) 497–505.

24. Nitti D, Wils J, Sahmoud T, et al. Final results of a phase III clinical trial on adjuvant intraportal infusion with heparin and 5FU in resectable colon cancer (EORTC-GITCCG 1983–1987). *Eur. J. Cancer*, **33** (1997) 1209–1215.

25. Rougier P, Sahmoud T, Nitti D, et al. Adjuvant portal-vein infusion of fluorouracil and heparin in colorectal cancer: a randomized trial. *Lancet*, **351** (1998) 1677–1681.

26. James RD. Intraportal 5FU (PVI) and peri-operative radiotherapy (RT) in the adjuvant treatment of colorectal cancer (CRCa)—3681 patients randomized in the UK Coordinating Committee on Cancer Research (UKCCCR) AXIS trial. *Proc. Am. Soc. Clin. Oncol.*, **18** (2000) 264a.

27. Labianca R, Boffi L, Marsoni S, et al. A randomized trial of intraportal (ip) versus systemic (sy) versus ip + sy adjuvant chemotherapy in patients (pts) with resected Dukes B-C colon carcinoma (CC). *Proc. Am. Soc. Clin. Oncol.*, **18** (1999) 264a (abstract).

28. Gunderson LL and Sosin H. Areas of failure found at reoperation (second or symptomatic look) following "curative surgery" for adenocarcinoma of the rectum: clinicopathologic correlation and implications for adjuvant therapy. *Cancer*, **34** (1974) 1278–1292.

29. Tong D, Russell AH, Dawson LE, and Wisbeck W. Second laparotomy for proximal colon cancer: sites of recurrence and implications for adjuvant therapy. *Am. J. Surg.*, **145** (1983) 382–386.

30. Cunliffe WJ and Sugarbaker PH. Gastrointestinal malignancy: rationale for adjuvant therapy using early postoperative intraperitoneal chemotherapy. *Br. J. Surg.*, **76** (1989) 1082–1090.

31. Speyer JL, Collins JM, Dedrick RL, et al. Phase I and pharmacological studies of 5-fluorouracil administered intraperitoneally. *Cancer Res.*, **40** (1908) 567–572.

32. Speyer JL, Sugarbaker PH, Collins JM, et al. Portal levels and hepatic clearance of 5-fluorouracil after intraperitoneal administration in humans. *Cancer Res.*, **41** (1981) 1916–1922.

33. Kerr DJ and Los G. Pharmacokinetic principles of locoregional chemotherapy. *Cancer Surv.*, **17** (1993) 105–122.

34. Sugarbaker PH, Gianola FJ, Speyer JC, et al. Prospective randomized trial of intravenous versus intraperitoneal 5-fluorouracil in patients with advanced primary colon or rectal cancer. *Surgery*, **98** (1985) 414–421.

35. Rougier P and Nordlinger B. Large scale trial for adjuvant treatment in high risk resected colorectal cancers: rationale to test the combination of locoregional and systemic chemotherapy and to compare l-leucovorin + 5-FU to levamisole + 5-FU. *Ann. Oncol.*, **4(Suppl. 2)** (1993) 21–28.

36. Archer SG, McCulloch RK, and Gray BN. A comparative study of the pharmacokinetics of continuous portal vein infusion versus intraperitoneal infusion of 5-fluorouracil. *Reg. Cancer Treat.*, **2** (1989) 105–111.

37. August DA, Sugarbaker PH, Ottow RT, et al. Hepatic resection of colorectal metastases: influences of clinical factors and adjuvant intraperitoneal 5-fluorouracil via Teckhoff catheter on survival. *Ann. Surg.*, **201** (1985) 210–218.

38. Ekberg H, Tranberg KG, Persson B, et al. Intraperitoneal infusion of 5-Fu in liver metastases from colorectal cancer. *J. Surg. Oncol.*, **37** (1988) 94–99.

39. Arbuck SG, Trave F, Douglass HO Jr, et al. Phase I and pharmacologic studies of intraperitoneal leucovorin and 5-fluorouracil in patients with advanced cancer. *J. Clin. Oncol.*, **4** (1986) 1510–1517.

40. Palermo JA, Richards F, Lohman KK, et al. Phase II trial of adjuvant radiation and intraperitoneal 5-fluorouracil for locally advanced colon cancer: results with follow-up. *Int. J. Radiat. Oncol. Biol. Phys.*, **47** (2000) 725–733.

41. Muggia FM, Chan KK, Russell C, et al. Phase I and pharmacological evaluation of intraperitoneal 5-fluoro-2'deoxyuridine. *Cancer Chemother. Pharmacol.*, **28** (1991) 241–250.

42. Reichmann B, Markman M, Tong WP, et al. Phase I trial of intraperitoneal FUDR and leucovorin given every other week. *Proc. Am. Soc. Clin. Oncol.*, **10** (1991) 100 (abstract).

43. Reichmann B, Markman M, Hakes T, et al. Phase I trial of concurrent intraperitoneal and continuous intravenous infusion of 5-fluorouracil in patients with refractory cancer. *J. Cin. Oncol.*, **6** (1988) 158–162.

44. Kelson DP, Saltz L, Cohen AM, et al. A phase I trial of immediate postoperative intraperitoneal floxuridine and leucovorin plus systemic 5-fluorouracil and levamisole after resection of high risk colon cancer. *Cancer*, **74** (1994) 2224–2233.

45. Scheithauer W, Kornek GV, Rosen H, et al. Combined intraperitoneal plus intravenous chemotherapy after curative resection for colonic adenocarcinoma. *Eur. J. Cancer*, **31A** (1995) 1981–1986.

46. Scheithauer W, Kornek GV, Marczell A, et al. Combined intravenous and intraperitoneal chemotherapy with fluorouracil + leucovorin vs fluorouracil + levamisole for adjuvant therapy of resected colon carcinoma. *Br. J. Cancer*, **77** (1998) 1349–1354.

47. Vaillant JC, Nordlinger B, Deuffic S, et al. Adjuvant intraperitoneal 5-fluorouracil in high-risk colon cancer: a multicenter phase III trial. *Ann. Surg.*, **231** (2000) 449–456.

48. Sugarbaker PH and Chang D. Results of treatment of 385 patients with peritoneal surface spread of appendiceal malignancy. *Ann. Surg. Oncol.*, **6** (1999) 727–731.

49. Markman M. Intraperitoneal chemotherapy in the management of colon cancer. *Semin. Oncol.*, **26** (1999) 536–539.

50. Stephens AD, Alderman R, Chang D, et al. Morbidity and mortality analysis of 200 treatments with cytoreductive surgery and hyperthermic intraoperative intraperitoneal chemotherapy using the coliseum technique. *Ann. Surg. Oncol.*, **6** (1999) 790–796.

51. Maruyama M, Nagahama T, and Yuasa Y. Intraperitoneal versus intravenous CPT-11 for peritoneal seeding and liver metastasis. *Anticancer Res.*, **19** (1999) 4187–4191.

52. Kerr DJ, Young AM, Neoptolemos JP, et al. Prolonged intraperitoneal infusion of 5-fluorouracil using a novel carrier solution. *Br. J. Cancer*, **74** (1996) 2032–2035.

34 Molecular Markers of Chemotherapy Resistance in Colorectal Cancer

Peter V. Danenberg

CONTENTS

1. INTRODUCTION

A major obstacle to successful treatment of gastrointestinal (GI) cancer with chemotherapy has been that the majority of tumors prove to be intrinsically resistant to the drugs. The commonly used drug 5-fluorouracil (5-FU), for example, when used as a single agent against colorectal cancer causes tumor shrinkage that would be classified as a response in only about 20–25% of patients *(1,2)*. Thus, the majority of patients not only do not derive any benefit from this drug, but the treatment often does direct harm to the patient in the form of severe toxicity to normal tissues. Nevertheless, without the ability to predict who will or will not respond in advance of the treatment, there has been no recourse but to place all patients suffering from cancer into standard treatment protocols with the full knowledge that many, if not most, will have an unsatisfactory outcome from the treatment.

The major strategy for overcoming the limitations of chemotherapy has been to develop new drugs that might elicit a higher response rate. This approach has been ongoing for a long time at much effort and expense, but only recently have some new drug combinations such as 5-FU and CPT-11 *(3)* or 5-FU plus oxaliplatin *(4,5)* been found to elicit significantly higher response rates than 5-FU alone. The 5-FU/CPT-11 combination, which produces a modestly longer survival than 5-FU/LV (leucovorin) alone, has recently become the "most common standard treatment" for colorectal cancer in the United States. To date, no one drug or combination of drugs has yet to come close to producing a response in all patients.

Another strategy for increasing response rates to chemotherapy is based on the theory that tumors are sensitive or resistant because they have different expressions of biochemical response determinants for a drug. Therefore, the efficacy of the drug should be improvable

From: *Colorectal Cancer: Multimodality Management*
Edited by: L. Saltz © Humana Press Inc., Totowa, NJ

by manipulating the biochemistry of the tumor cells in the appropriate manner *(6)*. The best known example of biochemical modulation is the use of leucovorin along with 5-FU, which increases the inhibition of the target enzyme thymidylate synthase by the active metabolite FdUMP *(7,8)*. Overall, this approach, although attractive in theory, has had limited success to date.

A third approach for improving cancer treatment, which is just in its infancy, is to attempt the prediction of tumor response by measuring biochemical response determinants in each patients' tumor tissue prior to treatment, so that patients judged as probable nonresponders to a drug could then be given alternate therapy immediately. The principal hypothesis behind this approach is that interindividual variations in responses and toxicities are the result of genetic alterations in drug-metabolizing enzymes and/or drug target gene expression. Thus, provided (1) that a number of different agents are available for a particular tumor type and (2) that sensitivity determinants can be identified for each agent and analyzed in patients, it should be possible to get a very high response rate by tailoring the chemotherapy to fit the chemosensitivity profile of the individual tumor. The recent development of ultrasensitive analytical technologies such as real-time polymerase chain reaction (PCR), immunohistochemistry, and DNA array chips makes it realistic to consider implementing the concept of tumor response prediction.

In the case of colorectal cancer, 5-FU-based therapy, either with 5-FU as a single agent or in combination with other drugs, has been a mainstay of the treatment for over 40 yr and serves as a paradigm. In this review, we will describe recent work on the prediction of tumor response to 5-FU-based therapy and how it has been developed using newly available technology, taking into account current knowledge of molecular mechanisms of resistance and sensitivity to the drug.

2. RESPONSE DETERMINANTS TO 5-FU-BASED THERAPY

2.1. Metabolism and Mechanism of 5-FU

Identification of candidate response determinants requires a knowledge of the mechanism of action of drugs, their intracellular targets, and metabolic and anabolic pathways. In the case of 5-FU, over 40 yr of work has elucidated its complex metabolic pathway, which involves multiple-step conversion to the nucleotide forms as well as several different potential sites of activity. This has been well described in previous reviews *(8,9)*. The main route of activation appears to be through direct transfer of a ribosephosphate group to 5-FU mediated by the enzyme orotate phosphoribosyltransferase to give 5-fluorouridine-5′-phosphate (FUMP). Ribonucleotide reductase then converts FUMP to the deoxyribonucleotide FdUMP, the tight-binding inhibitor of thymidylate synthase (TS). The other route of conversion of 5-FU to FdUMP is via the deoxyribonucleoside 5-fluoro-2′-deoxyuridine (FdUrd), catalyzed by the enzyme thymidine phosphorylase. FdUrd is then phosphorylated to FdUMP by thymidine kinase.

The major mechanism of 5-FU cytotoxicity is considered to be its inhibition of TS, resulting in deprivation of thymine nucleotides for DNA synthesis, leading to eventual DNA fragmentation and cell death *(7)*. However, several secondary mechanisms are possible. Because the ribonucleotide of 5-FU, FUTP, is incorporated into RNA, an RNA-directed toxicity has been proposed, although its exact nature is still not well defined. The main piece of evidence for an RNA-directed pathway of 5-FU activity is indirect and is based largely on the observation that thymidine, which should circumvent a blockage of TS, does not usually rescue cells from 5-FU cytotoxicity *(9)*. There is some evidence that RNA splicing may be impacted by incorporated 5-FU residues. 5-FU is also incorporated into DNA by way of its deoxyribonucleotide FdUTP. This can result in DNA fragmentation because of the enzyme uracoyl-DNA glycosylase, which searches for and removes uracil (and thereby also 5-FU) residues from DNA *(1)*. The enzyme dUTPase cleaves FdUTP back to FdUMP, thereby protecting DNA from 5-FU incorporation. In the catabolic pathway, the enzyme dihydropyrimidine dehydrogenase (DPD) reduces 5-FU to dihydro 5-FU, which is the first and rate-limiting step for eventual degradation of 5-FU to fluoro-β-alanine *(10)*. An appreciable number of other enzymes are involved in 5-FU metabolism and activity, but the bulk of the data implicates those listed above as the main candidate biochemical determinants of 5-FU activity. In the next sections, we will summarize the work that has been done to identify mechanisms of resistance to 5-FU in colorectal tumors.

3. GENE EXPRESSION MEASUREMENTS IN COLORECTAL CANCER

Tumor response prediction requires the analysis of the appropriate biochemical response determinants in pretreatment biopsies, which could be available either in the form of fresh–frozen tissue or formalin-fixed paraffin-embedded (FFPE) specimens. Thus, traditional methods of measuring enzyme activities or metabolite levels, which depend on the availability of a fairly large amount of fresh tissue, generally would not be feasible. However, the application of quantitative PCR to this problem made it possible to measure gene expressions in pretreatment biopsy specimens with great sensitivity and accuracy. In order to begin studies in this area, we developed a quantitative reverse transcription (RT)–PCR method *(11)* in which the gene of interest in a sample is amplified along with an internal reference gene, such as β-actin. The reference gene is selected on the basis that its expression is expected to remain at a reasonably constant (constitutive) expression level and thus should represent the cell number in the specimen as well as the total amount of RNA successfully isolated from the specimen. To obtain the gene expression values, the amount of the amplified PCR product of the gene of interest formed within the exponential phase of the PCR amplification is divided by that of the internal reference gene, thus giving the data in the form of a unitless ratio. Comparing the ratios between the gene of interest and the reference gene in different specimens gives the relative expressions of the gene of interest in those specimens. Recently, real-time PCR technology has been developed that uses this same principle, but instead of laborious gel electrophoretic separation of PCR products, it uses a the release of fluorescent probes at each PCR cycle to quantitate the amounts of PCR products *(12)*. This methodology has made quantitative PCR much more rapid and convenient and has made large-scale studies possible.

3.1. TS Gene Expression and Response to Protracted Infusion 5-FU/Leucovorin

Most of the work in the area of tumor response prediction to 5-FU-based therapy has centered on the target enzyme TS in colorectal cancer. In vitro work with cell lines had shown that acquired resistance to fluoropyrimidines, in spite of numerous possible mechanisms of resistance that could be envisaged from the metabolic chart, was most often accompanied by the elevation of TS levels as a result of gene amplification *(13)*. This observation demonstrated that drug resistance could be effectively attained by increasing the amount of the drug's target in the cell and led to the hypothesis that if untreated tumors had variable expressions of TS, the ones with the highest levels should be more resistant to 5-FU. This hypothesis was tested by measurement of TS gene expression (mRNA levels) by means of RT-PCR in pretreatment tumor biopsy specimens.

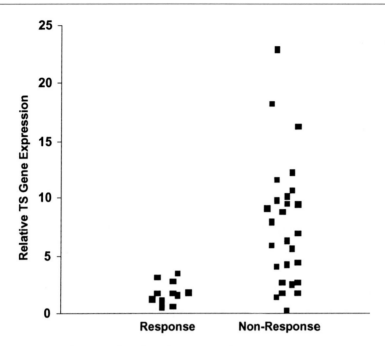

Fig. 1. TS gene expressions as a function of response of colorectal tumors treated with 5-FU/LV.

Leichman et al. *(14,15)* carried out a prospective clinical trial to correlate response with TS gene expression determined by RT-PCR in pretreatment biopsies from 42 measurable disseminated colorectal cancer treated with a 5-FU leucovorin protocol. All of the biopsies were from metastatic sites, mostly in the liver. In this group, 12 patients responded to the treatment and 34 patients were characterized as nonresponding, with 12 of these exhibiting stable disease and 22 who progressed immediately. The results are plotted in Fig. 1. There were two important results from this study: (1) a large overall range of TS gene expressions among these tumors of over 50-fold, which was necessary to have in order to be able to make correlations with clinical outcome, and (2) strikingly different ranges of TS gene expressions between responding and nonresponding tumors. The range of TS values of the responding groups (0.5–4.1) was narrower than that of the nonresponding groups (1.6–23), with the result that there was a "nonresponse cutoff" of TS expression above which there were nonresponders. Thus, patients with TS expression above this "nonresponse" cutoff could be positively identified as nonresponders prior to therapy. Dividing the "no response" classification, which includes all responses with <50% tumor shrinkage, into progressing (>25% increase) and nonprogressing (<50% shrinkage, no change, or <25% increase) categories showed that the progressing tumors had the highest TS values. Thus, high TS expression identifies especially resistant tumors.

In colorectal cancer, tumor response to chemotherapy generally is associated with longer survival *(16)*. In this case also, as shown in Table 1, survival of colorectal patients that showed a response (i.e., had low TS) was over threefold longer than for those that had disease progression.

3.2. TS Expression and Response in Hepatic Artery Infusion

Analysis of TS gene expression was also carried out at the University of Ulm in a set of colorectal cancer patients with liver metastases treated with 5-FU-based chemotherapy

Table 1
Survival of Colorectal Cancer Patients as a Function of Response Category and TS Expression

Response category	TS median and range	Median survival (mo)
Response	2.1 (0.5–3.5)	20
Minimal or no change	4.5 (1.6–9.4)	10
Progression	8.0 (0.3–23)	6

administered by hepatic artery infusion (HAI) *(17)*. All TS expression factors were remarkably similar to those of the set of tumors described in the previously cited study. TS expression values varied over a range of 135-fold and the median TS expression was 3.0. In spite of the fact that other drugs were included along with 5-FU, the nonresponse cutoff of TS expression was 4.2 compared to the value of 4.1 found previously for 5-FU as a single agent. Patients with TS levels below 4.2 were fourfold more likely to respond compared to patients with TS levels above this value. This study also showed that the highest TS values were associated with tumors that progressed under the therapy. Responding patients in this group also had a higher probability of survival (23.5 mo) compared to high-TS nonresponding patients (16.8 mo). In the case of HAI, an additional incentive for identifying nonresponsive patients is to avoid the surgery for device implantation.

3.3. TS Expression in Metastases of Colorectal Cancer

Gorlick et al. *(18)* measured TS expression in colorectal cancer metastases to the lung and the liver of patients. Figure 2 shows that TS expression was substantially higher in each of the lung metastases, which are known to be particularly refractory to treatment. The DNA refers to quantitation of the TS gene copy number relative to actin in the genomic DNA, indicating that transcriptional regulation rather than gene amplification is primarily responsible for the increase in TS mRNA levels.

3.4. p53 Status as a Marker for Response to 5-FU

One of the normal biological roles of the tumor suppressor p53 is to sense DNA damage and either initiate repair or trigger the apoptotic pathway when there is a sufficient level of damage to the cell. Earlier studies have shown that inactivation of p53 by mutation, deletion, or suppression results in cells being more resistant to many different agents, including 5-FU, cisplatin, and radiation *(19)*. Ju et al. *(20)* showed this directly by transfecting wt p53 into HL-60 cells and finding that the transfected cells became significantly more sensitive to 5-FU and FdUrd. Lenz et al. *(21)* tested whether the p53 was a response determinant for colorectal tumors treated with 5-FU/LV. The p53 status in 38 tumors was established by sequencing the p53 gene and by IHC staining with antibody DO-7. The data from this study, summarized in Table 2, show a lower response rate among tumors with mutant p53 than with wt p53. Interestingly, the p53 status appeared to be associated with TS expression: tumors with wt p53 had over a threefold lower average TS expression than among those with altered p53. Thus, it is not clear whether the better response rate of wt p53 tumors is the result of the activity of p53 or to lower TS levels. Most of the mutations were in the known "hotspots," with G273A being the most common mutation. This particular p53 mutant has demonstrated strong transactivating activity toward a p53 consensus binding sequence controlled CAT reporter gene *(22,23)*. All seven tumors with G273A had lower TS gene expression than in tumors with other p53 mutations.

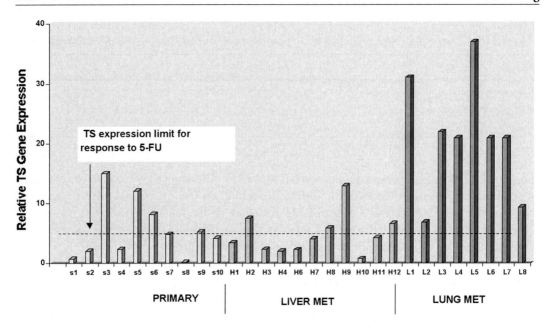

Fig. 2. TS gene expressions in primary, liver metastases, and lung metastases of colorectal cancer.

Table 2
Summary of Results for p53 Status, Tumor Response, and TS Expression

	wt p53	Altered p53
Number	10/38	28/38
(percentage)	(26%)	(74%)
Response to 5-FU/LV	5/10 (50%)	5/28 (18%)
Mean TS expression	1.9	7.1
(p = 0.035)		
Range of TS expression	0.5–6.3	0.3–39.1

The relationship between wt p53 and TS expression was also confirmed by Lenz et al. *(24)*. The original purpose of this study was to determine the association of tumor TS content and p53 status with recurrence, but in this case, instead of gene expression determinations, tumor biopsy specimens were IHC stained for contents of TS with antibody TS 106 and p53 with antibody DO-7. Recurrence was significantly associated with both high-intensity TS staining and with positive staining for p53. Although those tumors with both high TS and p53 overexpression had the highest probability of recurrence (85%), the relative risk from combining the two determinants was only slightly higher than for either one alone (6.0), indicating that p53 and TS expression are not independent risk factors. Indeed, of the 16 tumors that revealed high TS protein expression, 13 also had p53 overexpression in the same tumor sections, indicating a strong association between the p53 nuclear overexpression and the cytoplasmatic TS staining (Table 3).

Table 3
Association Between IHC Staining for p53 and TS in Tumors
from 44 Patients with Stage II Colon Cancer

	p53 positive	p53 negative	Number of patients
High TS staining (≥2)	13 (81%)	3 (19%)	16
Low TS staining (≤1)	5 (18%)	23 (82%)	28

3.5. Thymidine Phosphorylase

Thymidine phosphorylase (TP), which catalyzes the interconversion of thymine and thymidine using deoxyribose-1-phosphate as the second substrate, has been associated with fluoropyrimidine chemotherapy for over 30 yr. Early interest in TP centered on the design of inhibitors of this enzyme, because TP was thought to degrade the powerful drug FdUrd to the less potent 5-FU *(25)*. However, in vitro work has shown that TP can increase the potency of 5-FU by converting it to FdUrd in the presence of deoxyribose donor molecules *(26,27)*. In order to determine the role of TP in tumor response to 5-FU, Metzger et al. *(28)* measured TP gene expression in colorectal tumors treated with 5-FU/leucovorin. Unexpectedly, a pattern similar to that of TS expression was obtained; that is, higher levels of TP, instead of causing the tumors to be more responsive by activating the 5-FU to FdUrd, were actually associated with nonresponding tumors. This was explained on the basis that TP is also a angiogenic molecule, known in that role as platelet-derived endothelial cell growth factor (PD-ECGF) *(29)*, and therefore that high levels of TP may simply identify more aggressive and drug-resistant tumors. TP and TS gene expressions were shown to be independently regulated, and an important finding from this study was that if TP and TS were combined as response indicators, a much higher response prediction could be obtained. These data showed that whereas low TS expression (<4.1) predicts a response rate of 50%, patients with low TS and low TP (<18) could expect an 80% response rate.

3.6. Dihydropyrimidine Dehydrogenase

As discussed earlier, dihydropyrimide dehydrogenase (DPD) is a catabolic enzyme which reduces the 5,6 double bond of 5-FU, thus inactivating it as a cytotoxic agent. A number of previous studies had shown that DPD levels in normal tissues could influence the bioavailability of 5-FU, and thereby its pharmacokinetics and anti-tumor activity *(30)*. Evidence had been presented in earlier studies that DPD levels in tumors are also associated with sensitivity to 5-FU *(31,32)*. Salonga et al. *(33)* investigated gene expression of DPD as a response determinant for 5-FU/leucovorin in the same set of tumors in which TS and TP had already been determined. As with TS and TP, the range of DPD expression among the responding tumors was relatively narrow (0.6–2.5, 4.2-fold) compared with that of the nonresponding tumors (0.2–16, 80-fold). There were no responding tumors with a DPD expression > 2.5. Furthermore, DPD and TS expression values showed no correlation, indicating that they were independently regulated. Among the group of 12 tumors having both TS and DPD expressions below the respective nonresponse cutoff values, 11 were responders and only 1 was a nonresponder to 5-FU/LV, equivalent to a 92% response rate. The one tumor not predicted by TS and DPD was identified as a nonresponder by a high TP expression above its cutoff of 18. Thus, all of the responding tumors could be identified by

Table 4
Summary of Response Data for Tumors with Different Expressions of DPD, TS and TP Genes

Gene expression status (values × 10⁻³)	No. of responding patients	No. of nonresponding patients	p-Value (Fisher's two-tail exact test)
DPD < 2.5 (n = 22)	11	11	0.005
DPD > 2.5 (n = 11)	0	11	
DPD < 2.5, TS < 4.1, and TP < 18 (n = 11)	11	0	0.0001
DPD > 2.5 or TS > 4.1 or TP > 18 (n = 22)	0	22	

low expression values of DPD, TS, or TP, as summarized in Table 4. These data dramatically illustrate how combining more than one independent response determinant can increase the predictive power for clinical outcome.

Figure 3 is a graphical illustration of these data. Two striking observations emerge from an inspection of this graph: (1) The transition from responding to nonresponding tumors is accompanied by substantial disregulation of gene expression and (2) all of the tumors are quite different as to the pattern of expression of these three marker genes.

3.7. Alternative Treatments to 5-FU: CPT-11

The question can be raised of whether a high TS level in a tumor specifically predicts for resistance to 5-FU or if it is an indication of a generally refractory, multidrug resistant tumor. The alternative drug CPT-11 (irinotecan) is now available for treatment of colorectal cancer patients. CPT-11 is converted in vivo to an active form called SN-38, which then binds to the "cleavable complex" of topoisomerase I (topo I) and DNA *(34)*. SN-38 stabilizes the enzyme within the cleavable complex and inhibits the religation step, resulting eventually in single-strand DNA breaks *(34)*. The data in Fig. 3 show that four tumors with TS expression levels that would put them into the group not expected to respond to 5-FU or, indeed, have already been treated and have failed 5-FU, do respond to CPT-11 *(35)*. In fact, preliminary results form this laboratory suggest that high TS patients may even be predisposed to respond better to CPT-11: Among a group of patients that had failed 5-FU, the response rate of low TS (TS < 4.1) tumors to CPT-11 (as a single agent) was 15% (10/59), but the response rate of high TS tumors (TS > 4.1) was 43% (16/37) (Danenberg, unpublished results). One possible explanation for this observation is that the expressions of topo I and TS are coregulated. In that case, tumors with high TS would also tend to have high topo I. This should, in theory, increase the sensitivity of the tumors to CPT-11 because a greater number of potential topo I–DNA cleavable complex binding sites for CPT-11 would increase the possibility of DNA strand-breakage events. In fact, topo I activity was found to be higher in ovarian cancer patients responding to CPT-11 than in nonresponders *(36)*. The coregulation of TS and topo I may be mediated through the transcription factor protein E2F, which is thought to regulate the transcription of a number of genes involved in DNA synthesis *(37)*. In vitro studies have shown that transfection of the E2F gene into cells increased the levels of TS *(38)*. These cells acquired resistance to 5-FU because of the higher TS level but, interestingly,

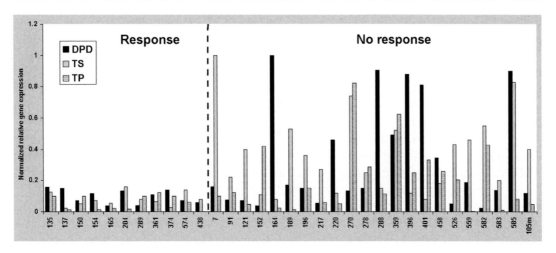

Fig. 3. Normalized TS, TP, and DPD gene expressions in advanced colorectal tumors as a function of response to 5-FU/LV.

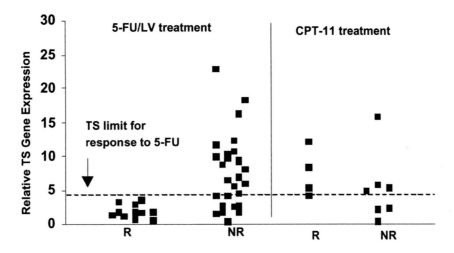

Fig. 4. TS gene expression as a function of response to 5-FU/LV (left panel) and to CPT-11 (right panel).

were more sensitive to CPT-11. The in vivo connection between TS and E2F is confirmed by a recent study *(39)* showing that E2F expression, just as TS expression, was elevated in pulmonary metastases of colorectal cancer and that the E2F and TS expressions correlated very closely in this tissue.

4. COLORECTAL CANCER CHEMOSENSITIVITY DETERMINANTS STUDIED BY IHC

4.1. TS Protein Expression and Response to 5-FU/LV

The development of TS-specific monoclonal antibody TS 106 by investigators at the National Cancer Institute *(40)* made it possible to detect femtomolar amounts of TS protein and to carry out correlative studies of TS protein content of tumors and response to fluoropyrimidines. In general, the results of measuring TS protein expression and TS gene expression have led to similar conclusions.

The first study using TS 106 to assess the association of TS protein level with chemotherapeutic benefit was carried out by Johnston et al. *(41)* in rectal cancer patients given either adjuvant treatment with 5-FU-based chemotherapy or no treatment. The results of this study showed that 38% of patients with high TS were disease-free after 5 yr when treated with chemotherapy compared to 17% of high TS patients treated with surgery alone, whereas in the low TS group, there was no difference in survival between the two groups. This result appears at first somewhat puzzling because, although TS expression was found to be an independent prognostic factor of disease-free survival (and overall survival), the effect seems to be the opposite of what might be predicted (i.e., that chemotherapy with 5-FU would have the greatest effect on patients with low TS tumors). The explanation for this observation probably lies in the fact that low TS patients overall with or without adjuvant therapy had such a dramatically better 5-yr disease-free survival than the high TS patients (49% vs 27%, respectively) that the administration of the drugs was not able to improve on an already optimal survival situation. A later study *(42)* confirmed that TS protein expression in rectal cancer was an independent prognostic factor for local recurrence, distant metastases disease-free survival, and overall survival in rectal cancer. Again, patients with low TS had a significantly better outcome than those with high levels of TS protein.

Thymidylate synthase protein expression was also shown to be a predictor of response of colorectal tumors to 5-FU-based therapy. Davies et al. *(43)* studied the association of colorectal liver metastasis staining for TS expression with antibody TS 106 with response to hepatic artery infusion (HAI) of FdUrd (floxuridine) infusion. TS staining intensity in this study was designated at only two levels: "low" or "high." The TS protein level was found to be associated with tumor response: 75% of patients with partial response had low TS compared to 29% of nonresponders. Among low TS patients, there were 9/16 responses, but only 3/20 among high TS staining tumors. Thus, although a statistically significant difference was seen in response rates among low and high TS staining tumors, these results nevertheless indicate that IHC staining cannot be used to reliably identify nonresponding patients on an individual basis because some tumors with high TS will be found among the responders.

Paradiso et al. *(44)* performed a study to determine the association of TS protein expression and p53 status with response of advanced colorectal tumors to chemotherapy with 5-FU modulated by methotrexate (MTX) (an example of the biochemical modulation approach mentioned in Section 1.). Objective responses occurring in 30% of the tumors staining negatively for TS had objective responses compared to 15% of tumors staining positively. In contrast to the previously cited study of Lenz et al. *(21,24)*, no relationship was seen solely between p53 status and tumor response. The response rate was 20% in tumors that stained positively for p53 and 23% in negatively staining tumors. However, when both TS and p53 status were combined, a dramatic improvement in tumor response prediction resulted: the response rate for p53-positive–TS-positive tumors was 7%, whereas for p53-positive–TS-negative tumors, it was 46%.

McKay et al. *(45)* obtained somewhat different results, at least with regard to TS. They employed an enrichment approach to the identification of tumor response markers. They selected the best and worst responders to a standard 5-FU/LV regimen from a population of cancer patients, such that a significantly different survival could be expected for these defined patient groups. Examination of a panel of candidate response determinants in metastatic deposits showed that bcl-2 status correlated with clinical response, whereas no clear association was seen between response and a number of other factors, including p53, TP, TS, Dukes' stage, or histological grade.

In a subset of the colorectal tumors studied by Leichman et al. *(14)*, TS protein was also analyzed by IHC staining with monoclonal antibody TS 106. There was a good correlation ($r^2 = 0.6$) between TS gene expression and TS protein when the latter was measured by Western blot analysis of tumor tissue lysates *(41)*. However, the correspondence of gene expression values with IHC staining of the corresponding FFPE specimens was not as good. Even in the small set of tumors studied, there were several cases in which no immunostaining was detected, even though the tumors showed both TS gene expression and TS protein detected by Western blotting. These results suggest that, in some cases, IHC staining for TS content can give false-negative results, and support the conclusion stated earlier that caution is indicated for using this methodology in making tumor response predictions on an individual basis.

5. SUMMARY

The approach of tumor response prediction prior to therapy by measuring tumor response determinants has been "built in" into the clinical protocol in only one published case—that of her2-neu expression as a marker for treatment of breast cancer with herceptin *(46)*. However, the work summarized here adequately demonstrates that it is possible to predict response to other drugs as well. The clinical implementation of this approach should be pursued vigorously in the interest of presenting the optimal treatment options for all patients.

REFERENCES

1. Grem JL. 5-Fluorouracil plus leucovorin in cancer therapy. In *Principles and Practice of Oncology*. De Vita VT Jr., Hellman S, and Rosenberg SA (eds.), UpdateSeries. JB Lippincott, Philadelphia, 1988, Vol. 2(7).
2. Moertel CG. Chemotherapy for colorectal cancer. *N. Engl. J. Med.*, **330** (1994) 1136–1142.
3. Saltz LB, Cox JV, Blanke C, Rosen LS. Fehrenbacher L, Moore MJ, et al. Irinotecan plus fluorouracil and leucovorin for metastatic colorectal cancer. Irinotecan Study Group. *N. Engl. J. Med.*, **343** (2000) 905–914.
4. Bleiberg H. and de Gramont A. Oxaliplatin plus 5-FU: clinical experience in patients with advanced colorectal cancer. *Semin. Oncol.*, **25** (1998) 32–39.
5. Raymond E, Faivre S, Woynarowski JM, and Chaney SG. Oxaliplatin: mechanism of action and antineoplastic activity. *Semin. Oncol.*, **25** (1998) 4–12.
6. Soros GA, Grogan LM, and Allegra CJ. Preclinical and clinical aspects of biomodulation of 5-fluorouracil. *Cancer Treat. Rev.*, **20** (1994) 11–49.
7. Danenberg PV. Thymidylate synthetase: a target enzyme in cancer chemotherapy. *Biochim. Biophys. Acta*, **473** (1977) 73–92.
8. Pinedo HM and Peters GF. Fluorouracil: biochemistry and pharmacology. *J. Clin. Oncol.*, **6** (1988) 16,753–16,764.
9. Heidelberger C, Danenberg PV, and Moran RG. Fluorinated pyrimidines and their nucleosides. *Adv. Enzymol. Related Areas Mol. Biol.*, **54** (1983) 58–119.
10. Naguib FNM, El Kouni AM, and Cha S. Enzymes of uracil catabolism in normal and neoplastic human tissues. *Cancer Res.*, **45** (1985) 5405–5412.
11. Horikoshi T, Danenberg KD, Stadlbauer THW, Volkenandt M, Shea LLC, Aigner K, et al. Quantitation of thymidylate synthase, dihydrofolate reductase, and DT-diaphorase gene expression in human tumors using the polymerase chain reaction. *Cancer Res.*, **52** (1992) 108–116.
12. Heid CA, Stevens J, Livak KJ, and Williams PPM. Real-time quantitative PCR. *Genome Res.*, **6** (1996) 995–1001.
13. Copur S, Aiba K, Drake JC, et al. Thymidylate synthase gene amplification in human colon cancer cell lines resistant to 5-fluorouracil. *Biochem. Pharmacol.*, **49** (1995) 1419–1426.
14. Leichman L, Lenz H-J, Leichman CG, Groshen S, Danenberg KD, Baranda J, et al. Quantitation of intratumoral thymidylate synthase expression predicts for resistance to protracted infusion of 5-fluorouracil and weekly leucovorin in disseminated colorectal cancers. *Eur. J. Cancer*, **31** (1995) 1306–1310.

15. Leichman CG, Lenz H-J, Leichman L, Danenberg K, Baranda J, Groshen S, et al. Quantitation of intratumoral thymidylate synthase expression predicts for disseminated colorectal cancer response and resistance to protracted infusion 5-fluorouracil and weekly leucovorin. *J. Clin Oncol.*, **15** (1997) 3223–3229.

16. Graf W, Pahlman L, Beregstrom R, and Glimelius B. The relationship between and objective response to chemotherapy and survival in colorectal cancer. *Br. J. Cancer*, **70** (1994) 559–563.

17. Kornmann M, Link KH, Lenz HJ, Pillasch J, Butzer U, Leder G, et al. Quantitation of intratumoral thymidylate synthase predicts response and resistance to hepatic artery infusion with fluoropyrimdines in patients with colorectal liver metastases. *Cancer Lett.*, **118** (1997) 29–35.

18. Gorlick R, Metzger R, Danenberg KD, Salonga D, Miles JS, Longo GSA, Fu J, et al. Higher levels of thymidylate synthase gene expression are observed in pulmonary as compared to heaptic metastases of colorectal adenocarcinoma. *J. Clin. Oncol.*, **16** (1998) 1465–1469.

19. Lowe SW, Bodis S, McClatchey A, et al. p53 Status and the efficacy of cancer therapy in vivo. *Science*, **266** (1994) 807–810.

20. Ju J-F, Banerjee D, Lenz H-J, Danenberg KD, Schmittgen TC, Spears CP, et al. Restoration of wild-type p53 activity in p53-null HL-60 cells confers multi-drug sensitivity. *Clin. Cancer Res.*, **4** (1998) 1315–1323.

21. Lenz HJ, Hayashi K, Metzger R, Danenberg K, Salonga D, Banerjee D, et al. p53 Point mutations and thymidylate synthase mRNA levels in disseminated colorectal cancer: an analysis of response and survival. *Clin. Cancer Res.*, **4** (1998a) 1243–1251.

22. Miller CW, Chumakow A, Said J, Chen DL, Aslo A, and Koeffler HP. Mutant p53 proteins have diverse intracellular abilities to oligomerize and activate transcription. *Oncogene*, **8** (1993) 1815–1824.

23. Park DJ, Nakamura H, Chumakov AM, Said JW, Miller CW, Chen DL, et al. Transactivational and DNA binding abilities of endogenous p53 in p53 mutant cell lines. *Oncogene*, **9** (1994) 1899–1906.

24. Lenz H-J, Danenberg KD, Leichman CG, Florentine B, Johnston PG, Groshen S, et al. p53 and thymidylate synthase expression in untreated stage II colon cancer: Associations with recurrence, survival and site. *Clin. Cancer Res.*, **4** (1998b) 1227–1235.

25. Birnie GD, Kroeger H, and Heidelberger C. Studies of fluorinated pyrimidines. XVIII. The degradation of 5-fluoro-2'-deoxyuridine and related compounds by nucleoside phosphorylase. *Biochemistry*, **2** (1963) 566–572.

26. Santelli G and Birnie F. In vivo potentiation of 5-fluorouracil toxicity against AKR leukemia by purines, pyrimidines, and their nucleosides and deoxynucleosides. *J. Natl. Cancer Inst.*, **64** (1980) 69–72.

27. Schwartz EL, Baptiste N, Wadler S, and Makower D. Thymidine phosphorylase mediates the sensitivity of colon carcinoma cells to 5-fluorouracil. *J. Biol. Chem.*, **270** (1995) 19,073–19077.

28. Metzger R, Danenberg KD, Leichman CG, Salonga D, Schwartz EL, Wadler S, et al. High basal level gene expression of thymidine phosphorylase (platelet-derived endothelial cell growth factor) in colorectal tumors is associated with non-response to 5-fluorouracil. *Clin. Cancer Res.*, **4** (1998) 2371–2376.

29. Usuki K, Saras J, Waltenberger J, Miyazono K, Pierce G, Thomason A, et al. Platelet-derived endothelial cell growth factor has thymidine phosphorylase activity. *Biochem. Biophys. Res. Commun.*, **184** (1992) 1311–1316.

30. Harris BE, Song R, He YJ, Soong SJ, and Diasio RB. Relationship between dihydropyrimidine dehydrogenase activity and plasma drug levels in cancer patients receiving 5-fluorouracil by protracted continuous infusion. *Cancer Res.*, **50** (1990) 197–201.

31. Beck A, Etienne MC, Cheradame S, Fischel JL, Formento P, Renee N, et al. A role for dihydropyrimidine dehydrogenase and thymidylate synthase in tumor sensitivity to 5-fluorouracil. *Eur. J. Cancer*, **30** (1994) 1517–1522.

32. Etienne MC, Cheradame S, Fischel JL, Formento P, Dassonville O, Renee N, et al. Response to fluorouracil therapy in cancer patients: the role of intratumoral dihydropyrimidine dehydrogenase activity. *J. Clin. Oncol.*, **13** (1995) 1663–1670.

33. Salonga D, Danenberg KD, Johnson M, Metzger R, Groshen S, Tsao-Wei DD, et al. Colorectal tumors responding to 5-fluorouracil have low gene expression levels of dihydropyrimidine dehydrogenase, thymidylate synthase, and thymidine phosphorylase. *Clin. Cancer Res.*, **6** (2000) 1322–1327.

34. Pommier Y. Cellular determinants of sensitivity and resistance to camptothecins. In *Camptothecins: New Anticancer Agents*. Potmesil M and Pinedo H (eds.), CRC, Boca Raton, FL, 1995.

35. Saltz L, Danenberg K, Paty P, et al. High thymidylate synthase (TS) expression does not preclude activity of CPT-11 in colorectal cancer (CRC). *Proc. Am. Soc. Clin. Oncol.*, **17** (1998) 281.

36. Kigawa J, Takahashi M, Minagawa Y, Oishi T, Sugiyama T, Yakushiji M, et al. Topoismerase-I activity and response to second-line chemotherapy consisting of camptothecin-11 and cisplatin in patients with ovarian cancer. *Int. J. Cancer*, **84** (1999) 521–524.

37. DeGregori J, Kowalik T, and Nevins JR. Cellular targets for activation by the E2F1 transcription factor include DNA synthesis and G1/S-regulatory genes. *Mol. Cell. Biol.*, **15** (1995) 4215–4224.

38. Banerjee D, Schnieders B, Fu JZ, Adhikari D, Zhao SC, and Bertino JR. Role of E2F-1 in chemosensitivity. *Cancer Res.*, **58(19)** (1998) 4292–4296.
39. Banerjee D, Gorlick R, Liefshitz A, Danenberg K, Danenberg PC, Danenberg PV, et al. Levels of E2F-1 expression are higher in lung metastasis of colon cancer as compared with hepatic metastasis and correlate with levels of thymidylate synthase. *Cancer Res.*, **60** (2000) 2365–2368.
40. Johnston PG, Liang CM, Henry S, Chabner BA, and Allegra CJ. Production and characterization of monoclonal antibodies that localize human thymidylate synthase in the cytoplasm of human cells and tissue. *Cancer Res.*, **51** (1991) 6668–6676.
41. Johnston PG, Fisher ER, Rockette HE, Fisher B, Wolmark N, Drake JC, et al. The role of thymidylate synthase expression in prognosis and outcome of adjuvant chemotherapy in patients with rectal cancer. *J. Clin. Oncol.*, **12** (1994) 2640–2647.
42. Edler D, Kressner U, Ragnhammar P, Johnston PG, Magnusson I, Glimelius B, et al. Immunohistochemically detected thymidylate synthase in colorectal cancer: an independent prognostic factor of survival. *Clin. Cancer Res.*, **6** (2000) 488–492.
43. Davies MM, Johnston PG, Kaur S, and Allen-Mersh TG. Colorectal liver metastasis thymidylate synthase staining correlates with response to hepatic arterial floxuridine. *Clin. Cancer Res.*, **5** (1999) 325–328.
44. Paradiso A, Simone G, Petroni S, Leone B, Vallejo C, Lacava J, et al. Thymidilate synthase and p53 primary tumour expression as predictive factors for advanced colorectal cancer patients. *Br. J. Cancer*, **82** (2000) 560–567.
45. McKay JA, Lloret C, Murray GI, Johnston PG, Bicknell R, Ahmed FY, et al. Application of the enrichment approach to identify putative markers of response to 5-fluorouracil therapy in advanced colorectal carcinomas. *Int. J. Oncol.*, **17** (2000) 153–158.
46. Stebbing J, Copson E, and O'Reilly S. Herceptin (trastuzamab) in advanced breast cancer. *Cancer Treat. Rev.*, **26** (2000) 287–290.

V   SUPPORTIVE MANAGEMENT

35 Cancer Pain Syndromes in Colorectal and Anal Cancers

Nathan I. Cherny

CONTENTS

1. INTRODUCTION

Patients with colorectal cancer are heterogeneous in their experience of pain and symptom distress. Clinicians who care for these patients must be prepared to manage a diverse spectrum of problems, ranging from the treatment of acute procedure-related pain to the management of chronic unremitting pain in patients with advanced disease *(1)*. Although established analgesic strategies can benefit most patients, undertreatment is common.

Surveys indicate that pain is experienced by 30–60% of cancer patients during active therapy and more than two-thirds of those with advanced disease *(2)*. This has been corroborated in a series of recent studies which identified a pain prevalence of 28% among patients with newly diagnosed cancer *(3)*, 50–70% among patients receiving active anti-cancer therapy *(4,5)* and 64–80% among patients with far advanced disease *(6–8)*.

Unrelieved pain is incapacitating and precludes a satisfying quality of life; it interferes with physical functioning and social interaction, and is strongly associated with heightened psychological distress. Persistent pain interferes with the ability to eat *(9)*, sleep *(10,11)*, think, and interact with others *(12,13)* and is correlated with fatigue in cancer patients *(14)*. The presence of pain can provoke or exacerbate existential distress *(15)* disturb normal processes of coping and adjustment *(16)* and augment a sense of vulnerability, contributing to a preoccupation with the potential for catastrophic outcomes *(16)*.

The high prevalence of acute and chronic pain among cancer patients, and the profound psychological and physical burdens engendered by this symptom, oblige all treating clinicians to be skilled in pain management *(17–21)*. Relief of pain in cancer patients is an ethical imperative and it is incumbent upon clinicians to maximize the knowledge, skill, and diligence needed to attend to this task.

From: *Colorectal Cancer: Multimodality Management*
Edited by: L. Saltz © Humana Press Inc., Totowa, NJ

The undertreatment of cancer pain, which continues to be common *(19,22)*, has many causes, among the most important of which is inadequate assessment *(23,24)*.

2. APPROACH TO CANCER PAIN ASSESSMENT

Assessment is an ongoing and dynamic process that includes evaluation of presenting problems, elucidation of pain syndromes and pathophysiology, and formulation of a comprehensive plan for continuing care. The objectives of cancer pain assessment include (1) the accurate characterization of the pain, including the pain syndrome and inferred pathophysiology and (2) the evaluation of the impact of the pain and the role it plays in the overall suffering of the patient.

This assessment is predicated on the establishment of a trusting relationship with the patient in which the clinician emphasizes the relief of pain and suffering as central to the goal of therapy, and encourages open communication about symptoms. The prevalence of pain is so great that an open-ended question about the presence of pain should be included at each patient visit in routine oncological practice. If the patient is either unable or unwilling to describe the pain, a family member may need to be questioned to assess the distress or disability of the patient.

2.1. Pain Syndromes

Cancer pain syndromes are defined by the association of particular pain characteristics and physical signs with specific consequences of the underlying disease or its treatment. Syndromes are associated with distinct etiologies and pathophysiologies, and have important prognostic and therapeutic implications. Pain syndromes associated with cancer can be either acute (Table 1) or chronic (Table 2). Whereas acute pains experienced by cancer patients are usually related to diagnostic and therapeutic interventions, chronic pains are most commonly caused by direct tumor infiltration. Adverse consequences of cancer therapy, including surgery, chemotherapy, and radiation therapy, account for 15–25% of chronic cancer pain problems, and a small proportion of the chronic pains experienced by cancer patients are caused by pathology unrelated to either the cancer or the cancer therapy.

2.2. Pain Characteristics

The evaluation of pain characteristics provides some of the data essential for syndrome identification. These characteristics include intensity, quality, distribution, and temporal relationships.

2.2.1. INTENSITY

The evaluation of pain intensity is pivotal to therapeutic decision-making *(25,26)*. It indicates the urgency with which relief is needed and influences the selection of analgesic drug, route of administration, and rate of dose titration *(25)*.

2.2.2. QUALITY

The quality of the pain often suggests its pathophysiology. Somatic nociceptive pains are usually well localized and described as sharp, aching, throbbing or pressure-like. Visceral nociceptive pains are generally diffuse and may be gnawing or crampy when resulting from obstruction of a hollow viscus, or aching, sharp or throbbing when resulting from involvement of organ capsules or mesentery *(27,28)*. Neuropathic pains may be described as burning, tingling or shock-like (lancinating).

Table 1
Acute Pain Syndromes in Colorectal and Anal Cancer

Acute pain associated with diagnostic and therapeutic interventions
    Acute pain associated with diagnostic interventions
        Arterial or venous blood sampling
        Lumbar puncture
        Colonoscopy
        Myelography
        Percutaneous biopsy
    Acute postoperative pain
    Acute pain caused by other therapeutic interventions
        Pleurodesis
        Tumor embolization
        Suprapubuc catheterization
        Intercostal catheter
        Nephrostomy insertion
    Acute pain associated with analgesic techniques
        Injection pain
        Opioid headache
        Spinal opioid hyperalgesia syndrome
        Epidural injection pain
Acute pain associated with anticancer therapies
    Acute pain associated with chemotherapy infusion techniques
        Intravenous infusion pain
        Hepatic artery infusion pain
        Intraperitoneal chemotherapy abdominal pain
    Acute pain associated with chemotherapy toxicity
        Mucositis
        Corticosteroid-induced perineal discomfort
        Steroid pseudorheumatism
        Colony stimulating factor-induced bone pain
        5-Flurouracil-induced anginal chest pain
    Acute pain associated with immunotherapy
        Interferon (IFN)-induced acute pain
    Acute pain associated with radiotherapy
        Incident pains
        Acute radiation enteritis and proctocolitis
        Subacute radiation myelopathy
Acute pain associated with infection
    Acute herpetic neuralgia
    Abdominal or pelvic abscess

2.2.3. Distribution

Patients with cancer pain commonly experience pain at more than one site *(5,29,30)*. The distinction between focal, multifocal and generalized pain may be important in the selection of therapy, such as nerve blocks, radiotherapy or surgical approaches. Focal pains can be distinguished from those that are referred to a site remote from the lesion. Familiarity with pain referral patterns is essential to target appropriate diagnostic and therapeutic maneuvers *(31,32)* (Table 3). For example, a patient who develops progressive shoulder pain and has no

Table 2
Chronic Pain Syndromes in Colorectal and Anal Cancer

Tumor-related pain syndromes
    Visceral pain syndromes
        Hepatic distention syndrome
        Midline retroperitoneal syndrome
        Chronic intestinal obstruction
        Peritoneal carcinomatosis
        Malignant perineal pain
        Malignant pelvic floor myalgia
        Ureteric obstruction
    Pain syndromes due to tumor involvement of the peripheral nervous system
        Malignant lumbosacral plexopathy and radiculopathy
    Bone pain syndromes
        Vertebral syndromes
        Back pain and epidural (spinal cord and cauda equina) compression
        Pain syndromes of the bony pelvis and hip
    Headache and facial pain syndromes
        Intracerebral tumor
        Leptomeningeal metastases
        Base of skull metastases
        Painful cranial neuralgias
Chronic pain syndromes associated with cancer therapy
    Post-chemotherapy pain syndromes
        Avascular necrosis of femoral or humeral head
        Plexopathy associated with intraarterial infusion
    Chronic post-surgical pain syndromes
        Phantom anus pain
        Postsurgical pelvic floor myalgia
    Chronic post-radiation pain syndromes
        Radiation-induced lumbosacral plexopathy
        Chronic radiation enteritis and proctitis
        Burning perineum syndrome
    Chronic radiation myelopathy
    Osteoradionecrosis

evidence of focal pathology needs to undergo evaluation of the region above and below the diaphragm to exclude the possibility of referred pain from diaphragmatic irritation.

2.2.4. TEMPORAL RELATIONSHIPS

Cancer-related pain may be acute or chronic. Acute pain is defined by a recent onset and a natural history characterized by transience. The pain is often associated with overt pain behaviors (such as moaning, grimacing, and splinting), anxiety, or signs of generalized sympathetic hyperactivity, including diaphoresis, hypertension, and tachycardia. Chronic tumor-related pain is usually insidious in onset, often increases progressively with tumor growth, and may regress with tumor shrinkage. Overt pain behaviors and sympathetic hyperactivity are often absent, and the pain may be associated with affective disturbances (anxiety and/or depression) and vegetative symptoms, such as asthenia, anorexia and sleep disturbance *(33–36)*.

Table 3
Common Patterns Of Pain Referral

Pain mechanism	Site of lesion	Referral site
Visceral	Diaphragmatic irritation	Shoulder
	Urothelial tract	Inguinal region and genitalia
Somatic	C7-T1 vertebrae	Interscapular
	L1-2	Sacroiliac joint and hip
	Hip joint	Knee
	Pharynx	Ipsilateral ear
Neuropathic	Nerve or plexus	Anywhere in the distribution of a peripheral nerve
	Nerve root	Anywhere in the corresponding dermatome
	Central nervous system	Anywhere in the region of the body innervated by the damaged structure

Transitory exacerbations of severe pain over a baseline of moderate pain or less may be described as "breakthrough pain" *(37)*. Breakthrough pains are common in both acute or chronic pain states. These exacerbations may be precipitated by volitional actions of the patient (so-called incident pains), such as movement, micturition, cough or defecation, or by nonvolitional events, such as bowel distention. Spontaneous fluctuations in pain intensity can also occur without an identifiable precipitant.

2.3. Inferred Pain Mechanisms

Inferences about the mechanisms that may be responsible for the pain are helpful in the evaluation of the pain syndrome and in the management of cancer pain. The assessment process usually provides the clinical data necessary to infer a predominant pathophysiology.

2.3.1. NOCICEPTIVE PAIN

"Nociceptive pain" describes pain that is perceived to be commensurate with tissue damage associated with an identifiable somatic or visceral lesion. The persistence of pain is thought to be related to ongoing activation of nociceptors. Nociceptive pain that originates from somatic structures (somatic pain) is usually well localized and described as sharp, aching, burning or throbbing. As previously described, pain that arises from visceral structures (visceral pain) is generally diffuse, and pain characteristics may differ depending on the involved structures. From the clinical perspective, nociceptive pains (particularly somatic pains) usually respond to opioid drugs *(38–40)* or to interventions that ameliorate or denervate the peripheral lesion.

2.3.2. NEUROPATHIC PAIN

The term "neuropathic pain" is applied when pain is due to injury to, or diseases of, the peripheral or central neural structures or is perceived to be sustained by aberrant somatosensory processing at these sites. It is most strongly suggested when a dysesthesia occurs in a region of motor, sensory or autonomic dysfunction that is attributable to a discrete neurological lesion. The diagnosis can be challenging, however, and is often inferred solely from the distribution of the pain and identification of a lesion in neural structures that innervate this region.

The diagnosis of neuropathic pain has important clinical implications. The response of neuropathic pains to opioid drugs is less predictable and generally less dramatic than the response of nociceptive pains *(41)*. Optimal treatment may depend on the use of so-called adjuvant analgesics *(42,43)* or other specific approaches, such as somatic or sympathetic nerve block *(32)*.

2.3.3. IDIOPATHIC PAIN

Pain that is perceived to be excessive for the extent of identifiable organic pathology can be termed idiopathic unless the patient presents with affective and behavioral disturbances that are severe enough to infer a predominating psychological pathogenesis, in which case a specific psychiatric diagnosis (somatoform disorder) can be applied *(44)*. When the inference of a somatoform disorder cannot be made, however, the label "idiopathic" should be retained, and assessments should be repeated at appropriate intervals. Idiopathic pain in general, and pain related to a psychiatric disorder specifically, are uncommon in the cancer population, notwithstanding the importance of psychological factors in quality of life.

2.4. A Stepwise Approach to the Evaluation of Cancer Pain

A practical approach to cancer pain assessment incorporates a stepwise approach that begins with data collection and ends with a clinically relevant formulation.

2.4.1. DATA COLLECTION

2.4.1.1. HISTORY. A careful review of past medical history and the chronology of the cancer are important to place the pain complaint in context. The pain-related history must elucidate the relevant pain characteristics, as well as the responses of the patient to previous disease-modifying and analgesic therapies. The presence of multiple pain problems is common, and if more than one is reported, each must be assessed independently.

The clinician should assess the consequences of the pain, including impairment in activities of daily living; psychological, familial and professional dysfunction, disturbed sleep, appetite, and vitality, and financial concerns. The patient's psychological status, including current level of anxiety or depression, suicidal ideation, and the perceived meaning of the pain, is similarly relevant. Pervasive dysfunctional attitudes, such as pessimism, idiosyncratic interpretation of pain, self-blame, catastrophizing, and perceived loss of personal control, can usually be detected through careful questioning. It is important to assess the patient–family interaction and to note both the kind and frequency of pain behaviors and the nature of the family response.

Most patients with cancer pain have multiple other symptoms. The clinician must evaluate the severity and distress caused by each of these symptoms. Symptom checklists and quality-of-life measures may contribute to this comprehensive evaluation *(45,46)*.

2.4.1.2. Examination. A physical examination, including a neurological evaluation, is a necessary part of the initial pain assessment. The need for a thorough neurological assessment is justified by the high prevalence of painful neurological conditions in this population *(47,48)*. The physical examination should attempt to identify the underlying etiology of the pain problem, clarify the extent of the underlying disease, and discern the relationship of the pain complaint to the disease.

2.4.1.3. Review of Previous Investigations. Careful review of previous laboratory and imaging studies can provide important information about the cause of the pain and the extent of the underlying disease.

2.4.2. PROVISIONAL ASSESSMENT

The information derived from these data provides the basis for a provisional pain diagnosis, an understanding of the disease status, and the identification of other concurrent concerns.

This provisional diagnosis includes inferences about the pathophysiology of the pain and an assessment of the pain syndrome. Additional investigations are often required to clarify areas of uncertainty in the provisional assessment *(47)*. The extent of diagnostic investigation must be appropriate to the patient's general status and the overall goals of care.

The lack of a definitive finding on an investigation should not be used to override a compelling clinical diagnosis. In the assessment of bone pain for example, plain radiographs provide only crude assessment of bony lesions and further investigation with bone scintigrams, computerized tomography (CT) or magnetic resonance imaging (MRI) may be indicated. To minimize the risk of error, the physician ordering the diagnostic procedures should personally review them with the radiologist to correlate pathologic changes with the clinical findings.

Pain should be managed during the diagnostic evaluation. Comfort will improve compliance and reduce the distress associate with procedures. No patient should be inadequately evaluated because of poorly controlled pain.

2.4.3. Formulation and Therapeutic Planning

The evaluation should enable the clinician to appreciate the nature of the pain, its impact, and concurrent concerns that further undermine quality of life. The findings of this evaluation should be reviewed with the patient and appropriate others. Through candid discussion, current problems can be prioritized to reflect their importance to the patient.

This evaluation may also identify potential outcomes that would benefit from contingency planning. Examples include evaluation of resources for home care, prebereavement interventions with the family, and the provision of assistive devices in anticipation of compromised ambulation.

2.4.4. The Measurement of Pain and Its Impact on Patient Well-being

Although pain measurement has generally been used by clinical investigators to determine the impact of analgesic therapies, it has become clear that it has an important role in the routine monitoring of cancer patients in treatment settings *(49–51)*. Because observer ratings of symptom severity correlate poorly with patient ratings and are generally an inadequate substitute for patient reporting *(24)*, patient self-report is the primary source of information for the measurement of pain.

3. ACUTE PAIN SYNDROMES

Cancer-related acute pain syndromes are most commonly the result of diagnostic and therapeutic interventions (Table 1). Although some tumor-related pains have an acute onset (such as pain from a pathological fracture), most of these will tend to be chronic or recurrent unless effective treatment for the underlying lesion is provided.

4. CHRONIC PAIN SYNDROMES (TABLE 2)

4.1. Pains Syndromes Resulting From Tumor Involvement of Viscera and Adjacent Structures

Pain may be caused by pathology involving the luminal organs of the gastrointestinal or genitourinary tracts, the parenchymal organs, the peritoneum, or the retroperitoneal soft tissues. Obstruction of hollow viscus, including intestine, biliary tract, and ureter, produce visceral nociceptive syndromes that are well described in the surgical literature. Pain arising from retroperitoneal and pelvic lesions may involve mixed nociceptive and neuropathic mechanisms if both somatic structures and nerve plexi are involved.

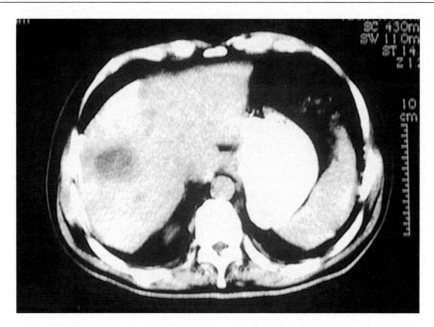

Fig. 1. CT scan demonstrating extensive hepatic metastases.

4.1.1. HEPATIC DISTENTION SYNDROME

The liver is the most common visceral site of metastases arising from colonic and rectal neoplasms. Pain sensitive structures in the region of the liver include the liver capsule, vessels, and biliary tract *(52)*. Nociceptive afferents that innervate these structures travel via the celiac plexus, the phrenic nerve, and the lower right intercostal nerves. Extensive intrahepatic metastases, or gross hepatomegaly associated with cholestasis, may produce discomfort in the right subcostal region and less commonly in the right mid-back or flank *(52–54)*. Referred pain may be experienced in the right neck or shoulder or in the region of the right scapula *(53)*. The pain, which is usually described as a dull aching, may be exacerbated by movement, pressure in the abdomen, and deep inspiration. Pain is commonly accompanied by symptoms of anorexia and nausea. Physical examination may reveal a hard irregular subcostal mass that descends with respiration and is dull to percussion. Other features of hepatic failure may be present. Imaging of the hepatic parenchyma by either ultrasound or CT will usually identify the presence of space-occupying lesions or cholestasis (Fig. 1).

Occasional patients who experience chronic pain due to hepatic distension develop an acute intercurrent subcostal pain that may be exacerbated by respiration. Physical examination may demonstrate a palpable or audible rub. These findings suggest the development of an overlying peritonitis, which can develop in response to some acute event, such as a hemorrhage into a metastasis.

4.1.2. MIDLINE RETROPERITONEAL SYNDROME

Retroperitoneal pathology involving the upper abdomen may produce pain by injury to deep somatic structures of the posterior abdominal wall, distortion of pain-sensitive connective tissue, vascular and ductal structures, local inflammation, and direct infiltration of the celiac plexus. Among patients with colorectal cancers the most common cause is retroperitoneal lymphadenopathy *(55–57)*, particularly celiac lymphadenopathy *(58)*. The pain is experienced in the epigastrium, in the low thoracic region of the back, or in both locations. It is often diffuse and poorly localized. It is usually dull and boring in character, exacerbated with recumbency and improved by sitting. The lesion can usually be demonstrated by CT, MRI, or ultrasound scanning of the upper abdomen. If a tumor is identified in the paravertebral space or vertebral body destruction is identified, consideration should be given to careful evaluation of the epidural space *(59)*.

4.1.3. Chronic Intestinal Obstruction

Abdominal pain is an almost invariable manifestation of chronic intestinal obstruction, which may occur in patients with abdominal or pelvic cancers *(60,61)*. The factors that contribute to this pain include smooth muscle contractions, mesenteric tension, and mural ischemia. Obstructive symptoms may result primarily from the tumor or, more likely, from a combination of mechanical obstruction and other processes, such as autonomic neuropathy and ileus from metabolic derangement or drugs. Both continuous and colicky pains occur, which may be referred to the dermatomes represented by the spinal segments supplying the affected viscera. Vomiting, anorexia, and constipation are important associated symptoms. Abdominal radiographs taken in both supine and erect positions may demonstrate the presence of air–fluid levels and intestinal distention. CT or MRI scanning of the abdomen can assess the extent and distribution of intrabdominal neoplasm, which has implication for subsequent treatment options.

4.1.4. Peritoneal Carcinomatosis

Colorectal cancer is among the most common causes of peritoneal carcinomatosis. Peritoneal carcinomatosis occurs most often by transcelomic spread of abdominal or pelvic tumor; hematogenous spread of an extra-abdominal neoplasm in this pattern is rare. Carcinomatosis can cause peritoneal inflammation, mesenteric tethering, malignant adhesions, and ascites, all of which can cause pain. Pain and abdominal distension are the most common presenting symptoms *(62–65)*. Mesenteric tethering and tension appears to cause a diffuse abdominal or low-back pain. Tense malignant ascites can produce diffuse abdominal discomfort and a distinct stretching pain in the anterior abdominal wall. Adhesions can also cause obstruction of hollow viscus with intermittent colicky pain *(66)*. CT scanning may demonstrate evidence of ascites, omental infiltration, and peritoneal nodules (Fig. 2) *(67)*.

4.1.5. Perineal Pain

Tumors of the colon or rectum, female reproductive tract, and distal genitourinary system are most commonly responsible for perineal pain *(68–71)*. Severe perineal pain following antineoplastic therapy may precede evidence of detectable disease and should be viewed as a potential harbinger of progressive or recurrent cancer *(68,69)*. There is evidence to suggest that this phenomenon is caused by microscopic perineural invasion by recurrent disease *(72)*. The pain, which is typically described as constant and aching, is often aggravated by sitting or standing and may be associated with tenesmus or bladder spasms *(68)*.

Tumor invasion of the musculature of the deep pelvis can also result in a syndrome that appears similar to the so-called tension myalgia of the pelvic floor *(73)*. The pain is typically described as a constant ache or heaviness that exacerbates with upright posture. When caused by tumor, the pain may be concurrent with other types of perineal pain. Digital examination of the pelvic floor may reveal local tenderness or palpable tumor.

4.1.6. Ureteric Obstruction

Carcinoma of the rectum is one of the most common tumors associated with this complication *(74,75)*. Less commonly, obstruction can be more proximal, associated with

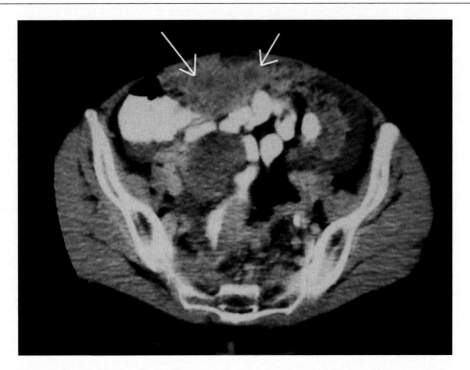

Fig. 2. Abdominal CT scan of a 52-yr-old woman with metastatic carcinoma of the colon presents with abdominal distension and persistant abdominal pain. The arrows indicate peritoneal implants.

retroperitoneal lymphadenopathy, an isolated retroperitoneal metastasis, mural metastases or intraluminal metastases. Pain may or may not accompany ureteric obstruction. When present, it is typically a dull chronic discomfort in the flank, which may radiate into the inguinal region or genitalia. If pain does not occur, ureteric obstruction may be discovered when hydronephrosis is discerned on abdominal imaging procedures or renal failure develops. Ureteric obstruction can be complicated by pyelonephritis or pyonephrosis, which often present with features of sepsis, loin pain and dysuria. Diagnosis of ureteric obstruction can usually be confirmed by the demonstration of hydronephrosis on renal sonography. The level of obstruction can be identified by pyelography, and CT scanning techniques will usually demonstrate the cause *(76)*.

4.2. Pains Syndromes Involving the Peripheral Nervous System

4.2.1. Lumbosacral Plexopathy

In the cancer population, lumbosacral plexopathy is usually caused by neoplastic infiltration or compression. Polyradiculopathy from leptomeningeal metastases or epidural metastases can mimic lumbosacral plexopathy, and the evaluation of the patient must consider these lesions as well (*see* Section 4.2.1.1.). Occasional patients develop lumbosacral plexopathy as a result of surgical trauma, radiation therapy, infarction, cytotoxic damage, infection in the pelvis or psoas muscle, abdominal aneurysm, or idiopathic lumbosacral neuritis *(77–82)*.

4.2.1.1. Malignant Lumbosacral Plexopathy. Colorectal cancer is among the most common causes of malignant lumbosacral plexopathy *(83,84)*. In general, tumors involve the plexus by direct extension from intrapelvic neoplasm; metastases account for only one-fourth of cases *(84)*. In one study, two-thirds of patients developed plexopathy within 3 yr of their primary diagnosis and one-third presented within 1 yr *(84)*.

Pain is the first symptom reported by most patients with malignant lumbosacral plexopathy. Pain is experienced by almost all patients during the course of the disease, and it is the only symptom in almost 20% of patients. The quality is usually aching, pressure-like, or stabbing; dysesthesias appear to be relatively uncommon. Most patients develop numbness, paresthesias, or weakness weeks to months after the pain begins. Common signs include leg weakness that involves multiple myotomes, sensory loss that crosses dermatomes, reflex asymmetry, focal tenderness, leg edema, and positive direct or reverse straight leg raising signs.

An upper plexopathy occurs in almost one-third of patients with lumbosacral plexopathy *(84)*. This lesion is usually the result of direct extension from a low abdominal tumor, most frequently colorectal. Pain may be experienced in the back, lower abdomen, flank or iliac crest, or the anterolateral thigh. Examination may reveal sensory, motor, and reflex changes in a L1–4 distribution. A subgroup of these patients presents with a syndrome characterized by pain and paresthesias limited to the lower abdomen or inguinal region, variable sensory loss and no motor findings. CT scan may show tumor adjacent to the L1 vertebra (the L1 syndrome) *(84)* or along the pelvic side wall, where it presumably damages the ilioinguinal, iliohypogastric, or genitofemoral nerves. Another subgroup has neoplastic involvement of the psoas muscle and presents with a syndrome characterized by upper lumbosacral plexopathy, painful flexion of the ipsilateral hip, and positive psoas muscle stretch test. This has been termed the malignant psoas syndrome *(85)*. Similarly, pain in the distribution of the femoral nerve has been observed in the setting of recurrent retroperitoneal sarcoma *(86)* and tumor in the iliac crest can compress the lateral cutaneous nerve of the thigh producing a pain that mimics meralgia parasthetica *(87)*.

A lower plexopathy occurs in just over 50% of patients with lumbosacral plexopathy *(84)*. This lesion is usually the result of direct extension from a pelvic tumor, most frequently rectal cancer, gynecological tumors or pelvic sarcoma. Pain may be localized in the buttocks and perineum, or referred to the posterolateral thigh and leg. Associated symptoms and signs conform to an L4–S1 distribution. Examination may reveal weakness or sensory changes in the L5 and S1 dermatomes and a depressed ankle jerk. Other findings include leg edema, bladder or bowel dysfunction, sacral or sciatic notch tenderness, and a positive straight leg raising test. A pelvic mass may be palpable.

Sacral plexopathy may occur from direct extension of a sacral lesion or a presacral mass. This may present with predominant involvement of the lumbosacral trunk, characterized by numbness over the dorsal medial foot and sole and weakness of knee flexion, ankle dorsiflexion, and inversion. Other patients demonstrate particular involvement of the coccygeal plexus, with prominent sphincter dysfunction and perineal sensory loss. The latter syndrome occurs with low pelvic tumors, such as those arising from the rectum or prostate.

A panplexopathy with involvement in a L1–S3 distribution occurs in almost one-fifth of patients with lumbosacral plexopathy *(84)*. Local pain may occur in the lower abdomen, back, buttocks or perineum. Referred pain can be experienced anywhere in distribution of the plexus. Leg edema is extremely common. Neurological deficits may be confluent or patchy within the L1–S3 distribution and a positive straight leg raising test is usually present.

Autonomic dysfunction, particularly anhydrosis and vasodilation, has been associated with plexus and peripheral nerve injuries. Focal autonomic neuropathy, which may suggest the anatomic localization of the lesion *(81)*, has been reported as the presenting symptom of metastatic lumbosacral plexopathy *(88)*.

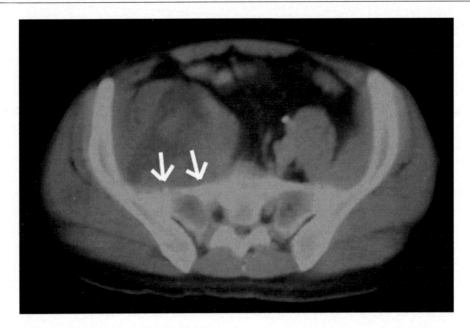

Fig. 3. Large pelvic lymphadenopathy compressing right lumbosacral plexus (arrow).

Cross-sectional imaging, with either CT or MRI, is the usual diagnostic procedure to evaluate lumbosacral plexopathy (Fig. 3) *(11)*. Scanning should be done from the level of the L1 vertebral body, through the sciatic notch. When using CT scanning techniques, images should include bone and soft tissue windows. Limited data suggests superior sensitivity MRI over CT imaging *(89)*. Definitive imaging of the epidural space adjacent to the plexus should be considered in the patient who has feature's indicative of a relatively high risk of epidural extension including bilateral symptoms or signs, unexplained incontinence, or a prominent paraspinal mass *(59,84)*.

4.3. Bone Pain

Bone metastases arising from carcinomas of the colon, rectum have a low incidence, but by virtue of the high prevalence of these conditions they accounted for over 20% of bone metastases observed an autopsy study *(90)*. Bone metastases could potentially cause pain by any of multiple mechanisms, including endosteal or periosteal nociceptor activation (by mechanical distortion or release of chemical mediators) or tumor growth into adjacent soft tissues and nerves *(91)*.

Bone pain caused by metastatic tumor needs to be differentiated from less common causes of chronic bone pain in cancer patients. Non-neoplastic causes in this population include osteoporotic pathological fractures and focal osteonecrosis which may be idiopathic or related to corticosteroids or radiotherapy.

In general, the vertebrae are the most common sites of bony metastases *(92,93)*. Vertebral metastases of colorectal tumors metastasize most commonly to the lumbosacral spine *(92,94)*. The early recognition of pain syndromes due to neoplastic invasion of vertebral bodies is essential, since pain usually precedes compression of adjacent neural structures and prompt primary therapy directed at the lesion may prevent the subsequent development of neurologic deficits. This recognition often requires substantial clinical acumen; referral of pain is common, and the associated symptoms and signs can mimic a variety of other disorders, both malignant (e.g., paraspinal masses) and nonmalignant.

4.3.1. SACRAL PAIN

Sacral invasion is common among patients with pelvic recurrence of colorectal cancer. Severe focal pain radiating to the buttocks, perineum, or posterior thighs may accompany destruction of the sacrum *(95–97)*. The pain is often exacerbated by sitting or lying and is relieved by standing or walking. The neoplasm can spread laterally to involve muscles that rotate the hip (e.g., the pyriformis muscle). This may produce severe incident pain induced by motion of the hip, or a malignant "pyriformis syndrome," characterized by buttock or posterior leg pain that is exacerbated by internal rotation of the hip. Local extension of the tumor mass may also involve the sacral plexus *(see* Section 4.2.1.).

4.3.2. BACK PAIN AND EPIDURAL CORD COMPRESSION

In general, epidural compression (EC) of the spinal cord or cauda equina is a common neurologic complication of cancer; tumors of the distal gastrointestinal tract account for less than 5% of these episodes *(92,94,98)*. Most EC is caused by posterior extension of vertebral body metastasis to the epidural space, others are caused by tumor extension from the posterior arch of the vertebra or infiltration of a paravertebral tumor through the intervertebral foramen.

Back pain is the initial symptom in almost all patients with EC, and in 10%, it is the only symptom at the time of diagnosis *(99)*. Because pain usually precedes neurologic signs by a prolonged period, it should be viewed as a potential indicator of EC, which could lead to treatment at a time that a favorable response is most likely.

Some pain characteristics are particularly suggestive of epidural extension *(100)*. Rapid progression of back pain in a crescendo pattern is an ominous occurrence *(101)*. Radicular pain, which can be constant or lancinating, has similar implications *(100)*. It is usually unilateral in the cervical and lumbosacral regions and bilateral in the thorax, where it is often experienced as a tight, belt-like band across the chest or abdomen *(100)*. The likelihood of EC is also greater when back or radicular pain is exacerbated by recumbency, cough, sneeze, or strain *(102)*.

Weakness, sensory loss, autonomic dysfunction and reflex abnormalities usually occur after a period of progressive pain *(100)*. Weakness may begin segmentally if related to nerve root damage or in a multisegmental or pyramidal distribution if the cauda equina or spinal cord, respectively, is injured. The rate of progression of weakness is variable; in the absence of treatment, following the onset of weakness one-third of patients will develop paralysis within 7 d *(103)*. Patients whose weakness progresses slowly have a better prognosis for neurologic recovery with treatment than those who progress rapidly *(104,105)*. Without effective treatment, sensory abnormalities, which may also begin segmentally, may ultimately evolve to a sensory level with complete loss of all sensory modalities below the site of injury. The upper level of sensory findings may correspond to the location of the epidural tumor or be below it by many segments *(104)*.

Bladder and bowel dysfunction occur late, except in patients with a conus medullaris lesion who may present with acute urinary retention and constipation without preceding motor or sensory symptoms *(100)*.

Other features that may be evident on examination of patients with EC include scoliosis, asymmetrical wasting of paravertebral musculature, and a gibbus (palpable step in the spinous processes). Spinal tenderness to percussion, which may be severe, often accompanies the pain.

Clinical and radiological findings that indicate a high likelihood of epidural encroachment or compression have been defined (Table 4). Patients with one or more of these clinical features have a high likelihood of EC and, unless a specific contraindication exist, require

Table 4
Clinical Features Suggestive of Epidural Spinal Cord and Cauda Equina Compression

Clinical features	Notes
Rapid progression of back pain	Ominous occurrence
Radicular pain	Can be intermittent, constant or lancinating
	Usually unilateral in cervical and lumbosacral regions
	Usually bilateral in the thorax
	Exacerbated by-recumbency, cough, sneeze or valsalva
Weakness	Segmental: suggestive of radiculopathy
	Lumbosacral multisegmental: suggestive of cauda equina compression
	Pyramidal distribution: suggestive of spinal cord compression
	Variable rate of progression
	After development of weakness, 30% develop paraplegia within 7 d
Sensory abnormalities	May also begin segmentally, may ultimately evolve to a sensory level
	Upper level of sensory findings may correspond to the location of the epidural tumor
Bladder and bowel dysfunction	Generally occurs late
	Early symptom of conus medullaris or corda equina lesion
Musculoskeletal features	Scoliosis
	Asymmetrical wasting of paravertebral musculature
	Gibbus (palpable step) in the dorsal spines
	Spinal tenderness to percussion

definitive imaging of the epidural space. Definitive imaging of the epidural space confirms the existence of EC (and thereby indicates the necessity and urgency of treatment), defines the appropriate radiation portals and determines the extent of epidural encroachment (which influences prognosis and may alter the therapeutic approach) *(106)*. The options for definitive imaging include MRI, myelography and CT-myelography or spiral CT without myelographic contrast.

4.3.3. Pain Syndromes of the Pelvis and Hip

The pelvis and hip are common sites of metastatic involvement. The weight bearing function of these structures, essential for normal ambulation, contributes to the propensity of disease at these sites to cause incident pain with ambulation.

4.3.3.1. Hip Joint Syndrome. Tumor involvement of the acetabulum or head of femur typically produces localized hip pain which is aggravated by weight bearing and movement of the hip. The pain may radiate to the knee or medial thigh, and occasionally this is the only site of pain *(107,108)*. Medial extension of acetabular tumor can involve the lumbosacral plexus as it traverses the pelvic side-wall. Plain radiographs and bone scintigraphy usually demonstrate bony involvement. CT and MRI tomographic techniques are more sensitive, and they also demonstrate the extent of adjacent soft tissue involvement *(109)*.

4.4. Headache and Facial Pain

Tumor-related headache is a relatively uncommon cancer pain problem in the colorectal and anal cancer population. Cancer-related headache results from traction, inflammation, or infiltration of pain-sensitive structures in the head and neck *(110)*.

4.4.1. BRAIN METASTASES

The incidence of cerebral metastases in patients with colorectal cancer is approx 5%. Headache is a common presenting symptom in patients with brain metastases, occurring in 60–90% of patients *(110,111)*. The headache is presumably produced by traction on pain-sensitive vascular and dural tissues. Patients with multiple metastases and those with posterior fossa metastases are more likely to report this symptom *(110)*. The pain may be focal, overlying the site of the lesion, or generalized. Headache has lateralizing value, especially in patients with supratentorial lesions *(111)*. Posterior fossa lesions often cause a bifrontal headache. The quality of the headache is usually throbbing or steady, and the intensity is usually mild to moderate *(111)*.

4.4.2. LEPTOMENINGEAL METASTASES

Leptomeningeal metastases, characterized by diffuse or multifocal involvement of the subarachnoid space by metastatic tumor, are rare in colorectal carcinoma. Leptomeningeal metastases present with focal or multifocal neurological symptoms or signs that may involve any level of the neuraxis *(112,113)*. The diagnosis of leptomeningeal metastases is often difficult. Cerebrospinal fluid (CSF) cytology and gadolinium enhanced spinal or brain MR imaging are complimentary since both are associated with significant false negative rates *(114)*.

4.4.3. BASE OF SKULL METASTASES

Bony metastases to the base of skull are associated with well described clinical syndromes *(115)*, named according to the site of metastatic involvement: orbital, parasellar, middle fossa, jugular foramen, occipital condyle, clivus and sphenoid sinus (Table 5). When base of skull metastases are suspected, CT scan with bone window settings is the diagnostic procedure of choice to evaluate bony disease *(115)*. MRI is most sensitive for assessing soft tissue extension. CSF analysis may be needed to exclude leptomeningeal metastases.

4.4.4. PAINFUL CRANIAL NEURALGIAS

Glossopharyngeal and trigeminal neuralgias can occur from metastases in the base of skull or leptomeninges. Each of these syndromes has a characteristic presentation *(116)*. Early diagnosis is critical to prevent progressive neurologic injury.

4.5. Chronic Pain Syndromes Associated with Cancer Therapy

Most treatment-related pains caused by tissue-damaging procedures are acute and are remarkable for their predictability and self-limited natural history. Chronic treatment-related pain syndromes are associated with either a persistent nociceptive complication of an invasive treatment, such as a postsurgical abscess, or, more commonly, to neural injury *(116)*. In some cases, these syndromes occur long after the therapy is completed, resulting in a difficult differential diagnosis between recurrent disease and a complication of therapy.

4.5.1. CHRONIC POST-CHEMOTHERAPY PAIN SYNDROMES

4.5.1.1. Oxaliplatin Peripheral Neuropathy. Oxaliplatin is a highly active cytotoxic agent in colorectal cancer *(117)*. Like *cis*-platinum, it is a neurotoxin and it commonly produces a sensory peripheral neuropathy characterized by numbness, cold sensitivity and painful dysesthesias. The neuropathy is cumulative; occuring in 10% of patients after six treatment cycles and in 50% after nine cycles of an oxaliplatin dosage of 130 mg/m^2 once every 3 wk *(117)*. In most cases, the neuropathy is slowly reversible on termination of therapy with resolution over several months.

Table 5
Pain Syndromes Associated with Base of Skull Metastases

Syndrome	Usual presentation
Orbital	Progressive ipsilateral retroorbital and supraorbital pain
Parasellar	Unilateral supraorbital and frontal headache
	May be associated with diplopia
	May be opthalmoparesis or papilledema
	May demonstrate hemianopsia or quadrantinopsia
Middle cranial fossa	Facial numbness in the distribution of second or third divisions of the trigeminal nerve
	Paresthesias or pain referred to the cheek or jaw
Jugular foramen	Hoarseness or dysphagia
	Pain referred to the ipsilateral ear or mastoid
	Occasionally glossopharyngeal neuralgia, with or without syncope
Occipital condyle	Unilateral occipital pain worsened with neck flexion
	Associated with stiffness of the neck
Clivus	Vertex headache, which is often exacerbated by neck flexion
	Lower cranial nerve (VI-XII) dysfunction (may become bilateral)
Sphenoid sinus	Bifrontal headache radiating to the temporal region, and intermittent retroorbital pain

4.5.2. CHRONIC POST-SURGICAL PAIN SYNDROMES

4.5.2.1. Phantom Anus Syndrome. Phantom pain is perceived to arise from a resected body structure, as if the structure were still contiguous with the body. A phantom anus pain syndrome occurs in approx 15% of patients who undergo abdomino-perineal resection of the rectum *(69,118)*. Phantom anus pain may develop either in the early postoperative period or after a latency of months to years. Late onset pain is almost always associated with tumor recurrence *(69,118)*.

4.5.2.2. Postsurgical Pelvic Floor Myalgia. Surgical trauma to the pelvic floor can cause a residual pelvic floor myalgia, which like the neoplastic syndrome described previously, mimics so-called tension myalgia *(73)*. The risk of disease recurrence associated with this condition is not known, and its natural history has not been defined. In patients who have undergone anorectal resection, this condition must be differentiated from the phantom anus syndrome (*see* above).

4.5.2.3. Post-Surgical Lumbosacral Plexopathy. Surgical trauma to the lumbosacral plexus during deep pelvic resection can result in persistent neurological dysfuntion and pain.

4.5.3. CHRONIC POST-RADIATION PAIN SYNDROMES

Chronic pain occurring as a complication of radiation therapy tends to occur late in the course of a patient's illness. These syndromes must always be differentiated from recurrent tumor.

4.5.3.1. Radiation-Induced Lumbosacral Plexopathy. Radiation fibrosis of the lumbosacral plexus is a rare complication that may occur from 1 to over 30 yr following radiation treatment. The use of intracavitary radium implants for carcinoma of the cervix may be an additional risk factor *(119)*. Radiation-induced plexopathy typically presents with progressive weakness and leg swelling; pain is not usually a prominent feature *(119,120)*.

Weakness typically begins distally in the L5–S1 segments and is slowly progressive. The symptoms and signs may be bilateral *(120)*. If CT scanning demonstrates a lesion, it is usually a nonspecific diffuse infiltration of the tissues. Electromyography may show myokymic discharges *(120)*.

4.5.3.2. Chronic Radiation Enteritis and Proctitis. Chronic enteritits and proctocolitis occur as a delayed complication in 2–10% of patients who undergo abdominal or pelvic radiation therapy *(121,122)*. The rectum and rectosigmoid are more commonly involved than the small bowel, a pattern that may relate to the retroperitoneal fixation of the former structures. The latency is variable (3 mo–30 yr) *(121,122)*. Chronic radiation injury to the rectum can present as proctitis (with bloody diarrhea, tenesmus, and cramping pain), obstruction from stricture formation, or fistulae to the bladder or vagina. Small bowel radiation damage typically causes colicky abdominal pain, which can be associated with chronic nausea or malabsorption. Barium studies may demonstrate a narrow tubular bowel segment resembling Crohn's disease or ischemic colitis. Endoscopy and biopsy may be necessary to distinguish suspicious lesions from recurrent cancer.

4.5.3.3. Burning Perineum Syndrome. Persistent perineal discomfort is an uncommon delayed complication of pelvic radiotherapy. After a latency of 6–18 mo, burning pain can develop in the perianal region; the pain may extend anteriorly to involve the vagina or scrotum *(123)*. In patients who have had abdomino-perineal resection, phantom anus pain and recurrent tumor are major differential diagnoses.

4.5.3.4. Chronic Radiation Myelopathy. Chronic radiation myelopathy is a late complication of spinal cord irradiation. The latency is highly variable but is most commonly 12–14 mo. The most common presentation is a partial transverse myelopathy at the cervicothoracic level, sometimes in a Brown–Sequard pattern *(124)*.

REFERENCES

1. Balch CM. The surgeon's expanded role in cancer care. *Cancer*, **65(3 Suppl.)** (1990) 604–609.
2. Bonica JJ, Ventafridda V, and Twycross RG. Cancer Pain. In *The Management of Pain*, 2nd ed. Bonica JJ (ed.). Philadelphia: Lea & Febiger, pp. 400–460, 1990.
3. Vuorinen E. Pain as an early symptom in cancer. *Clin. J. Pain*, **9(4)** (1993) 272–278.
4. Cleeland CS, Gonin R, Hatfield AK, Edmonson JH, Blum RH, Stewart JA, et al. Pain and its treatment in outpatients with metastatic cancer. *N. Engl. J. Med.*, **330(9)** (1994) 592–596.
5. Portenoy RK, Miransky J, Thaler HT, Hornung J, Bianchi C, Cibas-Kong I, et al. Pain in ambulatory patients with lung or colon cancer. Prevalence, characteristics, and effect. *Cancer*, **70(6)** (1992) 1616–1624.
6. Tay WK, Shaw RJ, Goh CR. A survey of symptoms in hospice patients in Singapore. *Ann. Acad. Med. Singapore*, **23(2)** (1994) 191–196.
7. Brescia FJ, Portenoy RK, Ryan M, Krasnoff L, and Gray G. Pain, opioid use, and survival in hospitalized patients with advanced cancer. *J. Clin. Oncol.*, **10(1)** (1992) 149–155.
8. Donnelly S and Walsh D. The symptoms of advanced cancer. *Semin. Oncol.*, **22(2 Suppl 3)** (1995) 67–72.
9. Feuz A and Rapin CH. An observational study of the role of pain control and food adaptation of elderly patients with terminal cancer. *J. Am. Diet. Assoc.*, **94(7)** (1994) 767–770.
10. Thorpe DM. The incidence of sleep disturbance in cancer patients with pain. In 7th World Congress on Pain: Abstracts. Seattle: I.A.S.P. Publications, Abstract p. 451, 1993.
11. Cleeland CS, Nakamura Y, Mendoza TR, Edwards KR, Douglas J, and Serlin RC. Dimensions of the impact of cancer pain in a four country sample: new information from multidimensional scaling. *Pain*, **67(2–3)** (1996) 267–273.
12. Ferrell BR. The impact of pain on quality of life. A decade of research. *Nurs. Clin. North Am.*, **30(4)** (1995) 609–624.
13. Massie MJ and Holland JC. The cancer patient with pain: psychiatric complications and their management. *J. Pain Symptom. Manage.*, **7(2)** (1992) 99–109.
14. Burrows M, Dibble SL, Miaskowski C. Differences in outcomes among patients experiencing different types of cancer-related pain. *Oncol. Nurs. Forum*, **25(4)** (1998) 735–741.

15. Strang P. Existential consequences of unrelieved cancer pain. *Palliat. Med.*, **11(4)** (1997) 299–305.

16. Fishman B. The cognitive behavioral perspective on pain management in terminal illness. *Hosp. J.*, **8(1–2)** (1992) 73–88.

17. Emanuel EJ. Pain and symptom control. Patient rights and physician responsibilities. *Hematol. Oncol. Clin. North Am.*, **10(1)** (1996) 41–56.

18. Haugen PS. Pain relief. Legal aspects of pain relief for the dying. *Minn. Med.*, **80(11)** (1997) 15–18.

19. Cherny NI and Catane R. Professional negligence in the management of cancer pain. A case for urgent reforms [editorial; comment]. *Cancer*, **76(11)** (1995) 2181–2185.

20. Wanzer SH, Federman DD, Adelstein SJ, Cassel CK, Cassem EH, Cranford RE, et al. The physician's responsibility toward hopelessly ill patients. A second look. *N. Engl. J. Med.*, **320(13)** (1989) 844–849.

21. Edwards RB. Pain management and the values of health care providers. In *Drug Treatment of Cancer Pain in a Drug Oriented Society*. Hill CS and Fields WS (eds.), New York, Raven Press, pp. 101–112, 1989.

22. Stjernsward J, Colleau SM, and Ventafridda V. The World Health Organization Cancer Pain and Palliative Care Program. Past, present, and future. *J. Pain Symptom Manage.*, **12(2)** (1996) 65–72.

23. Von Roenn JH, Cleeland CS, Gonin R, Hatfield AK, and Pandya KJ. Physician attitudes and practice in cancer pain management. A survey from the Eastern Cooperative Oncology Group. *Ann. Intern. Med.*, **119(2)** (1993) 121–126.

24. Grossman SA, Sheidler VR, Swedeen K, Mucenski J, and Piantadosi S. Correlation of patient and caregiver ratings of cancer pain. *J. Pain Symptom Manage.*, **6(2)** (1991) 53–57.

25. Cherny NJ, Chang V, Frager G, Ingham JM, Tiseo PJ, Popp B, et al. Opioid pharmacotherapy in the management of cancer pain: a survey of strategies used by pain physicians for the selection of analgesic drugs and routes of administration. *Cancer*, **76(7)** (1995) 1283–1293.

26. World Health Organization. *Cancer Pain Relief*, 2nd ed. Geneva: World Health Organization 1996.

27. Giamberardino MA and Vecchiet L. Visceral pain, referred hyperalgesia and outcome: new concepts. *Eur. J. Anaesthesiol. Suppl.*, **10** (1995) 61–66.

28. Cervero F. Visceral nociception: peripheral and central aspects of visceral nociceptive systems. *Philos. Trans. R. Soc. Lond. B. Biol. Sci.*, **308(1136)** (1985) 325–337.

29. Portenoy RK, Kornblith AB, Wong G, Vlamis V, Lepore JM, Loseth DB, et al. Pain in ovarian cancer patients. Prevalence, characteristics, and associated symptoms. *Cancer*, **74(3)** (1994) 907–915.

30. Grond S, Zech D, Diefenbach C, Radbruch L, and Lehmann KA. Assessment of cancer pain: a prospective evaluation in 2266 cancer patients referred to a pain service. *Pain*, **64(1)** (1996) 107–114.

31. Kellgren JG. On distribution of pain arising from deep somatic structures with charts of segmental pain areas. *Clin. Science*, **4** (1938) 35–46.

32. Cherny NI, Arbit E, and Jain S. Invasive techniques in the management of cancer pain. *Hematol. Oncol. Clin. North Am.*, **10(1)** (1996) 121–137.

33. McCaffery M and Thorpe DM. Differences in perception of pain and the development of adversarial relationships among health care providers. In *Drug Treatment of Cancer Pain in a Drug Oriented Society*, Hill CS and Fields WS (eds.), New York, Raven Press, p. 19–26, 1989.

34. Ventafridda V, Ripamonti C, De Conno F, Tamburini M, and Cassileth BR. Symptom prevalence and control during cancer patients' last days of life. *J. Palliat. Care*, **6(3)** (1990) 7–11.

35. Coyle N, Adelhardt J, Foley KM, and Portenoy RK. Character of terminal illness in the advanced cancer patient: pain and other symptoms during the last four weeks of life. *J. Pain Symptom Manage.*, **5(2)** (1990) 83–93.

36. Reuben DB, Mor V, and Hiris J. Clinical symptoms and length of survival in patients with terminal cancer. *Arch. Intern. Med.*, **148(7)** (1988) 1586–1591.

37. Portenoy RK and Hagen NA. Breakthrough pain: definition, prevalence and characteristics. *Pain*, **41(3)** (1990) 273–281.

38. Jadad AR, Carroll D, Glynn CJ, Moore RA, and McQuay HJ. Morphine responsiveness of chronic pain: double-blind randomised crossover study with patient-controlled analgesia. *Lancet*, **339(8806)** (1992) 1367–1371.

39. Arner S and Meyerson BA. Lack of analgesic effect of opioids on neuropathic and idiopathic forms of pain. *Pain*, **33(1)** (1988) 11–23.

40. Cherny NI, Thaler HT, Friedlander-Klar H, Lapin J, Foley KM, Houde R, et al. Opioid responsiveness of cancer pain syndromes caused by neuropathic or nociceptive mechanisms: a combined analysis of controlled, single-dose studies. *Neurology*, **44(5)** (1994) 857–861.

41. Hanks GW and Forbes K. Opioid responsiveness. *Acta. Anaesthesiol. Scand.*, **41(1 Pt 2)** (1997) 154–158.

42. McQuay HJ, Tramer M, Nye BA, Carroll D, Wiffen PJ, and Moore RA. A systematic review of antidepressants in neuropathic pain. *Pain*, **68(2–3)** (1996) 217–227.

43. Lipman AG. Analgesic drugs for neuropathic and sympathetically maintained pain. *Clin. Geriatr. Med.*, **12(3)** (1996) 501–515.
44. American Psychiatric Association. Somatoform disorders. In *Diagnostic and Statistical Manual of Mental Disorders (DSM-IV)*, 4th ed. Washington: American Psychiatric Association, p. 445–471, 1994.
45. Bruera E, Kuehn N, Miller MJ, Selmser P, and Macmillan K. The Edmonton Symptom Assessment System (ESAS): a simple method for the assessment of palliative care patients. *J. Palliat. Care*, **7(2)** (1991) 6–9.
46. Portenoy RK, Thaler HT, Kornblith AB, Lepore JM, Friedlander-Klar H, Kiyasu E, et al. The Memorial Symptom Assessment Scale: an instrument for the evaluation of symptom prevalence, characteristics and distress. *Eur. J. Cancer*, **30A(9)** (1994) 1326–1336.
47. Gonzales GR, Elliott KJ, Portenoy RK, and Foley KM. The impact of a comprehensive evaluation in the management of cancer pain. *Pain*, **47(2)** (1991) 141–144.
48. Clouston PD, DeAngelis LM, and Posner JB. The spectrum of neurological disease in patients with systemic cancer. *Ann. Neurol.*, **31(3)** (1992) 268–273.
49. Cleeland CS, Gonin R, Baez L, Loehrer P, and Pandya KJ. Pain and treatment of pain in minority patients with cancer. The Eastern Cooperative Oncology Group Minority Outpatient Pain Study. *Ann. Intern. Med.*, **127(9)** (1997) 813–816.
50. American Pain Society Quality of Care Committee. Quality improvement guidelines for the treatment of acute pain and cancer pain. American Pain Society Quality of Care Committee [see comments]. *JAMA*, **274(23)** (1995) 1874–1880.
51. Au E, Loprinzi CL, Dhodapkar M, Nelson T, Novotny P, Hammack J, et al. Regular use of a verbal pain scale improves the understanding of oncology inpatient pain intensity. *J. Clin. Oncol.*, **12(12)** (1994) 2751–2755.
52. Coombs DW. Pain due to liver capsular distention. In *Common Problems in Pain Management*, Ferrer-Brechner T (ed.), Chicago: Year Book Medical Publishers, p. 247–253, 1990.
53. Mulholland MW, Debas H, and Bonica JJ. Diseases of the liver, biliary system and pancreas. In *The Management of Pain*, Bonica JJ (ed.), Philadelphia: Lea & Febiger, p. 1214–1231, 1990.
54. De Conno F and Polastri D. Clinical features and symptomatic treatment of liver metastasis in the terminally ill patient. *Ann. Ital. Chir.*, **67(6)** (1996) 819–826.
55. Sponseller PD. Evaluating the child with back pain. *Am. Fam. Physician*, **54(6)** (1996) 1933–1941.
56. Neer RM, Ferrucci JT, Wang CA, Brennan M, Buttrick WF, and Vickery AL. A 77-year-old man with epigastric pain, hypercalcemia, and a retroperitoneal mass. *N. Engl. J. Med.*, **305(15)** (1981) 874–883.
57. Krane RJ and Perrone TL. A young man with testicular and abdominal pain. *N. Engl. J. Med.*, **305(6)** (1981) 331–336.
58. Schonenberg P, Bastid C, Guedes J, and Sahel J. [Percutaneous echography-guided alcohol block of the celiac plexus as treatment of painful syndromes of the upper abdomen: study of 21 cases]. *Schweiz. Med. Wochenschr.*, **121(15)** (1991) 528–531.
59. Portenoy RK, Galer BS, Salamon O, Freilich M, Finkel JE, Milstein D, et al. Identification of epidural neoplasm. Radiography and bone scintigraphy in the symptomatic and asymptomatic spine. *Cancer*, **64(11)** (1989) 2207–2213.
60. Ripamonti C. Management of bowel obstruction in advanced cancer. *Curr. Opin. Oncol.*, **6(4)** (1994) 351–357.
61. Baines MJ. Intestinal obstruction. *Cancer Surv.*, **21** (1994) 147–156.
62. Garrison RN, Kaelin LD, Galloway RH, and Heuser LS. Malignant ascites. Clinical and experimental observations. *Ann. Surg.*, **203(6)** (1986) 644–651.
63. Truong LD, Maccato ML, Awalt H, Cagle PT, Schwartz MR, and Kaplan AL. Serous surface carcinoma of the peritoneum: a clinicopathologic study of 22 cases. *Hum. Pathol.*, **21(1)** (1990) 99–110.
64. Fromm GL, Gershenson DM, and Silva EG. Papillary serous carcinoma of the peritoneum. *Obstet. Gynecol.*, **75(1)** (1990) 89–95.
65. Ransom DT, Patel SR, Keeney GL, Malkasian GD, and Edmonson JH. Papillary serous carcinoma of the peritoneum. A review of 33 cases treated with platin-based chemotherapy. *Cancer*, **66(6)** (1990) 1091–1094.
66. Averbach AM and Sugarbaker PH. Recurrent intraabdominal cancer with intestinal obstruction. *Int. Surg.*, **80(2)** (1995) 141–146.
67. Archer AG, Sugarbaker PH, and Jelinek JS. Radiology of peritoneal carcinomatosis. *Cancer Treat. Res.*, **82** (1996) 263–288.
68. Stillman M. Perineal pain: Diagnosis and management, with particular attention to perineal pain of cancer. In *Second International Congress on Cancer Pain*, Foley KM, Bonica JJ, and Ventafrida V (eds.), New York: Raven Press, p. 359–377, 1990.

69. Boas RA, Schug SA, and Acland RH. Perineal pain after rectal amputation: a 5-year follow-up. *Pain*, **52(1)** (1993) 67–70.

70. Miaskowski C. Special needs related to the pain and discomfort of patients with gynecologic cancer. *J. Obstet. Gynecol. Neonatal Nurs.*, **25(2)** (1996) 181–188.

71. Hagen NA. Sharp, shooting neuropathic pain in the rectum or genitals: pudendal neuralgia. *J. Pain Symptom Manage.*, **8(7)** (1993) 496–501.

72. Seefeld PH and Bargen JA. The spread of carcinoma of the rectum: invasion of lymphatics, veins and nerves. *Ann. Surgery*, **118** (1943) 76–90.

73. Sinaki M, Merritt JL, and Stillwell GK. Tension myalgia of the pelvic floor. *Mayo Clin Proc.*, **52(11)** (1977) 717–722.

74. Harrington KJ, Pandha HS, Kelly SA, Lambert HE, Jackson JE, and Waxman J. Palliation of obstructive nephropathy due to malignancy. *Br. J. Urol.*, **76(1)** (1995) 101–107.

75. Kontturi M and Kauppila A. Ureteric complications following treatment of gynaecological cancer. *Ann. Chir. Gynaecol.*, **71(4)** (1982) 232–238.

76. Greenfield A and Resnick MI. Genitourinary emergencies. *Seminars in Oncology*, **16** (1989) 516–520.

77. Chad DA and Bradley WG. Lumbosacral plexopathy. *Semin. Neurol.*, **7(1)** (1987) 97–107.

78. Lefebvre V, Leduc JJ, and Choteau PH. Painless ischaemic lumbosacral plexopathy and aortic dissection [letter]. *J. Neurol. Neurosurg. Psychiatry*, **58(5)** (1995) 641.

79. Cifu DX and Irani KD. Ischaemic lumbosacral plexopathy in acute vascular compromise: case report. *Paraplegia*, **29(1)** (1991) 70–75.

80. van Alfen N and van Engelen BG. Lumbosacral plexus neuropathy: a case report and review of the literature. *Clin. Neurol. Neurosurg.*, **99(2)** (1997) 138–141.

81. Evans RJ and Watson CPN. Lumbosacral plexopathy in cancer patients. *Neurology*, **35** (1985) 1392–1393.

82. Bradley WG, Chad D, Verghese JP, Liu HC, Good P, Gabbai AA, et al. Painful lumbosacral plexopathy with elevated erythrocyte sedimentation rate: a treatable inflammatory syndrome. *Ann. Neurol.*, **15(5)** (1984) 457–464.

83. Jaeckle KA. Nerve plexus metastases. *Neurol. Clin.*, **9(4)** (1991) 857–866.

84. Jaeckle KA, Young DF, and Foley KM. The natural history of lumbosacral plexopathy in cancer. *Neurology*, **35(1)** (1985) 8–15.

85. Stevens MJ and Gonet YM. Malignant psoas syndrome: recognition of an oncologic entity. *Australas. Radiol.*, **34(2)** (1990) 150–154.

86. Zografos GC and Karakousis CP. Pain in the distribution of the femoral nerve: early evidence of recurrence of a retroperitoneal sarcoma. *Eur. J. Surg. Oncol.*, **20(6)** (1994) 692–693.

87. Tharion G and Bhattacharji S. Malignant secondary deposit in the iliac crest masquerading as meralgia paresthetica. *Ann. Phys. Med. Rehabil.*, **78(9)** (1997) 1010–1011.

88. Dalmau J, Graus F, and Marco M. 'Hot and dry foot' as initial manifestation of neoplastic lumbosacral plexopathy. *Neurology*, **39(6)** (1989) 871–872.

89. Taylor BV, Kimmel DW, Krecke KN, and Cascino TL. Magnetic resonance imaging in cancer-related lumbosacral plexopathy. *Mayo Clin. Proc.*, **72(9)** (1997) 823–829.

90. Abrams HL, Spiro R, and Goldstein N. Metastases in carcinoma. Analysis of 1000 autopsied cases. *Cancer*, **23** (1950) 74–85.

91. Mercadante S. Malignant bone pain: pathophysiology and treatment. *Pain*, **69(1–2)** (1997) 1–18.

92. Gilbert RW, Kim JH, and Posner JB. Epidural spinal cord compression from metastatic tumor: diagnosis and treatment. *Ann. Neurol.*, **3(1)** (1978) 40–51.

93. Sorensen S, Borgesen SE, Rohde K, Rasmusson B, Bach F, Boge-Rasmussen T, et al. Metastatic epidural spinal cord compression. Results of treatment and survival. *Cancer*, **65(7)** (1990) 1502–1508.

94. Stark RJ, Henson RA, and Evans SJ. Spinal metastases. A retrospective survey from a general hospital. *Brain*, 105(Pt 1) (1982) 189–213.

95. Porter AD, Simpson AH, Davis AM, Griffin AM, and Bell RS. Diagnosis and management of sacral bone tumours [see comments]. *Can. J. Surg.*, **37(6)** (1994) 473–478.

96. Feldenzer JA, McGauley JL, and McGillicuddy JE. Sacral and presacral tumors: problems in diagnosis and management. *Neurosurgery*, **25(6)** (1989) 884–891.

97. Hall JH and Fleming JF. The "lumbar disc syndrome" produced by sacral metastases. *Can. J. Surg.*, **13(2)** (1970) 149–156.

98. Grant R, Papadopoulos SM, Sandler HM, and Greenberg HS. Metastatic epidural spinal cord compression: current concepts and treatment. *J. Neurooncol.*, **19(1)** (1994) 79–92.

99. Greenberg HS, Kim JH, and Posner JB. Epidural spinal cord compression from metastatic tumor: results with a new treatment protocol. *Ann. Neurol.*, **8(4)** (1980) 361–366.

100. Helweg-Larsen S and Sorensen PS. Symptoms and signs in metastatic spinal cord compression: a study of progression from first symptom until diagnosis in 153 patients. *Eur. J. Cancer*, **30A(3)** (1994) 396–398.

101. Rosenthal MA, Rosen D, Raghavan D, Leicester J, Duval P, Besser M, et al. Spinal cord compression in prostate cancer. A 10-year experience. *Br. J. Urol.*, **69(5)** (1992) 530–533.

102. Ruff RL and Lanska DJ. Epidural metastases in prospectively evaluated veterans with cancer and back pain. *Cancer*, **63(11)** (1989) 2234–2241.

103. Barron KD, Hirano A, Araki S, et al. Experience with metastatic neoplasms involving the spinal cord. *Neurology*, **9** (1959) 91–100.

104. Helweg-Larsen S. Clinical outcome in metastatic spinal cord compression. A prospective study of 153 patients. *Acta. Neurol. Scand.*, **94(4)** (1996) 269–275.

105. Helweg-Larsen S, Rasmusson B, and Sorensen PS. Recovery of gait after radiotherapy in paralytic patients with metastatic epidural spinal cord compression. *Neurology*, **40(8)** (1990) 1234–1236.

106. Portenoy RK, Lipton RB, and Foley KM. Back pain in the cancer patient: an algorithm for evaluation and management. *Neurology*, **37(1)** (1987) 134–138.

107. Graham DF. Hip pain as a presenting symptom of acetabular metastasis. *Br. J. Surg.*, **63(2)** (1976) 147–148.

108. Sim FH. Metastatic bone disease of the pelvis and femur. *Instr. Course Lect.*, **41** (1992) 317–327.

109. Beatrous TE, Choyke PL, and Frank JA. Diagnostic evaluation of cancer patients with pelvic pain: comparison of scintigraphy, CT, and MR imaging [see comments]. *AJR Am. J. Roentgenol.*, **155(1)** (1990) 85–88.

110. Forsyth PA and Posner JB. Headaches in patients with brain tumors: a study of 111 patients. *Neurology*, **43(9)** (1993) 1678–1683.

111. Suwanwela N, Phanthumchinda K, and Kaoropthum S. Headache in brain tumor: a cross-sectional study. *Headache*, **34(7)** (1994) 435–438.

112. Grossman SA and Moynihan TJ. Neoplastic meningitis. *Neurol. Clin.*, **9(4)** (1991) 843–856.

113. Wasserstrom WR, Glass JP, and Posner JB. Diagnosis and treatment of leptomeningeal metastases from solid tumors: experience with 90 patients. *Cancer*, **49(4)** (1982) 759–772.

114. DeAngelis LM. Current diagnosis and treatment of leptomeningeal metastasis. *J. Neurooncol.*, **38(2–3)** (1998) 245–252.

115. Greenberg HS, Deck MD, Vikram B, Chu FC, and Posner JB. Metastasis to the base of the skull: clinical findings in 43 patients. *Neurology*, **31(5)** (1981) 530–537.

116. Elliott K and Foley KM. Neurologic pain syndromes in patients with cancer. *Crit. Care Clin.*, **6(2)**, (1990) 393–420.

117. Wiseman LR, Adkins JC, Plosker GL, and Goa KL. Oxaliplatin: a review of its use in the management of metastatic colorectal cancer. *Drugs Aging*, **14(6)** (1999) 459–475; the above report in MacintoshPCUNIX TextHTML format.

118. Ovesen P, Kroner K, Ornsholt J, and Bach K. Phantom-related phenomena after rectal amputation: prevalence and clinical characteristics. *Pain*, **44(3)** (1991) 289–291.

119. Stryker JA, Sommerville K, Perez R, Velkley DE. Sacral plexus injury after radiotherapy for carcinoma of cervix. *Cancer*, **66(7)** (1990) 1488–1492.

120. Thomas JE, Cascino TL, and Earle JD. Differential diagnosis between radiation and tumor plexopathy of the pelvis. *Neurology*, **35(1)** (1985) 1–7.

121. Yeoh EK, Horowitz M. Radiation enteritis. *Surg. Gynecol. Obstet.*, **165(4)** (1987) 373–379.

122. Nussbaum ML, Campana TJ, and Weese JL. Radiation-induced intestinal injury. *Clin. Plast. Surg.*, **20(3)** (1993) 573–580.

123. Minsky BD and Cohen AM. Minimizing the toxicity of pelvic radiation therapy in rectal cancer. *Oncology (Huntingt.)*, **2(8)** (1988) 21–25, 28–29.

124. Schultheiss TE and Stephens LC. Invited review: permanent radiation myelopathy. *Br. J. Radiol.*, **65(777)** (1992) 737–753.

36   Pain Management in Colorectal and Anal Cancers

Nathan I. Cherny

CONTENTS

1. GENERAL CONSIDERATIONS

Optimal management of pain problems in this population requires familiarity with a range of therapeutic options, including antineoplastic therapies, analgesic pharmacotherapy, and anesthetic, neurosurgical, psychological, and physiatric techniques. Successful pain management is characterized by the implementation of the techniques with the most favorable therapeutic index for the prevailing circumstances along with provision for repeated evaluations so that a favorable balance between pain relief and adverse effects is maintained. Currently available techniques can provide adequate relief to a vast majority of patients.

2. PRIMARY THERAPY

The assessment process may reveal a cause for the pain that is amenable to disease-modifying primary therapy. For pain produced by tumor infiltration or compression, antineoplastic treatment with surgery, radiotherapy, chemotherapy, or other novel approaches may be considered. Pain caused by infections may be amenable to antibiotic therapy or drainage procedures. If successful, such primary therapy can have profound analgesic consequences.

2.1. Radiotherapy

Although it is generally true that radiotherapy has a pivotal role in the palliative treatment of bone metastases *(1)*, epidural spinal cord compression *(2)*, and cerebral metastases *(3)*, data specific to metastases arising from the colon, rectum, and anus are not available. Guidelines for the evaluation of the role of palliative radiotherapy have been described: A

From: *Colorectal Cancer: Multimodality Management*
Edited by: L. Saltz © Humana Press Inc., Totowa, NJ

high likelihood of efficacy should be anticipated, the treatment should not entail significant risk of adverse effects, and the duration of treatment should be short and it should offer a greater palliative index than other available therapeutic modalities *(4)*. There is a paucity of data regarding the efficacy of radiotherapy in the management of pelvic plexopathic pain. Limited but successful experience has been described among patients with malignant infiltration of the lumbosacral plexus *(5,6)*. The results with the perineal pain of low sacral plexopathy and the phantom anus syndrome are more encouraging *(7,8)*. Hepatic radiotherapy, with 2000–3000 rad, is generally well tolerated and can relieve the pain of hepatic capsular distension in 50–90% of patients *(9–13)*.

2.2. Chemotherapy

Despite a paucity of data concerning the specific analgesic benefits of chemotherapy, there is a strong clinical impression that tumor shrinkage is generally associated with relief of pain. Although there are some reports of analgesic value even in the absence of significant tumor shrinkage *(14–16)*, the likelihood of a favorable effect on pain is generally related to the likelihood of tumor response. Patients with advanced colonic or rectal cancer have a relatively low likelihood of objective tumor response (10–40%) to chemotherapy. Despite this, controlled data supports the conclusion that a substantial minority of patients will achieve clinically significant benefit *(17–19)*. Palliative chemotherapy for colorectal cancer should be administered as a trial of therapy, additional to specific analgesic treatment. Squamous cell cancer of the anus, in contrast, can be highly responsive to combined modality treatment, and an impressive cure rate is reported even with advanced disease *(20–22)*. The response to salvage chemotherapy for recurrent anal cancer is variable, and long duration of initial response duration is predictive of a higher likelihood of second response.

2.3. Surgery

Surgery may have a role in the relief of symptoms caused by specific problems, such as obstruction of a hollow viscus *(23–26)*, unstable bony structures *(27–29)*, and compression of neural tissues *(30–32)*. The potential benefits must be weighed against the risks of surgery, the anticipated length of hospitalization and convalescence, and the predicted duration of benefit *(33)*. Clinical experience suggests that the surgical interventions of high palliative index include the stabilization of pathological fractures, the relief of remediable bowel obstructions, and the drainage of symptomatic ascites. Paracentesis may provide prompt relief from the pain and discomfort of tense ascites. The duration of relief is generally short unless large volumes are drained. Large-volume (up to 5–10 L) paracentesis, for example, may provide prompt and prolonged relief from the pain and discomfort of tense ascites *(33,34)*, with a small risk of hypotension *(34,35)* or hypoproteinemia *(36)*. Radical surgery to excise locally advanced disease in patients with no evidence of metastatic spread may be palliative and potentially increase the survival of some patients *(37,38)*. Successful management of pain associated with uncontrollable recurrent pelvic tumors ulcerating through the perineum after radical surgical debridement with perineal reconstruction has been reported *(39,40)*.

2.4. Antibiotic Therapy

Antibiotics may be analgesic when the source of the pain involves infection. Illustrative examples include cellulitis, chronic sinus infections, pelvic abscess, pyonephrosis, and

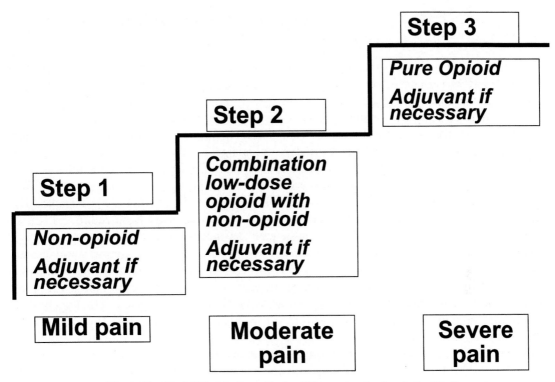

Fig. 1. The World Health Organization "Three-step Analgesic Ladder."

osteitis pubis *(41,42).* In some cases, infection may be occult and confirmed only by the symptomatic relief provided by empiric treatment with these drugs *(43–45).*

3. ANALGESIC THERAPY: AN OVERVIEW

For the large majority of patients, pain management involves the administration of specific analgesic approaches. Systemic pharmacological therapy is the mainstay and should be integrated with psychological and physiatric techniques. Anesthetic and neurosurgical techniques should be considered for the patient who has not obtained satisfactory pain relief. In all cases, these analgesic treatments must be skillfully integrated with the management of other symptoms.

There is universal agreement that analgesic pharmacotherapy remains the mainstay of cancer pain management. Controversy, however, has arisen regarding the validity and application of the "Three-step Analgesic Ladder" of the World Health Organization, which advocated three basic steps of therapy according to the severity of the presenting pain problem (Fig. 1) *(46).* Despite data from a series of validation studies that demonstrated that this approach, combined with appropriate dosing guidelines, provides adequate relief to 70–90% of patients *(47–52),* a review of these studies concluded that there was a lack of evidence for the long-term efficacy of this approach *(53).* Additionally, the recent production of low-dose formulations of pure opioid agonists traditionally used for severe pain and the introduction of other agents such as tramadol, has blurred the distinction between steps 2 and 3.

4. SYSTEMIC ANALGESIC PHARMACOTHERAPY

4.1. Nonopioid Analgesics

The nonopioid analgesics (aspirin, acetaminophen, and the nonsteroidal anti-inflammatory drugs [NSAIDs]) are useful alone for mild to moderate pain (step 1 of the analgesic ladder) and provide additive analgesia when combined with opioid drugs in the treatment of more severe pain *(54)*. They are useful in a broad range of pain syndromes of diverse mechanisms, but there are no data to support therapeutic superiority to alternative options in ant poarticular stetting other than inflamation *(54)*. Unlike opioid analgesics, the nonopioid analgesics have a "ceiling" effect for analgesia and produce neither tolerance nor physical dependence.

The nonopioid analgesics constitute a heterogeneous group of compounds that differ in chemical structure but share many pharmacological actions (Table 1). The NSAID drugs are competitive blockers of cyclooxygenase. It has recently been found that there are at least two isoforms of cylooxygenase with distinct roles in analgesia and toxicity *(55)*. Cyclooxygenase-1 is responsible for the synthesis of the protective prostaglandins, which preserve the integrity of the stomach lining and maintain normal renal function in a compromised kidney, and cyclooxygenase-2 is an inducable enxyme involved in inflammation, pain, and fever. Recently, a range of relatively selective cyclooxygenase-2 inhibitors, including meloxicam, nemesulide, rofecoxib, and celecoxib, have been introduced and approved as analgesics. These agents are equianalgesic with the nonselective inhibitors and they are associated with less mucosal and renal morbidity *(56–58)*.

Safely administering nonopioid analgesics requires familiarity with their potential adverse effects *(59–62)*. Aspirin and the other NSAIDs have a broad spectrum of potential toxicity; bleeding diathesis because of inhibition of platelet aggregation, gastroduodenopahy (including peptic ulcer disease), and renal impairment are the most common *(61)*. Less common adverse effects include confusion, precipitation of cardiac failure, and exacerbation of hypertension. Particular caution is required in the administration of these agents to patients at increased risk of adverse effects, including the elderly and those with blood-clotting disorders, predilection to peptic ulceration, impaired renal function, and concurrent corticosteroid therapy. Of the NSAIDs, the relatively cyclooxygenase-2-selective inhibitors (nimuselide, meloxicam, rofecoxib, and celecoxib) *(63)* or the nonacetylated salicylates (choline magnesium trisalicylate and salsalate) *(64)* are preferred in patients who have a predilection to peptic ulceration or bleeding; these drugs have less effect on platelet aggregation and no effect on bleeding time at the usual clinical doses. Data from randomized trials support the use of either omeprazole *(65)*, pantoprazole, misoprostol *(66)*, or high-dose famotidine (80 mg/d) *(67)* as the preferred agent for the prevention of NSAID-related peptic ulceration. In some countries, a combined formulation of diclofenac and misoprostol is available as a convenient and cost-effective option *(68,69)*.

Acetaminophen rarely produces gastrointestinal toxicity and there are no adverse effects on platelet function; hepatic toxicity is possible, however, and patients with chronic alcoholism and liver disease can develop severe hepatotoxicity at the usual therapeutic doses *(70)*.

The optimal administration of nonopioid analgesics requires an understanding of their clinical pharmacology. There is no certain knowledge of the minimal effective analgesic dose, ceiling dose, or toxic dose for any individual patient with cancer pain. Based on clinical experience, an upper limit for dose titration is usually set at 1.5–2 times the standard recommended dose of the drug in question. Because failure with one NSAID can be followed

Table 1
Commonly Used Nonopioid Analgesics

Chemical class	Generic name
Cox-2-specific	Meloxicam
	Nemesulide
	Rofecoxib
	Celecoxib
Nonacidic	Acetaminophen
Acidic	
Salicylates	Aspirin
	Diflunisal
	Choline magnesium trisalicylate
	Salsalate
Proprionic acids	Ibuprofen
	Naproxen
	Fenoprofen
	Ketoprofen
	Flurbiprofen
	Suprofen
Acetic acids	Indomethacin
	Tolmentin
	Sulindac
	Diclofenac
	Ketorolac
Oxicams	Piroxicam
Fenemates	Mefenamic acid
	Meclofenamic acid

by success with another, sequential trials of several NSAIDs may be useful in identifying a drug with a favorable balance between analgesia and side effects.

4.2. Opioid Analgesics: Basic Pharmacology

A trial of systemic opioid therapy should be administered to all cancer patients with pain of moderate or greater severity regardless of the pain mechanism. Although somatic and visceral pain appear to be relatively more responsive to opioid analgesics than neuropathic pain, a neuropathic mechanism does not confer "opioid resistance" and appropriate dose escalation will identify many patients with neuropathic pain who can achieve adequate relief *(71,72)*.

Optimal use of opioid analgesics requires a sound understanding of the general principles of opioid pharmacology, the pharmacological characteristics of each of the commonly used drugs, and principles of administration, including drug selection, routes of administration, dosing and dose titration, and the prevention and management of adverse effects.

4.3. Important Principles in Opioid Drug Therapy

4.3.1. CLASSIFICATION

Opioid compounds can be divided into agonist, agonist–antagonist, and antagonist classes based on their interactions with the various receptor subtypes (Table 2). In the

Table 2
Classification of Opioid Analgesics

Agonists	Partial agonists	Agonist–antagonists
Morphine	Buprenorphine	Pentazocine
Codeine	Dezocine	Butorphanol
Oxycodone		Nalbuphine
Heroin		
Oxymorphone		
Meperidine		
Levorphanol		
Hydromorphone		
Methadone		
Fentanyl		
Sufentanil		
Alfentanil		
Propoxyphene		

management of cancer pain, the pure agonists are most commonly used. The mixed agonist–antagonist opioids (pentazocine, nalbuphine, and butorphanol) and the partial agonist opioids (buprenorphine and probably dezocine) play a minor role in the management of cancer pain because of the existence of a ceiling effect for analgesia, the potential for precipitation of withdrawal in patients physically dependent to opioid agonists, and, in the case of mixed agonist–antagonists, the problem of dose-dependent psychotomimetic side effects that exceed those of pure agonist drugs *(73)*.

4.3.2. Dose-Response Relationship

The pure agonist drugs do not have a ceiling dose; as the dose is raised, analgesic effects increases in a semi log-linear function, until either analgesia is achieved or the patient develops dose-limiting adverse effects such as nausea, vomiting, confusion, sedation, myoclonus, or respiratory depression.

4.3.3. The Equianalgesic Dose Ratio

The relative analgesic potency of opioid is commonly expressed in terms of the equianalgesic dose ratio. This is the ratio of the dose of two analgesics required to produce the same analgesic effect. By convention, the relative potency of each of the commonly used opioids is based on a comparison to 10 mg of parenteral morphine *(74)*. Equianalgesic dose information (Table 3) provides guidelines for dose selection when the drug or route of administration is changed.

Several principles are critical in interpreting the data presented in equianalgesic dose tables. The commonly quoted values do not reflect the substantial variability that is observed in both single-dose and multidose crossover studies. Numerous variables may influence the appropriate dose for the individual patient, including pain severity, prior opioid exposure (and the degree of cross-tolerance this confers), age, route of administration, level of consciousness, and genetically determined metabolic or receptor heterogeneity. For most agents, the equianalgesic dose relationship to morphine is linear; for methadone, however, the relationship appears to be curvilinear with the equianalgesic dose ratio falling as the dose of prior morphine increases. At low doses of morphine (30–300 mg oral morphine),

Table 3
Opioid Agonist Drugs

Drug	Dose (mg) equianalgesic to 10 mg im morphine		Half-life (h)	Duration of action (h)	Comments
	im	*po*			
Codeine	130	200	2–3	2–4	Usually combined with a nonopioid.
Oxycodone	7–10	15–20	2–3	2–4	
Propoxyphene	100	50	2–3	2–4	Usually combined with nonopioid; norpropoxyphene toxicity may cause seizures.
Morphine	10	30	2–3	3–4	Multiple routes of administration and formulations available; M6G accumulation in renal failure.
Hydromorphone	2–3	7.5	2–3	2–4	Multiple routes of administration and formulations available.
Methadone	1–3	2–6	15–190	4–8	Plasma accumulation may lead to delayed toxicity; dosing should be initiated on a PRN basis.
Meperidine	75	300	2–3	2–4	Low oral bioavailability; normeperidine toxicity limits utility; contraindicated in patients with renal failure and those receiving MAO inhibitors.
Oxymorphone	1	10 (P.R.)*	2–3	3–4	No oral formulation available; less histamine release.
Levorphanol	2	4	12–15	4–8	Plasma accumulation may lead to delayed toxicity.
Fentanyl transdermal system		empirically transdermal fentanyl 100 μg/h = 2–4 mg/h intravenous morphine		48–72	Patches available to deliver 25, 50, 75, and 100 μg/h.

*P. R., per rectum.

the equianalgesic ratio for oral methadone to oral morphine is $1:4$ to $1:6$ and at high doses (> 300 mg oral morphine), it is $1:10$ to $1:12$ *(75)*.

4.3.4. OPIOID AGONISTS

4.3.4.1. Codeine. Codeine is the most commonly used opioid analgesic for the management of mild to moderate pain. It is generally formulated in combination with aspirin or acetaminophen. Its plasma half-life and duration of action is usually in the range of 2–4 h.

4.3.4.2. Dihydrocodeine. Dihydrocodeine is an equianalgesic codeine analog. In the United States, it is only available in combination with acetaminophen or aspirin. A single-agent sustained-release formulation is has been developed and is available in some countries *(76)*.

4.3.4.3. Oxycodone. Oral oxycodone has a high bioavailability (60%) and an analgesic potency that is 25–50% greater than morphine *(77)*. Oral oxycodone, in combination with aspirin or acetaminophen in products that provide 5 mg of oxycodone per tablet, is a useful drug for moderate pain in step II of the "analgesic ladder." Single-agent tablet or syrup formulations are also available, and doses of these can be adjusted to effectively manage severe pain *(78)*. Recently, sustained-release formulations in a wide dose range (10, 20, 40, and 80 mg) have been developed. These formulations have a duration of action of 8–12 h and are suitable for the management of both moderate and severe pain *(77,79)*.

4.3.4.4. Propoxyphene (Dextropropoxyphene). Propoxyphene is a congener of methadone. It is metabolized to norpropoxyphene, which has a long half-life and is associated with excitatory effects, including tremulousness and seizures *(80)*. These effects are dose related and are not a clinical problem at the doses of propoxyphene typically administered for moderate pain (50–100 mg every 4 h) *(81)*. In the United States, propxyphene is available in short-acting formulation in combination with acteominophen.

4.3.4.5. Morphine. Based on its availability and clinician familiarity with its use, morphine has been designated as the prototypical agent for step III of the "analgesic ladder" *(82)* and it is on the essential drug list of the WHO. It is available in a very wide range of formulations: injectable, immediate and controlled-release tablets, immediate and controlled-release rectal suppositories, immediate-release syrup, and controlled-release suspension. This very wide range of formulations is unique among the pure opioid agonists and contributes to the great flexibility of this agent.

Morphine usually has a half-life and duration of action of 2–4 h. Morphine undergoes hepatic glucuronidation at the 3- and 6-positions and the metabolites are excreted by the kidneys. Morphine-3-glucuronide (M3G) is the major metabolite *(83)*. M3G is not an analgesic, rather there are data to suggest a role in the production of dose-related adverse effects such as hyperalgesia/allodynia and myoclonus *(84)*. M6G excretion by the kidney is related to creatinine clearance *(85)*, and in some patients with impaired renal function, high concentrations of M6G have been associated with toxicity *(86–88)*, suggesting the need for enhanced vigilance when administering morphine to patients with renal impairment. The im to po relative potency is $1:3$ or $1:2$ *(89)*.

4.3.4.6. Hydromorphone. Hydromorphone is a versatile, short half-life opioid that can be administered by the oral, rectal, parenteral, and intraspinal routes *(90)*. Its solubility, high bioavailability by continuous subcutaneous infusion (78%) *(91)*, and the availability of a high-concentration preparation (10 mg/cm^3), make it particularly suitable for subcutaneous infusion. Orally, it is available in both immediate and controlled-relase formulations *(79,92)*. The equianalgesic ratio of parenteral morphine to hydromorphone is approx $4:1$ *(93,94)*.

4.3.4.7. Meperidine (Pethidine). Meperidine is a short half-life opioid agonist with a profile of potential adverse effects that limits its utility. Meperidine is N-demethylated to normeperidine, which is an active metabolite that is twice as potent as a convulsant and one-half as potent as an analgesic than its parent compound. The half-life of normeperidine is 12–16 h, approximately four to five times the half-life of meperidine. Accumulation of normeperidine after repetitive dosing of meperidine can result in central nervous system toxicity characterized by subtle adverse mood effects, tremulousness, multifocal myoclonus, and, occasionally, seizures *(95,96)*.

4.3.4.8. Methadone. Methadone is a synthetic opioid with a very long plasma half-life, which averages approximately 24 h (range from 13 to over 100 h) *(97)*. Despite this long half-life, many patients require dosing at a 4 to 8 h interval to maintain analgesic effects *(98)*. After treatment is initiated or the dose is increased, plasma concentration rises for a prolonged period, and this may be associated with delayed onset of side effects. Serious adverse effects can be avoided if the initial period of dosing is accomplished with "as needed" administration *(99,100)*. When steady state has been achieved, scheduled dose frequency should be determined by the duration of analgesia following each dose. Most patients can be well controlled on 8–12-h dosing. Oral and parenteral preparations of methadone are available. Subcutaneous infusion has been reported to cause local skin toxicity and is not recommended *(101)*.

The equianalgesic dose ratio of morphine to methadone has been a matter of confusion and controversy. Recent data from crossover studies with morphine and methadone, and hydromorphone and methadone indicate that methadone is much more potent than previously described in literature and that the ratio correlates with total opioid dose administered before switching to methadone *(102)*. Among patients receiving low doses of morphine, the ratio is 4:1; in contrast, for patients receiving more than 300 mg of oral morphine (or parenteral equivalent), the ratio is approx 10:1 *(103)*.

4.3.4.9. Oxymorphone. Oxymorphone is a potent, short-half-life lipophilic congener of morphine that is available as injectable and rectal formulations in the United States. Substantial experience has been reported using oxymorphone for intravenous or subcutaneous patient-controlled analgesia *(104–106)*. The rectal formulation is approximately equipotent with parenteral morphine.

4.3.4.10. Levorphanol. Levorphanol is a morphine congener with a long half-life (12–16 h) *(107)* that is available in both oral and parenteral formulations. It is five times more potent than morphine and has an oral to parenteral relative potency ratio of 2:1 *(108)*. Like methadone, drug accumulation may follow the initiation of therapy or dose escalation. Levorphanol is used commonly as a second-line agent in patients with chronic pain who cannot tolerate morphine.

4.3.4.11. Fentanyl. Fentanyl is a semisynthetic opioid characterized by high potency, lipophilicity, and a short half-life after bolus administration. The development of a transdermal system (*see* Section 4.5.) has broadened its clinical utility for the management of cancer pain *(109)*. Fentanyl is also used parenterally as a premedication for painful procedures *(110)* and in continual infusion either intravenously *(111)* or by the subcutaneous route *(112)*. A recently developed oral transmucosal formulation may be particularly useful in the management of "breakthrough" pain in the cancer population *(113)*.

4.4. Selecting an Appropriate Opioid

The factors that influence opioid selection in chronic pain states include pain intensity, pharmacokinetic and formulatory considerations, previous adverse effects, and the presence of coexisting disease.

Traditionally, patients with moderate pain have been conventionally treated with a combination product containing acetaminophen or aspirin plus codeine, dihydrocodeine, hydrocodone, oxycodone, and propoxyphene. The doses of these combination products can be increased until the maximum dose of the nonopioid coanalgesic is attained (e.g., 4000 mg acetaminophen). Recent years have witnessed the proliferation of new opioid formulations that may improve the convenience of drug administration for patients with moderate pain. These include controlled-release formulations of codeine, dihydrocodeine, oxycodone, morphine, and tramadol in dosages appropriate for moderate pain.

Patients who present with strong pain are usually treated with morphine, hydromorphone, oxycodone, oxymorphone, fentanyl, methadone, or levorphanol. Of these, the short-half-life opioid agonists (morphine, hydromorphone, fentanyl, oxycodone, or oxymorphone) are generally favored because they are easier to titrate than the long-half-life drugs, which require a longer period to approach steady-state plasma concentrations. Morphine is generally preferred because it has a short half-life and is easy to titrate in its immediate release form, and it is also available as a controlled-release preparation that allows an 8- to 12-h dosing interval.

If the patient is currently using an opioid that is well tolerated, it is usually continued unless difficulties in dose titration occur or the required dose cannot be administered conveniently. A switch to an alternative opioid is considered if the patient develops dose-limiting toxicity that precludes adequate relief of pain without excessive side effects or if a specific formulation, not available with the current drug, is either needed or may substantially improve the convenience of opioid administration. Some patients will require sequential trials of several different opioids before a drug that is effective and well tolerated is identified *(114,115)*. This strategy has been variably labeled opioid-rotation or opioid-switching. The existence of incomplete cross-tolerance to various opioid effects (analgesia and side effects) may explain the utility of these sequential trials. It is strongly recommended that clinicians be familiar with at least three opioid drugs used in the management of severe pain and have the ability to calculate appropriate starting doses using equianalgesic dosing data when switching between drugs.

4.5. Selecting the Appropriate Route of Systemic Opioid Administration

Opioids should be administered by the least invasive and safest route capable of providing adequate analgesia. Usually, the oral route is preferred. Alternative routes are necessary for patients who have impaired swallowing or gastrointestinal dysfunction, those who require a very rapid onset of analgesia, and those who are unable to manage either the logistics or side effects associated with the oral route.

The development of transdermal fentanyl has provided a convenient an noninvasive alternative to oral administration. Transdermal patches capable of delivering 25, 50, 75, and 100 µg/h are available. The dosing interval for each patch is usually 72 h *(116)*, but some patients require a 48-h schedule *(109)*. Recent data from controlled studies indicate that the transdermal administration of fentanyl is associated with a lesser incidence of constipation than oral morphine and is often preferred *(117–119)*. Multiple patches may be used simultaneously for patients who require higher doses. At the present time, the limitations of the transdermal delivery system include its cost and the requirement for an alternative short-acting opioid for breakthrough pain.

Other noninvasive routes are less commonly used. Rectal suppositories containing oxycodone, hydromorphone, oxymorphone, and morphine have been formulated, and controlled-release morphine tablets can also be administered per rectum *(120,121)*. The potency of opioids administered rectally is approximately equivalent to that achieved by the oral route *(89)*.

The sublingual route has limited value because of the lack of formulations, poor absorption of most drugs, and the inability to deliver high doses or prevent swallowing of the dose. Anecdotally, sublingual morphine has also been reported to be effective; however, this drug has poor sublingual absorption *(122)* and efficacy may be related, in part, to swallowing of the dose.

An oral transmucosal formulation of fentanyl, which incorporates the drug into a candy base, has recently been approved for use in the management of breakthrough pain *(123)*.

4.5.1. Invasive Routes

A parenteral route may be considered when the oral route is precluded or there is need for rapid onset of analgesia, or a more convenient regimen. Repeated parenteral bolus injections, which may be administered by the intravenous (iv), intramuscular (im) or subcutaneous (sc) routes, provides the most rapid onset and shortest duration of action. Parenteral boluses are most commonly used to treat very severe pain, in which case doses can be repeated at an interval as brief as that determined by the time to peak effect, until adequate relief is achieved *(124)*. Repeated bolus doses without frequent skin punctures can be accomplished through the use of an indwelling iv or sc infusion device such as a 25–27 gage infusion device (a "butterfly"), which can be left under the skin for up to a week *(125)*. Repetitive im injections are not recommended: they are painful and offer no pharmacokinetic advantage *(126)*.

Continuous parenteral infusions are useful for many patients who cannot be maintained on oral opioids. Long-term infusions may be administered iv or sc. In practice, the major indication for continuous infusion occurs among patients who are unable to swallow or absorb opioids. Continuous infusion is also used in some patients whose high opioid requirement renders oral treatment impractical. Ambulatory patients can easily use continuous sc infusion. A range of pumps is available varying in complexity, cost, and ability to provide patient-controlled "rescue doses" as an adjunct to a continuous basal infusion *(125)*. Opioids suitable for continuous sc infusion must be soluble, well absorbed, and nonirritant. Extensive experience has been reported with heroin, hydromorphone, oxymorphone, morphine, and fentanyl. Methadone appears to be relatively irritating and is not recommended. To maintain the comfort of an infusion site, the sc infusion rate should not exceed 3–5 cm^3/h. Patients who require high doses may benefit from the use of concentrated solutions. A high concentration hydromorphone (10 mg/cm^3) is available commercially and the organic salt of morphine, morphine tartrate, is available in some countries as an 80-mg/cm^3 solution. In selected cases, concentrated opioid solutions can be compounded specifically for continuous sc infusion.

Occasionally, patients develop focal erythematous swelling at the site of injection; this complication must be distinguished from injection-site abscess formation, which may require antibiotic therapy and, in some cases, surgical drainage.

In some circumstances, continuous iv infusion may be the most appropriate parenteral route. The need for very large doses, treatment with methadone, or the development of injection-site reactions may suggest the utility of this approach. If continuous iv infusion is to be continued on a long-term basis, a permanent central venous access is recommended.

4.5.2. Changing Routes of Administration

The switch between oral and parenteral routes should be guided by knowledge of relative potency (Table 3) to avoid subsequent overdosing or underdosing. In calculating the equianalgesic dose, the potencies of the iv, sc, and im routes are considered equivalent. In recognition of the imprecision in the accepted equianalgesic doses and the risk of toxicity from potential overdose, a modest reduction in the equianalgesic dose is prudent.

4.6. Scheduling of Opioid Administration

The schedule of opioid administration should be individualized to optimize the balance between patient comfort and convenience. "Around the clock" dosing and "as needed" dosing both have a place in clinical practice.

4.6.1. "Around the Clock" Dosing with "Rescue Doses"

"Around the clock" dosing provides the chronic pain patient with continuous relief by preventing the pain from recurring. Controlled-release preparations of opioids can lessen the inconvenience associated with the use of "around the clock" administration of drugs with a short duration of action. Currently, controlled-release formulations are available for administration by the oral, transdermal, and rectal routes. Patients should also be provided a so-called "rescue dose," which is a supplemental dose offered on an "as needed" basis to treat pain that breaks through the regular schedule (127). The frequency with which the rescue dose can be offered depends on the route of administration and the time to peak effect for the particular drug. Oral rescue doses are usually offered up to every 1–2 h and parenteral doses can be offered as frequently as every 15–30 min. Clinical experience suggests that the initial size of the rescue dose should be equivalent to approx 50–100% of the dose administered every 4 h for oral or parenteral bolus medications, or 50–100% of the hourly infusion rate for patients receiving continuous infusions. Alternatively, this may be calculated as 5–15% of the 24-h baseline dose. The magnitude of the rescue dose should be individualized and some patients with low baseline pain but severe exacerbations may require rescue doses that are substantially higher (128). The drug used for the rescue dose is usually identical to that administered on a scheduled basis.

This approach provides a method for safe and rational stepwise dose escalation, which is applicable to all routes of opioid administration. Patients who require more than four to six rescue doses per day should generally undergo escalation of the baseline dose. The quantity of the rescue medication consumed can be used to guide the dose increment. Alternatively, each dose increment can be set at 33–50% of the pre-existing dose. In all cases, escalation of the baseline dose should be accompanied by a proportionate increase in the rescue dose so that the size of the supplemental dose remains a constant percentage of the fixed dose.

4.6.2. "As-Needed" Dosing

Opioid administration on an "as needed" (PNR) basis, without an "around the clock" dosing regimen, may provide additional safety during the initiation of opioid therapy, particularly when rapid dose escalation is needed or therapy with a long-half-life opioid such as methadone or levorphanol is begun. "As needed" dosing may also be appropriate for patients who have rapidly decreasing analgesic requirement or intermittent pains separated by pain-free intervals.

4.6.3. Patient Controlled Analgesia

Patient-controlled analgesia (PCA) generally refers to a technique of parenteral drug administration in which the patient controls an infusion device that delivers a bolus of analgesic drug "on demand" according to parameters set by the physician. Long-term PCA in cancer patients is most commonly accomplished via the subcutaneous route using an ambulatory infusion device *(129)*. In most cases, PCA is added to a basal infusion rate and acts essentially as a rescue dose *(129)*. Rare patients have benefited from PCA alone to manage episodic pains characterized by an onset so rapid that an oral dose could not provide sufficiently prompt relief.

4.7. Dose Selection and Titration

4.7.1. SELECTING A STARTING DOSE

A patient who is relatively nontolerant, having had only some exposure to an opioid typically used on the second rung of the "analgesic ladder" for moderate pain, should generally begin one of the opioids typically used for severe pain at a dose equivalent to 5–10 morphine im every 4 h *(89)*. If morphine is used, a po to im relative potency ratio of 2:1–3:1 is conventional *(89)*. When patients on higher doses of opioids are switched to an alternative opioid drug, the starting dose of the new drug should be reduced to 50–75% of the equianalgesic dose to account for incomplete cross-tolerance.

4.7.2. DOSE ADJUSTMENT

Inadequate relief should be addressed through gradual escalation of dose until adequate analgesia is reported or excessive side effects supervene. Because opioid response increases linearly with the log of the dose, a dose increment of less than 30–50% is not likely to significantly improve analgesia. The absolute dose is immaterial as long as administration is not compromised by excessive side effects, inconvenience, discomfort, or cost.

4.7.3. RATE OF DOSE TITRATION

The rate of dose titration depends on the severity of the pain, the medical condition of the patient, and the goals of care. Patients who present with very severe pain are sometimes best managed by repeated parenteral administration of a dose every 15–30 min until pain is partially relieved. Patients with moderate pain may not require a loading dose of the opioid, but rather the initiation of a regular dose with provision for rescue doses and gradual dose titration. In this situation, dose increments of 30–50% can be administered at intervals greater than that required to reach steady state following each change. The dose of morphine (tablets or elixir), hydromorphone, or oxycodone can be increased on a twice-daily basis, and the dose of controlled-release oral morphine or transdermal fentanyl can be increased every 24–48 h.

4.7.4. THE PROBLEM OF TOLERANCE

When the need for dose escalation arises, disease progression *(130,131)*, increasing psychological distress or changes in the pharmacokinetics of an analgesic drug are much more common than true analgesic tolerance. Indeed, most patients who require an escalation in dose to manage increasing pain have demonstrable progression of disease. True analgesic tolerance, which could compromise the utility of treatment, can only be said to occur if a patient manifests the need for increasing opioid doses in the absence of other factors (e.g., progressive disease) that would be capable of explaining the increase in pain.

Together, these observations suggest several important conclusions:

1. That true pharmacological tolerance to the analgesic effects of opioids is not a common clinical problem.
2. Concern about tolerance should not impede the use of opioids early in the course of the disease.

3. Worsening pain in a patient receiving a stable dose of opioids should not be attributed to tolerance, but should be assessed as presumptive evidence of disease progression or, less commonly, increasing psychological distress.

4.8. Management of Opioid Adverse Effects

Successful opioid therapy requires that the benefits of analgesia and other desired effects clearly outweigh treatment-related adverse effects. Thus, a detailed understanding of adverse opioid effects and the strategies used to prevent and manage them are essential skills for all involved in cancer pain management.

4.8.1. ADVERSE DRUG INTERACTIONS

In patients with advanced cancer side effects resulting from drug combinations are common. The potential for additive side effects and serious toxicity from drug combinations must be recognized. The sedative effect of an opioid may add to that produced by numerous other centrally acting drugs, such as anxiolytics, neuroleptics, and antidepressants *(132)*. Likewise, drugs with anticholinergic effects probably worsen the constipatory effects of opioids. As noted previously, a severe adverse reaction, including excitation, hyperpyrexia, convulsions, and death, has been reported after the administration of meperidine to patients treated with a monoamine oxidase inhibitor *(133)*.

4.8.2. GASTROINTESTINAL SIDE EFFECTS

The gastrointestinal adverse effects of opioids are common. In general, they are characterized by having by having a weak dose-response relationship.

4.8.2.1. Constipation. Constipation is the most common adverse effect of chronic opioid therapy *(134)*. The likelihood of opioid-induced constipation is so great that laxative medications should be prescribed prophylactically to most patients.

4.8.2.2. Nausea and Vomiting. Opioids may produce nausea and vomiting through both central and peripheral mechanisms. These drugs stimulate the medullary chemoreceptor trigger zone, increase vestibular sensitivity and have effects on the gastrointestinal tract (including increased gastric antral tone, diminished motility, and delayed gastric emptying. With the initiation of opioid therapy, patients should be informed that nausea can occur and that it is usually transitory and controllable. Routine prophylactic administration of an antiemetic is not necessary, except in patients with a history of severe opioid-induced nausea and vomiting, but patients should have access to an antiemetic at the start of therapy if the need for one arises. Anecdotally, the use of prochlorperazine and metoclopromide has usually been sufficient.

4.8.3. CENTRAL NERVOUS SYSTEM SIDE EFFECTS

The CNS side effects of opioids are generally dose related. The specific pattern of CNS adverse effects is influenced by individual patient factors, duration of opioid exposure, and dose.

4.8.3.1. Sedation. Initiation of opioid therapy or significant dose escalation commonly induces sedation that persists until tolerance to this effect develops, usually in days to weeks. It is useful to forewarn patients of this potential and thereby reduce anxiety and encourage avoidance of activities, such as driving, that may be dangerous if sedation occurs *(135)*. Some patients have a persistent problem with sedation, particularly if other confounding factors exist. These factors include the use of other sedating drugs or coexistent diseases such as dementia, metabolic encephalopathy, or brain metastases. Both dextroamphetamine and methylphenidate have been widely used in the treatment of opioid-induced sedation *(136)*.

Table 4
Examples of Stepwise Dose Escalation of Morphine Sulfate
Administered as Oral Immediate Release Preparation,
Oral Controlled Release and Continuous Infusion

	Oral immediate release morphine sulfate		
Step[a]	*mg q 4 h* *ATC*	*Rescue dose (mg)*	
1	15	7.5	PRN q 1 h
2	30	15.0	PRN q 1 h
3	45	22.5	PRN q 1 h
4	60	30.0	PRN q 1 h
5	90	45.0	PRN q 1 h

	Oral controlled release morphine sulfate *(immediate-release rescue dose)*		
Step[a]	*mg ATC*	*Immediate release rescue dose (mg)*	
1	30 q 12	7.5	PRN q 1 h
2	30 q 8	15.0	PRN q 1 h
3	60 q 12	15.0	PRN q 1 h
4	100 q 12	30.0	PRN q 1 h
5	100 q 8	45.0	PRN q 1 h

	Continuous morphine infusion		
Step[a]	*mg/h*	*Rescue dose (mg)*	
1	3	2.0	PRN q 30 min
2	5	2.5	PRN q 30 min
3	7	3.5	PRN q 30 min
4	10	5.0	PRN q 30 min
5	15	7.5	PRN q 30 min

[a]Suggested indications for progression from one step to the next include (1) requirement of more than two rescue doses in any 4-h interval or (2) requirement of more than six rescue doses in 24 h.

Treatment with methylphenidate or dextroamphetamine is typically begun at 2.5–5 mg in the morning, which is repeated at midday if necessary to maintain effects until evening. Doses are then increased gradually if needed. Few patients require more than 40 mg/d in divided doses. This approach is relatively contraindicated among patients are with cardiac arrhythmias, agitated delirium, paranoid personality, and past amphetamine abuse.

4.8.3.2. Confusion and Delirium. Mild cognitive impairment is common following the initiation of opioid therapy or dose. Similar to sedation, however, pure opioid-induced encephalopathy appears to be transient in most patients, persisting from days to a week or two. Although persistent confusion attributable to opioid alone occurs, the etiology of persistent delirium is usually related to the combined effect of the opioid and other contributing factors, including electrolyte disorders, neoplastic involvement of the central nervous system, sepsis, vital-organ failure, and hypoxemia *(136)*. A stepwise approach to management (Table 4) often culminates in a trial of a neuroleptic drug. Haloperidol in low doses (0.5–1.0 mg po or 0.25–0.5 mg iv or im) is most commonly recommended because of its efficacy and low incidence of cardiovascular and anticholinergic effects.

4.8.3.3. Respiratory Depression. When sedation is used as a clinical indicator of CNS toxicity and appropriate steps are taken, respiratory depression is rare. When, however, it does occur, it is always accompanied by other signs of CNS depression, including sedation and mental clouding. Respiratory compromise accompanied by tachypnea and anxiety is never a primary opioid event.

With repeated opioid administration, tolerance appears to develop rapidly to the respiratory depressant effects of the opioid drugs; consequently, clinically important respiratory depression is a very rare event in the cancer patient whose opioid dose has been titrated against pain.

The ability to tolerate high doses of opioids is also related to the stimulus-related effect of pain on respiration in a manner that is balanced against the depressant opioid effect. Opioid-induced respiratory depression can occur, however, if pain is suddenly eliminated (such as may occur following neurolytic procedures) and the opioid dose is not reduced *(137)*.

When respiratory depression occurs in patients on chronic opioid therapy, administration of the specific opioid antagonist naloxone usually improves ventilation. This is true even if the primary cause of the respiratory event was not the opioid itself, but, rather, an intercurrent cardiac or pulmonary process. A response to naloxone, therefore, should not be taken as proof that the event was the result of the opioid alone and an evaluation for these other processes should ensue.

Naloxone can precipitate a severe abstinence syndrome and should be administered only if strongly indicated. If the patient is bradypneic but readily arousable and the peak plasma level of the last opioid dose has already been reached, the opioid should be withheld and the patient monitored until improved. If severe hypoventilation occurs (regardless of the associated factors that may be contributing to respiratory compromise) or the patient is bradypneic and unarousable, naloxone should be administered. To reduce the risk of severe withdrawal following a period of opioid administration, dilute naloxone (1:10) should be used in doses titrated to respiratory rate and level of consciousness. In the comatose patient, it may be prudent to place an endotracheal tube to prevent aspiration following administration of naloxone.

4.8.3.4. Multifocal Myoclonus. All opioid analgesics can produce myoclonus. Mild and infrequent myoclonus is common. In occasional patients, however, myoclonus can be distressing or contribute to breakthrough pain that occurs with the involuntary movement. If the dose cannot be reduced because of persistent pain, consideration should be given to either switching to an alternative opioid *(114)* or to symptomatic treatment with a benzodiazepine (particularly clonazepam or midazolam), dantrolene, or an anticonvulsant *(136)*.

4.9. Other Effects

Opioid analgesics increase smooth-muscle tone and can occasionally cause bladder spasm or urinary retention (because of an increase in sphincter tone). This is an infrequent problem that is usually observed in elderly male patients. Tolerance can develop rapidly but catheterization may be necessary to manage transient problems.

4.10. Dependence and Addiction

Confusion about physical dependence and addiction augment the fear of opioid drugs and contribute substantially to the undertreatment of pain *(138–144)*. To understand these phenomena as they relate to opioid pharmacotherapy for cancer pain, it is useful to first present a concept that might be called "therapeutic dependence." Patients who require a specific pharmacotherapy to control a symptom or disease process are clearly dependent on the therapeutic efficacy of the drugs in question. Examples of this "therapeutic dependence" include the requirements of patients with congestive cardiac failure for cardiotonic and diuretic medications or the reliance of insulin-dependent diabetics on insulin therapy. In these patients, undermedication or withdrawal of treatment results in serious untoward consequences for the patient, the fear of which could conceivably induce aberrant psychological responses and drug-seeking behaviors. Patients with chronic cancer pain have an analogous relationship to their analgesic pharmacotherapy. This relationship may or may not be associated with the development of physical dependence, but it is virtually never associated with addiction.

4.10.1. Physical Dependence

Physical dependence is a pharmacological property of opioid drugs defined by the development of an abstinence (withdrawal) syndrome following either abrupt dose reduction or administration of an antagonist. Despite the observation that physical dependence is most commonly observed in patients taking large doses for a prolonged period of time, withdrawal has also been observed in patients after low doses or short duration of treatment. Physical dependence rarely becomes a clinical problem if patients are warned to avoid abrupt discontinuation of the drug, a tapering schedule is used if treatment cessation is indicated, and opioid antagonist drugs (including agonist–antagonist analgesics) are avoided *(131)*. Occasionally, patients who are switched form a pure agonist opioid to transdermal fentanyl will develop an abstinence syndrome within the first 24 h, the mechanism of which is not understood *(118,145)*.

4.10.2. Addiction

The term "addiction" refers to a psychological and behavioral syndrome characterized by a continued craving for an opioid drug to achieve a psychic effect (psychological dependence) and associated aberrant drug-related behaviors, such as compulsive drug-seeking, unsanctioned use or dose escalation, and use despite harm to self or others. Addiction should be suspected if patients demonstrate compulsive use, loss of control over drug use, and continuing use despite harm.

The medical use of opioids is very rarely associated with the development of addiction *(131)*. In the largest prospective study, only 4 cases could be identified among 11,882 patients with no history of addiction who received at least 1 opioid preparation in the hospital setting *(146)*. In a prospective study of 550 cancer patients who were treated with morphine for a total of 22,525 treatment days, 1 patient developed problems related to substance abuse *(131)*. Health care providers, patients, and families often require vigorous and repeated reassurance that the risk of addiction is extremely small.

4.10.3. "Pseudoaddiction"

The distress engendered in patients who have a therapeutic dependence on analgesic pharmacotherapy but who continue to experience unrelieved pain is occasionally expressed in behaviors that are reminiscent of addiction, such as intense concern about opioid availability and unsanctioned dose escalation. Pain relief, usually produced by dose escalation, eliminates these aberrant behaviors and distinguishes the patient from the true addict. This syndrome has been termed "pseudoaddiction" *(147)*. Misunderstanding of these phenomena may lead the clinician to inappropriately stigmatize the patient with the label "addict," which may compromise care and erode the doctor–patient relationship. In the setting of unrelieved pain, aberrant drug-related behaviors require careful assessment, renewed efforts to manage pain, and avoidance of stigmatizing labels.

4.11. Adjuvant Analgesics

The term "adjuvant analgesic" describes a drug that has a primary indication other than pain but is analgesic in some conditions. In the cancer population, these drugs may be combined with primary analgesics in any of the three steps of the "analgesic ladder" to improve the outcome for patients who cannot otherwise attain an acceptable balance between relief and side effects. The potential utility of an adjuvant analgesic is usually suggested by the characteristics of the pain or by the existence of another symptom that may be amenable to a nonanalgesic effect of the drug.

There is great interindividual variability in the response to all adjuvant analgesics. Although patient characteristics, such as advanced age or coexistent major-organ failure, may increase the likelihood of some (usually adverse) responses, neither favorable effects nor specific side effects can be reliably predicted in the individual patient. Furthermore, there is remarkable intraindividual variability in the response to different drugs, including those within the same class. These observations suggest the potential utility of sequential trials of adjuvant analgesics. The process of sequential drug trials, like the use of low initial doses and dose titration, should be explained to the patient at the start of therapy to enhance compliance and reduce the distress that may occur if treatments fail.

In the management of cancer pain, adjuvant analgesics can be broadly classified based on conventional use. Four groups are distinguished:

1. Multipurpose adjuvant analgesics
2. Adjuvant analgesics used for neuropathic pain
3. Adjuvant analgesics used for bone pain
4. Adjuvant analgesics used for visceral pain

4.11.1. MULTIPURPOSE ADJUVANT MEDICATIONS

4.11.1.1. Corticosteroids. Corticosteroids are among the most widely used adjuvant analgesics *(148)*. They have been demonstrated to have analgesic effects, to significantly improve quality of life, and to have beneficial effects on appetite, nausea, mood, and malaise in the cancer population. Painful conditions that commonly respond to corticosteroids include raised intracranial pressure headache, acute spinal cord compression, superior vena cava syndrome, metastatic bone pain, neuropathic pain resulting from infiltration or compression by tumor, symptomatic lymphedema, and hepatic capsular distention *(148)*. The mechanism of analgesia produced by these drugs may involve anti-edema effects, anti-inflammatory effects, and a direct influence on the electrical activity in damaged nerves *(149)*. The most commonly used drug is dexamethasone, a choice that gains theoretical support from the relatively low mineralocorticoid effect of this agent. Dexamethasone also has been conventionally used for raised intracranial pressure and spinal cord compression.

Patients with advanced cancer who experience pain and other symptoms may respond favorably to a relatively small dose of corticosteroid (e.g., dexamethasone 1–2 mg twice daily). In some settings, however, a high-dose regimen may be appropriate. For example, patients with spinal cord compression, an acute episode of very severe bone pain, or neuropathic pain that cannot be promptly reduced with opioids may respond dramatically to a short course of relatively high doses (e.g., 100 mg dexamethasone, followed initially by 96 mg/d in divided doses) *(150)*. This dose can be tapered over weeks, concurrent with initiation of other analgesic approaches, such as radiotherapy.

Although the effects produced by corticosteroids in patients with advanced cancer are often very gratifying, side effects are potentially serious and increase with prolonged usage *(151)*. The most common adverse effects include oropharyngeal candidiasis, edema or cushingoid habitus, dyspepsia, weight gain, neuropsychological changes and ecchymoses, hyperglycemia, and myopathy. The risk of peptic ulcer is approximately doubled in patients chronically treated with corticosteroids, and coadministration of corticosteroid with aspirin or a NSAID further increases the risk of gastroduodenopahy and is not recommended *(152)*. Active peptic ulcer disease, systemic infection, and unstable diabetes are relative contraindications to the use of corticosteroids as adjuvant analgesics.

4.11.1.2. Topical Local Anesthetics. Topical local anesthetics can be used in the management of painful cutaneous and mucosal lesions and as a premedication prior to skin puncture. Eutectic mixture of 2.5% lidocaine and 2.5% prilocaine (EMLA) is effective in reducing pain associated with venipuncture, lumbar puncture, and arterial puncture. It has also been used for painful ulcerating skin lesions. Viscous lidocaine is frequently used in the management of oropharyngeal ulceration. Although the risk of aspiration appears to be very small, caution with eating is required after oropharyngeal anesthesia.

4.11.2. Adjuvants Used for Neuropathic Pain

Neuropathic pains are generally less responsive to opioid therapy than nociceptive pain and, in many cases, the outcome of pharmacotherapy may be improved by the addition of an adjuvant analgesic.

Antidepressant drugs are commonly used to manage continuous neuropathic pains and the evidence for analgesic efficacy is greatest for the tertiary amine tricyclic drugs, such as amitriptyline, doxepin, and imipramine *(153)*. The secondary amine tricyclic antidepressants (such as desipramine, clomipramine, and nortryptyline) have fewer side effects and are preferred when concern about sedation, anticholinergic effects, or cardiovascular toxicity is high *(153)*. The selective serotonin uptake inhibitor antidepressants are much less effective in the management of neuropathic pain and are generally not recommended for this purpose.

The starting dose of a tricyclic antidepressant should be low (e.g., 10 mg amitriptyline in the elderly and 25 mg in younger patients). Doses can be increased every few days and the initial dosing increments are usually the same size as the starting dose. When doses have reached the usual effective range (e.g., 75–150 mg amitriptyline), it is prudent to observe effects for a week before continuing upward dose titration. It is reasonable to continue upward dose titration beyond the usual analgesic doses in patients who fail to achieve benefit and have no limiting side effects. Plasma drug concentration, if available, may provide useful information and should be followed during the course of therapy.

Selected anticonvulsant drugs appear to be analgesic for the lancinating dysesthesias that characterize diverse types of neuropathic pain *(154)*. Although most practitioners prefer to begin with carbamazepine because of the very good response rate observed in trigeminal neuralgia *(154)*, this drug must be used cautiously in cancer patients with thrombocytopenia, those at risk for marrow failure (e.g., following chemotherapy), and those whose blood counts must be monitored to determine disease status. If carbamazepine is used, a complete blood count should be obtained prior to the start of therapy, after 2 and 4 wk, and then every 3–4 mo thereafter. A leukocyte count below 4000 is usually considered to be a contraindication to treatment, and a decline to less than 3000 or an absolute neutrophil count of less than 1500 during therapy should prompt discontinuation of the drug. Other anticonvulsant drugs may also be useful and published reports and clinical experience support trials with gabapentin, phenytoin, clonazepam, and valproate *(154)*. When anticonvulsant drugs are used as adjuvant analgesics, it is recommended that dosing follow the dosing guidelines customarily employed in the treatment of seizures.

Occasionally, systemically administered local anesthetic drugs may be useful in the management of neuropathic pains characterized by either continuous or lancinating dysesthesias. It is reasonable to undertake a trial with an oral local anesthetic in patients with continuous dysesthesias who fail to respond adequately or who cannot tolerate the tricyclic antidepressants and in patients with lancinating pains refractory to trials of anticonvulsant drugs and baclofen. Mexiletine is the safest of the oral local anesthetics *(155,156)* and is preferred. Analgesic response to a trial of intravenous lidocaine (5 mg/kg over 45 min) may predict for likelihood of response to oral mexiletine *(157)*. Dosing with mexiletine should usually be started at 100–150 mg/d. If intolerable side effects do not occur, the dose can be increased by a like amount every few days, until the usual maximum dose of 300 mg three times per day is reached.

Less compelling data support the use of clonidine, baclofen, calcitonin, and subcutaneously administered ketamine *(158)*.

4.11.3. Adjuvant Analgesics Used for Bone Pain

The management of bone pain frequently requires the integration of opioid therapy with multiple ancillary approaches. Although a meta-analysis of NSAID therapy in cancer pain that reviewed data from 1615 patients in 21 trials found no specific efficacy in bone pain and analgesic effects equivalent only to "weak" opioids *(54)*, some patients appear to benefit greatly from the addition of such a drug. Corticosteroids are often advocated in difficult cases *(148)*.

Bisphosphonates are analogs of inorganic pyrophosphate that inhibit osteoclast activity and reduce bone resorption in a variety of illnesses. Controlled and uncontrolled trials of intravenous pamidronate in patients with advanced cancer have demonstrated significant reduction of bone pain *(159)*. The analgesic effect of pamidronate appears to be dose and schedule dependant, a dose response is evident at doses between 15 and 30 mg/wk, and it has been noted that 30 mg every 2 wk is less effective than 60 mg every 4 wk *(159)*. Similar effects have been observed with orally administered clodronate *(160)*.

Radiolabeled agents that are absorbed into areas of high bone turnover have been evaluated as potential therapies for metastatic bone disease. It has the advantages of addressing all sites of involvement and relatively selective absorption, thus limiting radiation exposure to normal tissues. Excellent clinical responses with acceptable hematological toxicity have been observed with a range of radiopharmaceuticals. The best studied and most commonly used radionuclide is strontium-89. Large, prospectively randomized clinical trials have demonstrated its efficacy as a first-line therapy *(161)* or as an adjuvant to external beam radiotherapy *(162)*. This approach is contraindicated with patients who have a platelet count less than 60,000 or a WCC < 2.4 and is not advised for patients with very poor performance status *(163)*. Using another approach, bone-seeking radiopharmaceuticals that link a radioisotope with a bisphosphonate compound have been synthesized. Positive experience has been reported with samarium-153–ethylenediaminetetramethylene phosphonic acid, and rhenium-186–hydroxyethylidene diphosphonate.

4.11.4. Adjuvant Analgesics for Visceral Pain

There are limited data that support of the potential efficacy of a range of adjuvant agents for the management of bladder spasm, tenesmoid pain, and colicky intestinal pain. Oxybutynin chloride, a tertiary amine with anticholinergic and papaverine-like, direct muscular antispasmodic effects, is often helpful for bladder spasm pain *(164)*, as is flavoxate

(165). Based on limited clinical experience and in vitro evidence that prostaglandins play a role in bladder smooth-muscle contraction, a trial of NSAIDs may be justified for patients with painful bladder spasms *(166)*. Limited data support a trial of intravesical capsaicin *(167,168)*.

There is no well-established pharmacotherapy for painful rectal spasms. A recent double-blinded study demonstrated that nebulized salbutamol can reduce the duration and severity of attacks *(169)*. There is anecdotal support for trials of diltiazem *(170,171)*, clonidine *(172)*, chlorpromazine *(173)*,and benzodiazepines *(174)*.

Colicky pain as a result of inoperable bowel obstruction has been treated empirically with intravenous scopolamine (hyoscine) butylbromide *(175–177)* and sublingual scopolamine (hyoscine) hydrobromide *(178)*. Limited data support the use of octreotide for this indication *(179)*.

4.12. Other Noninvasive Analgesic Techniques

4.12.1. PSYCHOLOGICAL THERAPIES IN CANCER PAIN

Psychological approaches are an integral part of the care of the cancer patient with pain. All patients can benefit from psychological assessment and support and some are good candidates for specific psychological interventions, including those commonly used in the management of pain. Cognitive-behavioral interventions can help some patients decrease the perception of distress engendered by the pain through the development of new coping skills and the modification of thoughts, feelings, and behaviors *(180–182)*. Relaxation methods may be able to reduce muscular tension and emotional arousal or enhance pain tolerance *(183)*. Other approaches reduce anticipatory anxiety that may lead to avoidant behaviors or lessen the distress associated with the pain *(184)*. Successful implementation of these approaches in the cancer population requires a cognitively intact patient and a dedicated, well-trained physician *(182)*.

4.12.2. PHYSIATRIC TECHNIQUES

Physiatric techniques can be used to optimize the function of the patient with chronic cancer pain *(185,186)* or enhance analgesia through application of modalities such as electrical stimulation, heat, or cryotherapy. The treatment of lymphedema by use of wraps, pressure stockings, or pneumatic pump devices can both improve function and relieve pain and heaviness *(187,188)*. The use of orthotic devices can immobilize and support painful or weakened structures, and assistive devices can be of great value to patients with pain precipitated by weight bearing or ambulation.

4.12.3. TRANSCUTANEOUS ELECTRICAL NERVE STIMULATION

The mechanisms by which transcutaneous electrical stimulation (TENS) reduces pain are not well defined; local neural blockade and activation of a central inhibitory systems have been proposed as explanations *(189,190)*. Clinical experience suggests that this modality can be a useful adjunct in the management of mild to moderate musculoskeletal or neuropathic pain *(191)*.

4.13. Anesthetic and Neurosurgical Analgesic Techniques for Pain Refractory to Systemic Pharmacotherapy

Anesthetic and neurosurgical techniques are important for the patient who has not obtained satisfactory pain relief using systemically administered opioids and adjuvant analgesics. In the Italian validation study of the WHO analgesic ladder, anesthetic and

Table 5
Anesthetic and Neurosurgical Analgesic Techniques for Pain Refractory
to Systemic Pharmacotherapy and Their Indications

Technique	Clinical situation in which it should be considered
Spinal opioids	Systemic opioid analgesia complicated by unmangeable supraspinally mediated adverse effects
Celiac plexus block	Refractory malignant pain involving the upper abdominal viscera including the upper retroperitoneum, liver, small bowel, and proximal colon
Lumbar sympathetic blockade	Sympathetically maintained pain involving the legs
Chemical rhizotomy	Refractory bilateral pelvic or lumbosacral plexus pain in patient confined to bed and with urinary diversion
Transacral neurolysis	Refractory pain limited to the perineum
Cordotomy	Refractory unilateral pain arising below mid-thoracic level

neurosurgical techniques were required in less than 30% of patients. Even when these methods are implemented, concurrent systemic pharmacotherapy will be required *(192)*. The major indications for these techniques are presented in Table 5.

4.13.1. REGIONAL ANALGESIA

4.13.1.1. Epidural and Intrathecal Opioids. The delivery of low opioid doses near the sites of action in the spinal cord may decrease supraspinally mediated adverse effects. In the absence of randomized trials that compare the various intraspinal techniques with other analgesic approaches, the indications for the spinal route remain empirical *(193)*, but they are based on relative therapeutic index *(194)*. One survey reported that only 16 of 1205 cancer patients with pain required intraspinal therapy *(195)*. Compared to neuroablative therapies, spinal opioids have the advantage of preserving sensation, strength, and sympathetic function. Contraindications include bleeding diathesis, profound leukopenia, and sepsis. A temporary trial of spinal opioid therapy should be performed to assess the potential benefits of this approach before implantation of a permanent catheter.

Opioid selection for intraspinal delivery is influenced by several factors. Hydrophilic drugs, such as morphine and hydromorphone, have a prolonged half-life in cerebrospinal fluid and significant rostral redistribution *(196–198)*. Lipophilic opioids, such as fentanyl and sufentanil, have less rostral redistribution *(199–200)* and may be preferable for segmental analgesia at the level of spinal infusion. The addition of a low concentration of a local anesthetic, such as 0.125–0.25% bupivacaine, to an epidural *(201–203)* or intrathecal opioid *(204–206)* has been demonstrated to increase analgesic effect without increasing toxicity. Other agents have also been coadministered with intraspinal opioids, including clonidine *(207)*, octreotide *(208)*, ketamine *(109,210)*, and calcitonin *(211)*, but additional studies are required to assess their potential utility.

There are no trials comparing the intrathecal and epidural routes in cancer pain and extensive experience has been reported with both approaches *(204,212,213)*. Longitudinal studies of epidural or intrathecal opioid infusions for cancer pain suggest that the risks associated with these techniques are similar *(201,212,214)*. The potential morbidity for these procedures indicates the need for a well-trained clinician and long-term monitoring.

4.13.2. ANESTHETIC TECHNIQUES FOR SYMPATHETICALLY MAINTAINED PAIN AND VISCERAL PAIN

4.13.2.1. Celiac Plexus Block. Neurolytic celiac plexus blockade can be considered in the management of pain caused by neoplastic infiltration of the upper abdominal viscera, including the pancreas, upper retroperitoneum, liver, gallbladder, and proximal small bowel *(215–217)*. In addition to an extensive anecdotal experience, this technique is supported by two controlled studies of the percutaneous approach *(218,219)* and a controlled trial of intraoperative neurolysis *(220)*. Reported analgesic response rates in patients with pancreatic cancer are 50–90%, and the reported duration of effect is generally 1–12 mo *(216,218,221,222)*. Common transient complications include postural hypotension and diarrhea *(222–224)*. Rarely, the procedure can produce a paraplegia resulting from an acute ischemic myelopathy (probably caused by involvement of Adamkievicz's artery) *(225,226)*. Posterior spread of neurolytic solution can occasionally lead to involvement of lower thoracic and lumbar somatic nerves, which can potentially result in a neuropathic pain syndrome *(224)*. Other uncommon complications include pneumothorax and retroperitoneal hematoma *(227)*.

4.13.2.2. Superior Hypogastric Nerve Plexus Block. The superior hypogastric nerve plexus lies anterior to the sacral promontory and transmits sensation from pelvic visceral structures. Bilateral percutaneous neurolytic superior hypogastric plexus blocks with 10% phenol can relieve of chronic cancer arising from the descending colon and rectum and the lower genitourinary structures in 40–80% of patients *(228,229)*.

4.13.2.3. Ganglion Impar Block. The ganglion impar (ganglion of Walther) is a solitary retroperitoneal structure at the sacrococcygeal junction that marks the termination of the paired paravertebral sympathetic chains. Neurolysis of this structure can relieve visceral sensations referred to the rectum, perineum, or vagina caused by locally advanced cancers of the pelvic visceral structures *(230–232)*.

4.13.3. NEUROABLATIVE TECHNIQUES FOR SOMATIC AND NEUROPATHIC PAIN

4.13.3.1. Rhizotomy. Segmental or multisegmental destruction of the dorsal sensory roots (rhizotomy), achieved by surgical section, chemical neurolysis, or radio-frequency lesion, can be an effective method of pain control for patients with otherwise refractory localized pain syndromes. Satisfactory analgesia is achieved in about 50% of patients *(233)* and the average duration of relief is 3–4 mo but with a wide range of distribution. Adverse effects can be related to the injection technique (e.g., spinal headache, infection, and arachnoiditis) or to the destruction of non-nociceptive nerve fibers. Specific complications of the procedure depend on the site of neurolysis. The complications of lumbosacral neurolysis include paresis (5–20%), sphincter dysfunction (5–60%), impairment of touch and proprioception, and dysesthesias. Although neurological deficits are usually transient, the risk of increased disability through weakness, sphincter incompetence, and loss of positional sense suggests that these techniques should be reserved for patients with limited function and pre-existent urinary diversion. Patient counseling regarding the risks involved is essential.

4.13.3.2. Cordotomy. During cordotomy, the anterolateral spinothalamic tract is ablated to produce contralateral loss of pain and temperature sensibility *(234,235)*. The patient with severe unilateral pain arising in the torso or lower extremity is most likely to benefit from this procedure *(234,235)*. The percutaneous technique is generally preferred *(234,235)*; open cordotomy is usually reserved for patients who are unable to lie in the supine position or are not cooperative enough to undergo a percutaneous procedure. Significant pain relief is achieved in more than 90% of patients during the period immediately following cordotomy

(234,235). Fifty percent of surviving patients have recurrent pain after 1 yr *(236)*. Repeat cordotomy can sometimes be effective. The neurological complications of cordotomy include paresis, ataxia, and bladder and "mirror-image" pain *(235)*. The complications are usually transient, but they are protracted and disabling in approx 5% of cases *(235)*. Rarely, patients with a long duration of survival (>12 mo) develop a delayed-onset dysesthetic pain *(236)*. The most serious potential complication is respiratory dysfunction, which may occur in the form of phrenic nerve paralysis or as sleep induced *(237,238)*. Because of the latter concern, bilateral high cervical cordotomies or a unilateral cervical cordotomy ipsilateral to the site of the only functioning lung are not recommended.

4.13.4. Considerations in Selection of Invasive Techniques

Interpretation of data regarding the use of alternative analgesic approaches and extrapolation to the presenting clinical problem requires caution. The literature is characterized by the lack of uniformity in patient selection, inadequate reporting of previous analgesic therapies, inconsistencies in outcome evaluation, and paucity of long-term follow-up. Furthermore, reported outcomes in the literature may not predict the outcomes of a procedure performed on a medically ill patient by a physician who has more limited experience with the techniques involved.

When indicated, the use of invasive and neurodestructive procedures should be based on an evaluation of the likelihood and duration of analgesic benefit, the immediate and long-term risks, the likely duration of survival, the availability of local expertise, and the anticipated length of hospitalization.

For most pain syndromes, there exists a range of techniques that may theoretically be applied. In choosing among a range of procedures, the following principles are salient:

1. Ablative procedures are deferred as long as pain relief is obtainable by nonablative modalities.
2. The procedure most likely to be effective should be selected. If there is a choice, however, the one with the fewest and least serious adverse effects is preferred.
3. In progressive stages of cancer, pain is likely to be multifocal and a procedure aimed at a single locus of pain, even if completed flawlessly, is unlikely to yield complete relief of pain until death. A realistic and sound goal is a lasting decrease in pain to a level that is manageable by pharmacotherapy with minimal side effects.
4. Whenever possible, neurolysis should be proceeded by the demonstration of effective analgesia with a local anesthetic prognostic block.
5. Because there is a learning curve with all of the procedures, performance by a physician who is experienced in the specific intervention may improve the likelihood of a successful outcome.

In general, regional analgesic techniques such as intraspinal opioid and local anesthetic administration or intrapleural local anesthetic administration are usually considered first because they can achieve this end without compromising neurological integrity. Neurodestructive procedures, however, are valuable in a small subset of patients, and some of these procedures, such as celiac plexus blockade in patients with pancreatic cancer, may have a favorable enough risk to benefit ratio that early treatment is warranted.

Because individual clinician bias can influence decision-making, a case-conference approach is prudent when assessing a challenging case. This conference may involve the participation of oncologists, palliative care physicians, anesthesiologists, neurosurgeons and psychiatrists, nurses, social workers, and others. The discussion attempts to clarify the remaining therapeutic options and the goals of care. When local expertise is limited, telephone consultation with physicians who are expert in the management of cancer pain is encouraged.

4.14. Guidelines for the Selection of Invasive Techniques According to Pain Site

4.14.1. VISCERAL PAIN

In the management of visceral pain, the degree of relief achieved by invasive techniques can be variable and unpredictable. Thus, patient outcomes may be enhanced by familiarity with a range of options. For patients with upper abdominal visceral pain arising from the pancreas, upper retroperitoneum, liver, gallbladder, and proximal small bowel options include celiac plexus block, intrapleural local anesthetic infusion, and spinal opioid ± local anesthetic. Celiac plexus blockade is not a trivial intervention, and patient counseling should incorporate discussion of the small risk of paraplegia *(225,226)*. For patients with low visceral pain, neurolysis of the superior hypogastric plexus ganglion impar *(228,229)* can be considered. Although less responsive than somatic pain to opioids, many authors consider spinal opioids as the procedure of choice if a ganglionic block is unsuccessful.

4.14.2. UNILATERAL LOWER QUADRANT PAIN

The sensory afferents of the pelvis and lower limb are conducted through the lumbar and lumbosacral plexi to the dorsal spine nerve roots (L2-S2). Pain in the region is amenable to both regional anesthetic and ablative approaches. Because neuroablative approaches may occasionally result in significant neurological deficits, spinal opioid ± local anesthetic approaches are the first-line approach in this setting. If this approach is unsuccessful or contraindicated, then either cordotomy or chemical rhizotomy should be considered *(239)*. Of the neuroablative approaches, cordotomy is generally preferred over chemical rhizotomy because of the lower likelihood of motor deficit and sphincteric dysfunction.

4.14.3. PELVIC PERINEAL AND BILATERAL LOWER LIMB PAIN

The sensory afferents of the perineum are conducted through the lumbosacral plexi to the dorsal spine nerve roots (S2–4). Treatment is challenging because the neuroanatomy risks paralysis and sphincter dysfunction when neurodestructive approaches are used; thus, whenever possible spinal opioids with or without local anesthetic are the preferred approach for these patients.

For patients in whom this approach is either unsuccessful or contraindicated, neuroablative options should be considered. Somatic pain that is limited to the perineum may be amenable to a selective neurolysis of S4 via a transsacral approach or C1 midline myelotomy. For ambulatory patients with pain that is midline or bilateral who have intact sphincteric function, open upper thoracic bilateral cordotomy can control or C1 midline myelotomy should be considered. Patients with pre-existing motor and sphincter dysfunction are the optimal candidates for chemical rhizotomy.

4.15. Sedation as Pain Therapy

Through the vigilant application of analgesic care pain is often relieved adequately without compromising the sentience or function of the patient beyond that caused by the natural disease process itself. Occasionally, however, this cannot be achieved and pain is perceived to be "refractory" *(240)*. In deciding that a pain is refractory, the clinician must perceive that the further application of standard interventions are either (1) incapable of providing adequate relief, (2) associated with excessive and intolerable acute or chronic morbidity, or (3) unlikely to provide relief within a tolerable time frame. In this situation, sedation may be the only therapeutic option capable of providing adequate relief. This approach is described as "sedation in the management of refractory symptoms at the end of life" *(240)*.

The justification of sedation in this setting is that it is goal-appropriate and proportionate. At the end of life, when the overwhelming goal of care is the preservation of patient comfort, the provision of adequate relief of symptoms must be pursued, even in the setting of a narrow therapeutic index for the necessary palliative treatments *(241–243)*. In this context, sedation is a medically indicated and proportionate therapeutic response to refractory symptoms, which cannot be otherwise relieved. Appeal to patients' rights also underwrites the moral legitimacy of sedation in the management of otherwise intolerable pain at the end of life. Patients have a right, recently affirmed by the Supreme Court, to palliative care in response to unrelieved suffering *(241)*.

Once a clinical consensus exists that pain is refractory, it is appropriate to present this option to the patient or their surrogate. When presented to a patient with refractory symptoms, the offer of sedation can demonstrate the clinician's commitment to the relief of suffering. This can enhance trust in the doctor–patient relationship and influence the patient's appraisal of their capacity to cope. Indeed, patients commonly decline sedation, acknowledging that pain will be incompletely relieved but secure in the knowledge that if the situation becomes intolerable to them, this option remains available. Other patients reaffirm comfort as the predominating consideration and request the initiation of sedation.

The published literature describing the use of sedation in the management of refractory pain at the end of life is anecdotal and refers to the use of opioids, neuroleptics, benzodiazepines, barbiturates, and propofol *(240)*. In the absence of relative efficacy data, guidelines for drug selection are empirical. Irrespective of the agent or agents selected, administration initially requires dose titration to achieve adequate relief, followed by provision of ongoing therapy to ensure maintenance of effect.

5. CONCLUSION

Among patients with colorectal and anal cancer, the experience of acute pain is virtually universal, and a large proportion develop chronic pain in the setting of incurable disease. The illness experience of the patient with locally extensive or metastatic disease can be long, and adequate symptom control is a major clinical challenge that can extend over many months or years. The individual practitioner can effectively treat the majority of pain problems by attending to careful pain assessment and implementing analgesic therapy. Currently available analgesic techniques can provide adequate relief to a vast majority of patients, most of whom will respond to systemic pharmacotherapy alone. Comprehensive continuing care requires the integration of this expertise with management of other symptoms and the psychosocial needs of the patient. Cancer is a dynamic problem, and successful ongoing management requires a continuity of care that provides an appropriate level of monitoring and responds quickly, flexibly, and expertly to the changing needs of the patient. Patients with refractory pain or unremitting suffering related to other losses or distressing symptoms should have access to specialists in pain management or palliative medicine who can provide an approach capable of addressing these complex problems.

REFERENCES

1. Janjan NA. Radiation for bone metastases: conventional techniques and the role of systemic radiopharmaceuticals. *Cancer*, **80(8 Suppl.)** (1997) 1628–1645.
2. Bates T. A review of local radiotherapy in the treatment of bone metastases and cord compression. *Int. J. Radiat. Oncol. Biol. Phys.*, **23(1)** (1992) 217–221.

3. Vermeulen SS. Whole brain radiotherapy in the treatment of metastatic brain tumors. *Semin. Surg. Oncol.*, **14(1)** (1998) 64–69.

4. Myint AS. The role of radiotherapy in the palliative treatment of gastrointestinal cancer. *Eur. J. Gastroenterol. Hepatol.*, **12(4)** (2000) 381–390.

5. Russi EG, Pergolizzi S, Gaeta M, Mesiti M, D'Aquino A, and Delia P. Palliative-radiotherapy in lumbosacral carcinomatous neuropathy. *Radiother. Oncol.*, **26(2)** (1993) 172–173.

6. Ampil FL. Palliative irradiation of carcinomatous lumbosacral plexus neuropathy. *Int. J. Radiat. Oncol. Biol. Phys.*, **12(9)** (1986) 1681–1686.

7. Dobrowsky W and Schmid AP. Radiotherapy of presacral recurrence following radical surgery for rectal carcinoma. *Dis. Colon Rectum*, **28(12)** (1985) 917–919.

8. Bosch A and Caldwell WL. Palliative radiotherapy in the patient with metastatic and advanced incurable cancer. *Wis. Med. J.*, **79(4)** (1980) 19–21.

9. Leibel SA, Pajak TF, Massullo V, Order SE, Komaki RU, Chang CH, et al. A comparison of misonidazole sensitized radiation therapy to radiation therapy alone for the palliation of hepatic metastases: results of a Radiation Therapy Oncology Group randomized prospective trial. *Int. J. Radiat. Oncol. Biol. Phys.*, **13(7)** (1987) 1057–1064.

10. Mohiuddin M, Chen E, and Ahmad N. Combined liver radiation and chemotherapy for palliation of hepatic metastases from colorectal cancer. *J. Clin. Oncol.*, **14(3)** (1996) 722–728.

11. Sherman DM, Weichselbaum R, Order SE, Cloud L, Trey C, and Piro AJ. Palliation of hepatic metastasis. *Cancer*, **41(5)** (1978) 2013–2017.

12. Turek-Maischeider M and Kazem I. Palliative irradiation for liver metastases. *JAMA*, **232(6)** (1975) 625–628.

13. Borgelt BB, Gelber R, Brady LW, Griffin T, and Hendrickson FR. The palliation of hepatic metastases: results of the Radiation Therapy Oncology Group pilot study. *Int. J. Radiat. Oncol. Biol. Phys.*, **7(5)** (1981) 587–591.

14. Patt YZ, Peters RE, Chuang VP, Wallace S, Claghorn L, and Mavligit G. Palliation of pelvic recurrence of colorectal cancer with intra- arterial 5-fluorouracil and mitomycin. *Cancer*, **56(9)** (1985) 2175–2180.

15. Rothenberg ML. New developments in chemotherapy for patients with advanced pancreatic cancer. *Oncology (Huntingt.)*, **10(9 Suppl.)** (1996) 18–22.

16. Thatcher N, Anderson H, Betticher DC, and Ranson M. Symptomatic benefit from gemcitabine and other chemotherapy in advanced non-small cell lung cancer: changes in performance status and tumour-related symptoms. *Anticancer Drugs*, **6 (Suppl. 6)** (1995) 39–48.

17. Simmonds PC. Palliative chemotherapy for advanced colorectal cancer: systematic review and meta-analysis. Colorectal Cancer Collaborative Group [see comments]. *Br. Med. J.*, **321(7260)** (2000) 531–535.

18. Glimelius B, Graf W, Hoffman K, L Pa, Sjoden PO, and Wennberg A. General condition of asymptomatic patients with advanced colorectal cancer receiving palliative chemotherapy. A longitudinal study. *Acta Oncol.*, **31(6)** (1992) 645–651.

19. Glimelius B, Hoffman K, Graf W, Haglund U, Nyren O, L Pa, et al. Cost-effectiveness of palliative chemotherapy in advanced gastrointestinal cancer [see comments]. *Ann. Oncol.*, **6(3)** (1995) 267–274.

20. Johnson D, Lipsett J, Leong L, Wagman LD, and Terz JJ. Carcinoma of the anus treated with primary radiation therapy and chemotherapy. *Surg. Gynecol. Obstet.*, **177(4)** (1993) 329–334.

21. Svensson C, Kaigas M, and Goldman S. Induction chemotherapy with carboplatin and 5-fluorouracil in combination with radiotherapy in loco-regionally advanced epidermoid carcinoma of the anus—preliminary results. *Int. J. Colorect. Dis.*, **7(3)** (1992) 122–124.

22. Knecht BH. Combined chemotherapy and radiotherapy for carcinomas of the anus. *Am. J. Surg.*, **159(5)** (1990) 518–521.

23. Barbalias GA, Siablis D, Liatsikos EN, Karnabatidis D, Yarmenitis S, Bouropoulos K, et al. Metal stents: a new treatment of malignant ureteral obstruction. *J. Urol.*, **158(1)** (1997) 54–58.

24. Mainar A, Tejero E, Maynar M, Ferral H, and Castaneda-Zuniga W. Colorectal obstruction: treatment with metallic stents. *Radiology*, **198(3)** (1996) 761–764.

25. Parker MC and Baines MJ. Intestinal obstruction in patients with advanced malignant disease. *Br. J. Surg.*, **83(1)** (1996) 1–2.

26. Jong P, Sturgeon J, and Jamieson CG. Benefit of palliative surgery for bowel obstruction in advanced ovarian cancer. *Can. J. Surg.*, **38(5)** (1995) 454–457.

27. Tarn TS and Lee TS. Surgical treatment of metastatic tumors of the long bones. *Chung Hua I Hsueh Tsa Chih (Taipei)*, **54(3)** (1994) 170–175.

28. Algan SM and Horowitz SM. Surgical treatment of pathologic hip lesions in patients with metastatic disease. *Clin. Orthop.*, **332** (1996) 223–231.

29. Braun A and Rohe K. Orthopedic surgery for management of tumor pain. *Recent Results Cancer Res.*, **89** (1984) 157–170.

30. Harris JK, Sutcliffe JC, and Robinson NE. The role of emergency surgery in malignant spinal extradural compression: assessment of functional outcome. *Br. J. Neurosurg.*, **10(1)** (1996) 27–33.

31. Gokaslan ZL. Spine surgery for cancer. *Curr. Opin. Oncol.*, **8(3)** (1996) 178–181.

32. Sucher E, Margulies JY, Floman Y, and Robin GC. Prognostic factors in anterior decompression for metastatic cord compression. An analysis of results. *Eur. Spine J.*, **3(2)** (1994) 70–75.

33. Boraas MC. Palliative surgery. *Semin. Oncol.*, **12(4)** (1985) 368–374.

34. Ross GJ, Kessler HB, Clair MR, Gatenby RA, Hartz WH, and Ross LV. Sonographically guided paracentesis for palliation of symptomatic malignant ascites. *Am. J. Roentgenol.*, **153(6)** (1989) 1309–1311.

35. Cruikshank DP and Buchsbaum HJ. Effects of rapid paracentesis. Cardiovascular dynamics and body fluid composition. *JAMA*, **225(11)** (1973) 1361–1362.

36. Lifshitz S and Buchsbaum HJ. The effect of paracentesis on serum proteins. *Gynecol. Oncol.*, **4(4)** (1976) 347–353.

37. Avradopoulos KA, Vezeridis MP, and Wanebo HJ. Pelvic exenteration for recurrent rectal cancer. *Adv. Surg.*, **29** (1996) 215–233.

38. Estes NC, Thomas JH, Jewell WR, Beggs D, and Hardin CA. Pelvic exenteration: a treatment for failed rectal cancer surgery. *Am. Surg.*, **59(7)** (1993) 420–422.

39. Temple WJ and Saettler EB. Locally recurrent rectal cancer: role of composite resection of extensive pelvic tumors with strategies for minimizing risk of recurrence. *J. Surg. Oncol.*, **73(1)** (2000) 47–58.

40. Temple WJ and Ketcham AS. Surgical palliation for recurrent rectal cancers ulcerating in the perineum. *Cancer*, **65(5)** (1990) 1111–1114.

41. Hughes LL, Styblo TM, Thoms WW, Schwarzmann SW, Landry JC, Heaton D, et al. Cellulitis of the breast as a complication of breast-conserving surgery and irradiation. *Am. J. Clin. Oncol.*, **20(4)** (1997) 338–341.

42. Lopez MR, Stock JA, Gump FE, and Rosen JS. Carcinoma of the breast metastatic to the ureter presenting with flank pain and recurrent urinary tract infection. *Am. Surg.*, **62(9)** (1996) 748–752.

43. Coyle N and Portenoy RK. Infection as a cause of rapidly increasing pain in cancer patients. *J. Pain Symptom Manage.*, **6(4)** (1991) 266–269.

44. Gonzales GR, Elliott KJ, Portenoy RK, and Foley KM. The impact of a comprehensive evaluation in the management of cancer pain. *Pain*, **47(2)** (1991) 141–144.

45. Bruera E and MacDonald N. Intractable pain in patients with advanced head and neck tumors: a possible role of local infection. *Cancer Treat. Rep.*, **70(5)** (1986) 691–692.

46. World Health Organization. *Cancer Pain Relief.* World Health Organization, Geneva, 1986.

47. Takeda F. Japanese field-testing of WHO guidelines. *PRN Forum*, **4(3)** (1985) 4–5.

48. Ventafridda V, Tamburini M, Caraceni A, De Conno F, and Naldi F. A validation study of the WHO method for cancer pain relief. *Cancer*, **59(4)** (1987) 850–856.

49. Walker VA, Hoskin PJ, Hanks GW, and White ID. Evaluation of WHO analgesic guidelines for cancer pain in a hospital-based palliative care unit. *J. Pain Symptom Manage.*, **3(3)** (1988) 145–149.

50. Schug SA, Zech D, and Dorr U. Cancer pain management according to WHO analgesic guidelines. *J. Pain Symptom Manage.*, **5(1)** (1990) 27–32.

51. Goisis A, Gorini M, Ratti R, and Luliri P. Application of a WHO protocol on medical therapy for oncologic pain in an internal medicine hospital. *Tumori*, **75(5)** (1989) 470–472.

52. Grond S, Zech D, Schug SA, Lynch J, and Lehmann KA. Validation of World Health Organization guidelines for cancer pain relief during the last days and hours of life. *J. Pain Symptom Manage.*, **6(7)** (1991) 411–422.

53. Jadad AR and Browman GP. The WHO analgesic ladder for cancer pain management. Stepping up the quality of its evaluation [see comments]. *JAMA*, **274(23)** (1995) 1870–1873.

54. Eisenberg E, Berkey CS, Carr DB, Mosteller F, and Chalmers TC. Efficacy and safety of nonsteroidal antiinflammatory drugs for cancer pain: a meta-analysis. *J. Clin. Oncol.*, **12(12)** (1994) 2756–2765.

55. Vane JR, Bakhle YS, and Botting RM. Cyclooxygenases 1 and 2. *Annu. Rev. Pharmacol. Toxicol.*, **38** (1998) 97–120.

56. Lefkowith JB. Cyclooxygenase-2 specificity and its clinical implications. *Am. J. Med.*, **106(5B)** (1999) 43S–50S.

57. Ehrich EW, Dallob A, De Lepeleire I, Van Hecken A, Riendeau D, Yuan W, et al. Characterization of rofecoxib as a cyclooxygenase-2 isoform inhibitor and demonstration of analgesia in the dental pain model. *Clin. Pharmacol. Ther.*, **65(3)** (1999) 336–347.

58. Hawkey CJ. COX-2 inhibitors. *Lancet*, **353(9149)** (1999) 307–314.

59. Bennett WM, Henrich WL, and Stoff JS. The renal effects of nonsteroidal anti-inflammatory drugs: summary and recommendations. *Am. J. Kidney Dis.*, **28(1 Suppl. 1)** (1996) S56–S62.

60. Laine L. Nonsteroidal anti-inflammatory drug gastropathy. *Gastrointest. Endosc. Clin. North Am.*, **6(3)** (1996) 489–504.

61. Lehmann T, Day RO, and Brooks PM. Toxicity of antirheumatic drugs. *Med. J. Aust.*, **166(7)** (1997) 378–383.

62. Brooks PM and Day RO. Nonsteroidal antiinflammatory drugs—differences and similarities. *N. Engl. J. Med.*, **324(24)** (1991) 1716–1725.

63. Raskin JB. Gastrointestinal effects of nonsteroidal anti-inflammatory therapy. *Am. J. Med.*, **106(5B)** (1999) 3S–12S.

64. Johnson JR and Miller AJ. The efficacy of choline magnesium trisalicylate (CMT) in the management of metastatic bone pain: a pilot study. *Palliat. Med.*, **8(2)** (1994) 129–135.

65. Hawkey CJ. Progress in prophylaxis against nonsteroidal anti-inflammatory drug- associated ulcers and erosions. Omeprazole NSAID Steering Committee. *Am. J. Med.*, **104(3A)** (1998) 67S–74S; discussion 79S–80S.

66. Valentini M, Cannizzaro R, Poletti M, Bortolussi R, Fracasso A, Testa V, et al. Nonsteroidal antiinflammatory drugs for cancer pain: comparison between misoprostol and ranitidine in prevention of upper gastrointestinal damage. *J. Clin. Oncol.*, **13(10)** (1995) 2637–2642.

67. Taha AS, Hudson N, Hawkey CJ, Swannell AJ, Trye PN, Cottrell J, et al. Famotidine for the prevention of gastric and duodenal ulcers caused by nonsteroidal antiinflammatory drugs [see comments]. *N. Engl. J. Med.*, **334(22)** (1996) 1435–1439.

68. Plosker GL and Lamb HM. Diclofenac/misoprostol. Pharmacoeconomic implications of therapy. *Pharmacoeconomics*, **16(1)** (1999) 85–98.

69. McKenna F. Diclofenac/misoprostol: the European clinical experience. *J. Rheumatol.*, **51(Suppl.)** (1998) 21–30.

70. Makin AJ and Williams R. Acetaminophen-induced hepatotoxicity: predisposing factors and treatments. *Adv. Intern. Med.*, **42** (1997) 453–483.

71. Portenoy RK, Foley KM, and Inturrisi CE. The nature of opioid responsiveness and its implications for neuropathic pain: new hypotheses derived from studies of opioid infusions [see comments]. *Pain*, **43(3)** (1990) 273–286.

72. Hanks GW and Forbes K. Opioid responsiveness. *Acta Anaesthesiol. Scand.*, **41(1 Pt. 2)** (1997) 154–158.

73. Hanks GW. The clinical usefulness of agonist-antagonistic opioid analgesics in chronic pain. *Drug Alcohol Depend.*, **20(4)** (1987) 339–346.

74. Houde RW, Wallenstein SL, and Beaver WT. Evaluation of analgesics in patients with cancer pain. In *International Encycloped of Pharmacology and Therapeutics*. Lasagna L (ed.), Pergamon, New York, 1966, pp. 59–67.

75. Ripamonti C, Groff L, Brunelli C, Polastri D, Stravakis A, and De Conno F. Switching from morphine to oral methadone in treating cancer pain. What is the equianalgesic dose ratio? *J. Clin. Oncol.*, **16** (1998) 3216–3221.

76. Lloyd RS, Costello F, Eves MJ, James IG, and Miller AJ. The efficacy and tolerability of controlled-release dihydrocodeine tablets and combination dextropropoxyphene/paracetamol tablets in patients with severe osteoarthritis of the hips. *Curr. Med. Res. Opin.*, **13(1)** (1992) 37–48.

77. Heiskanen T and Kalso E. Controlled-release oxycodone and morphine in cancer related pain. *Pain*, **73(1)** (1997) 37–45.

78. Glare PA and Walsh TD. Dose-ranging study of oxycodone for chronic pain in advanced cancer. *J. Clin. Oncol.*, **11(5)** (1993) 973–978.

79. Hagen NA and Babul N. Comparative clinical efficacy and safety of a novel controlled-release oxycodone formulation and controlled-release hydromorphone in the treatment of cancer pain. *Cancer*, **79(7)** (1997) 1428–1437.

80. Inturrisi CE, Colburn WA, Verebey K, Dayton HE, Woody GE, and O'Brien CP. Propoxyphene and norpropoxyphene kinetics after single and repeated doses of propoxyphene. *Clin. Pharmacol. Ther.*, **31(2)** (1982) 157–167.

81. Mercadante S, Salvaggio L, Dardanoni G, Agnello A, and Garofalo S. Dextropropoxyphene versus morphine in opioid-naive cancer patients with pain. *J. Pain Symptom Manage.*, **15(2)** (1998) 76–81.

82. World Health Organization. *Cancer Pain Relief.* 2nd ed. World Health Organization, Geneva, 1996.

83. Sawe J, Svensson JO, and Rane A. Morphine metabolism in cancer patients on increasing oral doses—no evidence for autoinduction or dose-dependence. *Br. J. Clin. Pharmacol.*, **16(1)** (1983) 85–93.

84. Christrup LL. Morphine metabolites. *Acta Anaesthesiol. Scand.*, **41(1 Pt. 2)** (1997) 116–122.

85. Osborne R, Joel S, Grebenik K, Trew D, and Slevin M. The pharmacokinetics of morphine and morphine glucuronides in kidney failure [see comments]. *Clin. Pharmacol. Ther.*, **54(2)** (1993) 158–167.

86. Hagen NA, Foley KM, Cerbone DJ, Portenoy RK, and Inturrisi CE. Chronic nausea and morphine-6-glucuronide. *J. Pain Symptom Manage.*, **6(3)** (1991) 125–128.

87. Osborne RJ, Joel SP, and Slevin ML. Morphine intoxication in renal failure: the role of morphine-6-glucuronide. *Br. Med. J. (Clin. Res. Ed.)*, **292(6535)** (1986) 1548–1549.

88. Sjogren P, Dragsted L, and Christensen CB. Myoclonic spasms during treatment with high doses of intravenous morphine in renal failure. *Acta Anaesthesiol. Scand.*, **37(8)** (1993) 780–782.

89. European Association for Palliative Care. Morphine in cancer pain: modes of administration. Expert Working Group of the European Association for Palliative Care. *Br. Med. J.*, **312(7034)** (1996) 823–826.

90. Houde RW. Clinical analgesic studies of hydromorphone. In *Opioid Analgesics in the Management of Clinical Pain*. Foley KM and Inturrisi CE (eds.), Raven, New York, 1986, pp. 129–136.

91. Moulin DE, Kreeft JH, Murray-Parsons N, and Bouquillon AI. Comparison of continuous subcutaneous and intravenous hydromorphone infusions for management of cancer pain [see comments]. *Lancet*, **337(8739)** (1991) 465–468.

92. Bruera E, Sloan P, Mount B, Scott J, and Suarez-Almazor M. A randomized, double-blind, double-dummy, crossover trial comparing the safety and efficacy of oral sustained-release hydromorphone with immediate-release hydromorphone in patients with cancer pain. Canadian Palliative Care Clinical Trials Group. *J. Clin. Oncol.*, **14(5)** (1996) 1713–1717.

93. Collins JJ, Geake J, Grier HE, Houck CS, Thaler HT, Weinstein HJ, et al. Patient-controlled analgesia for mucositis pain in children: a three-period crossover study comparing morphine and hydromorphone. *J. Pediatr.*, **129(5)** (1996) 722–728.

94. Lawlor P, Turner K, Hanson J, and Bruera E. Dose ratio between morphine and hydromorphone in patients with cancer pain: a retrospective study. *Pain*, **72(1–2)** (1997) 79–85.

95. Szeto HH, Inturrisi CE, Houde R, Saal S, Cheigh J, and Reidenberg MM. Accumulation of normeperidine, an active metabolite of meperidine, in patients with renal failure of cancer. *Ann. Intern. Med.*, **86(6)** (1977) 738–741.

96. Eisendrath SJ, Goldman B, Douglas J, Dimatteo L, and Van Dyke C. Meperidine-induced delirium. *Am. J. Psychiatry*, **144(8)** (1987) 1062–1065.

97. Ripamonti C, Zecca E, and Bruera E. An update on the clinical use of methadone for cancer pain. *Pain*, **70(2–3)** (1997) 109–115.

98. Grochow L, Sheidler V, Grossman S, Green L, and Enterline J. Does intravenous methadone provide longer lasting analgesia than intravenous morphine? A randomized, double-blind study [see comments]. *Pain*, **38(2)** (1989) 151–157.

99. Mercadante S, Sapio M, Serretta R, and Caligara M. Patient-controlled analgesia with oral methadone in cancer pain: preliminary report. *Ann. Oncol.*, **7(6)** (1996) 613–617.

100. Sawe J, Hansen J, Ginman C, Hartvig P, Jakobsson PA, Nilsson MI, et al. Patient-controlled dose regimen of methadone for chronic cancer pain. *Br. Med. J. (Clin. Res. Ed.)*, **282(6266)** (1981) 771–773.

101. Bruera E, Fainsinger R, Moore M, Thibault R, Spoldi E, and Ventafridda V. Local toxicity with subcutaneous methadone. Experience of two centers. *Pain* **45(2)** (1991) 141–143.

102. Ripamonti C, De Conno F, Groff L, Belzile M, Pereira J, Hanson J, et al. Equianalgesic dose/ratio between methadone and other opioid agonists in cancer pain: comparison of two clinical experiences. *Ann. Oncol.*, **9(1)** (1998) 79–83.

103. Ripamonti C, Groff L, Brunelli C, Polastri D, Stavrakis A, and De Conno F. Switching from morphine to oral methadone in treating cancer pain: what is the equianalgesic dose ratio? [see comments]. *J. Clin. Oncol.*, **16(10)** (1998) 3216–3221.

104. Sinatra RS, Lodge K, Sibert K, Chung KS, Chung JH, Parker A Jr, et al. A comparison of morphine, meperidine, and oxymorphone as utilized in patient-controlled analgesia following cesarean delivery. *Anesthesiology*, **70(4)** (1989) 585–590.

105. Sinatra R, Chung KS, Silverman DG, Brull SJ, Chung J, Harrison DM, et al. An evaluation of morphine and oxymorphone administered via patient-controlled analgesia (PCA) or PCA plus basal infusion in postcesarean-delivery patients. *Anesthesiology*, **71(4)** (1989) 502–507.

106. Sinatra RS and Harrison DM. Oxymorphone in patient-controlled analgesia. *Clin. Pharm.*, **8(8)** (1989) 541–544.

107. Dixon R, Crews T, Inturrisi C, and Foley K. Levorphanol: pharmacokinetics and steady-state plasma concentrations in patients with pain. *Res. Commun. Chem. Pathol. Pharmacol.*, **41(1)** (1983) 3–17.

108. Wallenstein SL, Rogers AG, Kaiko RF, and Houde RW. Clinical analgesic studies of levorphanol in acute and chronic cancer pain: assay methodology. *Adv. Pain Res. Ther.*, **8(211)** (1986) 211–215.

109. Jeal W and Benfield P. Transdermal fentanyl. A review of its pharmacological properties and therapeutic efficacy in pain control. *Drugs*, **53(1)** (1997) 109–138.

110. Agency for Health Care Policy and Research: Acute Pain Management Panel. *Acute Pain Management: Operative or Medical Procedures and Trauma*. U.S. Department of Health and Human Services, Washington, DC, 1992.

111. Lenz KL and Dunlap DS. Continuous fentanyl infusion: use in severe cancer pain. *Ann. Pharmacother.* **32(3)** (1998) 316–319.

112. Paix A, Coleman A, Lees J, Grigson J, Brooksbank M, Thorne D, et al. Subcutaneous fentanyl and sufentanil infusion substitution for morphine intolerance in cancer pain management. *Pain*, **63(2)** (1995) 263–269.

113. Farrar JT, Cleary J, Rauck R, Busch M, and Nordbrock E. Oral transmucosal fentanyl citrate: randomized, double-blinded, placebo- controlled trial for treatment of breakthrough pain in cancer patients. *J. Natl. Cancer Inst.*, **90(8)** (1998) 611–616.

114. Cherny NJ, Chang V, Frager G, Ingham JM, Tiseo PJ, Popp B, et al. Opioid pharmacotherapy in the management of cancer pain: a survey of strategies used by pain physicians for the selection of analgesic drugs and routes of administration. *Cancer*, **76(7)** (1995) 1283–1293.

115. de Stoutz ND, Bruera E, and Suarez-Almazor M. Opioid rotation for toxicity reduction in terminal cancer patients. *J. Pain Symptom Manage.*, **10(5)** (1995) 378–384.

116. Varvel JR, Shafer SL, Hwang SS, Coen PA, and Stanski DR. Absorption characteristics of transdermally administered fentanyl. *Anesthesiology*, **70(6)** (1989) 928–934.

117. Ahmedzai S and Brooks D. Transdermal fentanyl versus sustained-release oral morphine in cancer pain: preference, efficacy, and quality of life. The TTS–Fentanyl Comparative Trial Group. *J. Pain Symptom Manage.*, **13(5)** (1997) 254–261.

118. Donner B, Zenz M, Tryba M, and Strumpf M. Direct conversion from oral morphine to transdermal fentanyl: a multicenter study in patients with cancer pain. *Pain*, **64(3)** (1996) 527–534.

119. Payne R, Mathias SD, Pasta DJ, Wanke LA, Williams R, and Mahmoud R. Quality of life and cancer pain: satisfaction and side effects with transdermal fentanyl versus oral morphine. *J. Clin. Oncol.*, **16(4)** (1998) 1588–1593.

120. Kaiko RF, Fitzmartin RD, Thomas GB, and Goldenheim PD. The bioavailability of morphine in controlled-release 30-mg tablets per rectum compared with immediate-release 30-mg rectal suppositories and controlled-release 30-mg oral tablets. *Pharmacotherapy*, **12(2)** (1992) 107–113.

121. Maloney CM, Kesner RK, Klein G, and Bockenstette J. The rectal administration of MS Contin: clinical implications of use in end stage cancer. *Am. J. Hosp. Care*, **6(4)** (1989) 34–35.

122. Weinberg DS, Inturrisi CE, Reidenberg B, Moulin DE, Nip TJ, Wallenstein S, et al. Sublingual absorption of selected opioid analgesics. *Clin. Pharmacol. Ther.*, **44(3)** (1988) 335–342.

123. Simmonds MA. Oral transmucosal fentanyl citrate produces pain relief faster than medication typically used for breakthrough pain in cancer patients. *Proc. Annu. Meet. Am. Soc. Clin. Oncol.*, **16** (1997) A180 (abstract).

124. Hagen NA, Elwood T, and Ernst S. Cancer pain emergencies: a protocol for management. *J. Pain Symptom Manage.*, **14(1)** (1997) 45–50.

125. Coyle N, Cherny NI, and Portenoy RK. Subcutaneous opioid infusions at home. *Oncology (Huntingt.)*, **8(4)** (1994) 21–27; discussion 31–2, 37.

126. Cooper IM. Morphine for postoperative analgesia. A comparison of intramuscular and subcutaneous routes of administration [see comments]. *Anaesth. Intens. Care*, **24(5)** (1996) 574–578.

127. Cleary JF. Pharmacokinetic and pharmacodynamic issues in the treatment of breakthrough pain. *Semin. Oncol.*, **24(5 Suppl. 16)** (1997) S16–S13–9.

128. Lyss AP. Long-term use of oral transmucosal fentanyl citrate (OTFC) for breakthrough pain in cancer patients. *Proc. Annu. Meet. Am. Soc. Clin. Oncol.*, (1997) p. A144 (abstract).

129. Ripamonti C and Bruera E. Current status of patient-controlled analgesia in cancer patients. *Oncology (Huntingt.)*, **11(3)** (1997) 373–80, 383–384; discussion 384–386.

130. Paice JA. The phenomenon of analgesic tolerance in cancer pain management. *Oncol. Nurs. Forum*, **15(4)** (1988) 455–460.

131. Schug SA, Zech D, Grond S, Jung H, Meuser T, and Stobbe B. A long-term survey of morphine in cancer pain patients. *J. Pain Symptom Manage.*, **7(5)** (1992) 259–266.

132. Pies R. Psychotropic medications and the oncology patient. *Cancer Pract.*, **4(3)** (1996) 164–166.

133. Browne B and Linter S. Monoamine oxidase inhibitors and narcotic analgesics. A critical review of the implications for treatment. *Br. J. Psychiatry*, **151** (1987) 210–212.

134. Fallon M and O'Neill B. ABC of palliative care. Constipation and diarrhoea. *Br. Med. J.*, **315(7118)** (1997) 1293–1296.

135. Vainio A, Ollila J, Matikainen E, Rosenberg P, and Kalso E. Driving ability in cancer patients receiving long-term morphine analgesia. *Lancet*, **346(8976)** (1995) 667–670.

136. Portenoy RK. Management of common opioid side effects during long-term therapy of cancer pain. *Ann. Acad. Med. Singapore*, **23(2)** (1994) 160–170.

137. Wells CJ, Lipton S, and Lahuerta J. Respiratory depression after percutaneous cervical anterolateral cordotomy in patients on slow-release oral morphine [letter]. *Lancet*, **1(8379)** (1984) 739.

138. Mortimer JE and Bartlett NL. Assessment of knowledge about cancer pain management by physicians in training. *J. Pain Symptom Manage.*, **14(1)** (1997) 21–28.

139. Hill CS Jr. Government regulatory influences on opioid prescribing and their impact on the treatment of pain of nonmalignant origin. *J. Pain Symptom Manage.*, **11(5)** (1996) 287–298.

140. Ward SE, Berry PE, and Misiewicz H. Concerns about analgesics among patients and family caregivers in a hospice setting. *Res. Nurs. Health*, **19(3)** (1996) 205–211.

141. Hill CS Jr. The barriers to adequate pain management with opioid analgesics. *Semin. Oncol.*, **20(2 Suppl. 1)** (1993) 1–5.

142. Ward SE, Goldberg N, Miller-McCauley V, Mueller C, Nolan A, Pawlik-Plank D, et al. Patient-related barriers to management of cancer pain. *Pain*, **52(3)** (1993) 319–324.

143. Bressler LR, Geraci MC, and Schatz BS. Misperceptions and inadequate pain management in cancer patients. *DICP.*, **25(11)** (1991) 1225–1230.

144. McCaffery M. Pain control. Barriers to the use of available information. World Health Organization Expert Committee on Cancer Pain Relief and Active Supportive Care. *Cancer*, **70(5 Suppl.)** (1992) 1438–1449.

145. Zenz M, Donner B, and Strumpf M. Withdrawal symptoms during therapy with transdermal fentanyl (fentanyl TTS)? *J. Pain Symptom Manage.*, **9(1)** (1994) 54–55.

146. Porter J and Jick H. Addiction rare in patients treated with narcotics. *N. Engl. J. Med.*, **302(2)** (1980) 123.

147. Weissman DE and Haddox JD. Opioid pseudoaddiction—an iatrogenic syndrome. *Pain*, **36(3)** (1989) 363–366.

148. Watanabe S and Bruera E. Corticosteroids as adjuvant analgesics. *J. Pain Symptom Manage.*, **9(7)** (1994) 442–445.

149. Devor M, Govrin-Lippmann R, and Raber P. Corticosteroids suppress ectopic neural discharge originating in experimental neuromas. *Pain*, **22(2)** (1985) 127–137.

150. Sorensen S, Helweg-Larsen S, Mouridsen H, and Hansen HH. Effect of high-dose dexamethasone in carcinomatous metastatic spinal cord compression treated with radiotherapy: a randomised trial. *Eur. J. Cancer*, **30A(1)** (1994) 22–27.

151. Twycross R. The risks and benefits of corticosteroids in advanced cancer. *Drug Safety*, **11(3)** (1994) 163–178.

152. Ellershaw JE and Kelly MJ. Corticosteroids and peptic ulceration. *Palliat. Med.*, **8(4)** (1994) 313–319.

153. McQuay HJ, Tramer M, Nye BA, Carroll D, Wiffen PJ, and Moore RA. A systematic review of antidepressants in neuropathic pain. *Pain*, **68(2–3)** (1996) 217–227.

154. McQuay H, Carroll D, Jadad AR, Wiffen P, and Moore A. Anticonvulsant drugs for management of pain: a systematic review. *Br. Med. J.*, **311(7012)** (1995) 1047–1052.

155. Ruskin JN. The cardiac arrhythmia suppression trial (CAST). *N. Engl. J. Med.*, **321(6)** (1989) 386–388.

156. (CAST) Cardiac Arrhythmia Suppression Trial Investigators. Preliminary report: effect of encainide and flecainide on mortality in a randomized trial of arrhythmia suppression after myocardial infarction. *N. Engl. J. Med.*, **321(6)** (1989) 406–412.

157. Galer BS, Harle J, and Rowbotham MC. Response to intravenous lidocaine infusion predicts subsequent response to oral mexiletine: a prospective study. *J. Pain Symptom Manage.*, **12(3)** (1996) 161–167.

158. Lipman AG. Analgesic drugs for neuropathic and sympathetically maintained pain. *Clin. Geriatr. Med.*, **12(3)** (1996) 501–515.

159. Strang P. Analgesic effect of bisphosphonates on bone pain in breast cancer patients: a review article. *Acta Oncol.*, **5(50)** (1996) 50–54.

160. Ernst DS, Brasher P, Hagen N, Paterson AH, MacDonald RN, and Bruera E. A randomized, controlled trial of intravenous clodronate in patients with metastatic bone disease and pain. *J. Pain Symptom Manage.*, **13(6)** (1997) 319–326.

161. Robinson RG, Preston DF, Schiefelbein M, and Baxter KG. Strontium 89 therapy for the palliation of pain due to osseous metastases. *JAMA*, **274(5)** (1995) 420–424.

162. Porter AT, McEwan AJ, Powe JE, Reid R, McGowan DG, Lukka H, et al. Results of a randomized phase-III trial to evaluate the efficacy of strontium-89 adjuvant to local field external beam irradiation in the management of endocrine resistant metastatic prostate cancer. *Int. J. Radiat. Oncol. Biol. Phys.*, **25(5)** (1993) 805–813.

163. Schmeler K and Bastin K. Strontium-89 for symptomatic metastatic prostate cancer to bone: recommendations for hospice patients. *Hosp. J.*, **11(2)** (1996) 1–10.

164. Paulson DF. Oxybutynin chloride in control of post-trasurethral vesical pain and spasm. *Urology*, **11(3)** (1978) 237–238.

165. Baert L. Controlled double-blind trail of flavoxate in painful conditions of the lower urinary tract. *Curr. Med. Res. Opin.*, **2(10)** (1974) 631–635.

166. Abrams P and Fenely R. The action of prostaglandins on smooth muscle of the human urinary tract in vitro. *Br. J. Urol.*, **(47)** (1976) 909–915.

167. Lazzeri M, Beneforti P, Benaim G, Maggi CA, Lecci A, and Turini D. Intravesical capsaicin for treatment of severe bladder pain: a randomized placebo controlled study. *J. Urol.*, **156(3)** (1996) 947–952.

168. Barbanti G, Maggi CA, Beneforti P, Baroldi P, and Turini D. Relief of pain following intravesical capsaicin in patients with hypersensitive disorders of the lower urinary tract. *Br. J. Urol.*, **71(6)** (1993) 686–691.

169. Eckardt VF, Dodt O, Kanzler G, and Bernhard G. Treatment of proctalgia fugax with salbutamol inhalation. *Am. J. Gastroenterol.*, **91(4)** (1996) 686–689.

170. Boquet J, Moore N, Lhuintre JP, and Boismare F. Diltiazem for proctalgia fugax [letter]. *Lancet*, **1(8496)** (1986) 1493.

171. Castell DO. Calcium-channel blocking agents for gastrointestinal disorders. *Am. J. Cardiol.*, **55(3)** (1985) 210B–213B.

172. Swain R. Oral clonidine for proctalgia fugax. *Gut*, **28(8)** (1987) 1039–1040.

173. Patt RB, Proper G, and Reddy S. The neuroleptics as adjuvant analgesics. *J. Pain Symptom Manage.*, **9(7)** (1994) 446–453.

174. Hanks GW. Psychotropic drugs. *Postgrad. Med. J.*, **60(710)** (1984) 881–885.

175. Ventafridda V, Ripamonti C, Caraceni A, Spoldi E, Messina L, and De Conno F. The management of inoperable gastrointestinal obstruction in terminal cancer patients. *Tumori*, **76(4)** (1990) 389–393.

176. De Conno F, Caraceni A, Zecca E, Spoldi E, and Ventafridda V. Continuous subcutaneous infusion of hyoscine butylbromide reduces secretions in patients with gastrointestinal obstruction. *J. Pain Symptom Manage.*, **6(8)** (1991) 484–486.

177. Baines MJ. ABC of palliative care. Nausea, vomiting, and intestinal obstruction. *Br. Med. J.*, **315(7116)** (1997) 1148–1150.

178. Baines MJ. Management of intestinal obstruction in patients with advanced cancer. *Ann. Acad. Med. Singapore*, **23(2)** (1994) 178–182.

179. Mercadante S. The role of octreotide in palliative care. *J. Pain Symptom Manage.*, **9(6)** (1994) 406–411.

180. Spiegel D and Moore R. Imagery and hypnosis in the treatment of cancer patients. *Oncology (Huntingt.)*, **11(8)** (1997) 1179–1189; discussion 1189–1195.

181. Loscalzo M. Psychological approaches to the management of pain in patients with advanced cancer. *Hematol. Oncol. Clin. North Am.*, **10(1)** (1996) 139–155.

182. Fishman B. The cognitive behavioral perspective on pain management in terminal illness. *Hosp. J.*, **8(1–2)** (1992) 73–88.

183. Arathuzik D. Effects of cognitive-behavioral strategies on pain in cancer patients. *Cancer Nurs.*, **17(3)** (1994) 207–214.

184. Turk DC and Feldman CS. Noninvasive approaches to pain control in terminal illness: the contribution of psychological variables. *Hosp. J.*, **8(1–2)** (1992) 1–23.

185. Williams FH and Maly BJ. Pain rehabilitation. 3. Cancer pain, pelvic pain, and age-related considerations. *Arch. Phys. Med. Rehabil.*, **75(5 Spec No)** (1994) S15–S20.

186. Gamble GL, Kinney CL, Brown PS, and Maloney FP. Cardiovascular, pulmonary, and cancer rehabilitation. 5. Cancer rehabilitation: management of pain, neurologic and other clinical problems. *Arch. Phys. Med. Rehabil.*, **71(4–S)** (1990) S248–S251.

187. Marcks P. Lymphedema. Pathogenesis, prevention, and treatment. *Cancer Pract.*, **5(1)** (1997) 32–38.

188. Brennan MJ, DePompolo RW, and Garden FH. Focused review: postmastectomy lymphedema. *Arch. Phys. Med. Rehabil.*, **77(3 Suppl.)** (1996) S74–S80.

189. Long DM. Fifteen years of transcutaneous electrical stimulation for pain control. *Stereotact. Funct. Neurosurg.*, **56(1)** (1991) 2–19.

190. Bushnell MC, Marchand S, Tremblay N, and Duncan GH. Electrical stimulation of peripheral and central pathways for the relief of musculoskeletal pain. *Can. J. Physiol. Pharmacol.*, **69(5)** (1991) 697–703.

191. Sykes J, Johnson R, and Hanks GW. ABC of palliative care. Difficult pain problems. *Br. Med. J.*, **315(7112)** (1997) 867–869.

192. Ventafridda V, Spoldi E, Caraceni A, and De Conno F. Intraspinal morphine for cancer pain. *Acta Anaesthesiol. Scand.*, **85(Suppl.)** (1987) 47–53.

193. Krames ES. Intrathecal infusional therapies for intractable pain: patient management guidelines. *J. Pain Symptom Manage.*, **8(1)** (1993) 36–46.

194. Devulder J, Ghys L, Dhondt W, and Rolly G. Spinal analgesia in terminal care: risk versus benefit. *J. Pain Symptom Manage.*, **9(2)** (1994) 75–81.

195. Hogan Q, Haddox JD, Abram S, Weissman D, Taylor ML, and Janjan N. Epidural opiates and local anesthetics for the management of cancer pain. *Pain*, **46(3)** (1991) 271–279.

196. Moulin DE, Inturrisi CE, and Foley KM. Epidural and intrathecal opioids: cerebrospinal fluid and plasma pharmacokinetics in cancer pain patients. In *Opioid Analgesics in the Management of Clinical Pain*. Foley KM and Inturrisi CE (eds.), Raven, NY, 1986, pp. 369–383.

197. Max MB, Inturrisi CE, Kaiko RF, Grabinski PY, Li CH, and Foley KM. Epidural and intrathecal opiates: cerebrospinal fluid and plasma profiles in patients with chronic cancer pain. *Clin. Pharmacol. Ther.*, **38(6)** (1985) 631–641.
198. Brose WG, Tanelian DL, Brodsky JB, Mark JB, and Cousins MJ. CSF and blood pharmacokinetics of hydromorphone and morphine following lumbar epidural administration. *Pain*, **45(1)** (1991) 11–15.
199. Grass JA. Sufentanil: clinical use as postoperative analgesic—epidural/intrathecal route. *J. Pain Symptom Manage.*, **7(5)** (1992) 271–286.
200. Grass JA. Fentanyl: clinical use as postoperative analgesic—epidural/intrathecal route. *J. Pain Symptom Manage.*, **7(7)** (1992) 419–430.
201. Nitescu P, Appelgren L, Linder LE, Sjoberg M, Hultman E, and Curelaru I. Epidural versus intrathecal morphine-bupivacaine: assessment of consecutive treatments in advanced cancer pain. *J. Pain Symptom Manage.*, **5(1)** (1990) 18–26.
202. Du Pen SL, Kharasch ED, Williams A, Peterson DG, Sloan DC, Hasche-Klunder H, et al. Chronic epidural bupivacaine-opioid infusion in intractable cancer pain [see comments]. *Pain*, **49(3)** (1992) 293–300.
203. Du Pen SL and Williams AR. Management of patients receiving combined epidural morphine and bupivacaine for the treatment of cancer pain. *J. Pain Symptom Manage.*, **7(2)** (1992) 125–127.
204. Nitescu P, Sjoberg M, Appelgren L, and Curelaru I. Complications of intrathecal opioids and bupivacaine in the treatment of "refractory" cancer pain. *Clin. J. Pain*, **11(1)** (1995) 45–62.
205. Sjoberg M, Nitescu P, Appelgren L, and Curelaru I. Long-term intrathecal morphine and bupivacaine in patients with refractory cancer pain. Results from a morphine : bupivacaine dose regimen of 0.5 : 4.75 mg/ml. *Anesthesiology*, **80(2)** (1994) 284–297.
206. Mercadante S. Intrathecal morphine and bupivacaine in advanced cancer pain patients implanted at home. *J. Pain Symptom Manage.*, **9(3)** (1994) 201–207.
207. Eisenach JC, DuPen S, Dubois M, Miguel R, Allin D. Epidural clonidine analgesia for intractable cancer pain. The Epidural Clonidine Study Group. *Pain*, **61(3)** (1995) 391–399.
208. Penn RD, Paice JA, and Kroin JS. Octreotide: a potent new non-opiate analgesic for intrathecal infusion [see comments]. *Pain*, **49(1)** (1992) 13–19.
209. Yang CY, Wong CS, Chang JY, and Ho ST. Intrathecal ketamine reduces morphine requirements in patients with terminal cancer pain. *Can. J. Anaesth.*, **43(4)** (1996) 379–383.
210. Yaksh TL. Epidural ketamine: a useful, mechanistically novel adjuvant for epidural morphine? *Reg. Anesth.*, **21(6)** (1996) 508–513.
211. Blanchard J, Menk E, Ramamurthy S, and Hoffman J. Subarachnoid and epidural calcitonin in patients with pain due to metastatic cancer. *J. Pain Symptom Manage.*, **5(1)** (1990) 42–45.
212. Gestin Y, Vainio A, and Pegurier AM. Long-term intrathecal infusion of morphine in the home care of patients with advanced cancer. *Acta Anaesthesiol. Scand.*, **41(1 Pt. 1)** (1997) 12–17.
213. Gourlay GK, Plummer JL, Cherry DA, Onley MM, Parish KA, Wood MM, et al. Comparison of intermittent bolus with continuous infusion of epidural morphine in the treatment of severe cancer pain. *Pain*, **47(2)** (1991) 135–140.
214. Hassenbusch SJ, Stanton-Hicks M, Covington EC, Walsh JG, and Guthrey DS. Long-term intraspinal infusions of opioids in the treatment of neuropathic pain. *J. Pain Symptom Manage.*, **10(7)** (1995) 527–543.
215. Caraceni A and Portenoy RK. Pain management in patients with pancreatic carcinoma. *Cancer*, **78(3)** (1996) 639–653.
216. Eisenberg E, Carr DB, and Chalmers TC. Neurolytic celiac plexus block for treatment of cancer pain: a meta-analysis [published erratum appears in *Anesth. Analg.*, **(81)1** (1995) 213, *Anesth. Analg.*, **80(2)** (1995) 290–295.
217. Brown DL. A retrospective analysis of neurolytic celiac plexus block for nonpancreatic intra-abdominal cancer pain. *Reg. Anesth.*, **14(2)** (1989) 63–65.
218. Kawamata M, Ishitani K, Ishikawa K, Sasaki H, Ota K, Omote K, et al. Comparison between celiac plexus block and morphine treatment on quality of life in patients with pancreatic cancer pain. *Pain*, **64(3)** (1996) 597–602.
219. Mercadante S. Celiac plexus block versus analgesics in pancreatic cancer pain. *Pain*, **52(2)** (1993) 187–192.
220. Lillemoe KD, Cameron JL, Kaufman HS, Yeo CJ, Pitt HA, and Sauter PK. Chemical splanchnicectomy in patients with unresectable pancreatic cancer. A prospective randomized trial. *Ann. Surg.*, **217(5)** (1993) 447–455; discussion 456–457.
221. Ischia S, Ischia A, Polati E, and Finco G. Three posterior percutaneous celiac plexus block techniques. A prospective, randomized study in 61 patients with pancreatic cancer pain. *Anesthesiology*, **76(4)** (1992) 534–540.

222. Brown DL, Bulley CK, and Quiel EL. Neurolytic celiac plexus block for pancreatic cancer pain. *Anesth. Analg.*, **66(9)** (1987) 869–873.

223. Chan VW. Chronic diarrhea: an uncommon side effect of celiac plexus block. *Anesth. Analg.*, **82(1)** (1996) 205–207.

224. Davies DD. Incidence of major complications of neurolytic coeliac plexus block. *J. R. Soc. Med.*, **86(5)** (1993) 264–266.

225. Hayakawa J, Kobayashi O, and Murayama H. Paraplegia after intraoperative celiac plexus block. *Anesth. Analg.*, **84(2)** (1997) 447–448.

226. Wong GY and Brown DL. Transient paraplegia following alcohol celiac plexus block. *Reg. Anesth.*, **20(4)** (1995) 352–325.

227. De Conno F, Caraceni A, Aldrighetti L, Magnani G, Ferla G, Comi G, et al. Paraplegia following coeliac plexus block. *Pain*, **55(3)** (1993) 383–385.

228. Plancarte R, de Leon-Casasola OA, El-Helaly M, Allende S, and Lema MJ. Neurolytic superior hypogastric plexus block for chronic pelvic pain associated with cancer. *Reg. Anesth.*, **22(6)** (1997) 562–568.

229. Plancarte R, Amescua C, Patt RB, and Aldrete JA. Superior hypogastric plexus block for pelvic cancer pain. *Anesthesiology*, **73(2)** (1990) 236–239.

230. Plancarte R, Velazquez R, and Patt RB. Neurolytic block of the sympathetic axis. In *Cancer Pain*. Patt RB (ed.), Lippincott, Philadelphia, 1993, pp. 377–425.

231. Wemm K Jr and Saberski L. Modified approach to block the ganglion impar (ganglion of Walther) [letter]. *Reg. Anesth.*, **20(6)** (1995) 544–545.

232. Nebab EG and Florence IM. An alternative needle geometry for interruption of the ganglion impar [letter]. *Anesthesiology*, **86(5)** (1997) 1213–1214.

233. Patt RB and Reddy S. Spinal neurolysis for cancer pain: indications and recent results. *Ann. Acad. Med. Singapore*, **23(2)** (1994) 216–220.

234. Stuart G and Cramond T. Role of percutaneous cervical cordotomy for pain of malignant origin. *Med. J. Aust.*, **158(10)** (1993) 667–670.

235. Sanders M and Zuurmond W. Safety of unilateral and bilateral percutaneous cervical cordotomy in 80 terminally ill cancer patients. *J. Clin. Oncol.*, **13(6)** (1995) 1509–1512.

236. Cowie RA and Hitchcock ER. The late results of antero-lateral cordotomy for pain relief. *Acta Neurochir. (Wien)*, **1(2)** (1982) 39–50.

237. Chevrolet JC, Reverdin A, Suter PM, Tschopp JM, and Junod AF. Ventilatory dysfunction resulting from bilateral anterolateral high cervical cordotomy. Dual beneficial effect of aminophylline. *Chest*, **84(1)** (1983) 112–115.

238. Polatty RC and Cooper KR. Respiratory failure after percutaneous cordotomy. *South. Med. J.*, **79(7)** (1986) 897–899.

239. Ischia S, Luzzani A, Ischia A, Magon F, and Toscano D. Subarachnoid neurolytic block (L5-S1) and unilateral percutaneous cervical cordotomy in the treatment of pain secondary to pelvic malignant disease. *Pain*, **20(2)** (1984) 139–149.

240. Cherny NI and Portenoy RK. Sedation in the management of refractory symptoms: guidelines for evaluation and treatment. *J. Palliat. Care*, **10(2)** (1994) 31–38.

241. Burt RA. The Supreme Court speaks—not assisted suicide but a constitutional right to palliative care. *N. Engl. J. Med.*, **337(17)** (1997) 1234–1236.

242. President's Commission for the Study of Ethical Problems in Medical and Biomedical and Behavioral Research. *Deciding to Forgo Life Sustaining Treatment: Ethical and Legal Issues in Treatment Decisions.* U.S. Government Printing Office, Washington, DC, 1983.

243. American Medical Association. Good care of the dying patient. Council on Scientific Affairs, American Medical Association. *JAMA*, **275(6)** (1996) 474–478.

37 Sexuality and Fertility in Patients with Colorectal Cancer

Megan P. Fleming

1. IMPORTANCE OF SEXUAL HEALTH AND EXPRESSION

Sexual health is often a neglected component of treatment for an individual diagnosed with cancer. Intimacy, closeness, and sexual expression are valued aspects of quality of life across the life-span for both men and women, with many individuals expressing a need for renewing closeness when threatened with impending loss. Maintaining intimate relationships and sexual functioning are important aspects of a patient's life that are frequently left unattended by oncology professionals.

Oncology professionals typically focus on the disease process and its treatment, and sexual functioning is often neglected from assessment. This omission may be the result of the provider's generalized feeling of discomfort discussing sexual issues, increased time constraints under managed care, and/or a lack of sufficient training and information regarding the impact of treatments on sexual functioning. Too often, practitioners judge a patient's psychosocial needs without asking the patient about their importance. Perhaps the assumption that sexuality is not important during cancer treatment and in survivorship prevents this important domain from being assessed. Contrary to this assumption, Vincent and colleagues *(1)* found that 80% of patients receiving cancer treatment wanted more information about sex, although 75% indicated they would not broach the subject themselves. Further validating patient concerns regarding sexual health, Singer et al. *(2)* reported the

From: *Colorectal Cancer: Multimodality Management*
Edited by: L. Saltz © Humana Press Inc., Totowa, NJ

results of a hypothetical query in which men expressed a willingness to trade survival time for preserved or improved sexual functioning.

Colorectal cancer is the third most common cancer in the United States for both men and women. In the year 2000, an estimated 130,200 individuals will be newly diagnosed, including 93,800 with colon cancer and 36,400 with rectal cancer. Sixty-one percent of these newly diagnosed individuals will survive for at least 5 yr *(3)*. With so many survivors who have undergone interventions with known risks of sexual morbidity, sexual health needs to be integrated as a rehabilitative component of assessment and treatment.

Despite the growing recognition of sexual expression as an important aspect of quality of life and the recognized psychosexual sequelae of ostomy surgery, a recent study of 1700 ostomates found that only 23% of patients had received any information about the possible consequences of treatment on their sexual functioning. Of this informed group, only 55% reported this information as adequate *(4)*. Chorost and colleagues *(5)* document a similar lack of information, reporting on the results of 52 patient charts by retrospective review. Seventy-one percent of patients who underwent curative procedures for rectal cancer had no documentation of a presurgical discussion regarding the risk of sexual dysfunction. Even among stoma care nurses, a recent study found only 11% of nurses routinely incorporated a sexual history into their practice and 84% of these nurses had received no formal training in how to carry out a sexual health assessment *(6)*. It is clear from the literature that discussing sexuality with patients is one of the most uncomfortable topics for the medical profession *(7)*.

There are no clear guidelines for addressing sexuality during the stages of disease and its treatment. From the time of diagnosis, cancer patients are faced with life-changing decisions and events: mortality, uncomfortable, disfiguring, and sometimes lengthy treatments, and emotional impact on their partner, family, and work. From the beginning of assessment, when therapeutic decisions are being made, providers should offer education and information to patients, ideally with their partner present, regarding the known risks of sexual morbidity associated with the proposed treatments.

Oncology professionals can assist patients and their partners by asking specific open-ended questions to validate the importance of sexual health concerns, thus providing an environment in which the patient/couple are encouraged and feel safe to express their own personal concerns. Providers should also examine their own thoughts and feelings regarding sexuality. If not comfortable addressing these issues, providers should not ignore or dismiss their patient's concerns, but offer referrals to alternate resources. Although some patients may not want to discuss their sexual health, providers should at least offer the option, conveying that sex is an appropriate topic to cover during future visits. This chapter outlines current knowledge of the impact of colorectal cancer and its treatment on sexual functioning, discusses psychosocial factors that affect sexual functioning, and provides information regarding the assessment and treatment of alterations in sexual functioning.

Sexuality is a complex, multidimensional phenomenon that incorporates biologic, psychologic, interpersonal, and behavioral dimensions. It is important to recognize that a wide range of "normal" sexual functioning exists. The National Health and Social Life Survey conducted in 1992 documented adult sexual behavior in the United States with a probability sample of 3432 men and women (representative of the general population) between the ages of 18 and 59 yr old *(8)*. A recently published analysis of these data documents, among the respondents who were sexually active, a 43% prevalence of sexual dysfunction in women and 31% rate of prevalence in men *(9)*. Given these statistics, it is important to consider an individual's premorbid level of sexual functioning prior to a diagnosis of cancer and its treatment. The patient and his/her partner within a context of factors such as gender, age, personal attitudes, and religious and cultural values ultimately defines their sexuality.

2. PHASES OF SEXUAL RESPONSE

Since the 1970s, sexual functioning has been conceptualized as a series of phases that are discrete and separate aspects of the human sexual response, yet interact and affect each other respectively. Masters and Johnson (10) were the first to study and describe the physical changes that take place in the body during a sexual experience. They proposed four stages in the sexual response cycle: excitement, plateau, orgasm, and resolution. Kaplan (11) added the conceptualization and delineation of a desire phase and has written extensively on a triphasic model (desire, arousal, orgasm) of sexual disorders. The triphasic model enables professionals and patients to qualify problems in sexual functioning, as sexual dysfunction occurs in the areas of desire (interest), arousal (excitement), and orgasm (tension release). Individuals often experience changes in more than one phase of sexual function. Resolution is not included in the triphasic model of sexual response, as it is not associated with dysfunction; rather, it is marked by the return to normal genital responses to sexual stimulation. The triphasic model is widely adopted in research and review of the sexual difficulties associated with cancer and its treatment (12–16).

2.1. Desire

Kaplan delineated sexual desire as the urge to seek out and respond to sexual activity (17). Desire is an individual's interest in being sexual and includes dreams, fantasies, and the frustration because of a lack of sex, the mental precedent, and accompaniment to physiological responses. Behaviorally, the individual initiates and/or is responsive to a partner's initiation for sexual activity such that desire can be influenced by visual, auditory, and/or tactile cues. For women, sexual desire often depends on emotional factors, including personal comfort level with their sexuality and feeling sexually attractive. Sexual desire is stimulated in both men and women by testosterone and other hormones (androgens) linked to sexual feelings. In women, testosterone is produced in both the ovaries and the adrenal glands; however, women have lower levels of androgens than men. Women also depend on the hormone estrogen to stimulate female characteristics and promote healthy genital function. Sexual desire waxes and wanes over time and is highly influenced by life stressors and major life changes.

2.2. Arousal (Excitement)

Arousal is a psychophysiological response by which sexual stimulation (psychological and physical) elicits neurological, vascular, muscular, and endocrine reactions. Other physiological parameters, including increased heart rate, blood pressure, and perspiration, often accompany arousal. The two major indicators of sexual arousal are myotonia and genital vasocongestion (10). For men, the perception of arousal is associated with the quality of their erection. In women, the vagina produces a natural lubrication with arousal as the vaginal walls expand, loosen, and widen. For women, however, physiological indications of arousal, namely lubrication, are often not well correlated with the cognitive, subjective perception of arousal (18). Overall sensitivity to sensation increases with vasocongestion in both men and women.

2.3. Orgasm

Orgasm is the climax of pleasure, a physical release, and emotional pleasure, followed by a period of resolution. For women, the orgasmic platform consists of 0.8-s rhythmic muscular contractions of the uterus and the rectal sphincter *(11)*. Most women need direct clitoral stimulation, which can be a part of intercourse, to reach orgasm; however, for a majority of women, orgasm does not occur with intercourse alone. Women, unlike men, are often capable of multiple orgasms within a single sexual experience. For men, the orgasmic platform is the experience of three to seven ejaculatory spurts at 0.8-s intervals. The rhythmic contractions of the penile urethra, the muscles of the penile base, and perineal muscles, which follow immediately after ejaculation, constitute the second component of orgasm. A specific period of time, the refractory period, must elapse before a man can ejaculate again *(11)*.

2.4. Resolution

Resolution, or the refractory phase, is defined by physiological changes and emotional responses following orgasm. Resolution marks a return to normal heart rate, respiration, body perspiration, and the genital response to decreasing blood supply. Most individuals also experience a state of relaxation.

3. HOW DOES TREATMENT OF COLORECTAL CANCER AFFECT SEXUALITY?

An individual's sexual response can be affected in a number of ways from the time of a colorectal cancer diagnosis through treatment. The causes of sexual difficulties are often both physiological and psychological. Many patients undergoing treatment experience loss of libido and interest in sexual expression. Men may experience sexual difficulties, including erectile dysfunction (difficulty attaining and maintaining an erection), anejaculation (absence of ejaculation), retrograde ejaculation (ejaculation going backward to the bladder), or the inability to reach orgasm. Most often, however, orgasm remains intact, although it may be delayed secondary to medications and/or anxiety. Women may experience change in genital sensations because of pain or a loss of sensation and numbness. Loss of sensation can be as distressing as painful sensation for some individuals. The experience of pain with intercourse (dyspareunia) is not uncommon, as well as a decreased ability to reach orgasm. Often, both men and women experience a decrease in sexual activity when undergoing management of their cancer *(19–21)*. Providers should recognize that the tremendous anticipatory anxiety often associated with the first attempt to resume sexual intercourse after treatment often leads to a rushed sexual experience with insufficient arousal. For many patients, this initial experience is uncomfortable, at best, and painful, at worst.

Research on treatments for colorectal cancer have identified several predictors of postoperative sexual functioning, including extent of surgery, patient's age, premorbid sexual and bladder functioning, and tumor size. Despite this knowledge, sexual response after colorectal cancer surgery remains an insufficiently understood and researched area; in particular, issues of sexual recovery in women have received too little clinical attention and research *(20,21)*. Review of the literature highlights the need for prospective studies with longer-term follow-up, validated measures, and larger sample sizes. A recent review of 54 articles on quality of life (with sexual function as a domain) after treatment for rectal cancer quantified some of these limitations *(21)*. Only 3 of the 54 studies measured global quality of life with a well-researched questionnaire, only 14 were prospective, and sample sizes ranged from 5 to 265, with the majority involving groups of less than 25 patients.

3.1. Impact of Specific Cancer Treatment Modalities

3.1.1. Surgery

The extent of surgery is an important factor relative to risk of sexual morbidity *(19,21,22)*. For patients with colon cancer, the biology of local tumor growth and associated lymphadenectomy determine the extent of surgical resection *(23)*, with en-bloc surgical resection being the primary technique. Anastomosis after resection, on average, removes 10–12 in. of bowel and introduces minor changes in bowel habits during a brief recovery period. The predominant research on sexual functioning has been on the outcomes after surgical management of rectal cancer *(19,24–39)*.

For rectal cancer, tumor size, its exact location within the rectum, and extent around the circumference of the rectum determine the most appropriate surgical treatment. The two main objectives of rectal surgery are cancer cure and preservation of fecal continence *(40)*. Sexual and urinary dysfunction are recognized complications of resection for rectal cancer. The main cause of sexual dysfunction from surgical resection appears to be injury to the autonomic nerves in the pelvis along the distal aorta from blunt pelvic resection or undefined cutting. Incidence of genitourinary dysfunction depends on the type of surgery performed (i.e., the plane of dissection, the degree of preservation of the autonomic nerves, and the extent of pelvic dissection) *(26)*. Nerve injury can occur via direct injury, by vascular damage to the vasa nervosa, or when the blood supply to the nerves that enter laterally are disrupted with traction or devascularization *(5)*.

The neuroanatomy for sexual functioning requires an intact autonomic nervous system, which includes an interaction between the parasympathetic and the sympathetic nervous systems. Erection, a parasympathetically mediated response, is governed by impulses traveling along the nervi erigentes that arise from the second, third, and fourth sacral nerves *(41)*, whereas ejaculation depends on sympathetic control. The sympathetic fibers originate from the lower thoracic and upper lumbar segments of the spinal cord. These fibers descend along the aorta, forming the superior hypogastric plexus near the aortic bifurcation. The plexus divides into two trunks, which enter the pelvis, along its lateral walls, as the hypogastric nerves. The parasympathetic fibers to the pelvis join the hypogastric nerves on each pelvic wall to form the pelvic plexuses *(41)*. Damage to the hypogastric (sympathetic) nerves or sacral splanchnic (parasympathetic) nerves, or both, during surgical resection are the most likely cause of urinary and sexual dysfunction *(27)*. Pelvic plexus preservation is necessary to maintain erectile functioning, and both hypergastric nerve and pelvic plexus preservation are necessary to maintain ejaculate function and orgasm *(30)*.

Many stage I and most stage II and stage III rectal cancers are removed by either lower anterior resection (LAR), or abdomino-perineal resection (APR). Since the introduction of the mechanical stapling instruments, more LAR resections have been performed, which enable the application of anal-sphincter-preserving techniques and, in most cases, render a permanent colostomy unnecessary *(20)*. Whereas LAR has become accepted as a viable surgical option for cancer of the upper and middle rectum, APR remains the standard surgical approach for patients with distal rectal cancers. Sexual morbidity is more common after APR than LAR *(26)*.

Recent advances in surgical techniques have brought attention to the preservation of the autonomic nerves to reduce the incidence of concomitant bladder and sexual dysfunction. Preservation of the autonomic nerves is accomplished through surgical techniques usually combined with total mesorectal excision (TME) or radical pelvic lymphadectomy *(19)*. In pelvic dissections that preserve hypogastric nerve trunks arising from the preaortic plexus and parasympathetic trunks arising from the sacral roots, postoperative sexual dysfunction rates have been reduced from more than 50% to a range of 10–28% *(22)*.

Havenga and colleagues *(19)* provide a review of the functional results for both conservative surgical and autonomic nerve-preserving techniques. The review examined the English, German, French, and Dutch medical literature on bladder and sexual dysfunction after resection for rectal cancer since 1980. Although bladder dysfunction and associated patient distress have implications for sexual expression and impact on sexual function, a detailed review of bladder complications is beyond the scope of this chapter. Nineteen studies were found to report on male sexual function after conventional resection for rectal cancer (*see* Table 1) *(24,25,29,31–34,36,38,39,42–50)*. Ignoring the inherent difficulties of comparing retrospective studies, examining the data from these studies together shows the number of men who developed complete erectile dysfunction (ED) is 25% (170/677). After APR, 34% (132/416) of men developed complete ED, and 20% after LAR (35/251). Loss of ejaculation occurred in 16% (107/677) of men, with 19% (64/416) after APR and 33% (36/25) after LAR.

Havenga and colleagues *(19)* reviewed seven studies regarding female sexual function after conventional resection, the results of which are found in Table 2 *(25,31,38,45,46,49,50)*. Only one study that examined quality of sexual function in women was prospective. For these women, decreased libido was found for 24% of all patients, dyspareunia was found in 38%, and diminished or no orgasm was found in 28%.

Sexual function after autonomic nerve-preserving resection for rectal cancer is reviewed in five Japanese studies, the results of which are summarized in Table 3 *(32,37,51–53)*. After preservation of both the parasympathetic nerves and the hypogastric nerves, "excellent" outcome in male sexual function was achieved. However, in those men for whom both hypogastric nerves were sacrificed, almost all reported an inability to ejaculate. Depending on the degree of nerve preservation, sexual dysfunction following surgical resection may still be significant *(54)*.

3.1.2. COLOSTOMY

An increasing number of patients have a temporary colostomy with later closure and reanastomosis of the bowel. In recent years, the rate of sphincter salvage in rectal cancer has increased to 70% and the need for APR and a permanent colostomy has been reported to be less than 10% in institutions with coloproctology specialization *(55)*. Despite these advances, patients with a cancer in the middle or lower one-third of the rectum are still confronted with the possibility of a permanent colostomy *(40)*. Whether temporary or permanent, the psychosocial consequences of stoma surgery are severe and are associated with a process of adjustment that extends over the first postoperative year and sometimes longer *(56,57)*.

Adapting to a changed body image and concern/embarrassment from potential odor or fecal leakage can greatly impact self-esteem. Women and younger patients frequently experience persistent problems with negative body image *(58)*. One year after stoma surgery, 18–25% of patients reported an increase in emotional problems such as depression, anxiety, anger, and irritation *(59)*. Frequently the postoperative psychological distress experienced by stoma patients goes undetected by professionals involved with surgery and stoma care *(57)*.

Recognizing that psychological distress is not uncommon, providers should be aware that negative, postoperative emotional reactions might also contribute to a pattern of sexual avoidance. A member of the oncology team (social worker, nurse, physician, or other health care professional) should offer support and education related to self-care of the ostomy.

Table 1
Male Sexual Function After Conventional Surgery for Rectal Cancer[a,b]

Author/reference	Year	Operation	Number of patients	Complete erectile dysfunction	Partial erectile dysfunction	Loss of ejaculation	Altered ejaculation	Retrograde ejaculation	Maximum age (yr)
Leo et al. (42)	1993	LAR with CAA	7	0	0	5 (71)			
Aghaji and Obiekwe (43)	1991	APR	26	8 (31)		2 (8)			40
Havenga and Welvaart (44)	1991	APR	9	5 (56)	3 (33)	7 (78)		1 (11)	80
		LAR	17	4 (24)	4 (24)	5 (29)		5 (29)	
Cunsolo et al. (45)	1990	APR	22	4 (18)	9 (41)		13 (59)		60
Hojo et al. (32)	1989	APR	11	5 (45)	4 (36)				
		LAR	29	10 (34)	4 (14)				
		APR-ext	14	11 (79)	1 (7)				
Zenico et al. (39)	1989	APR	18	1 (6)	3 (17)	8 (44)		3 (17)	65
Hellstrom (29)	1988	APR	2	1 (50)					
		LAR	10	1 (10)		3 (30)			
Santangelo et al. (36)	1987	APR	9	4 (44)	2 (20)	2 (22)			60
		LAR	12	12 (33)		3 (25)			
Cirino et al. (46)	1987	APR	28	7 (25)	5 (18)	2 (7)		3 (11)	65
Kinn and Ohman (33)	1986	APR or LAR	10	3 (30)	5 (50)	7 (70)		1 (10)	
Fegiz et al. (25)	1986	APR	30	(50)	(60)		(37)		
		LAR–sa	42	(20)	(57)		(15)		
		LAR–ma	31		(39)		(20)		
La Monica et al. (34)	1985	APR	20	7 (39)		(70)			70
		LAR	20	7 (35)		(40)			
Neal (47)	1984	APR	18		6 (33)	7 (39)			
		LAR	20		5 (25)	7 (35)			
Hjortrup et al. (31)	1984	LAR	21	1 (5)					65
Balslev and Harling (24)	1983	APR	93	17 (18)	10 (11)	3 (3)			70
		LAR	17		3 (18)	3 (18)			
Williams and Johnston (48)	1983	APR	17	8 (47)	3 (18)	1 (16)			
		LAR	20	4 (20)		2 (18)			
Von Segesser and Marti (49)	1983	APR	17	16 (94)		16 (94)			
Deixonne et al. (50)	1983	APR	92	38 (41)	19 (21)	10 (11)	1 (1)		60
Williams and Slack (38)	1980	APR	4	1 (25)	1 (25)				
		LAR	5			2 (40)			

[a]Havenga K, Maas CP, DeRuiter MC, Welvaart K, and Trimboos JB. Avoiding long-term disturbance to bladder and sexual function in pelvic surgery, particularly with rectal cancer. Sem. Surg. Onc., 18 (2000) 235–243. Copyright © 2000, John Wiley & Sons, Inc. Reprinted by permission of Wiley-Liss, Inc., a subsidiary of John Wiley & Sons, Inc. (19).

[b]Numbers in parentheses are percentages.

APR, abdominoperineal excision; LAR, low anterior resection; CAA, colo-anal anastomosis; est, wide iliopelvic lymphadenectomy, no attempt to preserve pelvic autonomic nerves; sa, staples anastomosis; ma, manual anastomosis.

Table 2
Female Sexual Function After Conventional Surgery for Rectal Cancer[a,b]

Author/reference	Year	Operation	Number of patients	Decreased libido	Dyspareunia	Altered orgasm	Maximum age (yr)
Cunsolo et al. *(45)*	1990	APR	8	2 (25)	4 (50)	2 (25)	
Cirino et al. *(46)*	1987	APR	18	15 (83)	6 (33)	1 (6)	64
Fegiz et al. *(25)*	1986	APR	15		(65)	(70)	
		LAR–sa	9		(65)	(24)	
		LAR–ma	17		(44)	(44)	
Hjortrup et al. *(31)*	1984	LAR	20		2 (10)	1 (5)	65
Von Segesser and Marti *(49)*	1983	APR	7		3 (43)		59
Deixonne et al. *(50)*	1983	APR	26	12 (46)	8 (31)	11 (42)	
Williams and Slack *(38)*	1980	APR	3				

[a]Havenga K, Maas CP, DeRuiter MC, Welvaart K, and Trimboos JB. Avoiding long-term disturbance to bladder and sexual function in pelvic surgery, particularly with rectal cancer. *Sem. Surg. Onc.*, **18** (2000) 235–243. Copyright © 2000, John Wiley & Sons, Inc. Reprinted by permission of Wiley-Liss, Inc., a subsidiary of John Wiley & Sons, Inc.
[b]Numbers in parentheses are percentages.
APR, abdominoperineal excision; LAR, low anterior resection; sa, staples anastomosis; ma, manual anastomosis.

Table 3
Male Sexual Function After Nerve Preserving Surgery for Rectal Cancer in Japan[a,b]

	Number of patients	Erection	Ejaculation
Complete preservation of the pelvic autonomic nerves			
Saito et al. *(51)*	29	22 (76)	16 (55)
Sugihara et al. *(37)*	27	26 (96)	19/26 (73)
Masui et al. *(52)*	98	(93)	(83)
Moriya et al. *(53)*	31	28 (90)	21 (60)
Hojo et al. *(32)*	10	8 (80)	6 (60)
Resection of hypogastric nerves and preservation of pelvic plexus			
Sugihara et al. *(37)*	9	9 (100)	0 (0)
Moriya et al. *(53)*	19	6 (32)	2 (11)
Hojo et al. *(32)*	1	1	0
Unilateral preservation of hypogastric nerve and pelvic plexus			
Saito et al. *(51)*	16	11 (69)	4 (25)
Masui et al. *(52)*	17	(82)	(47)
Resection of hypogastic nerves and partial or unilateral preservation of pelvic plexus			
Sugihara et al. *(37)*	13	11 (85)	0 (0)
Masui et al. *(52)*	19	(61)	0
Moriya et al. *(53)*	11	2 (18)	0 (0)
Complete resection of the pelvic autonomic nerves			
Sugihara et al. *(37)*	8	4 (50)	0 (0)
Hojo et al. *(32)*	11	0 (0)	0 (0)

[a]Havenga K, Maas CP, DeRuiter MC, Welvaart K, and Trimboos JB. Avoiding long-term disturbance to bladder and sexual function in pelvic surgery, particularly with rectal cancer. *Sem. Surg. Onc.*, **18** (2000) 235–243. Copyright © 2000, John Wiley & Sons, Inc. Reprinted by permission of Wiley-Liss, Inc., a subsidiary of John Wiley & Sons, Inc. *(19)*.
[b]Numbers in parentheses are percentages.

Anticipating the patient concerns and reactions will help them normalize and manage these initial emotional reactions and help the individual to regain his/her physical self-esteem.

Research on the prevalence of sexual dysfunction between stoma and nonstoma patients supports greater dysfunction in the stoma group *(25,34,36,58)*. The overall rate of sexual dysfunction among male stoma patients (66–100%), is consistently higher than in male patients whose sphincters have been left intact (30–75%) *(36,48,58)*. In the limited studies that have examined women, percentages of sexual dysfunction (i.e., dyspareunia and diminished orgasm) and reduced sexual activity were again higher among those women with stomas *(20,25,31,38,45,46,49,50,58)*. A recent study *(60)* examined quality of life in 391 stoma patients and reported that major stomal problems included rashes 51%, leakage 36%, and ballooning in those individuals with ileostomies 90%. The majority, 80% of patients, experienced some change in their lifestyle and more than 40% of patients reported problems with their sex lives. Although many of the addressed psychosocial issues for those individuals with a temporary colostomy will resolve, changes in sexual function will still likely require clinical attention.

To avoid the stigma associated with iliac colostomy, procedures have been developed to create a neoanus and neosphincter at the coloperineal anastomosis *(40)*. Gamagami and colleagues *(61)* conducted a prospective study on the functional outcome, morbidity, and degree of patient satisfaction with a continent perineal colostomy constructed from a colonic smooth-muscle cuff wrap in combination with colonic irrigation for 63 patients with distal rectal and anal tumors. Satisfactory continence (complete continence to stool and incontinence to gas) was achieved by 56% of patients by 6 mo and by 59% of patients at 12 mo. Eighty-five percent of patients were satisfied with their functional results; however, 72% were reported to be uneasey, at times, with their bowel function. Although avoidance of a permanent stoma is generally considered a favorable outcome, patients undergoing sphincter-preserving surgeries may develop a number of unpleasant symptoms, typically fecal soiling and urgency, especially with low anastomoses. As sexual and bowel functions may still be impaired despite advances in surgical techniques, it cannot be assumed that these patients will always fare better than patients in whom sphincter function must be sacrificed *(48,58,62)*.

3.1.3. Neoadjuvant/Adjuvant Treatments

Given the incidence of sexual dysfunction associated with the surgical management of colorectal cancer, it is difficult to ascertain the additional adverse effects on sexual function from adjuvant treatments. The following is a review of the literature that reports on the sexual morbidity associated with adjuvant treatments and often the impact of systemic effects of treatment on an individual's body image and experience of sexuality. The impact of these adjuvant treatments on reproductive potential is then addressed.

3.1.4. Chemotherapy

Common side effects experienced after chemotherapy include nausea, vomiting, diarrhea, constipation, mucositis, weight changes (gain or loss), and altered sense of taste and smell *(63)*. These symptoms often leave patients feeling asexual. Alopecia is often one of the most distressing side effects, as this loss, with its visible changes, is an outward reminder of cancer and its treatment with associated changes in body image. Loss of pubic hair can also be particularly uncomfortable, which, in turn, promotes feeling asexual.

Chemotherapy is associated with loss of desire and decreased frequency of intercourse for both men and women. For women, cytoxic agents are associated with vaginal dryness, dyspareunia, reduced ability to reach orgasm, and, for older women, greater risk of ovarian failure *(15)*.

Ovarian failure secondary to chemotherapy or radiation brings the sudden onset of menopausal symptoms and women who experience sudden loss of estrogen and androgen production from the ovaries experience a number of associated sexual changes. Sexual symptoms associated with menopause include thinning of the vulvar tissues and vagina, loss of tissue elasticity, decreased vaginal lubrication, hot flushes, increased frequency of urinary tract infections, mood swings, fatigue, and irritability. The impact of menopause on sexual functioning and the arousal phase of the sexual response in particular, are often not communicated to women who struggle to understand these changes in their sexual responsiveness.

For men, chemotherapy agents rarely play an obvious role in erectile dysfunction *(15)*. Some cytoxic agents may cause nerve damage, but few reports indicate permanent loss of erections upon completion of treatment. For those men who have temporary or permanent damage to the testicles from chemotherapy, testosterone replacement may be necessary to restore sexual function *(15)*.

3.1.5. RADIATION THERAPY

Radiation often irritates the intestinal lining and may cause diarrhea *(64)*. The fatigue and change in bowel habits associated with radiation likely contribute to loss of libido and decreased sexual activity reported for both men and women.

For women, pelvic radiation also causes changes to occur in the vagina. Both external beam radiation and implants damage the vaginal epithelium and basal layer of the mucosa, leading to vaginal stenosis and vascular fibrosis. These factors can then lead to long-term sexual dysfunction, painful pelvic examinations, dyspareunia, potential gonadal toxicity, and infertility. Women who receive radiation should be educated regarding the use of vaginal dilators. Vascular compromise can be temporary or permanent *(63)*. For men, radiation has been associated with difficulties attaining/maintaining erection. A recent study by Saito and colleagues *(51)* found no significant increase in rate of impotency among those patients who received radiation with nerve-sparing surgery versus those who received only nerve-sparing surgery. Seventy-six percent of advanced rectal cancer patients retained potency after preoperative radiation followed by nerve-sparing surgery.

The exact etiology of sexual dysfunction after radiation therapy remains unknown *(5)*. Proposed etiologies include pudendal or sympathetic nerve injury, vascular occlusion of penile arteries, or decreased levels of testosterone. Often, sexual changes are insidious, with changes over 6 mo to 1 yr after radiation as fibrosis develops. There is a greater risk of sexual morbidity in men who already have compromised quality of erections prior to cancer diagnosis. Other risk factors, which contribute to greater risk of sexual morbidity, include cigarette smoking, history of heart disease, hypertension, and/or diabetes.

4. FERTILITY ISSUES

As 93% of new diagnoses for colorectal cancer occur in individuals over the age of 50 *(65)*, many patients may have already lost their reproductive capacity, being infertile or sub-fertile, at the time of diagnosis. However, a number of individuals will have concerns regarding their reproductive potential following treatment. All patients who are fertile should be instructed about the general recommendation to continue birth control use during active adjuvant therapy and for at least 12 mo afterward *(63)*. Many patients who have experienced temporary loss of fertility fail to recognize the possibility of pregnancy during treatment.

Previously reviewed surgical treatments for colorectal cancer may lead to organic sexual dysfunction resulting from a resection that may impact the vascular supply and/or innervation to the pelvis. The adjuvant therapies of radiation and/or chemotherapy introduce higher risks of infertility in the treatment of colorectal cancer, and sterility from these therapies may be temporary or permanent. The occurrence of this toxicity is related to a number of factors, including the individual's gender, age at time of treatment, type of therapeutic agent, total dose, single vs multiple agents, and length of time since treatment.

With regard to chemotherapy, patient age is an important factor and the possibility of gonadal recovery improves with the length of time off chemotherapy. Patients younger than 35 are better able to tolerate higher doses of chemotherapy without resulting permanent infertility *(66)*. As an antimetabolite, 5-fluorouracil (5-FU) has documented deleterious effects on fertility, including amenorrhea, oligospermia, azoospermia, and ovarian failure *(67)*.

When the testes are exposed to radiation, sperm count begins to decrease and, depending on the dosage, may result in temporary or permanent sterility *(66)*. Men who receive radiation to the abdominal or pelvic region may still regain partial or full sperm production depending on the amount of injury to the testes. Effective dosing schedules for preoperative radiotherapy for rectal cancer include 20–25 Gy in 5 fractions and 40–45 Gy in 20–25 fractions *(64)*. Although the testicles are not the direct target of radiation for the treatment of rectal cancer, radiation tends to scatter so that the testicles may experience some radiation. Exposing the testes to ionizing radiation at a dose below 600 rad causes disturbances of spermatogenesis and altered spermatocytes with recovery periods dependent on dose *(68)*; doses above 600 rad cause permanent infertility by killing off all stem cells *(15)*. For men, gonadal toxicity can be evidenced by three measurements: testicular biopsy, serum hormone assays (levels), and semen analysis. When male infertility is the result of abnormal hormone production, the use of hormone manipulation may lead to the return of sperm production *(69)*.

For women, a dose of 5–20 Gy administered to the ovary is sufficient to completely impair gonadal function regardless of the patient's age; a dose of 30 Gy provokes premature menopause in 60% of women less than 26 yr of age *(70)*. Measurement of gonadal toxicity in women is more difficult to assess because of the relative inaccessibility of the ovary to biopsy (which would require laparoscopy). Therefore, menstrual and reproductive history, measurements of serum hormone levels, and clinical evidence of ovarian function are the criteria most commonly used to determine ovarian failure. Gradishar and Schilsky *(69)* provide a review of gonadal dysfunction in patients receiving chemotherapy; Yarbro and Perry *(68)* provide a more extensive review of the effect of cancer therapy on gonadal function.

As 2–8% of women with colorectal cancer have synchronous ovarian metastatases, prophylactic oophorectomy may be recommended. For premenopausal women, this possibility should be discussed preoperatively relative to their interest in childbearing. For those premenopausal and perimenopausal women who have no concern related to infertility and those women who are already postmenopausal, consideration should be given to remove grossly normal ovaries *(23)*.

4.1. Procreative Alternatives

When feasible and relative to the necessity of treatment, oncology professionals should discuss reproductive cell and tissue banking with patients, referring to a reproductive endocrinologist prior to chemotherapy and/or radiation. Men can store sperm from semen ejaculate, epididymal aspirate, testicular aspirate, and testicular biopsy *(72)*. Women can store ovarian tissue, ovarian follicles, and embryos *(73)*. In oocyte cryopreservation, which is still experimental *(74)*, reproductive cells/tissue are cryopreserved for future use in artificial insemination for patients who wish to protect their reproductive capacity. Donnez and Bassil *(70)* reviewed indications for cyropreservation of ovarian tissue, and Colon *(75)* reviewed current reproductive-assisted technologies.

However, these options are not appropriate for all patients. Counseling is an important part of the decision-making process for patients, as thinking through these decisions at a time when individuals are struggling with issues of life and potential death are often difficult. Patients need to consider costs, stress, time, emotions, and potential inclusion of another individual in the pregnancy process (i.e., a surrogate). For many patients, the financial costs associated with in vitro fertilization (IVF) and subsequent embryo cyropreservation is prohibitive. Consideration also needs to be given to current rate of failure to implant in IVF procedures and the potential adverse effect of malignancy on sperm parameters *(74)*. A recent retrospective analysis, with a limited sample size, reported the oocytes from patients with malignant disorders were of a poorer quality and exhibited a significantly impaired fertilization rate compared to age-matched controls *(74)*. For all patients who wish to be parents and have permanent infertility, adoption should be presented as a choice.

For men who experience retrograde ejaculation after treatment and remain fertile, it is often possible to retrieve live sperm cells. An infertility specialist can retrieve sperm cells from the testicles and from urine. Medication can sometimes be used to stimulate the remaining nerves around the prostate and seminal vesicles to convert a retrograde ejaculation to an antegrade ejaculation; in the United States, ephedrine sulfate is used most often; and in Europe, imipramine has also been used. Pharmacologic agents can also be used to induce an ejaculation (i.e., intrathecal neostigmine or subcutaneous physostigmine). When medication does not work, several other techniques are available and may be recommended, including vibratory stimulation, electroejaculation, direct aspiration of fluid from the vas deferens, perineal needle stimulation, and hypogastric nerve stimulator. Further review of these treatments and information regarding treatment of infertility and assisted reproductive technology is available *(15,72,76,77)*.

4.2. Preventative Strategies

For women, studies *(78)* have shown that movement of the ovaries out of the field of radiation (ovarioplexy), either to the iliac crest or behind the uterus, may help preserve fertility when high doses of radiation therapy are being applied. By relocating the ovaries laterally, it is possible to shield them during radiation of the para-aortic and femoral lymph nodes *(68)*. Pelvic radiation provokes an irradiation of 5–10% of the ovary, even if transposed outside the irradiation area *(70)*. Similar prevention strategies may be available for men; when possible, lead shields should be used to protect the testes *(66)*.

4.3. Colorectal Cancer in Pregnancy

Colon and rectal carcinoma diagnosed during pregnancy is rare. The incidence rate has been reported as high as 0.1% and as low as 0.001% of all pregnancies. The first reported case of rectal cancer in a woman who was pregnant was diagnosed in 1842. Since then, 245 cases of colorectal cancer have been reported in pregnancy. Medich and Fazio *(79)* compared the distribution of colon and rectal tumors among the 245 pregnant women to the general population and to patients less than 40 yr of age with colon or rectal cancer. Unlike the general population with a distribution of 73% colon and 27% rectum and patients under 40 yr of age with 68% colon and 32% rectum, the pregnant women had a significantly higher incidence of rectal cancer (83%) compared to colon (17%). Although a rare phenomenon in pregnancy, given the high incidence of rectal tumors in pregnant women, those pregnant women with unexplained rectal bleeding should be evaluated by anorectal examination and flexible sigmoidoscopy *(79)*. Bernstein and colleagues *(80)* have published the largest single series of these cases for review. Although the management of patients with colorectal tumors should be determined on an individual basis and is beyond the scope of this chapter, a review of treatment options and outcomes can be found in refs. *79* and *80*.

5. OTHER FACTORS ASSOCIATED WITH TREATMENT THAT IMPACT SEXUAL FUNCTIONING

Having reviewed the more direct impact of treatments on sexual functioning, oncology practitioners should also recognize the impact of other systemic treatment side effects on sexual function and expression.

Fatigue is a common medical condition for cancer patients and for patients undergoing chemotherapy; fatigue can be a chronic symptom that may significantly limit physical activity. Patients can benefit from education related to behavioral strategies (i.e., energy conservation), symptom management, and methods to minimize exertion in sexual activity if fatigue has been a limiting factor of expression *(15,63)*.

Pain can negatively impact an individual's receptivity to sexual stimulation and decrease sexual desire. Pain medications are also known to have deleterious effects on libido and arousal *(14,15,81)*.

Nausea and vomiting are frequently associated with cancer treatments. These symptoms can certainly decrease sexual desire. Antiemetics are often used to treat these symptoms, yet their sedative effects may also interfere with sexual function.

Range-of-motion difficulties can contribute to trouble finding positions that are comfortable for sexual intimacy and to asexual feelings.

Shortness of breath can be a deterrent to initiating sexual intimacy. Pulmonary hygiene before sexual activity may provide some benefit and keeping the affected partner's head and upper torso raised with pillows also may be helpful *(63)*.

6. ASSESSMENT OF SEXUAL FUNCTIONING

The literature contains a number of articles and resources that address sexual assessment *(14)*, with many specific to cancer patients *(12,14,15,63)*. Kaplan *(82)* provides a useful interview model to evaluate sexual problems in healthy and medically ill individuals, focusing on the chief complaint, sexual status, medical status, psychiatric status, family and psychosocial history, relationship assessment, summary, and recommendations. Auchincloss *(12,13)* applies Kaplan's model to oncology settings, briefly describing the assessment for each part of the interview. The P-LI-SS-IT model *(83)*, an acronym for the four levels of permission, limited information, specific suggestion, and intensive therapy, is another model of assessment and intervention commonly used as a framework for sexual rehabilitation in cancer care and medical illness *(7,63,83–85)*.

The following brief list of factors known to impact current sexual functioning should be included in an assessment. The patient's specific sexual concerns or needs at the time dictate the approach and content of the discussion.

6.1. General Factors Affecting Sexual Functioning to be Evaluated in Assessment

6.1.1. PREMORBID SEXUAL FUNCTIONING

An individual's past (preillness) sexual development, preferences, and experience are vital to assessment of sexual status. Level of sexual functioning prior to diagnosis and treatment, interest, satisfaction, and importance of sexual functioning in the relationship all influence the patient's potential distress related to current sexual status. Individuals who have already experienced sexual difficulties may be especially vulnerable to the effects of treatment. Clinicians should be careful not to make assumptions regarding the patient's previous sexual experience and importance of sexual expression.

6.1.2. PSYCHOSOCIAL ASPECTS OF SEXUALITY

6.1.2.1. Relationship Status. The patient may or may not have an available partner at the time of diagnosis. Sexuality should be taken no less seriously by the clinician or the patient in this circumstance. For patients with a partner, the clinician should consider and discuss the duration, quality, and stability of the relationship prior to diagnosis. Additionally, as many patients fear rejection and abandonment, the clinician should inquire about the partner's response to the illness and the patient's concerns of the treatment impact on the partner *(87)*. Partners share many of the same reactions as patients in that their most significant concerns typically relate to loss and fear of death. Moreover, the partner's physical, sexual, and emotional health should be considered relative to his/her previous and current sexual status in a complete assessment. A clinician should recognize that most couples experience difficulty discussing sexual preferences, concerns, and fears even under ideal circumstances and sexual communication problems tend to worsen with illness and threat of death.

Although little research in colorectal cancer examines the role of the partner, Northouse, Mood, Templin, Mellon and George *(88)*, recently conducted a longitudinal study to examine couple's patterns of adjustment to colon cancer during the first year following surgery. Both patients and spouses reported decreases in family functioning and social support, but also decreases in emotional stress over time. This study included no measure of sexual functioning.

6.1.2.2. Psychological Status. The affective spectrum during cancer treatment ranges from disbelief to clinical depression and typically changes over time. Anxiety and depression are the two most common affective (disruptions) among patients with cancer and both have been found to have deleterious effects on sexual functioning *(12,13,63,89,90)*. A clinician should be aware of current mental status and any history of depression or other psychiatric disorder, previous psychotherapy, treatment with psychotropic medication, and/or hospitalizations. Current use of psychotropic medications should also be reviewed with respect to impact on sexual function.

Cancer treatment produces changes to the body that negatively impacts body image and self-esteem *(63,91)*. Commonly patients have difficulty seeing themselves as sexually attractive during and after treatment. Identifying body-image disturbances is important to incorporate into goals of care and rehabilitation.

Frequently the couple experiences changes of social roles during treatment. An individual's identity and sense of worth may be threatened when role changes occur *(15,87)*. The partner's participation in the patient's physical care often negatively impacts feelings of sexuality. Younger couples, more than older couples, may be vulnerable to problems playing alternative or new domestic roles and experiencing the myriad of life and financial stressors associated with treatment *(15)*.

Table 4
Pharmacologic Agents that Affect Sexual Response

Cardiovascular Drugs
    Antihypertensive agents
    Antichollesterolemic agents
    Antiarrhythmic drugs
Psychotropic drugs
    Antidepressants (SSRIs)
    Anxiolytics/Sedatives-Hypnotics
    Neuroleptics (management of delerium)
    Stimulants/anorectics
Other medications
    Anticonvulsants
    Antiulcer drugs
    Anticancer drugs
    Narcotics
    Endocrine drugs, including hormones

6.1.3. MEDICAL ASPECTS OF SEXUALITY

The clinician should ascertain past medical history with a particular emphasis on other concurrent medical illnesses contributes to risk of sexual dysfunction, additional decrease in social and role functioning, mental health, and health perceptions. Medical illnesses that impact the endocrine, vascular, central nervous, and neurological systems are all well known to have a potential deleterious effects on the sexual response cycle *(92–94)*. Diabetes, hypertension, vascular disease, multiple sclerosis, and many others impact sexual function, particularly quality of erections in men. Two textbooks extensively review the impact of chronic illness and disability on sexual function *(92,94)*. Lifestyle factors, including smoking and substantial alcohol consumption are also risk factors of sexual morbidity. In men, cigarette smoking may induce vasoconstriction and penile venous leakage *(93)*; in larger amounts alcohol is a strong sedative-hypnotic producing decreasing libido, and transient erectile dysfunction *(93)*.

Pharmacology during treatment for cancer and chronic illness in general is an often necessary and integral component of health maintenance. However, some pharmacologic treatments may have direct or indirect deleterious effects on sexual function through multiple physiologic and psychologic pathways. Pharmacologic agents that may negatively affect sexual response are presented in Table 4. A number of resources provide further delineation of the mechanisms for changes in sexual function associated with these agents with listings of specific medications and known effects on sexual function *(15,95–97)*.

6.2. Time Constraints/Brief Screening

Recognizing that time constraints may limit the ability of any one provider in an oncology practice to adequately assess quality of sexual functioning, a few brief screening questions can easily be added to a more general follow-up and to identify those patients who will need further assessment *(14)*. Even one question—"Have you experienced any change in your sexual functioning since your diagnosis and treatment?"—can identify sexual concerns. Ideally, one sexual counseling specialist in an oncology practice (i.e., nurse, social worker, psychologist) can follow up on identified concerns. Dunn *(98)* and Schover *(99)* provide recommendations and strategies for establishing programs to treat sexual problems in medical settings. If no sexual counseling specialist is available, a referral network can be identified. Most individuals with sexual problems or concerns do not need extensive medical or psychological treatment. A review of 384 consultations for sexual rehabilitation in a cancer center indicated that 73% of patients were only seen once or twice *(100)*. The majority of patients can benefit from brief counseling and education.

7. TEACHING PATIENTS TO COPE: WAYS TO TREAT DIFFICULTIES IN SEXUALITY AND INTIMACY

Many patients are fearful or anxious of their first sexual experience after treatment and can often begin a pattern of sexual avoidance. As the patient is concerned about sending mixed signals to their partner, this can lead to avoidance of general intimacy and touch. The partner may also be contributing to generalized avoidance of intimacy through their reluctance to initiate any behavior that might be perceived as pressure to be more intimate or that may contribute to any potential physical discomfort from greater expression of physical intimacy. Providers need to reassure patients and their significant others that even when intercourse is difficult or impossible, their sex lives are not over. They can always give and receive pleasure and satisfaction because love and intimacy can be expressed by use of the hands, mouth, tongues, and lips. Providers should encourage the couple to express affection in alternative ways (hugging, kissing, nongenital touching) until they feel ready to resume sexual activity. The couple should be encouraged to communicate honest feelings and concerns and preferences.

If a man cannot possibly attain an erection firm enough for penetration and/or intercourse may be painful for a woman, some couples may be willing to find alternative ways to bring each other to orgasm and express sexual intimacy. "Sensate Focus" exercises of noncoital pleasuring were developed by Masters and Johnson *(10)*, and later enhanced by Kaplan *(11)*. These exercises, based on principles of sensuous massage, give couples an experience of sexual expression that allow them to be physically close and intimate without the pressure and anxiety that can be associated with anticipation of intercourse. The structure and ground rules of sensate focus can help bypass performance anxiety (self-consciousness and self-evaluation) and enable the couple to lose themselves in the current experience of pleasurable touch. These exercises also help the couple communicate about potentially problematic or emotionally sensitive areas of the body. Providers should determine a couple's openness to modification of their sexual technique.

As many patients will experience anticipatory anxiety about reestablishing sexual intimacy with their partner and potential uncertainty of their own sexual response, the potential advantages of self-stimulation can be explored. Self-stimulation has the advantage that it allows the individual to become comfortable with his/her sexual response and arousal without the added pressure of performance anxiety commonly heightened by concern for their partner's pleasure, reactions, concerns, and/or fears. For many individuals, a cognitive reframing of masturbation to self-stimulation or self-pleasuring allows the individual to accept this activity as part of the process in sexual rehabilitation. For others, this behavior may still be a resilient and persistent taboo for cultural and religious reasons.

For those couples who wish to have sexual intercourse, sexual positions that place no weight on a scar or ostomy and positions that allow for better control of depth of penetration can be explored. The side-by-side position (spooning) in which the man is behind the woman, or the L-shape position, with both partners lying down, torsos at right angles and legs entwined, are two possibilities. The American Cancer Society publishes two comprehensive pamphlets on sexuality and cancer, for both men *(101)* and women *(102)*, which provide illustration of sexual positions and other self-help information.

For patients with colostomies, or ileostomies, the United Ostomy Association prints several pamphlets related to resuming sexual activity, including sex and the female ostomate, sex and the male ostomate, and gay and lesbian ostomates. Providers can educate patients on limiting food intake prior to anticipated sexual activity, watching the types of food consumed, and planning times for intimacy when a bowel movement is less likely. Although the ostomy pouch is typically changed when about one-third full, patients should be taught to empty the pouch sooner when anticipating sexual intimacy, traveling, and exercising. Patients may fear that the ostomy bag will interfere with sexual intimacy, become dislodged, or cause damage to the stoma. An empty and flat ostomy bag will not become dislodged from the stoma and can be rolled up or taped down so that it will not get in the way of sexual intimacy. Decorative covers may also be worn *(71,103)*. A much greater selection of products for ostomates exists today, including disposable pouches, reusable pouches that empty from the bottom or top while still attached, pouches with filters to control odors, and pouches that hang sideways instead of down for physical activity. Patients concerned about potential odor can use deodorant tablets or liquids in the bottom of the pouch or as recommended by the manufacturer *(103)*.

A provider should help educate couples with practical suggestions to help overcome changes in responsiveness to sexual stimulation. Couples should allow plenty of time for sexual expression with sufficient foreplay to develop the fullest possible sexual arousal. For some couples, early morning may be a good restful time for sexual expression. Conditions that facilitate sexual pleasure should be explored and may include relaxation, dreams, fantasy, breathing, and recalling positive experiences with partner.

When women experience changes in arousal, most notably vaginal dryness, vaginal moisturizers and water-based lubricants should be suggested. If changes in arousal are also associated with the endocrine changes of menopause, the option and evaluation of hormone replacement should be discussed. Some women may experience discomfort with penetration around the vaginal entrance and can learn to relax the pubococcygeus (PC) muscles with Kegel exercises *(12,15,63)*. For women who have received radiation to the pelvis, instructions for use of a vaginal dilator and lubrication should be given; with regular use, considerable improvement in vaginal circumference and length can be obtained *(12)*. More specific information for the evaluation and treatment of female sexual dysfunction, including painful intercourse (dyspareunia), vaginismus, inhibited orgasm, sexual arousal and desire disorders is available in other resources *(12,15,17,82,91)*.

When erectile functioning is impaired, counseling should initially focus on obtaining sexual pleasure and satisfaction without erections or intercourse. Because the nerves damaged in surgery may potentially regenerate for up to 2.5 yr after the operation, postsurgical erectile dysfunction may improve over time *(103)*. Many men with erectile dysfunction are able to have orgasms with manual or oral stimulation; many partners are similarly satisfied and orgasmic with noncoital stimulation. Several treatment options are available depending on the cause and degree of dysfunction. If the desire for intercourse remains, treatment options include oral medication, topical or intraurethral medication, vacuum constriction device, intracavernous injection, and penile prosthesis. These treatment options should be discussed with professional consultation. Providers should educate patients that no medical intervention to restore erections is also a valid choice. Comprehensive reviews of the current management of erectile dysfunction are available *(15,82,93,104–106)*. Ducharme and Gill *(105)*, Kaplan *(82)*, and Zilbergeld *(107)*, provide further discussion on the management of inhibited sexual desire and other male sexual dysfunctions.

The goal of this chapter has been to highlight the sexuality and fertility issues that a person with colorectal cancer may experience. The oncology professional should educate patients of the sexual morbidity risks as therapeutic decisions are being made and should screen all patients at follow-up sessions to determine if changes in their sexual response have occurred. Routine screening will enable a clinician to determine whether further evaluation and intervention is necessary before long-term consequences, including relationship dysfunction, develop. More clinical attention and research is needed on the sexual functioning of both men and women treated for colorectal cancer.

REFERENCES

1. Vincent CE, Vincent B, Greiss FC, and Linton EB. Some marital-sexual concomitants of carcinoma of the cervix. *South. Med. J.*, **68** (1975) 552–558.
2. Singer PA, Tasch ES, Stocking C, et al. Sex or survival: trade-offs between quality and quantity of life. *J. Clin. Oncol.*, **9(2)** (1991) 328–334.
3. American Cancer Society. Cancer facts and figures—2000. American Cancer Society, Atlanta, 2000.
4. Van de Wiel HBM, Weijmar Shultz WCM, Hengeveld MW, and Staneke A. Sexual functioning after ostomy surgery. *J. Sex. Marital Ther.*, **6** (1991) 195–207.
5. Chorost MI, Weber TK, Lee J, Rodriguez-Bigas MA, and Petrelli NJ. Sexual dysfunction: informed consent and multimodal therapy for rectal cancer. *Am. J. Surg.*, **179** (2000) 271–274.
6. Borwell B. The psychosexual needs of stoma patients. *Profess. Nurse*, **12** (1997) 250–255.
7. Penson RT, Gallagher J, Gioiella ME, Wallace M, Borden K, Duska, LA, et al. Sexuality and cancer: conversation comfort zone. *Oncology*, **5(4)** (2000) 336–344.
8. Lauman EO, Gagnon JH, Michael RT, and Michaels S. *The Social Organization of Sexuality: Sexual Practices in the United States.* University of Chicago Press, Chicago, 1994.
9. Lauman EO, Paik A, and Rosen RC. Sexual dysfunction in the united states: prevalence and predictors. *JAMA*, **281(6)** (1999) 537–544.
10. Masters WH and Johnson VE. *Human Sexual Response.* Little, Brown, Boston, 1966.
11. Kaplan HS. *The New Sex Therapy: Active Treatment of Sexual Dysfunctions.* Random House, New York, 1974.
12. Auchincloss SS. Sexual dysfunction in cancer patients: issues in evaluation and treatment. In *Handbook of Psychooncology: Psychological Care of the Patient with Cancer.* Holland JC and Rowland JH (eds.), Oxford University Press, New York, 1989, pp. 383–413.
13. Auchincloss S. Sexual dysfunction after cancer treatment. *J. Psychosoc. Onc.*, **9(1)** (1991) 23–42.
14. Lamb MA and Woods NF. Sexuality and the cancer patient. *Can. Nurs.*, **4** (1981) 137–144.
15. Schover LR. *Sexuality and Fertility After Cancer.* Wiley, New York, 1997.
16. Beckham JC and Godding PR. Sexual dysfunction in cancer patients. *J. Psychosoc. Onc.*, **8(1)** (1990) 1–16.
17. Kaplan HS. *The Sexual Desire Disorders.* Simon & Schuster, New York, 1995.
18. Laan E, Everaerd W, van Bellen G, and Hanewald G. Women's sexual and emotional responses to male and female produced erotica. *Behav. Res. Ther.*, **23** (1994) 153–170.
19. Havenga K, Maas, CP, DeRutter, MC, Welvaart K, and Trimbos JB. Avoiding long-term disturbance to bladder and sexual function in pelvic surgery, particularly with rectal cancer. *Semin. Surg. Oncol.*, **18** (2000) 235–243.
20. Weijmar Schultz WCM, Van de Wiel, HBM, Hahn, DEE, and Van Driel MF. Sexuality and cancer in women. *Ann. Rev. Sex. Res.*, **3** (1992) 151–200.
21. Camilleri-Brennan J and Steele RJC. Quality of life after rectal cancer. *Br. J. Surg.*, **85** (1998) 1036–1043.
22. Ruo L and Guillem JG. Major 20th-century advancements in the management of colorectal cancer. *Dis. Colon Rectum*, **42** (1999) 563–578.
23. Cohen AM, Minsky BD, and Schilsky RL. *Colon Cancer.* In *Cancer: Principles & Practice of Oncology*, 5th ed., DeVita VT Jr, Hellman S, and Rosenberg SA (eds.), Lippincott, Philadelphia, 1997, pp. 929–967.
24. Balslev I and Harling H. Sexual dysfunction following operation for carcinoma of the rectum. *Dis. Colon Rectum*, **26** (1983) 785–788.
25. Fegiz G, Trenti A, Bezzi M, Ambrogi V, Papini Papi M, Tucci G, et al. Sexual and bladder dysfunctions following surgery for rectal carcinoma. *Ital. J. Surg. Sci.*, **16** (1986) 103–109.
26. Nesbakken A, Nygaard K, Bull-Njaa T, Carlsen E, and Eri LM. Bladder and sexual dysfunction after mesorectal excision for rectal cancer. *Br. J. Surg.*, **87(2)** (2000) 206–210.

27. Havenga K, Enker WE, McDermott K, Cohen AM, Minsky BD, and Guillem J. Male and female sexual and urinary function after total mesorectal excision with autonomic nerve preservation for carcinoma of the rectum. *J. Am. Coll. Surg.*, **182** (1995) 495–502.

28. Havenga K, Enker WE, McDermott K, et al. Male and female sexual and urinary function after total mesorectal excision with autonomic nerve preservation for carcinoma of the rectum. *J. Am. Coll. Surg.*, **182** (1996) 495–502.

29. Hellstrom P. Urinary and sexual dysfunction after rectosigmoid surgery. *Ann. Chir. Gynaecol.*, **77** (1988) 51–56.

30. Hidenobu M, Hideyuki I, Shigeki Y, Shigeo O, and Hiroshi S. Male sexual function after autonomic nerve-preserving operation for rectal cancer. *Dis. Colon Rectum*, **39(10)** (1996) 1140–1145.

31. Hjortrup A, Kirkegaard P, Friis J, Sanders S, and Anderson F. Sexual dysfunction after low anterior resection for midrectal cancer. *Acta Chir. Scand.*, **150** (1984) 687–688.

32. Hojo K, Sawada T, and Moriya Y. An analysis of survival and voiding, sexual function after wide iliopelvic lymphadenectomy in patients with carcinoma of the rectum, compared with conventional lymphadenectomy in patients with carcinoma of the rectum. *Dis. Colon Rectum*, **32** (1989) 128–133.

33. Kinn AC and Ohman U. Bladder and sexual function after surgery for rectal cancer. *Dis. Colon Rectum*, **29** (1986) 43–48.

34. LaMonica G, Audisio RA, Tamburini M, Filberti A, and Ventafridda V. Incidence of sexual dysfunction in male patients with treated surgically for rectal malignancy. *Dis. Colon Rectum*, **23** (1985) 937–940.

35. Leveckis J, Boucher NR, Parys BT, Reed MWR, Shorthouse AJ, and Anderson JB. Bladder and erectile dysfunction before and after rectal surgery for cancer. *Brit. J. Urol.*, **76** (1995) 752–756.

36. Santangelo ML, Romano G, and Sassaroli C. Sexual function after resection for rectal cancer. *Am. J. Surg.*, **154** (1987) 502–504.

37. Sugihara K, Moriya Y, Akasu T, and Fujita S. Pelvic autonomic nerve preservation for patients with rectal carcinoma: oncologic and functional outcome. *Cancer*, **78** (1996) 1871–1880.

38. Williams JT and Slack WW. A prospective study of sexual function after major colorectal surgery. *Br. J. Surg.*, **67** (1980) 772–774.

39. Zenico T, Neri W, Zoli M, Tamburini C, Fabri F, and Maltoni G. Sexual dysfunction after excision of the rectum. *Acta Urol. Belg.*, **57** (1989) 213–216.

40. Renner K, Rosen HR, Novi G, Holbling N, and Schiessel R. Quality of life after surgery for rectal cancer: do we still need a permanent colostomy? *Dis. Colon Rectum*, **42** (1999) 1160–1167.

41. Yeager E and Van Heerden JA. Sexual dysfunction following protocolectomy and abdominoperineal resection. *Ann. Surg.*, **191** (1980) 169–170.

42. Leo E, Belli F, Baldini MT, Vitellaro M, Santoro N, Mascheroni L, et al. Total rectal resection: colo-endoanal anastomosis and colic reservoir for cancer of the lower third of the rectum. *Eur. J. Surg. Oncol.*, **19** (1993) 283–293.

43. Aghaji MA and Obiekwe OM. Sexual function in males following abdomino-perineal resection in Nigeria. *Cent. Afr. J. Med.*, **37** (1991) 301–303.

44. Havenga K and Welvaart K. Sexual dysfunction in men following surgical treatment for rectosigmoid carcinoma. *Ned. Tijdschr. Geneeskd.*, **135** (1991) 710–713.

45. Cunsolo A, Bragaglia RB, Manara G, Poggioli G, and Gozzetti G. Urogenital dysfunction after abdomino-perineal resection for carcinoma of the rectum. *Dis. Colon Rectum*, **33** (1990) 918–922.

46. Cirino E, Pepe G, Pepe F, Panella M, Rizza G, and Cali V. Sexual complications after abdominoperineal resection. *Ital. J. Surg. Sci.*, **17** (1987) 315–318.

47. Neal DE. The effects on pelvic visceral function of anal sphincter ablating and anal sphincter preserving operations for cancer of the lower part of the rectum and or benign colo-rectal disease. *Ann. R. Coll. Surg. Engl.*, **66** (1984) 7–13.

48. Williams NS and Johnston D. The quality of life after rectal excision for low rectal cancer. *Br. J. Surg.*, **70** (1983) 460–462.

49. Von Segesser L and Marti MC. Abdomino-perineal amputation: socio-ocupational reintegration and late postoperative complications. *Schweiz. Med. Wochenschr.*, **113** (1983) 542–544 (in French).

50. Deixonne B, Baumel H, and Domergue J. Sexual disorders following abdominoperineal resection of the rectum. *Sem. Hop.*, **59** (1983) 677–682 (in French).

51. Saito N, Sarashina H, Nunomura M, Koda K, Takiguchi N, and Nakajima, N. Clinical evaluation of nerve sparing surgery combined with preoperative radiotherapy in advanced rectal cancer patients. *Am. J. Surg.*, **175** (1998) 277–282.

52. Masui H, Ike H, Yamaguchi S, Oki S, and Shimada H. Male sexual function after autonomic nerve-preserving operation for rectal cancer. *Dis. Colon Rectum*, **39** (1996) 1140–1145.

53. Moriya Y, Sugihara K, Akasu T, and Fujita S. Nerve-sparing surgery with lateral node dissection for advanced lower rectal cancer. *Eur. J. Cancer*, **31A** (1995) 1229–1232.

54. Pietrangeli A, Bove L, Innocenti P, Pace A, Tirelli C, Santoro E, et al. Neurophysiological evaluation of sexual dysfunction in patients operated for colorectal cancer. *Clin. Autonom. Res.*, **8** (1998) 353–357.

55. Leo E, Belli F, Baldini MT, et al. New perspectives in the treatment of low rectal cancer: total rectal resection and coloanal anastomosis. *Dis. Colon Rectum*, **37(Suppl.)** (1994) S62–S68.

56. Hurny C and Holland JC. Psychosocial sequelae of ostomies in cancer patients. *CA*, **36** (1985) 170–183.

57. Huish M, Kumar D, and Stones C. Stoma surgery and sexual problems in ostomates. *Sex. Mar. Ther.*, **13** (1998) 311–328.

58. Sprangers MAG, Taal BG, Aaronson NK, and te Velde A. Quality of life in colorectal cancer: stoma vs. nonstoma patients. *Dis. Colon Rectum*, **38** (1995) 361–369.

59. Bekkers MJTM, Van Knippenberg FCE, Van Dulmen AM, Van Den Borne HW, and Van Berge Henegouwen GP. Survival and psychosocial adjustment to stoma surgery and nonstoma bowel resection: a 4 year follow up. *J. Psychosom. Res.*, **42** (1997) 235–244.

60. Nugent K, Daniels P, Stewart SRN, Patankar R, and Johnson C: Quality of life in stoma patients. *Dis. Colon Rectum*, **42** (1999) 1569–1574.

61. Gamagami R, Chiotasso P, and Lazorthes F. Continent perineal colostomy after abdominoperineal resection: outcomes after 63 cases. *Dis. Colon Rectum*, **42** (1999) 626–631.

62. Parc R, Tiret E, Frilaux, P, Moszkowski E, and Loygue J. Resection and colo-anal anastomosis with colonic reservoir for rectal carcinoma. *Br. J. Surg.*, **84** (1997) 1449–1451.

63. Lamb MA. Sexuality and sexual functioning. In *Cancer Nursing: A Comprehensive Textbook* (2nd ed.). McCorkle R, Grant M, Frank-Stromberg M, and Baird SB (eds.), WB Saunders, Philadelphia, 1996, pp. 1105–1127.

64. Ooi BS, Tjundra JJ, and Green MD. Morbidities of adjuvant chemotherapy and radiotherapy for resectable rectal cancer: an overview. *Dis. Colon Rectum*, **42** (1999) 403–418.

65. Roll MG. Colon cancer. In *Oncology Nursing: Assessment and Clinical Care*. Miaskowski C and Buchsel P (eds.), Mosby, St. Louis, MO, 1999, pp. 697–719.

66. Krebs LU. Sexual and reproductive dysfunction. In *Cancer Nursing: Principles and Practice*. Baird SB, McCorkle R, and Grant M (eds.), Jones & Bartlett, Boston, 1993, pp. 697–719.

67. Lamb MA. Effects of chemotherapy on fertility in long-term survivors. *Dimens. Oncol. Nurs.*, **5(4)** (1991) 13–16.

68. Yarbro CH and Perry MC. The effect of cancer therapy on gonadal function. *Semin. Oncol. Nurs.*, **1(1)** (1985) 3–8.

69. Gradishar WJ and Schilsky RL. Effects of cancer treatment on the reproductive system. *Crit. Rev. Oncol. Hematol.*, **8(2)** (1988) 153–171.

70. Donnez J and Bassil S. Indications for cryopreservation of ovarian tissue. *Hum. Reprod. Update*, **4(3)** (1998) 248–259.

71. Grunberg KJ. Sexual rehabilitation of the cancer patient undergoing ostomy surgery. *J. Enterostomal. Ther.*, **13** (1986) 148–152.

72. Linsenmeyer TA. Management of male infertility. In *Sexual Function in People with Disability and Chronic Illness*. Sipski ML and Alexander CJ (eds.), Aspen Publishers, Gaithersburg, MD, 1997, pp. 487–510.

73. Welner SL. Management of female infertility. In *Sexual Function in People with Disability and Chronic Illness*. Sipski ML and Alexander CJ (eds.), Aspen Publishers, Gaithersburg, MD, 1997, pp. 537–556.

74. Pal L, Leykin L, Schifren JL, Isaacson KB, Chang YC, Nikruil N, et al. Malignancy may adversely influence the quality of behaviour of oocytes. *Euro. Soc. Hum. Reprod. Embryol.*, **13(7)** (1998) 1837–1840.

75. Colon JM. Assisted reproductive technologies. In *Sexual Function in People with Disability and Chronic Illness*. Sipski ML and Alexander CJ (eds.), Aspen Publishers, Gaithersburg, MD, 1997, pp. 557–576.

76. Schover LR and Thomas AJ. *Overcoming Male Infertility: Understanding its Causes and Treatments*. John Wiley, New York, 2000.

77. American Society for Reproductive Medicine. *Fertility After Cancer Treatment: A Guide for Patients*. Patient Information Series. American Society for Reproductive Medicine, Birmingham, AL, 1995.

78. Granai CO, Amando PM, and Goldstein AS. The effects of cancer therapy on fertility. *Clin. Adv. Oncol. Nurs.*, **3(1)** (1991) 7–9.

79. Medich DS and Fazio VW. Hemorrhoids, anal fissure, and carcinoma of the colon, rectum, and anus during pregnancy. *Surg. Clin. North Am.*, **75** (1995) 77–88.

80. Bernstein MA, Madoff RD, and Caushaj PF. Colon and rectal cancer in pregnancy. *Dis. Colon Rectum*, **36** (1993) 172–178.

81. Paice JA, Penn RD, and Ryan WG. Altered sexual function and decreased testosterone in patients receiving intraspinal opiods. *J. Pain Sym. Mgmt.*, **9(2)** (1994) 143–148.

82. Kaplan HS. *The Evaluation of Sexual Disorders: Psychological and Medical Aspects.* Brunner/Mazel, New York, 1983.

83. Annon JS. *Behavioral Treatment of Sexual Problems, Vol 1. Brief Therapy.* Enabling Systems, Honolulu, 1974.

84. Gallo-Silver L. The sexual rehabilitation of persons with cancer. *Cancer Pract.*, **8** (2000) 10–15.

85. Sipski ML and Alexander CJ. Impact of disability or sexual illness on sexual function. In *Sexual Function in People with Disability and Chronic Illness.* Sipski ML and Alexander CJ (eds.), Aspen Publishers, Gaithersburg, MD, 1997, pp. 3–9.

86. Waldman TL and Eliasof B. Cancer. In *Sexual Function in People with Disability and Chronic Illness.* Sipski ML and Alexander CJ (eds.), Aspen Publishers, Gaithersburg, MD, 1997, pp. 337–354.

87. McNeff EA. Issues for the partner of the person with a disability. In *Sexual Function in People with Disability and Chronic Illness.* Sipski ML and Alexander CJ (eds.), Aspen Publishers, Gaithersburg, MD, 1997, pp. 595–616.

88. Northouse LL, Mood D, Templin T, Mellon S, and George T. Couple's pattern of adjustment to colon cancer. *Soc. Sci. Med.*, **50** (2000) 271–284.

89. Anderson BL. Sexual functioning morbidity among cancer survivors. *CA*, **60(Suppl.)** (1985) 2123–2128.

90. Wise TN. Sexual functioning in neoplastic disease. *Med. Aspects Hum. Sex.*, **12** (1978) 16–23.

91. Whipple B and McGreer KB. Management of female sexual dysfunction. In *Sexual Function in People with Disability and Chronic Illness.* Sipski ML and Alexander CJ (eds.), Aspen Publishers, Gaithersburg, MD, 1997, pp. 511–536.

92. Schover LR and Jensen SB. *Sexuality and Chronic Illness: A Comprehensive Approach.* Guilford, New York, 1988.

93. Lue TF. *Contemporary Diagnosis and Management of Male Erectile Dysfunction.* Handbooks in Health Care, Newton, PA, 1999.

94. Sipski ML and Alexander CJ (eds.) *Sexual Function in People with Disability and Chronic Illness.* Aspen Publishers, Gaithersburg, MD, 1997.

95. Crenshaw TL and Goldberg JP. *Sexual Pharmacology: Drugs That Affect Sexual Functioning.* WW Norton, New York, 1996.

96. Weiner DN and Rosen RC. Medications and their impact. In *Sexual Function in People with Disability and Chronic Illness.* Sipski ML and Alexander CJ (eds.), Aspen Publishers, Gaithersburg, MD, 1997, pp. 85–118.

97. The Medical Letter. *Drugs That Cause Sexual Dysfunction.* New York. 2000.

98. Dunn KL. Sexuality education and the team approach. In *Sexual Function in People with Disability and Chronic Illness.* Sipski ML and Alexander CJ (eds.), Aspen Publishers, Gaithersburg, MD, 1997, pp. 381–402.

99. Schover LR. Counseling cancer patients about changes in sexual function. *Oncology*, **13(11)** (1999) 1585–1595.

100. Schover LR, Evans, RB, and von Eschenbach AC. Sexual rehabilitation in a cancer center: diagnosis and outcome in 384 consultations. *Arch. Sex. Behav.*, **16** (1987) 445–462.

101. Schover LR. *Sexuality and Cancer: For the Man Who Has Cancer and His Partner.* American Cancer Society, New York, 1998.

102. Schover LR. *Sexuality and Cancer: For the Woman Who Has Cancer and Her Partner.* American Cancer Society, New York, 1998.

103. Snow, B. The ostomist—self-image and sexual problems. *Sex. Dis.*, **3** (1980) 156–158.

104. Costabile RA. Cancer and male sexual dysfunction. *Oncology*, **14(2)** (2000) 195–205.

105. Ducharme SH and Gill KM. Management of other male sexual dysfunctions. In *Sexual Function in People with Disability and Chronic Illness.* Sipski ML and Alexander CJ (eds.), Aspen Publishers, Gaithersburg, MD, 1997, pp. 465–486.

106. Rivas DA and Chancellor MB. Management of erectile dysfunction. In *Sexual Function in People with Disability and Chronic Illness.* Sipski ML and Alexander CJ (eds.), Aspen Publishers, Gaithersburg, MD, 1997, pp. 429–464.

107. Zilbergeld B. *The New Male Sexuality.* Bantam Books, New York, 1992.

38 Complementary and Alternative Medicine Approaches in Colorectal Cancer

Andrew J. Vickers and Barrie R. Cassileth

CONTENTS

1. INTRODUCTION

Complementary and alternative medicine (CAM) is now a highly visible feature of contemporary health care. No longer restricted to the lay sector and the medical fringe, CAM practices can be found in conventional care settings. They are widely and increasingly being subject to research and there is now good evidence that at least some techniques are potentially effective. In the United States, as in other countries of the developed world, many millions of patients spend billions of dollars each year on CAM.

In this review, we will start by discussing the terminology and sociology of CAM, describe some of the main CAM approaches, and discuss relevant research evidence. We will conclude by reviewing sources of further information.

1.2. The Terminology of CAM

Complementary and alternative medicine is a general term used to describe techniques as diverse as chiropractic medicine and yoga, iridology and meditation, colonic irrigation, and spiritual healing. As such, it resists a simple definition. Most published terminologies define CAM simply as being anything that is not part of conventional medicine *(1)*.

A more important terminological point is the difference within CAM between "complementary" and "alternative" medicine. "Alternative" therapies are typically invasive and biologically active and are promoted for use *instead* of mainstream therapy. Conversely,

From: *Colorectal Cancer: Multimodality Management*
Edited by: L. Saltz © Humana Press Inc., Totowa, NJ

"complementary" therapies are used as adjuncts to mainstream care for symptom management and to enhance quality of life.

This distinction is especially important in oncology, where alternative methods are promoted as literal alternatives to conventional care, resulting in some patients selecting unproven methods instead of mainstream treatments following diagnosis. Most of these methods involve considerable travel and expense; furthermore, many are known to incur significant risks of adverse events.

1.3. Public Use of CAM

The most widely quoted survey of CAM use in the US general population reported prevalence rates increasing from one-third in 1991 to 42% in 1997 (2). Similar rates have been reported in other recent US surveys (3,4). Relaxation, massage, and chiropractic are the most widely utilized therapies; homeopathy, acupuncture, and folk remedies were the least used. Similar figures have been reported found for other industrialized countries such as the United Kingdom (5), western Europe (6), Australia (7), and Canada (8).

Surveys have also looked specifically at CAM use by cancer patients. A recent systematic review of relevant published data (9) located 26 surveys of cancer patients from 13 countries, including 5 from the United States. The average prevalence across all studies was 31%. Subsequent investigations have reported similar findings (10–12). All but one of the US surveys obtained information about specific therapies employed. There is some indication of a growth in CAM use by cancer patients in recent years. A secondary analysis of close to 3000 cancer patients estimates a 64% increase since 1997 (13).

Although research evidence is scant, the vast majority of CAM users seek complementary, not alternative, medicine; approx 8–10% of tissue-biopsy-diagnosed cancer patients eschew mainstream therapy and seek only alternative care (14).

1.4. CAM in Mainstream Medicine

Data on oncologists' referrals of patients to CAM practitioners are not available. However, there is evidence that nononcologists commonly make such referrals. A survey conducted in Massachusetts, Washington State, New Mexico, and Israel, for example, found that more than 60% of physicians had referred patients to alternative providers in the previous year (15). Primary care physicians were more likely than other specialists to use and to refer patients for complementary and alternative therapies, a finding also reported in other studies (16,17).

Referral for and delivery of CAM by doctors is probably more common abroad than in the United States. There are, for example, over 10,000 doctors practicing homoeopathy in France and Germany and nearly 2000 doctors practicing acupuncture in the United Kingdom (18). It is likely that application of these therapies to patients with cancer is infrequent and limited to symptom control.

Elective courses in CAM and portions of required courses are taught in at least 75 medical schools in the United States (19). This degree of activity displays broad interest, although an academic physician's analysis of the quality of courses found that almost all present material uncritically (20).

1.5. Regulation of CAM

1.5.1. REGULATION OF CAM PRACTITIONERS

Regulation of CAM practitioners varies by therapy and by state. The most consistently regulated are chiropractors, who undergo a 4-yr training and are licensed in all 50 states.

Naturopaths are currently licensed in 11 states after 4 yr of post-B.A. training. Practitioners of acupuncture and herbal medicine are trained for 3 yr and licensed in 34 states; three additional jurisdictions permit practice under a medical doctor's supervision. Regulation of massage practitioners also varies from state to state. While more than 30 states demand a state licensure, asking therapists to meet particular requirements, criteria, and exams, other states ask for less formal training, such as a certificate program, and others have no regulation at all. Many of those who practice hypnosis or relaxation techniques have conventional qualifications (e.g., nursing, clinical psychology). However, many without such qualification also practice these techniques and regulation of these practitioners appears to be highly inconsistent. Music therapists are voluntarily regulated by the Certification Board for Music Therapists. The title "Board-Certified Music Therapist" is legally protected, but there is no state licensure.

1.5.2. REGULATION OF CAM PRODUCTS

No legal standards currently exist for the processing or packaging of botanicals in the United States. The content of botanicals often differs widely from one bottle to the next, even within the same brand. For example, samples of St. John's Wort were analyzed recently by an independent laboratory commissioned by the *Los Angeles Times*. Three of 10 brands tested contained less than half the potency listed on the label *(21)*.

Poor quality control standards also lead to contamination of botanical products. Typical examples of such contamination are steroids in Chinese herbs *(22)*, heart problems resulting from digitalis-contaminated supplements *(23)* and atropine in herbal tea *(24)*. Contamination appears to be a particular problem with products imported from outside the United States and Europe.

2. ALTERNATIVE (UNPROVEN) CANCER TREATMENTS

A large number of unproven, and often unusual, treatments have been recommended for the treatment of cancer. Many of these are promoted as alternatives to conventional care. For example, the chapter on cancer in the popular book *Alternative Medicine* criticizes chemotherapy, radiation, and surgery as "highly invasive" interventions that "may shorten the patient's life" and recommends that therapy instead address the entire body and employ a "non-toxic approach…incorporating treatments that rely on biopharmaceutical, immune enhancement, metabolic, nutritional, and herbal, non-toxic methods" *(25)*.

Such unusual and possibly dangerous ideas are in surprisingly wide circulation, particularly with the advent of the Internet. A sophisticated search for alternative medicine for cancer typically results in between 250,000 and 500,000 hits. Many of the retrieved pages list dubious information, even though they appear to be from reputable sources. An article on alternative medicine for cancer published on Lycos's "Web M.D.," for instance, promotes a number of unusual and disproved therapies, advises against many common uses of chemotherapy, and accuses the conventional oncology community of extreme prejudice *(26)*. A Boston University website claims that the Livingston-Wheeler regimen, a disproved alternative therapy (*see* Section 2.4.), leads to a "seventy to ninety-five percent rate of remission" in early cancer and a 20% remission rate in terminal cancer *(27)*.

Alternative medicine is a worldwide problem. A recent survey conducted by the International Union Against Cancer *(28)* reported alternative cancer treatments in all participating nations, even though these were as varied as the United States, the United Kingdom, Israel, China, Zimbabwe, Brazil, Latvia, Malaysia, and Japan. A large number of different and unusual therapies were reported, including traditional medical systems such as curanderismo, botanicals such as aloe vera, unconventional drugs such as shark cartilage, combination regimes such as DiBella, and dietary approaches such as the "Breuss" diet. Some treatments were restricted to a single clinic in just one country.

Given the enormous range of alternative cancer treatments, it is beyond the scope of any text to give a comprehensive review. Described in the following subsections is a small selection of some of the more popular alternative cancer treatments.

2.1. Burzynski

Some alternative remedies for cancer are the invention of a single individual and are offered at a single site. An example is antineoplastons, developed by Stanislaw Burzynski, M.D. Initial laboratory analyses found no evidence that antineoplastons normalize tumor cells (29) and subsequent clinical trials have either failed to accrue patients or have been uninterpretable. Nonetheless, this remains a popular alternative therapy, especially for children with brain malignancies.

2.2. Di Bella

The Di Bella regimen, consisting of melatonin, bromocriptine, retinoids, and either somatostatin or octreotide, generated intense public interest in Italy in the late 1990s. In a rare example of strategically planned and rapidly implemented research in alternative medicine, two studies were completed. Both showed no benefit for this treatment (30,31).

2.3. Laetrile

Laetrile is an interesting "alternative" cancer medicine because, like many conventional chemotherapeutics, it consists of a single compound isolated from a natural substance (in this case, apricot pits or almonds). Yet, unlike taxol, for example, it is promoted as natural. Proponents claim that laetrile is actually "vitamin B17," an apparently fictitious nutrient, proper use of which could eradicate cancer entirely (32). This is despite a phase II trial showing no benefit, and some toxicity, to laetrile (33). Although laetrile waned in popularity following that study, it was revived recently by new promoters who dismissed the study, along with the general efforts of conventional regulatory bodies, as the result of pressure exerted by vested interests trying to protect their profits in the cancer industry (32).

2.4. Livingston-Wheeler

Alternative cancer treatments appear subject to fashion and often rise and fall in popularity. A good example of a therapy that was popular in the 1980s but less so now is Livingston-Wheeler. On the basis of an hypothesis tested and discarded in the 1930s, Virginia C. Livingston-Wheeler believed that cancer is caused by a bacterium, *Progenitor cryptocides*, an entity that has not been described outside of her work. The cancer treatment offered at the Livingston-Wheeler clinic in San Diego, CA consisted of efforts to strengthen the immune system by "detoxification" through diet and enemas and by the administration of special vaccines. A case-control study matched patients with advanced cancer treated at the Livingston-Wheeler clinic with those at a conventional cancer center. No difference in survival was found between the two sites, and Livingston-Wheeler patients had poorer quality of life (34).

2.5. Macrobiotics

Many diets have been suggested as cancer cures, with different diets popular in different countries. The macrobiotic diet, which is a common cancer diet in the United States has three features that make it typical of many alternative cancer diets: First, unless followed to extremes, in which case it is nutritionally deficient, macrobiotics is a relatively healthy diet, being high in fiber and low in fat; second, although following such a diet may help to prevent cancer, there is no reason to believe that is of value as a cancer treatment; third, the diet is bulky and difficult to digest and so may be inappropriate for many cancer patients.

2.6. Megadose Vitamin C

Nobel Laureate Linus Pauling claimed that massive doses of vitamin C could cure cancer, most effectively in patients who had not received chemotherapy. A randomized trial was conducted that failed to support vitamin C for cancer (35). This was criticized by Pauling who claimed that the inclusion of patients who had prior chemotherapy invalidated the results. A further trial, this time including only patients without prior chemotherapy, similarly found no survival benefit from vitamin C (36). Nonetheless, proponents still advocate vitamin C, apparently on the basis of epidemiological evidence, animal studies, and accusations of bias in the cancer research community (37).

2.7. Metabolic Therapy

Metabolic therapies are based on the belief that cancer and other illnesses result from an accumulation of toxins in the colon, which leads to liver failure and death. Treatment aims to counteract liver damage with a practitioner-specific low-salt, high-potassium diet, high doses of vitamins, minerals and enzymes, 1 gal of fruit and vegetable juice daily, and "detoxification" using high colonic irrigation with herbs, coffee, or enzymes. Research purportedly showing a survival benefit of "Gerson" metabolic therapy was grossly flawed by nonrandomized comparisons and subgroup analysis (38). A more recent case-series of 11 patients who received another variation of metabolic therapy reported encouraging findings (39) and serves as the basis for an ongoing controlled trial.

2.8. Shark Cartilage

The clinical basis for the use of shark cartilage in cancer appears to be the erroneous belief that, in the words of a popular book, "sharks don't get cancer." Advocates base their therapy on its putative antiangiogenic properties, but a recent phase I–II trial of shark cartilage found no clinical benefit (40). A study sponsored by the National Center for Complementary and Alternative Medicine is currently underway.

2.9. 714-X

A liquid medicine made from camphor, 714-X, contains nitrogen, ammonium salts, sodium chloride, and ethanol. It is generally given by injection. The treatment is based on an unusual set of theories about the biology of cancer, such as the importance of "somatids," particles essential to life that can be seen only with a special microscope, and a substance called "cocancerogenic K factor," which is said to protect cancer cells from immune attack. There does not appear to be any systematic human research on 714-X.

3. COMPLEMENTARY THERAPIES FOR SYMPTOM CONTROL AND ENHANCED QUALITY OF LIFE

A number of complementary therapies are recommended for adjunctive use to treat the side effects of cancer and cancer treatments.

3.1. Pain

3.1.1. MIND–BODY MEDICINE

A wide variety of complementary therapies claim to relieve stress and enhance quality of life by producing relaxation. One popular relaxation technique, known as progressive muscle relaxation, involves sequential tensing and relaxing of muscles. Another is hypnosis, the induction of a deeply relaxed state, with increased suggestibility and suspension of critical faculties. Once in this state, sometimes called a hypnotic trance, patients are given therapeutic suggestions to encourage changes in behavior or symptom relief. Visualization and imagery techniques involve the induction of a relaxed state followed by use of a visual image, such as a pastoral scene, that enhances the sense of relaxation. Several randomized trials have shown effects of hypnosis on pain related to malignancy and to treatment procedures such as bone marrow aspiration. Both a recent systematic review *(41)* and an NIH technology assessment panel *(42)* have supported the use of hypnosis for cancer-related pain. There is also randomized trial evidence that relaxation and imagery reduce pain in cancer patients *(43)*.

3.1.2. ACUPUNCTURE

Although details of practice may differ between individual schools, all traditional Chinese medical theory is based in the Taoist concept of *yin* and *yang* and the flow of *Qi* (energy) along hypothesized channels in the body. Many health professionals who practice acupuncture dispense with such traditional concepts. Instead, they view acupuncture points as corresponding to physiological and anatomical features such as peripheral nerve junctions, and diagnoses are developed in purely conventional terms. Many randomized trials have examined, and largely supported, the use of acupuncture for both acute pain such as dental surgery *(44)* and chronic pain, such as migraine *(45)*. As yet, there is no controlled study in the Western literature for cancer-related pain, and the value of acupuncture in reducing cancer pain remains to be documented.

3.1.3. MUSIC THERAPY

Music therapy is the controlled use of music to effect clinical benefit. Although it is ideally provided live by trained therapists, music therapy often takes the form of recorded music, particularly in the research setting. There is randomized evidence that music therapy is of benefit for acute pain, such as postoperative pain *(46)*. However, there are insufficient data specifically for cancer-related pain. A small trial of 15 patients reported that improvements in cancer pain scores during music were twice those found with nonmusic sound *(47)*.

3.1.4. MASSAGE

Therapeutic massage involves manipulation of the soft tissue of whole or partial body areas to induce general improvements in health, such as relaxation or improved sleep, or specific physical benefits, such as relief of muscular aches and pains. Despite many anecdotal reports that massage reduces pain, current research evidence is limited. One small randomized trial has been published that showed some benefits for pain in cancer patients *(48)*, but the trial was underpowered for meaningful analysis.

3.2. Anxiety and Depression

3.2.1. MIND–BODY MEDICINE

A number of randomized trials have examined the effects of relaxation therapy on anxiety, depression, or mood in cancer patients. Bindemann et al., for example, randomized newly diagnosed patients to relaxation training or control *(49)*. Anxiety and psychiatric morbidity increased significantly more in controls than in treated patients. There was also a positive effect on depression scores in women *(49)*. In studies using similar designs in breast cancer, relaxation training has been shown to lead to better mood *(50)* and general quality of life *(51)*. Relaxation training and hypnosis have been shown to have an effect on anxiety during treatment procedures, such as chemotherapy or bone marrow aspiration, in most *(52–54)* but not all *(55)* randomized trials.

3.2.2. Massage

A number of randomized trials suggest that massage reduces anxiety, in the short term at least, in groups as varied as adolescent psychiatric patients *(56)*, intensive care unit patients *(57)*, elderly people in care homes *(58)*, and children suffering posttraumatic stress disorder *(59)*. A high-quality trial of massage for patients undergoing autologous bone marrow transplantation found clinically and statistically significant improvements in anxiety compared to controls. There were also improvements in nausea, fatigue and general well-being *(60)*.

3.2.3. Music Therapy

In a study of the effects of music therapy on the mood of hospitalized cancer patients, 50 patients were randomly assigned to receive either a live-music therapy session or a tape-recorded music. Patients receiving live music reported significantly reduced anxiety scores *(61)*.

3.3. Nausea and Vomiting

3.3.1. Mind–Body Medicine

Hypnosis has been found effective for the treatment of anticipatory nausea in children *(62)*. Trials have also generally found hypnosis and relaxation training to be beneficial against chemotherapy-induced nausea in adults *(63,64)*, although some studies find no differences between groups *(65)*. One of the more effective methods seems to be "systematic desensitization." Patients describe situations that cause anticipatory nausea and place these in a hierarchy (e.g., driving to the hospital is placed lower than sitting in the treatment room). Patients are then placed in a relaxed state and asked to imagine the nausea-inducing situations, which are presented in ascending order of intensity, while remaining relaxed *(64)*. Hypnosis and relaxation techniques do not seem to be effective for reducing nausea associated with bone marrow transplantation *(66)*.

3.3.2. Acupuncture

There is some good evidence that acupuncture can reduce nausea and vomiting in certain circumstances. A systematic review of acupuncture point stimulation for nausea and vomiting related to chemotherapy, pregnancy, or anaesthetics reported that 11 of 12 placebo-controlled, randomized, double-blind studies favored acupuncture *(67)*. A more recent meta-analysis combined data from 19 randomized trials of postoperative nausea and vomiting in 1679 patients *(68)*. For adults, statistically significant effects were found for both nausea and vomiting within 6 h of surgery. Acupuncture was also superior for vomiting within 48 h of surgery, but wide confidence intervals failed to exclude no difference between groups. Acupuncture did not seem to be effective for postoperative nausea and vomiting in children. Despite these promising results, the role of acupuncture antiemesis in cancer is not fully understood. Trials of chemotherapy-related nausea tend to be of lower methodological quality *(67)*, and the best method of providing acupuncture antiemesis for chemotherapy sickness remains to be established.

3.3.3. MUSIC THERAPY

Music has been investigated for the treatment of nausea and vomiting in bone marrow transplant patients, who receive particularly high doses and emetogenic regimens. Patients randomized to pharmacological antiemetics plus music distraction reported significantly less nausea and vomiting than those receiving antiemetics alone *(69)*.

3.4. Other Symptoms

3.4.1. DYSPNEA

In an uncontrolled study *(70)*, 14 of a series of 20 patients treated for cancer-related breathlessness with acupuncture reported marked symptomatic improvement. Subjective feelings of breathlessness reduced by about a third within 5 min of needle insertion. These results suggest that further hypothesis-testing research would be of value.

3.4.2. PERIOPERATIVE SYMPTOMS

3.4.2.1. Acupuncture. Acupuncture is the CAM modality perhaps most strongly associated with surgery, particularly after the publication of photographs showing operations in China being conducted apparently under acupuncture anesthesia. Acupuncture is not used as a stand-alone anesthetic technique in the West and its main role in surgery appears to be the treatment of postoperative pain and vomiting. There is good evidence from randomized controlled trials that acupuncture can be effective for both of these conditions.

The data for vomiting are described earlier. In the case of postoperative pain, most trials have taken place in dental surgery, in particular, third molar extraction. This is a good research model because of limited comorbidity, standardized treatment, and large patient population. A systematic review of 16 randomized trials concluded that acupuncture was better than placebo for postoperative pain *(71)*. Studies of acupuncture for pain following pelvic surgery have come to similar conclusions. Randomized trials of electrical stimulation of acupuncture points have reported significantly reduced use of analgesics, and associated side effects such as dizziness in women undergoing pelvic surgery *(72,73)*. A trial of electroacupuncture for postoperative pain in cancer patients undergoing pelvic or abdominal surgery had comparable findings *(74)*. However, one trial of acupuncture following hysterectomy found no significant difference between groups *(75)*.

3.4.2.2. Music Therapy. One of the first recorded uses of music in the clinical setting was that of the surgeon Evan O'Neill Kane, who, in 1914, used a phonograph in the operating room for calming patients prior to the application of anesthesia. Recent clinical research has broadly supported the use of music for surgery. Typical findings have been that music can reduce medication requirements during spinal anesthesia for urological procedures *(76)* or that music, particularly when combined with a relaxation procedure, reduces postoperative pain *(77)*. A trial in which guided imagery was combined with music found reduced pain, anxiety, opioid use, and time to first bowel movement in the treatment group compared to controls *(78)*.

3.4.2.3. Hypnosis and Relaxation Techniques. A number of techniques have been used to reduce preoperative and postoperative anxiety and pain by attempting to promote relaxation. In a typical study, patients scheduled for day-case gynecological operations were randomized to a short hypnotic induction or an educational intervention. Patients undergoing hypnosis had lower anxiety scores and required less medication for induction of anesthesia *(79)*. Similarly, a trial of a brief, nonhypnotic relaxation procedure reported lower anxiety, more rapid induction of anesthesia and less anesthetic required to maintain anesthesia *(80)*.

3.4.2.4. Massage. There is preliminary evidence that massage is of benefit in the postoperative period. In one study *(81)*, 30 gynecologic oncology patients were randomly assigned to receive either standard postsurgical care alone or standard care plus a daily 45-min therapeutic massage. Anxiety, depression, pain ratings, and patient-controlled analgesia use were lower, although not significantly so, during hospital stays in the massage group. Additionally, no additional medical services were used by the massage treatment group during the 4-wk follow-up period, whereas 5 out of 15 standard care patients utilized additional physician visits ($p = 0.02$). A replication of this trial, of sufficient size to permit adequately powered analyses, is warranted.

4. BOTANICALS

Many chemotherapeutic agents in contemporary clinical use were derived from natural products, predominantly from plants. One authority estimates that approximately two-thirds of anticancer drugs approved worldwide up to 1994 were derived from natural, and predominantly plant, sources *(82)*. Well-known examples include vincristine and vinblastine (from the Madagascan periwinkle) and paclitaxel (from the Pacific yew tree).

The standard method of developing anticancer agents from botanicals has been to isolate single active compounds that can be chemically synthesized. However, there are several reasons why whole botanical extracts may be of benefit in cancer treatment. First, different components in a single complex mixture may have complementary activities. For instance, some components of sho-saiko-to, a traditional medicine consisting of several different botanicals, show antiproliferative effects on cancer cells *(83)*, whereas a different set of components display moderate cytotoxic properties *(84)*. Moreover, there is evidence that the remedy as a whole improves immune function *(85)*. Any single compound isolated from sho-saiko-to may not retain the cytostatic, cytotoxic, and immune stimulant properties of the whole. It is also possible that separate components of botanical medicines act synergistically. The major component of huanglian, an extract from *Coptis chinensis*, is berberine. Although berberine shows antiproliferative effects on cancer cells, this effect is not as strong as whole huanglian, suggesting that different components of huanglian contribute to an anticancer effect *(86)*.

Botanicals are attractive to cancer patients because they generally have low toxicity, particularly when compared with plant-derived chemotherapy agents. Described in the following subsections is a selection of botanical cancer treatments, chosen either because they appear in wide use among patients or because there is important scientific data concerning their value.

4.1. Popular Botanicals

4.1.1. ESSIAC

Essiac was developed initially by a native Canadian healer and popularized by a nurse, Rene Caisse. This product consists of four botanicals: burdock, Turkey rhubarb, sorrel, and slippery elm. A review reported in the *Canadian Medical Association Journal* reported no published research on essiac *(87)*, but it remains in popular use.

4.1.2. MISTLETOE

Mistletoe extracts, which are more widely known by the trade names Iscador, Helixor, and Eurixor, are popular cancer treatments in Europe and are available in some mainstream

European cancer clinics. Unlike many herbal treatments, mistletoe extracts have been subject to randomized trials in cancer. A systematic review of these trials *(88)* reported serious methodological shortcomings in most studies. A more recent large and methodologically rigorous trial found no survival benefit in patients with head and neck cancer *(89)*.

4.1.3. NONI

A botanical currently of particular popularity among cancer patients in noni (*Morinda citrifolia*). In many ways, it is a typical unproven therapy: It is a natural product; it is said to have been used for "thousands of years" by "traditional Polynesian healers"; the discovery of its use in cancer is somewhat colorful, involving a miraculous cure of a pet dog, claims made for noni are ambiguous and implausible, such as it being a "strong blood purifier" and "cleans(ing) the body of harmful bacteria" *(90)*. Interestingly, there is at least some scientific evidence in favor of noni. Noni has been shown to increase the life-span of syngeneic mice implanted with Lewis lung carcinoma *(91)*. Moreover, a compound has been extracted from noni that shows potent tyrosine kinase inhibition *(92)*; an immunomodulatory polysaccharide has also been identified *(93)*. However, there do not appear to have been any human trials of this agent.

4.1.4. PAU D'ARCO TEA

Pau d'arco tea is said to be an old Inca Indian remedy for many illnesses, including cancer. Made from the bark of an indigenous South American evergreen tree, its active ingredient, lapachol, has been isolated. Although lapachol showed antitumor activity in animal studies *(94)*, it does not appear to affect human malignancies *(95)*. The tea can induce nausea and vomiting.

4.2. Botanicals of Promising Scientific Interest

4.2.1. KAMPO

Kampo medicines are traditional Japanese botanical formulas, each consisting of 5–12 different botanicals. Two kampo medicines of particular interest in cancer are sho-saiko-to and juzen-taiho-to. Sho-saiko-to has demonstrated marked antiproliferative effects on various cancer lines, particularly hepatoma (*see*, for example, ref. *96*) and has been shown to inhibit development and metastasis of lung carcinoma *(97)* and melanoma *(98)*. It is known to have immune stimulant properties in humans *(99,100)*. In a phase III randomized trial, 260 patients with cirrhosis were randomized to treatment with sho-saiko-to or control *(101)*. At 5 yr, sho-saiko-to led to a one-third reduction in the incidence of hepatocellular carcinoma (23% vs 34%) and a 40% reduction in deaths (24% vs 40%). Analyses of these data suggests that sho-saiko-to has multifactorial action, both reducing the incidence of hepatic cancer and acting as a hepatoprotective.

It is not known whether sho-saiko-to can prevent or treat colorectal metastases to the liver. However, juzen-taiho-to has demonstrated this effect in mouse models *(102,103)*. Juzen-taiho-to has additionally been shown to reduce the toxicity of platinum agents, apparently without compromising their antitumor effects *(104–106)*.

4.2.2. β-GLUCAN MUSHROOM EXTRACTS

Many mushrooms used in Oriental botanical medicine contain β-glucans, a class of polysaccharide molecule. The anticancer effects of these agents have been widely studied. Almost all of this research has taken place in Japan, where several mushroom extracts are licensed and used for cancer.

Mushroom-derived β-glucans appear to have strong immune stimulant effects in both animal *(107–110)* and human models *(111,112)*. There are a large number of animal studies showing anticancer activity. Typical studies have found that mushroom extracts reduce tumor weight of both breast carcinoma *(113)* and sarcoma *(114)*, prevent metastasis of prostate cancer *(115)*, reduce hepatic and colon tumors in combination with cyclophosphamide *(116)*, and prevent induced bladder *(117)* and liver *(118)* tumors. An overview of these studies given by Borchers *(119)*. There have been several reports of synergism between vaccine therapies and β-glucans. In one model, suppression of in vivo growth of a colon cancer line by a monoclonal antibody was enhanced by concurrent treatment with a mushroom extract *(120)*.

Most human phase III trials of mushroom-derived β-glucans have studied PSK, an extract of *Coriolus versicolor*, or SPG, which is extracted from the culture medium of *Schizophyllum commune* Fries. Trials typically compared chemotherapy or radiotherapy plus β-glucan or conventional treatment alone. Trials have found superior survival on PSK compared to controls in both gastrectomy *(121,122)* and esophagectomy patients *(123)*. Results have been less encouraging in breast cancer *(124,125)* and leukemia *(126)*. SPG was slightly but not significantly superior to control for gastrectomy, although in a subgroup analysis, improved survival was seen in patients with curative resection *(127,128)*. The most encouraging results for SPG are for cervical cancer, with trials demonstrating improvements in survival *(129)* and increased rates of tumor response *(130)*.

There have been two randomized trials of mushroom extracts in colorectal cancer. In the first, 120 patients with advanced colorectal cancer (Dukes' C) undergoing curative resection were randomized to PSK or placebo starting 10–15 d after surgery. The 111 evaluable patients were followed-up for up to 10 yr. There were statistically significant differences between groups for both disease-free and overall survival. Median survival in the PSK group was approx 5 yr compared to just over 4 yr in controls *(131)*. A subsequent trial randomized 462 colorectal cancer patients scheduled for curative resection to chemotherapy (mitomycin C and 5-fluorouracil [5-FU]) alone or chemotherapy plus PSK *(132)*. This trial included a wider range of patients, with approximately half being Dukes' A or B. Both disease-free and overall survival were significantly higher in the PSK group (3-yr rates 77.2% vs 67.7% and 85.8% vs 79.25, respectively). Given these promising results, it is unclear why mushroom derived β-glucans such as PSK are not more widely studied, and possibly brought to clinical use, outside of Japan.

4.2.3. HUANGLIAN

An extract of *Coptis chinensis*, known as huanglian, has been shown to inhibit topoisomerase I at levels comparable to camptothecins *(133)*. It has potent effects on growth and colony formation of gastric and colon lines, apparently by inhibiting cyclin B_1 *(86)*. A phase I trial of huanglian is currently underway at Memorial Sloan–Kettering Cancer Center.

4.2.4. GREEN TEA

Interest in green tea as an anticancer botanical originally stemmed from epidemiological studies demonstrating lower rates of various cancers, particularly colorectal cancer, in Chinese and Japanese green tea drinkers *(134)*. In a typical study, tea consumption was compared in cancer patients and matched controls in Shanghai: Odds ratios for colon and rectal cancer among those with the highest consumption were 0.6–0.8 compared to those who did not consume tea regularly *(135)*. Green tea has been shown to prevent induced colorectal tumors in animals models *(136,137)* and to have a direct, although moderate, inhibitory effect on cell growth *(138,139)*. Although green tea is being actively pursued for a possible chemopreventive role *(140)*, its activity as a cancer treatment has yet to be defined.

4.3. Botanicals for Treatment of Cancer Symptoms

Botanicals are used for a very wide range of indications and it is not surprising that at least some of these overlap with cancer or treatment-related symptoms. For example, a meta-analysis of relevant trials incidates that St John's Wort can be of benefit in the treatment of mild to moderate depression *(141)*, a condition that is not uncommon in cancer patients. In this report, it was found to be superior to placebo and of similar efficacy to tricyclic antidepressants, although with a superior adverse effect profile. Accordingly, at least one oncologist has recommended the use of St John's Wort for depressed cancer patients *(142)*.

There are two important problems with using botanicals for symptomatic treatment in cancer. The first is that the biology of a particular symptom may vary between cancer and noncancer populations. Extrapolating from traditional use to use in cancer may therefore be invalid. For instance, there is evidence from randomized trials that aloe vera is effective for psoriatic dermatitis *(143)* and, apparently on this basis, it is recommended radiation-induced dermatitis. However, a randomized trial found no effect of aloe vera for this indication in radiotherapy patients *(144)*. Similarly, although there is evidence that echinacea, a botanical with putative immunostimulant properties, may be effective in preventing respiratory infections in the general population *(145)*, a small trial in women receiving radiotherapy found no effect on infection rates *(146)*.

The second problem concerns interactions between botanicals and cancer drugs. There is evidence that St John's Wort leads to the induction of cytochrome P-450. This results in increased metabolism of drugs metabolized on the P-450 pathway. There are experimental data showing reduced concentrations of indinavir resulting from St John's Wort use *(147)*. Decreased levels of chemotherapy agents such as taxanes has not been empirically demonstrated, but remains a worrying possibility. Botanicals and chemotherapy agents may also interact directly. For example, pretreatment of colon cancer lines with berberine, the main constituent of huanglian, markedly reduces Paclitaxel-induced apoptosis and cell-cycle effects *(148)*. In short, botanicals may reduce the effectiveness of chemotherapy. This suggests that cancer patients should avoid using botanicals before and during conventional cancer treatment.

5. INTEGRATIVE MEDICINE

Some complementary therapies, such as acupuncture, traditionally have been available only outside of mainstream hospitals or cancer centers. Others, such as psychological support, humor therapy, or spiritual care, have been made available for decades as "supportive" care in oncology and other mainstream settings. In this sense, complementary medicine may be seen as an extension and an expansion of supportive care. In recent years, however, substantially greater integration of complementary and conventional medicine has occurred, often with both provided at the same site, and many additional therapies have been introduced.

At Memorial Sloan–Kettering Cancer Center, practitioners of massage, music therapy, mind–body relaxation therapies, and acupuncture work with inpatients following self-referral or referral by an oncologist or other health professional. These therapies and others are also available at outpatient sites, along with nutritional counseling and classes in yoga, tai chi, art therapy, and various exercise programs. Similar units have been established at other cancer centers in the United States and elsewhere.

The availability of complementary therapies within the walls of mainstream cancer centers affords the added benefit of integration at the academic and scientific level. Academic medical facilities provide a research infrastructure previously absent from CAM research. This has led, for example, to high-quality basic and clinical research in botanical cancer remedies for the first time. A small number of botanicals show promise as anticancer agents. It is of interest that few of these have been promoted as cancer cures by alternative practitioners. Instead, they were developed through laboratory and epidemiologic research conducted by conventionally trained scientists. These considerations suggest that CAM is best researched as well as used clinically as an integrated component of oncology care.

6. CONCLUSION

This distinction between complementary and alternative medicines is an important one. Both the helpful and the problematic components of CAM are likely to persist in cancer medicine. The literature indicates that popular alternative therapies—cures promoted for use instead of mainstream treatment—do not improve survival and, indeed, they may reduce survival or quality of life when patients fail to receive needed care in a timely fashion. Conversely, many complementary therapies, when used in conjunction with mainstream medicine, have demonstrable, important benefits, including decreased symptoms and enhanced quality of life. The challenge for the physician and for the patient is to promote and utilize the beneficial complementary therapies and to discard disproved or implausible alternatives. The challenge to the research community is to provide the data through controlled, high-quality studies, to allow us to make evidence-based decisions regarding the use of these therapies.

REFERENCES

1. Zollman C and Vickers A. ABC of complementary medicine. What is complementary medicine? *Br. Med. J.*, **319(7211)** (1999) 693–696.
2. Eisenberg DM, Davis RB, Ettner SL, Appel S, Wilkey S, Van Rompay M, et al. Trends in alternative medicine use in the United States, 1990–1997: results of a follow-up national survey. *JAMA*, **280** (1998) 1569–1575.
3. Elder NC, Gillcrist A, and Minz R. Use of alternative health care by family practice patients. *Arch. Fam. Med.*, **6(2)** (1997) 181–84.
4. The Landmark Report. November 1997. http://www.landmarkhealthcare.com
5. Vickers A. Use of complementary therapies. *Br. Med. J.*, **309** (1994) 1161.
6. Fisher P and Ward A. Complementary medicine in Europe. *Br. Med. J.*, **309** (1994) 107–111.
7. MacLennan AH, Wilson DH, and Taylor AW. Prevalence and cost of alternative medicine in Australia. *Lancet*, **347** (1996) 569–573.
8. Millar WJ. Use of alternative health care practitioners by Canadians. *Can. J. Public Health*, **88** (1997) 154–158.
9. Ernst E and Cassileth BR. The prevalence of complementary/alternative medicine in cancer: A systematic review. *Cancer*, **83** (1998) 777–782.
10. Crocetti E, Crotti N, Feltrin A, Ponton P, Geddes M, and Buiatti E. The use of complementary therapies by breast cancer patients attending conventional treatment. *Eur. J. Cancer*, **34(3)** (1998) 324–328.
11. Miller M, Boyer MJ, Butow PN, Gattellari M, Dunn SM, and Childs A. The use of unproven methods of treatment by cancer patients. Frequency, expectations and cost. *Support. Care Cancer*, **6(4)** (1998) 337–347.
12. Rees RW, Feigel I, Vickers A, Zollman C, McGurk R, and Smith C. Prevalence of complementary therapy use by women with breast cancer. A population-based survey. *Eur. J. Cancer*, **36(11)** (2000) 1359–1364.
13. Abu Realh MH, Magwood G, Narayan MC, Rupprecht C, and Suraci M. The use of complementary therapies

by cancer patients. *Nurs. Connect.*, **9(4)** (1996) 3–12.

14. Cassileth BR, Lusk EJ, Strouse TB, and Bodenheimer BJ. Contemporary unorthodox treatments in cancer medicine: a study of patients, treatments and practitioners. *Ann. Intern. Med.*, **101** (1984) 105–112.

15. Borkan J, Neher JO, Anson O, and Smoker B. Referrals for alternative therapies. *J. Fam. Pract.*, **39(6)** (1994) 545–550.

16. Perkin MR, Pearcy RM, and Fraser JS. A comparison of the attitudes shown by general practitioners, hospital doctors and Med students towards alternative medicine. *J. Roy. Soc. Med.*, **87(9)** (1994) 523–525.

17. Berman BM, Singh BK, Lao L, Singh BB, Ferentz KS, and Hartnoll SM. Physicians' attitudes toward complementary or alternative medicine: a regional survey. *J. Am. Board Fam. Pract.*, **8(5)** (1995) 361–366.

18. Zollman CE and Vickers AJ. ABC of complementary medicine: complementary medicine in conventional practice. *Br. Med. J.*, **319** (1999) 901–904.

19. Wetzel MS, Eisenberg DM, and Kaptchuk TJ. Courses involving complementary and alternative medicine at US Med schools. *JAMA*, **280(9)** (1998) 784–787.

20. Sampson W. The need for educational reform in teaching about alternative therapies. *Acad. Med.*, **76** (2001) 248–250.

21. Monmaney T. Remedy's sales zoom, but quality control lags; St. John's Wort: regulatory vacuum leaves doubt about potency, effects of herb used for depression. *Los Angeles Times*, August 31, 1998, p. A1.

22. Graham Brown RA, Bourke JF, and Bumphrey G. Chinese herbal remedies may contain steroids. *Br. Med. J.*, **308(6926)** (1994) 473.

23. Slifman NR, Obermeyer WR, Aloi BK, Musser SM, Correll WA Jr, Cichowicz SM, et al. Contamination of botanical dietary supplements by Digitalis lanata. *N. Engl. J. Med.*, **339(12)** (1998) 806–811.

24. Routledge PA and Spriggs TL. Atropine as possible contaminant of comfrey tea. *Lancet*, **1(8644)** (1989) 963–964.

25. Burton Goldberg Group. *Alternative Medicine: The Definitive Guide.* Future Publishing, Puyallup, WA, 1993.

26. http://webmd.lycos.com/content/dmk/dmk_article_57225 accessed 08/31/00.

27. http://www.bu.edu/cohis/cancer/about/alttx/i accesssed 09/07/00.

28. Cassileth BR, Schraub S, Robinson E, and Vickers A. Alternative medicine use worldwide: the International Union Against Cancer survey. *Cancer*, **91** (2001) 1390–1393.

29. Green S. Antineoplastons: an unproved cancer therapy. *JAMA*, **267** (1992) 2924–2928.

30. Anonymous. Evaluation of an unconventional cancer treatment (the Di Bella multitherapy): results of phase II trials in Italy. Italian Study Group for the Di Bella Multitherapy Trials. *Br. Med. J.*, **318(7178)** (1999) 224–228.

31. Buiatti E, Arniani S, Verdecchia A, and Tomatis L. Results from a historical survey of the survival of cancer patients given Di Bella multitherapy. *Cancer*, **86(10)** (1989) 2143–2149.

32. http://www.worldwithoutcancer.com; http://www.sumeria.net/health/laetrile.html (accessed 06/29/00).

33. Moertel CG, Fleming TR, Rubin J, Kvols LK, Sarna G, Koch R, et al. A clinical trial of amygdalin (Laetrile) in the treatment of human cancer. *N. Engl. J. Med.*, **306(4)** (1982) 201–206.

34. Cassileth BR, Lusk EJ, Guerry D, Blake AD, Walsh WP, Kascius L, et al. Survival and quality of life among patients receiving unproven compared with conventional cancer therapy. *N. Engl. J. Med.*, **324(17)** (1991) 1180–1185.

35. Creagan ET, Moertel CG, O'Fallon JR, Schutt AJ, O'Connell MJ, Rubin J, et al. Failure of high-dose vitamin C (ascorbic acid) therapy to benefit patients with advanced cancer. A controlled trial. *N. Engl. J. Med.*, **301(13)** (1979) 687–690.

36. Moertel CG, Fleming TR, Creagan ET, Rubin J, O'Connell MJ, and Ames MM. High-dose vitamin C versus placebo in the treatment of patients with advanced cancer who have had no prior chemotherapy. A randomized double-blind comparison. *N. Engl. J. Med.*, **312(3)** (1985) 137–141.

37. http://www.positivehealth.com/permit/Articles/Cancer/good2.htm; http://www.vitamincfoundation.org/.

38. Hildenbrand GL, Hildenbrand LC, Bradford K, and Cavin SW. Five-year survival rates of melanoma patients treated by diet therapy after the manner of Gerson: a retrospective review. *Altern. Therap. Health Med.*, **1(4)** (1995) 29–37.

39. Gonzalez NJ and Isaacs LL. Evaluation of pancreatic proteolytic enzyme treatment of adenocarcinoma of the pancreas, with nutrition and detoxification support. *Nutr. Cancer*, **33(2)** (1999) 117–124.

40. Miller DR, Anderson GT, Stark JJ, Granick JL, and Richardson D. Phase I/II trial of the safety and efficacy of shark cartilage in the treatment of advanced cancer. *J. Clin. Oncol.*, **16(11)** (1998) 3649–3655.

41. Sellick SM and Zaza C. Critical review of 5 nonpharmacologic strategies for managing cancer pain. *Cancer Prev. Control*, **2(1)** (1998) 7–14.

42. NIH Technology Assessment Panel on Integration of Behavioral and Relaxation Approaches into the Treatment of Chronic Pain and Insomnia. Integration of behavioral and relaxation approaches into the treatment of chronic pain and insomnia. *JAMA*, **276** (1996) 313–318.

43. Syrjala KL, Donaldson GW, Davis MW, Kippes ME, and Carr JE. Relaxation and imagery and cognitive-behavioral training reduce pain during cancer treatment: a controlled clinical trial. *Pain*, **63(2)** (1995) 189–198.

44. Lao L, Bergman S, Langenberg P, Wong RH, and Berman B. Efficacy of Chinese acupuncture on postoperative oral surgery pain. *Oral Sur. Oral Med. Oral Pathol. Oral Radiol. Endodont.*, **79(4)** (1995) 423–428.

45. Melchart D, Linde K, Fischer P, White A, Allais G, Vickers A, et al. Acupuncture for recurrent headaches: a systematic review of randomized controlled trials. *Cephalalgia*, **19(9)** (1999) 779–786.

46. Locsin RG. The effect of music on the pain of selected post-operative patients. *J. Adv. Nurs.*, **6(1)** (1981) 19–25.

47. Beck SL. The therapeutic use of music for cancer-related pain. *Oncol. Nurs. Forum*, **18(8)** (1991) 1327–1337.

48. Weinrich SP and Weinrich MC. The effect of massage on pain in cancer patients. *Appl. Nurs. Res.*, **3(4)** (1990) 140–145.

49. Bindemann S, Soukop M, and Kaye SB. Randomised controlled study of relaxation training. *Eur. J. Cancer*, **27(2)** (1991) 170–174.

50. Bridge LR, Benson P, Pietroni PC, and Priest RG. Relaxation and imagery in the treatment of breast cancer. *Br. Med. J.*, **297(6657)** (1988) 1169–1172.

51. Walker LG, Walker MB, Ogston K, Heys SD, Ah-See AK, Miller ID, et al. Psychological, clinical and pathological effects of relaxation training and guided imagery during primary chemotherapy. *Br. J. Cancer*, **80(1–2)** (1999) 262–268.

52. Burish TG and Lyles JN. Effectiveness of relaxation training in reducing adverse reactions to cancer chemotherapy. *J. Behav. Med.*, **4(1)** (1981) 65–78.

53. Kazak AE, Penati B, Boyer BA, Himelstein B, Brophy P, Waibel MK, et al. A randomized controlled prospective outcome study of a psychological and pharmacological intervention protocol for procedural distress in pediatric leukemia. *J. Pediatr. Psychol.*, **21(5)** (1996) 615–631.

54. Zeltzer L and LeBaron S. Hypnosis and nonhypnotic techniques for reduction of pain and anxiety during painful procedures in children and adolescents with cancer. *J. Pediatr.*, **101(6)** (1982) 1032–1035.

55. Wall VJ and Womack W. Hypnotic versus active cognitive strategies for alleviation of procedural distress in pediatric oncology patients. *Am. J. Clin. Hypn.*, **31(3)** (1989) 181–191.

56. Field T. Morrow C. Valdeon C. Larson S. Kuhn C. Schanberg S. Massage reduces anxiety in child and adolescent psychiatric patients. *J. Am. Acad. Child Adolesc. Psychiatry*, **31(1)** (1992) 125–131.

57. Stevensen C. The psychophysiological effects of aromatherapy massage following cardiac surgery. *Complement. Therap. Med.*, **2(1)** (1994) 27–35.

58. Fraser J and Kerr JR. Psychophysiological effects of back massage on elderly institutionalized patients. *J. Adv. Nurs.*, **18(2)** (1993) 238–245.

59. Field T, Seligman S, Scafidi F, and Schanberg S. Alleviating posttraumatic stress in children following Hurricane Andrew. J. Appl. Devel. Psychol., **17(1)** (1996) 37–50.

60. Ahles TA, Tope DM, Pinkson B, Walch S, Hann D, Whedon M, et al. Massage therapy for patients undergoing autologous bone marrow transplantation. *J. Pain Symptom Manage.*, **18(3)** (1999) 157–163.

61. Bailey LM. The effects of live music versus tape-recorded music on hospitalized cancer patients. *Music Therapy*, **3** (1983) 17–28.

62. Zeltzer LK, Dolgin MJ, LeBaron S, and LeBaron C. A randomized, controlled study of behavioral intervention for chemotherapy distress in children with cancer. *Pediatrics*, **88(1)** (1991) 34–42.

63. Vasterling J, Jenkins RA, Tope DM, and Burish TG. Cognitive distraction and relaxation training for the control of side effects due to cancer chemotherapy. *J. Behav. Med.*, **16(1)** (1993) 65–80.

64. Morrell C. Behavioral treatment for the anticipatory nausea and vomiting induced by cancer chemotherapy. *N. Engl. J. Med.*, **307(24)** (1982) 1476–1480.

65. Arakawa S. Use of relaxation to reduce side effects of chemotherapy in Japanese patients. *Cancer Nurs.*, **18(1)** (1995) 60–66.

66. Syrjala KL, Cummings C, and Donaldson GW. Hypnosis or cognitive behavioral training for the reduction of pain and nausea during cancer treatment: a controlled clinical trial. *Pain*, **48(2)** (1992) 137–146.

67. Vickers AJ. Can acupuncture have specific effects on health? A systematic review of acupuncture antiemesis trials. *J. R. Soc. Med.*, **89(6)** (1996) 303–311.

68. Lee A and Done ML. The use of nonpharmacologic techniques to prevent postoperative nausea and vomiting: a meta-analysis. *Anesth. Analg.*, **88(6)** (1999) 1362–1369.

69. Ezzone S, Baker C, Rosselet R, and Terepka E. Music as an adjunct to antiemetic therapy. *Oncol. Nurs. Forum*, **25(9)** (1998) 1551–1556.

70. Filshie J, Penn K, Ashley S, and Davis CL. Acupuncture for the relief of cancer-related breathlessness. *Palliat. Med.*, **10(2)** (1996) 145–150.

71. Ernst E and Pittler MH. The effectiveness of acupuncture in treating acute dental pain: a systematic review. *Br. Dental J.*, **184(9)** (1998) 443–447.

72. Wang B, Tang J, White PF, Naruse R, Sloninsky A, Kariger R, et al. Effect of the intensity of transcutaneous acupoint electrical stimulation on the postoperative analgesic requirement. *Anesth, Analg.*, **85(2)** (1997) 406–413.

73. Chen L, Tang J, White PF, Sloninsky A, Wender RH, Naruse R, et al. The effect of location of transcutaneous electrical nerve stimulation on postoperative opioid analgesic requirement: acupoint versus nonacupoint stimulation. *Anesth. Analg.*, **87(5)** (1998) 1129–1134.

74. Poulain P, Pichard Leandri E, Laplanche A, Montange F, Bouzy J, and Truffa Bachi J. Electroacupuncture analgesia in major abdominal and pelvic surgery: a randomised study. *Acupunct. Med.*, **15(1)** (1997) 10–13.

75. Christensen PA, Rotne M, Vedelsdal R, Jensen RH, Jacobsen K, and Husted C. Electroacupuncture in anaesthesia for hysterectomy. *Br. J. Anaesth.*, **71(6)** (1993) 835–838.

76. Koch ME, Kain ZN, Ayoub C, and Rosenbaum SH. The sedative and analgesic sparing effect of music. *Anesthesiology*, **89(2)** (1998) 300–306.

77. Good M, Stanton Hicks M, Grass JA, Cranston Anderson G, Choi C, Schoolmeesters LJ, et al. Relief of postoperative pain with jaw relaxation, music and their combination. *Pain*, **81(1-2)** (1999) 163–172.

78. Tusek DL, Church JM, Strong SA, Grass JA, and Fazio VW. Guided imagery: a significant advance in the care of patients undergoing elective colorectal surgery. *Dis. Colon Rectum*, **40(2)** (1997) 172–178.

79. Goldmann L, Ogg TW, and Levey AB. Hypnosis and daycase anaesthesia. A study to reduce pre-operative anxiety and intra-operative anaesthetic requirements. *Anaesthesia*, **43(6)** (1988) 466–469.

80. Markland D and Hardy L. Anxiety, relaxation and anaesthesia for day-case surgery. *Br. J. Clin. Psychol.*, **32(4)** (1993) 493–504.

81. Menard MB. The effect of therapeutic massage on post surgical outcomes. *Dissert. Abstr. Int.*, **57(1)** (1996) 276.

82. Cragg GM, Newman DJ, and Weiss RB. Coral reefs, forests, and thermal vents: the worldwide exploration of nature for novel antitumor agents. *Semin. Oncol.*, **24(2)** (1997) 156–163.

83. Okita K, Li Q, Murakamio T, and Takahashi M. Anti-growth effects with components of Sho-saiko-to (TJ-9) on cultured human hepatoma cells. *Eur. J. Cancer Prev.*, **2(2)** (1993) 169–175.

84. Yano H, Mizoguchi A, Fukuda K, Haramaki M, Ogasawara S, Momosaki S, et al. The herbal medicine sho-saiko-to inhibits proliferation of cancer cell lines by inducing apoptosis and arrest at the G0/G1 phase. *Cancer Res.*, **54(2)** (1994) 448–454.

85. Kok LD, Wong CK, Leung KN, Tsang SF, Fung KP, and Choy YM. Activation of the anti-tumor effector cells by Radix bupleuri. *Immunopharmacology*, **30(1)** (1995) 79–87.

86. Li X, Motwani M, Tong W, Bornmann W, and Schwartz GK. Huanglian, Chinese herbal extract, inhibits cell growth by suppressing the expression of cyclin B1 inhibiting CDC2 kinase activity in human cancer cells. *Mol. Pharmacol.*, **58** (2000) 1287–1293.

87. Kaegi E. Unconventional therapies for cancer: 1. Essiac. The Task Force on Alternative Therapies of the Canadian Breast Cancer Research Initiative. *Can. Med. Assoc. J.*, **158(7)** (1998) 897–902.

88. Kleijnen J and Knipschild P. Mistletoe treatment for cancer. Review of controlled trials in humans. *Phytomedicine*, **1** (1994) 255–260.

89. Steuer-Vogt MK, Bonkowsky V, Ambrosch P, Scholz M, Neiss A, Strutz J, et al. The effect of an adjuvant mistletoe treatment programme in resected head and neck cancer patients: a randomised controlled clinical trial. *Eur. J. Cancer*, **37** (2001) 23–31.

90. http://www.go-symmetry.com/Noni.htm (accessed 08/04/00).

91. Hirazumi A, Furusawa E, Chou SC, and Hokama Y. Anticancer activity of Morinda citrifolia (noni) on intraperitoneally implanted Lewis lung carcinoma in syngeneic mice. *Proc. West. Pharmacol. Soc.*, **37** (1994) 145–146.

92. Hiwasa T, Arase Y, Chen Z, Kita K, Umezawa K, Ito H, et al. Stimulation of ultraviolet-induced apoptosis of human fibroblast UVr-1 cells by tyrosine kinase inhibitors. *FEBS Lett.*, **444(2–3)** (1999) 173–176.

93. Hirazumi A and Furusawa E. An immunomodulatory polysaccharide-rich substance from the fruit juice of *Morinda citrifolia* (noni) with antitumour activity. *Phytother. Res.*, **13(5)** (1999) 380–387.

94. da Consolacao M, Linardi F, de Oliveira MM, and Sampaio MR. A lapachol derivative active against mouse lymphocytic leukemia P-388. *J. Med. Chem.*, **18(11)** (1975) 1159–1161.

95. Block JB, Serpick AA, Miller W, and Wiernik PH. Early clinical studies with lapachol (NSC-11905). *Cancer Chemother. Rep. (2)*, **4(4)** (1974) 27–28.

96. Yano H, Mizoguchi A, Fukuda K, Haramaki M, Ogasawara S, Momosaki S, et al. The herbal medicine sho-saiko-to inhibits proliferation of cancer cell lines by inducing apoptosis and arrest at the G0/G1 phase. *Cancer Res.*, **54(2)** (1994) 448–454.

97. Ito H and Shimura K. Effects of a blended Chinese medicine, xiao-chai-hu-tang, on Lewis lung carcinoma growth and inhibition of lung metastasis, with special reference to macrophage activation. *Jpn. J. Pharmacol.*, **41(3)** (1986) 307–314.

98. Kato M, Liu W, Yi H, Asai N, Hayakawa A, Kozaki K, et al. The herbal medicine Sho-saiko-to inhibits growth and metastasis of malignant melanoma primarily developed in ret-transgenic mice. *J. Invest. Dermatol.*, **111(4)** (1998) 640–644.

99. Kaneko M, Kawakita T, Tauchi Y, Saito Y, Suzuki A, and Nomoto K. Augmentation of NK activity after oral administration of a traditional Chinese medicine, xiao-chai-hu-tang (shosaiko-to). *Immunopharmacol. Immunotoxicol.*, **16(1)** (1994) 41–53.

100. Yamashiki M, Kosaka Y, Nishimura A, Takase K, and Ichida F. Efficacy of a herbal medicine "sho-saiko-to" on the improvement of impaired cytokine production of peripheral blood mononuclear cells in patients with chronic viral hepatitis. *J. Clin. Lab. Immunol.*, **37(3)** (1992) 111–121.

101. Oka H, Yamamoto S, Kuroki T, Harihara S, Marumo T, Kim SR, et al. Prospective study of chemoprevention of hepatocellular carcinoma with Sho-saiko-to (TJ-9). *Cancer*, **76(5)** (1995) 743–749.

102. Ohnishi Y, Fujii H, Hayakawa Y, Sakukawa R, Yamaura T, Sakamoto T, et al. Oral administration of a Kampo (Japanese herbal) medicine Juzen-taiho-to inhibits liver metastasis of colon 26-L5 carcinoma cells. *Jpn. J. Cancer Res.*, **89(2)** (1998) 206–213.

103. Onishi Y, Yamaura T, Tauchi K, Sakamoto T, Tsukada K, Nunome S, et al. Expression of the anti-metastatic effect induced by Juzen-taiho-to is based on the content of Shimotsu-to constituents. *Biol. Pharm. Bull.*, **21** (1998) 761–765.

104. Kiyohara H, Matsumoto T, Komats Y, and Yamada H. Protective effect of oral administration of a pectic polysaccharide fraction from a Kampo (Japanese herbal) medicine "Juzen-Taiho-To" on adverse effects of cis-diaminedichloroplatinum. *Planta. Med.*, **61** (1995) 531–534.

105. Sugiyama K, Ueda H, and Ichio Y. Protective effect of juzen-taiho-to against carboplatin-induced toxic side effects in mice. *Biol. Pharm. Bull.*, **18** (1995) 544–548.

106. Sugiyama K, Ueda H, Ichio Y, and Yokota M. Improvement of cisplatin toxicity and lethality by juzen-taiho-to in mice. *Biol. Pharm. Bull.*, **18** (1995) 53–58.

107. Adachi K, Nanba H, and Kuroda H. Potentiation of host-mediated antitumor activity in mice by beta-glucan obtained from Grifola frondosa (maitake). *Chem. Pharm. Bull. (Tokyo)*, **35(1)** (1987) 262–270.

108. Suzuki I, Hashimoto K, Oikawa S, Sato K, Osawa M, and Yadomae T. Antitumor and immunomodulating activities of a beta-glucan obtained from liquid-cultured Grifola frondosa. *Chem. Pharm. Bull. (Tokyo)*, **37(2)** (1989) 410–413.

109. Suzuki I, Hashimoto K, Ohno N, Tanaka H, and Yadomae T. Immunomodulation by orally administered beta-glucan in mice. *Int. J. Immunopharm.*, **11(7)** (1989) 761–769.

110. Abel G and Czop JK. Stimulation of human monocyte beta-glucan receptors by glucan particles induces production of TNF-alpha and IL-1 beta. *Int. J. Immunopharm.*, **14(8)** (1992) 1363–1373.

111. Kato M, Hirose K, Hakozaki M, et al. Induction of gene expression for immunomodulating cytokines in peripheral blood mononuclear cells in response to orally administered PSK , an immunomodulating protein-bound polysaccharide. *Cancer Immunol. Immunother.*, **40** (1995) 152–156.

112. Kano Y, Kakuta H, and Hashimoto J. Effect of sizofiran on regional lymph nodes in patients with head and neck cancer. *Biotherapy*, **9(4)** (1996) 257–262.

113. Yamada Y, Nanba H, and Kuroda H. Antitumor effect of orally administered extracts from fruit body of Grifola frondosa (Maitake). *Chemotherapy*, **38(8)** (1990) 790–796.

114. Hishida I, Nanba H, and Kuroda H. Antitumor activity exhibited by orally administered extract from fruit body of *Grifola frondosa* (maitake). *Chem. Pharm. Bull. (Tokyo)*, **36(5)** (1988) 1819–1827.

115. Kobayashi H, Matsunaga K, and Oguchi Y. Antimetastatic effects of PSK (Krestin), a protein-bound polysaccharide obtained from basidiomycetes: an overview. *Cancer Epidemiol. Biomarkers Prev.*, **4(3)** (1995) 275–281.

116. Abe S, Tsubouchi J, Takahashi K, Yamazaki M, and Mizuno D. Combination therapy of murine tumors with lentinan plus lipopolysaccharide plus cyclophosphamide. *Gann*, **73(6)** (1982) 961–967.

117. Kurashige S, Akuzawa Y, Endo F,, Kurashige S, Akuzawa Y, and Endo F. Effects of *Lentinus edodes*, *Grifola frondosa* and *Pleurotus ostreatus* administration on cancer outbreak, and activities of macrophages and lymphocytes in mice treated with a carcinogen, *N*-butyl-*N*-butanolnitrosoamine. *Immunopharmacol. Immunotoxicol.*, **19(2)** (1997) 175–183.

118. Nanba H. Activity of maitake D-fraction to inhibit carcinogenesis and metastasis. *Ann NY Acad. Sci.*, **768** (1995) 243–245.

119. Borchers AT, Stern JS, Hackman RM, Keen CL, and Gershwin ME. Mushrooms, tumors, and immunity. *Proc. Soc. Exp. Biol. Med.*, **221(4)** (1999) 281–293.

120. Kanoh T, Saito K, Matsunaga K, Oguchi Y, Taniguchi N, Endoh H, et al. Enhancement of the antitumor effect by the concurrent use of a monoclonal antibody and the protein-bound polysaccharide PSK in mice bearing a human cancer cell line. *In Vivo*, **8(2)** (1994) 241–245.

121. Niimoto M, Hattori T, Tamada R, Sugimachi K, Inokuchi K, and Ogawa N. Postoperative adjuvant immunochemotherapy with mitomycin C, futraful, and PSK for gastric cancer. An analysis of data on 579 patients followed for five years. *Jpn. J. Surg.*, **18(6)** (1988) 681–686.

122. Nakazato H, Koike A, Saji S, Ogawa N, and Sakamoto J. Efficacy of immunochemotherapy as adjuvant treatment after curative resection of gastric cancer. *Lancet*, **343** (1994) 1122–1126.

123. Ogoshi K, Satou H, Isono K, Mitomi T, Endoh M, and Sugita M. Immunotherapy for esophageal cancer. A randomized trial in combination with radiotherapy and radiochemotherapy. Cooperative Study Group for Esophageal Cancer in Japan. *Am. J. Clin. Oncol.*, **18(3)** (1995) 216–222.

124. Toi M, Hattori T, Akagi M, Inokuchi K, Orita K, Sugimachi K, et al. Randomized adjuvant trial to evaluate the addition of tamoxifen and PSK to chemotherapy in patients with primary breast cancer. 5-Year results from the Nishi–Nippon Group of the Adjuvant Chemoendocrine Therapy for Breast Cancer Organization. *Cancer*, **70(10)** (1992) 2475–2483.

125. Iino Y, Yokoe T, Maemura M, Horiguchi J, Takei H, Ohwada S, et al. Immunochemotherapies versus chemotherapy as adjuvant treatment after curative resection of operable breast cancer. *Anticancer Res.*, **15(6B)** (1995) 2907–2911.

126. Ohno R, Yamada K, Masaoka T, et al. A randomized trial of chemoimmunotherapy of acute nonlymphocytic leukemia in adults using a protein-bound polysaccharide preparation. *Cancer Immunol. Immunother.*, **18** (1984) 149–154.

127. d001132 Fujimoto S, Furue H, Kimura T, Kondo T, Orita K, Taguchi T, et al. Clinical evaluation of schizophyllan adjuvant immunochemotherapy for patients with resectable gastric cancer—a randomized controlled trial. *Jpn. J. Surg.*, **14(4)** (1984) 286–292.

128. d001089 Fujimoto S, Furue H, Kimura T, Kondo T, Orita K, Taguchi T, et al. Clinical outcome of postoperative adjuvant immunochemotherapy with sizofiran for patients with resectable gastric cancer: a randomised controlled study. *Eur. J. Cancer*, **27(9)** (1991) 1114–1118.

129. Okamura K, Suzuki M, Chihara T, Fujiwara A, Fukuda T, Goto S, et al. Clinical evaluation of sizofiran combined with irradiation in patients with cervical cancer. A randomized controlled study; a five-year survival rate. *Biotherapy*, **1(2)** (1989) 103–107.

130. Noda K, Takeuchi S, Yajima A, Akiya K, Kasamatsu T, Tomoda Y, et al. Clinical effect of sizofiran combined with irradiation in cervical cancer patients: a randomized controlled study. Cooperative Study Group on SPG for Gynecological Cancer. *Jpn. J. Clin. Oncol.*, **22(1)** (1992) 17–25.

131. Torisu M, Hayashi Y, Ishimitsu T, et al. Significant prolongation of disease-free period gained by oral polysaccharide K (PSK) administration after curative surgical operation of colorectal cancer. *Cancer Immunol. Immunother.*, **31** (1990) 261–268.

132. Mitomi T, Tsuchiya S, Iijima N, Aso K, Suzuki K, Nishiyama K, et al. Randomized, controlled study on adjuvant immunochemotherapy with PSK in curatively resected colorectal cancer. The Cooperative Study Group of Surgical Adjuvant Immunochemotherapy for Cancer of Colon and Rectum (Kanagawa). *Dis. Colon Rectum*, **35(2)** (1992) 123–130.

133. Kobayashi Y, Yamashita Y, Fujii N, Takaboshi K, Kawakami T, Kawamura M, et al. Inhibitors of DNA topoisomerase I and II isolated from the Coptis rhizomes. *Planta Med.*, **61(5)** (1995) 414–418.

134. Kohlmeier L, Weterings KG, Steck S, and Kok FJ. Tea and cancer prevention: an evaluation of the epidemiologic literature. *Nutr. Cancer*, **27(1)** (1997) 1–13.

135. Ji BT, Chow WH, Hsing AW, McLaughlin JK, Dai Q, Gao YT, et al. Green tea consumption and the risk of pancreatic and colorectal cancers. *Int. J. Cancer*, **70(3)** (1997) 255–258.

136. Hirose M, Hoshiya T, Akagi K, Takahashi S, Hara Y, and Ito N. Effects of green tea catechins in a rat multi-organ carcinogenesis model. *Carcinogenesis*, **14(8)** (1993) 1549–1553.

137. Hirose M, Takahashi S, Ogawa K, Futakuchi M, Shirai T, Shibutani M, et al. Chemoprevention of heterocyclic amine-induced carcinogenesis by phenolic compounds in rats. *Cancer Lett.*, **143(2)** (1999) 173–178.

138. Yang GY, Liao J, Kim K, Yurkow EJ, and Yang CS. Inhibition of growth and induction of apoptosis in human cancer cell lines by tea polyphenols. *Carcinogenesis*, **19(4)** (1998) 611–616.

139. Chen ZP, Schell JB, Ho CT, and Chen KY. Green tea epigallocatechin gallate shows a pronounced growth inhibitory effect on cancerous cells but not on their normal counterparts. *Cancer Lett.*, **129(2)** (1998) 173–179.
140. Kelloff GJ, Crowell JA, Steele VE, Lubet RA, Malone WA, Boone CW, et al. Progress in cancer chemoprevention: development of diet-derived chemopreventive agents. *J. Nutr.*, **130(2S Suppl.)** (2000) 467S–471S.
141. Linde K, Ramirez G, Mulrow CD, Pauls A, Weidenhammer W, and Melchart D. St John's Wort for depression—an overview and meta-analysis of randomised clinical trials. *Br. Med. J.*, **313(7052)** (1996) 253–258.
142. Moyad MA. Alternative therapies for advanced prostate cancer. What should I tell my patients? *Urol. Clin. North Am.*, **26(2)** (1999) 413–417.
143. Syed TA, Ahmad SA, Holt AH, Ahmad SA, Ahmad SH, and Afzal M. Management of psoriasis with aloe vera extract in a hydrophilic cream: a placebo-controlled, double-blind study. *Trop. Med. Intl. Health*, **1** (1996) 505–509.
144. Williams MS, Burk M, Loprinzi CL, Hill M, Schomberg PJ, Nearhood K, et al. Phase III double-blind evaluation of an aloe vera gel as a prophylactic agent for radiation-induced skin toxicity. Int. J. Radiat. Oncol. Biol. Phys., **36(2)** (1996) 345–349.
145. Melchart D, Linde K, and Fischer P. Echinacea for the prevention and treatment of the common cold (Cochrane Review). *Cochrane Libr.*, (1998) Issue 4.
146. Bendel R, Bendel V, Renner K, and Stolze K. Supplementary treatment with Esberitox of female patients undergoing curative adjuvant irradiation following breast cancer. *Strahlenther. Onkol.*, **164(5)** (1988) 278–283.
147. Piscitelli SC, Burstein AH, Chaitt D, Alfaro RM, and Falloon J. Indinavir concentrations and St John's Wort. *Lancet*, **355(9203)** (2000) 547–548.
148. Lin HL, Liu TY, Wu CW, and Chi CW. Berberine modulates expression of mdr1 gene product and the responses of digestive track cancer cells to Paclitaxel. *Br. J. Cancer*, **81(3)** (1999) 416–422.

VI   NEW AGENTS IN COLORECTAL CANCER

39 Angiogenesis and Colorectal Cancer
From the Laboratory to the Clinic

Lee S. Rosen and William W. Li

CONTENTS

FROM THE LABORATORY
THE ANGIOGENIC CASCADE
ANGIOGENESIS AND COLORECTAL CANCER
TOWARD THE CLINIC
CLINICAL TRIAL DESIGN
CLASSES OF ANGIOGENESIS INHIBITORS
TRIALS SPECIFIC TO COLORECTAL CANCER
CONCLUSION
REFERENCES

1. FROM THE LABORATORY

When in 1998 a *New York Times* front-page article declared that a new class of drugs could potentially cure cancers by cutting off their blood supply, the eyes of the world turned to the field of angiogenesis *(1)*. Actually, it had been in 1966 when Folkman and his colleagues first observed that in order to grow beyond a size of 1–2 mm^3, tumors depended on new blood vessel growth, a process termed angiogenesis. Over 30 yr later, and after the expansion of this work in several laboratories around the world, more is known about angiogenesis and tumor biology and several drugs have been developed that interfere with various parts of this process. Although much of the success in 1998 was limited to preclinical models and the occasional anecdotal patient, currently large-scale human clinical trials are underway, some with quite promising results. Whatever we learn from this ongoing set of studies will undoubtedly help us understand the process by which new vessels are created, what mechanisms of resistance to therapy exist, if any, and whether existing anticancer therapy will work synergistically or in competition with these new agents. We will hopefully learn whether angiogenesis is a central part of all tumor growth or whether it might be restricted to certain disease types and stages. Above all, we will gain in our understanding of clinical trial design, as these agents have very different characteristics from conventional cytotoxic chemotherapy. This chapter attempts to summarize the current knowledge base with regards to these very challenging questions.

From: *Colorectal Cancer: Multimodality Management*
Edited by: L. Saltz © Humana Press Inc., Totowa, NJ

Table 1
Endogenous Regulators of Angiogenesis

Angiogenic factors	*Antiangiogenic factor*
Vascular endothelial growth factor (VEGF)	Angiostatin
Platelet-derived growth factor (PDGF)	Endostatin
Acidic and basic fibroblast growth factor (FGF)	Vasculostatin
Angiogenin	Interferon α, β
Hepatocyte growth factor	Maspin
Interleukin-8 (IL-8)	METH-1, -2
Placental growth factor	Platelet factor 4
Platelet-derived endothelial cell growth factor	Prolactin fragment
Transforming growth factor α, β	Thrombospondin
Tumor necrosis factor α	TIMP
Insulin growth factor (IGF)	Others
Others	

Source: Modified from *Drug Discov. Today*, **2** (1997) 50–63.

2. THE ANGIOGENIC CASCADE

Our understanding of how tumors cause new blood vessels to be created has deepened over the past several years. This grouping of cellular and molecular events, although seemingly well characterized, may, in fact, be only part of as yet undiscovered processes. Table 1 lists known proangiogenic and antiangiogenic factors and Fig. 1 depicts key steps of the angiogenesis cascade.

2.1. Angiogenic Growth Factor Production and Release

In response to tissue hypoxia among other stimuli, tumors secrete various angiogenic growth factors that bind to receptors on the endothelial cells of pre-existing capillaries and venules *(2)*. Vascular endothelial growth factor (VEGF) and its receptors (VEGFR-1/Flt-1, VEGFR-2/KDR/Flk-1, VEGFR-3/KDR/Flt-1, VEGFR-3/Flt-4, VEGFR-4/neuropilin-1) have been extensively studied *(3)*. Either the adult endothelial cells or circulating endothelial progenitor cells may be recruited to form new vessels *(4)*.

2.2. Endothelial Receptor Binding and Activation

Once a growth factor binds to its receptor, a series of cellular events occurs. Receptor dimerization and the phosphorylation of tyrosine and other kinases are components of key signal transduction pathways that alter endothelial gene expression and cell proliferation *(5–7)*. Antiapoptotic pathways (e.g., Bcl-2 and survivin) are also activated when VEGF and basic fibroblast growth factor (bFGF) bind to their respective receptors, promoting prolonged endothelial cell survival *(8,9)*. Angiopoietin-1, attaching to the Tie-2 receptor and activating the phosphatidylinositol 3′-kinase/Akt signal transduction pathway, can also prolong cell survival *(10)*.

2.3. Formation of Angiogenic Mother Vessel

Parent vessels change morphologically once the endothelial cells are activated. They will enlarge in cross-sectional area to form what can be called "mother vessels" *(11)*. In preparation for neovascular sprouting, the "mother vessels" possess thinned endothelial cell lining, increased endothelial cell number, decreased numbers of pericytes with pericyte

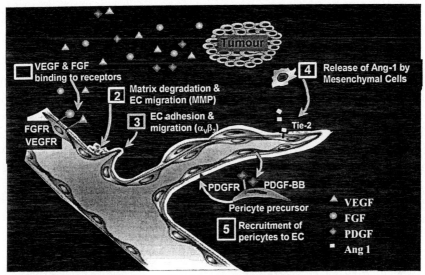

Modified based on Klagsbrun & Moses, Chemistry & Biology 1999;6:R217

Fig. 1. The Angiogenesis Cascade.

detachment, and early degradation of the basement membrane. The "mother vessels" also become hyperpermeable in response to VEGF, with increased fenestrae and prominent collections of vesiculovacuolar organelles *(12)*. The local microvascular dilatation, hyper-permeability, extravascular fibrin deposition, and edema are among the earliest signs of angiogenesis.

2.4. Morphogenesis of the Mother Vessel

These "mother vessels" last only a few days. From there, growth occurs by at least four divergent morphological pathways: (1) muscular artery or vein formation (occurring in 1–3 mo); (2) vascular bridging (occurring in 3 d to 3 wk); (3) intussusceptive microvascular growth (occurring in days to weeks); and (4) sprouting of "capillary-like" microvessels (occurring in days) *(12)*. Through these mechanisms, the "mother vessels" can evolve into medium-sized arteries and veins or can eventually divide into smaller, separate well-differentiated channels known as "daughter vessels." The "mother vessels" can also split longitudinally (termed "intussusception") following local invagination of connective tissue pillars within the vessels themselves *(13,14)*. FGF can mediate this vascular branching *(15)*. However, the most well-characterized process of tumor angiogenesis is an actual sprouting of the endothelial cells themselves *(16)*.

2.5. Basement Membrane Dissolution

In order for the sprouting to occur, the basement membrane must dissolve in areas of activated endothelium. The endothelium can secret a number of proteolytic enzymes, including plasminogen activator and matrix metalloproteinases, which enable the endothelial cells to exit the vessel abluminally *(17)*.

2.6. Endothelial Cell Proliferation

Activated endothelial cells can proliferate rapidly, in contradistinction to the endothelial cells of nonpathologic blood vessels, which do not. This difference can be exploited to design drugs that interfere with the angiogenic process in cancers, while not harming the normal vasculature.

2.7. Endothelial Cell Migration

The proliferating endothelial cells migrate out of the "mother vessel" into the extracellular matrix and toward the angiogenic stimulus *(18)*. In the presence of VEGF, angiopoietin-2 binds to the Tie-2 receptor, competitively displacing angiopoietin-1. This new ligand–receptor interaction leads to a decoupling of endothelial cells, pericytes, smooth-muscle cells, and components of the extracellular matrix in these angiogenic regions *(19,20)*. The angiogenic endothelial cells express adhesion molecules (the $\alpha_v\beta_3$ and $\alpha_v\beta_5$ integrins) that facilitate migration and improve vascular survival *(21,22)*. As the new vessels continue to grow, the endothelial cells will secrete matrix metalloproteinases that enhance the ability to invade *(23,24)*.

2.8. Vascular Tube Formation

For the sprouting endothelial cells to form a lumen, there must be interactions between cell-associated surface proteins and the extracellular matrix. Hybrid oligosaccharides galectin-2, PECAM-1 and VE-cadherin are among the identified cell surface proteins *(25–27)*. Three populations of endothelial cells must migrate together as a single cordlike structure in order to create these vascular lumina. A second cell population containing numerous intracellular vacuoles surrounds an initial internal endothelial population. The internal population disappears within 12 h of formation. The surrounding vacuoles of the second population fuse with the plasma membrane and are secreted, resulting in extensive remodeling of the center of a solid vascular cord into a lumen. The third endothelial population combines with the newly formed endothelial outer layer and expands the luminal circumference *(28)*. Tumors are reported to form vascular channels without endothelial cells, but this theory of "vasculogenic mimicry" remains poorly understood and controversial *(29,30)*. If tumors are capable of a more direct means of increasing their blood supply, this might explain the observed resistance to therapy with several existing angiogenesis inhibitors in clinical testing.

2.9. Arterial–Venous Differentiation

The vascular tubes fuse to become vascular loops and define functional arterial and venous components of the neovasculature. From knowledge of embryonic vascular development, it is suggested that molecular cues on the afferent and efferent arms of differentiating vessels are provided by the ephrin-B2 transmembrane ligand (arterial endothelium) and its receptor, Eph-B4 (venous endothelium) *(31,32)*. The ephrin ligand–receptor interactions occur at the cell–cell juncture of arterio-venous anastamoses and along the length of a newly forming arterial vessel and an adjacent vein *(33)*. The ephrin-B2/EphB4 interaction is thought to guide patterned development of arterial and venous boundaries *(34)*.

2.10. Vascular Stabilization

Smooth-muscle cells and pericytes must be recruited by the developing blood vessel before blood flow can begin. These periendothelial cells are found in varying degrees throughout the vasculature. Binding of ephrin-Eph mediates signals between endothelial cells and these mesenchymal cells *(35)*. The angiopoietins also play a role as angiopoietin-1 binds to the Tie-2 receptor on angiogenic endothelium. This interaction leads to promotion of vascular tube formation, endothelial survival, and the secretion of PDGF and other chemokines that recruit the smooth-muscle cells and pericytes to support the new vessel architecture *(36–38)*. Pericytes or smooth-muscle cells grown together with endothelial cells in culture engage in paracrine signaling. Once the two populations of cells come into contact, activated tumor growth factor-β (TGF-β), itself an angiogenesis inhibitor, is secreted and endothelial cell proliferation is suppressed *(39)*. Vascular stabilization can thus downregulate angiogenesis at a terminal maturation phase of new blood vessel growth. Angiopoietin-2 is a competitive ligand for the Tie-2 receptor and, when bound, can destabilize vessels by uncoupling the periendothelial cells from the endothelial cells *(40)*. In the presence of VEGF, angiopoietin-2 allows angiogenesis. If VEGF is withdrawn from the system, however, Ang-2/Tie-2 binding leads to endothelial cell apoptosis and regression of the neovasculature.

3. ANGIOGENESIS AND COLORECTAL CANCER

Experimental models that characterize the angiogenesis cascade ought to be generic to several tumor types. Specific evidence that angiogenesis is involved in or even required for colorectal cancer growth and spread has been generated from animal models of the disease and from studies of human tumor specimens. Several studies suggest correlations between angiogenic phenotypes and patient prognosis. However, considerable debate exists about how to measure angiogenesis, whether the measurements are reproducible, and how precisely the information can be used clinically.

3.1. Microvessel Density

Engel and colleagues examined a small series of resected colorectal cancer patients and concluded that tumor microvessel counts were an important predictor of tumor recurrence, even when controlled for Dukes' staging *(41)*. Others have used angiogenesis scores in order to standardize vessel counting, and have shown that higher scores (higher amounts of new blood vessel growth) are associated with higher recurrence rates and diminished survival *(42)*. These angiogenesis scores have not yet been validated in examining metastases from colorectal cancer and it is not yet known if a correlation exists between primary lesions and metastases in the same patient. Contradictory reports have been published showing no significant correlation between microvessel density and clinical outcome, although, at times, different techniques for measuring the microvessel density can account for the different conclusions in different studies *(43)*. Until histopathologic techniques are standardized or image analysis algorithms are validated and used uniformly, microvessel density will remain a subjective measurement. Tumors are not uniform in microvessel density and the existence of so-called "angiogenic hot spots" is well known to pathologists. Current best practice studies of tumor microvessel density employ measurements of angiogenesis within these hot spots, which may vary even within a given tumor. Microvessel density analysis still requires tumor biopsies, which are clearly available at the time of surgical resection but may not be feasible to monitor the effects of treatment and subject patients to multiple serial biopsies. Although microvessel density measurements may provide some pathologic insights into the colorectal cancer disease process, they have not yet been fully validated as a clinical technique for evaluation or management of the disease.

3.2. VEGF Levels

The presence or level of VEGF in the serum, plasma, or expressed in the tumor is associated with patient prognosis, probability of recurrence and survival *(44)*. Serum VEGF levels appeared to increase as tumor size increased in a group of untreated advanced colorectal cancer patients receiving serial radiographic scanning *(45)*. Preoperative VEGF levels were shown to be predictive of colorectal cancer staging *(45)*. Plasma VEGF levels appeared to correlate with serum VEGF levels in a study of gastrointestinal cancers *(46)*.

In patients not yet diagnosed with colorectal cancer, serum VEGF levels do not appear to be useful as a diagnostic marker on their own *(47)*. Sensitivity can increase by combining the VEGF level with the carcinoembryonic antigen (CEA) blood marker in one small series. However, once the patient carried the colorectal cancer diagnosis, the VEGF levels here, too, did correlate with clinical stage and outcome.

The pathophysiologic role of VEGF in colorectal cancer is being investigated. Kondo et al. hypothesized that new blood vessels appeared to develop as tumors progressed from adenomas to noninvasive carcinomas, mediated in part as a result of VEGF *(48)*. His group found no evidence of VEGF mRNA or protein in dysplastic adenomas, but 62% of the carcinomas did demonstrate VEGF protein. These observations suggest a rationale for using an anti-VEGF therapy to prevent colorectal cancer by intervening at an early stage of pathogenesis. The use of the COX-2 inhibitor celecoxib (Celebrex®, Pharmacia, Inc.) to prevent polyp formation in familial adenomatous polyposis coli (FAP) further supports this approach *(49)*. Recent studies have shown that the COX-2 pathway mediates VEGF expression *(50)*. Furthermore, COX-2 inhibition can inhibit angiogenesis *(51)*.

VEGF, also known as vascular permeability factor (VPF), may play a role in the development of malignant ascites by increasing the permeability between endothelial cells *(52)*. When compared to ascites in cirrhotic patients, the fluid in those with metastatic colorectal cancer induced vascular hyperpermeability in vitro, using an assay of human umbilical vein endothelial cells (HUVEC). This activity was reversed by the addition of a neutralizing antibody to VEGF.

The VEGF levels in clinical specimens of serum and plasma are easy to measure using widely available commercial assay kits. However, larger clinical studies are needed to validate the role of VEGF measurements in assessing prognosis, staging or response to treatment in colorectal cancer.

4. TOWARD THE CLINIC

As scientists learn more about the angiogenesis cascade, new targets for drug development become readily apparent. The challenge of course lies in identifying drugs that are specific and learning how to overcome possible mechanisms of resistance. Since interferon-α2a was first used in children in 1988 to treat pulmonary hemangiomatosis, more than 60 agents have been developed to interfere with the angiogenesis pathways *(53)*. A list of agents now in various stages of clinical testing is listed in Table 2. The discussion that follows focuses on how angiogenesis inhibitors are being developed before describing the clinical data from human trials themselves.

5. CLINICAL TRIAL DESIGN

As a new class of anticancer agents, the angiogenesis inhibitors pose many challenges to investigators designing appropriate clinical trials to test hypotheses about efficacy, mechanisms of action, and long-term safety. Some challenges are unique to this class of drugs and others are shared with different types of novel agent. Table 3 highlights some of the differences between conventional chemotherapy drugs, termed "cytotoxic" here, and the angiogenesis inhibitors termed "cytostatic" *(54)*. This brief discussion can help the

Table 2
Angiogenesis Drugs in Clinical Testing, 2001

Drug	Sponsor
Rhu Mab Anti-VEGF	Genentech
Avicine	AVI Biopharma
Carboxyamidotriazole (CAI)	NCI
IM862 (Glufanide disodium)	Cytran/Alza
Interferon alpha	Hoffman-LaRoche
LDI-200	Milkhaus Laboratory
Neovastat AE-941	Aeterna Laboratories
Octreotide (Somatostatin)	Novartis
SU5416	Sugen/Pharmacia
Tetrathiomolybdate (TM)	U Michigan Comprehensive Cancer Center
Thalomid (Thalidomide)	Celgene
Viraldon	ML Labs
Prinomastat (AG-3340)	Agouron/Pfizer
SU101 (Leflunomide)	SUGEN
Angiozyme (RP4610)	Ribozyme/Chiron
Aplidine	PharmaMar
Apra(CT-2584)	Cell Therapeutics
BMS275291	Bristol-Myers Squibb
CEP-701	Cephalon
EMD 121974 (cilengitide)	Merck/ImClone
Flavopiridol	NCI
GBC-590	SafeScience
Green Tea Extract (GTE)	NCI
ImmTher	Endorex
Interferon-alpha gene therapy	Valentis
Interleukin-12 (Edodekin-alfa)	Genetics Institute/Hoffman-LaRoche
Metaret (Suramin hexasodium)	NCI
Panzem (2Methoxyestradiol)	EntreMed
Penicillamine	NCI
PI-88	Progen Industries, Ltd.
Solimastat (BB-3644)	British Biotech
Suramin hexasodium	NCI
Squalamine (MSI 1256F)	Genaera
Suradista (FCE 26644)	Pharmacia
TPA + Captopril	Dana Farber Cancer Institute
Vitaxin II	MedImmune
Angiostatin	EntreMed
CC4047	Celgene Corporation
CC5013	Celgene Corporation
CC7085	Celgene Corporation
CDC801	Celgene Corporation
CGP-41251 (PKC412)	Novartis
CM101	CarboMed
Col-3 (Metastat)	CollaGenex
Combretastatin A-4 Prodrug	OXiGENE/Bristol-Myers Squibb
CP-564,959	OSI Pharmaceuticals
Endostatin	EntreMed
Genistein (GCP)	Amino Up
INGN 241	Introgen Therapeutics
IMC 1C11	ImClone
Interleukin-12	NCI
NM-3	ILEX Oncology
Panzem (2-methoxyestradiol)	EntreMed
PTK787A (ZK2254)	Novartis
RO317453	Hoffman-LaRoche
SMART Anti-VEGF	Protein Design Labs
Solimastat	British Biotech/Schering-Plough
SU6668	Sugen/Pharmacia
UCN-01	NCI
ZD6126	AstraZeneca
ZD6474	AstraZeneca

Source: The Angiogenesis Foundation, Cambridge, MA.

Table 3
Developing Cytotoxic and Cytostatic Drugs

Cytotoxic drugs	Cytostatic drugs
Target = tumor	Target may not be tumor
Acquired/intrinsic resistance	Resistance may not be a concern
Traditional response criteria	Need for surrogate markers
Intent to cure	Intent to delay progression
Traditional dose escalation	More may not be better
Maximum tolerated dose based on toxicity	Maximum tolerated dose based on chronicity
Short-term tolerability	Long-term tolerability
Cautious dose escalation	Rapid dose escalation

Source: Adapted from ref. *54.*

reader interpret information released in the early stages (phase I and II) of an antiangiogenic drug's development.

Traditionally, oncology drugs are evaluated based on their ability to induce complete or partial remission, an activity evaluated with serial radiographic testing or clinical examinations. Treatment response has been used as a surrogate marker for survival, the end point that probably matters most to an individual patient. Recently, other end points such as quality of life, needs for pain medication, time to tumor progression or to treatment failure have been recognized as clinically meaningful as well. Angiogenesis inhibitors target the tumor vasculature, not the cancer cells directly. Thus, the predicted biologic response is the halting or delay of further tumor growth and not necessarily tumor shrinkage on a given X-ray or computed tomography (CT) scan. Accordingly, a classical definition of tumor response may not help investigators accurately determine a drug's worthiness for further development in phase II or III studies. The use of principles originally designed to evaluate cytotoxic drugs may be inappropriate for evaluating cytostatic ones and lead to a premature discontinuation of an agent's development *(55,56)*. For this reason, an increasing emphasis is being placed on demonstrating a drug's biological efficacy at the preclinical stage of development, using surrogate markers that demonstrate that a drug is achieving its designated target or radiographic evidence that the drug is altering blood flow to a tumor through functional imaging studies. Clinical trials of an angiogenesis inhibitor should incorporate correlative studies that can help investigators accept or reject hypotheses about an agent's biological efficacy and help plan for the further development of that agent or class of drugs. Finally, the agent's biological efficacy must be correlated with easily measured parameters of clinical efficacy to show patient benefit.

Although the scientific principles of angiogenesis have been characterized for more than 30 yr, the clinical study of angiogenesis inhibitors is still at its infancy. The first antiangiogenic agents were placed into clinical trial in the early 1990s, with only preliminary knowledge of the mechanism of action of these agents, even less knowledge about required adaptations in clinical trial design, and virtually no information about safety, tolerability, and efficacy. Early clinical efforts were principally guided by experimental studies in mice showing tumor suppression and, in some cases, tumor shrinkage, following treatment with angiogenesis inhibitors. From the last decade of trial experience in over 50 different agents, it is becoming clear that antiangiogenic therapy (1) is generally safer and better tolerated than conventional cytotoxic chemotherapy, (2) results more often in disease stabilization (cytostatic effect) than tumor regression when given as monotherapy, and (3) is compatible when coadministered with standard chemotherapy agents. With regard to establishing therapeutic efficacy, there is more complexity ahead. Efforts are now underway to learn more about each agent's mechanism of action, the possibilities for matching agents with specific molecular targets found in an individual cancer patient, or newer molecularly targeted therapy. Importantly, studies have been initiated to examine patterns of failure as well as success in antiangiogenic drug development. In this way, the next generation of compounds can be designed to be more specific and effective. Also, we can determine if we need only one type of angiogenesis inhibitor or several.

Cytostatic drugs, like the angiogenesis inhibitors, challenge our traditional notions of drug development in other ways as well. Lifelong, chronic treatment using angiogenesis inhibitors may be the norm for cancer patients. Accordingly, the routes of drug administration (e.g., oral, intravenous) and dosing schedule take on new importance. Studies of chronic toxicity and compliance must be conducted. The ability of the drug to achieve its target over longer courses of therapy must be assessed as well.

The development of acquired drug resistance is an important consideration in the field of antiangiogenic therapy. The endothelial cells, because of their relative genomic stability, are thought to be less susceptible to the development of resistance compared to tumor cells. However, the redundancy of angiogenic mechanisms in both normal and neoplastic tissue makes it highly likely that resistance to antiangiogenic therapy is possible, at least to certain antiangiogenic strategies. Moreover, Kerbel and colleagues have recently demonstrated that hypoxic regions within experimental tumors may become less dependent on a vascular supply for growth *(57)*. Other studies have suggested that clonal expansion of tumor-specific endothelial cells may yield blood vessels that are resistant to certain antiangiogenic agents, such as endostatin *(58)*.

Once the longer-term safety issues of angiogenesis inhibitors and their effects on the normal vasculature are clarified, it is likely that antiangiogenic therapy will be tested in increasingly earlier disease stages and even in chemoprevention. Presently, however, virtually all agents are tested in advanced disease populations, making it difficult to tell in a negative trial whether the drug was not efficacious or if the patient population was simply too advanced for the drug to be effective. Similar challenges were faced in the early development of antibiotics for the treatment of life-threatening infections.

6. CLASSES OF ANGIOGENESIS INHIBITORS

Antiangiogenic agents can be classified according to their reported mechanism of action (Table 4). A more comprehensive list of drugs currently in various stages of clinical testing is presented in Table 2.

6.1. Growth Factor Antagonists

These agents are characterized by their antagonism of growth factor production, transport, or receptor binding. Several drugs such as suramin, interferon-α, Neovastat, IM-862 and Angiozyme suppress growth factor production *(59–61)*. Others have developed monoclonal antibodies and soluble receptors against VEGF (discussed in Section 7.1.) *(62–64)*. VEGF targeting may also suppress production of paracrine survival factors and lead to endothelial cell apoptosis *(65,66)*.

Table 4
Classes of Angiogenesis Inhibitors

Growth factor antagonists
 • Inhibition of angiogenic factor production
 • Anti-growth-factor ribozymes
 • Soluble growth factor receptors
 • Monoclonal antibodies directed against angiogenic factors
Endothelial cell signal transduction inhibition
 • Receptor tyrosine kinase inhibition
 • Protein kinase C inhibition
Inhibitors of endothelial cell proliferation
 • Cell-cycle inhibitors
Matrix Metalloproteinase (MMP) inhibition
 • Selective inhibitors of MMP-2 and MMP-9
 • Nonselective MMP inhibition
Endothelial surface marker targeting
 • Anti-integrin antibodies or cyclic peptides
Endothelial cell subpopulation inhibitors
 • Suppression of endothelial progenitor cells
Endothelial cell destruction
 • Vascular targeting agents

Source: From Li WW. Tumor angiogenesis. *Acad. Radiol.*, **7** (2000) 800–811.

6.2. Endothelial Cell Signal Transduction Inhibition

With advanced techniques in drug discovery, it is now possible to design small molecule inhibitors of endothelial cell signal transduction by interfering with ligand–receptor binding or kinase phosphorylation. Selective (against a single growth factor) and nonselective (against multiple growth factors) agents are in clinical trials. Examples of such agents include SU5416, SU6668, and ZD 6474.

6.3. Inhibitors of Endothelial Cell Proliferation

TNP-470 and squalamine are examples of drugs that inhibit endothelial cell proliferation. In the average adults, endothelial cells probably remain quiescent and, therefore, only tumor-associated vasculature is proliferating.

6.4. Matrix Metalloproteinase Inhibition

Inhibiting matrix metalloproteinase (MMP) activity interferes with both endothelial and tumor cell invasion into the extracellular matrix at primary and metastatic sites. There are at least 20 distinct enzymes in this family of proteins, of which MMP-2 and MMP-9 are thought to be most closely associated with angiogenesis *(67–69)*. Selective and nonselective MMP inhibitors are now in advanced trials, with only one agent, Neovastat, showing benefit in advanced clinical trials for non-small-cell lung cancer and renal cell carcinoma. Numerous MMP inhibitors have failed in phase III clinical trials including Marimastat, AG3349 (Prinomostat), BAY129566 (Tamomastat), and MMI270.

6.5. Endothelial Surface Marker Targeting

Tumor angiogenesis may be interrupted by targeting markers specific to the tumor vasculature such as the integrins, cell surface adhesion receptors selectively expressed

Table 5
Major Antiangiogenic Agents Being Developed for Colorectal Cancer, 2001

Drug	Phase	Sponsor
Angiozyme	I	Ribozyme Pharmaceuticals
Anti-VEGF recombinant human monoclonal antibody	III	Genentech
Avicine	III	AVI Biopharma
Celecoxib	I	Pharmacia Oncology
Combretastatin A4Prodrug	I	OXiGENE
CP1C11	I	ImClone
GBC-590	II	SafeScience
IM862	II	Cytran
ImmTher*	I	Endorex
Interferon alpha*	II	Hoffman-LaRoche
Octreotide (somatostatin)*	III	U.S. National Cancer Institute
Metastat (Col-3)	I	CollaGenex
SU5416	III	Sugen
Thalidomide*	II	Celgene Corporation

*Not pure angiogenesis inhibitors.
Source: The Angiogenesis Foundation Clinical Trials Database, 2001, Cambridge, MA.

on angiogenic endothelial cells *(70)*. In addition to anti-migratory effects, disrupting the $\alpha_v\beta_3$ integrins with monoclonal antibodies or cyclic peptides can activate the p53 tumor suppressor gene and cause endothelial cell apoptosis *(71)*. Vitaxin II (humanized LM609) and EMD121974 (cilentigitide) are two integrin antagonists in clinical development.

6.6. Suppression of Endothelial Progenitor Cells

Bone-marrow-derived endothelial progenitor cells contribute to tumor angiogenesis. The endogenous angiogenesis inhibitor angiostatin appears to target preferentially the endothelial progenitor cells over mature endothelial cells, although this molecule is thought to have other mechanism of action as well *(72)*.

7. TRIALS SPECIFIC TO COLORECTAL CANCER

Presented in Table 5 is a list of angiogenesis inhibitors being tested specifically in colorectal cancer. Most of the agents are being tested in patients with advanced disease. Many are in phase I or early phase II testing, with no published results to date. As a class of drugs, the matrix metalloproteinase (MMP) inhibitors were the first to reach phase III testing. In colorectal cancer in particular, the VEGF-based strategies are furthest along in clinical development and the available data will be discussed at length. Specifically excluded from this chapter's discussion are the agents that inhibit the epidermal growth factor receptor (EGFR), such as IMC C225 and Iressa, which belong to their own distinct therapeutic class, although some EGF receptor inhibitors may indeed possess antiangiogenic properties.

7.1. VEGF-Based Antiangiogenic Strategies

Two different anti-VEGF molecules, the recombinant monoclonal antibody to VEGF (rhuMAb VEGF or Avastin®, Genentech) and SU5416 (Semaxanib®, Pharmacia/Sugen) are being studied in patients with advanced untreated colorectal cancer, comparing conventional chemotherapy with or without the experimental agent. The preliminary phase I and II studies

Table 6
Phase II Trial of RhuMAb VEGF in Advanced Colorectal Cancer

	Control N = 36	5 mg/kg rhuMAb VEGF N = 35	10 mg/kg rhuMAb VEGF N = 33
Median time to progression (mo)	5.2	9.0 ($p = 0.005$)	7.2 ($p = 0.217$)
Median survival (mo)	13.8	>17.3 ($p = 0.083$)	16.1 ($p = 0.97$)
Response rate	17%	40% ($p = 0.03$)	24% ($p = 0.43$)

Source: ref. 76.

with these agents showed encouraging results and the field awaits the results of these ongoing phase III trials to determine if these agents improve survival, time to progression, or quality of life when compared to standard chemotherapy alone.

7.1.1. RHUMAB VEGF

rhuMAb VEGF (Avastin, Genentech) was created by combining a human immunoglobulin IgG1 framework with a murine neutralizing the antibody's VEGF-binding complementarity-determining regions *(73)*. It is a humanized monoclonal antibody that blocks the binding of all VEGF isoforms to their receptors. Anti-VEGF antibodies have been extensively studied in the laboratory and have inhibited a wide variety of tumor types, in a dose-dependent manner *(74)*. Phase I studies reported the safety and tolerability of rhuMAb VEGF in patients with advanced cancers *(75,76)*. The first, using the antibody alone, reported that of 25 patients with advanced cancers treated with doses ranging from 0.1 to 10.0 mg/kg on d 0, 28, 35, and 42, no dose-limiting toxicities were observed. Gordon and colleagues described minor elevations in subjects' blood pressure and two cases of serious bleeding at the 3.0-mg/kg dose that appear to have been disease related rather than drug related. No patients developed antibodies to rhuMAb VEGF during the 70-d study period. Although no objective responses were seen, there were two minor responses and disease stabilization was noted, consistent with cytostatic activity. The second trial, reported by Margolin et al., evaluated weekly doses of rhuMAb VEGF given concurrently with each of four different cytotoxic chemotherapy regimens. One cohort of four patients received 500 mg/m^2 fluorouracil (5-FU) with 20 mg/m^2 leucovorin (LV) weekly, for 6 wk out of 8 wk. There were no observed drug–drug interactions between the antibody and the chemotherapy agents (on any arm) and no bleeding or thrombotic events were seen. Of the four colorectal cancer patients treated, one received the equivalent of 40 total doses of rhuMAb VEGF and five 6-wk cycles of chemotherapy before disease progression occurred.

Based on these encouraging results, a randomized phase II trial was conducted comparing 5-FU/LV alone (doses of 500 mg/m^2 5-FU and 500 mg/m^2 LV given weekly for 6 wk out of 8 wk) to 5-FU/LV with low dose (5 mg/kg) rhuMAb VEGF to 5FU/LV with higher dose antibody (10 mg/kg) *(77)*. One hundred four patients with untreated advanced colorectal cancer were enrolled, with results (Table 6) showing that patients treated with both 5-FU/LV and rhuMAb VEGF had a statistically significant improvement in response rate and time to tumor progression, with a trend toward an increased survival. With longer follow-up, the survival advantage may become significant. The principal safety concern in this small trial was for thrombotic events, as 9% of the patients treated with chemotherapy alone

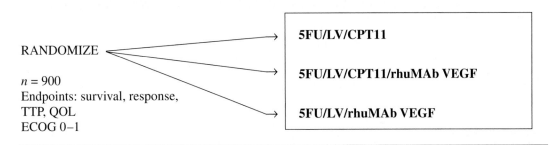

RANDOMIZE

n = 900
Endpoints: survival, response,
TTP, QOL
ECOG 0–1

5FU/LV/CPT11

5FU/LV/CPT11/rhuMAb VEGF

5FU/LV/rhuMAb VEGF

experienced such events, compared to 26% of the patients receiving 5 mg/kg rhuMAb VEGF and 13% of the patients receiving 10 mg/kg of the antibody (only some thromboses were classified as grade 3 or 4 adverse events). The relationship between dose and efficacy or dose and thromboses, if any, is not yet clear. However, based on these encouraging results, two larger trials are now underway (Table 7), comparing chemotherapy alone with chemotherapy plus rhuMAb VEGF in patients with advanced, untreated colorectal cancer.

7.1.2. SU5416

SU5416 (Semaxanib, Pharmacia/Sugen) is a selective inhibitor of the tyrosine kinase activity of the flk-1/KDR receptor binding to VEGF *(78)*. The drug competes directly with ATP at the intracellular kinase domain of flk-1/KDR, preventing tyrosine phosphorylation and effective transduction of the extracellular signal *(79)*. This agent was also found to be effective against a broad range of tumor types in vitro. Sixty-nine patients with advanced cancers were enrolled in the first phase I trial of SU5416 *(80)*. Two objective responses were seen, and 12 patients had stable disease for greater than 90 d. The drug was well tolerated, with observed toxicities including mild–moderate headaches, nausea, and vomiting (more severe forms of which were dose limiting). Thrombotic events were also seen, two of which were fatal, but the relationship to the antiangiogenic drug remains unclear. With more than 600 patients worldwide now having received SU5416, alone or with various conventional chemotherapy agents, the incidence of clotting events appears below that which is reported for all cancer patients *(81–83)*. Because clotting events were noted and because SU5416 requires intravenous administration through a central venous access device, patients in subsequent studies have been placed on prophylactic low-dose (1 mg) warfarin to reduce the incidence of catheter-related deep venous thromboses *(84–86)*.

Promising results from the phase I trial combined with preclinical studies showing that the combination of cytotoxic chemotherapy with SU5416 in colorectal cancer models was superior to either agent alone, led to a second phase I trial in patients with advanced and untreated colorectal cancer *(87,88)*. In that study, 28 patients received 5-FU/LV on either the Mayo Clinic or Roswell Park chemotherapy regimens. Patients were able to tolerate full doses of all agents given simultaneously, with no observed drug–drug interactions. Results showed no adverse effects on response rate and some evidence for improved time to disease progression and overall survival (first column in Table 8). This was not a randomized trial, so comparison with chemotherapy alone was made with historical controls. The small number of patients is another limiting factor in the interpretation of these results.

To place these results in context, this group of 28 patients has been compared with 1000 randomized subsets of 28 patients from a large (600+ patient) multicenter phase III trial's

Table 8
Phase I/II Trial of SU5416/5-FU/LV in Advanced Colorectal Cancer
(Compared to Historical Controls with 5-FU/LV and 5-FU/LV/CPT11)

End Point	SU-5416/ 5-FU/LV[a]	CPT-11/ 5-FU/LV[b]	5-FU/LV[b]
Overall RR (%)	35.7	60.7	28.6
95% CI	18.0–54.0	42.6–78.8	11.9–45.3
Median TTP (mo)	9.0	9.3	5.1
95% CI	7.2–10.2	6.4–12.1	3.2–6.9
Median survival (mo)	22.6	26.4	16.2
95% CI	18.8+	18.7–34.1	11.3–21.0

[a]Phase I/II study ($N = 28$).
[b]Means from 1000 random subsets ($N = 28$) from phase III study.
Source: ref. *89.*

irinotecan (CPT-11)/5-FU/LV and 5-FU/LV arms *(90).* To match for critical prognostic factors, subsets from the phase III study were chosen with the same baseline performance status (PS) and LDH distribution as in the pilot 5-FU/LV/SU5416 trial *(91).* The results depicted in Table 8 demonstrate the potential for SU5416-mediated tumor growth delay. The median time to tumor progression (TTP) with 5-FU/LV/SU5416 was similar to that of the now standard combination 5-FU/LV/CPT11 and was improved relative to the TTP seen with 5-FU/LV alone. The median survival with the small group of 5-FU/LV/SU5416 patients has not yet been reached at this writing and approaches the median survival seen in the randomized subsets of patients treated with 5-FU/LV/CPT11 and exceeds the survival of those treated with 5-FU/LV alone.

Two phase III trials are now underway (Table 9). The first compares 5-FU/LV, administered on the Roswell Park schedule, with or without SU5416 in patients with advanced, untreated colorectal cancer. This trial, begun in early 2000, has nearly completed accrual. However, because of the change in practice patterns in many countries to adopt 5-FU/LV/CPT11 as the standard of care for this patient population, a second phase III trial has been initiated comparing this combination with or without SU5416.

The emergence of yet other new molecularly targeted and traditional therapies and their impact on the standard of care in colorectal cancer and for clinical trial design is yet another challenge faced by developers of antiangiogenic drugs.

8. CONCLUSION

Three years have passed since the *New York Times* article prompted so much interest by the public, the oncology community, and the pharmaceutical industry in angiogenesis inhibition as a new approach to cancer therapy. Although extensive basic laboratory work has been conducted in this field, relatively little is known about the therapeutic effects of angiogenesis inhibitors in cancer patients and how to optimize any clinical benefit. Phase III trials of several agents are nearly completed in colorectal cancer and there is reason for optimism that early promising results from phase I and II trials will be validated in the larger, randomized, controlled setting. Even if they are not, various groups are already beginning to piece together patterns of failure with patterns of success, so that the current experience in antiangiogenic drug development will be analyzed to advance the field's next-generation agents and to bring direct benefit to the patient. Based on the progress made so far, both

Table 9
Phase III Trials of SU5416 in Advanced Untreated Colorectal Cancer

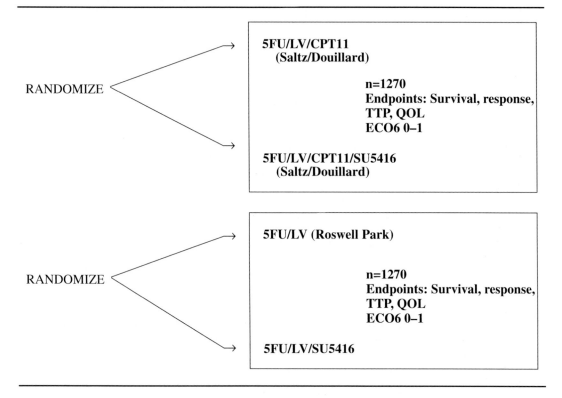

participants and followers of the angiogenesis field can anticipate the future treatment of colorectal cancer to incorporate new strategies aimed at the tumor vasculature.

REFERENCES

1. Kolata G. HOPE IN THE LAB: A special report; a cautious awe greets drugs that eradicate tumors in mice, *New York Times*, May 3, 1998.
2. Shweiki D, Itin A, Soffer D, et al. Vascular endothelial growth factor induced by hypoxia may mediate hypoxia-initiated angiogenesis. *Nature*, **359** (1992) 843–845.
3. Veikkola T, Karkkainen M, Claesson-Welsh L, and Alitalo K. Regulation of angiogenesis via vascular endothelial growth factor receptors. *Cancer Res.*, **60** (2000) 203–212.
4. Asahara T, Murohara T, Sullivan A., et al. Isolation of putative progenitor endothelial cells for angiogenesis. *Science*, **275** (1997) 964–967.
5. Waltenberger J, Claesson-Welsh L, Siegbahn A, Shibuya M, and Heldin C.-H. Different signal transduction properties of KDR and Flt-1, two receptors for vascular endothelial growth factor. *J. Biol. Chem.*, **269** (1994) 26,988–26,995.
6. Landgren E, Schiller P, Cao Y, and Claesson-Welsh L. Placenta growth factor stimulates MAP kinase and mitogenicity but not phospholipase C-g and migration of endothelial cells expressing Flt-1. *Oncogene*, **16** (1998) 359–367.
7. D'Angelo G, Struman I, Martial J, and Winer RI. Activation of mitogen-activated proteinase kinases by vascular endothelial growth factor and basic fibroblast growth factor in capillary endothelial cells is inhibited by the antiangiogenic factor 16-kDa N-terminal fragment of prolactin. *Proc. Natl. Acad. Sci. USA*, **92** (1995) 6374–6378.
8. Nor JE, Christensen J, Mooney DJ, and Polverini PJ. Vascular endothelial growth factor (VEGF)-mediated angiogenesis is associated with enhanced endothelial cell survival and induction of Bcl-2 expression. *Am. J. Pathol.*, **154** (1999) 375–384.

9. O'Conner DS, Schechner JS, Adida C, et al. Control of apotosis during angiogenesis by surviving expression in endothelial cells. *Am. J. Pathol.*, **156** (2000) 393–398.

10. Kim I, Kim HG, So J-N, Kim JH, Kwak HJ, and Koh GY. Angiopoietin-1 regulates endothelial cell survival through the phosphatidylinositol 3'-kinase/Akt signal transduction pathway. *Circ. Res.*, **86** (2000) 24–29.

11. Paku S and Paweletz N. First steps of tumor-related angiogenesis. *Lab. Invest.*, **65** (1991) 334–346.

12. Pattersson A, Nagy JA, Brown LF, et al. Heterogeneity of the angiogenic response induced in different normal adult tissues by vascular permeability factor/vascular endothelial growth factor. *Lab. Invest.*, **80** (2000) 99–115.

13. Djonov V, Schmid M, Tschanz SA, and Burri PH. Intussusceptive angiogenesis: its role in embryonic vascular network formation. *Circ. Res.*, **86** (2000) 286–292.

14. Patan S, Munn LL, and Jain RK. Intussusceptive microvascular growth in a human colon adenocarcinoma xenograft: a novel mechanism of tumor angiogenesis. *Microvasc. Res.*, **51** (1996) 260–272.

15. Metzger RJ and Krasnow MA. Genetic control of branching morphogenesis. *Science*, **284** (1999) 1635–1639.

16. Ausprunk D and Folkman J. Migration and proliferation of endothelial cells in preformed and newly formed blood vessels during tumor angiogenesis. *Microvasc. Res.*, **14** (1977) 43–65.

17. Pepper MS, Ferrara N, Orci L, and Montesano R. Vascular endothelial growth factor (VEGF) induces plasminogen activators and plasminogen activator inhibitor-1 in microvascular endothelial cells. *Biochem. Biophys. Res. Commun.*, **181** (1991) 902–906.

18. Zetter BR. Migration of capillary endothelial cells is stimulated by tumor-derived factors. *Nature*, **285** (1980) 41–43.

19. Asahara T, Chem D, Takahashi T, et al. Tie2 receptor ligands, angiopoietin-1 and angiopoietin-2, modulated VEGF-induced postnatal neovascularization. *Circ. Res.*, **83** (1998) 233–240.

20. Maisonpierre PC, Suri C, Jones PF, et al. Angiopoietin-2, a natural antagonist for Tie2 that disrupts in vivo angiogenesis. *Science*, **277** (1997) 55–60.

21. Friedlander M, Brooks PC, Shaffer RW, Kincaid CM, Varner JA, and Cheresh DA. Definition of two angiogenic pathways by distinct alpha v integrins. *Science*, **270** (1995) 1500–1502.

22. Brooks PC, Montgomery AM, Rosenfeld M, et al. Integrin alpha v beta 3 antagonists promote tumor regression by inducing apoptosis of angiogenic blood vessels. *Cell*, **79** (1994) 1157–1164.

23. Nelson AR, Fingleton B, Rothenberg ML, and Martrisian LM. Matrix metalloproteinases: biologic activity and clinical implications. *J. Clin. Oncol.*, **18** (2000) 1135–1149.

24. Sang QXA. Complex role of matrix metalloproteinases in angiogenesis. *Cell Res.*, **8** (1998) 171–177.

25. Nangio-Makker P, Honjo Y, Sarvis R, et al. Galectin-3 induces endothelial cell morphogenesis and angiogenesis. *Am. J. Pathol.*, **156** (2000) 899–909.

26. Gamble J, Meyer G, Noack L, et al. B1 integrin activation inhibits in vitro tube formation: effects of cell migration, vacuole coalescence and lumen formation. *Endothelium*, **7** (1999) 23–34.

27. Yang S, Graham J, Kahn J, Schwartz EA, and Gerritsen ME. Functional roles for PECAM-1 (CD31) and VE-cadherin (CD144) in tube assembly and lumen formation in three-dimensional collagen gels. *Am. J. Pathol.*, **155** (1999) 887–895.

28. Meyer GT, Matthias LJ, Noack L, Vadas MA, and Gamble JR. Lumen formation during angiogenesis in vitro involves phagocytic activity, formation and secretion of vacuoles, cell death, and capillary tube remodeling by different populations of endothelial cells. *Anat. Rec.*, **249** (1997) 327–340.

29. Maniotis AJ, Folberg R, Hess A, et al. Vascular channel formation by human melanoma cells in vivo and in vitro: vasculogenic mimicry. *Am. J. Pathol.*, **155** (1999) 739–752.

30. McDonald DM, Munn L, and Jain RK. Vasculogenic mimicry: how convincing, how novel and how significant? *Am. J. Pathol.*, **156** (2000) 383–388.

31. Wang HU, Chen ZF, and Anderson DJ. Molecular distinction and angiogenic interaction between embryonic arteries and veins revealed by ephrin-B2 and its receptor Eph-B4. *Cell*, **93** (1998) 741–753.

32. Adams RH, Wilkinson GA, Weiss C, et al. Roles of ephrinB ligands and EphB receptors in cardiovascular development: demarcation of arterial/venous domains, vascular morphogenesis, and sprouting angiogenesis. *Genes Dev.*, **13** (1999) 295–306.

33. Yancopoulos GD, Klagsbrun M, and Folkman J. Vasculogenesis, angiogenesis and growth factors: ephrins enter the fray at the border. *Cell*, **93** (1998) 661–664.

34. Mellitzer G, Xu Q, and Wilkinson DG. Eph receptors and ephrins restrict cell intermingling and communication. *Nature*, **400** (1999) 77–81.

35. Adams RH, Wilkinson GA, Weiss C, et al. Roles of ephrinB ligands and EphB receptors in cardiovascular development: demarcation of arterial/venous domains, vascular morphogenesis, and sprouting angiogenesis. *Genes Dev.*, **13** (1999) 295–306.

36. Folkman J and D'Amore PA. Blood formation: what is its molecular basis? *Cell*, **87** (1996) 1153–1155.

37. Darland DC and D'Amore PA. Blood vessel maturation: vascular development comes of age. *J. Clin. Invest.*, **103** (1999) 157–158.

38. Hayes AJ, Huang WQ, Mallah J, Yang D, Lippman ME, and Li LY. Angiopoietin-1 and its receptor Tie-2 participate in the regulation of capillary-like tubule formation and survival of endothelial cells. *Microvasc. Res.*, **58** (1999) 224–237.

39. Antonelli-Orlidge A, Saunders KB, Smith SR, and D'Amore PA. An activated form of transforming growth factor beta is produced by cocultures of endothelial cells and pericytes. *Proc. Natl. Acad. Sci. USA*, **86** (1989) 4544–4548.

40. Maisonpierre PC, Suri C, Jones PF, et al. Angiopoietin-2, a natural antagonist for Tie2 that disrupts in vivo angiogenesis. *Science*, **277** (1997) 55–60.

41. Engel CJ, Bennett ST, Chambers AF, Doig GS, Kerkvliet N, and O'Malley FP. Tumor angiogenesis predicts recurrence in invasive colorectal cancer when controlled for Dukes staging. *Am. J. Surg. Pathol.*, **20** (1996) 1260–1265.

42. Saclarides TJ. Angiogenesis in colorectal cancer. In *New and Controverial Issues in the Management of Colorectal Diseases.* 1997, vol. 77, pp. 253–260.

43. Pietra N, Sarli L, Caruana P, Cabras A, Costi R, Gobbi S, et al. Is tumour angiogenesis a prognostic factor in patients with colorectal cancer and no involved nodes? *Eur. J. Surg.*, **166** (2000) 552–556.

44. Takahashi YT, Tucker SL, Kitadai Y, et al. Vessel counts and expression of vacular endothelial growth factors as prognostic factors in node-negative colon cancer. *Arch. Surg.*, **132** (1997) 541–546.

45. Dirix LY, Vermeulen PB, Hubens G, et al. Serum basic fibroblast growth factor and vascular endothelial growth factor and tumour growth kinetics in advanced colorectal cancer. *Ann. Oncol.*, **7** (1996) 843–848.

46. Hyodo I, Doi T, Endo H, et al. Clinical significance of plasma vascular endothelial growth factor in gastrointestinal cancer. *Eur. J. Cancer*, **34** (1998) 2041–2045.

47. Broll R, Erdmann H, Duchrow M, Oevermann E, Schwandner O, Market U, et al. Vascular endothelial growth factor (VEGF)—a valuable serum tumour marker in patients with colorectal cancer? *Eur. J. Surg. Oncol.*, **27** (2001) 37–42.

48. Kondo Y, Aril S, Furutani M, Isigami S-I, Mori A, Onodera H, et al. Implication of vascular endothelial growth factor and p53 status for angiogenesis in noninvasive colorectal carcinoma. *Cancer*, **88** (2000) 1820–1827.

49. Steinbach G, Lynch PM, Phillips RK, Wallace MH, Hawk E, Gordon GB, et al. The effect of celecoxib, a cyclooxygenase-2 inhibitor, in familial adenomatous polyposis. *N. Engl. J. Med.*, **342(26)** (2000) 1946–1952.

50. Gallo O, Franchi A, Magnelli L, Sardi I, Vannacci A, Boddi V, et al. Cyclooxygenase-2 pathway correlates with VEGF expression in head and neck cancer. *Neoplasia*, **3(1)** (2001) 53–61.

51. Masferrer JL, Leahy KM, Koki AT, Zweifel BS, Settle SL, Woerner BM, et al. Antiangiogenic and antitumor activities of cyclooxygenase-1 inhibitors. *Cancer Res.*, **60(5)** (2000) 1306–1311.

52. Zebrowski BK, Liu W, Ramirez K, Akagi Y, Mills GB, and Ellis LM. Markedly elevated levels of vascular endothelial growth factor in malignant ascites. *Ann. Surg. Oncol.*, **6** (1999) 373–378.

53. White CW, Sondheimer HM, Crouch EC, Wilson H, and Fan LL. Treatment of pulmonary hemangiomatosis with recombinant interferon alpha-2a. *N. Engl. J. Med.*, **320** (1989) 1197–1200.

54. Carter SK. Clinical strategy for the development of angiogenesis inhibitors. *Oncologist*, **5(Suppl. 1)** (2000) 51–54.

55. Thompson WD, Li WW, and Maragoudakis M. The clinical manipulation of angiogenesis: pathology, side-effects, surprises, and opportunities with novel human therapies. *J. Pathol.*, **187** (1999) 503–510.

56. Li WW, Li VW, and Casey R. Clinical trials of angiogenesis-based therapies: overview and new guiding principles. In *Angiogenesis: Models, Modulators, and Clinical Applications.* Maragoudakis M (ed.), New York, Plenum, 1998, pp. 475–492.

57. Yu JL, Rak JW, Carmeliet P, Nagy A, Kerbel RS, and Coomber BL. Heterogenous vascular dependence of tumor cell populations. *Am. J. Pathol.*, **158** (2001) 1325–1334.

58. Boye E, Yu Y, Paranya G, Mulliken JB, Olsen BR, and Bischoff J. Clonality and altered behavior of endothelial cells from hemangiomas. *J. Clin. Invest.*, **107** (2001) 745–752.

59. Dinney CP, Bielenberg DR, Perrotte P, et al. Inhibition of basic fibroblast growth factor expression, angiogenesis, and growth of human bladder carcinoma in mice by systemic interferon-alpha administration. *Cancer Res.*, **58** (1998) 808–814.

60. Takano S, Gately S, Neville ME, et al. Suramin, an anticancer and angiosuppressive agent, inhibits endothelial cell binding of basic fibroblast growth factor, migration, proliferation, and reduction of urokinase-type plasminogen activator. *Cancer Res.*, **54** (1994) 2654–2660.

61. Sandberg JA, Bouhana KS, Gallegos AM, et al. Pharmacokinetics of an antiangiogenic ribozyme (ANGIO-ZYME) in the mouse. *Antisense Nucleic Acid Drug Dev.*, **9** (1999) 271–277.

62. Li CY, Shan S, Huang Q, et al. Initial stages of tumor cell-induced angiogenesis: evaluation via skin window chambers in rodent models. *J. Natl. Cancer Inst.*, **92** (2000) 143–147.

63. Borgstrom P, Gold DP, Hillan KJ, and Ferrara N. Importance of VEGF for breast cancer angiogenesis in vivo: implications from intravital microscopy of combination treatments with an anti-VEGF neutralizing monoclonal antibody and doxorubicin. *Anticancer Res.*, **19** (1999) 4203–4214.

64. Roeckl W, Hecht D, Sztajer H, Waltenberger J, Yayon A, and Weich HA. Differential binding characteristics and cellular inhibition by soluble VEGF receptors 1 and 2. *Exp. Cell Res.*, **241** (1998) 161–170.

65. Nor JE, Christensen J, Mooney DJ, and Polverini PJ. Vascular endothelial growth factor (VEGF)-mediated angiogenesis is associated with enhanced endothelial cell survival and induction of Bcl-2 expression. *Am. J. Pathol.*, **154** (1999) 375–384.

66. O'Conner DS, Schechner JS, Adida C, et al. Control of apotosis during angiogenesis by surviving expression in endothelial cells. *Am. J. Pathol.*, **156** (2000) 393–398.

67. Nelson AR, Fingleton B, Rothenberg ML, and Martrisian LM. Matrix metalloproteinases: biologic activity and clinical implications. *J. Clin. Oncol.*, **18** (2000) 1135–1149.

68. Itoh T, Tanioka M, Yoshida H, Yoshioka T, Nishimoto H, and Itohara S. Reduced angiogenesis and tumor progression in gelatinase A-deficient mice. *Cancer Res.*, **58** (1998) 1048–1051.

69. Vu TH, Shipley JM, Bergers G, et al. MMP-9/gelatinase B is a key regulator of growth plate angiogenesis and apoptosis of hypertrophic chondrocytes. *Cell*, **93** (1998) 411–422.

70. Gaincotti FG and Ruoslahti E. Integrin signaling. *Science*, **285** (1999) 1028–1032.

71. Cheresh DA. Death to a blood vessel, death to a tumor. *Nat. Med.*, **4** (1998) 395–396.

72. Ito H, Rovira II, Bloom ML, Takeda K, Ferrans VJ, Quyyumi AA, et al. Endothelial progenitor cells as putative targets for angiostatin. *Cancer Res.*, **59** (1999) 5875–5877.

73. Kim KJ, Li B, Houck K, et al. The vascular endothelial growth factor proteins: Identification of biologically relevant regions by neutralizing monoclonal antibodies. *Growth Factors*, **7** (1992) 53–64.

74. Kim K, Li B, Winer J, et al. Inhibition of vascular endothelial growth factor-induced angiogenesis suppresses tumour growth in vivo. *Nature*, **362** (1993) 841–844.

75. Gordon MS, Margolin K, Talpaz M, Sledge GW Jr, Holmgren E, Benjamin R, et al. Phase I safety and pharmacokinetic study of recombinant human anti-vascular endothelial growth factor in patients with advanced cancer. *J. Clin. Onc.*, **19** (2001) 843–850.

76. Margolin K, Gordon MS, Holmgren E, Gaudreault J, Novotny W, Fyfe G, et al. Phase Ib trial of intravenous recombinant humanized monoclonal antibody to vascular endothelial growth factor in combination with chemotherapy in patients with advanced cancer: pharmacologic and long-term safety data. *J. Clin. Onc.*, **19** (2001) 851–856.

77. Bergsland E, Hurwitz H, Fehrenbacher L, Meropol NJ, Novotny WF, Gaudreault J, et al. A randomized phase II trial comparing rhuMAb VEGF (recombinant humanized monoclonal antibody to vascular endothelial cell growth factor) plus 5-fluorouracil/leucovorin (FU/LV) to FU/LV alone in patients with metastatic colorectal cancer. *Am. Soc. Clin. Sci.*, **19:242a** (2000) 939 (abstract).

78. Fong TAT, Shawver LK, Sun L, et al. SU5416 is a potent and selective inhibitor of the vascular endothelial growth factor receptor (Flk-1/KDR) that inhibits tyrosine kinase catalysis, tumor vascularization, and growth of multiple tumor types. *Cancer Res.*, **59** (1999) 99–106.

79. Mendel DB, Laird AD, Smolich BD, et al. Development of SU5416, a selective small molecule inhibitor of VEGF receptor tyrosine kinase activity, as an angiogenesis agent. *Anticancer Drug Des.*, **15** (2000) 29–41.

80. Rosen LS, Kabbinavar F, Rosen P, Mulay M, Quigley S, and Hannah AL. Phase I trial of SU5416. A novel angiogenesis inhibitor in patients with advanced malignancies. *Proc. Amer. Soc. Oncol.* (1998) 218a.

81. Levine M, Hirsh J, Gent M, et al. Double-blind randomized trial of a very-low-dose warfarin for prevention of thromboembolism in stage IV breast cancer. *Lancet*, **343(8902)** (1994) 886–889.

82. Bern MM, Lokich JJ, Wallach SR, et al. Very low doses of warfarin can prevent thrombosis in central venous catheters. A randomized prospective trial. *Ann. Intern. Med.*, **112(6)** (1990) 423–428.

83. Monreal M, Alastrue A, Rull M, et al. Upper extremity deep venous thrombosis in cancer patients with venous access devices—prophylaxis with a low molecular weight heparin (Fragmin) *Thromb. Haemost.*, **75(2)** (1996) 251–253.

84. Kamphaus GD, Colorado PC, Panka DJ, Hopfer H, Ramchandran R, Torre A, et al. Canstatin, a novel matrix-derived inhibitor of angiogenesis and tumor growth. *J. Biol. Chem.*, **275** (2000) 1209–1215; Lucas R, Holmgren L, Garcia I, et al. Multiple forms of angiostatin induce apoptosis in endothelial cells. *Blood*, **92** (1998) 4730–4741.

85. Lucas R, Holmgren L, Garcia I, et al. Multiple forms of angiostatin induce apoptosis in endothelial cells. *Blood*, **92** (1998) 4730–4741.

86. Dhanabal M, Ramchandran R, Waterman JM, et al. Endostatin induces endothelial cell apoptosis. *J. Biol. Chem.*, **274** (1999) 11,721–11,726.

87. SU5416 Investigator brochure, SUGEN, Inc., South San Francisco, CA.

88. Rosen, P, Amado R, Hecht JR, Chang D, Mulay M, Parson M, et al. A phase I/II study of SU5416 in combination with 5-FU/leucovorin in patients with metastatic colorectal cancer. *Am. Soc. Clin. Oncol.*, **19** (2000) 3a (abstract).

89. Miller LL, Elfring GL, Hannah AL, Allred R, Scigalla P, and Rosen LS. Efficacy results of a phase I/II study of SU5416 (S)/5-fluorouracil (F)/leucovorin (L) relative to results in random subsets of similar patients (Pts) from a phase III study of irinotecan (C)/F/L or F/L alone in the therapy of previously untreated metastatic colorectal cancer (MCRC). *Am. Soc. Clin. Oncol.*, **20** (2001) 144a (abstract).

90. Saltz LB, Box JV, Blanke C, Rosen LS, Fehrnabacher L, Moore MJ, et al. for the Irinotecan Study Group. Irinotecan plus fluorouracil and leucovorin for metastatic colorectal cancer. *N. Eng. J. Med.*, **343** (2000) 905–914.

40

Selected Targets and Rationally Designed Therapeutics for Patients with Colorectal Cancer

Future Drug Development

Eric K. Rowinsky

CONTENTS

1. INTRODUCTION

There have been clear improvements in the outcome of patients with colorectal cancer, largely the result of the adjuvant use of "nonselective" cytotoxic chemotherapeutics such as the fluoropyrimidines and the recent development and incorporation of new classes of "nonselective" cytotoxic agents (e.g., topoisomerase I inhibitors) into conventional treatment regimens. However, the overall clinical impact of these therapeutics has been modest and a point of "diminishing returns" has been reached.

Among the many new types of rationally designed agents are therapeutics targeting various strategic facets of growth signal transduction, malignant angiogenesis, survival, metastasis, and cell-cycle regulation. However, because the most common antitumor effects noted following targeting of these processes in preclinical studies is a decreased rate of tumor growth, the predominant clinical outcome of treatment is likely to be delayed tumor growth. This may not be readily detected or quantified using the methodologies traditionally used in early nonrandomized studies of nonselective cytotoxics *(1)*. Additionally, the results of preclinical studies of these therapeutics suggest that dose–toxicity relationships are not likely to be as steep as with nonselective cytotoxics, indicating that these agents may be usable with less toxicity. Therefore, both regulatory and clinical practice end points such as

From: *Colorectal Cancer: Multimodality Management*
Edited by: L. Saltz © Humana Press Inc., Totowa, NJ

increased time to progression and improvements in disease-related symptoms and quality of life, which are generally considered secondary end points, may evolve into primary end points for target-based therapeutics. The evaluation of these agents will likely require radical departure from the traditional paradigms in order to realize their full potential. At this time, it is difficult to predict which targets and associated therapeutic candidates will yield the most promising results in the treatment of colorectal cancer. This chapter will discuss several of the most promising targets for therapeutic development, particularly those related to cancer self-sufficiency, growth signal transduction, and evasion of cell death.

2. TARGETING "SELF-SUFFICIENCY" IN GROWTH SIGNALING

Normal cells require mitogenic signals before they can transition from a quiescent state to an active proliferating state. These signals are transmitted into cells by transmembrane receptors that bind distinct classes of signaling ligands such as diffusible growth factors, extracellular matrix components, and cell-to-cell adhesion/interaction molecules. Unlike normal cells, which cannot proliferate in the absence of exogenous stimulatory signals, cancer cells have activated oncogenes and other aberrant components that lead to mimicking of normal growth signaling *(2)*. In essence, cancer cells generate many of their own growth signals, thereby reducing dependence on stimulation from the microenvironment and disrupting a homeostatic mechanism that operates to ensure the proper behavior of the various cell types in any given tissue. Growth signaling pathways may be dysregulated in most human tumors *(2–4)*. Human colon cancer is perhaps the best studied tumor with regard to dysregulated signaling and oncogenic mutations that confer self-sufficiency.

2.1. The ErbB Growth Factor Receptor Family as a Target

2.1.1. GENERAL RELEVANCE

Binding of growth factors to their receptors induces receptor activation, initiating or modifying signal transduction processes. These growth-regulating molecules and their receptors modulate cell proliferation and differentiation in normal tissues. In many malignancies, including colorectal cancer, growth factors or their receptors are overexpressed or aberrantly expressed. Such abnormal stimulation of growth factor signaling pathways results in unregulated cell signaling, which contributes to growth dysregulation, tumor initiation/promotion, and metastases. The degree to which tumors capitalize on these signaling pathways is illustrated by the large number of oncogenes related to cellular genes encoding growth factors (e.g., *sis*, *hst*), growth factor receptors (kit, trk, ErbB2), and tyrosine *kinases (abl, src, lck) (5).*

The ErbB growth factor receptor family is the best characterized of the tumor-related growth factor receptor families. Epidermal growth factor (EGF) receptor (EGFR; also know as ErbB1 or HER1) is one of four members of the ErbB family that also includes ErbB2 *(neu* or HER2), ErbB3 (HER3), and ErbB4 (HER4) *(6)*. All members of the ErbB family, particularly ErbB1 and ErbB2, are expressed by human colorectal cancer; however, the relative expression and functional importance of each type of receptor is unclear. Following ligand binding, all ErbB receptors, except ErbB3, undergo either homodimerization or preferential heterodimerization with other members of the ErbB receptor family, autophosphorylation, and activation of the receptor tyroisine kinase (TK) (RTK) (Fig. 1). These events lead to signal transduction through multiple intracellular pathways, resulting in the transcription of genes that modulate proliferation, survival, angiogenesis, motility, and invasion.

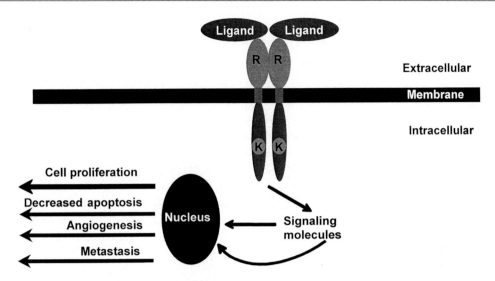

Fig. 1. The epidermal growth factor receptor (EGFR). The EGFR is a 170-kDa membrane-spanning glycoprotein composed of an extracellular ligand-binding domain, a transmembrane region, and a cytoplasmic TK domain. Binding of specific ligands, such as EGF and TGF-α, to the extracellular domain results in EGFR autophosphorylation, activation of the receptor TK, and initiation of various signal transduction events that lead to gene transcription in the nucleus and stimulation of proliferative, antiapoptotic, metastatic, and angiogenic events.

The EGFR is the best characterized ErbB receptor. The EGFR gene encodes a 170-kDa membrane-spanning glycoprotein composed of an extracellular ligand-binding domain, a transmembrane region, and a cytoplasmic TK domain. Binding of specific ligands, such as EGF, to the extracellular domain results in EGFR autophosphorylation, activation of the receptor's cytoplasmic TK domain, and initiation of multiple signaling events that lead to gene transcription.

The EGFR is expressed on the cell surface of many normal tissues, and elevated numbers of receptors (overexpression) have been detected on colorectal cancers and other epidermoid malignancies. EGFR expression or overexpression has been documented in 25–77% of human colon cancers *(7,8)*. With regard to the clinical relevance of EGFR expression in patients with colorectal cancer, the percentage of EGFR-expressing cells has been inversely related to prognosis *(8)*. Similarly, EGFR expression has been inversely related to sensitivity to chemotherapy and survival in patients with many other types of epidermoid malignancies.

2.1.2. EGFR and EGFR Ligands

Ligands for EGFR include EGF, transforming growth factor-α (TGF-α), amphiregulin, heparin binding EGF, and betacellulin *(7)*. EGFR and TGF-α appear to be the principal endogenous ligands that result in EGFR-mediated stimulation, although TGF-α may be more important in promoting angiogenesis *(9)*. EGFR overexpression renders tumor cells more sensitive to low concentrations of growth factors *(10)*. Ligands can be secreted by tumors in an autocrine manner and many cancers depend on EGFR stimulation for survival and proliferation. These observations support the concept that ligand binding to EGFR and subsequent TK activation may play a role in tumor promotion and progression *(11)*.

Consequently, inhibition of EGFR expression and/or function may potentially block one or more critical events in the growth and progression of tumors.

2.1.3. Cell Survival and Apoptosis

In addition to modulating proliferation, experimental data indicate that the EGFR pathway regulates cell survival. Many EGFR-expressing tumors depend on EGF or TGF-α stimulation for survival. In some cell lines that overexpress, EGF has been demonstrated to prevent apoptosis and promote survival *(12)*, which may be the result of cross-talk between pathways such as the PI3K survival pathway *(see* Section 2.2.2.) *(4)*. Furthermore, EGF stimulation has been shown to protect against apoptosis triggered by Fas, a cell death receptor activated by many types of cytotoxic agents *(13)*. In contrast, inhibition of EGFR through anti-EGFR antibodies, receptor tyrosine kinase (RTK) inhibitors, and EGFR antisense oligonucleotides (ASONs) induce arrest in the G1 phase of the cell cycle and apoptosis in human cancer cell lines and xenografts, including those derived from human colorectal carcinoma *(12–18)*.

2.1.4. Angiogenesis

Experimental data suggest that both EGF and EGFR play roles in angiogenesis. Coexpression of TGF-α and EGFR is highly correlated with microvessel density *(19)*, and TGF-α promotes expression of vascular endothelial growth factor (VEGF) that induces proliferation and permeability of blood vessels *(20,21)*. In patients with stages I–III non-small-cell lung cancer, gender, nodal status, stage, tumor size, microvessel count, and EGFR overexpression are independent determinants of survival, with a lower probability in patients whose tumors express high levels of amphiregulin and have high microvessel counts *(22)*. Conversely, blocking EGF binding by treating cells with anti-EGFR antibodies (e.g., IMC-C225; Imclone) and RTK inhibitors block malignant angiogenesis, as manifested in vitro by decreased production of VEGF, interleukin-9 (IL-9), and basic fibroblast growth factor (bFGF), and in vivo by tumor regression, inhibition of metastases, and reduced formation of microvessels *(23,24)*.

2.1.5. Cell Motility and Metastases

The epidermal growth factor receptor is involved in regulating tumor cell motility and metastases. Treatment of EGFR-transfected tumor cells in vitro with TGF-α increases cell motility, whereas treatment with EGF leads to invasiveness. EGF has also been demonstrated to enhance the motility of cancer cells in a concentration-dependent manner in vitro *(25)*. Some of these effects may be mediated by matrix metalloproteinases (MMPs), particularly MMP-9 *(26)*. For example, treatment of nude mice bearing orthotopic transitional cell bladder carcinoma with the EGFR antibody IMC-C225 results in inhibition of tumor growth and metastases and decreased MMP-9 expression *(27)*. EGFR TK inhibitors have also been demonstrated to downregulate the expression of MMP-9 in vitro. Furthermore, heregulin stimulation promotes physical attractions between p21-activated kinase 1, actin, and HER2, promoting cellular invasion via modifications in the actin cytoskeleton *(28)*.

2.1.6. Therapeutics Targeting EGFR and other ErbB Family Members

2.1.6.1. General. Because the ErbB family of receptors are integral components of the principal signaling cascade involved in regulating solid tumor growth, a rational therapeutic approach to treating colorectal and other epidermoid maligancies is to block ErbB function, thereby inhibiting cancer cell proliferation and tumor progression. As shown in Table 1, several therapeutic approaches to target ErbB are being pursued. One of the most attractive approaches are monoclonal antibodies (MAbs) directed against the extracellular domain

Table 1
Therapeutic Approaches Targeting EGFR

Anti-EGFR Antibodies (Chimeric, Humanized, Bispecific)
- Antibody binds to EGFR on cell surface
- Ligand binding to receptor blocked
- Signal transduction cascade blocked
- Receptor–antibody complex internalized

Small-Molecule Inhibitors of Tyrosine Kinase (EGFR and Pan-ErbB)
- Inhibitors bind intracellularly to EGFR tyrosine kinase
- Receptor tyrosine kinase activity inhibited
- Signal transduction cascade blocked

Ligand Conjugates
- EGFR ligand (e.g., EGF, TGF-α) conjugated to a toxin (ricin, *Pseudomonas exotoxin*)

Immunoconjugates
- Anti-EGFR antibody complexed to a toxin

Antisense Oligonucleotides
- EGFR or TGF-α antisense oligonucleotides bind to DNA or RNA
- May be delivered using liposome technology

of the ErbB receptor to block ligand binding (EGF or TGF-α) and receptor-activated cell growth. Another approach involves small-molecule inhibitors of RTKs that act directly on the cytoplasmic domain of the ErbB receptor, preventing transduction of proliferative signals to the nucleus. Another effort involves synthesis of ligand conjugates, which bind specifically to the ErbB receptor and induce direct toxicity following internalization. To date, most efforts have been directed toward ErbB1 (EGFR) and ErbB2, but therapeutics targeting all members of the ErbB receptor family are also being evaluated.

2.1.6.2. Anti-EGFR Antibodies. Based on the clinical success of MAbs targeting ErbB2, MAbs directed against the EGFR are being evaluated. These antibodies block ligand binding to the EGFR and inhibit EGF-stimulated RTK activity *(14–16,22–24,29–31)*. Initially, the EGFRs from epidermoid cancers were used to immunize mice to raise MAbs against the EGFR. Two such antibodies, M225 and M528, were found to compete with EGF binding to the EGFR, inhibit EGF-induced TK-dependent phosphorylation, and downregulate EGFR expression by inducing receptor internalization. These MAbs block EGF-induced anchorage-dependent and anchorage-independent growth of the EGFR-expressing cells and inhibit tumor growth, presumably by blocking signal transduction cascades required for survival. Early clinical trials using murine MAbs revealed that some patients develop a human anti-mouse antibody immune response against these foreign proteins, resulting in accelerated clearance and limited therapeutic utility. However, chimeric or partially "humanized" MAbs that retain only the small portion of the murine sequences responsible for antigen binding, with the remainder of the molecule composed of the human immunoglobulin, have been developed. IMC-225, a chimeric MAb with a binding affinity 10-fold greater than that of the natural EGFR ligand, has been shown to inhibit the growth of established tumor xenografts *(29)*. Although IMC-C225 induces receptor dimerization, EGF-induced activation, autophosphorylation, and receptor internalization are also blocked *(6)*. IMC-C225 and totally humanized (ABX-EGFR; Abgenex) and bispecific (MDX-447; Medrinex) MAbs against the EGFR also inhibit the growth of EGFR-expressing human tumor xenografts of pancreatic, colorectal, prostate, renal, and breast origin, with induction of apoptosis in some studies *(6,15,22–24,29–31)*.

There is also evidence that MAbs to EGFR enhance the cytotoxic effects of many types of nonselective chemotherapeutics and radiation. One possible explanation for these favorable interactions is that alterations in the expression or activity of the EGFR or downstream molecular signals potentate the damage caused by these therapeutics and/or inhibit repair of cell damage *(32)*. Enhanced cytotoxicity and inhibition of tumor growth have been noted following treatment with MAbs against the EGFR and cisplatin, doxorubicin, topotecan, and paclitaxel *(6,17,33–35)*. Similar interactions between radiation and MAbs against EGFR have also been noted, and these effects have been associated with enhanced radiation-induced apoptosis and decreased EGFR autophosphorylation *(36–38)*. Because DNA damage caused by many cytotoxic agents and radiation results in cell-cycle arrest in G1, in which cells repair damage, followed by apoptosis if DNA repair does not occur, growth factor restriction and treatment with DNA-damaging agents may preferentially enhance apoptosis in tumor cells *(39)*.

In addition to EGFR overexpression, other common genetic mutations, such as those involving the p53 suppressor gene, may alter the cellular response to chemotherapy or radiation *(40)*. Inhibition of EGFR TK activity by MAbs and small molecules also blocks activation of downstream cell signaling along the mitogen-activated protein kinase (MAPK) and PI3K pathways. In many tumor cell lines, inhibition of MAPK or PI3K enhances radiosensitivity, radiation-induced DNA damage, and apoptosis *(40–43)*. There is also evidence indicating that the pathway from EGFR to MAPK serves not only as a proliferation pathway but also as a survival pathway. In tumor cells that depend on stimulation of the EGFR, inhibition of these pathways by specific MAbs or small-molecule inhibitors of RTK may abrogate these survival signals, thereby sensitizing cells to radiation. Because of the strong preclinical evidence for favorable interactions between MAbs against EGFR and traditional cytotoxic therapeutics, IMC-C225 is being developed in combination with radiation (head and neck cancer) and irinotecan (colorectal cancer) *(44)*.

2.1.6.3. Receptor Tyrosine Kinase Inhibitors. Another approach to blocking the EGFR involves small-molecule inhibitors of RTK. Inhibition of RTK prevents receptor autophosphorylation and phosphorylation of downstream proteins. This approach may inhibit signaling induced by EGF and TGF-α, as well as signaling that is independent of growth factors. For example, deletion mutations resulting in constitutively active EGFR have been reported in several types of cancers *(45–47)*. Many small-molecule inhibitors of EGFR have significant antitumor activity, blocking both the proliferation of EGFR-overexpressing cells in vitro and growth of EGFR-expressing xenografts.

An important new class of RTK inhibitors is the quinazoline derivatives *(48)*. These compounds are highly selective for EGFR, more selective for EGFR than for other ErbB RTKs, and competitive inhibitors of ATP. ZD1839 (Iressa®; AstraZeneca) is an oral anilinoquinazoline with an IC_{50} of 20 nM for the EGFR TK. The agent inhibits EGFR autophosphorylation and EGF-stimulated growth of cancer cells in vitro. ZD1839 has demonstrated significant antitumor activity, both tumoricidal and tumoristatic, against many types of human tumor xenograft, including lung, colon, and prostate tumors *(48–51)*. The agent has also been demonstrated to induce regression of several well-established human tumor xenografts, but regrowth of the tumors generally occurs following cessation of treatment *(50,51)*. OSI-774 (formerly CP-358,774 [Pfizer]; OSI Pharmaceuticals Inc.) is another oral quinazoline analog with a nanomolar IC_{50} for inhibition of EGFR activity and has high specificity for the receptor *(48,49)*. The agent inhibits proliferation of DiFi colorectal cells and leads to cell-cycle arrest *(18)*. Both ZD1839 and OSI-774 have demonstrated tolerable safety profiles in early clinical trials, with skin toxicity and diarrhea precluding dose escalation on continuous daily oral schedules *(52–54)*. Thus far, ZD1839 has demonstrated prominent clinical activity in phase I evaluations, with major regressions observed in previously treated patients with non-small-cell lung cancer, whereas patients with previously treated non-small-cell lung, head and neck, and renal cancers have had major responses following treatment with OSI-774 in phase I and II studies. Phase I studies of OSI-774 and ZD1839 in combination with a variety of cytotoxic agents, including 5-fluorouracil (5-FU)/leukovorin and/or irinotecan, are ongoing. In addition, other selective inhibitors of EGFR TK, such as PKI-166 (Novartis), are in early-stage clinical evaluations *(48,50)*. The ErbB TK inhibitors CI-1033 (Pfizer) and EKB-549 (Wyeth-Genetics Institute) are also potent inhibitors of the EGFR TK , but these agents also inhibit the RTKs of other ErbB family members, particularly ErbB2, which may confer broader antitumor activity. Both agents are undergoing phase I evaluations.

2.1.6.4. Other Therapeutic Modalities Against EGFR. In addition to MAbs and RTK inhibitors, other approaches have been used to target the EGFR. A gene encoding a single-chain antibody that specifically binds to EGFR has been constructed and shown to inhibit EGF-induced activation and growth of EGFR-transformed 3T3 fibroblasts in vitro *(55)*. Antisense therapy using DNA or RNA oligonucleotides has been designed to block translation of the specific mRNA transcripts into proteins. ASONs directed at oncogenes and/or growth factors have been demonstrated to inhibit the growth of several human cancers in experimental systems. When mice bearing EGFR-positive tumor xenografts have been treated with EGFR antisense RNA sequences, EGFR expression and tumor growth have been suppressed, whereas treatment with EGFR sense constructs has been ineffective *(56)*. Other EGFR ASONs that have demonstrated prominent antitumor activity in preclinical studies include ASONs in folate–polyethylene glycol liposomes, antisense constructs directed against mRNAs of TGF-α, and the EGF-related peptides amphiregulin and cripto *(57–59)*.

Immunoconjugates linking toxins and immunomodulators to anti-EGFR antibodies have also demonstrated antitumor activity in preclinical studies. Conjugates of the anti-EGFR MAbs IMC-C225 and 528 with ricin A chain, a potent protein synthesis inhibitor, have been shown to preferentially inhibit the growth of EGFR-expressing tumor cells in vitro *(60,61)*. Because normal cells express the EGFR, selectivity may be problematic in the clinic, but the therapeutic index of these therapeutics may ultimately relate to the magnitude of EGFR expression in the tumor. Conjugates of toxins and EGFR ligands have been designed with the aim of specifically targeting EGFR-expressing tumors while minimizing nonselective toxicity. A conjugate composed of EGF and Pseudomonas endotoxin (PE) has been demonstrated to be toxic against the EGFR-expressing tumor cells in vitro *(60–63)*. Other conjugates against EGFR that had been demonstrated to inhibit tumor growth, induce apopotosis, and/or improve survival in preclinical studies include the following: a genetically engineered TGF-α–PE hybrid toxin; genistein, a soybean-derived general TK inhibitor coupled to EGF; a ligand fusion toxin, consisting of human EGF fused to the active moiety of diphtheria toxin (DAB389EGF), which kills cells by inhibiting protein synthesis; and an immunotoxin, in which an anti-EGFR antibody (B4G7) is conjugated to gelonin, a ribosome-inactivating protein *(64–66)*. Of the aforementioned conjugates, only DAB389EGF has been evaluated in a clinical trial *(66)*.

2.2. Rapamycin-Sensitive Signal Transduction as a Therapeutic Target

2.2.1. RAPAMYCIN

Rapamycin (sirolimus; Rapimmune®; Wyeth Ayerst-Genetics Institute), a macrolide first identified as a fungicide produced by the bacterium *Streptomyces hygroscopicus*, possesses antimicrobial, immunosuppressive, and antitumor properties. These properties are the result of its effects on signal transduction pathways that link mitogenic stiumuli to the synthesis of proteins involved in G_1 to S cell-cycle traverse. In addition, a branch of the pathway also affects the phosphorylation (activation) status of key proteins involved in survival and apoptosis. Rapamycin has received regulatory approval as an immunsuppressant in the setting of organ transplantation; however, its effects on the PI3K pathway have served as an impetus for evaluations of rapamycin-related therapeutics in the treatment of cancer.

Rapamycin initially demonstrated antiproliferative activity in a variety of murine tumor systems, including B16 melanoma and P388 leukemia, in the late 1970s and was later shown to broadly inhibit growth of solid tumors *(67–70)*. In addition to its growth inhibitory actions, rapamycin induces *p53*-independent apoptosis, augments the apoptotic effects of traditional cytotoxic agents, blocks cyclin D1 expression, and inhibits the proliferation of several types of malignant tumors, suggesting that it may affect essential components of the cell survival pathway and enhance the efficacy of cytotoxic agents *(70–72)*.

2.2.2. THE RAPAMYCIN-SENSITIVE SIGNAL TRANSDUCTION PATHWAY

2.2.2.1. General. A schematic representation of the principal rapamycin-sensitive signal transduction pathway is shown in Fig. 2. Similar to other natural immunosuppressants, rapamycin binds to members of the ubiquitous immunophilin family of FK506 binding proteins (FKBPs), inhibiting their enzymatic activity as prolyl isomerases *(73)*. Although these enzymes plays an important role in altering protein conformation, this function is irrelevant to the effects of rapamycin. Instead, several lines of evidence suggest that FKBP12 is the principal binding protein of rapamycin and that the rapamycin-FKBP12 complex is the principal active intermediate *(74)*. The rapamycin–FKBP12 complex blocks the activity of a large, highly conserved polypeptide kinase termed, mammalian target of rapamycin (mTOR) *(74)*. Both mammalian and yeast mTOR are members of the PI3K-related kinases (PIKKs) family of protein kinases, which are involved in many essential cellular functions integral to cell-cycle progression, checkpoint control, DNA repair, and DNA recombination *(75)*.

Following stimulation of quiescent cells by growth factors, there is an increase in translation of a subset of mRNAs, whose protein products are required for cell-cycle traverse through G_1 *(76)*, and mTOR regulates key pathways affecting the efficiency of protein translation. PI3K/protein kinase B (Akt) appears to be the key modulatory factor in the upstream pathway by which growth factor–growth factor receptor interactions affect mTOR's phosphorylation state *(77)*. Both PI3K and Akt are likely protooncogenes, and the pathway is inhibited by the tumor supressor gene *PTEN*, which is often mutated in human cancer *(78)*. Although other signaling pathways are activated downstream of PI3K, the Akt pathway is of interest because of its role in inhibiting apoptosis and promoting cell proliferation *(78,79)*. In mammalian cells, activated mTOR signals two separate sets of mRNAs, including the 40S ribosomal protein S6 kinase (p70[s6k]) and the eukaryotic initiation factor (e1F)-4E-binding protein-I (4E-BP1; also known as PHAS-I) *(20,80,81)*. Among subset mRNAs regulated by these pathways are the encoding components of the protein synthesis machinery itself. Treatment of activated PI3K- or Akt-expressing cells with rapamycin blocks p70[s6k] and 4E-BP1/PHAS-I phosphorylation, indicating that mTOR is required for these responses *(81–84)*. Akt also appears to phosphorylate mTOR, contributing to its activation *(82,83)*.

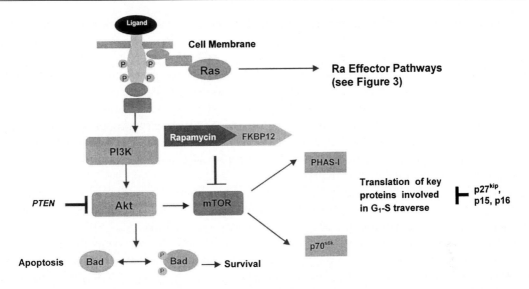

Fig. 2. Rapamycin-sensitive signal transduction pathways. Binding of rapamycin and/or rapamycin analogs to FKBP-12 forms a complex that inhibits kinase activity of mTOR and, consequently, its downstream mediators 4E-BP1/PHAS and p70^{s6k}. This results in inhibition of proliferative signals mediated through the PI3K/Akt signal transduction pathway that leads to activation of antiapoptotoic (survival) proteins and translation of proteins that facilitate G_1 to S phase traverse. Inhibitory proteins *PTEN*, p27^{kip}, p15, and p16 are shown.

2.2.2.2. Downstream Effects. The downstream effects of mTOR on protein translation have also been well characterized *(85–89)*. Inhibition of these critical signaling pathways leads to inefficient translation of the mRNAs of proteins that are necessary for G1 traverse (e.g., cyclin D1, ornithine decarboxylase). Rapamycin also accelerates the turnover of cyclin D1, both at the mRNA and protein levels, resulting in a deficiency of active cdk4/cyclin D1 complexes required for pRB phosphorylation, release of E2F transcription factor, and increased association of p27^{kip1} with cyclin E/cdk2. These two events, along with the inhibition of translation of other mRNAs, explain inhibition at the G_1/S phase transition *(89–92)*. There is also evidence that cells in which the *p27* gene has been disrupted are only partially resistant to rapamycin, indicating that rapamycin can inhibit cell-cycle progression by *p27*-independent mechanisms *(93)*.

2.2.3. RAPAMYCIN ANALOG DEVELOPMENT

2.2.3.1. CCI-779. Because poor aqueous solubility and instability compromised the development of rapamycin as an anticancer agent, soluble ester analogs were evaluated by Wyeth-Ayerst and CCI-779 was selected for development based on its mechanism of action and favorable preclinical efficacy and toxicity data. In the National Cancer Institute human tumor cell-line screen, CCI-779 and rapamycin demonstrated similar profiles and potencies (Pearson correlation coefficient, 0.86), with IC$_{50}$ values frequently less than 0.01 μM *(94)*. Platelet-derived growth factor stimulation of the human glioblastoma line T98G was markedly inhibited, consistent with its proposed mechanism of action as an inhibitor of signal transduction, and growth-inhibited cells were arrested in G_1 *(94)*. Several intermittent dosing regimens were effective in human tumor xenografts, and the immunosuppressive effects of CCI-779 were resolved within 24 h following treatment.

Two treatment schedules have been evaluated in phase I trials: a weekly schedule and a daily × 5-d every-2-wk schedule *(95,96)*. Doses levels ranging from 7.5 to 60 mg/m^2/wk have been well tolerated on the weekly schedule, and toxicity has generally been in the form of modest cutaneous and mucosal toxicity. On the daily × 5-d every-2-wk schedule, doses above 24 mg/m^2/d have been associated with moderate myelosuppression and fatigue. Hyperlipidemia, elevated serum lactate dehydrogenase, hypophosphatemia, hypocalcemia, and hyokalemia have been observed. Partial responses in patients with non-small-cell lung and renal cell cancers have been documented and minor regressions in patients with other types of malignancies have been noted. Broad phase II evalutions, including studies in patients with colorectal cancer, are planned.

Given the current understanding of the mechanism of action of rapamycin and CCI-779 and their spectra of activity, it is possible that drug-sensitive tumors may be those that rely on paracrine or autocrine stimulation of receptors that trigger the PI3K/Akt/mTOR pathway, or tumors with mutations that cause constitutive activation of the PI3/Akt pathway may depend on rapamycin-sensitive pathways for growth. In fact, abnormal activation of this pathway is relatively common because mutations of the tumor suppressor gene *PTEN*, which encodes for a lipid phosphatase that inhibits PI3K-dependent activation of PKB/Akt, occur in many tumor types with a frequency approaching that of *p53* mutations.

2.3. Targeting Ras: Farnesylprotein Transferases and Other Modalities

2.3.1. WHAT IS RAS AND WHY TARGET IT?

Ras is critical intermediate in signal transduction pathways that mediate proliferative signals largely from upstream of RTK to a downstream cascade of protein kinases that control growth and regulatory processes that are aberrant in malignant cells *(97–99)*. Because of its central role in regulating these processes, Ras and Ras effector pathways provide opportunities to develop novel therapeutics that specifically target the aberrant signaling pathways of malignant cells. Three *ras* protooncogenes have been identified: the H-*ras* gene, the K-*ras* gene, and the N-*ras* gene, which encode four 21-kDa proteins, called p21^{ras} or Ras (H-Ras, N-Ras, and K-Ras4A and K-Ras4B), that are localized to the inner surface of the plasma membrane *(97–101)*. All Ras proteins have a specific amino acid sequence motif at the carboxyl (C) terminus that specifies the intracellular localization of the Ras protein. This C-terminal motif is commonly referred to as the CA1A2X box, in which C represents a cysteine residue, A_1 and A_2 represent aliphatic amino acids, usually valine, leucine, or isoleucine, and X is either methionine or serine.

Ras proteins are an extended family of guanosine triphosphatases (GTPases), which are involved in protein synthesis and signal transduction *(102)*. Ras functions as a chemical switch, cycling between inactive guanosine diphosphate (GDP)-bound and active guanosine triphosphate (GTP)-bound states. The processes by which Ras is activated and functions in intracellular signaling are depicted in Fig. 3. Ras is synthesized as an inactive cytosolic peptide and is localized to the inner surface of the plasma membranes only after it undergoes a series of posttranslational modifications at the C-terminus, which increases its hydrophobicity and facilitates association with the cell membrane *(100–104)*. The first and most critical step, farnesylation, catalyzed by the enzyme protein farnesyltransferase (FTase), adds a 15-carbon farnesyl isoprenoid group to H-, K-, and N-Ras.

Ras transmits extracellular signals from cell surface receptors to the cytoplasm and nucleus, initiating a cascade of protein kinases that ultimately regulate nuclear, cytoskeletal, and cytoplasmic processes. Considerable progress has been made in characterizing the signaling pathways upstream of Ras, but less is known about downstream signaling. In

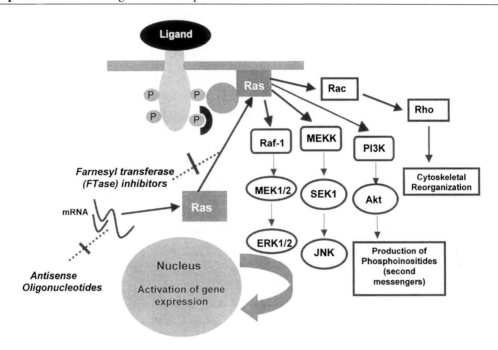

Fig. 3. Ras pathways. Ras is synthesized in the cytoplasma and undergoes a series of posttranslational modifications that increase protein hydrophobicity and facilitate its association with the inner surface of the plasma membrane where Ras cycles from an inactive GDP-bound state to an active GTP-bound state. The first posttranslational modification is catalyzed by Ftase, which results in the covalent addition of a farnesyl group from FDP onto the cysteine residue of the CAAX box of Ras. This reaction is the target of several classes of FTase inhibitors. Ras mRNAs are also being targeted with specific antisense oligonucleotides. In response to growth factor ligands and receptor stimulating, GTP is exchanged for GDP. Ras-GTP then activates multiple effector pathways, including Raf-1, MAPK pathway, Rac/Rho, and PI3K. Ras-GTP is then converted back it to an inactive Ras-GDP state; however, the stability of Ras-GTP is governed by the mutational status of Ras.

its wild-type state, Ras-GDP is rapidly and transiently converted to Ras-GTP in response to diverse extracellular stimuli, including growth factors such as those that stimulate (1) fibroblasts and related cells (e.g., EGFR, ErbB2, PDGF), (2) lymphocytes and hematopoietic cells (e.g., IL-2, IL-3, GM-CSF), (3) hormones (e.g., insulin), and (4) neurotransmitters (e.g., carbachol) *(105,106)*. Typically, the cell surface receptors for these growth factors proximal to Ras are RTKs *(107,108)*. In a similar manner, cytokines and other transmitters may bind to receptors that activate nonreceptor TKs *(105,107)*. When stimulated by a cascade of events following phosphorylation of both RTKs and nonreceptor TKs, Ras becomes activated by binding GTP and is capable of promoting proliferation and other effects.

2.3.2. EFFECTORS OF RAS

During normal cell growth, stimulation by extracellular growth factors is required to maintain wild-type Ras in an activated state; otherwise, it reverts rapidly to its inactive form. Although wild-type Ras has low intrinsic GTPase activity, GTPase activator proteins enhance the hydrolysis of bound GTP to GDP, converting Ras to an inactive form. Biochemical studies suggest that although mutant Ras exhibits slightly less intrinsic GTPase activity than wild-type Ras, the principal functional effect conferred by mutant Ras is a marked decrease in the ability of Ras to interact with GAP *(108)*. Instead of reverting to its inactive GDP-bound state, mutant Ras remains in an active GTP-bound state and continues to activate downstream effectors despite the absence of growth factor stimulation. In its GTP-bound state, Ras activates several downstream effector pathways, particularly the Raf-1 serine–threonine kinase pathway. Once activated, Raf-1 phosphorylates two mitogen-activated protein (MAP) kinase kinases, MEK_1 and MEK_2, which, in turn, phosphorylates the MAP kinases extracellular signal-regulated kinases 1 (ERK1) and 2 (ERK2). Upon activation, ERK1 and ERK2 translocate to the nucleus, where they phosphorylate several substrates, including the Elk1 nuclear transcription factor, ultimately leading to the activation of other kinases, transcription factors, c-*fos*, and other downstream target genes associated with proliferation *(109)*.

There are multiple branch points in the Ras pathway and Raf is only one of many effectors of Ras signaling *(104,105,109)*. Other effectors include the small GTP-binding proteins Rac and Rho, and PI3K, and MAP kinase kinase kinase (MEKK). Ras-GTP also activates the G-proteins Rac and Rho through an activation pathway often referred to as the cell morphology pathway *(36–38)*. A principal function of Rho is to regulate the actin cytoskeleton *(110)*. The activation of Rac and Rho by oncogenic Ras may lead to morphologic changes that increase the invasiveness properties of transformed cells *(111–115)*. Ras also activates the downstream effector PI3K that plays a role in controling the actin cytoskeleton, motility, invasiveness, survival, and suppression of apoptosis (*see* Section 2.2.) *(116,117)*.

2.3.3. RAS MUTATIONS IN CANCERS

In a large percentage of human tumors, one of the three *ras* genes harbor a point mutation that confers an aberrant protein with a single altered amino acid *(97–99)*. Mutations of *ras* occur in about 30% of all human cancers, including a significant proportion of colorectal (approx 50%) and pancreatic (approx 70%) cancers *(1,13)*. Most mutationally activated forms of *ras* in tumors result in disrupted guanine nucleotide regulation and constitutive activation of Ras *(3)*. Of the three *ras* genes, mutation of K-*ras* is most commonly found in human tumors, whereas N-*ras* mutations are encountered less often, and H-*ras* mutations rarely *(97–99)*. The clinical significance of these different mutations is not completely understood, although there is evidence that each Ras isoform leads to distinct biochemical consequences because of differences in activation of the many downstream effector pathways. The type of *ras* mutation seems to correlate with tumor type *(1,13,67,105)*.

For Ras to transduce the extracellular signals provided by growth factors and cytokines, the protein must be associated with the inner surface of the plasma membrane, which is facilitated by a series of posttranslational chemical modifications. Following its synthesis, Ras is sequentially modified at the C-terminus. In the first step of the process, farnesylation, FTase recognizes the CAAX motif and transfers a 15-carbon farnesyl isoprenoid from farnesyl diphosphate (FDP) to form a thioether bond with the Ras cysteine of the CAAX box *(100,103,104,118–123)*. In another prenylation reaction relevant to cell signaling and many posttranslational protein processes, geranylgeranylation, protein geranylgeranyl transferases (GGTases) I and II transfer either one or two 20-carbon geranylgeranyl isoprenoids from geranylgeranyl diphosphate (GGDP) to proteins. The proteins modified by GGTases-I and -II are more hydrophobic than those modified by farnesylation, and geranylgeranylation may also serve as part of a recognition sequence for protein–protein interactions. Strategies that are capable of blocking FTase and preventing farnesylation may inhibit the maturation of Ras into a biologically active molecule, thus turning off signal transduction. An in-depth understanding of other posttranslational processes related to Ras is emerging, along with studies designed to determine whether they have a role as strategic therapeutic targets.

2.3.4. TYPES OF RAS INHIBITORS

2.3.4.1. FTase Inhibitors. The acquisition of detailed kinetic information about the FTase reaction from the elucidation of the crystalline structure of FTase has led to the rational design of FTase inhibitors *(100,124–128)*. Four general types of small molecule inhibitors of FTase have been designed and evaluated: (1) FDP analogs that compete with the FTase substrate FDP (FDP analog FTase inhibitors); (2) peptidomimetics or CAAX mimetics that compete with the CAAX portion of Ras for FTase (peptidomimetics and nonpeptidomimetics); (3) bisubstrate analogs that combine the features of both FDP analogues and peptidomimetics; and (4) nonpeptidomimetic inhibitors. Most of the efforts targeting FTase have sought to selectively develop inhibitors that are more than 1000-fold more potent at inhibiting FTase than either GGTase-I or GGTase-II. It can be argued that selectivity is desirable to avoid toxicities that might result from GGTase inhibition, because a far greater number of physiologic proteins are known to be substrates for GGTase-I. Selective GTase inhibitors might be useful in determining the role of GGTase in cells *(125–129)*. The coordinate use of inhibitors of GGTase and FTase may be more effective against cells harboring mutated K-*ras*, which is a substrate for GGTase-I.

2.3.4.2. Antisense Compounds. Although most efforts aimed at blocking the activation of mutant Ras have focused on inhibiting FTase, ASONs that block Ras function have also been designed. Most research efforts have focused on short ASONs to target H-*ras* and K-*ras* RNA. ASONs against H-*ras* have selective activity against the mutant H-*ras* genes in vitro *(130,131)*. One ASON reduced Ras expression in H-Ras transformed NIH 3T3 cells by greater than 90% and in vitro treatment for 3 d led to suppression of tumor growth for up to 14 d after inoculation of the antisense-treated cells. Direct in vivo antitumor activity has also been reported for some of the mutant *ras* selective constructs as well. The expression of mutant H-Ras can be inhibited by ASONs that interact with H-*ras* mRNA codon 12, where mutations most frequently occur *(132)*. These ASONs were shown to inhibit the growth of tumors with mutant Ras implanted in nude mice. Another antisense construct, ISIS 2503 (Isis Pharmaceuticals), which is being evaluated alone and in combination with chemotherapy, does not selectively target the point mutations at codon 12,13, or 61 *(133,134)*. Instead, it targets the initiation region of the H-*ras* message. In targeting H-*ras* broadly, the molecule seems to deliver antitumor activity in human tumor xenografts irrespective of *ras* gene status. Antitumor activity has been reported against pancreatic MiaPACA2 tumors, which bear K-*ras*B mutations and HT-29 colon tumors without *ras* muations. This broad activity, similar to that seen with pharmacological modulators of FTase, suggests an important role for the H-ras isoform in malignant signal transduction. In contrast to H-*ras* antisense strategies, most of the successful strategies targeting K-*ras* have not involved short ASONs, but large constructs that could be delivered as plasmids or in viral vectors *(135,136)*. In early studies, a 2-kb antisense sequence of the K-*ras* gene was electroporated into H460A lung cancer cells, a cell line that bears a mutant (codon 61) K-*ras* gene *(136)*. Cell proliferation, anchorage-independent growth, and growth of the in vitro transfected cells, as well as murine xenografts, were all suppressed by transfection of the K-*ras* plasmid. In addition to the biological responses, expression of the antisense RNA and reduction of K-*ras* mRNA were observed. The 2-kb K-*ras* antisense was also incorporated into an adenoviral vector, which was effective in generating the K-*ras* antisense RNA to levels which reduced K-Ras protein and inhibited proliferation and anchorage-independent growth of the H460a lung cancer cell line *(137)*. Although the adenovirus K-*ras* construct was targeted for a codon 61 mutation, the adenovirus was also highly active in a cell line bearing a K-*ras* codon 12 mutation.

Transfection of H460A cells in cell culture with the K-*ras* adenovirus prior to inoculation in mice inhibited the growth of tumor cells implanted in an orthotopic intratracheal tumor model *(138)*.

The AOSNs can also be used against other signaling proteins activated by Ras proteins, such as Raf *(139–141)*. Although an advantage of this approach is specificity of the ASON to the target gene, blocking only one of the downstream proteins will likely be insufficient to reverse the full effect of activated Ras expression.

2.3.5. ANTITUMOR EFFECTS OF FTASE INHIBITORS

FTase inhibitors block farnesylation of Ras in a dose-dependent manner in cancer cells in vitro, although most studies have been performed in tumor cells in which the substrate is a mutated form of H-Ras. FTase inhibitors also block farnesylation of many other protein substrates of FTase, but generally higher concentrations of FTase inhibitors are required. One caveat is that inhibitors of FTase are generally less effective at modulating the processing of K-Ras, whose gene is the most frequently mutated ras in human cancer *(134)*. This phenomenon may reflect the ability of GGTase-I to alternatively prenylate K-Ras in cells treated with FTase inhibitors *(142,143)*. FTase inhibitors have been effective against a broader range of cancer cells than originally anticipated, including tumors whose growth rates were not solely dependent on the status of ras; however, their optimal activity has generally been against tumors expressing H-*ras* > N-*ras* >> K-*ras*, which may reflect the ability of K-Ras to alternatively be prenylated by GGTase-I when farnesylation is blocked *(144)*. Alternatively, the incomplete correlation between Ras mutational status and sensitivity to FTase inhibitors suggests that not all cells with *ras* gene mutations depend on Ras for transformed growth. Indeed, these cells may have other mutations that make mutant Ras functionally redundant. Another possible explanation that may have far-reaching ramifications is that farnesylation of other proteins, in addition to Ras, is important for cancer cell growth and that the cytotoxic actions of the FTase inhibitors are unrelated to their effects on Ras. Supporting this hypothesis is evidence that many other critical proteins are targets for FTase inhibitors and may play a role in conferring tumor sensitivity to FTase inhibitors. One putative target is RhoB, which is both farnesylated and geranylgeranylated in vivo; however, RhoB appears to be farnesylated primarily by GGTase-I in vitro *(144)*.

Investigations of alternative or complementary mechanisms by which FTase inhibitors cause tumor regression are warranted. In ras-transformed cells, the peptidomimetic L-739,749 (Merck) induces massive DNA degeneration and cell death that is independent of *p53* but inhibited by the apoptosis suppressor Bcl-xl *(145)*. Other FTase inhibitors have been demonstrated to augment the expression of the apoptosis-promoting proteins Bax and Bcl-xs and induce apoptosis in human ovarian cancer cells, suggesting that FTase inhibitors may inhibit tumor growth under certain conditions by promoting apoptosis.

Many types of FTase inhibitors have been demonstrated to block the growth of human tumor xenografts. Several agents that inhibit growth of tumors with and without activated ras oncogenes in vitro have shown impressive activity against a wide array of human tumor xenografts, including colon, lung, pancreas, prostate, and bladder cancers *(116,146)*. FTase inhibitors have demonstrated efficacy against human tumors expressing K-*ras* mutations, including LoVo human colon and CAPAN-2 pancreatic tumor xenografts *(147,148)*. The nonpeptidomimetic FTase inhibitor R115777 (Janssen) predominantly inhibits malignant angiogenesis in LoVo tumors, whereas the principal effect in the CAPAN-2 tumors is growth arrest *(145,147–149)*. These results indicate that FTase inhibitors block tumor growth by several mechanisms. The bisubstrate FTase inhibitor BMS-214662 (Bristol-Myers Squibb), has also shown activity against human tumor xenografts of colon, bladder, pancreas, and lung origin *(149)*.

Tumors arising in transgenic mice more closely resemble human tumors with regard to the cellular environment and natural history of tumor development than do xenograft models. One such transgenic mouse model that is ideal for the evaluation of FTase inhibitors is the mouse mammary tumor virus (MMTV)–H-ras transgenic mouse that develops both mammary and salivary adenocarcinomas at about 8 mo *(150,151)*. Many FTase inhibitors have demonstrated substantial tumor growth inhibition and reduction of well-established tumors in this model *(152)*.

2.3.6. TOXICITY IN PRECLINICAL STUDIES

An unexpected, but desirable, aspect of FTase inhibitors is their apparent lack of growth inhibitory activity against nonmalignant cells in vitro and their tolerance in both animal and human studies. Histologic examination of the tissues of animals treated with the peptidomimetics L-744,832 (Merck) and L-739,749 (Merck) for protracted periods has revealed no abnormalities in rapidly dividing tissues (e.g., bone marrow and gastrointestinal tissue) or in tissues in which farnesylated proteins appear to play critical physiologic roles (e.g., eyes and skeletal muscle) *(150,153)*.

2.3.7. THE CHALLENGE OF EVALUATING FTASE INHIBITORS IN THE CLINIC

2.3.7.1. Single-Agent Phase I Studies. Several FTase inhibitors have entered early clinical evaluations. A major challenge in developing these compounds is the selection of an optimal dose for disease-directed studies, because antitumor activity may not correlate with toxicity, unlike conventional cytotoxic therapy, in which toxicity and antitumor activity are related, albeit weakly. Toxicity may not be evident at doses that inhibit Ras farnesylation or may not be quantifiable or even related to FTase inhibition. Pharmacologically guided studies may be used to assess whether biologically relevant plasma concentrations associated with maximal inhibition of Ras farnesylation and antitumor activity in preclinical studies are being achieved in patients. The development and validation of assays of protein prenylation in accessible tissues that reflect farnesylation of Ras in tumors will facilitate the ability to define the optimal doses of FTase inhibitors in phase I studies. Both immunohistochemical and gel mobility shift assays have been used to quantify prenylation of proteins that might be associated with a desirable target effects (e.g., lamin A, the hDJ2 chaperone protein) *(139)*. Inhibition of ERK phosphorylation and/or basal ERK phosphorylation have also been related to antitumor activity in leukemia patients in a phase I study of R115777 *(154)*.

Determining the optimal schedule of administration of FTase inhibitors is an important challenge. There is experimental evidence indicating that continuous drug exposure, perhaps optimally achieved with continuous treatment, is required for maximal efficacy. The use of protracted dosing schedules, however, raises concerns about both acquired drug resistance and toxicity. Preliminary clinical safety data for several different FTase inhibitors administered on various chronic treatment schedules are available.

R115777 (Janssen), the orally bioavailable methyl-quinolone nonpeptidomimetic inhibitor sharing structural similarities to the CAAX motif of Ras, was the first FTase inhibitor to enter clinical evaluations. In a phase I study of patients with advanced solid malignancies, R115777 was administered twice daily for 5 d every 2 wk at escalating doses as a solution (25–850 mg twice orally) or as pellet capsules (500–1300 mg twice orally) *(155)*. In this study, biologically relevant steady-state plasma concentrations were achieved within 2–3 d of initiating treatment. At doses below 1300 mg twice daily, R115777 was well tolerated, although an unacceptably high rate of dose-limiting toxicity, consisting of neuropathy, fatigue with decreased performance status, and gastrointestinal complaints, were observed at the 1300-mg twice daily dose level. One patient with metastatic colorectal cancer treated at the 500-mg twice daily dose level had a 46% decrease in carcinoembryonic antigen (CEA), which was associated with improvement in symptoms and stable disease for 5 mo. In contrast, neutropenia and thrombocytopenia were the principal dose-limiting side effects when R115777 was administered twice daily for 3 wk at doses ranging from 60 to 420 mg/m^2, with the maximum tolerated dose being 240 mg/m^2 twice daily (156). Biologically relevant steady-state plasma concentrations were achieved within 3 d of beginning treatment. Neutropenia and thrombocytopenia were the principal dose-limiting toxicities. Stable disease of greater than 6 mo duration was noted in two patients with advanced carcinomas of the parotid gland and prostate.

The membrane permeable peptidomimetic L-778,123 (Merck) with a benzylimidazole core and low nanomolar activity against FTase has been administered as a continuous 7-d intravenous infusion in phase I trials, with a view toward proceeding to a protracted administration schedule (157,158). Continuous intravenous administration of this agent at doses ranging from 35 to 1120 mg/m^2/d for 7 d resulted in QTc prolongation and severe thrombocytopenia at 1120 mg/m^2/d; the recommended phase II dose was 560 mg/m^2/d. Plasma concentrations, capable of inhibiting Ras processing and growth of tumors with ras mutations in experimental studies, were achieved at the recommened phase II dose. Inhibition of farnesylation of a marker protein hDJ-2 in peripheral blood mononuclear cells was related to dose and plasma concentrations. Maximal inhibition of farnesylation was achieved between d 4 and 8, with rapid reversal following treatment.

Similarly, the tolerability and pharmacokinetic profile of SCH66336 (Schering-Plough), an orally bioavailable tricyclic nonpeptidomimetic FTase inhibitor, are being evaluated (159–161). In a phase I study, in which SCH66336 was administered daily twice daily for 7 d every 3 wk, dose-limiting diarrhea, nausea, vomiting, and fatigue were noted at the 400-mg bid dose level. Inhibition of farnesylation of prelamin A was also demonstrated in buccal mucosal cells (159). There was one partial response lasting 9 mo in a patient with previously treated non-small-cell lung carcinoma. The recommended phase II dose on this schedule was 350 mg twice daily. In another phase I trial, in which SCH66336 was administered twice daily for 2 wk every month (doses of 25–300 mg twice daily), the dose-limiting toxicities were also diarrhea, nausea, vomiting, and fatigue (160). The recommended phase II dose was 200 mg twice daily. In phase I studies of SCH66336 administered on a twice daily continuous dosing schedule, vomiting, diarrhea, myelosuppression, fatigue, confusion, and disorientation were the principal toxicities at the 300- and 400-mg twice-daily dose levels, and the recommended phase II dose was 240 mg twice daily (159–161). Stable disease lasting longer than 9 mo was noted in patients with pseudomyxoma peritonei and thyroid carcinoma.

Phase I studies of the bisubstrate inhibitor BMS-214662 are evaluating single intravenous administration every 3 wk and five daily intravenous treatments repeated every 3 wk (140). To date, toxicities have included fatigue, nausea, vomiting, anorexia, hepatic transaminase elevations, and ataxia. The half-life is short (range, 2–4 h) and biologic correlative studies have demonstrated dose-related inhibition of FTase catalytic activity in peripheral blood mononuclear cells, with regeneration within 24 h.

Phase I studies of ASONs against H-Ras and K-Ras are also in progress. Thus far, pharmacodynamic assays reveal biological activity, but the overall development and assessment of these therapies are complex, particularly in patients with advanced disease.

2.3.7.2. Combination Studies with Other Agents and Therapeutic Modalities. Given the importance of multiple pathways in malignant transformation, it is likely that combination therapies will be more effective than single-agent regimens. These studies may be quite relevant, particularly because the nonpeptidomimetic R115777 has demonstrated prominent activity in patients with metastatic breast cancer, and the ErbB2 is expressed in both colorectal and breast cancer, establishing a rationale for evaluating combinations of ErbB2- and FTase-targeting therapetuics *(141)*. The FTase inhibitors may complement the activity of other anticancer therapeutics that may or may not affect Ras-mediated pathways. Additionally, although FTase inhibitors have the capacity to rapidly reduce the size of tumors in some preclinical studies (rather than simply decreasing the rate of tumor growth, which is their predominant preclinical effect), residual tumors generally proliferate following discontinuation of treatment. Therefore, FTase inhibitors combined with cytotoxic agents may produce greater cytoreduction and reduce the need for protracted therapy. The overlapping antitumor spectra and nonoverlapping toxicity profiles of FTase inhibitors and cytotoxic agents also provide support for evaluations of combination regimens. The FTase inhibitor L-744,832 and inhibitors of tubulin depolymerization, such as the taxanes and epothilones, have been demonstrated to inhibit the growth of several breast cancer cell lines in vitro in a synergistic manner, whereas interactions between the FTase inhibitor and antimicrotubule agents that induce tubulin depolymerization are much less pronounced, but still additive *(162)*. Furthermore, the results of mechanistic studies have indicated that L-744,832 enhances the mitotic block induced by agents that prevent tubulin polymerization. The combination of paclitaxel or cisplatin with minimally effective concentrations of R115777 was demonstrated to produce additive antiproliferative activity against human MCF-7 (breast), CAPAN-2 (pancreatic), and C32 (melanoma) cells in vitro, as well as established tumor xenografts and tumors implanted into Wap-*ras* transgenic mice *(162)*. In another study, the combination of the FTase inhibitor SCH66336 and paclitaxel demonstrated either synergistic or additive activity against a broad panel of human tumor cell lines and human tumor xenografts *(163,164)*.

Combinations of FTase inhibitors and cytotoxic agents are being evaluated in early clinical trials. For example, the peptidomimetic FTase inhibitor L-778,123 has been combined with paclitaxel in a phase I trial *(153,165)*. The maximum tolerated doses were 280 mg/m^2/d L-778,124 as a 7-d continuous infusion and 175 mg/m^2 paclitaxel on d 1 every 3 wk. The combination of R115777 with 5-FU and leucovorin has been evaluated in patients with advanced colorectal and pancreatic cancers. Patients received R115777 at doses ranging from 200–500 mg twice daily, with a bimonthly fixed dose of 5-FU/leucovorin (leucovorin mg/m^{2}200/2 h, 400 mg/m^2 5-FU intravenous bolus, 600 mg/m^2 5-FU over 22 h on d 1 and 2). Severe myelosuppression was observed at the 500-mg twice-daily dose level. The combination of R115777 with gemcitabine has also been studied. In one study, patients received R115777 at escalating doses from 100 to 300 mg twice daily, with gemcitabine at a fixed dose (1000 mg/m^2 on d 1, 8 and 15 every 4 wk). Neutropenia was the dose-limiting toxicity, and the recommended phase II doses were 200 mg R115777 twice daily with 1000 mg/m^2 gemcitabine on d 1, 8, and 15 every 4 wk. No drug–drug interactions were observed.

Oncogenic Ras is known to be involved in pathways of angiogenesis, and FTase inhibitors are capable of inhibiting angiogenesis *(166,167)*. In one study, the peptidomimetic FTase inhibitor L-739,749 blocked expression of VEGF in H-*ras* transformed cells. H-*ras* and other oncogenes have also been demonstrated to confer resistance to the cytotoxic effects of radiation, and FTase inhibitors have demonstrated radiation-sensitizing properties in tumors in vitro and in vivo *(168)*. Furthermore, the radiosensitivity of normal cells is not enhanced, indicating a selective radiosensitizing effect, which provides a rationale for evaluations of FTase inhibitors and radiation, which are currently ongoing in patients with advanced neoplasms.

3. THERAPEUTICS TARGETING ABERRANT CELL DEATH AND DEGRADATION

Because some cancer cells do not differ from normal cells in their rates of proliferation, but differ in their rates of turnover, agents targeting cellular features related to the proliferative index may have limited value. The complexity of cell death has recently become better understood, leading to the characterization of multiple pathways of cell death and development of therapeutics targeting pathways that govern cell death.

3.1. Targeting Proteosomes

3.1.1. UBIQUITIN PROTEOSOME PATHWAY

The regulation of protein activities by the proactive synthesis and degradation of specific protein molecules is vital to cellular metabolic integrity and proliferation. The ubiquitin proteasome pathway (UPP) consists of two distinct biochemical steps, which lead to cellular protein degradation *(169–172)*. In a highly regulated cascade of enzymatic reactions, ubiquitin is covalently linked to ε-amine moieties of lysine residues in proteins in a processive manner, leading to multiubiquinated chains. Once a protein has been marked with ubiquitin conjugates, it is destined to be degraded by the 26S proteosome, a multicatalytic protease. The 26S proteosome, a large multimeric protease complex, plays a central role in cellular protein regulation through catabolism of a wide variety of proteins, resulting in activation of certain pathways and blocking of others *(173–177)*. Although the UPP was previously believed to be merely a disposal system for damaged intracellular proteins, it now appears to be critical for regulating the amount of activated signal transduction proteins and protein activation of transcription *(178)*. In addition, the UPP may play a role in the processing and presentation of MHC class-I-restricted antigens. Furthermore, the ubiquitin-proteasome pathway processes the p105 nuclear factor-κB precursor into the active p50 subunit of the transcriptional activator. Finally, there is also evidence that the UPP may be critical in cell-cycle regulation by degrading cyclins that act at several cell-cycle checkpoints *(146,179–181)*.

Both naturally occurring and synthetic inhibitors of the UPP have been identified *(182–189)*. The most promising class of UPP inhibitors for therapeutic development are boronic acid dipeptide derivatives, which have a high degree of selectivity for the proteasome and do not inhibit many common proteases. One specific boronic acid dipeptide derivative, PS-341 (Millenium), has a K_i of 0.6 nM. Early studies using a hollow-fiber tumor-screening assay revealed that PS-341 and other boronic-acid-based proteasome inhibitors are bioactive and exhibit significant activity against many types of malignancy *(190)*. Further investigations demonstrated that PS-341 is capable of significantly reducing growth of both murine tumors (B16 melanoma, Lewis lung carcinoma) and human (HT-29 colon and PC-3 prostate) cancer xenografts *(190,191)*. Negligible adverse effects on body weight were noted at doses capable of significantly reducing tumor growth. The rationale for evaluating PS-341 as a candidate for cancer therapy also include the fact that it is a poor substrate for multidrug transporter proteins, it has not been associated with acquired drug-induced resistance in preclinical studies, and it has prominent activity against chemoresistant tumors that overexpress bcl-2 *(190,192)*.

To assist in evaluating the potential inhibition of target activity in clinical trials, an ex vivo biassay of 20S proteosome activity has been developed *(190,193)*. This assay may be useful in determining the effects of proteasome inhibitors on their principal biochemical target, the proteosome, in biopsies of both tumors and normal tissues. It may also be useful for pharmacokinetic profiling. By following the inhibition of proteasome activity in blood, it may be possible to determine whether the drug is exerting its biochemical effects at any particular time and when drug effects have receded. Using this information, it may be possible to design treatment schedules associated with optimal therapeutic indices.

The rationale for combining traditional nonselective chemotherapeutics with proteosome inhibitors is supported by the preliminary preclinical results. The topoisomerase-I-targeting agent irinotecan is known to increase NFκB activity in tumor cells in vitro, which, in turn, may augment transcription of various antiapoptotic factors *(194)*. Such activity may hypothetically nullify the antitumor activity of irinotecan elicited through inhibition of its target enzyme, topoisomerase I. By blocking NFκB activity, PS-341 and other proteasome inhibitors may enhance the antitumor activity of irinotecan. Because PS-341 alone has antitumor activity, then its addition to irinotecan-based regimens might result in favorable, possibly synergistic, antitumor activity. Such results have been demonstrated in preclinical studies, in which both agents significantly reduce the growth of human LoVo colon xenografts *(195)*. Furthermore, proteasomes have been shown to degrade toposomerase I–camptothecin complexes, thereby releasing the enzyme from the critical intermediate complex and limiting drug activity *(196)*. PS-341 could, therefore, enhance the antitumor activity of irinotecan by reducing the degradation of intermediate complexes and, hence, increasing the duration of its activity. Similar positive interactions have been shown with PS-341 and other chemotherapeutics, including 5-FU, paclitaxel, cisplatin, and doxorubicin *(191)*.

Several dosing schedules of PS-341 as a single agent are being evaluated in phase I trials *(197,198)*. In addition to defining the maximum tolerated dose, pharmacokinetics, and the toxicity profile of PS-341, these studies are also examining the magnitude of proteasome inhibition in blood, which will be related to antitumor activity and toxicity. Broad phase II evaluations of PS-341 and phase I combination studies are also planned.

3.2. Targeting Bcl-2 Apoptotic Pathway

One molecular pathway that is commonly altered in colorectal cancer and other malignancies is the bcl-2 apoptotic pathway, with either overexpression of the *bcl-2* gene, or inactivating mutations of the *bax* gene *(199–202)*. The *bcl-2* protooncogene, which was originally identified at the chromosomal breakpoint of the translocation of a portion of chromosome 18–14 in B-cell lymphomas, belongs to a growing family of related genes whose proteins regulate programmed cell death in both normal and abnormal cells *(200)*. The family of apoptotic regulatory gene products may be either death antagonists (bcl-2, bcl-x$_1$, bcl-W, bfl-1, brag-1, Mcl-1) or death agonists (bax, bak, bcl-x$_s$, bad, bid, bik, hrk) *(201)*. The ratio of death antagonists to agonists is a determinant of cell sensitivity to apoptotic signals. The death/survival balance is mediated, at least in part, by the selective and competitive dimerization between pairs of antagonists (bcl-2) and agonists (bax). An excess of bcl-2 protein expression relative to that of bax inhibits apoptosis resulting from many types of proapoptotic signals, including those generated by cytoxics and radiation *(201)*. In addition, bcl-2 expression confers a multidrug-resistant phenotype and bcl-2 transfection results in tumor cells that are resistant to radiation and many cytotoxic agents including irinotecan *(202,203)*.

Bcl-2 overexpression has been reported in 30–94% of pathologic specimens of human colorectal cancer, whereas bcl-2 is only weakly expressed in the basal proliferative layer of normal colonic epithelium *(203–206)*. Furthermore, bcl-2 overexpression in primary colon cancer specimens has been reported to be a negative prognostic factor with respect to recurrence and survival. Bax expression or function may be reduced in colorectal cancer resulting from inactivating mutations within the *bax* gene *(203–211)*. Colorectal cancers with the microsatellite mutator phenotype (MMP) frequently contain somatic frameshift mutations within the BAX gene. MMP is characterized by genomic instability that leads to deletions and muational insertions at simple repeat sequences *(208–211)*. The majority of tumors of the hereditary nonpolyposis colon cancer syndrome and up to 10–15% of sporadic colon cancer exhibit the MMP *(209–212)*. These tumors exhibit a high degree of bax mutations (51%) and concomitant reduction in bax protein expression or function *(209–212)*.

Strategies directed at downregulation of bcl-2 may modulate resistance to chemotherapy. A specific strategy uses a bcl-2 ASON to hybridize to bcl-2 mRNA. One such ASON, G3139 (Genta), an 18-mer ASON, targets the first six codons of the bcl-2 mRNA open reading frame sequence 5′-tctcccagcgtgcgccat *(213)*. Following hybridization, the mRNA undergoes degradative cleavage mediated through RNase H, which leads to a decrease in bcl-2 protein expression and significant enhancement of chemosensitivity in vitro and in vivo *(214)*. This effect is sequence-specific and does not occur with either 2-base mismatched or reverse-polarity ASON contols. The results of preclinical and early clinical evaluations also indicate that G3139 enhances the chemosensitivity of malignant melanoma to dacarbazine *(215)*.

The feasibility of administering G3139 and irinotecan is currently being evaluated in phase I and II studies in patients with advanced colorectal malignancies at the Cancer Therapy and Research Center (San Antonio). In the study, G3139 is administered as continuous intravenous infusion for 7 d, with irinotecan administered on d 6. Preliminary results indicate significant downregulation of bcl-2 in peripheral blood mononuclear cells.

3.3. Targeting Death Receptors

3.3.1. Apo2 Ligand/TRAIL

Apo2 ligand (Apo2L; also called TRAIL), a member of the tumor necrosis factor (TNF) gene superfamily, was discovered concurrently by scientists at Genentech and Immunex on the basis of sequence homology to Fas/Apo1 ligand (Fas/Apo1L) and TNF *(216,217)*. TNF and its relatives interact with corresponding members of the TNF superfamily to regulate diverse biological functions, including cell proliferation, differentiation, and apoptosis *(218–223)*. Interestingly, many human tissues express Apo2L mRNA, suggesting that normal cells may be resistant to Apo2L *(222,223)*.

Apo2L binds to death receptors (DR) 4 and 5, decoy receptors (DcR) 1 and 2, and osteoprotegerin (OPG). These receptors belong to the TNF receptor gene superfamily. DR4, DR5, DcR1, and DcR2 are closely related, and their encoding genes map together to human chromosome 8. DR4 and 5 are type 1 transmembrane proteins that contain a cytoplasmic death domain, through which they signal apoptosis. DcR2 is a type 1 transmembrane protein that contains a truncated cytoplasmic death domain that is not capable of apoptosis signaling. Upon expression, DcR1 and DcR2 inhibit the apoptosis-inducing activity of Apo2L, suggesting that they act as decoys that compete with DR4 and DR5 for ligand binding. OPG, a secreted soluble protein, is less closely related in sequence to the other receptors and appears to be an inhibitory molecule *(223)*.

Several factors may contribute to the relative safety of Apo2L. First, Apo2L is a weak activator of the proinflammatory transcription factor NF-κB in comparison to TNF *(224)*. Second, unlike expression of TNF and Fas/Apo1L mRNA, which is restricted mainly to activated leukocytes and to immune-privileged sites, many tissues constitutively express

Apo2L mRNA *(216,217)*. This suggests the existence of endogenous mechanisms that can protect normal cells against the cytotoxic effects of Apo2L. One such mechanism appears to be the decoy receptors, which are expressed in certain normal tissues, but infrequently in tumor cells. Other mechanisms that control sensitivity to Apo2L involve intracellular factors that can modulate the apoptosis-inhibitory protein FLIP whose expression seems to correlate with resistance of melanoma cell lines, but not colon cancer cell lines, to Apo2L *(225)*. Most of the 60 cell lines in the National Cancer Institute tumor screen were sensitive to Apo2L, including leukemia, melanoma, and lung, colon, central nervous system cancer, ovarian, renal, prostate, and breast cancers *(226)*. Sensitivity was independent of p53 status. Consistent with its p53 independence with regard to apoptosis induction, Apo2L produces favorable cytotoxic interactions in vitro when combined with traditional cytotoxic agents *(226–228)*. Apo2L has demonstrated significant growth inhibition against several types of human tumor xenografts and compares favorably with 5-FU in an HCT16 colon cancer model *(225)*. Following treatment of athymic mice bearing HCT116 human colon carcinoma with Apo2L, tumor homogenates showed clear evidence of Apo2L-dependent cleavage of the caspase-3 substrate poly-ADP ribose polymerase (PARP). There was also a ninefold increase in the number of apoptotic cells in histologic sections of tumors taken from mice 3 h posttreatment compared to treatment with the vehicle alone *(225)*. The agent has also been demonstrated to induce regression of well-established HCT116 colon xenografts and other human colon tumor xenografts *(225)*. Favorable interactions between Apo2L and 5-FU and irinotecan have also been observed in preclinical studies.

Based on the unique mechanism of Apo2L and the potential diminished susceptibility of normal compared with malignant tissues, scientists at Genentech have developed methods to produce a soluble recombinant version of human Apo2L that will likely enter clinical evaluations in the near future.

3.3.2. Nuclear Death Receptors

SR-45023A is a novel diphosphonate compound (Symphar), representing a new class of anticancer agents that activate the farnasoid X receptor (FXR). FXR is a nuclear receptor involved in the intracellular signaling and transcriptional control of processes that include cell proliferation, apoptosis, and reduction of HMG-CoA reductase activity. SR-45023A and several analogs activate FXR up to 3- to 40-fold more than the known standard, farnesol. Initially developed as a antihypercholesterolemic agent, SR-45023A reduces the activity of HMG-CoA to 8% of its original activity at concentrations of 0.6 μM. Broad screening conducted by Symphar and the National Cancer Institute demonstrated that SR-45023A has broad antiproliferative activity in a number of cell lines, including HT-29 (colon) and HOP 92 and PC3 (prostate) *(229–231)*. Preliminary investigations have demonstrated that the agent is not a substrate for common multidrug transporters and may enhance the cytotoxic effects of many types of chemotherapeutics *(232)*. Moveover, SR-45023A possesses antioxidant activity, inhibits slow calcium channels, and inhibits DNA synthesis in smooth-muscle cells following mitogenic stimuli. These factors suggest a possible role for the agent in combination with other cytotoxic agents, as well as in chemoprevention. The agent is currently undergoing phase I evaluations in patients with multiple types of advanced cancer.

4. TARGETING ABERRANT CELL-CYCLE AND CHECKPOINT CONTROL MECHANISMS

Cell-cycle traverse is very tightly regulated phases *(233–239)*. Following a commitment to cell-cycle progression during the G_1 phase, the genome is replicated during S phase.

This is followed by a second gap phase, G_2, after which cells enter mitosis and divide. Over the last several years, many central features of the cell-cycle machinery, particularly cyclin-dependent kinases (CDKs), which are the enzymes that regulate transition between the cell-cycle phases, have been elucidated. CDK activity is controlled at multiple levels, and deregulated CDK activity occurs universally in human cancer *(233–237)*.

Another hallmark of the transformed cell is aberrant cell-cycle checkpoint control *(233–239)*. Following DNA damage, traverse through the cell cycle in normal cells will be delayed at critical checkpoints at the G_1–S and G_2–M boundaries to undergo DNA repair, avoiding replication of damaged DNA, whereas cancer cells frequently lack such vital checkpoint control features. If checkpoint control is compromised, the replication of damaged DNA can promote genetic instability and the eventual emergence of malignant clones. Cytotoxics that damage DNA and microtubules exploit defective checkpoint control mechanisms in cancer cells because unchecked cell-cycle progression in the presence of massive damage is frequently lethal *(233–239)*.

The elucidation of the events regulating cell-cycle and checkpoint control has provided many molecular targets for novel drug design. One strategy is to treat specific errors that occur in transformed cells to restore cell-cycle control and halt tumor growth *(238,239)*. An alternative strategy is to disrupt components of cell-cycle checkpoints that remain intact in cancer cells to render cancer cells even more susceptible to the damage caused by cytotoxic agents and radiation *(238,239)*. These mechanism-based strategies may result in treatment that is more selective for tumor cells and less toxic to proliferating tissues with normal control functions.

4.1. Restoring Cell-Cycle Control with CDK Inhibitors

Among the strategic targets are those involved in the regulation of the activity of the retinoblastoma-susceptibility gene product, Rb *(233–239)*. In its active, or hypophosphory-lated, form, Rb prevents the progression from the G_1 to the S phase by interacting with members of the E2F transcription factor family. To traverse the G_1–S boundary, Rb must be inactivated. This is accomplished by the activity of several CDKs. As their name implies, CDKs are positively regulated by cyclins. D-Type cyclins pair with CDKs 4 and 6, and cyclin E complexes with CDK2 to sequentially phosphorylate Rb. This ultimately results in E2F activation, allowing the transcription of the genes required to progress through S phase. In addition, CDKs are regulated by their interactions with inhibitors, including members of the INK4 and Cip/Kip protein families.

Nearly all human cancers have an abnormality in at least one component of the Rb control pathway. Although a few cancers such as retinoblastoma and small-cell lung cancer lose Rb, most cancers retain wild-type Rb but have defects elsewhere in the pathway. For example, overexpression of cyclins D1 and E in mantle cell lymphoma and in breast and esophageal cancer promotes cell-cycle progression by maintaining CDK activity. Similarly, amplification of CDK4 has been described in sarcomas and glioblastomas. However, the most common cell-cycle regulation defect in cancer is loss of CDK inhibitors. In tumor cells expressing wild-type Rb, the gene encoding p16[INK4A] is frequently inactivated by deletion, mutation, or promoter hypermethylation. Expression of p21[Waf1/Cip1] and p27[Kip1] is often compromised as well.

Pharmacologic replacement of lost CDK inhibitory activity is a rational therapeutic approach to cancer treatment. However, because normal cells retain CDK inhibitory activity, CDK inhibitors may have little effect on normal cells. Furthermore, genetic replacement of CDK inhibitors, including p16[INK4A] and p27[Kip1], in tumor cells that lack the function of these genes has resulted in cell-cycle arrest and, in some cases, cell death or apoptosis *(233–239)*. This suggests that reconstituting CDK inhibitory activity may have cytotoxic as well as cytostatic effects on tumor cells. Also, because CDKs phosphorylate targets needed for cell-cycle progression in addition to Rb, inhibition of their activity also may be useful in tumor cells that lack Rb.

Many approaches to inhibiting CDK activity are feasible. Although several direct inhibitors are in preclinical development, only flavopiridol and UCN-01, to date, have been studied in clinical trials (reviewed in refs. *238* and *240*). Experience with these first-generation agents indicates what may be expected in the future. Flavopiridol is the first CDK inhibitor to enter clinical trials in the United States. Flavopiridol inhibits the activities of CDKs 1, 2, 4, and 6 involved in the G1–S and G2–M transitions, and it can also inhibit the activation of CDKs and repress transcription of the cyclin D1 gene. In the National Cancer Institute antitumor drug screen, flavopiridol showed potent antiproliferative activity against a broad range of tumor cell lines, causing G_1 and G_2 cell-cycle arrest. Flavopiridol can also induce apoptosis in many types of cells, although this frequently requires prolonged exposure to high concentrations and may be the result of actions on targets other than the CDKs. Based on preclinical experience in which frequent administration was necessary for maximal antitumor effects, a 72-h continuous infusion every-2-wk schedule was adopted for phase I trials. The principal toxicity was manageable diarrhea. Drug concentrations potentially able to inhibit CDK activity were achieved during the infusion. In phase I trials, a complete response occurred in a patient with gastric cancer, and partial and minor responses occurred in patients with renal cell cancer, non-Hodgkin's lymphoma, and colon cancer. Phase II trials are ongoing. Flavopiridol is synergistic with many standard chemotherapy agents (reviewed in refs. *238* and *239*). Although the precise mechanisms are not clear, CDK inhibition following cell-cycle disruption with DNA or microtubule-damaging drugs may drive cells down apoptotic pathways. Combination trials of flavopiridol with paclitaxel, cisplatin, and gemcitabine and irinotecan are currently underway. Other trials are investigating dose and schedule modifications of flavopiridol to optimize its activity.

4.2. Abrogation of Checkpoint Control

Another approach to therapy is potentiation of the effects of DNA-damaging agents by forcing damaged cancer cells through cell-cycle checkpoints before lethal errors can be repaired. Normal cells respond to DNA damage by arresting the cell cycle for DNA repair at the G_1–S or G_2–M boundary. The tumor suppressor p53 is involved in both of these checkpoints through activation of the CDK inhibitor p21[Waf1/Cip1]. Whereas most cancers have lost p53 function, other components of the checkpoints remain intact. Therefore, even p53-deficient tumor cells exposed to DNA damage will transiently arrest at these boundaries as the cancer cell attempts to avoid entering S phase or mitosis with damaged DNA *(238,240,241)*.

Arrest at the G_2–M boundary following DNA damage involves a complicated cascade of events that results in the inactivation of cyclin B–CDK1(CDC2) (reviewed in refs. *238* and *239*). UCN-01, an analog of staurosporine, prevents the inactivation of cyclin B–CDK1 in response to DNA damage, promoting the early entry of cells into mitosis. This results in the onset of apoptotic cell death. Therefore, when UCN-01 is combined with a DNA-damaging agent, such as cisplatin, cell death is enhanced. Enhancement of cell death occurs only in cells lacking p53 function, because cells expressing wild-type p53 will arrest at the G2 boundary following DNA damage. This approach is therefore selectively toxic to transformed cells lacking p53 function. Nontransformed cells, in which p53 function is preserved, will simply arrest at the G2 boundary in response to this therapy *(237,240,241)*.

In phase I clinical studies, UCN-01 has shown an unexpectedly long half-life (approx 30 d), 100 times longer than that observed in preclinical models, because of an avid species-specific binding to $\alpha_1$acid glycoprotein (reviewed in ref. *239*). Phase I studies also showed a relative lack of myelotoxicity or gastrointestinal toxicity, which were the DLTs in the animal models, despite high plasma concentrations of UCN-01. DLTs were nausea, vomiting, hyperglycemia as a result of induction of insulin resistance, and pulmonary toxicity. At the recommended phase II dose, plasma concentrations of UCN-01 were adequate to achieve G2 checkpoint abrogation. Clinical trials of UCN-01 combined with DNA-damaging chemotherapeutic agents are under way.

5. SELECTIVE IMMUNOCONJUGATES FOR COLORECTAL CANCER

Conventional chemotherapeutic agents are limited in their therapeutic effectiveness by severe toxicity because of their poor selectivity for tumors. The identification of strategic tumor antigens and development of MAbs against these targets may enhance the selectivity of anticancer agents on the basis of selective delivery. However, several attempts using MAbs linked to many anticancer drugs (e.g., doxorubicin, methotrexate, *Vinca* alkaloids) have been unsuccessful because these conjugates are only moderately potent and usually less cytotoxic than the corresponding unconjugated drugs *(233–244)*. In fact, antigen-specific cytotoxicity against tumor cells in vitro has rarely been demonstrated, and therapeutic effects in human tumor xenografts have been generally noted only when the treatment is commenced before the tumors are well established or when exceedingly large doses are used *(244–246)*. Intracellular concentrations of drugs necessary to kill the target cells are difficult to achieve with antibody–drug conjugates for the following reasons: (1) most commonly used anticancer drugs are only moderately cytotoxic; (2) the antigen targets are present on cell surfaces often in limited numbers; (3) the internalization processes for antigen–antibody complexes are generally inefficient; and (4) most linkers that have been used for the conjugation of drugs to antibodies do not efficiently release drug inside tumor cell.

5.1. Targeting C242 with hC242–DM1

Conjugates of toxins and potent cytotoxics (*Pseudomonas* endotoxin [PE]), TGF-α–PE hybrid toxin, genistein, diphtheria toxin, gelonin) to the EGFR ligands and MAbs to EGFR designed for specificity against EGFR overexpressing tumors, have been discussed previously (*see* Section 2.1.6.). The immunoconjugate SB-408075 (huC242–DM1) consists of an extremely potent cytotoxic agent linked to an MAb against an antigen found in most gastrointestinal and epithelial malignancies. In essence, SB-408075 is a tumor-activated prodrug created by the conjugation of a derivative of maytansine (DM1), an extremely potent antimicrotubule agent, to a humanized version of the murine monoclonal antibody C242. Maytansine and DM1, which inhibit tubulin polymerization and microtubule assembly, have approx 100-fold more cytotoxic potency in vitro than most conventional anticancer agents. IC_{50} values for DM1 in a panel of human tumor cell lines have been reported to range from 10 to 40 pM, which are 3- to 10-fold less values for maytansine.

The huC242 antibody is a genetically engineered humanized form of the parent complement-binding MAb C242 *(245)*, which defines an epitope that is sialidase sensitive, but otherwise structurally unknown. The epitope is found on the CanAg antigen, a mucin-type glycoprotein expressed to varying degrees by virtually all human colorectal and pancreatic cancers and to a lesser degree by non-small-cell lung, renal, and cerival cancers *(246–250)*.

In animal tissue distribution studies using the C242 antibody and SB-408075, binding is predominantly to the surface epithelium of gastrointestinal tissue and the secretory ducts of various organs, largely the result of binding to secreted mucin. Early pilot studies evaluated the therapeutic efficacy of a form of SB-408075, composed of a murine C242 MAb antibody instead of the humanized huC242 MAb, against human colon tumor xenografts in SCID mice *(250)*. At doses which induced negligible toxicity, C242–DM1 cured mice bearing well-developed (200–500 mm^3) subcutaneous COLO 205 tumor xenografts. Tumors in animals treated with mixtures of equivalent doses of "naked" antibody and free maytansinoid grew at the same rate as untreated controls. A nonbinding conjugate made with an irrelevant antibody had little effect, further supporting the antigen specificity of the therapeutic effect. C242–DM1 has also induced complete remissions in subcutaneous LoVo and HT-29 colon tumor xenografts, although the tumors express the target antigen in a heterogenous manner; only 20–30% of these cells demonstrate antigen-positivity by immunohistochemical staining *(250)*. The SB-408075 immunoconjugate has demonstrated similar activity, as well as an excellent therapeutic window, as the curative dose was below the toxic dose range. SB-408075 was also very effective in models of antigen-homogenous and antigen-heterogeneous tumors, which simulates human tumors in the clinical setting. In addition, irinotecan and 5-FU plus leucovorin used at their maximum tolerated doses were less effective than SB-408075, with no complete remissions noted in the two aforementioned models. This background has served as the rationale to develop and evaluate SB-408075 in patients with tumors expressing the C242 epitope and the agent is currently in phase I clinical evaluations at the Cancer Therapy and Research Center in San Antonio and the University of Chicago; several patients with colorectal cancer who had been previously treated with 5-FU and irinotecan had decrements in carinembryonic antigen levels following treatment *(251)*.

5.2. Immunocytokines

Several immunocytokines are also being developed to target colorectal and other relevant cancers *(252)*. These compounds consist of antibodies to antigens, usually cell membrane receptors, membrane glycoproteins (EpCAM/17-A), or components of the extracellular matrix (e.g., ganglioside GD2), fused to cytokines like TNF-α and IL-2. In vitro and in vivo studies have demonstrated that huKS-IL-2, IL-2 fused to an antibody against EpCAM/17-A (Merck KgaA), a membrane glycoprotein overexpressed in many colorectal and many other cancers, is active against colorectal tumors. This agent is currently in phase I clinical trials.

REFERENCES

1. Rowinsky EK. The pursuit of optimal outcomes in cancer therapy in a new age of antiproliferative therapies: shifting paradigms for therapeutic evaluation and cancer treatment. *Drugs*, **80** (Suppl. 1) (2000), 1–14.
2. Hanahan D and Weinberg RA. The hallmarks of cancer. *Cell*, **100** (2000) 57–70.
3. Medema RH and Bos JL. The role of p21-ras in receptor tyrosine kinase signaling. *Crit. Rev. Oncol.*, **4** (1993) 615–661.
4. Downward J. Mechanisms and consequences of activation of protein kinase B/Akt. *Curr. Opin. Cell. Biol.*, **10** (1998) 262–267.
5. Powis G. Signaling pathways as targets for anticancer drug development. *Pharmacol. Ther.*, **62** (1994) 57–95.
6. Grandis JR, Melhem MF, Barnes EL, et al. Quantitative immunohistochemical analysis of transforming growth factor-α and epidermal growth factor receptor in patients with squamous cell carcinoma of the head and neck. *Cancer*, **78** (1996) 1284–1292.
7. Salomon DS, Brandt R, Ciadiello F, et al. Epidermal growth factor-related peptides and their receptors in human malignancies. *Crit. Rev. Oncol. Hematol.*, **19** (1995) 183–232.

8. Mayer A, Takimoto M, Fritz E, et al. The prognostic significance of proliferating cell nuclear antigen, epidermal growth factor receptor, and *mdr* gene expression in colorectal cancer. *Cancer*, **71** (1993) 2454–2460.

9. Schreiber AB, Winkler ME, and Derynck R. Transforming growth factor-α: a more potent angiogenic mediator than epidermal growth factor. *Science*, **232** (1986) 1250–1253.

10. Ennis BW, Lippman ME, and Dickson RB. The EGF receptor system as a target for antitumor therapy. *Cancer Invest.*, **9** (1991) 553–562.

11. Kiyokawa N, Karunagaran D, Lee EK, et al. Involvement of cdc2-mediated phosphorylation in the cell cycle-dependent regulation of p185^{neu}. *Oncogene*, **15** (1997) 2633–2641.

12. Rodeck U, Jost M, Kari C, et al. EGFR-dependent regulation of keratinocyte survival. *J. Cell Sci.*, **110** (1997) 113–121.

13. Gibson S, Tu S, Oyer R, et al. Epidermal growth factor protects epithelial cells against Fas-induced apoptosis. Requirement for Akt activation. *J. Biol. Chem.*, **274** (1999) 17,612–17,618.

14. Modjahedi H, Affleck K, Stubberfield C, et al. EGFR blockade by tyrosine kinase inhibitor or monoclonal antibody inhibits growth, directs terminal differentiation and induces apoptosis in human squamous cell carcinoma HN5. *Int. J. Oncol.*, **13** (1998) 335–342.

15. Wu X, Fan Z, Masui H, et al. Apoptosis induced by an anti-epidermal growth factor receptor monoclonal antibody in a human colorectal carcinoma cell line and its delay by insulin. *J. Clin. Invest.*, **95** (1995) 1897–1905.

16. Fan Z, Baselga J, Masui H, et al. Antitumor effect of anti-epidermal growth factor receptor monoclonal antibodies plus cis-diammine-dichloroplatinum on well established A431 cell xenografts. *Cancer Res.*, **53** (1993) 4637–4642.

17. Moyer JD, Barbacci EG, Iwata KK, et al. Induction of apoptosis and cell cycle arrest by CP-358,774, an inhibitor of epidermal growth factor receptor tyrosine kinase. *Cancer Res.*, **57** (1997) 4838–4848.

18. Karnes WE Jr, Weller SG, Adjei PN, et al. Inhibition of epidermal growth factor receptor kinase induces protease-dependent apoptosis in human colon cancer cells. *Gastroenterology*, **114** (1998) 930–939.

19. De Jong JS, van Diest PJ, van der Valk P, et al. Expression of growth factors, growth-inhibiting factors, and their receptors in invasive breast cancer. II: correlations with proliferation and angiogenesis. *J. Pathol.*, **184** (1998) 53–57.

20. Dvorak HF, Brown LF, Detmar M, et al. Vascular permeability factor/vascular endothelial growth factor, microvascular hyperpermeability, and angiogensis. *Am. J. Pathol.*, **146** (1995) 1029–1039.

21. Hanahan D and Folkman J. Patterns and emerging mechanisms of the angiogenic switch during tumorigenesis. *Cell*, **86** (1996) 353–364.

22. Fontanini G, De Laurentiis M, Vignati S, et al. Evaluation of epidermal growth factor-related growth factors and receptors and of neoangiogenesis in completely resected stage I-IIIA non-small-cell lung cancer: amphiregulin and microvessel count is independent prognostic indicators of survival. *Clin. Cancer Res.*, **4** (1998) 241–249.

23. Viloria Petit AM, Rak J, Hung M-C, et al. Neutralizing antibodies against epidermal growth factor and Erbb-2/*neu* receptor tyrosine kinases down-regulate vascular endothelial growth factor production by tumor cell in vitro and in vivo: angiogenic implications for signal transduction therapy of solid tumors. *Am. J. Pathol.*, **151** (1997) 1523–1530.

24. Perrotte P, Matsumoto T, Inoue K, et al. Chimeric monoclonal antibody (Mab) C225 to the epidermal growth factor receptor (EGF-R) antibody inhibits angiogenesis in human transitional cell carcinoma (TCC). *Proc. Am. Assoc. Cancer Res.*, **39** (1998) 316 (abstract).

25. Shibata T, Kawano T, Nagayasu H, et al. Enhancing effects of epidermal growth factor on human squamous cell carcinoma motility and matrix degradation but not growth. *Tumor Biol.*, **17** (1996) 168–175.

26. Kondapaka SB, Fridman R, and Reddy KB. Epidermal growth factor and amphiregulin up-regulate matrix matalloproteinase-9 (MMP-9) in human breast cancer cells. *Int. J. Cancer*, **70** (1997) 722–726.

27. Matsumoto T, Perrotte P, Bar-Eli M, et al. Blockade of EGF-R signaling with anti-EGF-R monoclonal antibody C225 inhibits matrix metalloproteinase-9 expression and invasion of human transitional cell carcinoma in vitro and in vivo. *Proc. Am. Assoc. Cancer Res.*, **39** (1998) 565 (abstract).

28. Adam L, Vadlamudi R, Kondapaka, SB, et al. Heregulin regulates cytoskeletal reorganization and cell migration through the p21-activated kinase-1 via phosphatidylinositol-3 kinase. *J. Biol. Chem.*, **273** (1998) 28,238–28,246.

29. Goldstein NI, Prewett M, Zuklys K, et al. Biological efficacy of a chimeric antibody to the epidermal growth factor receptor in a human tumor xenograft model. *Clin. Cancer Res.*, **1** (1995) 1311–1318.

30. Prewett M, Overholser J, Hooper A, et al. Growth inhibition of human pancreatic in vitro and in vivo by chimeric anti-EGF receptor monoclonal antibody C225. *Proc. Am. Assoc. Cancer Res.*, **40** (1999) 4818 (abstract).

31. Etessami A and Bourhis J. Cetuximab. *Drugs Future*, **25** (2000) 895–899.
32. Mendelsohn J and Fan Z. Epidermal growth factor receptor family and chemosensitization. *J. Natl. Cancer Inst.*, **89** (1997) 341–343.
33. Baselga J, Norton L, Masui H, et al. Antitumor effects of doxorubicin in combination with anti-epidermal growth factor receptor monoclonal antibodies. *J. Natl. Cancer Inst.*, **85** (1993) 1327–1333.
34. Woodburn JR, Kendrew J, Fennell M, et al. ZD1839 ("IRESSA"), a selective epidermal growth factor receptor tyrosine kinase inhibitor (EGFR-TKI): inhibition of c-fos mRNA, an intermediate marker of EGFR activation, correlates with tumor growth inhibition. *Proc. Am. Assoc. Cancer Res.*, **41** (2000) 2552 (abstract).
35. Wen X, Li C, Wu Q-P, et al. Potentiation of antitumor activity of PG-TXL with anti-EGFR monoclonal antibody C225 in MDA-MB-468 human breast cancer xenograft. *Proc. Am. Assoc. Cancer Res.*, **41** (2000) 2052 (abstract).
36. Huang S-M, Bock JM, and Harari PM. Epidermal growth factor receptor blockade with C225 modulates proliferation, apoptosis, and radiosensitivity in squamous cell carcinoma of the head and neck. *Cancer Res.*, **59** (1999) 1935–1940.
37. Trummel HQ, Raisch, Ahmed A, et al. The biological effects of anti-epidermal growth factor and ionizing radiation in human head and neck tumor cell lines. *Proc. Am. Assoc. Cancer Res.*, **40** (1999) 958 (abstract).
38. Rao GS and Ethier SP. Potentiation of radiation-induced breast cancer cell death by inhibition of epidermal growth factor family of receptors. *Int. J. Radiat. Biol.*, **45** 162.
39. Thompson CB. Apoptosis in the pathogenesis and treatment of disease. *Science*, **267** (1995) 1456–1462.
40. Sartor C. Biological modifiers as potential radiosensitizers: targeting the epidermal growth factor receptor family. *Semin. Oncol.*, **6** (Suppl. 11) (2000) 15–20.
41. Carter S, Auer KL, Reardon DB, et al. Inhibition of the mitogen activated protein (MAP) kinase cascade potentiates cell killing by low dose ionizing radiation in A431 human squamous carcinoma cells. *Oncogene*, **16** (1998) 2787–2796.
42. Balaban N, Moni J, Shannon M, et al. The effect of ionizing radiation on signal transduction: antibodies to EGF receptor sensitize A431 cells to radiation. *Biochem. Biophys. Acta*, **1314** (1996) 147–156.
43. Price BD and Youmell MB. The phosphatidylinositol 3-kinase inhibitor wortmannin sensitizes murine fibroblasts and human tumor cells to radiation and blocks induction of *p53* following DNA damage. *Cancer Res.*, **56** (1996) 246–250.
44. Bonner JA, Ezekiel MP, Robert F, et al. Continued response following treatment with IMC-C225, an EGFr MoAb combined with RT in advanced head and neck malignancies. *Proc. Am. Soc. Clin. Oncol.*, **19** (2000) 4 (abstract).
45. Chu CT, Everiss KD, Wikstrand CJ, et al. Receptor dimerization is not a factor in the signalling activity of a transforming variant epidermal growth factor receptor (EGFRvIII). *Biochem. J.*, **324** (1997) 855–861.
46. Olapade-Olaopa EO, Moscatello DK, MacKay EH, et al. Evidence for the differential expression of a variant EGF receptor protein in human prostate cancer. *Br. J. Cancer*, **82** (2000) 186–194.
47. Wickstrand CJ, McLendon RE, Friedman AH, et al. Cell surface localization and density of the tumor-associated variant of the epidermal growth factor receptor, EGFRvIII. *Cancer Res.*, **57** (1997) 4130–4140.
48. Levitt ML and Koty PP. Tyrosine kinase inhibitors in preclinical development. *Invest. New Drugs*, **17** (1999) 213–226.
49. Woodburn JR. The epidermal growth factor receptor and its inhibition in cancer therapy. *Pharmacol. Ther.*, **82** (1999) 241–250.
50. Klohs WD, Fry DW, and Kraker AJ. Inhibitors of tyrosine kinase. *Curr. Opin. Oncol.*, **9** (1997) 562–568.
51. Woodburn JR, Kendrew J, Fennell M, et al. ZD1839 ("IRESSA"), a selective epidermal growth factor receptor tyrosine kinase inhibitor (EGFR-TKI): inhibition of c-fos mRNA, an intermediate marker of EGFR activation, correlates with tumor growth inhibition. *Proc. Am. Assoc. Cancer Res.*, **41** (2000) 2552 (abstract).
52. Hidalgo M, Siu LL, Nemunaitis J, et al. Phase I and pharmacologic study of OSI-774, an epidermal growth factor receptor tyrosine kinase inhibitor, in patients with advanced solid malignancies. *J. Clin. Oncol.*, **19** (2001) 3267–3279.
53. Ferry D, Hammond L, Ranson M, et al. Intermittent oral ZD1839 (Iressa), a novel epidermal growth factor receptor tyrosine kinase inhibitor (egfr-tki) shows evidence of good tolerability and activity: final results from a phase I study. *Proc. Am. Soc. Clin. Oncol.*, **19** (2000) 3 (abstract).
54. Baselga J, Herbst R, LoRusso P, et al. Continuous administration of ZD1839 (Iressa), a novel oral epidermal growth factor receptor tyrosine kinase inhibitor (EGFR-TKI), in patients with five selected tumor types: evidence of activity and good tolerability. *Proc. Am. Soc. Clin. Oncol.*, **19** (2000) 177 (abstract).
55. Beerli RR, Wels W, and Hynes NE. Autocrine inhibition of the epidermal growth factor receptor by intracellular expression of a single-chain antibody. *Biochem. Biophys. Res. Commun.*, **204** (1994) 666–672.

56. Lei W, Mayotte JE, and Levitt ML. EGF-dependent and independent programmed cell death pathways in NCI-H596 nonsmall cell lung cancer cells. *Biochem. Biophys. Res. Commun.*, **24** (1998) 939–945.

57. Wang S, Lee RJ, Cauchon G, et al. Delivery of antisense oligo- deoxyribonucleotides against the human epidermal growth factor receptor into cultured KB cells with liposomes conjugated to folate via polyethylene glycol. *Proc. Natl. Acad. Sci. USA*, **92** (1995) 3318–3322.

58. Normanno N, Bianco C, Damiano V, et al. Growth inhibition of human colon carcinoma cells by combinations of anti-epidermal growth factor-related growth factor antisense oligonucleotides. *Clin. Cancer Res.*, **2** (1996) 601–609.

59. Normanno N, De Luca A, Salomon DS, et al. Epidermal growth factor-related peptides as targets for experimental therapy of human colon carcinoma. *Cancer Detect. Prev.*, **22** (1998) 62–67.

60. Taetle R, Honeysett JM, and Houston LL. Effects of anti-epidermal growth factor (EGF) receptor antibodies and an anti-EGF receptor recombinant-rich A chain immunoconjugate on growth of human cells. *J. Natl. Cancer Inst.*, **80** (1988) 1053–1059.

61. Masui H, Kamrath H, Apell G, et al. Cytotoxicity against human tumor cells mediated by the conjugate of anti-epidermal growth factor receptor monoclonal antibody to recombinant ricin A chain. *Cancer Res.*, **49** (1989) 3482–3488.

62. FitzGerald DJ, Padmanabhan R, Pastan I, et al. Adenovirus-induced release of epidermal growth factor and *Pseudomonas* toxin into the cystol of KB cells during receptor-mediated endocytosis. *Cell*, **32** (1983) 607–617.

63. Xu Y-H, Chaudhary VK, et al. Cytotoxic activities of a fusion protein comprised of TGFα and *Pseudomonas* exotoxin. *FASEB J.*, **3** (1989) 2647–2652.

64. Genersch E, Schneider DW, Sauer G, et al. Prevention of EGF-modulated adhesion of tumor cells to matrix proteins by specific EGF receptor inhibition. *Int. J. Cancer*, **75** (1998) 205–209.

65. Uckun FM, Narla RK, Zeren T, et al. In vivo toxicity, pharmacokinetics, and anticancer activity of genistein linked to recombinant human epidermal growth factor. *Clin. Cancer Res.*, **4** (1998) 1125–1134.

66. Theodoulou M, Baselga J, Scher H, et al. Phase I dose-escalation study of the safety, tolerability, pharmacokinetics and biologic effects of DAB389EGF in patients with solid malignancies that express EGF receptors. *Proc. Am. Soc. Clin. Oncol.*, **14** (1995) 480 (abstract).

67. Eng CP, Sehgal SN, and Vezina C. Activity of rapamycin (AY-22,989) against transplanted tumors. *J. Antibiot.* (Tokyo), **37** (1984) 1231–1237.

68. Muthukkumar S, Ramesh TM, and Bondada S. Rapamycin, a potent immunosuppressive drug, causes programmed cell death in B lymphoma cells. *Transplantation*, **60** (1995) 264–270.

69. Seufferlein T and Rozengurt E. Rapamycin inhibits constitutive p70s6k phosphorylation, cell proliferation, and colony formation in small cell lung cancer cells. *Cancer Res.*, **56** (1996) 3895–3897.

70. Hosoi H, Dilling MB, Shikata T, et al. Rapamycin causes poorly reversible inhibition of mTOR and induces p53-independent apoptosis in human rhabdomyosarcoma cells. *Cancer Res.*, **59** (1999) 886–894.

71. Grewe M, Gansauge F, Schmid RM, et al. Regulation of cell growth and cyclin D1 expression by the constitutively active FRAP-p70s6K pathway in human pancreatic cancer cells. *Cancer Res.*, **59** (1999) 3581–3587.

72. Shi Y, Frankel A Radvanyi LG, et al. Rapamycin enhances apoptosis and increases sensitivity to cisplatin in vitro. *Cancer Res.*, **55** (1995) 1982–1988.

73. Koltin Y, Faucette L, Bergsma DJ, et al. Rapamycin sensitivity in Saccharomyces cerevisiae is mediated by a pep-tidyl-prolyl cis-trans isomerase related to human FK506-binding protein. *Mol. Cell. Biol.*, **11** (1991) 1718–1723.

74. Sabers CJ, Martin MM, Brunn GJ, et al. Isolation of a protein target of the FKBP12-rapamycin complex in mammalian cells. *J. Biol. Chem.*, **270** (1995) 815–822.

75. Keith CT and Schreiber SL. PIK-related kinases. DNA repair, recombination, and cell cycle checkpoints. *Science*, **270** (1995) 50–51.

76. Brown EJ and Schreiber SL. A signaling pathway to translational control. *Cell*, **86** (1996) 517–520.

77. Nav BT, Ouwens M, Withers DJ, et al. Mammalian target of rapamycin is a direct target for protein kinase B: identification of a convergence point for opposing effects of insulin and amino-acid deficiency on protein translation. *Biochem. J.*, **344** (1999) 427–431.

78. Cantley LC and Neel BG. New insights into tumor suppression: PTEN suppresses tumor formation by restraining the phosphoinositide 3-kinase B/Akt. *Proc. Natl. Acad. Sci. USA*, **96** (1999) 4240–4245.

79. Downward J. Mechanisms and activation of protein kinase B/Akt. *Curr. Opin. Cell. Biol.*, **10** (1998) 262–267.

80. Brunn GJ, Hudson CC, Sekulic A, et al. Phosphorylation of the translational repressor PHAS-I by the mammalian target of rapamycin. *Science*, **277** (1997) 99–101.

81. Gingras AC, Kennedy SG, O'Leary MA, et al. 4E-BP1, a repressor of mRNA translation, is phosphorylated and inactivated by the akt(PKB) signaling pathway. *Genes Dev.*, **12** (1998) 502–513.

82. Chung J, Grammer TC, Lemon KP, et al. PDGF- and insulin-dependent pp70S6k activation mediated by phosphatidylinositol-3-OH kinase. *Nature*, **370** (1994) 71–75.

83. Petritsch C, Woscholski R, Edelman HM, et al. Activation of p70 S6 kinase and erk-encoded mitogen-activated protein kinases is resistant to high cyclic nucleotide levels in Swiss 3T3 fibroblasts. *J. Biol. Chem.*, **270** (1995) 26,619–26,625.

84. Burgering BM and Coffer PJ. Protein kinase B (c-Akt) in phosphatidylinositol-3-OH kinase signal transduction. *Nature*, **376** (1995) 599–602.

85. Sonenberg N. Remarks on the mechanism of ribosome binding to eukaryotic mRNAs. *Gene Expr.*, **3** (1993) 317–323.

86. Sonenberg N and Gingras AC. The mRNA 5′ cap-binding protein eIF4E and control of cell growth. *Curr. Opin. Cell. Biol.*, **10** (1998) 268–275.

87. Metcalfe SM, Canman CE, Milner J, et al. Rapamycin and p53 act on different pathways to induce G1 arrest in mammalian cells. *Oncogene*, **15** (1997) 1635–1642.

88. Molnar-Kimber KL. Mechanism of action of rapamycin (Sirolimus, Rapamune). *Transplant. Proc.*, **28** (1996) 964–969.

89. Hashemolhosseini S, Nagamine Y, Morley SJ, et al. Rapamycin inhibition of the G1 to S transition is mediated by effects on cyclin D1 mRNA and protein stability. *J. Biol. Chem.*, **273** (1998) 14,424–14,429.

90. Sherr CJ and Roberts JM. Inhibitions of mammalian G1 cyclin-dependent kinases. *Genes Dev.*, **9** (1995) 1149–1163.

91. Morgan DO. Principles of CDK regulation. *Nature*, **374** (1995) 131–134.

92. Nourse J, Firpo E, Flanagan WM, et al. Interleukin-2-mediated elimination of the p27Kip1 cyclin-dependent kinase inhibitor prevented by rapamycin. *Nature*, **372** (1994) 570–573.

93. Luo Y, Marx SO, Kiyokawa H, et al. Rapamycin resistance tied to defective regulation of p27Kip1. *Mol. Cell. Biol.*, **16** (1996) 6744–6751.

94. Gibbons JJ, Discafani C, Peterson R, et al. The effect of CCI-779, a novel macrolide anti-tumor agent, on the growth of human tumor cells in vitro and in nude mouse xenografts in vivo. *Proc. Am. Assoc. Cancer Res.*, **40** (1999) 301 (abstract).

95. Raymond E, Alexander J, Depenbrock H, et al. CCI-779, a rapamycin analog with antitumor activity: a phase I study utilizing a weekly schedule. *Proc. Am. Soc. Clin. Oncol.*, **40** (2000) 187 (abstract).

96. Hidalgo M, Rowinsky E, Erlichman C, et al. CCI-779, a rapamycin analog and multifaceted inhibitor of signal transduction: a phase I study. *Proc. Am. Soc. Clin. Oncol.*, **19** (2000) 187 (abstract).

97. Boguski MS and McCormick F. Proteins regulating Ras and its relatives. *Nature*, **366** (1993) 643–654.

98. Rowinsky EK, Windle JJ, and Von Hoff DD. Ras protein franesyltransferase: a strategic target for anticancer drug development. *J. Clin. Oncol.*, **17** (1999) 3631–3652.

99. Lowy DR and Willumsen BM. Function and regulation of Ras. *Annu. Rev. Biochem.*, **62** (1993) 851–891.

100. Leonard DM. Ras farnesyltransferase: a new therapeutic target. *J. Med. Chem.*, **40** (1997) 2971–2990.

101. Shimizu K, Goldfarb M, Suard Y, et al. Three human transforming genes are related to the viral oncogenes. *Proc. Natl. Acad. Sci. USA*, **80** (1983) 2112–2116.

102. Gibbs JB. Lipid modifications of proteins in the Ras superfamily. In *GTPases in Biology*. Birnbaumer L and Dickey B (eds.), Springer-Verlag, New York, 1993, pp. 335–344.

103. Kato K, Cox AD, Hisaka MM, et al. Isoprenoid addition to Ras protein is the critical modification for its membrane association and transforming activity. *Proc. Natl. Acad. Sci. USA*, **89** (1992) 6403–6407.

104. Khosravi-Far R and Der CJ. The Ras signal transduction pathway. *Cancer Metastasis Rev.*, **13** (1994) 67–89.

105. McCormick F. Activators and effectors of ras p21 proteins. *Curr. Opin. Genet. Dev.*, **4** (1994) 71–76.

106. Pazin MJ and Williams LT. Triggering signaling cascades by receptor tryosine kinases. *Trends Biochem. Sci.*, **17** (1992) 374–378.

107. Clark GJ and Der CJ. Ras proto-oncogene activation in human malignancy. In *Cellular Cancer Markers*. Sell S (ed.), Humana, Totowa, NJ, 1995, pp. 17–52.

108. Khosravi-Far R, Campbell S, Rossman KL, and Der CJ. Increasing complexity of Ras signal transduction: involvement of Rho family members. *Adv. Cancer Res.*, **72** (1998) 57–107.

109. McCormick F. Ras biology in atomic detail. *Nature Struct. Biol.*, **3** (1996) 653–655.

110. Ridley AJ and Hall A. The small GTP-binding protein Rho regulates the assembly of focal adhesions and actin stress fibers in response to growth factors. *Cell*, **70** (1992) 389–399.

111. Rodriguez-Viciana P, Warne PH, Dhand R, et al. Phosphatidylinositol-3-OH kinase as a direct target of Ras. *Nature*, **370** (1994) 527–532.

112. Carpenter CL and Cantley LC. Phosphoinositide kinases. *Curr. Opin. Cell. Biol.*, **8** (1996) 153–158.

113. Yan J, Roy S, Apolloni A, et al. Ras isoforms vary in their ability to activate Raf-1 and phosphoinositide 3-kinase. *J. Biol. Chem.*, **273** (1998) 24,052–24,056.

114. Kennedy SG, Wagner AJ, Conzen SD, et al. The PI 3-kinase/Akt signaling pathway delivers an anti-apoptitic signal. *Genes Dev.*, **11** (1997) 701–713.

115. Kauffman-Zeh A, Rodriguez-Viciana P, Ulrich E, et al. Suppression of c-Myc-induced apoptosis by Ras signalling through PI(3)K and PKB. *Nature*, **385** (1997) 544–548.

116. Joneson T, White MA, Wigler MH, et al. Stimulation of membrane ruffling and MAP kinase activation by distinct effectors orf Ras. *Science*, **271** (1996) 810–812.

117. Ridley AJ, Paterson HF, Johnston CL, et al. The small GTP-binding protein Rac regulates growth-factor induced membrane ruffling. *Cell*, **70** (1992) 401–410.

118. Casey PJ. p21 Ras is modified by a farnesyl isoprenoid. *Proc. Natl. Acad. Sci. USA*, **86** (1989) 8323–8327.

119. Cox AD, Hisaka MM, Buss JE, et al. Specific isoprenoid modification is required for function of normal, but not oncogenic, Ras protein. *Mol. Cell. Biol.*, **12** (1992) 2606–2615.

120. Gibbs JB, Oliff A, and Kohl NE. Farnesyltransferase inhibitors: Ras research yields a potential cancer therapeutic. *Cell*, **77** (1994) 177–178.

121. Symons M. The Rac and Rho pathways as a source of drug targets for Ras-mediated malignancies. *Curr. Opin. Biotechnol.*, **6** (1995) 668–774.

122. Hancock JF, Cadwallader K, and Marshall CJ. A Caax or a Caal motif and a second signal are sufficient for plasma membrane targeting of ras proteins. *EMBO J*, **110** (1991) 641–646.

123. Casey PJ and Seabra MC. Protein prenyltransferases. *Biol. Chem.*, **271** (1996) 5289–5292.

124. Gibbs JB, and Oliff A. The potential of farnesyltransferase inhibitors as cancer chemotherapeutics. *Ann. Rev. Pharmacol. Toxicol.*, **37** (1997) 143–166.

125. Sebti SM and Hamilton AD. New approaches to anticancer drug design based on the inhibition of farnesyltransferase. *Drug Discov. Today*, **3** (1998) 26–33.

126. Heimbrook DC and Oliff A. Therapeutic intervention and signaling. *Curr. Opin. Cell. Biol.*, **10** (1998) 284–288.

127. Pompliano DL, Rands E, Schaber MD, et al. Steady-state kinetic mechanism of Ras farnesyl:protein transferase. *Biochemistry*, **31** (1992) 3800–3807.

128. Park HW, Boduluro SR, Moomaw JF, et al. Crystal structure of protein farnesyltransferase at 2.25 angstrom resolution. *Science*, **275** (1997) 1800–1804.

129. Vogt A, Sun J, Qian Y, et al. The geranylgeranyltransferase-I inhibitor GGTI-298 arrests human tumor cells in B_0/G_1 and induces p1$^{WAF/CIP/SDII}$ in a p53-independent manner. *J. Biol. Chem.*, **272** (1997) 27,224–27,229.

130. Monia BP, Johnston JF, Ecker DJ, et al. Selective inhibition of mutant Ha-ras mRNA expression by antisense oligonucleotides. *J. Biol. Chem.*, **267** (1992) 19,954–19,962.

131. Gray GD, Hernandez OM, Hebel D, et al. Antisense DNA inhibition of tumor growth induced by c-Ha-ras oncogene in nude mice. *Cancer Res.*, **53** (1993) 577–580.

132. Schwab G, Chavany C, Duroux I, et al. Antisense oligonucleotides absorbed to polyalkylcyanoacrylate nanoparticles specifically inhibit mutated Ha-ras-mediated cell proliferation and tumorigenicity in nude mice. *Proc. Natl. Acad. Sci. USA*, **91** (1994) 10,460–10,464.

133. Dorr A, Burce J, Monia B, et al. Phase I and pharmacokinetic trial of ISIS 2503, a 20-mer antisense olignucleotide against H-ras by 14-day continous infusion (CIV) in patients with advanced cancer. *Proc. Am. Soc. Clin. Oncol.*, **18** (1999) 603 (abstract).

134. Adjei A, Erlichman C, Sloan J, et al. A phase I trial of Isis 2503, an antisense inhibitor of H-Ras in combination with gemcitabine in patients with advanced cancer. *Proc. Am. Soc. Clin. Oncol.*, **19** (2000) 186 (abstract).

135. Mikhopadhyay T, Tainsky M, Cavendar AC, et al. Specific inhibition of K-ras expression and tumorigenicity of lung cancer cells by antisense RNA. *Cancer Res.*, **51** (1991) 1744–1748.

136. Georges R, Mukhopadyay T, Zhang Y, et al. Prevention of orthotopic human lung cancer growth by intrateracheal instillation of a retroviral antisense K-ras construct. *Cancer Res.*, **53** (1993) 1743–1746.

137. Alemany R, Ruan S, Masafumi K, et al. Growth inhibitory effect of anti-K-ras adenovirus on lung cancer cells. *Cancer Gene Ther.*, **3** (1996) 296–301.

138. Aoki K, Yoshida T, Sugimura T, and Terada M. Liposome mediated transfer of antisense K-ras construct inhibits pancreatic tumor dissemination in the murine peritoneal cavity. *Cancer Res.*, **55** (1995) 3810–3816.

139. Adjei AA, Davis JN, Erlichman C, et al. Comparison of potential surrogate markers of farnesyltransferase inhibition. *Clin. Cancer Res.*, **6** (2000) 2318–2325.

140. Sonnichsen D, Damle B, Manning J, et al. Pharmacokinetics and pharmacodynamics of the farnesyltransferase inhibitor BMS-214662 in patients with advanced solid tumors. *Proc. Am. Soc. Clin. Oncol.*, **19** (2000) 178 (abstract).

141. Johnston SR, Ellis PA, Houston S, et al. A phase II study of the farnesyl transferase inhibitor R115777 in patients with advanced breast cancer. *Proc. Am. Soc. Clin. Oncol.*, **19** (2000) 318.

142. Whyte DB, Kirschmeier P, Hockenberry TN, et al. K- and N-Ras are geranylgeranylated in cells treated with farnesyl protein transferase inhibitors. *J. Biol. Chem.*, **272** (1997) 14,459–14,464.

143. Rowell CA, Kowalczyk JJ, Lewis MD, et al. Direct demonstration of geranylgeranylation and farnesylation of Ki-Ras in vivo. *J. Biol. Chem.*, **272** (1997) 14,093–14,097.

144. Lebowitz PF, Davide JP, and Prendergast GC. Evidence that farnesyltransferase inhibitors suppress Ras transformation by interfering with Rho activity. *Mol. Cell. Biol.*, **15** (1995) 6613–6622.

145. Hung W-C and Chaung L-Y. The farnesyltransferase inhibitor FPT inhibitor III upregulates Bax and Bcl-xs expression and induces apoptosis in human ovarian cancer cells. *Int. J. Oncol.*, **12** (1998) 137–140.

146. Yaglom J, Goldberg A, Finley D, et al. The molecular chaperone Ydj1 is required for the p34CDC28-dependent phosphorylation of the cyclin Cln3 that signals its degradation. *Mol. Cell. Biol.*, **15** (1996) 3679–3684.

147. Smets G, Xhonneux B, Cornelissen F, et al. R115777, a selective farnesyl protein transfease inhibitor (FTI), induces antiangiogenic, apoptotic and anti-proliferative activity in CAPAN-2 and LoVo tumor xenografts. *Proc. Am. Assoc. Cancer Res.*, **39** (1998) 2170 (abstract).

148. Feldkamp M, Lau N, and Guha A. The farnesyl transferase inhibitor SCH66336 inhibits the growth of human astrocytoma cell lines and xenografts implanted in NOD-SCID mice. *Proc. Am. Assoc. Cancer Res.*, **41** (2000) 2834 (abstract).

149. Rose WC, Arico MA, Burke CL, et al. Preclinical antitumor activity of BMS-214662, a novel farnesyl transferase inhibitor. *Proc. Am. Assoc. Cancer Res.*, **41** (2000) 2835 (abstract).

150. Kohl NE, Omer CA, Conner MW, et al. Inhibition of farnesyltransferase induces regression of mammary and salivary carcinomas in ras transgenic mice. *Nature Med.*, **1** (1995) 792–799.

151. Sinn E, Muller W, Pattengale P, et al. Coexpression of MMTV/v-Ha-ras and MMTV/c-myc genes in transgenic mice. Synergistic action of oncogenes in vivo. *Cell*, **49** (1987) 465–475.

152. Barrington RE, Subler MA, Rands E, et al. A farnesyltransferase inhibitor induces tumor regression in transgenic mice harboring multiple oncogenic mutations by mediating alterations in both cell cycle control and apoptosis. *Mol. Cell. Biol.*, **18** (1998) 85–92.

153. Sharma S, Britten C, Spriggs D, et al. A phase I and pharmacokinetic study of farnesyl transferase inhibitor L-778,123 administered as a seven day continuous infusion in combination with paclitaxel. *Proc. Am. Soc. Clin. Oncol.*, **19** (2000) 184a (abstract).

154. Lancet J, Rosenblott J, Lieveld JL, et al. Use of farnesyltransferase inhibitor R1157777 in relapsed and refractory leukemia. Preliminary results of a phase I trial. *Proc. Am. Soc. Clin. Oncol.*, **19** (2000) 58 (abstract).

155. Zujewski J, Horak ID, Bol CJ, et al. A phase I study of farnesyl protein transferase inhibitor, R115777, in advanced cancer. *J. Clin. Oncol.*, **18** (2000) 927–934.

156. Hudes G, Schol J, Baab, et al. Phase I clinical and pharmacokinetic trial of the farnesyltransferase inhibitor R115777 on a 21-day dosing schedule. *Proc. Am. Soc. Clin. Oncol.*, **18** (1999) 156a (abstract).

157. Britten CD, Rowinsky E, Yao S-L, et al. A phase I and pharmacologic study of the farnesyl protein transferase inhibitor L-778,123 in patients with solid cancers. *Proc. Am. Soc. Clin. Oncol.*, **18** (1999) 597 (abstract).

158. Rubin E, Abbruzzese J, Morrison B, et al. Phase I trial of the farnesyl transferase (FPTase) inhibitor L-778,123 on a 14 or 28-day dosing schedule. *Proc. Am. Soc. Clin. Oncol.*, **19** (2000) 689 (abstract).

159. Adjei AA, Davis JN, Erlichman C, et al. A phase I and pharmacologic study of the farnesyl protein transferase inhibitor SCH66336: evidence for biological and clinical activity. *Cancer Res.*, **60** (2000) 1871–1877.

160. Hurwitz HI, Colvin OM, Petros WP, et al. A phase I and pharmacokinetic study of SCH 66336, a novel FPTI using a 2-week on, 2-week off schedule. *Proc. Am. Soc. Clin. Oncol.*, **18** (1999) 599 (abstract).

161. Eskens F, Awada A, Verweijj J, et al. Phase I and pharmacologic study of continuous daily oral SCH66336, a novel farnesyl transferase inhibitor, in patients with solid tumors. *Proc. Am. Soc. Clin. Oncol.*, **18** (1999) 156a (abstract).

162. Moasser MM, Sepp-Lorenzino L, Kohl NE, et al. Farnesyl transferase inhibitors cause enhanced mitotic sensitivity to taxol and epothilones. *Proc. Natl. Acad. Sci. USA*, **95** (1998) 1369–1374.

163. Liu M, Bryant MS, Chen J, et al. Antitumor activity of SCH66336, and orally bioavailable tricylic inhibitor of farnesyl protein transferase, in human tumor xenograft models and wap-ras transgenic mice. *Cancer Res.*, **58** (1998) 4947–4956.

164. Nielsen LL, Shi B, Hajian G, et al. Combination therapy with the farnesyl protein transferase inhibitor SCH66336 and SCH5850 (p53 adenovirus) in preclinical cancer models. *Cancer Res.*, **59** (1999) 5896–5901.

165. Patnaik A, Eckhardt SG, Izbicka E, et al. A phase I and pharmacologic (PK) study of the farnesyltransferanse inhibitor, R115777 in combination with Gemcitabine. *Proc. Am. Soc. Clin. Oncol.*, **19** (2000) 5 (abstract).

166. Grugel S, Finkenzeller G, Weindel K, et al. Both v-Ha-Ras and v-Raf stimulate expression of the vascular endothelial growth factor in NIH 3T3 cells. *J. Biol. Chem.*, **270** (1995) 25,915–25,919.

167. Rak J, Mitsuhashi Y, Bayko L, et al. Mutant ras oncogenes upregulate VEGF/VPF expression: Implications for induction and inhibition of tumor angiogenesis. *Cancer Res.*, **55** (1995) 4575–4580.

168. Bernhard EJ, Kao G, Cox AD, et al. The farnesyl transferase inhibitor FTI-277 radiosensitizes H-Ras transformed rat embryo fibroblasts. *Cancer Res.*, **56** (1996) 1727–1730.

169. Peters JM, Harris JR, and Finley D (eds.). *Ubiquitin and the Biology of the Cell.* Plenum, New York, 1998, Chaps. 1–6.

170. Ciechanover A. The ubiquitin-proteasome pathway: on protein death and cell life. *EMBO J.*, **24** (1998) 7151–7160.

171. Lee DH and Goldberg AL. Proteasome inhibitors: valuable new tools for cell biologists. *Trends Cell Biol.*, **8** (1998) 397–403.

172. Spataro V, Norbury C, and Harris AL. The ubiquitin-proteasome pathway in cancer. *Br. J. Cancer*, **77** (1998) 448–455.

173. Hilt W and Wolf D. Proteasomes: destruction as a programme. *Trends Biochem. Sci.*, **21** (1996) 96–102.

174. Maki C, Huibregtse J, and Howley P. In vivo ubiquitination and proteasome-mediated degradation of p53. *Cancer Res.*, **56** (1996) 2649–2654.

175. Rousset R, Desbois C, Bantignies F, and Jalinot P. Effects on NF-kB1/p105 processing of the interaction between the HTLV-1 transactivator Tax and the proteasome. *Nature*, **381** (1996) 328–331.

176. Palombella VJ, Rando OJ Goldberg AL, and Maniatis T. The ubiquitin–proteasome pathway is required for processing the NF-κB1 precursor protein and the activation of NF-κB. *Cell*, **78** (1994) 773–785.

177. Jensen TJ, Loo MA, Pind S, et al. Multiple proteolytic systems, including the proteasome, contribute to CFTR processing. *Cell*, **83** (1995) 129–135.

178. Kim T and Maniatis T. Regulation of interferon-γ-activated STAT1 by the ubiquitin–proteasome pathway. *Science*, **273** (1996) 1717–1719.

179. Deshaies R, Chau V, and Kirschner M. Ubiquitination of the G1 cyclin Cln2p by a Cdc34p-dependent pathway. *EMBO J.*, **14** (1995) 303–312.

180. Seufert W, Futcher B, and Jentsch S. Role of a ubiquitin conjugating enzyme in degradation of S- and M-phase cyclins. *Nature*, **373** (1995) 78–81.

181. Ritcher-Ruoff B and Wolf D. Proteasome and cell cycle. Evidence for a regulatory role of the protease on mitotic cyclins in yeast. *FEBS Lett.*, **336** (1993) 34–36.

182. Adams J and Stein R. Novel inhibitors of the proteasome and their therapeutic use in inflammation. *Annual Rep. Med. Chem.*, **31** (1996) 279–288.

183. Bogyo M, McMaster JS, Gaczynska M, et al. Covalent modification of the active site threonine of proteasomal B subunits and the Escherichia coli homologue Hs1V by a new class of inhibitors. *Proc. Natl. Acad. Sci.*, **94** (1997) 6629–6634.

184. Groettrup M and Schmidtke G. Selective proteasome inhibitors. *Proc. Natl. Acad. Sci. USA*, **94** (1997) 6629–6634.

185. Crews CM, Sin N, and Meng L. Natural products as molecular probes of angiogenesis. Book of Abstracts, 215th ACS Natl Mtg, Dallas, 1998, MEDI 208.

186. Figueiredo-Pereira ME, Chen WE, Li J, and Johdo O. The antitumor durg aclacinmonycin A which inhibits the degadration of ubiquitinated proteins, shows selectively for the chymotrypsin like activity of the bovine pituitary 20S proteasome. *J. Biol. Chem.*, **271** (1996) 16,455–16,459.

187. Meyer S, Kohler NG, and Joy A. Cyclosporine A is an uncompetitive inhibitor of proteasome activity and prevents NF-κB activation. *FEBS Lett.*, **413** (1997) 354–358.

188. Wang X, Omura S, Szweda LI, et al. Rapamycin inhibits proteasome activator expression and proteasome activity. *Eur. J. Immunol.*, **27** (1997) 2781–2786.

189. Andre P, Groettrup M, Klenerman P, et al. An inhibitor of HIV-1 protease modulates proteasome activity, antigen presentation, and T cell responses. *Proc. Natl. Acad. Sci. USA*, **95** (1998) 13,120–13,124.

190. Adams J, Palombella VJ, Sausville EA, et al. Proteasome inhibitors: a novel class of potent and effective anti-tumor agents. *Cancer Res.*, **59** (1999) 2615–2622.

191. Teicher BA, Ara G, Herbst R, et al. The Proteasome inhibitor PS-341 in cancer therapy. *J. Clin. Cancer Res.*, **5** (1999) 2638–2645.

192. Herrmann JL, Briones F Jr, Brisbay S, et al. Prostate carcinoma cell death resulting from inhibition of proteasome activity is independent of functional bcl-2 and p53. *Oncogene*, **17** (1998) 2889–2899.

193. Orlowski M, Cardozo C, and Michaud C. Evidence for the presence of five distinct proteolytic components in the pituitary multicatalytic proteinase complex. Properties of two components cleaving bonds on the carboxyl side of branched chain and small neutral amino acids. *Biochemistry,* **32** (1993) 1563–1572.

194. Wang CY, Cusack JC, Liu R, and Baldwin AS Jr. Control of inducible chemoresistance: enhanced anti-tumor therapy via increased apoptosis through inhibition of NF-kB. *Nature Med.*, **5** (1999) 412–417.

195. Adams J, Palombella VJ, and Elliott PJ. Proteasome inhibition: a new strategy in cancer treatment. *Invest. New Drugs*, **18** (2000) 109–121.

196. Shibatani T, Nazir M, and Ward W. Alteration of rat liver 20S proteasome activities by age and food restriction. *J. Gerontol.*, **51A** (1996) B316–B322.

197. Aghajanian C, Elliot P, Adams J, et al. Phase I trial of the proteasome inhibitor PS-341 in advanced malignancy. *Proc. Am. Soc. Clin. Oncol.*, **736** (2000) 189a.

198. Papandreou CN, Pagliaro L, Millkan R, et al. Phase I study of PS-341, a novel proteasome inhibitor, in patients with advanced malignancies. *Proc. Am. Soc. Clin. Oncol.*, **738** (2000) 190a.

199. Fearon ER and Vogelstein B. A genetic model for colorectal tumorigenesis. *Cell*, **61(5)** (1990) 759–767.

200. Tsujimoto Y, Ikegaki N, and Croce CM. Characterization of the protein product of bcl-2, the gene involved in human follicular lymphoma. *Oncogene*, **2** (1987) 3–7.

201. Reed JC. Bcl-2 and the regulation of programmed cell death. *J. Cell Biol.*, **124** (1994) 1–6.

202. Ohmori T, Podack ER, Nishio K, et al. Apoptosis of lung cancer cells caused by some anti-cancer agents (MMC, CPT-11, ADM) is inhibited by bcl-2. *Biochem. Biophys. Res. Comm.*, **192** (1993) 30–36.

203. Walton MI, Whysong D, O'Connor PM, et al. Constitutive expression of human Bcl-2 modulates nitrogen mustard and camptothecin induced apoptosis. *Cancer Res.*, **53** (1993) 1853–1861.

204. Nakamura T, Nomura S, Sakai T, and Nariya S. Expression of bcl-2 oncoprotein in gastrointestinal and uterine carcinomas and their premalignant lesions. *Hum. Pathol.*, **28** (1997) 309–315.

205. Valassiadou KE, Stefanaki K, Tzardi M, et al. Immunohistochemical expression of p53, bcl-2, mdm2 and wafl/p21 proteins in colorectal adenocarcinomas. *Anticancer Res.*, **17** (1997) 2571–2576.

206. Sinicrope FA, Ruan SB, Cleary KR, et al. bcl-2 and p53 oncoprotein expression during colorectal tumorigenesis. *Cancer Res.*, **55** (1995) 237–241.

207. Mueller J, Mueller E, Hoepnr I, et al. Expression of bcl-2 and p53 in de novo and ex-adenoma colon carcinoma: a comparative immunohistochemical study. *J. Pathol.*, **180** (1996) 259–265.

208. Teixeira C, Reed JC, and Pratt MA. Estrogen promotes chemotherapeutic drug resistance by a mechanism involving Bcl-2 proto-oncogene expression in human breast cancer cells. *Cancer Res.*, **55** (1995) 3902–3907.

209. Ionov Y, Peinado MA, Malkhosyan S, et al. Ubiquitous somatic mutations in simple repeated sequences reveal a new mechanism for colonic carcinogenesis. *Nature*, **363** (1993) 558–561.

210. Thibodeau SN, Bren G, and Schaid D. Microsatellite instability in cancer of the proximal colon. *Science*, **260** (1993) 816–819.

211. Yamamoto H, Sawai H, Weber TK, et al. Somatic frameshift mutations in DNA mismatch repair and proapoptosis genes in hereditary nonpolyposis colorectal cancer. *Cancer Res.*, **58** (1998) 997–1003.

212. Rampino N, Yamamoto H, Ionov, et al. Somatic frameshift mutations in the BXA gene in colon cancers of the microsatellite mutator phenotype. *Science*, **275** (1997) 967–969.

213. Tolcher A, Gleave M, Brown B, et al. Antisense bcl-2 oligonucleotides inhibit the progession to androgen-independence (AI) after castration in the LNCaP tumor model. *Proc. Am. Assoc. Cancer Res.*, **39** (1998) 417 (abstract).

214. Miyake H, Tolcher A, and Gleave ME. Antisense Bcl-2 oligodeoxynucleotides inhibit progression to androgen-independence after castration in the Shionogi tumor model. *Cancer Res.*, **59** (1999) 4030–4034.

215. Janse B, Schlagbauer-Wadl H, Brown BD, et al. bcl-2 antisense therapy chemosensitizes human melanoma in SCID mice. *Nature Med.*, **4** (1998) 232–234.

216. Pitti, RM, Masters SA, Ruppert S, et al. Induction of apoptosis by Apo-2 ligand, a new member of the tumor nevrosis factor receptor family. *J. Biol. Chem.*, **271** (1996) 12,687–12,690.

217. Wiley SR, Schooley K, Smolak PJ, et al. Identification and characterization of a new member of the TNF family that induces apoptosis. *Immunity*, **3** (1995) 673–682.

218. Smith CA, Farrah T, and Goodwin RG. The TNF receptor superfamily of cellular and viral proteins: activation, costimulation, and death. *Cell*, **76** (1994) 959–962.

219. Gruss HJ and Dower SK. Tumor necrosis factor ligand superamily: involvement in the pathology of malignant lymphomas. *Blood*, **85** (1995) 3378–3404.

220. Ashkeazi A and Dixit VM. Death receptors: signaling and modulation. *Science*, **281** (1998) 1305–1308.

221. Walczak H, Miller RE, Ariail K, et al. Tumoricidal activity of tumor necrosis factor-related apoptosis-inducing ligand in vivo. *Nature Med.*, **5** (1999) 157–163.
222. Ashkenazi A, Pai RC, Fong S, et al. Safety and anti-tumor activity of recombinant soluble Apo2 ligand. *J. Clin. Invest.*, **104** (1999) 155–162.
223. Emery JG, McDonnell P, Burke MB, et al. Osteoprotegerin is a receptor for the cytotoxic ligand TRIAL. *J. Biol. Chem.*, **273** (1998) 14,363–14,367.
224. Griffith TS, Chin WA, Jackson GC, et al. Intracellular regulation of TRAIL-induced apoptosis in human melanoma cells. *J. Immunol.*, **161** (1998) 2833–2840.
225. Ashkenazi A and Dixit VM. Apoptosis control by death and decoy receptors. *Curr. Opin. Cell Biol.*, **5** (1999) 156–163.
226. Rieger J, Naumann U, Glaser T, et al. Apo2 ligand: a novel lethal weapon against malignant glioma? *FEBS Lett.*, **427** (1998) 124–128.
227. Keane M, Ettenberg S, Nau MM, et al. Chemotherapy augments TRAIL-induced apoptosis in breast cell lines. *Cancer Res.*, **59** (1999) 734–741.
228. Mori S, Murakami-Mori K, Nakamura S, et al. Sensitization of AIDS-Kaposi's sarcoma cells to Apo2 ligand-induced apoptosis by actinomycin D. *J. Immumol.*, **162** (1999) 5616–5623.
229. Niesor E, Gillespie A, Antoni I, et al. SR-45023A is a new anticancer agent which inhibits cell proliferation and specifically triggers apoptosis in tumor cells. *Proc. Am. Assoc. Cancer Res.*, **39** (1998) 314.
230. Niesor E, Flach J and Bentzen C. A new class of potential anticancer agents acting on the mevalonate-isoprenoid regulatory pathway. 10th NCI–EORTC Symposium, 1998, p. 413.
231. Weinberger C, Katzenellenbogen J, Niesor E, et al. The nuclear receptor FXR as a potential target for drugs regulating mevalonate-isoprenoid biosynthesis and cell growth. 10th NCI–EORTC Symposium, 1998, p. 414.
232. Flach J, Antoni I, Villemin P, et al. SR-45023A overcomes multidrug resistance and restores sensitivity to taxol in the p-glycoprotein expressing cell line MCF7/ADR. *Proc. Am. Assoc. Cancer Res.*, **39** (1998) 171.
233. Sausville EA. Cyclin-dependent kinases: novel targets for cancer treatment. In *American Society of Clinical Oncology 1999 Yearbook of Oncology.* Perry MC (ed.), American Society of Clinical Oncology, Alexandria, VA, 2000, pp. 9–76.
234. Senderowicz AM and Sausville EA. Preclinical and clinical development of cyclin-dependent kinase modulators. *J. Natl. Cancer Inst.*, **92** (2000) 376–387.
235. Shapiro GI and Harper JW. Anticancer drug targets: cell cycle and checkpoint control. *J. Clin. Invest.*, **104** (1999) 1645–1653.
236. Sherr CJ. Cancer cell cycles. *Science*, **274** (1996) 1672–1677.
237. Lundberg AS and Weinberg RA. Control of the cell cycle and apoptosis. *Eur. J. Cancer*, **35** (1999) 1886–1894.
238. Sielecki TM, Boylan JF, Benfield PA, and Trainor GL. Cyclin-dependent kinase inhibitors: useful targets in cell cycle regulation. *J. Med. Chem.*, **43** (2000) 1–18.
239. Kaubisch A and Schwartz G. Cyclin-dependent kinase and protein kinase C inhibitors: a novel class of antineoplastic agents in clinical development. *Cancer J.*, **6** (2000) 192–212.
240. El-Deiry WS. Role of oncogenes in resistance and killing by cancer therapeutic agents. *Curr. Opin. Oncol.*, **9** (1997) 79–87.
241. Lowe SW and Lin AW. Apoptosis in cancer. *Carcinogenesis*, **21** (2000) 485–495.
242. Trail PA, Willner D, Lasch SJ, et al. Cure of xenografted human carcinomas by BR96–doxorubicin immunoconjugates. *Science*, **261** (1993) 212–215.
243. Kanellos J, Pietersz GA, and McKenzie IE. Studies of methotrexate-monoclonal antibody conjugates for immunotherapy. *J. Natl. Cancer Inst.*, **75** (1985) 319–332.
244. Starling JJ, Maciak RS, Law KL, et al. In vivo antitumor activity of a monoclonal antibody-Vinca alkaloid immunoconjugate directed against a solid tumor membrane antigen characterized by heterogeneous expression and noninternaliation of antibody-antigen complexes. *Cancer Res.*, **51** (1991) 2965–2972.
245. Johansson C, Nilsson O, Baeckstrom D, et al. Novel epitope on the CA50-carrying antigen: chemical and immunochemical studies. *Tumor Biol.*, **12** (1991) 159–170.
246. Calvete JA, Newell DR, Wright AF, et al. ICI D0490: a potent and selective immunotoxin for the treatment of colorectal cancer. *Cancer Res.*, **54** (1994) 4684–4690.
247. Calvete JA, Newell DR, Charlton CJ, et al. Pharmacokinetic studies in mice with ICI D0490, a novel recombinant ricin A-chain immunotoxin. *Br. J. Cancer*, **67** (1993) 1310–1315.
248. Johansson C, Nilsson O, and Lindholm L. Comparison of serological expression of different epitopes on the CA50-carrying antigen CanAg. *Int. J. Cancer*, **48** (1991) 757–763.

249. Haglund C, Lindgren J, Roberts PJ, et al. Tissue expression of the tumor associated antigen CA242 in benign and malignant pancreatic lesions. A comparison with CA 50 and CA 19-9. *Br. J. Cancer*, **60** (1989) 845–851.
250. Liu C, Tadayoni BM, Bourret LA, et al. Eradication of large colon tumor xenografts by targeted delivery of maytansinoids. *Proc. Natl. Acad. Sci. USA*, **93** (1996) 8618–8623.
251. Tolcher AW, Ochoa L, Patnaik A, et al. SB-4087945, a maytansinoid immunoconjugate directed to the C242 antigen: a phase I, pharmacokinetic, and biologic correlative study. Proc NCI–EORTC–AACR Meeting, Amsterdam, 2000, p. 128.
252. Lode HN, Xiang R, Becker JC, et al. Immunocytokines: a promising approach to cancer immunotherapy. *Pharmacol. Ther.*, **80** (2000) 277–292.

41 Vaccine Strategies for Colorectal Cancer

Kenneth A. Foon

1. INTRODUCTION

Immune approaches to the therapy of colorectal cancer have substantially evolved over the past years, from treating patients with nonspecific immune stimulants to a focus on the use of tumor-associated antigens (TAA) either by passive immune therapy with antibodies targeted directly against tumor cells or by active immune therapy in which the patient's own immune system is stimulated to attack the cancer, either via vaccination with tumor cells or tumor cell lysates, vaccination with peptides, carbohydrates, or gene constructs encoding proteins, or via the use of anti-idiotype antibodies that mimic tumor-associated antigens. A study from Germany in Dukes' C patients who were randomized to a monoclonal antibody, designated 171A, demonstrated improved survival by 30% over patients on the observation control arm *(1)*. One hypothesis to explain this result is that 171A may activate the idiotype network and thus, through activation of the immune response against the 171A antigen, generate a clinical response. A recent report refutes this hypothesis, however, and suggests that another immunologic mechanism, perhaps the stimulation of antibody-dependent cellular toxicity, may be involved *(2)*. The opportunity to improve results in Dukes' B2, C, and D patients with this passive immunotherapeutic approach in addition to chemotherapy is under investigation, and clinical results of these trials are eagerly awaited. This chapter, however, will focus primarily on vaccine approaches in colorectal cancer.

2. VACCINES

2.1. Specific Active Immunotherapy

Specific active immunotherapy differs from nonspecific immune-based therapies such as bacillus Calmette–Guérin (BCG), in that the goal is specific targeted activation to eliminate only the tumor cells and not affect surrounding normal tissue. Specific immunotherapy through vaccines activates a unique lymphocyte response (B- and/or T-cell), which has

From: *Colorectal Cancer: Multimodality Management*
Edited by: L. Saltz © Humana Press Inc., Totowa, NJ

both an immediate antitumor effect as well as a memory response against future tumor challenge.

The first and most obvious type of vaccines are autologous or allogeneic whole tumor cell preparations. Alternatively, membrane preparations alone from tumor cells have been used. With advances in molecular biology, gene-modified tumor cells that express antigens designed to increase immunogenicity or cells that have been gene modified to secrete cytokines have been actively investigated. In addition, increase in our knowledge of TAA biology has led to the use of purified TAAs, DNA-encoding protein antigens, and/or protein-derived peptides. All of these approaches are being tested in the clinic.

2.2. Structure of the Immune System

Mechanistically, the ultimate aim of a vaccine is to activate a component of the immune system, such as antibodies or lymphocytes, against TAAs presented by the tumor. Antibodies must recognize antigens in the native protein state at the cell surface. Once bound, these molecules can mediate antibody-dependent cellular cytotoxicity (ADCC) or complement-mediated cytotoxicity (CMC). T-Lymphocytes, on the other hand, recognize fragments of proteins, or peptides, presented in the context of major histocompatibility complex (MHC) antigens on the surface of the cells being recognized (3,4). The proteins from which the peptides are derived may be cell surface or cytoplasmic proteins (5,6). MHC antigens are highly polymorphic, and different alleles have distinct peptide binding capabilities. The sequencing of peptides derived from MHC molecules has led to the discovery of allele-specific motifs that correspond to anchor residues that fit into specific pockets on MHC class I or II molecules (7,8).

There are two types of T-lymphocytes, helper and cytotoxic, which recognize antigens through a specific T-cell receptor (TCR). The TCR is composed of both α- and β-subunits arranged in close conjunction to the CD3 molecule, which is responsible for signaling (Fig. 1). CD4 helper T-cells secrete lymphokines and cytokines that enhance immunoglobulin production as well as activate CD8 cytotoxic T-lymphocytes (CTL). CD4 helper T-cells are activated by binding via their TCR to class II molecules, which contain 14–25 amino acid (mer) peptides in their antigen-binding cleft (9–11). Extracellular proteins are endocytosed and degraded (exogenous processing) into 14–25-mer peptides in endocytic compartments (acidified endosomes) and bind to newly synthesized MHC class II molecules. The MHC peptide complex is transported to the cell membrane where it can be recognized by specific CD4 helper T-cells. In most cases, the MHC class II antigen containing peptide is presented to the CD4 helper T-cells by a specialized cell called an antigen-presenting cell (APC). A variety of cells are capable of processing and presenting exogenous antigen, including B-cells, monocytes, macrophages, and the bone-marrow-derived dendritic cell (DC). DCs are the most efficient APC and express high levels of MHC class I and II molecules, costimulatory molecules such as CD80 and CD86, and specific markers such as CD83. Following antigen uptake, DCs migrate peripherally to lymph nodes, where antigen presentation to CD4 helper T-cells takes place (12,13).

There are two types of CD4 helper T-cells capable of generating either an antibody or a cell-mediated immune response. Th1 CD4 helper T-cells stimulate cell-mediated immunity (CMI) by activating CTLs through the release of lymphocytokines such as interleukin-2 (IL-2). Th2 CD4 helper T-cells mediate an antibody response through the release of lymphocytokines such as IL-4 and IL-10. In some instances, the generation of one type of response may serve to inhibit the generation of the other (14) (i.e., IL-10 secretion by Th2 helper T-cells inhibits the generation of CTLs).

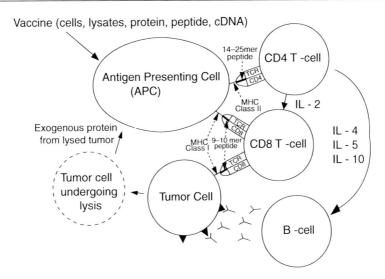

Fig. 1. T-Cell activation. T-Cells recognize antigens as fragments of proteins (peptides) presented with major histocompatibility complex (MHC) molecules on the surface of cells. The antigen-presenting cell processes exogenous protein from the vaccine or from the lysed tumor cell into a peptide and presents the 14/25-mer peptide to CD4 helper T-cells on a class II molecule. There are also data that suggests that exogenous proteins can be processed into 9/10-mer peptides that may be presented on MHC class I molecules to CD8 cytotoxic T-cells. Activated Th1 CD4 helper T-cells secrete Th1 cytokines such as IL-2 that upregulate CD8 cytotoxic T-cells. Activated Th2 CD4 helper T-cells secrete Th2 cytokines such as IL-4, IL-5, and IL-10 that activate B-cells.

CD8-positive CTLs are activated in most cases by peptides derived from intracellular proteins that are cleaved to 9–10-mer peptides in the cytosol of tumor cells or APCs by protesomes. The peptides are then transported via specialized transporter molecules called TAP proteins to the endoplasmic reticulum, where they become associated with newly synthesized MHC class I molecules *(15)*. The complex is then transported via the Golgi apparatus to the cell surface membrane, where the complex is recognized by CD8 cytotoxic T-cells via a specific TCR. Any endogenously processed protein can be presented to the immune system in this way. Several reports suggest that a subset of APCs can present exogenously processed proteins on MHC class I molecules to CTLs *(16–20)*.

2.3. Vaccine Strategies

2.3.1. WHOLE TUMOR CELL VACCINES

The most straightforward means of immunization is the use of whole tumor cell preparations (either autologous or allogeneic tumor cells). The advantage to this approach is that all potential TAA are presented to the immune system for processing and presentation to the appropriate T-cell precursors. The difficulty with this approach lies in the availability of fresh autologous tumor material and in the sparcity of well-characterized long-term tumor cell lines that are HLA typed and express high levels of MHC antigens. Regardless, whole tumor cell vaccines have been an area of intense interest.

In a prospective randomized trial, 98 patients with Dukes' stage B2 through stage C3 colon or rectal cancer were treated by resection alone or resection plus active specific immunotherapy with a whole tumor cell preparation *(21)*. This study design was based on a highly successful guinea pig model *(22–26)*. Vaccine administration consisting of 10^7

viable irradiated autologous tumor cells and 10^7 viable BCG organisms began 4–5 wk after tumor resection, beginning with one intradermal vaccination per week for 2 wk. In the third week, patients received 1 vaccination of 10^7 irradiated tumor cells alone. Overall and disease-free survival did not show a statistically significant difference for the 80 eligible patients. However, the rectal cancer patients received postimmunotherapy radiation, which may have blunted the immune response. When these patients were separated from the colon cancer patients, with a median follow-up of 93 mo, a significant improvement in overall and disease-free survival was seen in the colon cancer patients who received active specific immunotherapy. Correlations with immune responses were not reported.

In a recent phase III trial (27), 412 patients with colon cancer (297 with stage II disease, 115 with stage III disease) were randomized to observation versus intradermal injections of irradiated autologous tumor cells mixed with BCG after surgical resection. After a 7.6-yr median follow-up, there were no statistically significant differences in clinical outcomes between the treatment arms. However, there were disease-free survival ($p = 0.78$) and overall survival ($p = 0.12$) trends in favor of the vaccine arm for patients who received the intended treatment.

In another study, freshly thawed autologous colon cancer cells were inactivated with radiation and infected with Newcastle disease virus or mixed with BCG (28). All patients had resected Dukes' B or C colorectal cancer. The 2-yr survival rate for patients treated with cells containing Newcastle disease virus was 98%, versus 67% for those treated with cells mixed with BCG. Delayed-type hypersensitivity skin reactions to Newcastle-virus-infected cells were reported in 68% of patients studied.

2.3.2. GENETICALLY MODIFIED TUMOR CELLS

Another approach to tumor cell vaccines is the introduction into tumor cells of foreign genes encoding cytokines such as IL-2, granulocyte-macrophage colony-stimulating factor (GM-CSF), tumor necrosis factor (TNF), or interferon-γ (29,30). Alternatively, molecules designed to increase tumor cell immunogenicity, such as CD80 and CD86, have proven to be very effective in murine models and are showing promise in vitro in allowing the generation of tumor-specific CTL (31–35). Gene transfer can be accomplished by transfection of plasmid constructs (electroporation, lipofectamine) or transduction utilizing a viral vehicle such as retroviruses or adenoviruses.

Retroviruses have been most widely used for gene transfer into fresh human tumor cells. Retroviral vectors have a high efficiency of gene transfer as well as stable insertion and expression of the protein in the target cell (29,36). However, because retroviral vectors require actively proliferating cells for stable gene transfer, their usefulness in human clinical trials has been hampered. In most cases, this approach is most successful using tumor cell lines because they more readily take up foreign DNA and express the protein product than do fresh tumor cells.

Alternative gene delivery has been tested using other viral delivery systems such as adenovirus and poxviruses, where cell division is not a prerequisite for gene transfer, however, specificity of binding of the virus to the target cell becomes an issue. In addition, other possible adverse effects of these viruses include potential adverse effects on antigen presentation through the downregulation of class I molecules and induction of antiviral responses that may limit subsequent immunization. There are also the safety concerns inherent in the use of attenuated viruses in human patients.

Another option that has been tested for gene transfer is physical gene delivery in which plasmid or "naked" DNA is delivered directly into tumor cells. Liposomes can serve as gene carriers. Use of a "gene gun," electroporation, and calcium-phosphate-mediated gene transfer are all alternative methodologies that have been evaluated for the physical delivery of genes into tumor cells. The primary problem with a nonviral gene delivery system is that gene expression in the transfected cells tends to be transient.

A murine colon carcinoma cell line that was transduced with the IL-2 gene generated active specific tumor immunity (bypassing T-helper function); implanted tumors were promptly rejected *(37)*. In another animal model, recombinant vaccinia virus encoding the gene for GM-CSF (rV-GM-CSF) was used to transfect the MC38 murine colon carcinoma cell line *(38)*. The rV-GM-CSF infected MC38 cell line suppressed the growth of MC38 primary tumors, with long-lasting immunity that was dependent on the presence of both CD4 and CD8 T-cells. MC38 cells infected with recombinant vaccinia virus expressing IL-2 or IL-6 did not mediate protection.

Overall, the tumor cell approach is most interesting in that the vaccine can have a profound effect on the inflammatory infiltrate. The granulocytes and macrophages that are contained therein serve to begin the rejection and destruction of tumor cells. Macrophages and DC precursors contained in the infiltrate phagocytyze tumor debris and begin the presentation to TAA-specific lymphocyte precursors (Fig. 1). All of these activities may be enhanced in the presence of the cytokine delivered by the tumor cells. Alternatively, tumor cells gene modified with lymphocyte costimulatory molecules (CD80/86) present TAAs directly to lymphocyte precursors. Ultimately, one looks for a localized antitumor response, that, if properly propagated, develops into a potent systemic antitumor immunity.

2.3.3. PEPTIDES, MUCINS, AND CARBOHYDRATES

An alternative to the above-described vaccine strategies is the use of purified protein or peptide molecules as immunogens. The molecules themselves code for the relevant TAA. In most instances, these molecules can be manufactured in large quantities, and if delivered properly, they can result in a potent antitumor immune response. Whole proteins, as opposed to peptides, can be processed and presented by a wider array of class I and II molecules. Peptide vaccines have a potential advantage in that they can be more easily synthetically generated in a reproducible fashion. The major disadvantage of peptides, however, is that they are restricted to a single HLA molecule and are not, of themselves, very immunogenic *(39)*. To increase their immunogenicity, peptides may be injected with adjuvants, cytokines, or liposomes or may be presented on dendritic cells *(40–48)*. An extensive literature is beginning to amass on class I and II restricted protein antigens in melanoma *(2,49–57)*. Unfortunately, a less extensive literature exists for epithelial tumors, including colon cancer *(58–65)*.

Mucins, such as MUC1, are heavily glycosylated high-molecular-weight proteins abundantly expressed on human cancers of epithelial origin *(66–70)*. The MUC1 gene is overexpressed and aberrantly glycosylated on a variety of cancers, including colorectal cancer. Much of the glycosylation is found within regions of tandemly repeated sequences of 20 amino acids per repeat *(70–72)*. Tumors derived from cells of epithelial origin often lose the carbohydrate side chains, exposing the tandemly repeated protein core of the mucin, resulting in antigenically active epitopes being exposed to the cell surface membrane *(70)*.

Numerous mucin-specific antibodies have been generated following immunization of animals with epithelial cells *(70,73,74)*. MHC-restricted and unrestricted recognition of mucin by T-cells has also been reported *(75,76)*. In one study, patients were vaccinated with a 105 amino acid polypeptide that included 5 repetitions of the entire conserved tandem repeat of the MUC1 peptide *(77)*. Sixty-three patients were vaccinated with 100 μg of the mucin peptide mixed with BCG. Two additional vaccinations were given at 3-wk intervals. Toxicity included local ulceration at the site of the vaccination. Delayed-type hypersensitivity reactions were evaluated at 48 h and intense T-cell infiltration was reported in the majority of patients. A limited number of patients had a twofold to fourfold increase in mucin-specific CTL precursors in the peripheral blood after vaccination. A 9-mer peptide spanning the MUC1 tandem repeat with an HLA-A11 MHC class I restriction association has been identified. CTLs specific for this peptide have been identified from peripheral blood of HLA-A11 donors *(78)*.

The "Holy Grail" for successful tumor immunotherapy has been the induction of CTL rather than the generation or use of antibodies. In a recent study, however, it was determined that humans immunized with MUC1 produce good antibody responses, but poor CTL responses. This appears to be the result of the fact that humans do not express gal$^\alpha$ (1,3)gal on their tissues and, therefore, produce natural antibodies against exogenous gal$^\alpha$ (1,3)gal present in bacteria and food. These antibodies cross-react with MUC1 *(79)*, causing the CTL response to switch to an antibody response. Mice do not produce these natural antibodies because they express gal$^\alpha$ (1,3)gal and, thus, generate CTL in response to MUC1.

Authors working on this approach have expressed disappointment in not being able to generate anti-MUC1 CTL in patients. In an accompanying editorial, Houghton and Lloyd *(80)* take issue with the general tone of negativism by these authors. They point out that the current era of "CTL chauvinism" is largely based on experiments in transplantable tumor models in mice, usually tumors produced by mutagens, which are rejected following CTL responses. They argue that although these models are extremely valuable for our understanding of tumor immunology in general, the direct relevance to slowly progressing cancers in humans is not clear. They point out that vaccines against infectious agents act through antibodies, not CTL. These antibodies likely prevent blood-borne dissemination to compensate for limited efficacy against infection at tissue sites. They propose that antibodies may play an important role in preventing metastasis, which could be critical in the postsurgical adjuvant setting.

Immunization against tumor-associated carbohydrate antigen has also been attempted. Vaccine studies have been reported using the GM-2 disialoganglioside primarily associated with melanoma, sarcoma, and neural-derived tumors *(81–83)*. Carbohydrate antigens typically bypass T-cell help for B-cell activation. Investigators have demonstrated that some carbohydrates may activate an alternative T-cell pathway *(84–87)*. Thomsen-Friedenreich (TF) and Sialyl-Tn (sTn) antigens are blood-group-related disaccharides that are O-linked to serine and threonine residues of mucins on epithelial cancers including colorectal cancer *(88–94)*. In normal tissues, TF and sTn antigens are restricted to the luminal surface of secretory cells, which is largely inaccessible to the immune system. Similar to the case with MUC-1, altered glycosylation leads to exposure of these core structures in malignant tissues. However, TF and sTn are poor immunogens because they are carbohydrates and autoantigens. It has also been hypothesized that altered mucins shed by cancer cells induce a T-suppressor lymphocyte response *(94)*. Postsurgical patients who were disease-free but at high risk for recurrence were immunized with synthetic TF and sTn covalently linked to keyhole limpet hemocyanin (KLH), without adjuvant or mixed with the adjuvants Detox or QS-21 *(95)*. The QS-21 mixture was most potent in inducing IgM and IgG titers against the respective synthetic disaccharide epitopes. However, the antibodies only weakly reacted against the natural antigens.

2.3.4. Recombinant Vaccines Expressing CEA

The carcinoembryonic antigen (CEA) gene has been sequenced. It is part of the human immunoglobulin supergene family located on chromosome 19 *(96,97)*. CEA is highly expressed on colorectal cancer and a variety of other epithelial tumors and is thought to be involved in cell–cell interactions. CEA is considered an adhesion molecule and may play an important role in the metastatic process by mediating attachment of tumor cells to normal cells *(98,99)*. For all of the above reasons, we and others have found CEA to be a very attractive target antigen for immunotherapy. The immunogenic nature of CEA in humans is unclear, and there has been no evidence of cell-mediated responses to CEA in humans. Copresentation of CEA with a strong immunogen such as the vaccinia virus would be one logical approach to inducing an anti-CEA response. Vaccinia viruses are highly immunogenic and stimulate both humoral and cell-mediated responses. A recombinant vaccinia virus expressing human CEA (rV-CEA) was shown to stimulate T-cell responses in animal species, including nonhuman primates *(100–102)*. A variety of CEA peptides selected to conform to human HLA-A2 motifs have been established. One 9-mer peptide designated CAP-1 stimulated T-cell lines from the peripheral blood of patients vaccinated with rV-CEA *(103)*. T-Cell lines were demonstrated to lyse HLA-A2-positive colon carcinoma cell lines. This study was important for a number of reasons. First, it was the first to demonstrate human CTL responses to specific CEA epitopes. Second, it demonstrated class I HLA-A2-restricted T-cell-mediated lysis. Third, it demonstrated the ability of human tumor cells to endogenously process CEA to present a specific CEA peptide in the context of a major histocompatibility complex for T-cell-mediated lysis.

In order to enhance the induced immune response, low-dose IL-2 was administered in a murine tumor model with rV-CEA *(104)*. The addition of low-dose IL-2 enhanced immunity and resulted in complete tumor regression in the majority of animals. A DNA plasmid has also been constructed that encodes the full-length complementary DNA for CEA and can function as a polynucleotide vaccine *(105)*. Following lingual injections in mice, this polynucleotide vaccine generated humoral and/or cellular immune responses specific for CEA. Clinical trials of this approach are in progress.

2.3.5. ANTI-IDIOTYPE ANTIBODIES

The idiotype network hypothesis of Lindenmann and Jerne offers an elegant approach to transforming epitope structures into idiotypic determinants expressed on the surface of antibodies *(106,107)*. According to the network concept, immunization with a given tumor-associated antigen will generate production of antibodies against this tumor-associated antigen, which are termed Ab1; Ab1 is then used to generate a series of anti-idiotype antibodies against the Ab1, termed Ab2. Some of these Ab2 molecules can effectively mimic the three-dimensional structure of the original tumor-associated antigen identified by the Ab1. These antibodies, called Ab2β, fit into the paratopes of Ab1 and express the internal image of the tumor-associated antigen. The Ab2β can induce specific immune responses similar to those induced by the original tumor-associated antigen and, therefore, can be used as a surrogate for tumor-associated antigens. Immunization with Ab2β can lead to the generation of anti-anti-idiotypic antibodies (Ab3) that recognize the corresponding original tumor-associated antigen identified by Ab1. Because of this Ab1-like reactivity, the Ab3 is also called Ab1′ to indicate that it might differ in its other idiotopes from Ab1. The anti-idiotype antibody represents an exogenous protein that should be endocytosed by antigen-presenting cells, degraded to 14–25-mer peptides, and presented by class II antigens to activate CD4 helper T-cells (Fig. 2). Activated Th2 CD4 helper T-cells secrete cytokines such as IL-4 that stimulate B-cells that have been directly activated by the Ab3 to produce antibody that binds to the original antigen identified by the Ab1. In addition, activation of Th1 CD4 helper T-cells secrete cytokines that activate T-cells, macrophages, and NK cells,

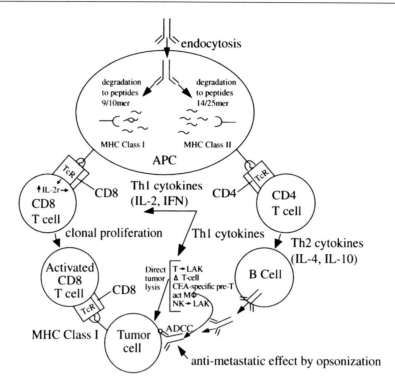

Fig. 2. Potential immune pathways for anti-idiotype vaccines. Anti-idiotype antibodies are endocytosed by antigen presenting cells. They may be degraded to 14/25-mer peptides and presented on MHC class II molecules to CD4 helper T-cells. Activated Th2 CD4 helper T-cells secrete Th2 cytokines that stimulate B-cells that have been directly activated by the anti-idiotype antibody to produce the anti-anti-idiotypic antibody or Ab3 (Ab1) that binds directly to tumor cells. This antibody can mediate complement and antibody-dependent cellular cytotoxicity as well as a direct antimetastatic effect by opsonization. In addition, Th1 CD4 helper T-cells secrete Th1 cytokines that activate T-cells, NK cells, and macrophages. The activated macrophages and LAK cells may also serve as effector cells for antibody-dependent cellular cytotoxicity. All of these cells may mediate direct tumor lysis. There are also data to suggest that exogenously processed proteins can be degraded to 9/10-mer peptides that can be presented by MHC class I molecules to activate CD8 cytotoxic T-cells. This is enhanced by Th1 cytokines such as interleukin-2. Activated CD8 cytotoxic T-cells make contact with tumor cells leading to direct tumor cell lysis.

which directly lyse tumor cells and, in addition, contribute to ADCC. Th1 cytokines such as IL-2 also contribute to the activation of a CD8 cytotoxic T-cell response. This represents a second putative pathway of endocytosed anti-idiotype antibody. The anti-idiotype antibody may be degraded to 9/10-mer peptides to present in the context of class I antigens to activate CD8 cytotoxic T-cells (13–17), which are also stimulated by the IL-2 from Th1 CD4 helper T-cells.

Several anti-idiotype antibodies that mimic tumor-associated antigens on colorectal cancer cells have been reported. One such antibody was generated against the murine 17-1A antibody, previously described. Following surgery for colorectal cancer, six patients were immunized with this human anti-idiotype antibody, which mimicks the GA733-2 antigen (108). All of the patients developed a long-lasting T-cell immunity against GA733-2 and five mounted a specific IgG antibody response against GA733. Another group, using a rat anti-idiotype antibody generated to the 17-1A antibody, immunized nine colorectal cancer patients with aluminum-hydroxide-precipitated 17-1A; none of the nine patients developed

Table 1
Resected Dukes' B, C, and D Patients Treated with CeaVac

Stage	No.	Without progression		With progression		Death	
		No.	Months	No.	Months	No.	Months
B2	4	3	26–28	1	18 (lung CA)	0	
C1	3	2	18, 23	1	35	0	
C2	8	6	21–47	2	19, 24	1	48
D_R	8	5	17–40	3	9–24	0	
D_{IR}	9	1	21	8	6–31	4	14–34

specific antibodies, although four patients developed delayed-type hypersensitivity *(109)*. Another group of investigators has developed both murine and human monoclonal anti-idiotype antibodies that mimic the gp72 antigen *(110–113)*. They demonstrated delayed-type hypersensitivity reactions when murine anti-idiotype antibody was injected without adjuvant *(113)*. When the anti-idiotype was linked to KLH in the presence of Freund's adjuvant, anti-gp72 antibodies were detected. Using the human equivalent anti-idiotype antibody precipitated in aluminum hydroxide, 9 of 13 patients with advanced colorectal cancer produced blastogenic responses to gp72-expressing tumor cells or produced detectable levels of IL-2 in their plasma *(111)*. They suggested that survival correlated with immune responses. In another study, with the same human anti-idiotype antibody, six patients with rectal cancer were immunized preoperatively *(112)*. This study demonstrated significant killing of autologous tumor cells using cryopreserved lymphocytes or lymph node cells from patients 1–2 wk postimmunization.

We have had a major interest in an anti-idiotype antibody designated 3H1, or CeaVac *(114)*. We generated the CeaVac anti-idiotype murine monoclonal antibody to an antibody designated 8019 that identifies a specific epitope on CEA that is highly restricted to tumor cells and not found on normal tissues. We demonstrated that the CeaVac anti-idiotype antibody functioned as an internal image of CEA by generating anti-idiotypic (Ab3) responses that recognize CEA in mice, rabbits, and monkeys and had a major antitumor effect in a murine tumor model *(115)*. Among 23 patients with advanced colorectal cancer, 17 generated anti-anti-idiotypic Ab3 responses and 13 of these responses were proven to be true anti-CEA responses (Ab1′) *(116,117)*. The antibody response was polyclonal and sera from 11 patients mediated antibody-dependent cellular cytotoxicity. Ten patients had idiotypic T-cell responses and five had specific T-cell responses to CEA. None of the patients had objective clinical responses, but overall median survival for the 23 evaluable patients was 11.3 mo, with 44% 1-yr survival (95% confidence interval: 23–64). Toxicity was limited to local swelling and minimal pain. The overall survival of 11.3 mo was comparable to other phase II data with advanced colorectal cancer patients treated with a variety of chemotherapy agents, including irinotecan, and had considerably less toxicity.

Thirty-two patients with resected colorectal cancer were randomized to treatment with 2 mg of aluminum-hydroxide-precipitated CeaVac intracutaneously or 2 mg of CeaVac mixed with 100 µg of the QS-21 adjuvant subcutaneously every other week times four, then monthly until recurrent disease (Table 1) *(118)*. Four patients were Duke's B, 11 were Duke's C, 8 were completely resected Duke's D, and 9 were completely resected Duke's D with minimal residual disease (MRD). Fifteen of the patients received 5-fluorouracil (5-FU)-based chemotherapy regimens simultaneously with CeaVac vaccine. Fifteen patients have relapsed or demonstrated disease progression at 6–35 mo (1 Duke's B developed a secondary lung cancer, 3 Duke's C, and 11 Duke's D). All 32 patients had high-titer polyclonal anti-CEA responses that mediated ADCC. The predominant Ab3 immunoglobulin was IgG, and the major subclass was IgG1. All 32 patients generated idiotypic-specific T-cell responses and 75% were CEA-specific. A linear peptide derived from the CDR2 light-chain region stimulated a CD4 proliferative response *(119)*. These data demonstrate that 5-FU-based chemotherapy regimens do not adversely effect the immune response to CeaVac. In addition, this immune response can be maintained indefinitely with monthly boosts with CeaVac. Injections were well tolerated with only minor local reactions and minimal systemic side effects. Although longer follow-up is required, there appears to be a biological effect on tumor progression suggested by one patient with MRD who continues on study without progression at 21 mo, and eight MRD patients who did not show signs of progression until 6–31 mo. A planned phase III trial conducted by the American College of Surgeons Oncology Group will randomize Duke's C patients to 5-FU and leucovorin vs 5-FU, leucovorin, and CeaVac.

Anti-idiotype vaccines are capable of inducing prophylactic and therapeutic immunity in animal models *(120,121)*. It has been suggested that they may not be ready for the clinic because murine antibodies induce neutralizing antibody responses in humans, idiotype vaccines do not induce long-lasting immunity, and the predominant immune response to anti-idiotypes is IgM *(122)*. Our data, however, clearly demonstrate that monthly injections of murine anti-idiotype antibodies can generate and maintain high titer IgG antibody and proliferative T-cell responses *(123)*.

REFERENCES

1. Riethmuller G, Holz E, Schlimok G, Schmiegel W, Raab R, Hoffken K, et al. Monoclonal antibody therapy for resected Dukes' C colorectal cancer: seven-year outcome of a multicenter randomized trial. *J. Clin. Oncol.*, **16** (1998) 1788–1794.
2. Gruber R, van Haarlem LJ, Warnaar SO, Holz E, and Riethmuller G. The human antimouse immunoglobulin response and the anti-idiotypic network have no influence on clinical outcome in patients with minimal residual colorectal cancer treated with monoclonal antibody CO17-1A. *Cancer Res.*, **60** (2000) 1921–1926.
3. Brodsky FM and Guagliardi LD. The cell biology of antigen processing and presentation. *Annu. Rev. Immunol.*, **9** (1991) 707–744.
4. Parham P. Antigen processing. Transporters of delight. *Nature (Lond.)*, **348** (1990) 674–675.
5. Townsend A and Bodmer H. Antigen recognition by class 1 restricted T lymphocytes. *Annu. Rev. Immunol.*, **7** (1989) 601–624.
6. Monaco J. A molecular model of MHC class-1-restricted antigen processing. *Immunol. Today*, **13** (1992) 173–179.
7. Falk K, Rotzchke O, Stevanovic J, et al. Allele-specific motifs revealed by sequencing of self-peptides eluted from MHC molecules. *Nature*, **351** (1991) 290–294.
8. Falk K and Rotzchke O. Consensus motifs and peptide ligands of MHC class I molecules. *Semin. Immunol.*, **5** (1993) 81–87.
9. Keene J and Forman J. Helper activity is required for the in vitro generation of cytotoxic T lymphocytes. *J. Exp. Med.*, **150** (1982) 1134–1142.
10. Raulet D and Bevan M. Helper T cells for cytotoxic T lymphocytes need not be region restricted. *J. Exp. Med.*, **155** (1982) 1766–1784.
11. Kast W, Bronklhorst, DeWaal L, et al. Cooperation between cytotoxic and helper T lymphocytes in protection against lethal Sendai virus infection. *J. Exp. Med.*, **164** (1986) 723–738.
12. Steinman RM. The dendritic cell system and its role in immunogenicity. *Annu. Rev. Immunol.*, **9** (1991) 271–296.
13. Allison JP, Hurwitz AA, and Leach DR. Manipulation of co-stimulatory signals to enhance antitumor T-cell responses. *Curr. Opin. Immunol.*, **7** (1995) 682–686.
14. Fitch FW, Laneki DW, and Gajewski TF. T-cell mediated immune regulation: help and suppression. In *Fundamental Immunology*. Paul W. and Nita E. (eds.), Raven, New York, 1993, pp. 733–761.

15. Zinkernagel R and Doherty P. MHC-restricted cytotoxic cell: studies on the biological role of polymorphic major transplantation antigens determining T cell restriction-specificity, function and responsiveness. *Adv. Immunol.*, **27** (1979) 51–106.

16. Rock KL, Gamble S, and Rothstein L. Presentation of exogenous antigen with class I major histocompatibility complex molecules. *Science*, **249** (1990) 918–921.

17. Grant EP and Rock KL. MHC class I-restricted presentation of exogenous antigen by thymic antigen-presenting cells in vitro and in vivo. *J. Immunol.*, **148** (1992) 13–18.

18. Rock KL, Rothstein L, Gamble S, et al. Characterization of antigen-presenting cells that present exogenous antigens in association with class I MHC molecules. *J. Immunol.*, **150** (1993) 438–446.

19. Harding CV and Song R. Phagocytic processing of exogenous particulate antigens by macrophages for presentation by class I MHC molecules. *J. Immunol.*, **153** (1994) 4925–4933.

20. Kovacsovic-Bankowski M and Rock KL. A phagosome-to-cytosol pathway for exogenous antigens presented on MHC class I molecules. *Science*, **267** (1995) 243–245.

21. Hoover HC Jr, Brandhorst JS, Peters LC, Surdyke MG, Takeshita Y, Madariaga J, et al. Adjuvant active specific immunotherapy for human colorectal cancer: 6.5-year median follow-up of a phase III prospectively randomized trial. *J. Clin. Oncol.*, **11** (1993) 390–399.

22. Hanna MG Jr., Pollack VA, Peters LC, et al. Active-specific immunotherapy of established micrometastases with BCG plus tumor cell vaccines: effective treatment of BCG side effects with isoniazid. *Cancer*, **49** (1982) 659–664.

23. Hoover HC Jr, Peters LC, Brandhorst JS, et al. Therapy of spontaneous metastases with an autologous tumor vaccine in a guinea pig model. *J. Surg. Res.*, **30** (1981) 409–415.

24. Key ME and Hanna MG Jr. Mechanism of action of BCG-tumor cell vaccines in the generation of systemic tumor immunity: 1. Synergism between BCG and line 10 tumor cells in the induction of an inflammatory response. *J. Natl. Cancer Inst.*, **67** (1981) 853–861.

25. Peters LC and Hanna MG Jr. Active-specific immunotherapy of established micrometastasis: effect of cryopreservation procedures on tumor cell immunogenicity in guinea pigs. *J. Natl. Cancer Inst.*, **64** (1980) 1521–1525.

26. Peters LC, Brandhorst JS, Hanna MG Jr. Preparation of immunotherapeutic autologous tumor cell vaccines from solid tumors. *Cancer Res.*, **39** (1979) 1353–1360.

27. Harris JE, Ryan L, and Hanna MG Jr, et al: Adjuvant active specific immunotherapy for stage II and III colon cancer with an autologous tumor cell vaccine: Eastern Cooperative Oncology Group Study E5283. *J. Clin. Oncol.*, **18** (2000) 148–157.

28. Ockert D, Schirrmacher V, Beck N, Stoelben E, Ahlert T, Flechtenmacher J, et al. Newcastle disease virus-infected intact autologous tumor cell vaccine for adjuvant active specific immunotherapy of resected colorectal carcinoma. *Clin. Cancer Res.*, **2** (1996) 21–28.

29. Gilboa E and Lyerly HK. Specific active immunotherapy of cancer using genetically modified tumor vaccines. *Biol. Ther. Cancer*, **6** (1994) 1–16.

30. Yannelli JR, Hyatt C, Johnson S, Hwu P, and Rosenberg SA. Characterization of human tumor cell lines with the cDNA encoding either tumor necrosis factor-alpha (TNF-α or interleukin-2 (IL-2). *J. Immunol. Methods,* **161** (1993) 77–90.

31. Bixby DL and Yannelli JR. CD80 expression in an HLA-A2 positive human non-small cell lung cancer cell line enhances tumor-specific cytotoxicity of HLA-A2-positive T-cells derived from normal donors and patients with non-small cell lung cancer. *Int. J. Cancer*, **78** (1998) 685–694.

32. Chen T, Linsley PS, and Hellström KE. Costimulation of T-cells for tumor immunity. *Immunol. Today*, **14** (1993) 483–486.

33. Chen L, McGown P, Ashe S, Johnson J, Li Y, Hellström I, and Hellström KE. Tumor Immunogenicity determines the effect of B7 costimulation on T-cell mediated tumor immunity. *J. Exp. Med.*, **179** (1994) 523–532.

34. Townsend SE and Allison JP. Tumor rejection after direct costimulation of CD8+ T-cells by B7-transfected melanoma cells. *Science*, **259** (1993) 368–370.

35. Yang S, Darrow TL, and Seigler HF. Generation of primary tumor specific cytotoxic lymphocytes from autologous and human lymphocyte antigen class I matched allogeneic peripheral blood lymphocytes by B7 gene modified melanoma cells. *Cancer Res.*, **57** (1997) 1561.

36. Jaffee E, Dranoff G, Cohen L, et al. High efficiency gene transfer into primary human tumor explants without cell selection. *Cancer Res.*, **53** (1993) 2221–2226.

37. Fearon E, Pardoll D, Itaya T, et al. Interleukin-2 production by tumor cells bypasses T helper function in the generation of an antitumor response. *Cell*, **60** (1990) 397–403.

38. McLaughlin JP, Abrams S, Kantor J, Dobrzanski MJ, Greenbaum J, Schlom J, et al. Immunization with a syngeneic tumor infected with recombinant vaccinia virus expressing granulocyte-macrophage colony-

stimulating factor (GM-CSF) induces tumor regression and long-lasting systemic immunity. *J. Immunother.*, **20(6)** (1997) 449–459.

39. Kubo RT, Sett A, Grey HM, et al. Definition of specific peptide motifs for four major HLA-A alleles. *J. Immunol.*, **152** (1994) 3913–3924.

40. Vitiello A, Ishioka G, Grey H, et al. Development of a lipopeptide-based therapeutic vaccine to treat chronic HBV infection. *J. Clin. Invest.*, **95** (1995) 341–349.

41. Mayordomo JL, Zorina T, Storkus WJ, et al. Bone marrow-derived dendritic cells pulsed with synthetic tumour peptides elicit protective and therapeutic antitumour immunity. *Nature Med.*, **1** (1995) 1297–1302.

42. Young JW and Inaba K. Dendritic cells as adjuvants for class I major histocompatibility complex-restricted antitumor immunity. *J. Exp. Med.*, **183** (1996) 7–11.

43. Zitvogel L, Mayordomo JI, Tjandrawan T, et al. Therapy of murine tumors with tumor peptide-pulsed dendritic cells: dependence on T cell, B7 co-stimulation, and T helper cell 1-associated cytokines. *J. Exp. Med.*, **183** (1996) 87–97.

44. Porgador A, Snyder D, and Gilboa E. Induction of antitumor immunity using bone-marrow generated dendritic cells. *J. Immunol.*, **156** (1996) 2918–2926.

45. Marchand M, Weynants P, Rankin E, et al. Tumor regression responses in melanoma patients treated with a peptide encoded by the gene MAGE-3. *Int. J. Cancer*, **63** (1995) 883–885.

46. Parkhurst MR, Salgaller ML, Southwood S, et al. Improved induction of melanoma reactive CTL with peptides from melanoma antigen gp100 modified at HLA-A*0201 binding residues. *J. Immunol.*, **157** (1995) 2539–2548.

47. Mukherji B, Chakraborty NG, Yamasaki S, et al. Induction of antigen-specific cytolytic T cells in situ in human melanoma by immunization with synthetic peptide-pulsed autologous antigen-presenting cells. *Proc. Natl. Acad. Sci. USA*, **92** (1995) 8078–8082.

48. Rosenberg SA, Yang JC, Schwartzentruber DJ, Hwu P, Marincola FM, Topalian SL, et al. Immunologic and therapeutic evaluation of a synthetic peptide vaccine for the treatment of patients with metastatic melanoma. *Nature Med.*, **4** (1998) 321–332.

49. Kawakami Y, Eliyahu S, Sakaguchi K, et al. Identification of the immunodominant peptides of the MART-1 human melanoma antigen recognized by the majority of HLA-A2 restricted tumor infiltrating lymphocytes. *J. Exp. Med.*, **180** (1994) 347–352.

50. Kawakami Y, Eliyahu S, Sakaguchi K, et al. Recognition of multiple epitopes in the human melanoma antigen gp100 associated with in vivo tumor regression. *J. Immunol.*, **154** (1995) 3961–3968.

51. Bakker A, Schreurs M, Tafazzul G, et al. Identification of a novel peptide derived from the melanocyte-specific gp100 antigen as the dominant epitope recognized by an HLA-A2.1-restricted anti-melanoma CTL line. *Int. J. Cancer*, **62** (1995) 97–102.

52. Kawakami Y, Eliyahu S, Delgado CH, et al. Identification of a human melanoma antigen recognized by tumor infiltrating lymphocytes associated with in vivo tumor rejection. *Proc. Natl. Acad. Sci. USA*, **91** (1994) 6458–6462.

53. Castelli C, Storkus WJ, Maeurer MJ, et al. Mass spectrometric identification of a naturally processed melanoma peptide recognized by CD8+ cytotoxic T lymphocytes. *J. Exp. Med.*, **181** (1995) 363–368.

54. Brichard V, Van Pel A, Wölfel T, et al. The tyrosinase gene codes for an antigen recognized by autologous cytolytic T-lymphocytes on HLA-A2 melanomas. *J. Exp. Med.*, **178** (1993) 759–764.

55. Traversari C, Van der Bruggen P, Luescher F, et al. A non-apeptide encoded by human gene MAGE-1 is recognized on HLA-A1 by cytolytic T-lymphocytes directed against tumor antigen-MZ2-E. *J. Exp. Med.*, **176** (1992) 1453–1457.

56. Boel P, Wildmann C, Sensi ML, et al. BAGE: a new gene encoding an antigen recognized on human melanomas by cytolytic T lymphocytes. *Immunity*, **2** (1995) 167–175.

57. Coulie PG, Lehmann F, Lethe B, et al. A mutated intron sequence codes for an antigenic peptide recognized by cytolytic T lymphocytes on a human melanoma. *Proc. Natl. Acad. Sci. USA*, **92** (1995) 7976–7980.

58. Fisk B, Blevins TL, and Wharton JT. Identification of an immunodominant peptide of HER-2/neu protoon-cogene recognized by ovarian tumor-specific cytotoxic T lymphocytes lines. *J. Exp. Med.*, **181** (1995) 2109–2117.

59. Linehan DC, Goedegebuure PS, Peoples GE, et al. Tumor-specific and HLA-A2-restricted cytolysis by tumor-associated lymphocytes in human metastatic breast cancer. *J. Immunol.*, **155** (1995) 4486–4491.

60. Ressing ME, Van Driel W, Celis E, et al. Occasional memory CTL responses of patients with human papillomavirus type 16 positive cervical lesions against a human leukocyte antigen A*0201 restricted E7 encoded epitope. *Cancer Res.*, **56** (1996) 582–588.

61. Tsang KY, Zaremba S, Nieroda CA, et al. Generation of human cytotoxic T cells specific for human carcinoembryonic antigen epitopes from patients immunized with recombinant vaccina-CEA vaccine. *J. Natl. Cancer Inst.*, **87** (1995) 982–990.

62. Disis ML, Calenoff E, McLaughlin G, et al. Existent T-cell and antibody immunity to HER-2/neu protein in patients with breast cancer. *Cancer Res.*, **54** (1994) 16–20.

63. Disis NL, Gralow JR, Bernhard H, et al. Peptide-based, but not whole protein, vaccines elicit immunity to HER-2/neu, an oncogenic self-protein. *J. Immunol.*, **156** (1996) 3151–3158.

64. Kast WM, Brandt RPM, Sidney J, et al. Role of HLA-A motifs in identification of potential CTL epitopes in human papillomavirus type 16 E6 and E7 proteins. *J. Immunol.*, **152** (1994) 3904–3912.

65. Feltkamp MCW, Smits HL, Vierboom MPM, et al. Vaccination with cytotoxic T lymphocyte epitope-containing peptide protects against a tumor induced by human papillomavirus type 16-transformed cells. *Eur. J. Immunol.*, **23** (1993) 2242–2249.

66. Kotera Y, Fontenot JD, Pecher G, Metzgar RS, and Finn OJ. Human immunity against a tandem repeat epitope of human mucin MUC-1 in sera from breast, pancreatic and colon cancer patients. *Cancer Res.*, **54** (1994) 2856–2860.

67. Devine PL, Layton GT, Clark BA, Birrell GW, Ward BG, Xing PX, et al. Production of MUC1 and MUC2 mucins by human tumor cell lines. *Biochem. Biophys. Res. Commun.*, **178** (1991) 593–599.

68. Hollingsworth MA, Strawhecker JM, Caffrey TC, and Mack DR. Expression of MUC1, MUC2, MUC3 and MUC4 mucin mRNAs in human pancreatic and intestinal tumor cell lines. *Int. J. Cancer*, **57** (1994) 198–203.

69. Hareuveni M, Gautier C, Kieny M-P, Wreschner D, Chambon P, and Lathe R. Vaccination against tumor cells expressing breast cancer epithelial tumor antigen. *Proc. Natl. Acad. Sci. USA*, **87** (1990) 9498–9502.

70. Gendler SJ, Spicer AP, Lalani E-N, Duhig T, Peat N, Burchell J, et al. Structure and biology of a carcinoma-associated mucin, MUC1. *Am. Rev. Respir. Dis.*, **144** (1991) S42–S47.

71. Burchell J, Taylor-Papadimitriou J, Boshell M, Gendler S, and Duhig T. A short sequence, within the amino acid tandem repeat of a cancer-associated mucin, contains immunodominant epitopes. *Int. J. Cancer*, **44** (1989) 691–696.

72. Fontenot JD, Tjandra N, Bu D, Ho C, Montelaro RC, and Finn OJ. Biophysical characterization of one-, two-, and three-tandem repeats of human mucin (muc-1) protein core. *Cancer Res.*, **53** (1993) 5386–5394.

73. Perez L, Hayes DF, Maimonis P, Abe M, O'Hara C, and Kufe DW. Tumor selective reactivity of a monoclonal antibody prepared against a recombinant peptide derived from the DF3 human breast carcinoma-associated antigen. *Cancer Res.*, **52** (1992) 2563–2568.

74. Ding L, Lalani E-N, Reddish M, Koganty R, Wong T, Samuel J, et al. Immunogenicity of synthetic peptides related to the core peptide sequence encoded by the human MUC1 mucin gene: effect of immunization on the growth of murine mammary adenocarcinoma cells transfected with the human *MUC1* gene. *Cancer Immunol. Immunother.*, **36** (1993) 9–17.

75. Barnd DL, Lan M, Metzgar R, and Finn OJ. Specific MHC-unrestricted recognition of tumor associated mucins by human cytotoxic T cells. *Proc. Natl. Acad. Sci. USA*, **86** (1989) 7159–7163.

76. Jerome KR, Barnd DL, Bendt KM, et al. Cytotoxic T-lymphocytes derived from patients with breast adenocarcinoma recognize an epitope present on the protein core of a mucin molecule preferentially expressed by malignant cells. *Cancer Res.*, **51** (1991) 2908–2916.

77. Goydos JS, Elder E, Whiteside TL, Finn OJ, and Lotze MT. A phase I trial of a synthetic mucin peptide vaccine: induction of specific immune reactivity in patients with adenocarcinoma. *J. Surg. Res.*, **63** (1996) 298–304.

78. Doménech N, Henderson RA, and Finn OJ. Identification of an HLA-A11-restricted epitope from the tandem repeat domain of the epithelial tumor antigen mucin. *J. Immunol.*, **155** (1995) 4766–4774.

79. Apostolopoulos V, Osinski C, and McKenzie IFC. MUC1 cross-reactive Galalpha(1,3)Gal antibodies in humans switch immune responses from cellular to humoral. *Nature Med.*, **4** (1998) 315–320.

80. Houghton AN and Lloyd KO. Stuck in the MUC on the long and winding road: antibodies that cross react with the tumor antigen MUC1 switch a cellular immune response to a humoral one with implications for the immunotherapy of cancer. *Nature Med.*, **4** (1998) 270–271.

81. Livingston PO, Ritter F, Srivastava P, Padavan M, Calves MJ, Oettgen HF, et al. Characterization of IgG and IgM antibodies induced in melanoma patients by immunization with purified GM2 ganglioside. *Cancer Res.*, **49** (1984) 7045–7050.

82. Livingston PO, Natoli EJ Jr, Calves MJ, Stockert E, Oettgen HF, and Old LJ. Vaccines containing purified GM2 ganglioside elicit GM2 antibodies in melanoma patients. *Proc. Natl. Acad. Sci. USA*, **84** (1987) 2911–2915.

83. Livingston PO, Wong GYC, Adluri S, Tao Y, Padavan M, Parente R, et al. Improved survival in stage III melanoma patients with GM2 antibodies: a randomized trial of adjuvant vaccination with GM2 ganglioside. *J. Clin. Oncol.*, **12** (1994) 1036–1044.

84. Sieling PA, Chatterjee D, Porcelli SA, Prigozy TI, Mazzaccaro RJ, Soriano T, et al. CD1-restricted T-cell recognition of microbial lipoglycan antigens. *Science*, **269** (1985) 227–230.

85. Moody DB, Reinhold BB, Guy MR, Beckman EM, Frederique DE, Furlong ST, et al. Structural requirements for glycolipid antigen recognition by CD1b-restricted T-cells. *Science*, **278** (1997) 283–286.

86. Haurum JS, Arsequell G, Lellouch AC, Wong SYC, Dwek RA, McMichael AJ, et al. Recognition of carbohydrate by major histocompatability complex class I-restricted, glycopeptide-specific cytotoxic T lymphocytes. *J. Exp. Med.*, **180** (1994) 739–744.

87. Beckman EM, Porcelli SA, Morita CT, Behar SM, Furlong ST, and Brenner MB. Recognition of a lipid antigen by CD1-restricted $\alpha\beta^+$ T cells. *Nature*, **372** (1994) 691–694.

88. Springer GF. T and Tn, general carcinoma antoantigens. *Science*, **224** (1984) 1198–1206.

89. Longenecker BM, Willan DJ, MacLean GD, et al. Monoclonal antibodies and synthetic tumor-associated glycoconjugates in the study of the expression of Thomsen–Friedenreich-like and Tn-like antigens on human cancers. *J. Natl. Cancer Inst.*, **78** (1987) 489–496.

90. Samuel J, Noujaim AA, MacLean GD, et al. Analysis of human tumor associated Thomsen-Friedenreich antigen. *Cancer Res.*, **50** (1990) 4801–4808.

91. Springer GF, Taylor CR, Howard DR, et al. Tn, a carcinoma associated antigen, reacts with anti-Tn of normal human sera. *Cancer*, **55** (1995) 561–569.

92. Itzkowitz SH, Bloom EJ, Kokal WA, et al. Sialosyl-Tn. A novel mucin antigen associated with prognosis in colorectal cancer patients. *Cancer*, **66** (1990) 1960–1966.

93. Itzkowitz S, Yuan M, Montgomery CK, et al. Expression of Tn, sialosyl-Tn, and T antigens in human colon cancer. *Cancer Res.*, **49(1)** (1989) 197–204.

94. MacLean GD, Reddish MA, Bowen-Yacshyn MB, Poppema S, and Longenecker BM. Active specific immunotherapy against adenocarcinomas. *Cancer Invest.*, **12(1)** (1994) 46–56.

95. Adluri S, Helling F, Ogata S, Zhang S, Itzkowitz SH, Lloyd KO, et al. Immunogenicity of synthetic TF-KLH (keyhole limpet hemocyanin) and sTn-KLH conjugates in colorectal carcinoma patients. *Cancer Immunol. Immunother.*, **41** (1995) 185–192.

96. Thompson J and Zimmerman W. The carcinoembryonic antigen gene family: structure, expressions, and evolution. *Tumour Biol.*, **9** (1988) 63–83.

97. Paxton RJ, Mooser G, Pande H, Lee TD, and Shivley JE. Sequence analysis of carcinoembryonic antigen: identification of glycosylation sites and homology with the immunoglobulin super-gene family. *Proc. Natl. Acad. Sci. USA*, **84** (1987) 920–924.

98. Benchimol S, Fuks A, Jothy S, Beauchemia N, Shirota K, and Stanners C. Carcinoembryonic antigen, a human tumor marker, functions as an intercellular adhesion molecule. *Cell*, **57** (1989) 327–334.

99. Oikawa S, Inuzuka C, Kuroki M, Matsuoka Y, Kosaki G, and Nakazato H. Cell adhesion activity of non-specific cross-reacting antigen (NCA) and carcinoembryonic antigen (CEA) expressed on CHO cell surface: homophilic and heterophilic adhesion. *Biochem. Biophys. Res. Commun.*, **164** (1989) 39–45.

100. Kaufman H, Schlom J, and Kantor J. A recombinant vaccinia virus expressing human carcinoembryonic antigen (CEA). *Int. J. Cancer*, **48** (1991) 900–907.

101. Kantor J, Irvine K, Abrams S, Kaufman H, DiPietro J, and Schlom J. Antitumor activity and immune response induced by a recombinant carcinoembryonic antigen-vaccinia virus vaccine. *J. Natl. Cancer Inst.*, **84** (1992) 1084–1091.

102. Kantor J, Irvine K, Abrams S, Snoy P, Olsen R, Greiner J, et al. Immunogenicity and safety of a recombinant vaccinia virus vaccine expressing the carcinoembryonic antigen gene in a nonhuman primate. *Cancer Res.*, **52** (1992) 6917–6925.

103. Tsang KY, Zaremba S, Nieroda CA, Zhu MZ, Hamilton JM, and Schlom J. Generation of human cytotoxic T-cells specific for human carcinoembryonic antigen (CEA) epitopes from patients immunized with recombinant vaccinia-CEA (rV-CEA) vaccine. *J. Natl. Cancer Inst.*, **87** (1995) 982–990.

104. McLaughlin JP, Schlom J, Kantor JA, and Greiner JW. Improved immunotherapy of a recombinant carcinoembryonic antigen vaccinia vaccine when given in combination with interleukin-2. *Cancer Res.*, **56** (1996) 2361–2367.

105. Conry RM, LoBuglio AF, Kantor J, Schlom J, Loechel F, Moore SE, et al. Immune response to a carcinoembryonic antigen polynucleotide vaccine. *Cancer Res.*, **54** (1994) 1164–1168.

106. Lindenmann J. Speculations on idiotypes and homobodies. *Ann. Immunol. (Paris)*, **124** (1973) 171–184.

107. Jerne NK. Towards a network theory of the immune system. *Ann. Immunol. (Paris)*, **125C** (1974) 373–389.

108. Fagerberg J, Steinitz M, Wigzell H, Askelöf P, and Mellstedt H. Human anti-idiotypic antibodies induced a humoral and cellular immune response against a colorectal carcinoma-associated antigen in patients. *Proc. Natl. Acad. Sci. USA*, **92** (1995) 4773–4777.

109. Herlyn D, Harris D, Zaloudik J, Sperlagh M, Maruyama H, Jacob L, et al. Immunomodulatory activity of monoclonal anti-idiotypic antibody to anti-colorectal carcinoma antibody CO17-1A in animals and patients. *J. Immunother.*, **15** (1994) 303–311.

110. Robins RA, Denton GWL, Hardcastle JD, Austin EB, Baldwin RW, and Durrant LG. Antitumor immune response and interleukin 2 production induced in colorectal cancer patients by immunization with human monoclonal anti-idiotypic antibody. *Cancer Res.*, **51** (1991) 5425–5429.

111. Denton GWL, Durrant LG, Hardcastle JD, Austin EB, Sewell HF, and Robins RA. Clinical outcome of colorectal cancer patients treated with human monoclonal anti-idiotypic antibody. *Int. J. Cancer*, **57** (1994) 10–17.

112. Durrant LG, Buckey TJD, Denton GWL, Hardcastle JD, Sewell HF, and Robins RA. Enhanced cell-mediated tumor killing in patients immunized with human monoclonal anti-idiotypic antibody 105AD7. *Cancer Res.*, **54**, (1994) 4837–4840.

113. Durrant LG, Doran M, Austin EB, and Robins RA. Induction of cellular immune responses by a murine monoclonal anti-idiotypic antibody recognizing the 791Tgp72 antigen expressed on colorectal, gastric and ovarian human tumours. *Int. J. Cancer*, **61** (1995) 62–66.

114. Bhattacharya-Chatterjee M, Mukerjee S, Biddle W, Foon KA, and Köhler H. Murine monoclonal anti-idiotype antibody as a potential network antigen for human carcinoembryonic antigen. *J. Immunol.*, **145** (1990) 2758–2765.

115. Pervin S, Chakraborty M, Bhattacharya-Chatterjee M, Zeytin H, Foon KA, and Chatterjee S. Induction of antitumor immunity by an anti-idiotype antibody mimicking carcinoembryonic antigen. *Cancer Res.*, **57** (1997) 728–734.

116. Foon KA, Chakraborty M, John WJ, Sherratt A, Köhler H, and Bhattacharya-Chatterjee M. Immune response to the carcinoembryonic antigen in patients treated with an anti-idiotype antibody vaccine. *J. Clin. Invest.*, **96** (1995) 334–342.

117. Foon KA, John WJ, Chakraborty M, Sherratt A, Garrison J, Flett M, et al. Clinical and immune responses in advanced colorectal cancer patients treated with anti-idiotype monoclonal antibody vaccine that mimics the carcinoembryonic antigen. *Clin. Cancer Res.*, **3** (1997) 1267–1276.

118. Foon KA, John WJ, Chakraborty M, Das R, Teitelbaum A, Garrison J, et al. Clinical and immune responses in resected colorectal cancer patients treated with anti-idiotype monoclonal antibody vaccine that mimics the carcinoembryonic antigen. *J. Clin. Oncol.*, **17** (1999) 2889–2895.

119. Chatterjee SK, Tripathi PK, Chakraborty M, Yannelli J, Wang H, Foon KA, Molecular mimicry of carcinoembryonic antigen by peptides derived from the structure of an anti-idiotype antibody. *Cancer Res.*, **58** (1998) 1217–1224.

120. Magliani W, Polonelli L, Conti S, et al. Neonatal mouse immunity against group B streptococcal infection by maternal vaccination with recombinant anti-idiotypes. *Nature Med.*, **4** (1998) 705–709.

121. Ruiz PJ, Wolkowicz R, Waisman A, et al. Immunity to mutant p53 and tumor rejection induced by idiotypic immunization. *Nature Med.*, **4** (1998) 710–712.

122. Bona CA. Idiotype vaccines: forgotten but not gone. *Nature Med.*, **4** (1998) 668–669, 1998.

123. Foon KA and Bhattacharya-Chatterjee M. Idiotype vaccines in the clinic. *Nature Med.*, **4** (1998) 870.

42

Gene Therapy Strategies for Colorectal Cancer

Anand G. Menon, Marjolijn M. van der Eb,
Peter J. K. Kuppen, and Cornelis J. H. van de Velde

CONTENTS

1. INTRODUCTION

Gene therapy is a relatively young and rapidly developing field in which, classically, the aim is to treat a disease, which is caused by an error in a particular gene, by replacing the defective gene with the correct DNA sequence. Early gene therapy applications were mainly focused on monogenic, inheritable diseases such as adenosine deaminase deficiency, hemophilia, or familial hypercholesterolemia, but now more than half of the gene therapy clinical trials focus on cancer. In spite of the fact that (colorectal) cancer encompasses a multitude of changes in key regulatory genes, targeting only one of those essential genes can already result in an impressive reduction of tumor size and even in complete responses in preclinical models, giving hope that this will also occur in clinical practice. In addition to attacking tumors at the root of the problem (i.e., defective gene replacement), two other strategies can also be used. The first strategy aims at localizing antitumor drugs (e.g., 5-fluorouracil [5-FU]) in tumor tissue by transfecting tumor cells with "suicide genes" that will convert a nontoxic prodrug into a toxic metabolite that will kill these cells. Commonly, systemic chemotherapy is limited by systemic side effects. Gene therapy offers opportunities to deliver chemotherapy more specifically to tumor cells. In addition, normal cells, such as the hematopoietic stem cell lines in the bone marrow, that are susceptible to chemotherapy, can be armored with "chemoprotective genes" in order to prevent toxicity from high-dose systemic chemotherapy *(1)*.

From: *Colorectal Cancer: Multimodality Management*
Edited by: L. Saltz © Humana Press Inc., Totowa, NJ

The second strategy aims at enhancing the body's own antitumor defense (i.e., immune modulation). Although, tumor cells harbor a wide variety of genetic alterations, which result in the production of potentially immunogenic proteins, tumor cells also use a number of mechanisms to evade the immune system. Gene therapy can aid by vaccinating against certain altered proteins, by making the immune system more potent, or by enhancing the immunogenicity of tumor cells.

In this chapter, we will discuss the backgrounds of gene therapy, the different strategies in cancer treatment, achievements in colorectal cancer patients, and future prospects.

2. GENE THERAPY

2.1. The History of Gene Therapy

A number of historical landmarks are important on the road that has led to the present stage of gene therapy *(2)*. One of the early clues that alterations or transformation of genetic information is possible stemmed from a study on DNA-mediated change in phenotype of pneumococci by Avery et al. *(3)*. This eventually led to the technique of bacterial transformation, which is the basis for recombinant technology. However, stable transformation of mammalian cells was impossible until the early seventies, when the calcium phosphate-precipitation technique was developed *(4)*. With this method, it became possible to genetically transform cultured mammalian cells with DNA fragments *(5)*. The discovery that infection of mammalian cells with viruses could lead to stable integration of viral DNA or of a DNA copy of a retroviral RNA genome, led to the idea that viruses could serve as a vehicle of genetic information *(6,7)*. Another important milestone in the development of gene therapy was the establishment of recombinant DNA techniques (i.e., techniques to purify and manipulate specific parts of DNA). The combination of recombinant DNA techniques and viruses as vectors led to the concept of gene therapy as a feasible alternative or addition to the classical armamentum for treatment of various genetic diseases, which could now be approached curatively for the first time. Although the early gene therapy trials showed disappointing results and certain experiments caused severe criticism from academic, political, and ethical institutions and from the general public, the proof of principle was demonstrated and further research into this up to then science-fiction-held field of technology increased tremendously.

2.2. The Techniques of Gene Therapy

Minute flaws in the coding DNA sequences (e.g., mutations, translocations, or deletions) can have profound impact on the structure and function of the encoded protein. Many flaws in a variety of genes have been identified using sophisticated biochemical techniques and these errors are, in principle, correctable by introducing a correct copy of the gene to the affected cell. This immediately highlights the two most important challenges in gene therapy: (1) targeting the genes to the affected cells and (2) regaining physiological expression of the gene of interest. A number of techniques exist to transduce genetic information to a target cell (*see* Table 1). These can be roughly divided into nonviral and viral delivery methods. This distinction is of importance, because of the implications for using genetically modified viruses that are potentially pathogenic to humans. The recent death of a youngster after treatment with virus-based gene therapy for a metabolic disorder further stresses this point *(8)*. Although the nonviral delivery methods do not have these stringent concerns for safety, and in spite of the fact that these nonviral vectors can be produced safely, at low cost and

Table 1
Transduction Methods in Gene Therapy

Nonviral
    Direct injection of DNA
    $CaPO_4$
    Liposomes
    Cationic lipids
    Ligand
    Electroporation
    DNA–polylysine–cell receptor conjugates
Viral
    Retrovirus
    Adenovirus
    AAV
    Herpesvirus
    Poxviruses (ALVAC, NYVAC, vaccinia)
    Lenti virus
    Polyoma virus

in high, purified batches, viral vectors are most commonly used in colorectal cancer, and, therefore, these will be focused on in this chapter.

2.2.1. Nonviral Delivery Methods

Direct injection into the target cells or tissues was the earliest and simplest method for gene transfer, but, as can be imagined, not many target cells are suitable for transfection by this method *(9)*. An improvement was obtained with the introduction of the calcium phosphate technique *(4)*. Unfortunately, permanent incorporation into the host-cell genome is only seen in less than 1% of the target cells and the method works best with cultured cells.

Another approach is the use of synthetic compounds that consist of DNA together with molecules that ensure the DNA delivery to target cells and protection from degradation once taken up inside a cell. For instance, liposomes consist of lipid "balloons," which contain a plasmid with the DNA sequence of interest. They are especially useful when receptor-mediated endocytosis is possible. Although transfection with liposomes or cationic lipids has led to an increase in the transfection of DNA, this is usually only transient and only low levels of expression are attained, which are mainly restricted to in vitro experiments. Nevertheless, progress is being made and the absence of potentially pathogenic particles, such as viral vectors, and the fact that they can be produced safely, inexpensively, and in highly purified batches, make these nonviral delivery methods an important asset to gene therapy.

2.2.2. Viral Vectors

The first clinical use of viral vectors was performed in a noncancer setting using a Shope papilloma virus. This virus was assumed to encode an argininase that could cure hyperarginaemic patients, but, unfortunately, the trial failed *(10)*. Since then, the retroviruses have received much attention, because of the discovery that parts of their genome integrate into target cells, thus offering potential to add genes of interest to these viruses.

2.2.2.1. Retroviral Vectors. These enveloped single-stranded RNA viruses cause a variety of biological effects in their hosts, ranging from benign, asymptomatic infections to lethal diseases such as the acquired immune deficiency syndrome and cancer. These viruses consist of seven genera that all have a similar structure: a lipid envelope and a nucleocapsid (core), consisting of an RNA genome encoding a distinct set of genes *gag*, *pol*, and *env*, of which *pol* encodes the essential enzymes reverse transcriptase and integrase *(7)*. The viral life cycle can be divided into two stages. In the first stage, the virus adheres to a specific receptor on the target cell and enters the cell. Subsequently, the RNA is reversely transcribed into double-stranded DNA by the enzyme reverse transcriptase, which is then transported to the nucleus and (randomly) integrated into the host cell genome by the enzyme integrase. The integrated viral genome is called the provirus, which, upon transcription, results in the assembly of new virions, which leave the cell by a budding process.

Interest in these viruses mainly stem from their ability to transduce almost 100% of the target cells if they are in the cell cycle. To construct a retroviral vector for gene therapy, the *gag*, *pol*, and *env* genes are removed from the viral genome and replaced by a gene of interest. By deletion of *gag*, *pol*, and *env*, it is virtually impossible for the virus to replicate in normal host cells. To multiply the viral vector, helper or packaging cells are used (i.e., host cells in which the viral genes *gag*, *pol*, and *env* are stably integrated. The viral proteins produced by these packaging cells will lead to the formation of progeny vector virus that contains viral proteins provided by the packaging cell and the genome containing the gene of interest. No replication-competent (wild-type) virus can be formed because no genetic information for viral reproduction is transferred from the packaging cell line. However, one must always remain cautious for spontaneous recombinations through which new replication-competent virus can be produced. A number of advantages and disadvantages are associated with the retroviruses. For instance, advantages include the high transduction efficiency of almost 100% of target cells, that the viruses can be produced in fairly high titers, and the integration of the genome results in stable gene expression. Disadvantages include, among others, the random integration of the provirus into the host-cell genome, which raises concern with respect to oncogenicity. Indeed, lymphomas have been demonstrated in monkeys after infection with replication-competent retroviruses *(11)*. In addition, the use of the retrovirus is restricted to dividing cells. There is also a size limitation for the inserted gene (7–8 kb), the virus is "labile" (loss of infectivity during purification), it is rapidly inactivated in vivo, and it lacks target cell specificity *(12)*.

2.2.2.2. Adenoviral Vectors. These viruses were first isolated and characterized as the etiologic agents of acute respiratory infections in the early 1950s. Since then, more than 50 serotypes have been discovered, which can be divided into 6 subgroups based on their hemagglutination capability. Adenoviruses not only cause "the common cold" but also conjunctivitis and gastroenteritis in children.

The virion consists of a double-stranded, linear DNA genome encapsidated in an icosahedral protein shell. The genome is made up of five early genes (*E1A*, *E1B*, *E2*, *E3*, and *E4*), two delayed genes (*IX*, *IVa2*), and five late genes (*L1–L5*) with distinct functions. For instance, the *E1A* gene, aided by *E1B*, is of importance in inducing the cell to enter the cell cycle. Other regions have functions to modulate the immune response of the host to the adenovirus and to regulate transcription and DNA replication.

The viral cycle can be divided into two parts, which are separated by the onset of viral DNA replication. The first phase is primarily concerned with the infection of a host cell and expression of early viral genes, which prepare the infected host cell to produce new viral particles. In the second phase, viral DNA is replicated and the late genes are expressed followed by the production of progeny virions.

Adenoviruses for gene therapy are made by replacing *E1A*, *E1B*, and *E3* from the genome and replacing it with 7–8 kb of the foreign DNA of interest. High titers are obtained in a fashion similar to that used for the production of retroviruses, namely with a packaging or helper cell line (e.g., 293, 911, or perC6 cells), which express the *E1A* and *E1B* gene but do not pass these genes to the produced virions *(13–15)*. The *E3* gene is a nonessential gene and is not included in the packaging cell line.

The adenoviruses have a number of advantages; among others are the ability to infect dividing as well as nondividing cells, the fact that viruses can be grown to high titers, and gene expression is maintained for a long time. In addition, the virus is relatively stable and can be easily purified and concentrated. However, the DNA does not integrate into the genome, but stays in an episomal state. A potential problem is that the viruses have transforming potential and that the transformed cells are oncogenic in immune-deficient animals (nude mice, rats). This holds also true for human Ad5, the virus from which Ad vectors are usually derived. Other drawbacks include the fact that humans often carry anti-adenovirus antibodies (which may crossreact with the injected vector and inactivate it soon after injection), the rapid induction of antiadenovirus antibodies, and the capacity to replicate under certain conditions in spite of the E1 deletion. Nevertheless, the adenoviruses are attractive as vectors for gene therapy studies.

2.2.2.3. Other Viral Vectors. Less well-studied viral vectors include vectors based on the adeno-associated virus (AAV), herpesvirus, vaccinia, poxviruses, and several others (e.g., lentivirus, polio virus, sindbis virus) *(16)*.

The adeno-associated virus is a small virus that can integrate its genome in both dividing and nondividing cells and has the advantage that it is not known to cause a particular disease. Of particular interest is the observation that it barely causes an anti-virus immunological reaction in the host organism and that its genome seems to have a preference to integrate in chromosome 19, a region that has been associated with chromosomal rearrangements in chronic B-cell leukemias *(17)*. This is potentially worrysome, but none of the constructed vectors have so far been shown to keep this property.

Herpesvirus has a unique specificity for the central nervous system, but difficulties in producing replication-incompetent viral stocks hinder its use in clinical studies.

Poxviruses, such as the canarypoxvirus, are DNA viruses that replicate in the cytoplasm of vertebrate and invertebrate cells. In terms of safety and efficiency, the canarypox virus is very attractive, because after infection of human cells, the virus undergoes abortive replication while the inserted genes are readily expressed. Indeed, a number of studies have shown positive results in the absence of significant side effects, as will be discussed later.

3. PRECLINICAL MODELS AND CLINICAL TRIALS FOR GENE THERAPY IN COLORECTAL CANCER

Basic research aimed at understanding the etiology of cancer has revealed a wide range of disrupted fundamental regulatory mechanisms of cellular homeostasis in cancer cells, varying from defects in oncogenes and tumor suppressor genes to the employment of various immune-escape mechanisms. Each of these pathophysiological defects can be potential targets for gene therapy. In the following subsection, the schematic interaction between tumor cell and the host in the process of tumorigenesis, as illustrated in Fig. 1, will be used to give an overview of the most commonly employed gene therapy strategies in colorectal neoplasms. Figure 1 schematically represents the attack of tumor cells by utilizing three

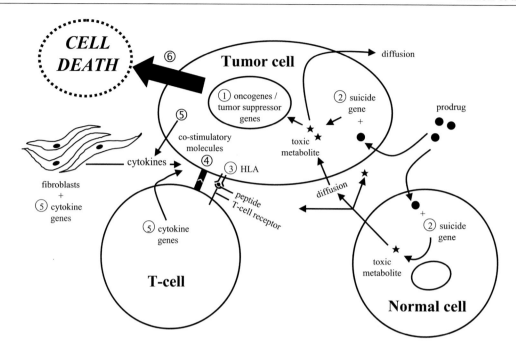

Fig. 1. Schematic interaction between tumor cell and the host in the process of tumorigenesis.

strategies: (1) gene replacement, (2) enhancement of chemotherapy and radiation therapy, and (3) augmentation of immunogenicity of tumor cells. Many other targets can also be used in gene therapy, such as the inappropriate activation of certain genes that are thought to promote cancer cell metastasis *(uPA/uPA-R) (18)*, *tPA (19)*, *PT-1 (20)*, *MIP-1 (21)*, *BCL-X (22)*, or the genes involved in the hereditary syndromes such as the Li–Fraumeni syndrome (germline mutation in one p53 allele) and the hereditary nonpolyposis colon cancer syndrome (HNPCC or Lynch syndrome), which consist of errors at the mismatch repair genes.

3.1. Gene Replacement Strategies

Advanced techniques in molecular biology and recombinant DNA have provided us with tools to study carcinogenesis at the basic level of our genetic information. Currently, many critical changes in tumor DNA have been detected and their pathophysiological effects elucidated. For instance, the pioneering adenoma–carcinoma model as proposed by Vogelstein and co-workers show specific changes (e.g., alterations at important genes such as *p53*, *K-ras*, deleted in colorectal carcinoma *(DCC)* and adenomatous polyposis coli *(APC) (23)* that occur at different stages of carcinogenesis, although not always in the same order. Oncogenes and tumor suppressor genes are the faulty counterparts of genes that normally orchestrate activation and inhibition of cellular proliferation in response to intracellular and extracellular signals. Defects in these normal genes will lead to uncontrolled cellular proliferation and are, by themselves, not sufficient to sustain malignant transformation, but they make them more susceptible to additional damage in other crucial genes, which can provide them with new properties of the malignant phenotypes, such as migration through the extracellular matrix, invasion of lymph and vascular structures, and evasion and suppression of the immune system. A number of important genes and their replacement strategies will be discussed in the following subsections.

3.1.1. P53

Originally thought to be an oncogene, because overexpression of this nuclear 53-kDa phosphoprotein was associated with malignant transformation, this gene has, in fact, turned out to be a tumor suppressor gene *(24)*. Also referred to as "the guardian of the genome" *(25)*, p53 performs its tumor-suppressive function in at least two ways: First, when a cell has incurred DNA damage (e.g., as a result of ultraviolet light, carcinogens, hypoxia, etc.), the damage is recognized, resulting in activation of *p53* (accompanied by an increase in p53 levels). As a result, the cell cycle is arrested at the G1–S interphase, so that the DNA damage can be repaired and the cell can continue the cell cycle subsequently. Second, if the DNA damage is too extensive to repair, p53 can activate an alternative route and the cell is driven into apoptosis, thereby preventing erroneous DNA from being passed on to the progeny *(26)*. When *p53* is mutated or lost, damaged cells fail to arrest the cell cycle or induce apoptosis, which will lead to the accumulation of mutations and uncontrolled growth. It should be noted that both *p53* genes must be inactivated before a cell can attain a growth advantage. This generally occurs by loss of one allele and a mutation in the remaining allele. The mutations occur almost exclusively within the conserved exons 5–8, and within those exons, there are approximately five mutational hotspots (codons 175, 245, 248, 273, and 282) *(27)*. Because of its essential role in controlling the integrity of the genome and taking into account the fact that *p53* alterations are among the most common detected alterations in various types of malignancies (in up to 70% of colorectal cancers), restoring p53 function is an attractive target in cancer gene therapy.

A large amount of data has been collected with preclinical studies on *p53* gene therapy in different malignancies. Several investigators have reported substantial growth-inhibitory effects using adenovirus–p53 constructs in head and neck cancer, breast *(28)*, lung cancer *(29)*, prostate carcinoma *(30)*, and ovarian cancer *(31)*. Similarly, in colorectal cancer, studies on cell lines and animals have demonstrated anti-tumor effects using *p53*, without negatively affecting healthy cells *(32,33)*. p53-based strategies can be roughly divided into four categories:

1. Gene replacement/restoration of p53 wild-type function
2. Gene replacement as a sensitizer for chemotherapy/radiation therapy
3. Selective replication in p53-deficient/mutated tumor cells
4. Immunotherapy against p53

3.1.1.1. Restoration of p53 Wild-Type Function. This strategy represents true gene therapy, which can be achieved in different ways. For instance, in one of the earlier studies, a colorectal cancer cell line was transfected with wild-type (wt) *p53* using the calcium phosphate procedure. Although this approach is not feasible in patients, the approach resulted in regression of established tumors in vivo *(32)*. Viruses are more applicable as vectors in humans. Almost all studies in colorectal cancer using *p53* in a gene replacement strategy use adenovirus, because of its potential to infect proliferating and quiescent tumor cells and because of the ability to produce highly purified batches of recombinant virus. Experiments on colorectal cancer cell lines and in vivo have demonstrated the efficacy of adeno-p53 to reduce tumor virulence and increase survival. Interestingly, in those cases in which tumor progressed, wild-type *p53* was not detected or it was inactivated by rearrangement *(34,35)*. Adeno-p53 has also shown similar effects in other malignancies, such as hepatocellular carcinoma, osteosarcoma, ovarian carcinoma, breast carcinoma, nonsmall-cell lung carcinoma, and chronic myeloid leukemia *(36)*.

It is tempting to attribute all of these exciting results to the single action of reintroduced wild-type *p53*, but part of these results can be attributed to release of cytokines (tumor necrosis factor [TNF], interferon [IFN]) after infection of monocytes with adenovirus *(37,38)*. In addition, it has been shown that part of p53 effects are mediated by downregulation of vascular endothelial growth factor (VEGF) in tumors, thereby inducing hypoxia and tumor necrosis *(39)*. In spite of these aspecific reactions, we gratefully make use of them, because a persistent problem with viral vectors is the ability to transduce all of the tumor cells. Using higher viral loads might have a dual action in being able to transduce more tumor cells and producing higher amounts of cytokines in the tumor tissue. In contrast to chemotherapy—which is the current standard treatment for disseminated colorectal cancer and is notorious for its negative affects on quality of life and limited gain in life expectancy—this p53-directed gene therapy has the advantage that it leaves nontransformed cells with wild-type *p53* unharmed and, therefore, has side effects that are limited to the symptoms associated with a viral infection (i.e., fever and mild malaise).

These approaches seem simple and straightforward, but others have postulated that the net effect of the transfected wt-*p53* depends on the extent of DNA alterations that the target cells have already undergone. Experiments by Vinyals and colleagues showed that the presence of mutated *p53* causes the transfected *wt-p53* soon to be mutated or deleted and thereby allows these cells to escape the effects of exogenous *wt-p53 (31)*. Vice versa, this also implies that tumor cells that have wild-type *p53* are also not attacked. This "dominant-negative" theory is indeed seen in a study by Wills and co-workers in which adenovirus-p53 infection of transformed cells with wild-type *p53* failed to display any form of tumor regression *(36)*.

This approach has been continued in a phase I clinical study in which virus was administered via the hepatic artery, but in spite of transduction of the hepatic metastases, no tumor regression was documented after treatment *(40)*. However, in other studies in patients with hepatocellular carcinoma *(41)*, head and neck carcinoma *(42,43)*, and nonsmall-cell lung cancer *(29,44)*, major tumor regressions have been documented objectively *(45)*. Currently, a phase I/II study is ongoing in which the safety and efficacy of hepatic artery infusion of adeno-p53-wt is evaluated in patients with colorectal liver metastases *(46)*.

3.1.1.2. Gene Replacement as a Sensitizer for Chemotherapy and Radiation Therapy. An important mechanism of chemotherapy- and radiation therapy-induced cell death is activation of the p53 apoptosis pathway *(47–49)*. Therefore, another approach in the anti-cancer battle could include the reintroduction of wild-type p53 into cancer cells, followed by cycles of chemotherapy or radiation therapy. In vitro experiments *(50)* on colorectal cancer cell lines using adenovirus-p53 (Adp53) demonstrated that Adp53 and chemotherapy or radiation therapy *(51)* had a synergistic antitumor effect on the tumor cells compared to single treatments, with a demonstrable increase in apoptosis. Furthermore, experiments in tumor-bearing mice showed that the combination therapy of Adp53 and chemotherapy also had a significant synergistic growth-suppressive effect. However, no complete growth inhibition was observed, which is probably the result of the limitations of gene delivery to all tumor cells by local injection. Similar results with Adp53 have been obtained in an in vivo model of lung carcinoma and cisplatin *(52)*.

Translation of these preclinical data of gene replacement to patients has not shown similar beneficial results. In a phase I study, Venook et al. infused adeno-p53 in the hepatic artery of colorectal cancer liver metastasis patients, which failed to result in tumor regression radiographically, but, interestingly, some patients also received subsequent intra-arterial chemotherapy and a majority of patients showed a partial response, possibly reflecting the previously mentioned hypothesis of synergistic effects between chemotherapy and p53 gene therapy *(40)*.

3.1.1.3. Selective Replication in p53-Deficient/Mutated Tumor Cells. A relatively new application that makes use of the *absence* of *wild-type p53* is the use of an *E1B*-defective adenovirus. Adenoviruses contain a number of genes that interact with important tumor suppressor genes of its target cells. For instance, *E1A* inactivates the retinoblastoma protein (a tumor suppressor protein), which results in S-phase entry, necessary for viral replication. The 55-kb E1B gene product binds to p53 and prevents p53-mediated apoptosis, which is probably induced by E1A. By making a deletion and a point mutation in the E1B gene, this virus is unable to replicate in p53-positive cells, as the cells go into apoptosis, but it has acquired the ability to selectively proliferate and display its cytopathic effects in p53-deficient or p53-mutant cells. A study performed by Bischoff and colleagues indeed demonstrated how infection with the described E1B mutant adenovirus, dl1520 (ONYX-015), resulted in slightly better or sometimes similar lysis of tumor cells as compared to infection with wild-type adenovirus. However, the mutant adenovirus clearly has an advantage, because normal cells with wild-type *p53* are unable to support viral replication *(53)*. Using this approach, promising results in phase I/II clinical trials have been obtained *(54)*.

3.1.2. RAS

The family of human *RAS* genes consists of three members, *NRAS*, *HRAS* and *KRAS*, that each encode related 21-kDa proteins *(55)*. They are involved in the transduction of extracellular growth signals to the nucleus. A variety of human malignancies have demonstrated abnormal activation of one or more of the *RAS* genes because of specific mutations in three hot spots *(56,57)*. As a result, the transduction pathway is constitutively activated; thus, cell proliferation is continuously stimulated. The frequency and nature of specific mutations in these hot spots are often characteristic for certain tissue types or mutagens. Mutations can be detected in approx 90% of pancreatic cancers, but only 10% of gastric cancers and about 50% of colorectal cancers.

Inhibition of the mutated function or replacement of the defective *KRAS* gene are the targets of gene therapy in colorectal cancer *(58)*. Sakakura and colleagues treated colorectal cancer cell lines with antisense oligonucleotides complementary to messenger RNA of K-ras, Only those cell lines with an activated *KRAS* gene showed dose-dependant inhibition of K-ras protein and inhibition of cell growth *(59)*. Problems encountered in this approach include the low levels of uptake of the antisense oligonucleotides and the variability in growth-inhibiting effects of different oligonucleotides. No in vivo studies or phase I studies have been initiated to further test these promising results.

3.2. Suicide Gene Therapy

Limitations of currently therapies include, among others, the nontargeted action of the used agents, thereby also harming innocent normal cells. To circumvent these problems, it would be ideal to have a drug that would be restricted to the malignant tissue and would only perform its anticancer effects there, while leaving the healthy cells unharmed. Selectively transducing nonmammalian, prodrug-converting enzymes into malignant cells offers such a possibility, thereby enabling these enzymes to convert the nontoxic prodrug into an effective anti-cancer agent in or near cancer cells. Transduction of all malignant cells has thus far been the Achilles heel of gene therapy, but it has been observed that although only a small fraction of the tumor cells are transduced with a suicide gene, the effects of the produced toxic metabolite traverse cellular boundaries and kill adjacent cells too. This effect, also known as the "bystander effect," is thought to be effectuated by the diffusion of the produced toxic metabolite to neighboring cells through the gap junctions, the activation of the immune system, diffusion of apoptotic vesicles, or a combination of these mechanisms.

A number of prodrug-converting enzyme systems are currently in use, such as herpes simplex–thymidine kinase, cytosine–deaminase, thymidine phosphorylase *(60)*, nitro-reductase *(61)*, carboxypeptidase G2 *(62)*, and UPRT *(63)*. Thymidine kinase and cytosine–deaminase are most commonly used and will be discussed in further detail.

3.2.1. HERPES SIMPLEX–THYMIDINE KINASE

The herpes simplex type 1 (HSV)–*thymidine kinase (TK)* gene has thus far been the most studied suicide gene. Expression of the HSV-*TK* gene renders cells susceptible to the anti-herpetic drugs ganciclovir (GCV) and acyclovir by converting them into toxic nucleotide analogs that inhibit DNA replication. Upon entry into cells, ganciclovir is phosphorylated to ganciclovir phosphates (GCV-P). The initial step yields ganciclovir monophosphate; this step is rate limiting and is catalyzed by the thymidine kinases derived from herpesviruses. Subsequent further phosphorylation is catalyzed by cellular kinases. The triphosphate form of ganciclovir inhibits DNA synthesis. Although GCV is presumed to act as a chain terminator, there is compelling evidence demonstrating the presence of GCV, but not of acyclovir, incorporated internally into the DNA, leaving the precise mechanism by which GCV inhibits DNA replication enigmatic *(64,65)*.

Cycling cells (e.g., tumor cells) are effectively killed by such an approach, whereas quiescent cells (e.g., hepatocytes, neurons) that express HSV-*TK* purportedly are hardly affected *(66)*. This enzyme–prodrug system could therefore be ideal for the rapidly cycling tumor cells of colorectal metastases within the quiescent liver parenchyma.

Ex vivo transduction of colorectal tumor cells with HSV-*TK* transplanted into syngeneic rat livers failed to give rise to tumors in combination with systemic GCV treatment. Control rats with HSV-TK-transduced tumor cells in the liver treated with buffer instead of GCV all grew tumors *(67)*. Also, intra-peritoneal or intra-tumoral treatment of mice bearing colorectal cancer metastases with HSV-*TK* has been shown to induce significant tumor regression and even total eradication of liver metastases. Interestingly, many of these tumors were infiltrated with large amounts of CD-4- and CD-8-positive lymphocytes and significantly less lung metastases were observed in the mice treated with HSV-*TK* as compared to control mice (either not treated or treated with wt virus) *(68,69)*. These observations have led to the hypothesis that by using suicide genes, tumor-associated antigens are revealed once tumor cells are lysed, which are able to induce effective immune responses and, therefore, could potentially be further enhanced by additional immune stimulation. Chen et al. used a combination of suicide gene therapy and immunotherapy for the treatment of these hepatic metastases. The bystander effect was demonstrated: As few as 3.3% of tumor cells transduced with HSV-*TK* resulted in the death of over 90% of tumor cells. Additionally, they showed that the addition of interleukin (IL-2) to HSV-TK resulted in a statistically significant extra reduction in tumor size and in a 100% protection to subsequent tumor challenge with parental tumor cells at a different site. This latter effect is associated with a specific increase in cytotoxic T lymphocyte (CTL) activity against the parental tumor cells in the HSV-TK/IL-2-treated animals only, and not in HSV-TK-treated animals or those treated with adeno-IL-2 alone *(70)*. Not all reports are in agreement with each other on the subject of side effects and the amount of bystander effect. Toxicity has been reported by several investigators in mice and rats with HSV-*TK* and GCV treatment, leading to the death of a considerable number of animals. High doses of recombinant adenovirus carrying the HSV-*TK* gene in combination with systemic GCV leads to severe liver toxicity *(67,71)*. Options to further improve HSV-*TK* responses include pharmacological enhancement of the bystander effect *(72)*, the use of replication-competent vectors *(73,74)*, the use of more active HSV-*TK* mutants *(75)*, and combination treatment with other modalities (e.g., immunotherapy, combination of suicide genes with chemotherapy).

The HSV-*TK* suicide gene strategy has not yet been tested in colorectal cancer patients. Clinical trials have been undertaken for other cancer types such as mesothelioma and brain cancer. Encouraging results have been found in a phase I clinical trial for mesothelioma *(76)*. However, disappointing results have been found in a large phase III multicenter study in malignant brain tumors *(77)*.

3.2.2. Cytosine–Deaminase

Cytosine–deaminase (CD) is a nonmammalian enzyme, which converts cytosine to uracil and the nontoxic prodrug 5-fluorocytosine (5-FC) into the toxic 5-fluorouracil (5-FU) (*see* Chapter 25). The expression of CD in bacteria and yeasts but not mammals makes the use of 5-FC an effective therapy for bacterial and fungal infections. This also gives opportunities to create a large therapeutic window if this gene can be transfected into malignant cells and subsequently treated with 5-FC *(78)*. This is even more so because the CD/5-FC system is also known to have a bystander effect, which some believe is more potent than that observed with the HStk/GCV system *(79)*. Furthermore, it is able to induce an immune reaction that is able to inhibit the growth of and even eradicate synchronous, untransduced liver metastases and inhibit subsequent rechallenges with untransduced parental tumor cells *(80)*. Similar distant bystander effects have also been obtained in head and neck cancers *(81)* and breast cancers *(82)*.

Three strategies can be employed to attack tumor cells using the CD/5-FC system. It can either be transduced into (1) tumor cells or (2) healthy, tumor-surrounding cells or (3) it can act as a sensitizer for chemotherapy or radiation therapy *(83)*. In the first approach, selective expression of the CD gene in tumor cells only can lead to a high concentration of 5-FU in these cells, without affecting healthy cells, because they do not proliferate or they proliferate at a considerably slower pace than tumor cells. In one of the first studies applying the CD/5-FC to malignancies, CD-containing capsules were placed near subcutaneously implanted glioma cells and anti-neoplastic effects were observed after 5-FC treatment *(84)*. This strategy was improved by using a retroviral vector to colorectal cancer with success in vitro *(85)*. Further translation of these data to animal experiments showed prolongation of survival, evidence of the bystander effect in vivo, and eradication of nontransduced tumors by activation of the immune system *(85)*. Similar results have been reported by others with impressive bystander effects (significant effects when only 2–4% of cancer cells were transduced!) and negligible toxicity *(86,87)*. Alternatively, other viral vectors can be used, such as vaccinia, which has more affinity for tumor cells than normal surrounding liver tissue, or adenovirus, which has distinct hepatotropic characteristics. Both viruses that encode CD have demonstrated effectivity in vitro and in vivo, although overall survival of rV-CD treated mice is still limited *(88–90)*.

The second approach was born out of the experience of some investigators that tumor cells were more difficult to transduce than normal tissue. Therefore, it was hypothesized that transducing the healthy cells surrounding the tumor cells with CD would result in a high local production of 5-FU after treatment with FC, practically drenching tumor cells in high concentrations of 5-FU. This second approach can be utilized in a metastasis model (e.g., liver metastases) in which there is a difference in proliferation rate between tumor cells and the surrounding normal cells. The quiescent state of the hepatocytes causes them to hardly incorporate any of the produced toxic metabolite, so that it can diffuse to the rapidly proliferating tumor cells. Animal experiment with this approach show complete suppression of tumor growth and tumor necrosis in the treated mice, in the absence of significant liver toxicity, measured histologically and serologically (91). Targeting hepatocytes has been achieved by taking advantage of the hepatotrophic characteristics of adenoviruses (92,93). Applications using the cytosine–deaminase/5-FC system have not yet moved into phase I studies in patients in spite of impressive antitumor effects without grave side effects.

3.2.3. Other Prodrug Therapies

Other prodrug therapies include uracil phosphoribosyltransferase (UPRT, which enhances the ability of transduced cancer cells to metabolize 5-FU) (63), nitroreductase {which reduces CB1954 [5-(aziridin-1-yl)-2,4-dinitrobenzamide] to the cytotoxic 4-hydroxy-lamino derivate (61,94)}, thymidine phosphorylase [activation of 5-FU (60,95)], carboxypeptidase G2 {activated the prodrug 4-[(2-chloroethyl)(2-mesyloxyethyl)amino]benzo-L-glutamic acid [CMDA] that crosslinks DNA (62)}. These systems have shown promising results in vitro and some have moved in phase I trials (96).

4. IMMUNOMODULATION

The immune-surveillance theory was postulated in the late 1960s by Burnett and states that the host's immune system scrutinizes its cells for (pre-)malignant transformations and is capable of eliminating these (pre-)malignant cells (97). Two types of immune reaction can be discriminated: (1) the humoral (or antibody) response and (2) the cellular (or cytotoxic T-cell response). Three "ingredients" are essential to cook up an effective immune response: (1) human leucocyte antigen (HLA) with a peptide, (2) stimulatory cytokines, and (3) co-stimulatory signals. This immune-surveillance theory is opposed to the long-held paradigm that the body will not mount an immune reaction to self-antigens under normal conditions because of (central and peripheral) tolerance. However, there is evidence that for a host to react to a self-antigen, the microenvironment (especially the *type* of cytokine) in which it is presented to the immune system, directs the immune response to that particular antigen into a "real" immune response (IL-2, IL-12, IFN-γ, TNF-α), or to a state in which the immune system will no longer be able to mount an immune reaction to that antigen (IL-4, IL-5, IL-10, TGF-β) (i.e., *anergy* or *tolerance*) (98).

On one hand, the mere fact that cancers arise and progress to a detectable stage indicates that these transformed cells have deployed certain mechanisms to escape recognition by the immune system, but, on the other hand, several studies have demonstrated an improved clinical outcome in patients with marked lymphocytic tumor infiltrate in colorectal cancer (99–101). In addition, other studies have demonstrated that stimulation of the immune system in these patients can improve survival (102–105). Therefore, immuno-gene therapy can be a feasible treatment option for colorectal cancer and this can be realized through different approaches:

1. Enhance HLA expression
2. Ensure appropriate cytokine production (IL-2, IL-12, IFN-γ, GM-CSF)
3. Provide adequate co-stimulatory signals (B7.1, B7.2)
4. Vaccination against (tumor-associated) antigens

4.1. Enhance HLA Expression

HLA downregulation is frequently observed in malignancies; it prevents the induction of humoral and cellular immune responses. In theory, this downregulation would activate nonspecific immune cells, such as natural killer (NK) cells (because certain HLA elements that inhibit NK cells are no longer present). However, it has also been acknowledged that partial downregulation of HLA can keep these NK-cell-inhibiting HLA fragments intact while deleting the required HLA fragments for T-cell activation. Reintroduction of (allogeneic) HLA is thought to improve the immunogenicity of tumor cells. This has been performed successfully with allogeneic HLA using liposomes in vivo, and even although the transduction efficiency was very poor (<1%), specific CTLs were induced and systemic immunity against the nontransduced parental cells was present. Unfortunately, this was not accompanied by an improved survival in these mice *(106)*. A phase I/II trial has shown effectivity in melanoma patients but not in colorectal cancer and renal carcinoma patients *(107,108)*.

4.2. Ensure Appropriate Cytokine Production

Cytokines comprise a variety of molecules that play a crucial role in directing the immune system into either a stimulatory response or an inhibitory response. It is known that this process is deregulated in patients with malignancies, with either insufficient production of stimulatory cytokines or inappropriate expression of inhibitory cytokines. Therefore, it is thought that increasing the production of stimulatory cytokines at the tumor site will result in immune stimulation and tumor eradication. A number of cytokines are thought to be able to enhance or induce antitumor immune reactions.

4.2.1. INTERLEUKIN-2

Interleukin-2 is a potent immunostimulant, which is capable of, among others, stimulating the proliferation of NK cells, lymphokine-activated killer (LAK) cells and helper (T_H) and cytotoxic T-cells (T_C). However, systemic use of IL-2 in man is associated with considerable toxic side effects, and this, in combination with the short half-life of IL-2, limits the dose and therefore efficacy. Limiting IL-2 expression to its place of action is essential and can be achieved with gene therapy. Two approaches are possible to enhance IL-2 concentrations locally, namely transduction of the tumor cells or transduction of tumor-adjacent cells (e.g., fibroblasts). Fearon et al. transduced a poorly immunogenic colorectal cancer cell line with *IL-2* and observed that subcutaneous implantation of these tumor cells resulted in rejection of the transduced tumor cells and, moreover, a rechallenge with nontransduced, wild-type, parental tumor cells *(109)*.

This approach has been tested in murine and human colorectal cancer in vitro and in vivo. The majority of studies demonstrate that IL-2 expression by tumor cells or tumor-adjacent cells (e.g., fibroblasts) leads to prevention of growth in tumor-challenge studies or to complete disappearance of tumor deposits. Even distant lesions and rechallenges with nontransduced (wild type) tumor cells are eliminated. Although not all investigators found as encouraging results, alternatives such as the addition of other cytokines (IL-12, GM-CSF) or co-stimulatory signals (B7.2) can overcome these disappointing results *(110–118)*.

A number of phase I studies have been executed in which safety is clearly demonstrated, but almost no colorectal cancer patients benefit from this approach. Similar results have been shown in renal cell carcinoma, melanoma, and glioblastoma. However, a complete response has also been documented in a patient with a lymphoma and it must be borne in mind that the investigated patient population is severely impaired immunologically and has a tremendous tumor burden *(119–123)*.

4.2.2. INTERLEUKIN-12

Interleukin-12 is a heterodimeric 70-kDa cytokine composed of a 35-kDa subunit and two 40-kDa subunits and is mainly produced by antigen-presenting cells and is known to enhance cytolytic activity of macrophages, LAK cells, NK cells, and T cells through stimulating IFN-γ production by NK cells and T-cells *(124,125)*. Preclinical studies have demonstrated anti-neoplastic effects in different tumors *(126,127)*. However, systemic use of IL-12 in humans has produced serious toxicity in the majority of patients and even mortality in some patients *(128)*. Therefore, limiting IL-12 production to the site of action by gene therapy is a major focus of attention.

The IFN-γ mediated effects of IL-12 make the liver an ideal target for this approach, because of a large pool of NK cells in the liver. Testing adeno-*IL-12* in a liver metastases model indeed resulted in long-term survival in several mice *(129)*. The inability to cure all mice probably results in part from the inability to infect all tumor cells, but also from the selection of NK-sensitive tumor cells. The NK-resistant cells might be more sensitive to T_C-mediated kill, which can be augmented by IL-2. This approach is under investigation. Further improvements can be expected by specifically depleting CD4+ lymphocytes because these are known to inhibit the efficacy of IL-12 *(130)*.

4.2.3. OTHER CYTOKINES

Other cytokines that are frequently used in (immuno-) gene therapy include granulocyte–macrophage–colony-stimulating factor (GM-CSF) *(131,132)*, IFN-γ *(133)*, IL-4 *(134)*, TNF *(135)*, and IFN-α *(136)*.

4.3. Provide Adequate Co-Stimulatory Signals

In addition to HLA with a peptide in its peptide-binding groove and the right cytokines, co-stimulatory signals are important for an effective immune response to ensue. A number of these receptor–ligand pairs have been identified (CD11/18-CD54, CD2-CD58, CD29/49-CD106, CD28-CD80/CD86). Of these, the B7.1/B7.2 have been investigated most thoroughly. B7.1 (CD80) and B7.2 (CD86) interact with the CD28 receptor on T-cells and provide additional signals for an incipient immune reaction. In addition, it can bind to CTLA-4 (CD152), which inhibits T-lymphocytes *(137–139)*. Unfortunately, tumor cells and antigen-presenting cells present in the colorectal cancer stroma hardly express these costimulatory molecules, so that instead of an immune response being initiated, the T-cells become unresponsive to the presented (tumor) antigens *(140)*. It is hypothesized that transduction of genes encoding these co-stimulatory signals into cancer cells will overcome T-cell anergy and initiate a potent anti-tumor response. This has indeed been shown in a number of pioneering studies in among others melanoma, in which rechallenges with unmodified tumor cells were also effectively attacked *(141–144)*.

Similar studies in colorectal cancer have also shown the induction of tumor-specific immune reactions mediated by CD8+ lymphocytes *(145)*. However, others were not able to confirm these findings *(146,147)*. Options to further improve these results lie in the addition of extra (co-) stimulatory signals, such CD54 (which not only increases CD28 expression but also improves CD80–CD28-mediated costimulations and directly induces co-stimulatory signals), or the addition of IL-2, IL-12, GM-CSF, or B7.2 *(145,148,149)*.

4.4. Vaccination Against (Tumor-Associated) Antigens

Mutation occurring in many genes during carcinogenesis results in the production of abnormal proteins that could be immunogenic. However, the immunosuppressed condition of cancer patients and the utilization of all kinds of immune-escape mechanisms prevent adequate immune responses to be initiated. Vaccination strategies against specific genes that are overexpressed in many colorectal cancers during carcinogenesis are attractive targets for the immune system. Although different vaccination targets exist (mutated ras, APC, p53, CEA), we will discuss p53 and CEA in the following subsections.

4.4.1. P53

In addition to the gene replacement strategy (with or without subsequent chemotherapy or radiation therapy) and the p53-alteration-selection-strategy (adenovirus dl1520 [ONYX-015]), another way to attack p53 is immunologically. Although p53 is an autoantigen, studies have shown that tolerance to p53 is not absolute, illustrated, for instance, by the presence of circulating p53 antibodies in approx 25% of colorectal cancer patients *(150)*. *p53* mutations (which are present in up to 70% of colorectal cancers) result in overexpression of p53, making it a distinguishable target from p53 in normal cells, in which it has a rapid turnover rate and very low expression levels. Roth and colleagues showed that vaccination with p53 using an attenuated canarypox virus (ALVAC-p53) as vector resulted in a prevention of tumor outgrowth after challenging with p53-overexpressing tumors in mice. Similarly, the reverse situation in which tumor vaccinations were given prior to vaccination also resulted in total regression of the established tumors, albeit that only small tumor loads could be eradicated *(151)*. This study has recently moved into a phase I/II clinical trial with end-stage colorectal cancer patients.

4.4.2. CEA

The carcinoembryonic antigen (CEA) gene was first described in 1965 *(152)*. It has been mapped to chromosome 19 and encodes a 180,000-kDa protein. It is a member of the human immunoglobulin gene superfamily and therefore shares some homology with other molecules found on normal human tissues, for instance with nonspecific crossreacting antigen (NCA), which is expressed on granulocytes *(153,154)*. It is thought that it plays a role in intercellular recognition and as an adhesion molecule *(155)*. During fetal development, it is expressed in abundance in epithelial tissues of the digestive tract, breast, lung, and ovaries, but in the adult, the expression is almost totally downregulated.

Almost all adenocarcinomas of the colon and rectum show overexpression of CEA, making it an attractive target for immunotherapy (in spite of the fact that it is a self-antigen) *(156–158)*. Although immunotherapy is the aim of most CEA-related studies, gene therapy is used often to reach this goal. So far, the *CEA* gene (with or without other genes) has been cloned into two related vectors, vaccinia virus and avipox virus (ALVAC) and it has been possible to overcome tolerance to CEA *(159,160)*.

Preclinical studies using recombinant vaccinia–CEA (rV-CEA) have been performed in mice and rhesus monkeys. Vaccinations with rV-CEA in mice followed by tumor challenge with CEA-expressing tumors resulted in tumor protection in 50% of mice, whereas all control mice developed tumors *(161–163)*. This model is artificial in several ways, among others because CEA is not expressed in rodents, mouse major histocompatibility complex (MHC)-binding motifs are different from human MHC-binding motifs, and humans are tolerant to CEA. Therefore, additional experiments were performed in which vaccinations with rV-CEA were only performed after fairly large tumors had developed in mice. In these

Table 2
Gene Therapy Studies with CEA in Colorectal Cancer Patients

n	Vector	Route of injection[a]	Clinical response[b]	CEA level[c]	Immune response[d]	Ref.
20	Adeno-CEA ALVAC-CEA	sc, im	All PD	Majority ↑	Humoral + Cellular +	164
17	Vaccinia–CEA	id	1 SD 16 PD	na	Cellular +	159
20	Vaccinia–CEA	id, sc	4 SD	All ↑	Humoral – Cellular –	165
17	Vaccinia–CEA	id	All PD	↓ in a few patients	na	166
20	ALVAC–CEA	im	All PD		+	104,170

[a]id: intradermal injection; im: intramuscular; sc: subcutaneous injection.
[b]PD: progressive disease, SD: stable disease.
[c]↓: declining CEA, ↑: rising CEA.
[d]na: not available.

latter experiments, a significant delay in tumor growth was observed with CEA-expressing tumors, which corresponded with the induction of a humoral and cellular immune response against CEA (expressing tumors). Similar results have been demonstrated by Kass and co-workers (163).

The first clinical trial with recombinant vaccinia–CEA was conducted in 1993 with 26 patients, of whom 17 had colon cancer. All patients had been inoculated with vaccinia in childhood against smallpox and now received three 4-weekly dermal scarifications with varying doses (2×10^5, 2×10^6, 1×10^7 pfu (plaque-forming units). Adverse effects consisted of mild local (pustules and erythema) and systemic inflammatory reactions (fever, fatigue). On follow-up, only 1 patient had stable disease, whereas 13 out of 14 patients who received the first two dose levels demonstrated progressive disease (164). Their results failed to show a proliferative response against CEA protein following vaccination, but additional experiments demonstrated the possibility of inducing cytotoxic T-cells capable of lysing autologous tumor cells in a peptide-specific, MHC-restricted manner (159). Other phase I studies failed to demonstrate effectivity as well (see Table 2) (165,166). These disappointing results are not entirely surprising for a number of reasons. First, it is a well known that cancer patients are immune compromised and are severely set back when stimulated to induce a new immune response. This is even more compelling when the target antigen is a self-antigen, to which tolerance usually exists. In addition, even if tolerance were not present, tumor cells are poor antigen-presenting cells, often lacking essential prerequisites, such as class I HLA and co-stimulatory molecules, and are known to produce immune-suppressive cytokines. Finally, the "average" colorectal cancer patient will have been exposed to vaccinia in childhood as part of the WHO smallpox eradication program. This will undoubtfully have produced memory immune cells against vaccinia that will inactivate the recombinant vaccinia virus well before it has been able to do its job of inducing an immune response against CEA. Therefore, alternative strategies have been employed, such as using different less immunogenic vectors, priming the immune response with one vector and boosting with another vector, the addition of co-stimulatory molecules or immune-enhancing cytokines to the vaccine (167), or a combination of these strategies. For instance, in one study, the immune reaction against CEA was primed with vaccinia–CEA mixed with a co-stimulatory molecule (vaccinia–B7.1) and boosted with a different vector, attenuated canarypox virus (ALVAC) encoding *CEA* and *B7.1*. Indeed, this approach has shown superior effects after one vaccination (as compared to the use of both constructs separately), resulting in enhanced CEA-specific, cellular, long-term antitumor immunity *(168)*. Likewise, similar exciting results have been documented in such a prime and boost strategy using vaccinia and ALVAC, with both vectors encoding *CEA (169)*.

A powerful alternative for vaccinia-based gene transfer is the availability of an attenuated canarypox virus that can be produced to encode several genes and has several advantages such as the fact that hardly anyone will have pre-existing antibodies to ALVAC and that it is a nonhuman pathogen. Moreover, there is evidence that once ALVAC has been administered to a patient, additional vaccinations with ALVAC can still further enhance an immune response against the encoded gene of interest, in spite of possible negative effects of an induced anti-ALVAC immune response. A phase I study using ALVAC–CEA was safe and induced an immune response, but this was of no clinical avail (*see* Table 2) *(104,170)*.

In summary, encouraging preclinical and clinical data have been obtained to justify further investigations, for instance in cancer patients with minimal residual disease (i.e., as adjuvant treatment after "curative" colorectal cancer surgery). This effect could be even more specific when used in combination with a CEA promotor and can be used to treat the primary tumor as well as metastases *(171,172)*.

5. CONCLUSION AND FUTURE PROSPECTS

Since the discovery of DNA by Watson and Crick in 1953, the possibilities of using these molecules for the diagnosis and treatment of human diseases have been increasing exponentially. The human genome project and recent advances in the field of technology and molecular biology will offer even more possibilities for the identification and treatment of diseases. In the past 10–15 yr, these possibilities have slowly moved from the laboratory testing phase to use in the clinic. Future research will have to focus on remaining challenges in several fields such as the safety and efficacy of viral and nonviral vector systems and the decreasing impedement of viral vectors by the immune system. Other fields that deserve attention include the identification of new vectors or the production of improved vectors that are able to carry large genes and can facilitate long-term expression. Although there are still many obstacles to overcome, progress is being made rapidly and the general attitude toward gene therapy is one of optimism.

REFERENCES

1. Niitsu Y, Takahashi Y, Ban N, Takayama T, Saito T, Katahira T, et al. A proof of glutathione *S*-transferase-pi-related multidrug resistance by transfer of antisense gene to cancer cells and sense gene to bone marrow stem cell. *Chem. Biol. Interact.*, **111–112** (1998) 325–332.
2. Friedmann T. A brief history of gene therapy. *Nat. Genet.*, **2(2)** (1992) 93–98.
3. Avery OT, McLeod CM, and McCarthy M. Studies on the chemical nature of the substance inducing transformation of pneumococcal types. *J. Exp. Med.*, **79** (1944) 137–158.
4. Graham FL and van der Eb AJ. A new technique for the assay of infectivity of human adenovirus 5 DNA. *Virology*, **52(2)** (1973) 456–467.
5. Graham FL, Abrahams PJ, Mulder C, Heijneker HL, Warnaar SO, De Vries FA, et al. Studies on in vitro transformation by DNA and DNA fragments of human adenoviruses and simian virus 40. *Cold Spring Harbor Symp. Quant. Biol.*, **39 (Pt. 1)** (1975) 637–650.
6. Abrahams PJ and van der Eb AJ. In vitro transformation of rat and mouse cells by DNA from simian virus 40. *J. Virol.*, **16(1)** (1975) 206–209.

7. Temin HM and Mizutani S. RNA-dependent DNA polymerase in virions of Rous sarcoma virus. *Nature*, **226(252)** (1970) 1211–1213.

8. Curiel D and Reynolds P. Gene therapy death highlights the remaining challenges. *Helix*, **9** (2000) 21–25.

9. Anderson WF, Killos L, Sanders HL, Kretschmer PJ, and Diacumakos EG. Replication and expression of thymidine kinase and human globin genes microinjected into mouse fibroblasts. *Proc. Natl. Acad. Sci. USA*, **77(9)** (1980) 5399–5403.

10. Rogers S, Lowenthal A, Terheggen HG, and Columbo JP. Induction of arginase activity with the Shope papilloma virus in tissue culture cells from an argininemic patient. *J. Exp. Med.*, **137(4)** (1973) 1091–1096.

11. Donahue RE, Kessler SW, Bodine D, McDonagh K, Dunbar C, Goodman S, et al. Helper virus induced T cell lymphoma in nonhuman primates after retroviral mediated gene transfer. *J. Exp. Med.*, **176(4)** (1992) 1125–1135.

12. Cornetta K, Moen RC, Culver K, Morgan RA, McLachlin JR, Sturm S, et al. Amphotropic murine leukemia retrovirus is not an acute pathogen for primates. *Hum. Gene Ther.*, **1(1)** (1990) 15–30.

13. Jones N and Shenk T. Isolation of adenovirus type 5 host range deletion mutants defective for transformation of rat embryo cells. *Cell*, **17(3)** (1979) 683–689.

14. Fallaux FJ, Kranenburg O, Cramer SJ, Houweling A, van Ormondt H, Hoeben RC, et al. Characterization of 911: a new helper cell line for the titration and propagation of early region 1-deleted adenoviral vectors. *Hum. Gene Ther.*, **7(2)** (1996) 215–222.

15. Fallaux FJ, Bout A, van de Velde I, van den Wollenberg DJ, Hehir KM, Keegan J, et al. New helper cells and matched early region 1-deleted adenovirus vectors prevent generation of replication-competent adenoviruses. *Hum. Gene Ther.*, **9(13)** (1998) 1909–1917.

16. Mulligan RC. The basic science of gene therapy. *Science*, **260(5110)** (1993) 926–932.

17. McKeithan TW, Rowley JD, Shows TB, and Diaz MO. Cloning of the chromosome translocation breakpoint junction of the t(14;19) in chronic lymphocytic leukemia. *Proc. Natl. Acad. Sci. USA*, **84(24)** (1987) 9257–9260.

18. Li H, Lu H, Griscelli F, Opolon P, Sun LQ, Ragot T, et al. Adenovirus-mediated delivery of a uPA/uPAR antagonist suppresses angiogenesis-dependent tumor growth and dissemination in mice. *Gene Ther.*, **5(8)** (1998) 1105–1113.

19. Hayashi S, Yokoyama I, Namii Y, Emi N, Uchida K, and Takagi H. Inhibitory effect on the establishment of hepatic metastasis by transduction of the tissue plasminogen activator gene to murine colon cancer. *Cancer Gene Ther.*, **6(4)** (1999) 380–384.

20. Su Z, Goldstein NI, and Fisher PB. Antisense inhibition of the PTI-1 oncogene reverses cancer phenotypes. *Proc. Natl. Acad. Sci. USA*, **95(4)** (1998) 1764–1769.

21. Nakashima E, Oya A, Kubota Y, Kanada N, Matsushita R, Takeda K, et al. A candidate for cancer gene therapy: MIP-1 alpha gene transfer to an adenocarcinoma cell line reduced tumorigenicity and induced protective immunity in immunocompetent mice. *Pharm. Res.*, **13(12)** (1996) 1896–1901.

22. Clarke MF, Apel IJ, Benedict MA, Eipers PG, Sumantran V, Gonzalez GM, et al. A recombinant bcl-x s adenovirus selectively induces apoptosis in cancer cells but not in normal bone marrow cells. *Proc. Natl. Acad. Sci. USA*, **92(24)** (1995) 11,024–11,028.

23. Hargest R and Williamson R. Expression of the APC gene after transfection into a colonic cancer cell line. *Gut*, **37(6)** (1995) 826–829.

24. Lane DP and Crawford LV. T antigen is bound to a host protein in SV40-transformed cells. *Nature*, **278(5701)** (1979) 261–263.

25. Lane DP. Cancer. p53, guardian of the genome. *Nature*, **358(6381)** (1992) 15–16.

26. Levine AJ, Momand J, and Finlay CA. The p53 tumour suppressor gene. *Nature*, **351(6326)** (1991) 453–456.

27. Hollstein M, Sidransky D, Vogelstein B, and Harris CC. p53 mutations in human cancers. *Science*, **253(5015)** (1991) 49–53.

28. Casey G, Lo HM, Lopez ME, Vogelstein B, and Stanbridge EJ. Growth suppression of human breast cancer cells by the introduction of a wild-type p53 gene. *Oncogene*, **6(10)** (1991) 1791–1797.

29. Roth JA, Nguyen D, Lawrence DD, Kemp BL, Carrasco CH, Ferson DZ, et al. Retrovirus-mediated wild-type p53 gene transfer to tumors of patients with lung cancer. *Nature Med.*, **2(9)** (1996) 985–991.

30. Yang C, Cirielli C, Capogrossi MC, and Passaniti A. Adenovirus-mediated wild-type p53 expression induces apoptosis and suppresses tumorigenesis of prostatic tumor cells. *Cancer Res.*, **55(19)** (1995) 4210–4213.

31. Vinyals A, Peinado MA, Gonzalez GM, Monzo M, Bonfil RD, and Fabra A. Failure of wild-type p53 gene therapy in human cancer cells expressing a mutant p53 protein. *Gene Ther.*, **6(1)** (1999) 22–33.

32. Shaw P, Bovey R, Tardy S, Sahli R, Sordat B, and Costa J. Induction of apoptosis by wild-type p53 in a human colon tumor-derived cell line. *Proc. Natl. Acad. Sci. USA*, **89(10)** (1992) 4495–4499.

33. Zhang WW, Alemany R, Wang J, Koch PE, Ordonez NG, and Roth JA. Safety evaluation of Ad5CMV–p53 in vitro and in vivo. *Hum. Gene Ther.*, **6(2)** (1995) 155–164.

34. Baker SJ, Markowitz S, Fearon ER, Willson JK, and Vogelstein B. Suppression of human colorectal carcinoma cell growth by wild-type p53. *Science*, **249(4971)** (1990) 912–915.

35. Harris MP, Sutjipto S, Wills KN, Hancock W, Cornell D, Johnson DE, et al. Adenovirus-mediated p53 gene transfer inhibits growth of human tumor cells expressing mutant p53 protein. *Cancer Gene Ther.*, **3(2)** (1996) 121–130.

36. Wills KN, Maneval DC, Menzel P, Harris MP, Sutjipto S, Vaillancourt MT, et al. Development and characterization of recombinant adenoviruses encoding human p53 for gene therapy of cancer. *Hum. Gene Ther.*, **5(9)** (1994) 1079–1088.

37. Gooding LR and Wold WS. Molecular mechanisms by which adenoviruses counteract antiviral immune defenses. *Crit. Rev. Immunol.*, **10(1)** (1990) 53–71.

38. Hock H, Dorsch M, Kunzendorf U, Qin Z, Diamantstein T, and Blankenstein T. Mechanisms of rejection induced by tumor cell-targeted gene transfer of interleukin 2, interleukin 4, interleukin 7, tumor necrosis factor, or interferon gamma. *Proc. Natl. Acad. Sci. USA*, **90(7)** (1993) 2774–2778.

39. Bouvet M, Ellis LM, Nishizaki M, Fujiwara T, Liu W, Bucana CD, et al. Adenovirus-mediated wild-type p53 gene transfer down-regulates vascular endothelial growth factor expression and inhibits angiogenesis in human colon cancer. *Cancer Res.*, **58(11)** (1998) 2288–2292.

40. Venook AP, Bergsland EK, Ring E, Nonaka-Wong S, Horowitz JA, Rybak ME, and Warren RS. Gene therapy of colorectal liver metastases using a recombinant adenovirus encoding WT p53 via hepatic artery infusion. *ASCO Proc.*, **17** (1998) 431a.

41. Habib NA, Ding SF, el Masry R, Mitry RR, Honda K, Michail NE, et al. Preliminary report: the short-term effects of direct p53 DNA injection in primary hepatocellular carcinomas. *Cancer Detect. Prev.*, **20(2)** (1996) 103–107.

42. Clayman GL, Frank DK, Bruso PA, and Goepfert H. Adenovirus-mediated wild-type p53 gene transfer as a surgical adjuvant in advanced head and neck cancers. *Clin. Cancer Res.*, **5(7)** (1999) 1715–1722.

43. Clayman GL, El Naggar AK, Lippman SM, Henderson YC, Frederick M, Merritt JA, et al. Adenovirus-mediated p53 gene transfer in patients with advanced recurrent head and neck squamous cell carcinoma. *J. Clin. Oncol.*, **16(6)** (1998) 2221–2232.

44. Swisher SG, Roth JA, Nemunaitis J, Lawrence DD, Kemp BL, Carrasco CH, et al. Adenovirus-mediated p53 gene transfer in advanced non-small-cell lung cancer. *J. Natl. Cancer Inst.*, **91(9)** (1999) 763–771.

45. Roth JA and Cristiano RJ. Gene therapy for cancer: what have we done and where are we going? *J. Natl. Cancer Inst.*, **89(1)** (1997) 21–39.

46. Habib NA, Hodgson HJ, Lemoine N, and Pignatelli M. A phase I/II study of hepatic artery infusion with wtp53–CMV–Ad in metastatic malignant liver tumours. *Hum. Gene Ther.*, **10(12)** (1999) 2019–2034.

47. Lowe SW, Ruley HE, Jacks T, and Housman DE. p53-Dependent apoptosis modulates the cytotoxicity of anticancer agents. *Cell*, **74(6)** (1993) 957–967.

48. Kinzler KW and Vogelstein B. Cancer therapy meets p53. *N. Engl. J. Med.*, **331(1)** (1994) 49–50.

49. Yang B, Eshleman JR, Berger NA, and Markowitz SD. Wild-type p53 protein potentiates cytotoxicity of therapeutic agents in human colon cancer cells. *Clin. Cancer Res.*, **2(10)** (1996) 1649–1657.

50. Ogawa N, Fujiwara T, Kagawa S, Nishizaki M, Morimoto Y, Tanida T, et al. Novel combination therapy for human colon cancer with adenovirus-mediated wild-type p53 gene transfer and DNA-damaging chemotherapeutic agent. *Int. J. Cancer*, **73(3)** (1997) 367–370.

51. Spitz FR, Nguyen D, Skibber JM, Meyn RE, Cristiano RJ, and Roth JA. Adenoviral-mediated wild-type p53 gene expression sensitizes colorectal cancer cells to ionizing radiation. *Clin. Cancer Res.*, **2(10)** (1996) 1665–1671.

52. Fujiwara T, Grimm EA, Mukhopadhyay T, Zhang WW, Owen-Schaub LB, and Roth JA. Induction of chemosensitivity in human lung cancer cells in vivo by adenovirus-mediated transfer of the wild-type p53 gene. *Cancer Res.*, **54(9)** (1994) 2287–2291.

53. Bischoff JR, Kirn DH, Williams A, Heise C, Horn S, Muna M, et al. An adenovirus mutant that replicates selectively in p53-deficient human tumor cells. *Science*, **274(5286)** (1996) 373–376.

54. Korn WM. Cancer therapy based on p53: the adenovirus mutant dl1520 (ONYX-015). First International Symposium on Genetic Anticancer Agents, Amsterdam, 2000.

55. Barbacid M. ras genes. *Annu. Rev. Biochem.*, **56** (1987) 779–827.

56. Bos JL. ras oncogenes in human cancer: a review [published erratum appears in *Cancer Res.*, **50(4)** (1990) 1352], *Cancer Res.*, **49(17)** (1989) 4682–4689.

57. Bos JL. The ras gene family and human carcinogenesis. *Mutat. Res.*, **195(3)** (1988) 255–271.

58. Calabretta B. Inhibition of protooncogene expression by antisense oligodeoxynucleotides: biological and therapeutic implications. *Cancer Res.*, **51(17)** (1991) 4505–4510.

59. Sakakura C, Hagiwara A, Tsujimoto H, Ozaki K, Sakakibara T, Oyama T, et al. Inhibition of colon cancer cell proliferation by antisense oligonucleotides targeting the messenger RNA of the Ki-ras gene. *Anticancer Drugs*, **6(4)** (1995) 553–561.

60. Evrard A, Cuq P, Robert B, Vian L, Pelegrin A, and Cano JP. Enhancement of 5-fluorouracil cytotoxicity by human thymidine–phosphorylase expression in cancer cells: in vitro and in vivo study. *Int. J. Cancer*, **80(3)** (1999) 465–470.

61. Friedlos F, Court S, Ford M, Denny WA, and Springer C. Gene-directed enzyme prodrug therapy: quantitative bystander cytotoxicity and DNA damage induced by CB1954 in cells expressing bacterial nitroreductase. *Gene Ther.*, **5(1)** (1998) 105–112.

62. Marais R, Spooner RA, Light Y, Martin J, and Springer CJ. Gene-directed enzyme prodrug therapy with a mustard prodrug/carboxypeptidase G2 combination. *Cancer Res.*, **56(20)** (1996) 4735–4742.

63. Kanai F, Kawakami T, Hamada H, Sadata A, Yoshida Y, Tanaka T, et al. Adenovirus-mediated transduction of *Escherichia coli* uracil phosphoribosyltransferase gene sensitizes cancer cells to low concentrations of 5-fluorouracil. *Cancer Res.*, **58(9)** (1998) 1946–1951.

64. Cheng YC, Grill SP, Dutschman GE, Frank KB, Chiou JF, Bastow KF, et al. Effects of 9-(1,3-dihydroxy-2-propoxymethyl)guanine, a new antiherpesvirus compound, on synthesis of macromolecules in herpes simplex virus-infected cells. *Antimicrob. Agents Chemother.*, **26(3)** (1984) 283–288.

65. Frank KB, Chiou JF, and Cheng YC. Interaction of herpes simplex virus-induced DNA polymerase with 9-(1,3-dihydroxy-2-propoxymethyl)guanine triphosphate. *J. Biol. Chem.*, **259(3)** (1984) 1566–1569.

66. Culver KW, Ram Z, Wallbridge S, Ishii H, Oldfield EH, and Blaese RM. In vivo gene transfer with retroviral vector-producer cells for treatment of experimental brain tumors. *Science*, **256(5063)** (1992) 1550–1552.

67. van der Eb MM, Cramer SJ, Vergouwe Y, Schagen FH, van Krieken JH, van der Eb AJ, et al. Severe hepatic dysfunction after adenovirus-mediated transfer of the herpes simplex virus thymidine kinase gene and ganciclovir administration. *Gene Ther.*, **5(4)** (1998) 451–458.

68. Hayashi S, Emi N, Yokoyama I, Uchida K, and Takagi H. Effect of gene therapy with the herpes simplex virus-thymidine kinase gene on hepatic metastasis in murine colon cancer. *Surg. Today*, **27(1)** (1997) 40–43.

69. Caruso M, Panis Y, Gagandeep S, Houssin D, Salzmann JL, and Klatzmann D. Regression of established macroscopic liver metastases after in situ transduction of a suicide gene. *Proc. Natl. Acad. Sci. USA*, **90(15)** (1993) 7024–7028.

70. Chen SH, Chen XH, Wang Y, Kosai K, Finegold MJ, Rich SS, et al. Combination gene therapy for liver metastasis of colon carcinoma in vivo. *Proc. Natl. Acad. Sci. USA*, **92(7)** (1995) 2577–2581.

71. Brand K, Arnold W, Bartels T, Lieber A, Kay MA, Strauss M, et al. Liver-associated toxicity of the HSV-tk/GCV approach and adenoviral vectors. *Cancer Gene Ther.*, **4(1)** (1997) 9–16.

72. Touraine RL, Vahanian N, Ramsey WJ, and Blaese RM. Enhancement of the herpes simplex virus thymidine kinase/ganciclovir bystander effect and its antitumor efficacy in vivo by pharmacologic manipulation of gap junctions. *Hum. Gene Ther.*, **9(16)** (1998) 2385–2391.

73. Wildner O, Morris JC, Vahanian NN, Ford H, Ramsey WJ, and Blaese RM. Adenoviral vectors capable of replication improve the efficacy of HSVtk/GCV suicide gene therapy of cancer. *Gene Ther.*, **6(1)** (1999) 57–62.

74. Wildner O, Blaese RM, and Morris JC. Therapy of colon cancer with oncolytic adenovirus is enhanced by the addition of herpes simplex virus–thymidine kinase. *Cancer Res.*, **59(2)** (1999) 410–413.

75. Black ME, Newcomb TG, Wilson HM, and Loeb LA. Creation of drug-specific herpes simplex virus type 1 thymidine kinase mutants for gene therapy. *Proc. Natl. Acad. Sci. USA*, **93(8)** (1996) 3525–3529.

76. Sterman DH, Treat J, Litzky LA, Amin KM, Coonrod L, Molnar KK, et al. Adenovirus-mediated herpes simplex virus thymidine kinase/ganciclovir gene therapy in patients with localized malignancy: results of a phase I clinical trial in malignant mesothelioma. *Hum. Gene Ther.*, **9(7)** (1998) 1083–1092.

77. Rainov NG. Herpes-simplex thymidine kinase gene/ganciclovir gene therapy for primary malignant glioma. Results of a phase III study. First International Symposium on Genetic Anticancer Agents, Amsterdam, 2000.

78. Andersen L, Kilstrup M, and Neuhard J. Pyrimidine, purine and nitrogen control of cytosine deaminase synthesis in *Escherichia coli* K 12. Involvement of the glnLG and purR genes in the regulation of codA expression. *Arch. Microbiol.*, **152(2)** (1989) 115–118.

79. Trinh QT, Austin EA, Murray DM, Knick VC, and Huber BE. Enzyme/prodrug gene therapy: comparison of cytosine deaminase/5-fluorocytosine versus thymidine kinase/ganciclovir enzyme/prodrug systems in a human colorectal carcinoma cell line. *Cancer Res.*, **55(21)** (1995) 4808–4812.

80. Pierrefite CV, Baque P, Gavelli A, Mala M, Chazal M, Gugenheim J, et al. Cytosine deaminase/5-fluorocytosine-based vaccination against liver tumors: evidence of distant bystander effect. *J. Natl. Cancer Inst.*, **91(23)** (1999) 2014–2019.

81. Bi W, Kim YG, Feliciano ES, Pavelic L, Wilson KM, Pavelic ZP, et al. An HSVtk-mediated local and distant antitumor bystander effect in tumors of head and neck origin in athymic mice. *Cancer Gene Ther.*, **4(4)** (1997) 246–252.

82. Wei MX, Bougnoux P, Sacre SB, Peyrat MB, Lhuillery C, Salzmann JL, et al. Suicide gene therapy of chemically induced mammary tumor in rat: efficacy and distant bystander effect. *Cancer Res.*, **58(16)** (1998) 3529–3532.

83. Gabel M, Kim JH, Kolozsvary A, Khil M, and Freytag S. Selective in vivo radiosensitization by 5-fluorocytosine of human colorectal carcinoma cells transduced with the *E. coli* cytosine deaminase (CD) gene. *Int. J. Radiat. Oncol. Biol. Phys.*, **41(4)** (1998) 883–887.

84. Nishiyama T, Kawamura Y, Kawamoto K, Matsumura H, Yamamoto N, Ito T, et al. Antineoplastic effects in rats of 5-fluorocytosine in combination with cytosine deaminase capsules. *Cancer Res.*, **45(4)** (1985) 1753–1761.

85. Mullen CA, Coale MM, Lowe R, and Blaese RM. Tumors expressing the cytosine deaminase suicide gene can be eliminated in vivo with 5-fluorocytosine and induce protective immunity to wild type tumor. *Cancer Res.*, **54(6)** (1994) 1503–1506.

86. Huber BE, Austin EA, Good SS, Knick VC, Tibbels S, and Richards CA. In vivo antitumor activity of 5-fluorocytosine on human colorectal carcinoma cells genetically modified to express cytosine deaminase. *Cancer Res.*, **53(19)** (1993) 4619–4626.

87. Huber BE, Austin EA, Richards CA, Davis ST, and Good SS. Metabolism of 5-fluorocytosine to 5-fluorouracil in human colorectal tumor cells transduced with the cytosine deaminase gene: significant antitumor effects when only a small percentage of tumor cells express cytosine deaminase. *Proc. Natl. Acad. Sci. USA*, **91(17)** (1994) 8302–8306.

88. Gnant MF, Puhlmann M, Bartlett DL, and Alexander HRJ. Regional versus systemic delivery of recombinant vaccinia virus as suicide gene therapy for murine liver metastases. *Ann. Surg.*, **230(3)** (1999) 352–360.

89. Gnant MF, Puhlmann M, Alexander HRJ, and Bartlett DL. Systemic administration of a recombinant vaccinia virus expressing the cytosine deaminase gene and subsequent treatment with 5-fluorocytosine leads to tumor-specific gene expression and prolongation of survival in mice. *Cancer Res.*, **59(14)** (1999) 3396–3403.

90. Hirschowitz EA, Ohwada A, Pascal WR, Russi TJ, and Crystal RG. In vivo adenovirus-mediated gene transfer of the *Escherichia coli* cytosine deaminase gene to human colon carcinoma-derived tumors induces chemosensitivity to 5-fluorocytosine. *Hum. Gene Ther.*, **6(8)** (1995) 1055–1063.

91. Ohwada A, Hirschowitz EA, and Crystal RG. Regional delivery of an adenovirus vector containing the *Escherichia coli* cytosine deaminase gene to provide local activation of 5-fluorocytosine to suppress the growth of colon carcinoma metastatic to liver. *Hum. Gene Ther.*, **7(13)** (1996) 1567–1576.

92. Huard J, Lochmuller H, Acsadi G, Jani A, Massie B, and Karpati G. The route of administration is a major determinant of the transduction efficiency of rat tissues by adenoviral recombinants. *Gene Ther.*, **2(2)** (1995) 107–115.

93. Topf N, Worgall S, Hackett NR, and Crystal RG. Regional "pro-drug" gene therapy: intravenous administration of an adenoviral vector expressing the *E. coli* cytosine deaminase gene and systemic administration of 5-fluorocytosine suppresses growth of hepatic metastasis of colon carcinoma. *Gene Ther.*, **5(4)** (1998) 507–513.

94. Green NK, Youngs DJ, Neoptolemos JP, Friedlos F, Knox RJ, Springer CJ, et al. Sensitization of colorectal and pancreatic cancer cell lines to the prodrug 5-(aziridin-1–yl)-2,4-dinitrobenzamide (CB1954) by retroviral transduction and expression of the *E. coli* nitroreductase gene. *Cancer Gene Ther.*, **4(4)** (1997) 229–238.

95. Evrard A, Cuq P, Ciccolini J, Vian L, and Cano JP. Increased cytotoxicity and bystander effect of 5-fluorouracil and 5-deoxy-5-fluorouridine in human colorectal cancer cells transfected with thymidine phosphorylase. *Br. J. Cancer*, **80(11)** (1999) 1726–1733.

96. Crystal RG, Hirschowitz E, Lieberman M, Daly J, Kazam E, Henschke C, et al. Phase I study of direct administration of a replication deficient adenovirus vector containing the *E. coli* cytosine deaminase gene to metastatic colon carcinoma of the liver in association with the oral administration of the pro-drug 5-fluorocytosine. *Hum. Gene Ther.*, **8(8)** (1997) 985–1001.

97. Burnett FM. The concept of immunological surveillance. *Prog. Exp. Tumor Res.*, **13** (1970) 1–27.

98. Matzinger P. Tolerance, danger, and the extended family. *Annu. Rev. Immunol.*, **12** (1994) 991–1045.

99. Svennevig JL, Lunde OC, Holter J, and Bjorgsvik D. Lymphoid infiltration and prognosis in colorectal carcinoma. *Br. J. Cancer*, **49(3)** (1984) 375–377.

100. Ropponen KM, Eskelinen MJ, Lipponen PK, Alhava E, and Kosma VM. Prognostic value of tumour-infiltrating lymphocytes (TILs) in colorectal cancer. *J. Pathol.*, **182(3)** (1997) 318–324.

101. Naito Y, Saito K, Shiiba K, Ohuchi A, Saigenji K, Nagura H, et al. CD8+ T cells infiltrated within cancer cell nests as a prognostic factor in human colorectal cancer. *Cancer Res.*, **58(16)** (1998) 3491–3494.

102. Hoover HC, Brandhorst JS, Peters LC, Surdyke MG, Takeshita Y, Madariaga J, et al. Adjuvant active specific immunotherapy for human colorectal cancer: 6.5-year median follow-up of a phase III prospectively randomized trial. *J. Clin. Oncol.*, **11(3)** (1993) 390–399.

103. Vermorken JB, Claessen AM, van Tinteren H, Gall HE, Ezinga R, Meijer S, et al. Active specific immunotherapy for stage II and stage III human colon cancer: a randomised trial. *Lancet*, **353(9150)** (1999) 345–350.

104. Marshall JL, Hawkins MJ, Tsang KY, Richmond E, Pedicano JE, Zhu MZ, et al. Phase I study in cancer patients of a replication-defective avipox recombinant vaccine that expresses human carcinoembryonic antigen. *J. Clin. Oncol.*, **17(1)** (1999) 332–337.

105. Riethmuller G, Schneider Gadicke E, Schlimok G, Schmiegel W, Raab R, Hoffken K, et al. Randomised trial of monoclonal antibody for adjuvant therapy of resected Dukes' C colorectal carcinoma. German Cancer Aid 17-1A Study Group. *Lancet*, **343(8907)** (1994) 1177–1183.

106. Plautz GE, Nabel EG, Fox B, Yang ZY, Jaffe M, Gordon D, et al. Direct gene transfer for the understanding and treatment of human disease. *Ann. NY Acad. Sci.*, **716** (1994) 144–153.

107. Vogelzang NJ, Sudakoff G, Hersh EM, Stopacek, A, Rubin J, Galanis E, et al. Clinical experience in a phase I and phase II testing of direct intratumoral administration with allovectin-7: a gene-based immunotherapeutic agent. *ASCO Proc.*, **15** (1996) 235.

108. Nabel GJ, Gordon D, Bishop DK, Nickoloff BJ, Yang ZY, Aruga A, et al. Immune response in human melanoma after transfer of an allogeneic class I major histocompatibility complex gene with DNA-liposome complexes. *Proc. Natl. Acad. Sci. USA*, **93(26)** (1996) 15,388–15,393.

109. Fearon ER, Pardoll DM, Itaya T, Golumbek P, Levitsky HI, Simons JW, et al. Interleukin-2 production by tumor cells bypasses T helper function in the generation of an antitumor response. *Cell*, **60(3)** (1990) 397–403.

110. Gansbacher B, Zier K, Daniels B, Cronin K, Bannerji R, and Gilboa E. Interleukin 2 gene transfer into tumor cells abrogates tumorigenicity and induces protective immunity. *J. Exp. Med.*, **172(4)** (1990) 1217–1224.

111. Lindauer M, Schackert HK, Gebert J, Rudy W, Habicht A, Siebels M, et al. Immune reactions induced by interleukin-2 transfected colorectal cancer cells in vitro: predominant induction of lymphokine-activated killer cells. *J. Mol. Med.*, **74(1)** (1996) 43–49.

112. Iwanuma Y, Kato K, Yagita H, and Okumura K. Induction of tumor-specific cytotoxic T lymphocytes and natural killer cells by tumor cells transfected with the interleukin-2 gene. *Cancer Immunol. Immunother.*, **40(1)** (1995) 17–23.

113. Sivanandham M, Shaw P, Bernik SF, Paoletti E, and Wallack MK. Colon cancer cell vaccine prepared with replication-deficient vaccinia viruses encoding B7.1 and interleukin-2 induce antitumor response in syngeneic mice. *Cancer Immunol. Immunother.*, **46(5)** (1998) 261–267.

114. Fakhrai H, Shawler DL, Gjerset R, Naviaux RK, Koziol J, Royston I, et al. Cytokine gene therapy with interleukin-2-transduced fibroblasts: effects of IL-2 dose on anti-tumor immunity. *Hum. Gene Ther.*, **6(5)** (1995) 591–601.

115. Diaz RM, Todryk S, Chong H, Hart IR, Sikora K, Dorudi S, et al. Rapid adenoviral transduction of freshly resected tumour explants with therapeutically useful genes provides a rationale for genetic immunotherapy for colorectal cancer. *Gene Ther.*, **5(7)** (1998) 869–879.

116. Patry Y, Douillard JY, Meflah K, and Le Pendu J. Immunization against a rat colon carcinoma by sodium butyrate-treated cells but not by interleukin 2-secreting cells. *Gastroenterology*, **109(5)** (1995) 1555–1565.

117. Sivanandham M, Scoggin SD, Tanaka N, and Wallack MK. Therapeutic effect of a vaccinia colon oncolysate prepared with interleukin-2-gene encoded vaccinia virus studied in a syngeneic CC-36 murine colon hepatic metastasis model. *Cancer Immunol. Immunother.*, **38(4)** (1994) 259–264.

118. Rodolfo M, Zilocchi C, Melani C, Cappetti B, Arioli I, Parmiani G, et al. Immunotherapy of experimental metastases by vaccination with interleukin gene-transduced adenocarcinoma cells sharing tumor-associated antigens. Comparison between IL-12 and IL-2 gene-transduced tumor cell vaccines. *J. Immunol.*, **157(12)** (1996) 5536–5542.

119. Sobol RE, Fakhrai H, Shawler D, Gjerset R, Dorigo O, Carson C, et al. Interleukin-2 gene therapy in a patient with glioblastoma. *Gene Ther.*, **2(2)** (1995) 164–167.

120. Belli F, Arienti F, Sule SJ, Clemente C, Mascheroni L, Cattelan A, et al. Active immunization of metastatic melanoma patients with interleukin-2-transduced allogeneic melanoma cells: evaluation of efficacy and tolerability [published erratum appears in *Cancer Immunol. Immunother.*, **45(2)** (1997) 119]. *Cancer Immunol. Immunother.*, **44(4)** (1997) 197–203.

121. Veelken H, Mackensen A, Lahn M, Kohler G, Becker D, Franke B, et al. A phase-I clinical study of autologous tumor cells plus interleukin-2-gene-transfected allogeneic fibroblasts as a vaccine in patients with cancer. *Int. J. Cancer*, **70(3)** (1997) 269–277.

122. Schmidt WI, Finke S, Trojaneck B, Denkena A, Lefterova P, Schwella N, et al. Phase I clinical study applying autologous immunological effector cells transfected with the interleukin-2 gene in patients with metastatic renal cancer, colorectal cancer and lymphoma. *Br. J. Cancer*, **81(6)** (1999) 1009–1016.

123. Gilly FN, Beaujard A, Bienvenu J, Trillet LV, Glehen O, Thouvenot D, et al. Gene therapy with Adv-IL-2 in unresectable digestive cancer: phase I–II study, intermediate report. *Hepatogastroenterology*, **46 (Suppl. 1)** (1999) 1268–1273.

124. Trinchieri G. Interleukin-12: a proinflammatory cytokine with immunoregulatory functions that bridge innate resistance and antigen-specific adaptive immunity. *Annu. Rev. Immunol.*, **13** (1995) 251–276.

125. Colombo MP, Vagliani M, Spreafico F, Parenza M, Chiodoni C, Melani C, et al. Amount of interleukin 12 available at the tumor site is critical for tumor regression. *Cancer Res.*, **56(11)** (1996) 2531–2534.

126. Brunda MJ, Luistro L, Warrier RR, Wright RB, Hubbard BR, Murphy M, et al. Antitumor and antimetastatic activity of interleukin 12 against murine tumors. *J. Exp. Med.*, **178(4)** (1993) 1223–1230.

127. Nastala CL, Edington HD, McKinney TG, Tahara H, Nalesnik MA, Brunda MJ, et al. Recombinant IL-12 administration induces tumor regression in association with IFN-gamma production. *J. Immunol.*, **153(4)** (1994) 1697–1706.

128. Lamont AG and Adorini L. IL-12: a key cytokine in immune regulation. *Immunol. Today*, **17(5)** (1996) 214–217.

129. Caruso M, Pham NK, Kwong YL, Xu B, Kosai KI, Finegold M, et al. Adenovirus-mediated interleukin-12 gene therapy for metastatic colon carcinoma. *Proc. Natl. Acad. Sci. USA*, **93(21)** (1996) 11,302–11,306.

130. Martinotti A, Stoppacciaro A, Vagliani M, Melani C, Spreafico F, Wysocka M, et al. CD4 T cells inhibit in vivo the CD8-mediated immune response against murine colon carcinoma cells transduced with interleukin-12 genes. *Eur. J. Immunol.*, **25(1)** (1995) 137–146.

131. Colombo MP, Ferrari G, Stoppacciaro A, Parenza M, Rodolfo M, Mavilio F, et al. Granulocyte colony-stimulating factor gene transfer suppresses tumorigenicity of a murine adenocarcinoma in vivo. *J. Exp. Med.*, **173(4)** (1991) 889–897.

132. Dranoff G, Jaffee E, Lazenby A, Golumbek P, Levitsky H, Brose K, et al. Vaccination with irradiated tumor cells engineered to secrete murine granulocyte–macrophage colony-stimulating factor stimulates potent, specific, and long-lasting anti-tumor immunity. *Proc. Natl. Acad. Sci. USA*, **90(8)** (1993) 3539–3543.

133. Stoppacciaro A, Melani C, Parenza M, Mastracchio A, Bassi C, Baroni C, et al. Regression of an established tumor genetically modified to release granulocyte colony-stimulating factor requires granulocyte–T cell cooperation and T cell-produced interferon gamma. *J. Exp. Med.*, **178(1)** (1993) 151–161.

134. Tepper RI, Pattengale PK, and Leder P. Murine interleukin-4 displays potent anti-tumor activity in vivo. *Cell*, **57(3)** (1989) 503–512.

135. de Vries MR, Rinkes IH, van de Velde CJ, Wiggers T, Tollenaar RA, Kuppen PJ, et al. Isolated hepatic perfusion with tumor necrosis factor alpha and melphalan: experimental studies in pigs and phase I data from humans. *Recent Results Cancer Res.*, **147** (1998) 107–119.

136. Sabaawy HE, Farley T, Ahmed T, Feldman E, and Abraham NG. Synergetic effects of retrovirus IFN-alpha gene transfer and 5-FU on apoptosis of colon cancer cells. *Acta Haematol.*, **101(2)** (1999) 82–88.

137. Janeway CA and Bottomly K. Signals and signs for lymphocyte responses. *Cell*, **76(2)** (1994) 275–285.

138. Schwartz RH. Costimulation of T lymphocytes: the role of CD28, CTLA-4, and B7/BB1 in interleukin-2 production and immunotherapy. *Cell*, **71(7)** (1992) 1065–1068.

139. Gimmi CD, Freeman GJ, Gribben JG, Gray G, and Nadler LM. Human T-cell clonal anergy is induced by antigen presentation in the absence of B7 costimulation. *Proc. Natl. Acad. Sci. USA*, **90(14)** (1993) 6586–6590.

140. Chaux P, Moutet M, Faivre J, Martin F, and Martin M. Inflammatory cells infiltrating human colorectal carcinomas express HLA class II but not B7-1 and B7-2 costimulatory molecules of the T-cell activation. *Lab. Invest.*, **74(5)** (1996) 975–983.

141. Townsend SE and Allison JP. Tumor rejection after direct costimulation of CD8+ T cells by B7-transfected melanoma cells. *Science*, **259(5093)** (1993) 368–370.

142. Hellstrom KE, Hellstrom I, and Chen L. Can co-stimulated tumor immunity be therapeutically efficacious? *Immunol. Rev.*, **145** (1995) 123–145.

143. Baskar S, Ostrand RS, Nabavi N, Nadler LM, Freeman GJ, and Glimcher LH. Constitutive expression of B7 restores immunogenicity of tumor cells expressing truncated major histocompatibility complex class II molecules. *Proc. Natl. Acad. Sci. USA*, **90(12)** (1993) 5687–5690.

144. Chen L, Ashe S, Brady WA, Hellstrom I, Hellstrom KE, Ledbetter JA, et al. Costimulation of antitumor immunity by the B7 counterreceptor for the T lymphocyte molecules CD28 and CTLA-4. *Cell*, **71(7)** (1992) 1093–1102.

145. Miyazono Y, Kamogawa Y, Ryo K, Furukawa T, Mitsuhashi M, Yamauchi K, et al. Effect of B7.1-transfected human colon cancer cells on the induction of autologous tumour-specific cytotoxic T cells. *J. Gastroenterol. Hepatol.*, **14(10)** (1999) 997–1003.

146. Habicht A, Lindauer M, Galmbacher P, Rudy W, Gebert J, Schackert HK, et al. Development of immuno- genic colorectal cancer cell lines for vaccination: expression of CD80 (B7.1) is not sufficient to restore impaired primary T cell activation in vitro. *Eur. J. Cancer*, **31A(13-14)** (1995) 2396–2402.

147. Chong H, Hutchinson G, Hart IR, and Vile RG. Expression of co-stimulatory molecules by tumor cells decreases tumorigenicity but may also reduce systemic antitumor immunity. *Hum. Gene Ther.*, **7(14)** (1996) 1771–1779.

148. Chong H, Todryk S, Hutchinson G, Hart IR, and Vile RG. Tumour cell expression of B7 costimulatory molecules and interleukin-12 or granulocyte–macrophage colony-stimulating factor induces a local antitumour response and may generate systemic protective immunity. *Gene Ther.*, **5(2)** (1998) 223–232.

149. Lindauer M, Rudy W, Guckel B, Doeberitz MV, Meuer SC, and Moebius U. Gene transfer of costimulatory molecules into a human colorectal cancer cell line: requirement of CD54, CD80 and class II MHC expression for enhanced immunogenicity. *Immunology*, **93(3)** (1998) 390–397.

150. Houbiers JG, Nijman HW, van der Burg SH, Drijfhout JW, Kenemans P, van de Velde CJ, et al. In vitro induction of human cytotoxic T lymphocyte responses against peptides of mutant and wild-type p53. *Eur. J. Immunol.*, **23(9)** (1993) 2072–2077.

151. Roth J, Dittmer D, Rea D, Tartaglia J, Paoletti E, and Levine AJ. p53 as a target for cancer vaccines: recombinant canarypox virus vectors expressing p53 protect mice against lethal tumor cell challenge. *Proc. Natl. Acad. Sci. USA*, **93(10)** (1996) 4781–4786.

152. Gold P and Freedman SO. Demonstration of tumor-specific antigens in human colonic carcinomata by immunological tolerance and absorption techniques. *J. Exp. Med.*, **121** (1965) 439–462.

153. Thompson JA, Grunert F, and Zimmermann W. Carcinoembryonic antigen gene family: molecular biology and clinical perspectives. *J. Clin. Lab. Anal.*, **5(5)** (1991) 344–366.

154. Oikawa S, Imajo S, Noguchi T, Kosaki G, and Nakazato H. The carcinoembryonic antigen (CEA) contains multiple immunoglobulin-like domains. *Biochem. Biophys. Res. Commun.*, **144(2)** (1987) 634–642.

155. Benchimol S, Fuks A, Jothy S, Beauchemin N, Shirota K, and Stanners CP. Carcinoembryonic antigen, a human tumor marker, functions as an intercellular adhesion molecule. *Cell*, **57(2)** (1989) 327–334.

156. Sikorska H, Shuster J, and Gold P. Clinical applications of carcinoembryonic antigen. *Cancer Detect. Prev.*, **12(1–6)** (1988) 321–355.

157. Muraro R, Wunderlich D, Thor A, Lundy J, Noguchi P, Cunningham R, et al. Definition by monoclonal antibodies of a repertoire of epitopes on carcinoembryonic antigen differentially expressed in human colon carcinomas versus normal adult tissues. *Cancer Res.*, **45(11 Pt. 2)** (1985) 5769–5780.

158. Fuchs C, Krapf F, Kern P, Hoferichter S, Jager W, and Kalden JR. CEA-containing immune complexes in sera of patients with colorectal and breast cancer—analysis of complexed immunoglobulin classes. *Cancer Immunol. Immunother.*, **26(2)** (1988) 180–184.

159. Tsang KY, Zaremba S, Nieroda CA, Zhu MZ, Hamilton JM, and Schlom J. Generation of human cytotoxic T cells specific for human carcinoembryonic antigen epitopes from patients immunized with recombinant vaccinia-CEA vaccine [see comments]. *J. Natl. Cancer Inst.*, **87(13)** (1995) 982–990.

160. Foon KA, John WJ, Chakraborty M, Sherratt A, Garrison J, Flett M, et al. Clinical and immune responses in advanced colorectal cancer patients treated with anti-idiotype monoclonal antibody vaccine that mimics the carcinoembryonic antigen. *Clin. Cancer Res.*, **3(8)** (1997) 1267–1276.

161. Kaufman H, Schlom J, and Kantor J. A recombinant vaccinia virus expressing human carcinoembryonic antigen (CEA). *Int. J. Cancer*, **48(6)** (1991) 900–907.

162. Kantor J, Irvine K, Abrams S, Kaufman H, DiPietro J, and Schlom J. Antitumor activity and immune responses induced by a recombinant carcinoembryonic antigen-vaccinia virus vaccine [see comments]. *J. Natl. Cancer Inst.*, **84(14)** (1992) 1084–1091.

163. Kass E, Schlom J, Thompson J, Guadagni F, Graziano P, and Greiner JW. Induction of protective host immunity to carcinoembryonic antigen (CEA), a self-antigen in CEA transgenic mice, by immunizing with a recombinant vaccinia–CEA virus. *Cancer Res.*, **59(3)** (1999) 676–683.

164. Hamilton JM, Chen AP, Nguyen B, Grem J, Abrams S, Chung Y, et al. Phase I study of recombinant vaccinia virus (rV) that expresses human carcinoembryonic antigen (CEA) in adult patients with adenocarcinomas. *ASCO Proc.*, **13** (1994) 295.

165. Conry RM, Khazaeli MB, Saleh MN, Allen KO, Barlow DL, Moore SE, et al. Phase I trial of a recombinant vaccinia virus encoding carcinoembryonic antigen in metastatic adenocarcinoma: comparison of intradermal versus subcutaneous administration. *Clin. Cancer Res.*, **5(9)** (1999) 2330–2337.

166. McAneny D, Ryan CA, Beazley RM, and Kaufman HL. Results of a phase I trial of a recombinant vaccinia virus that expresses carcinoembryonic antigen in patients with advanced colorectal cancer. *Ann. Surg. Oncol.*, **3(5)** (1996) 495–500.

167. McLaughlin JP, Schlom J, Kantor JA, and Greiner JW. Improved immunotherapy of a recombinant carcinoembryonic antigen vaccinia vaccine when given in combination with interleukin-2. *Cancer Res.*, **56(10)** (1996) 2361–2367.

168. Hodge JW, McLaughlin JP, Abrams SI, Shupert WL, Schlom J, and Kantor JA. Admixture of a recombinant vaccinia virus containing the gene for the costimulatory molecule B7 and a recombinant vaccinia virus containing a tumor-associated antigen gene results in enhanced specific T-cell responses and antitumor immunity. *Cancer Res.*, **55(16)** (1995) 3598–3603.

169. Hodge JW, McLaughlin JP, Kantor JA, and Schlom J. Diversified prime and boost protocols using recombinant vaccinia virus and recombinant non-replicating avian pox virus to enhance T-cell immunity and antitumor responses. *Vaccine*, **15(6–7)** (1997) 759–768.

170. Zhu MZ, Marshall J, Cole D, Schlom J, and Tsang KY. Specific cytolytic T-cell responses to human CEA from patients immunized with recombinant avipox-CEA vaccine. *Clin. Cancer Res.*, **6(1)** (2000) 24–33.

171. Richards CA, Austin EA, and Huber BE. Transcriptional regulatory sequences of carcinoembryonic antigen: identification and use with cytosine deaminase for tumor-specific gene therapy. *Hum. Gene Ther.*, **6(7)** (1995) 881–893.

172. Austin EA and Huber BE. A first step in the development of gene therapy for colorectal carcinoma: cloning, sequencing, and expression of Escherichia coli cytosine deaminase. *Mol. Pharmacol.*, **43(3)** (1993) 380–387.

INDEX

A

Abdominal colectomy and ileorectal anastomosis, familial adenomatous polyposis management, 101, 103, 104

Abdomino-perineal resection (APR), rectal cancer, 341, 343, 351, 357–359

Aberrant crypt foci (ACF), cancer pathogenesis, 6, 82

ACF, *see* Aberrant crypt foci

Acrylonitrile, occupational risks of colorectal cancer, 36

Acupuncture,
 nausea and vomiting management, 723, 724
 pain therapy, 722
 perioperative symptom management, 724

Adeno-associated virus, gene therapy vectors, 815

Adenovirus, gene therapy vectors, 814, 815

AG2009, aminoimidazole carboxamide ribonucleotide formyltransferase inhibition, 579

AG2034, glycinamide ribonucleotide formyltransferase inhibition and trials, 579

AICARFT, *see* Aminoimidazole carboxamide ribonucleotide formyltransferase

Alcohol, colorectal cancer risks, 37, 38, 53, 54

Aminoimidazole carboxamide ribonucleotide formyltransferase (AICARFT), AG2009 inhibition, 579

Analgesia,
 adjuvant analgesics,
  bone pain, 678
  classification, 676
  corticosteroids, 676, 677
  definition, 676
  neuropathic pain, 677, 678
  topical local anesthetics, 677
  visceral pain, 678, 679
 neurosurgical analgesia,
  celiac plexus block, 681
  cordotomy, 681, 682
  epidural analgesia, 680
  ganglion impar block, 681
  intrathecal analgesia, 680
  rhizotomy, 681
  selection of technique,
   guidelines, 682, 683
   pelvic perineal and bilateral lower limb pain, 683
   unilateral lower quadrant pain, 683

   visceral pain, 683
  superior nypogastric nerve plexus block, 681

nonopioid analgesics,
 adverse effects, 662, 663
 mechanism of action, 662
 types, 662, 663

opioids,
 adverse effects,
  addiction, 674, 675
  bladder spasm, 674
  confusion and delirium, 673, 674
  dependence, 674, 675
  drug interactions, 672
  gastrointestinal side effects, 672
  multifocal myoclonus, 674
  pseudoaddiction, 675, 676
  respiratory depression, 674
  sedation, 672, 673
 agonist drugs,
  codeine, 666
  dihydrocodeine, 666
  dosing, 665
  fentanyl, 667
  hydromorphone, 666
  levorphanol, 667
  meperidine, 666, 667
  methadone, 667
  morphine, 666
  oxycodone, 666
  oxymorphone, 667
  propoxyphene, 666
 classification, 663, 664
 dose-response, 664
 dosing,
  adjustment, 671
  starting dose, 671
  titration, 671
  tolerance, 671, 672
 equianalgesic dose ratio, 664, 666
 pharmacology, 663
 scheduling,
  around the clock dosing, 670
  as-needed dosing, 670
  patient controlled analgesia, 670, 671
 selection of drug, 667, 668
 systemic administration route,
  invasive routes, 669
  selection, 668, 669
  switching, 669, 670